Syndromes
of the Head and Neck

CONTRIBUTORS

Jaroslav Cervenka, M.D.
Robert Desnick, M.D.
Bryan Hall, M.D.
Heidi Pantke, D.D.S.
Olaf Pantke, D.D.S., M.D.
William Reed, M.D.
Charles Scott, M.D.
Heddie Sedano, D.D.S.
Burton Shapiro, D.D.S.
Jürgen Spranger, M.D.

SYNDROMES
OF THE HEAD AND NECK

SECOND EDITION

ROBERT J. GORLIN, D.D.S., M.S.
Professor and Chairman
Department of Oral Pathology
School of Dentistry
Professor of Pathology, Pediatrics,
Obstetrics and Gynecology, Otolaryngology, Dermatology
School of Medicine
University of Minnesota

JENS J. PINDBORG, D.D.S., DR. ODONT., ODONT. DR. H.C.
Professor and Chairman
Department of Oral Pathology
Royal Dental College
Chairman
Dental Department
University Hospital

M. MICHAEL COHEN, JR., D.M.D.
Associate Professor
Department of Oral and Maxillofacial
Surgery, Orthodontics, and Pediatrics
School of Dentistry and Medicine
University of Washington

McGRAW-HILL BOOK COMPANY
A Blakiston Publication

New York   St. Louis   San Francisco   Auckland   Düsseldorf   Johannesburg
Kuala Lumpur   London   Mexico   Montreal   New Delhi   Panama   Paris
São Paulo   Singapore   Sydney   Tokyo   Toronto

SYNDROMES OF THE HEAD AND NECK

Copyright © 1976, 1964 by McGraw-Hill, Inc.
All rights reserved. Printed in the United States of America.
No part of this publication may be reproduced, stored in a retrieval system,
or transmitted, in any form or by any means, electronic,
mechanical, photocopying, recording, or otherwise,
without the prior written permission of the publisher.

234567890 VHVH 7832109

This book was set in Trump Mediaeval by Progressive Typographers.
The editors were Joseph J. Brehm and J. W. Maisel;
the designer was Anne Canevari Green;
the production supervisor was Leroy A. Young.
Von Hoffmann Press, Inc., was printer and binder.

Library of Congress Cataloging in Publication Data

Gorlin, Robert J
Syndromes of the head and neck.

"A Blakiston publication."
Includes bibliographies and index.
1. Semiology. 2. Head—Diseases. 3. Neck—Diseases. I.
Pindborg, Jens Jørgen, date, joint author. II. Cohen, Meyer Michael, date,
joint author. III. Title. [DNLM: 1. Head—Abnormalities. 2.
Neck—Abnormalities. 3. Nomenclature. WB15 G669s]
RC69.G64   1976   617'.51'072   75-9774
ISBN 0-07-023790-5

To those who treasure the exceptional,
we dedicate this book.

"All cases are unique, and very similar to others."
T. S. Eliot, *The Cocktail Party.*

Contents

Foreword

The first edition of this book was the pioneering text for this segment of medicine. I vividly recall the excitement upon first reading the book in 1964. At last!—here was a cohesive authoritative text which portrayed the majority of syndromes which had been recognized at that time. Though entitled *Syndromes of the Head and Neck*, it covered all known features of each disorder in a nonspecialized and balanced manner, including the natural history, etiology, differential diagnosis, and pertinent references for each disorder. The field of syndromology has expanded since that time. The number of recognized disorders set forth in the book has more than doubled, and the knowledge has been updated on the original syndromes. A third person, M. Michael Cohen, Jr., has been added to the authorship of this expanded work on syndromes. Thus, this second edition is a most welcome addition for all those who work with, or are interested in, syndromes of malformation. Many children and their parents will be the indirect beneficiaries of this text. For our own patients, we sincerely thank the authors for this monumental work.

David W. Smith, M.D.
Professor of Pediatrics
Dysmorphology Unit
Department of Pediatrics
University of Washington
School of Medicine
Seattle, Washington

Introduction

"I shouldn't know you again if we did meet," Humpty Dumpty replied in a discontented tone, giving her one of his fingers to shake: "you're so exactly like other people."

"The face is what one goes by, generally," Alice remarked in a thoughtful tone.

"That's just what I complain of," said Humpty Dumpty. "Your face is the same as everybody has — the two eyes, so —" (marking their places in the air with his thumb) "nose in the middle, mouth under. It's always the same. Now if you had the two eyes on the same side of the nose, for instance — or the mouth at the top — that would be some help."

"It wouldn't look nice," Alice objected. But Humpty Dumpty only shut his eyes, and said, "Wait till you've tried."

Through the Looking Glass,
Lewis Carroll

There is something metaphysical about naming and recognizing a disorder. Not that it has directly helped the patient one scintilla! Nevertheless, all concerned — the patient, the clinician, the parents — seem to feel a certain satisfaction or sense of security from the fact that the condition is defined. In part this is valid, since understanding has its incipience in definition. Once the condition has been measured and its extent limned, its recognition is made easier and concentration and interest can therefore be more easily focused upon it. This in turn may lead to increased clinical and basic research, with ultimate understanding and even treatment.

Much of the current pediatric literature has been devoted to so-called "funny-looking kid" syndromes. This term disturbs us for personal as well as for scientific reasons. The use of the term "funny looking" is certainly pejorative. We strongly suspect that the clinician who would use such a term would not be flattered were he to be referred to as a "funny-looking doctor." Furthermore, we are disquieted since there is no precision in describing a child with manifold anomalies as being "funny-looking." This is not something that we alone have felt, but has been the concern of many persons all over the world.

The face is an area of interest which involves many disciplines: medicine, dentistry, physical anthropology, biomathematics, genetics, radiology, developmental biology, photography, and the arts. The face of man is observed by all about him. It is the part that manifests most clearly the stamp of the individual's reactions.

What is it that distinguishes the unusual-looking child from all those within the range of variation that constitutes the norm? Since we are concerned primarily with the face, we must consider many things. Do facial characteristics, present at birth in various genetic disorders, remain characteristic throughout life? Or do they change as the child grows older? Furthermore, does age either accentuate or minimize the stigmata that one considers characteristic for a given clinical entity? What specific measurements do we have for appraising the norm?

Various fanciful terms have been employed to describe the faces of infants, viz., elfin, leprechaun-like, etc. Precision is obviously not the forte of this technique, since, we suspect, few can be consonant regarding the appearance of imaginary creatures. Often erroneous is the statement that the patient has ocular hypertelorism when, in fact, no measurement of interocular distance was ever attempted, the clinician having depended on gestalt alone. It is easy to be misled by clinical impression, since the distance between the eyes may appear to be abnormal depending upon the width of the face, the form of the glabellar area, the presence of epicanthal folds, the shape and width of the nose, etc. Furthermore, one must accurately define what one means by ocular hypertelorism. Does one refer to bony interorbital distance, interpupillary distance, or inter-inner-canthal distance? How accurate is the latter if the patient has marked epicanthal folds? How accurate is measurement of interpupillary distance in an uncooperative patient? While few would question the precision of bony interorbital distance as measured in an infant cephalostat, how many clinicians have one at their disposal or consider sedating the patient justified for such a procedure?

Accurate facial description has been deficient, partly because of the lack of availability of precise standards. These data have been published over the years in various anthropologic, genetic, and pediatrics journals—unfortunately incomplete in many cases for various populations—but only recently has effort been made to establish rigorous standards, putting them in readily available source books.

Some of these measurements, no doubt, have ease of duplication, such as head circumference, ear length, palatal dimensions, interpupillary distance, and especially cephalometric distances and angles ascertained from radiographs. Other measurements, such as philtrum length and the intercommissural (interangular) length of the oral aperture, are less reliable, since they represent soft-tissue measurements which require the mouth to be completely at rest.

In spite of all these data, one commonly reads that a patient has "low-set ears," "high palatal vault," "wide-spaced eyes," or "funny-looking nose" when, in fact, as pointed out above, none of these findings was actually documented. In part, the difficulties inherent in such sloppy verbal descriptions can be neutralized by excellent clinical photographs. Nevertheless, the impression received by a photograph or even clinical examination of the patient, can be misleading. Posterior rotation, for example, can make the pinna look low-set. Abnormal palatal form may give the observer the impression of abnormally high palate. Sunken nasal bridge and epicanthal folds cause the child with Down syndrome to appear to have wide set eyes when, in fact, ocular hypotelorism (often as much as 5 mm below the norm) is usually found.

With all the sophisticated armamentarium at hand during this age of computerization, how can we approach the problem of abnormal facial form? While description of an object in nearly all fields is initiated by simple words of common parlance, the end point is analytic, i.e., defined in the precise language of mathematics. This concept was voiced most eloquently over 50 years ago by D'Arcy Thompson, who stated that "if the difficulties and representation could be overcome, it is by means of such coordinates in space that we should at last obtain an adequate and satisfying picture of the process of deformation and direction of growth."

Computerization of cephalometric roentgenograms can be quite rapid and accurate as a means of assessing both shape and growth. Conceivably, by means of grenz ray (x-ray) or other techniques, soft-tissue form may also be analyzed.

Biostereometrics, which is essentially contour mapping of various forms, is another technique which employs spatial and spatiotemporal analysis of biologic form and function based on principles of analytic geometry. When exposed under carefully controlled conditions, photographs, holographs, radiographs, infrared radiographs, and other forms of imagery can provide convenient, noncontact means of measuring organic form in three dimensions and changes in form, such as movement or growth. Thereby, the shape of the structure, be it the face or one of its component parts, can be characterized digitally, using Cartesian or other coordinate systems, and analogically by contour maps, cross sections, or physical replicas. A modification of this technique has been employed by projecting a grid onto the face of parents of a child with facial clefting, comparing their photographs with those of parents of normal children.

Another problem that concerns the dysmorphologist is the constancy of clinical aspects of a syndrome. Do the features of the disorder alter with time? In infants with the cri-du-chat syndrome, the mewing cry and the full round face disappear within the first year of life. With the disappearance of these hallmarks, the clinician is faced with a mentally retarded, microcephalic child who exhibits ocular hypertelorism and who "vanishes in the crowd" of undeciphered mental retardates unless described on the basis of karyotypic screening.

Conversely, we have other lacunae of ignorance. Is a facies as striking as that of the Williams syndrome one which is invariant with time? All pictures of individuals with this disorder that we have seen have been of children ranging in age from a year or so to adolescence, nary an adult. We became curious as to whether the overlong philtrum and the retroussé nose with anteverted nostrils so characteristic in the child metamorphose into far less subtle changes in the older patient. A short trip to an institution for the mentally retarded demonstrated that the facies does, in fact, remain constant with age, since we were able to obtain childhood pictures of adults with this condition.

The variability of expression of traits is, however, destined not to be conquered. For example, if one chooses to consider disorders in which one facet is a "thin nose," it should become apparent that not all thin noses are thin in the same way. Some are "thin" because of a markedly narrowed dorsum, others because of hypoplasia of the nasal alae, or extension of the nasal tip far below the columellar base. To complicate matters further by taking a specific example, the nasal alar

hypoplasia in the Waardenburg syndrome may be quite variable in its expression. Thus, while there may be a typical "Waardenburg nose," not all patients with the syndrome possess this attribute, nor do those who possess it have it to the same degree—a problem common enough to make any quantifier go gray!

In the clinical delineation of human malformation syndromes, a formidable vocabulary has rapidly evolved to designate various syndromes. With the exception of specialists in the field, most clinicians are baffled by the wide assortment of terms used, such as oculoauriculovertebral dysplasia, chondrodysplasia punctata, pseudoachondroplasia, Dubowitz syndrome, Hallermann-Streiff syndrome, Smith-Lemli-Opitz syndrome, and BBB syndrome. With the discovery of new syndromes almost daily, the number of designations is expanding to the point where even specialists can no longer remember all the syndrome designations or their phenotypic features.

Because a syndrome designation permits the collection of data, it is much more than just a label. As a syndrome becomes further delineated, its name connotes (a) its phenotypic spectrum, (b) its natural history, and (c) its mode of inheritance or risk of recurrence. If a syndrome designation can stand for such clinically relevant information where previously none existed, the designation can hardly be called "superficial" or "an exercise in merely applying labels."

Though the use of special terms for various human malformation syndromes is completely justified, there is no question that designations used are frequently cumbersome, unwieldy, unscientific, confusing, or inaccurate. The reasons for this will become apparent as we consider the various ways that have been used to designate malformation syndromes.

Unquestionably, the ideal way is to name the basic defect, such as an enzymatic or chromosomal abnormality, when this is known. "Cystathionine synthase deficiency" scientifically names a disorder. The term is certainly more accurate than the more commonly used designation "homocystinuria," since the latter is a consequence of the former and, as such, is both secondary and nonspecific. For example, homocystinuria can also occur with methylmalonic aciduria in defective coenzyme B_{12} synthesis. The basic defect in the Sanfilippo syndrome A is heparin sulfate sulfatase deficiency, which is also a suitable name for the disorder. Occasionally, the name of the basic defect can be unwieldy, as in hypoxanthine-guanine-phosphoribosyl-transferase deficiency. In this instance, it seems easier to use the terms "HGPRT deficiency" or "Lesch-Nyhan syndrome."

Microscopically detectable chromosomal defects associated with human malformation syndromes can be properly designated, such as trisomy 13 syndrome, $5p^-$ syndrome, $18q^-$ syndrome, XXY syndrome, and so forth.

In the future, we can probably anticipate elucidation of at least some heritable disorders of connective tissue at the molecular level—and hence proper designations for them. However, since the basic defect in the overwhelming majority of true multiple congenital anomaly syndromes is unknown, we are confronted by a bewildering salmagundi which must be designated by some other method.

Because different systems of nomenclature have been employed, a single syndrome may be known by several terms, thus causing confusion. For example, the hypertelorism-hypospadias syndrome is also known as Opitz syndrome and the BBB syndrome. Or to take another example, the inaccurately designated infantile hypercalcemia-peculiar facies-supravalvular aortic stenosis syndrome is synonymous with the elfin facies syndrome and the Williams syndrome.

In general, a new syndrome has been denoted by (a) an eponym, (b) one or more striking features, (c) an acronym, (d) a numeral, (e) geographic location or name of the original patients, or (f) some combination of the above. None of these systems of nomenclature is without fault. Let us consider the advantages and disadvantages of each.

Eponyms are frequently used to designate various malformation syndromes, e.g., Seckel syndrome, Russell-Silver syndrome, and Klippel-Trénaunay-Weber syndrome. McKusick has argued against using the possessive form of an eponym, since other persons have often contributed to our understanding of a given syndrome. Thus, "Apert's syndrome" is incorrect since the disorder had been described before Apert's paper and became more fully under-

stood subsequently because of the work of others. Furthermore, to paraphrase Warkany, Apert neither had nor owned the syndrome he described. Thus, the term "Apert syndrome" or "the Apert syndrome" seems preferable.

Two or more names are found in some eponyms and may indicate various things. The Smith-Lemli-Opitz syndrome indicates collaboration. The Morquio-Brailsford syndrome indicates independent simultaneous discovery. The Peutz-Jeghers syndrome indicates revival by Jeghers of Peutz's earlier observations. Some eponyms honor clinicians who have added new facets to an already established syndrome, e.g., Laurence-Moon-Biedl-Bardet syndrome, which subsequently was found to be heterogeneous and is now considered to be Laurence-Moon syndrome and Biedl-Bardet syndrome. In some instances, an eponym seems briefer than the accepted scientific term. For example, it seems easier to say Osler-Rendu-Weber syndrome than hereditary hemorrhagic telangiectasia. Finally, some eponyms are introduced because an alternative term has become etiologically heterogeneous since it was first described. For example, the Conradi syndrome used to be synonymous with chondrodystrophia calcificans congenita (now changed to chondrodysplasia punctata). Since there are now two distinct genetic forms of chondrodysplasia punctata, the term "Conradi syndrome" is restricted to the autosomal dominant type.

Error has often crept in. Family names, usually British, have led to the erroneous hyphenation of Ramsay Hunt, Treacher Collins, Parkes Weber, and Bence Jones. Robin's first name, Pierre, when coupled with his last, has been too often hyphenated. The European continental custom of coupling the parents' names as surname, e.g., Brown-Séquard, Duran-Reynals, Albers-Schönberg, Szent-Györgyi, has resulted in compound names which, if coupled with a co-worker's name, may cause the reader to assume a three-pronged authorship.

There are several advantages in using eponyms. Since eponyms avoid anatomic description, the syndrome can be expanded as new facets are recognized without changing its name. Furthermore, eponyms do not bias the phenotypic spectrum of future reports because there are no features of the syndrome in the designation. Nor do eponyms suggest a false etiology, prejudge the search for the basic defect, or conceal our ignorance of the nature of the disorder. The Hurler syndrome used to be known as lipochondrodystrophy, erroneously suggesting a basic defect in fat metabolism. Obviously, "the Hurler syndrome" was a better name. Furthermore, when the basic defect became known (α-L-iduronidase deficiency), this designation could be substituted for the interim term, Hurler syndrome.

One major disadvantage of eponyms is that more than one syndrome may be named after the same individual. This is especially true in the study of malformation syndromes, since a single clinician often discovers more than one syndrome. Thus, the Albright syndrome refers to pseudohypoparathyroidism on the one hand and to polyostotic fibrous dysplasia with café-au-lait spots and endocrine abnormalities on the other. This dilemma can be resolved by referring to the former as Albright hereditary osteodystrophy and to the latter as the McCune-Albright syndrome. Hanhart has four syndromes named in his honor. They can be distinguished as types I through IV. de Lange has two syndromes named after her—the well-known malformation syndrome and an unrelated condition, consisting of congenital muscular hypertrophy, extrapyramidal motor dysfunction, and mental deficiency. It is usually assumed that the term "de Lange syndrome" refers to the former unless otherwise specified.

These examples illustrate the confusion that confronts the neophyte who attempts to master nosology in the field irrespective of what device is used to separate various syndromes whose designations include the same name.

Another disadvantage briefly alluded to earlier is that frequently the individual for whom the syndrome was named was not the first to describe it. For example, the Down syndrome was reported earlier by Seguin. The Apert syndrome was reported by no less than seven different individuals prior to Apert's paper. The Williams syndrome was described earlier in three separate papers. The so-called "Roberts syndrome" was described earlier by no less than five different authors.

In some instances, it is argued that credit should be given not to the first author who described a syndrome, but to the author who recognized it as an entity or in some way illuminated the disorder. For example, although the de Lange syndrome was reported earlier by Brachmann, retention of the designation de Lange syndrome has been suggested rather than Brachmann-de Lange syndrome because of the illuminating quality of de Lange's contribution. If clear recognition of a syndrome entity be the criterion for using an eponym, then Appelt, Gerken, and Lenz should be credited for the so-called Roberts syndrome, rather than Roberts or the five other authors who described this syndrome prior to Roberts' paper.

In other instances, it is argued that any author who contributes to our understanding of a given syndrome should be included in the eponym. This, of course, can reach ridiculous extremes, as in the Laurence-Moon-Bardet-Biedl-Solis-Cohen-Weiss syndrome. Furthermore, because of chauvinism, the same syndrome may have entirely different names in two or more countries.

That whim enters into the assignment and persistence—or lack of persistence—of an eponym is evident. We retain the term "Marfan syndrome," although Marfan's original patient probably had congenital contractural arachnodactyly, not the Marfan syndrome. In 1956 Prader, Labhart, and Willi reported the syndrome of hypotonia, hypomentia, hypogonadism, and obesity. Today, however, the condition is known as the Prader-Willi syndrome. Labhart's name has mysteriously vanished from the designation.

Some syndromes have been designated by one or more of their features. In some cases, a single striking aspect provides a name by which the syndrome can be remembered with ease, as in the whistling-face syndrome, thanatophoric (death-bearing) dwarfism, diastrophic (twisted) dwarfism, and geleophysic (pleasing-face) dwarfism. Sometimes anatomic designations include two or more features of a syndrome, as in the hypertelorism-hypospadias syndrome or trichorhinophalangeal syndromes. Because such terms are descriptive, they can aid the clinician in remembering some of the presumably prominent features of a given syndrome.

However, there are several disadvantages in using syndrome features as designations. First, the name may be too general and nonspecific, as in the term "arachnodactyly" for the Marfan syndrome. Arachnodactyly is a feature of several other disorders. Furthermore, the feature may not be especially striking in some instances of the Marfan syndrome. The term "cerebrohepatorenal syndrome" has been used as a designation for the Zellweger syndrome. However, since "cerebrohepatorenal" is nonspecific, the designation could apply equally well to the Wilson disease.

Second, some designations are simply incorrect. "Adenoma sebaceum syndrome" is an inaccurate term for tuberous sclerosis, since angiofibromas, not sebaceous adenomas, are features of the disorder. The name "achondroplasia" is misleading because cartilage is formed in the disorder. Although "hypochondroplasia" would be better suited to this condition, the term is used to designate another, probably allelic chondrodysplasia. However, achondroplasia is so firmly entrenched that a name change is unlikely.

Third, introducing anatomic terminology into the designation biases the phenotypic spectrum of future reports. In fact, anatomic features honored in the designation tend to become obligatory rather than facultative, resulting in the danger that some clinicians will not diagnose a syndrome unless such features are present. The original use of the term "multiple lentigines (leopard) syndrome" biased further reports in favor of patients with dermatologic manifestations. Now, however, the majority of patients with this syndrome are known to lack lentigines. Patients with the macroglossia-omphalocele (Beckwith-Wiedemann) syndrome may lack both macroglossia and omphalocele. Most patients with the infantile hypercalcemia–supravalvular aortic stenosis Williams syndrome lack both features. An occasional patient with the broad thumbs (Rubinstein-Taybi) syndrome does not have broad thumbs.

Fourth, anatomic designations do not allow for further syndrome delineation within the name itself. For example, if we report a new syndrome which we designate as the auriculodigitorenal syndrome and, with further delineation, it becomes apparent that ocular and cardiac defects are also striking features of the disorder, in fact more common than either the digital or renal anomalies, then the original designation no longer fits the syndrome. To change the already established name to auriculooculocardiodigitorenal syndrome is confusing as well as frightfully unwieldy.

Finally, some designations may have unpleasant connotations for the affected individual or his family or both. Terms such as "bird-headed dwarfism," "gargoylism," and many others should be discarded for this reason.

Acronyms have been used to designate some malformation syndromes. They may serve as useful mnemonic devices, as in the LEOPARD syndrome (multiple *l*entigines, *e*lectrocardiographic conduction abnormalities, *o*cular hypertelorism, *p*ulmonic stenosis, *a*trial septal defect, *r*etardation of growth, and sensorineural *d*eafness) and the SHORT syndrome (*s*hort stature, *h*yperextensibility of joints, *o*cular depression, *R*ieger anomaly, and delayed *t*eething).

Acronyms based on the initials of the original patients' surnames have been proposed, e.g., BBB, G, SC, and RSH syndromes, although they have not been accepted by most workers in this field. Such designations (a) readily lend themselves to computer diagnosis and information retrieval systems, and (b) do not bias the phenotypic spectrum of future reports.

Other syndrome designations have been abbreviated by using various combinations of letters, e.g., EvC (Ellis-van Creveld syndrome, CHH (cartilage-hair hypoplasia), EMG (exomphalos-macroglossia-gigantism or Beckwith-Wiedemann syndrome, HHHO (hypotonia-hypomentia-hypogonadism-obesity or Prader-Willi syndrome), and EEC (ectrodactyly-ectodermal dysplasia–clefting syndrome).

Designations with numerals have been used (a) to subclassify various syndromes when knowledge expands, as in mucopolysaccharidoses (MPS I through VII); (b) to separate quite different disorders with the same eponym, as in the Hanhart syndromes (types I through IV); and (c) to separate quite different disorders with the same descriptive label, as in achondrogenesis (types I and II). Generally speaking, numerical nomenclature has found its most important use in those areas where knowledge at the biochemical level has rapidly demonstrated etiologic heterogeneity, as in the mucopolysaccharidoses. Numerals are easy to use, allow for the discovery of additional subtypes, and have no built-in phenotypic biases in their designations.

Two major disadvantages are inherent in this approach. First, it is difficult to remember syndrome designations with numerals, and it becomes more difficult as the number of such designations increases.

A second disadvantage is that numerical changes other than additions are likely to occur as our understanding of various syndromes is enhanced. For example, in 1966, the mucopolysaccharidoses were classified simply as MPS I, MPS II . . ., MPS VI. By 1972, MPS I as a simple designation no longer existed. In its place were MPS I-H (Hurler syndrome), MPS I-S (Scheie syndrome), and MPS I H/S (Hurler-Scheie compound). Furthermore, MPS V, which used to be employed for Scheie syndrome, is a vacant designation in McKusick's new classification.

The least common way to designate malformation syndromes is by geographic location of the original patients. Thus, de Lange evaluated her patients in the city of Amsterdam and called the syndrome which now bears her name "typus amstelodamensis." A second example is Brazilian-type achondrogenesis, a term introduced because most cases had been ascertained in central Brazil. In general, geographic designations have not been favorably received by students of malformation syndromes.

Finally, compound designations of various types may be used. In many instances such terms can help clarify which syndrome is under discussion. For example, the Hurler syndrome may be designated as α-L-iduronidase deficiency (Hurler syndrome) or as Hurler syndrome (MPS I-H). Subtyping descriptive terms with eponyms has been used in the International Nomenclature for Constitutional Diseases of Bone. For example, metaphyseal chondrodysplasia is classified as Jansen, Schmid, or McKusick type.

With regard to format of presentation, we have generally maintained the same approach that we employed in the first edition. We have alphabetically listed the syndromes under their most commonly employed names and have utilized the International Nomenclature for Constitutional Disorders of Bone whenever possible. For the sake of uniformity we have used terms employed by McKusick (1971) in his catalog of genetic conditions. Most syndromes have a chapter of their own. Some entities have been grouped in single chapters (miscellaneous cleft syndromes, oromandibular-limb hypogenesis, craniotubular bone dysplasias, mucopolysaccharidoses, etc.). Finally, we have placed a group of miscellaneous, mostly unique orofacial syndromes at the end of the text.

In the Appendix, we have presented a farrago of apposite normal metric data which should be useful to the reader.

We have attempted (not always successfully) to follow the suggestions made by an international committee which met at the National Institutes of Health, Bethesda, Maryland, on February 10 and 11, 1975, under the guidance of Dr. Richard L. Christiansen. The following definitions were agreed upon:

1 Malformation: a primary structural defect that results from a localized error of morphogenesis, e.g., cleft lip. It is distinguished from deformation, an alteration in shape and/or structure of a previously normally formed part, e.g., torticollis.
2 Anomalad: a malformation together with its subsequently derived structural changes, e.g., Robin anomalad.
3 Malformation syndrome: recognized pattern of malformation presumably having the same etiology and currently not interpreted as the consequence of a single localized error in morphogenesis, e.g., Down syndrome.
4 Association: a recognized pattern of malformations which currently is not considered to constitute a syndrome or an anomalad. As knowledge advances, an association may be reclassified as a syndrome or as an anomalad, e.g., hemihypertrophy with Wilms tumor.

In this second edition we used an eclectic approach to nomenclature. We chose a primary designation for each syndrome on the basis of how it was most commonly known. We also chose a second designation on the basis of the next most commonly used term. Designations were selected without regard for consistency of nomenclature. We agree with Emerson: "Consistency is the hobgoblin of little minds."

We wish to express our sincere appreciation to Drs. William Boggs (oral genetics), Judith G. Hall (medicine and pediatrics), James R. Hooley (oral and maxillofacial surgery), Leonard O. Langer (radiology), Jules Leroy (pediatrics), Ray Lewandowski, Jr. (pediatrics), Irving Shapiro (ophthalmology), David B. Shurtleff (pediatrics), David B. Smith (pediatrics), Robert A. Vickers (oral pathology), Susanne Ullman (dermatology), Carl Witkop (oral genetics), and Jorge Yunis (pathology) for providing encouragement and suggestions concerning various sections of this text. Finally,

we would like to gratefully acknowledge the United States Public Health Service both for providing a Career Development Award and for financial aid in grant DE-1770.

Furthermore, we wish to express our thanks to Mrs. Bridget Stellmacher for the tender loving care with which she has typed and retyped this manuscript; and to Virginia Hansen for her diligent job of proofreading the manuscript.

REFERENCES

Cohen, M. M., Jr., Syndrome Designations. *J. Med. Genet.* (in press).

Herrmann, J., and Opitz, J. M., Naming and Nomenclature of Syndromes. *Birth Defects* **10**(7):69–86, 1974.

Maroteaux, P., A Nomenclature for Constitutional (Intrinsic) Diseases of Bone. *Ann. Radiol.* (Paris. **13**:455–464, 1970; *J. Pediatr.* **78**:177–179, 1971.

McKusick, V. A., *Mendelian Inheritance in Man.* 4th ed. Johns Hopkins, Baltimore, 1975.

Smith, D. W., Nomenclature of Syndromes. *Birth Defects* **10**(7):65–67, 1974.

Warkany, J., Syndromes. *Am. J. Dis. Child.* **121**:365–370, 1971.

Warkany, J., *Congenital Malformations. Notes and Comments.* Year Book, Chicago, 1971, pp. 43–48.

The interested reader is referred to various texts which we believe will be helpful:

Becker, P. E. (ed.), *Humangenetik.* Thieme, Stuttgart, 1964–1972.

Bergsma, D., *Birth Defects. Atlas and Compendium.* National Foundation, Williams & Wilkins, Baltimore, 1973.

Konigsmark, B. and Gorlin, R. J., *Genetic and Metabolic Deafness,* W. B. Saunders, Philadelphia, 1976.

Leiber, B., and Olbrich, G., *Die klinischen Syndrome.* 5th ed. Urban & Schwarzenberg, Munich/Berlin, 1972.

McKusick, V. A., *Mendelian Inheritance in Man.* 4th ed., Johns Hopkins, Baltimore, 1975.

McKusick, V. A., *Heritable Disorders of Connective Tissue.* 4th ed., Mosby, St. Louis, 1973.

Poznanski, A. K., *The Hand in Radiologic Diagnosis.* Saunders, Philadelphia, 1974.

Rimoin, D. L., and Schimke, R. N., *Genetic Disorders of the Endocrine Glands.* Mosby, St. Louis, 1971.

Smith, D. W., *Recognizable Patterns of Human Malformation.* Saunders, Philadelphia, 1970.

Spranger, J., Langer, L. O., Jr., and Wiedemann, H. R., *Bone Dysplasias: An Atlas of Constitutional Disorders of Skeletal Development.* Saunders, Philadelphia, 1974.

Warkany, J., *Congenital Malformations.* Year Book, Chicago, 1971.

Aarskog Syndrome

(Facial-Digital-Genital Syndrome)

The disorder described by Aarskog (1) in 1970 and Scott (7) in 1971 is characterized by (a) short stature, (b) genital anomalies, and (c) unusual facies. It appears to have X-linked inheritance. The female heterozygote tends to be short and may exhibit minor stigmata (1, 3).

SYSTEMIC MANIFESTATIONS

Facies. The forehead is broad, with prominent ridging of the metopic suture (3, 7). Commonly there is a widow's peak (7). Ocular hypertelorism with ptosis of the upper eyelids combined with a short, broad, somewhat stubby nose with anteverted nostrils and a broad but not depressed nasal bridge characterize the face. The corneas may be somewhat large (3). The philtrum may be long, and the pinnas poorly modeled and rotated. There may be a linear curved depression below the lower lip. The earlobes are thick (8) and the upper helices malformed. Facial hair may be sparse (4) (Fig. 1-1*A*, *B*).

Musculoskeletal system. Although birth size has been normal, growth retardation has usually become evident between the ages of two to four years. Most patients have been below the 3d percentile in height. Adults rarely exceed 160 cm in height. Muscle tone usually remains poor throughout life. Small hands and feet, short fifth fingers, mild cubitus valgus, internal tibial tor-

sion, metatarsus varus, pigeon-toed gait, pes planus, "tree-frog toes," pectus excavatum, and hyperextensibility of interphalangeal joints have been noted (1–8) (Fig. 1-2). Inguinal hernia has been noted in over 60 percent of cases.

Radiographically, striking changes are generally limited to the cervical area of the spine and to the hands (3, 6, 8). Scott (7) described hypoplasia of the first cervical vertebra with an unfused posterior arch. On extension, it entered the foramen magnum. With flexion, there was subluxation of the first and second cervical vertebras. We have observed a patient with fusion of the second and third cervical vertebras. The terminal phalanges of the fingers and the middle phalanx of the fifth finger are hypoplastic. Hanley et al. (5) noted osteochondritis dissecans.

Genital anomalies. The scrotum appears bifid, with the scrotal fold extended ventrally around the base of the penis, somewhat resembling a shawl thrown about the neck (Fig. 1-2). Presumably this results from failure of caudal shift of the fused labioscrotal folds. In about 65 percent one or both testes are undescended (1). Fertility may be reduced (5).

Other findings. Bilateral simian creases and a single crease in the fifth fingers are frequent (3). Atrial septal defect has also been described (7).

Oral manifestations. Furukawa et al. (4) and Kunze and Spranger (6) noted hypoplastic narrow maxilla with relative mandibular prognathism.

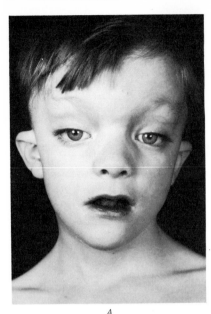 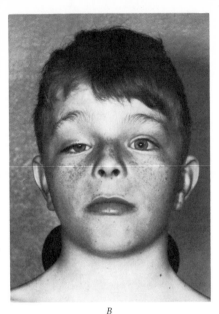

A   B

Figure 1-1. (*A*). *Aarskog syndrome.* Facies is characterized by broad forehead, hypertelorism, bilateral ptosis of upper eyelids, and low-set ears. (*From C. I. Scott*, Birth Defects **7**(6):240, 1971.) (*B*). Similar facies in patient from different family. Note unilateral ptosis.

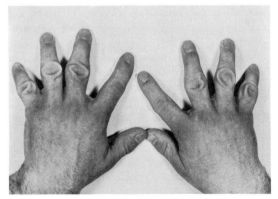

Figure 1-2. The hands are short and wide with frequent webbing of the fingers, hypermobility, and subluxation of the proximal interphalangeal joints. (*Courtesy of P. Berman, Montreal, Canada.*)

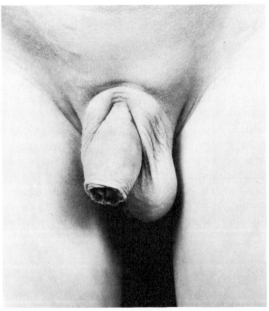

Figure 1-3. Abnormal penoscrotal configuration due to scrotal folds joining ventrally over base of penis. Note left inguinal hernia. (*From C. I. Scott*, Birth Defects **7**(6):240, 1971.)

DIFFERENTIAL DIAGNOSIS

The *Noonan syndrome* and the *leopard syndrome* share with this disorder such features as short stature, ocular hypertelorism, ptosis of upper eyelids, and hypogonadism.

LABORATORY AIDS

None is known.

REFERENCES

1 Aarskog, D., A Familial Syndrome of Short Stature Associated with Facial Dysplasia and Genital Anomalies. *J. Pediatr.* **77:**856–861, 1970; *Birth Defects* **7**(6):235–239, 1971.
2 Ainley, R. G., Hypertelorism (Greig's Syndrome). *J. Pediatr. Ophthalmol.* **5:**148–150, 1968.
3 Berman, P., et al., Inheritance of the Aarskog Syndrome. *Birth Defects* **10**(7):151–159, 1974.
4 Furukawa, C. T., et al., The Aarskog Syndrome. *J. Pediatr.* **81:**1117–1122, 1972.
5 Hanley, W. B., et al., Osteochondritis Dissecans and Associated Malformation in Brothers. *J. Bone Joint Surg.* **49A:**925–937, 1967.
6 Kunze, J., and Spranger, J., *Aarskog-Syndrom. Klin. Pediät.* **185:**490–494, 1973.
7 Scott, C. I., Jr., Unusual Facies, Joint Hypermobility, Genital Anomaly and Short Stature: A New Dysmorphic Syndrome. *Birth Defects* **7**(6):240–246, 1971.
8 Sugarman, G. I., et al., The Facial-Digital-Genital (Aarskog) Syndrome. *Am. J. Dis. Child.* **126:**248–252, 1973.

Acanthosis Nigricans and Adenocarcinoma

Although Pollitzer (35) and Janovsky (25) independently described acanthosis nigricans in 1890, it was Pollitzer (35), in 1909, who made the first extensive study of cases previously reported and who emphasized the relationship of the skin disease to abdominal malignancy. During the next 60 years, over 900 cases were reported, most of which have been associated with adenocarcinoma, principally of the stomach. Several excellent surveys (3, 30, 32) have been carried out, probably the greatest contributions being the numerous and extensive studies of Curth (7–15).

Acanthosis nigricans has been divided into four categories: (a) benign, a genodermatosis resembling ichthyosis hystrix, which may be present at birth or may begin later, either in childhood or, more often, at puberty, at which time it becomes more active; (b) pseudo, acquired and secondary to another disturbance, is most often seen in brunettes and associated with and dependent upon obesity which may be of endocrine origin (24); (c) malignant, which almost always arises in persons over twenty years of age and is always associated with an internal malignant tumor (14); and (d) acanthosis nigricans as part of a syndrome such as congenital lipodystrophy, Prader-Willi syndrome, the Crouzon syndrome, or Bloom syndrome (5, 13, 36). Rarely, acanthosis nigricans may be associated with lupoid hepatitis or ingestion of diethylstilbestrol. The benign and pseudo types occur with greater frequency than the malignant form.

Brown and Winkelmann (3), on the other hand, classified acanthosis nigricans into malignant and benign forms, further subdividing the latter into (a) idiopathic, (b) inherited, (c) endocrine-associated, and (d) drug-induced types. The patients with pseudo-acanthosis nigricans were included in the idiopathic group. The authors argue that weight reduction does not alter the presence of the acanthosis nigricans and that the patients with endocrine disorders are not necessarily obese.

Genetic studies on acanthosis nigricans have revealed that only the benign type shows a familial incidence and that an irregular dominant inheritance pattern is most common (7, 17, 21). The discussion that follows will be concerned largely with the malignant, or adult, type.

SYSTEMIC MANIFESTATIONS

Skin. Involvement of the skin may precede, accompany, or follow the detection of the cancer. It parallels the cancer in proportion to the degree of spread; it may regress with radiation therapy or surgical removal of the tumor and may reflourish with recurrence of the adenocarcinoma (12, 14).

In approximate order of frequency of pigmentation and papillomatous changes are the axillas, neck, genitalia, groin and inner thighs, umbilicus, perianal area, other flexural surfaces, and areolas. In addition to these changes, there is an

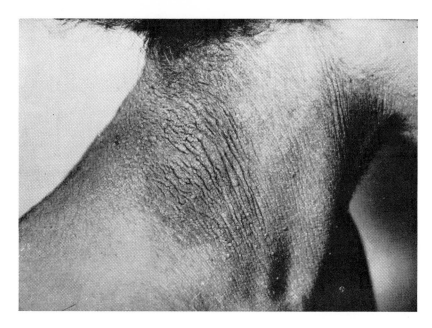

Figure 2-1. *Acanthosis nigricans—malignant form.* Pigmentations and papillomatosis of cervical region associated with gastric adenocarcinoma. (*From H. O. Curth, New York, New York.*)

exaggeration of normal skin markings. The axillas or neck usually become pigmented before other areas are involved (Figs. 2-1, 2-2). Generalized skin hyperpigmentation and pruritus occur in about 40 percent of cases of the malignant type (3). Palmar and plantar hyperkeratosis ac-

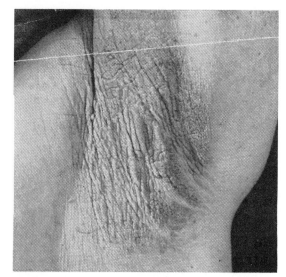

Figure 2-2. Pigmentation and papillomatosis of axillary area associated with gastric adenocarcinoma.

companies the malignant form in about 25 percent of the cases (3). More than 80 percent of affected persons are over forty years of age at the onset (27).

Microscopically, the skin exhibits the following features: increased thickness of stratum corneum, irregular acanthosis and atrophy of stratum spinosum, elongated, narrow papillary bodies, dense melanin deposits in the basal layer, and a few pigment-laden chromatophores in the papillary bodies (31). Increased numbers of mast cells may also be seen in the corium. In pseudo-acanthosis nigricans, the histologic changes are less severe than those in true acanthosis nigricans.

Adenocarcinoma. Curth and coworkers (12, 14) presented impressive evidence that nearly all associated tumors are adenocarcinomas. Furthermore, they indicated (7–10) that 92 percent of these tumors arise in the stomach (about 60 to 65 percent) or abdominal cavity (14, 17, 32). The uterus, ovary, gallbladder, pancreas, and intestines may also be the primary site. The other 8 percent arise in the breast, lung, etc.

Adenocarcinoma associated with acanthosis nigricans is extremely malignant. The mortality rate is 100 percent, and the average survival period after discovery is less than 2 years. Brown and Winkelmann (3) and Ackerman and Lantis (1) argue that although adenocarcinomas predominate, other tumors such as lymphomas may be associated with the malignant form. Garrott (19) has suggested that when acanthosis nigricans is associated with osteosarcoma, the distribution of skin lesions is different (extensor surfaces) and it affects young individuals.

Oral manifestations. Possibly the earliest description of oral lesions in acanthosis nigricans was made by Pollitzer (35) in 1909. Since then numerous authors have mentioned the occurrence of oral involvement, but, in most cases, description has been meager. Masson and Montgomery (27) and Fladung and Heite (17) suggested that at least 50 percent of patients with the adult form have oral lesions. On the other hand, the present authors, on the basis of a survey of over 200 reported malignant cases, think that a truer value is probably about 30 to 40 percent. A similar figure was reported by Brown and Winkelmann (3). Unfortunately, the oral mucosa is seldom thoroughly inspected in the course of a general examination.

Of all oral tissue, the tongue and lips are involved most frequently and to the greatest degree. The dorsum of the tongue, or at times the lateral border, exhibits hypertrophy and elongation of papillae. These give the tongue, marked by deep fissures or furrows, a shaggy or prickly appearance. In addition, one may see papillomatous growths studding its surface (7, 20, 27–29, 35, 39–41). In contrast to growths on the skin, these growths are rarely pigmented (2, 3).

The lips, especially the upper lip, may be markedly enlarged and covered by filiform or papillomatous growths which are especially marked at the angles of the mouth (12, 22, 27, 28, 35, 41) (Figs. 2-3, 2-4).

The buccal mucosa is usually less severely involved. One generally finds a diffuse unevenness of its surface and a velvety white appearance. Occasionally, single fungiform growths are observed (6, 12, 27, 39, 40). The palate may be similarly affected (28, 35). The gingiva, especially the interdental papillae, may become so much enlarged as almost to cover the teeth, resembling idiopathic fibromatosis. Although the teeth have been noted to loosen and to be

shed, the frequency of this phenomenon is yet to be determined (4, 6, 27).

There is insufficient evidence to suggest the frequency of oral involvement in the benign form of the disease, but it would not appear to be great (3, 20, 33, 42). Fladung and Heite (17) estimated the incidence of this form at 14 percent. The vaginal and conjunctival mucous membranes may also be the site of verrucous lesions (37). Readett (personal communication, 1961) indicated that the pharynx, esophagus, and large intestines may be involved as well.

DIFFERENTIAL DIAGNOSIS

Regarding endogenous pigmentation, one should consider Addison's disease, arsenic poisoning, and hemochromatosis, but in none of these conditions is there an associated papillomatosis. Ichthyosis hystrix, the *multiple hamartoma*

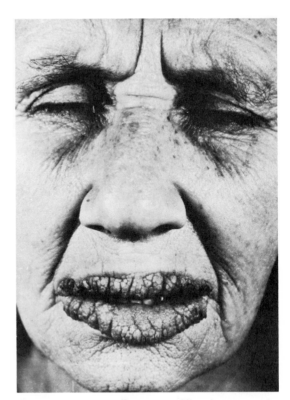

Figure 2-3. Note papillomatosis of lips. (*Courtesy of N. Danbolt, Oslo, Norway.*)

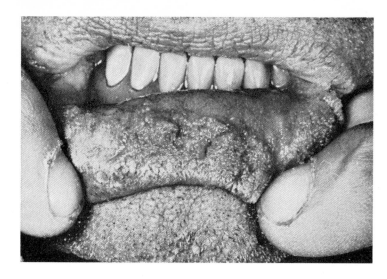

Figure 2-4. Thickening of labial mucosa and papillomatosis. Pigmentation of oral mucosa is characteristically absent. (*From A. Proppe, Kiel, Germany.*)

and neoplasia syndrome, bromoderma, pemphigus vegetans, *hyalinosis cutis et mucosae,* condyloma acuminatum, and hairy tongue must all be ruled out as well. In Afro-Americans, one should exclude dermatosis papulosa nigra. Hirschowitz et al. (23) recently described acanthosis nigricans in a syndrome of nerve deafness, absent gastric motility, small intestine diverticulitis, and progressive sensory neuropathy. Autosomal recessive inheritance appeared likely. Also see Chap. 144, Miscellaneous Syndromes.

LABORATORY AIDS

None is known.

REFERENCES

1 Ackerman, A. B., and Lantis, L. R., Acanthosis Nigricans with Hodgkin's Disease. *Arch. Dermatol.* **95:**202–205, 1967.

2 Andreev, V. C., et al., Acanthosis Nigricans of Oral Mucosa. *Dermatologica (Basel)* **126:**25–29, 1963.

3 Brown, J., and Winkelmann, R. K., Acanthosis Nigricans: A Study of 90 Cases. *Medicine* **47:**33–51, 1968.

4 Brown, J., et al., Acanthosis Nigricans and Pituitary Tumors. *J.A.M.A.* **198:**619–623, 1966.

5 Brubaker, M. M., et al., Acanthosis Nigricans and Congenital Lipodystrophy. *Arch. Dermatol.* **91:**320–325, 1965.

6 Cochrane, T., and Alexander, J. O'D., Acanthosis Nigricans. *Br. J. Dermatol.* **63:**225–230, 1951.

7 Curth, H. O., Benign Type of Acanthosis Nigricans. *Arch. Dermatol. Syph.* **34:**353–366, 1936.

8 Curth, H. O., Cancer Associated with Acanthosis Nigricans: Review of Literature and Report of a Case of Acanthosis Nigricans with Cancer of the Breast. *Arch. Surg.* **47:**517–552, 1943.

9 Curth, H. O., Acanthosis Nigricans and Its Association with Cancer. *Arch. Dermatol. Syph.* **57:**158–170, 1948.

10 Curth, H. O., Pseudo-acanthosis Nigricans. *Ann. Dermatol. Syphiligr. (Paris)* **78:**417–429, 1951.

11 Curth, H. O., Significance of Acanthosis Nigricans. *Arch. Dermatol. Syph.* **66:**80–100, 1952.

12 Curth, H. O., Pigmentary Changes of the Skin Associated with Internal Disease. *Postgrad. Med.* **41:**439–444, 1967.

13 Curth, H. O., The Necessity of Distinguishing Four Types of Acanthosis Nigricans, in *XIIIth International Congress on Dermatology, Munich, 1967.* Springer-Verlag, New York, 1968.

14 Curth, H. O., and Aschner, B. M., Genetic Studies on Acanthosis Nigricans. *Arch. Dermatol. Syph.* **79:**55–66, 1959.

15 Curth, H. O., et al., The Site and Histology of the Cancer Associated with Malignant Acanthosis Nigricans. *Cancer* **15:**364–382, 1962.

16 Dornbush, F. J., Acanthosis Nigricans, Adult Type (with Involvement of the Mucous Membranes of the Mouth, Eyes, and Vagina). *Arch. Dermatol.* **75:**765, 1957.

17 Fladung, G., and Heite, H. J., Häufigkeitsanalytische Untersuchungen zur Frage der symptomologischen Abgrenzung verschiedener Formen der Acanthosis nigricans. *Arch. Klin. Exp. Dermatol.* **205:**282–311, 1957.

18 Fox, H., and Gunn, A. D. G., Acanthosis Nigricans and Bronchial Carcinoma. *Br. J. Dis. Chest* **59:**47–50, 1965.

19 Garrott, T. C., Malignant Acanthosis Nigricans Associated with Osteogenic Sarcoma. *Arch. Dermatol.* **106**:384–385, 1972.

20 Hellerström, S., Zur Kenntnis der Acanthosis nigricans. *Acta Derm. Venereol. (Stockh.)* **14**:86–98, 1933.

21 Hermann, H., Zur Erbpathologie der Acanthosis nigricans. *Z. Menschl. Vererb. Konstit. Lehre* **33**:193–202, 1055.

22 Herold, W. C., et al., Acanthosis Nigricans: Its Occurrence in Association with Gastric Carcinoma in a Seventeen-year-old Girl. *Arch. Dermatol. Syph.* **44**:789–799, 1941.

23 Hirschowitz, B. I., et al., Hereditary Nerve Deafness in Three Sisters with Absent Gastric Mobility, Small Bowel Diverticulitis and Ulceration and Progressive Sensory Neuropathy. *Birth Defects* **8**(2):27–41, 1972.

24 Hollingsworth, D. R., and Amatruda, T. T., Jr., Acanthosis Nigricans and Obesity. *Arch. Intern. Med.* **124**:481–487, 1969.

25 Janovsky, V., in P. G. Unna et al. (eds.), *Internationaler Atlas seltener Hautkrankheiten.* Leopold Voss, Leipzig, 1890, plate II.

26 Krebs, A., Acanthosis nigricans mit Befall des Oesophagus und Mangel an Vitamin A. *Schweiz. Med. Wochenschr.* **92**:545–552, 1962.

27 Masson, J. C., and Montgomery, H., Relationship of Acanthosis Nigricans to Abdominal Malignancy. *Am. J. Obstet. Gynecol.* **32**:716–726, 1936.

28 Matras, A., Acanthosis nigricans mit Schleimhautveränderungen. *Zentralbl. Haut-Geschl.-Kr.* **63**:410, 1940.

29 McKenna, R. M. B., and Roxburgh, I., Acanthosis Nigricans. *Br. J. Dermatol.* **61**:251–252, 1949.

30 Moncorps, C., Acanthosis Nigricans, in J. Jadassohn (ed.), *Handbuch der Haut-und Geschlechtskrankheiten.* Springer-Verlag, Berlin, 1931.

31 Montgomery, H., and O'Leary, P. A., Pigmentation of the Skin in Addison's Disease, Acanthosis Nigricans and Hemochromatosis. *Arch. Dermatol. Syph.* **21**:970–984, 1930.

32 Mukai, F., see (30).

33 Pindborg, J. J., and Gorlin, R. J., Oral Changes in Acanthosis Nigricans: Juvenile Type. *Acta Derm. Venereol. (Stockh.)* **42**:63–71, 1962.

34 Pollitzer, S., in P. G. Unna et al. (eds.), *Internationaler Atlas seltener Hautkrankheiten.* Leopold Voss, Leipzig, 1890, plate 10.

35 Pollitzer, S., Acanthosis Nigricans: A Symptom of a Disorder of the Abdominal Sympathetic. *J.A.M.A.* **53**:1369–1373, 1909.

36 Reed, W. B., et al., Acanthosis Nigricans in Association with Various Genodermatoses. *Acta Derm. Venereol. (Stockh.)* **48**:465–473, 1968.

37 Scheer, M., Acanthosis Nigricans. *Arch. Dermatol. Syph.* **28**:118–119, 1933.

38 Schwartz, B., Acanthosis Nigricans. *Br. J. Dermatol.* **64**:462–463, 1952.

39 Schwartz, J. H., and Miller, E. C., Acanthosis Nigricans. *Arch. Dermatol. Syph.* **18**:534–538, 1928.

40 Scott, O. L. S., Acanthosis Nigricans. *Br. J. Dermatol.* **64**:461–462, 1952.

41 Shindelka, H., *Hautkrankheiten bei Haustiere.* W. Braunmüller, Leipzig, 1898, p. 415.

42 Tolmach, J. A., Acanthosis Nigricans: Juvenile Type. *Arch. Dermatol. Syph.* **40**:819–820, 1939.

43 Winkelmann, R. K., et al., Acanthosis Nigricans and Endocrine Disease. *J.A.M.A.* **174**:1145–1152, 1960.

3

Achondrogenesis

Separated by Parenti (16) in 1936 from achondroplasia, achondrogenesis is characterized by (a) lethality, (b) disproportionately large head, and (c) severe shortening of limbs and trunk (Fig. 3-1). This disorder should be distinguished clearly from the condition described by Grebe and Quelce-Salgado (achondrogenesis, Brazilian type) (17).

There is no sex predilection. The disorder is probably inherited as an autosomal recessive trait, affected sibs having been described (3a, 6, 20, 21) as well as parental consanguinity (20). It is likely that achondrogenesis is a heterogeneity (see Skeletal Alterations).

SYSTEMIC MANIFESTATIONS

Achondrogenesis is incompatible with life; the infant is born dead or survives but a few days. There may be a history of hydramnios (20, 22).

Facies. The head is disproportionately enlarged, the infant often erroneously being labeled as hydrocephalic. In fact, it is common for the head to exceed 40 percent of body length. The nose is usually flattened, and there appears to be no neck.

Skeletal alterations. The chest is short and dwarfed by the rotund belly (13, 22). The limbs are exceedingly abbreviated and bowed, in most cases rarely exceeding 20 cm in length. Total body length at term rarely exceeds 36 cm (range 25 to 38 cm).

Radiologically, the trunk appears squatter and the thorax wider than in thanatophoric dwarfism. The clavicles are often overlong. The ribs are short and horizontal, and sternal ossification is absent. The vertebral bodies are inadequately mineralized, at times appearing totally absent, especially in the lumbar and cervical regions. The interpediculate distance of the lumbar vertebras is not reduced. The sacral, pubic, and ischial bones are not ossified. The ilia are small with crescent-shaped inner and inferior edges. The vertebral column is proportionately shorter in achondrogenesis than in thanatophoric dwarfism. The talus and calcaneus are not ossified (Fig. 3-2).

The degree of ossification of long bones is quite variable. In Parenti's patient, virtually no ossification of long bones was evident, and the vertebras of Bremer's patient seem to lack ossification. In contrast to its condition in thanatophoric dwarfism, the femur is not bowed and rarely exceeds 3 cm in length. The metaphysis of the humerus is widened and cupped. Periosteal spurs give a cuspid appearance to the metaphyses. The phalanges are exceedingly small.

Histopathologic studies have demonstrated disorganized matrix synthesis or secretion. The resting cartilage from all sites is markedly hypercellular, consisting primarily of large ballooned chondrocytes with little intervening matrix (18, 23). A different histopathologic picture has been

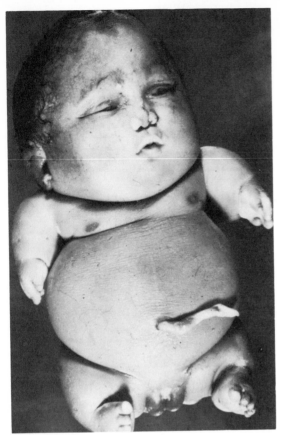

Figure 3-1. *Achondrogenesis.* An infant with this lethal dwarfism has a disproportionately large head, disproportionately short limbs, and pot belly. The head appears to sit directly on the thorax.

described in the so-called Houston-type dwarf (8).

In the so-called Houston or "Saskatoon" lethal achondrogenesis, also having autosomal recessive inheritance, the ribs are thinner and manifest multiple intrauterine fractures with callus formation. The iliac bones, scapulas, and long bones are even more shortened and bowed than in achondrogenesis (4, 7, 8). One of the infants described by Ryan and Kozlowski (19) also may have had this disorder.

Other findings. Inguinal hernia (9, 20) and patent ductus arteriosus (20) have been noted.

DIFFERENTIAL DIAGNOSIS

The clinical appearance alone should allow the clinician to separate this disorder from *thanatophoric dwarfism* (11, 21) and a rare autosomal recessive lethal disorder as yet unnamed (3).

Saldino (20) and Ryan and Kozlowski (19) described infants with achondrogenesis who exhibited only mild abbreviation of the extremities.

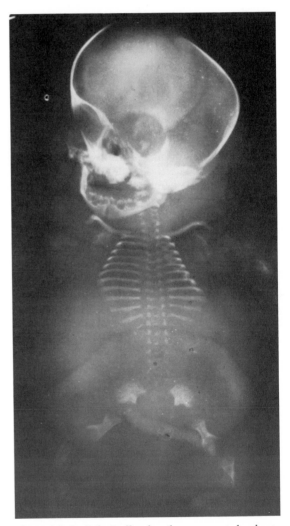

Figure 3-2. Radiologically, the ribs are seen to be short and horizontal. The vertebral bodies are inadequately mineralized, especially in the lumbar region. The sacral, pubic, and ischial bones are not ossified. Note severe shortening of long bones.

REFERENCES

1 Bremer, K., Eine seltene Missbildung aus dem Formenkreis der Chondrodystrophie. *Z. Geburtshilfe Gynäkol.* **140**:198–202, 1953.

2 Canton, E., Sobre tres fetos acondroplasicos y sus radiografías respectivas. *Sem. Med. (Buenos Aires)* **10**:489–505 (case 2), 1903.

3 Chapelle, A. de la, et al., Une rare dysplasie osseuse léthale de transmission recessive autosomique. *Arch. Fr. Pédiatr.* **29**:759–770, 1972.

3a Curran, J. P., et al., Lethal Forms of Chondrodysplastic Dwarfism. *Pediatrics* **53**:76–85, 1974.

4 Fraccaro, M., Contributo allo studio delle malattie del mesenchima osteopoietico: L'acondrogenesi. *Folia Hered. Pathol. (Milano)* **1**:190–198, 1952.

5 Gorlin, R. J., and Sedano, H. O., Achondrogenesis. *Mod. Med. (Minneapolis)* **38**:144–145, 1970.

6 Harris, R., and Patton, J. T., Achondroplasia and Thanatophoric Dwarfism in the Newborn. *Clin. Genet.* **2**:61–72 (cases 7, 8), 1971.

7 Harris, R., et al., Pseudo-achondrogenesis with Fractures. *Clin. Genet.* **3**:435–441, 1972.

8 Houston, C. S., et al., Fatal Neonatal Dwarfism. *J. Can. Assoc. Radiol.* **23**:45–61, 1972.

9 Jurczok, F., and Schollmeyer, R., Zur Frage des gehäuften Auftretens von Extremitätenmissbildungen bei Neugeborenen. *Geburtshilfe Frauenheilkd.* **22**:400–421 (case 3), 1962.

10 Krueger, R., *Die Phocomelie und ihre Übergange*, August Hirschwald, Berlin, 1906, pp. 58–59, 86–89 (cases 83, 84).

11 Langer, L. O., Thanatophoric Dwarfism: A Condition Confused with Achondroplasia in the Neonate, with Brief Comments on Achondrogenesis and Homozygous Achondroplasia. *Radiology* **92**:285–294, 1969.

12 Laquiere et al., Un cas d'achondroplasie. *Bull. Soc. Obstet. Gynecol. (Paris)* **23**:623–626, 1934.

13 Legrand, J., Un cliché de foetus achondroplasique "in utero." *J. Radiol. Électrol. Med. Nucl.* **37**:82–84, 1956.

14 Levi, L., and Bouchacourt, L., Radiographies de foetus achondroplases. *Rev. Hyg. Méd. Inf.* **3**:517–528 (case 2), 1904.

15 Maroteaux, P., and Lamy, M., Le diagnostic des nanismes chondro-dystrophiques chez les nouveau-nés. *Arch. Fr. Pédiatr.* **25**:241–262, 1968.

16 Parenti, G. C., La anosteogenesi: Una varietà della osteogenesi imperfetta. *Pathologica* **28**:447–462, 1936.

17 Quelce-Salgado, A., A New Type of Dwarfism with Various Bone Aplasias and Hypoplasias of the Extremities. *Acta Genet. (Basel)* **14**:63–66, 1964.

18 Rimoin, D., Histopathology and Ultrastructure of Cartilage in the Chondrodystrophies. *Birth Defects* **10**(9):1–18, 1974.

19 Ryan, J., and Kozlowski, K., Radiology of Stillborn Infants. *Australas. Radiol.* **15**:213–226, 1971.

20 Saldino, R. M., Lethal Short-limbed Dwarfism: Achondrogenesis and Thanatophoric Dwarfism. *Am. J. Roentgenol.* **112**:185–197, 1971.

21 Silverman, F., Personal communication, 1971.

22 Tonkes, E., Achondroplasia. *Gynaecologia (Basel)* **122**:327–337, 1946.

23 Xanthokos, E., and Rejent, M. M., Achondrogenesis. *J. Pediatr.* **82**:658–663, 1973.

4

Achondroplasia

The term "achondroplasia" was first used by Parrot (21) in 1878 to describe (a) a rhizomelic form of short-limbed dwarfism associated with (b) enlarged head, (c) depressed nasal bridge, and (d) short, stubby, trident hands, (e) lordotic lumbar spine, (f) prominent buttocks, and (g) protuberant abdomen. Achondroplasia is a misleading term because cartilage is, in fact, formed in the disorder. However, the term is well established in the medical literature. Until relatively recently, a variety of chondrodystrophies were frequently confused with achondroplasia (11, 12, 28). Achondroplasia and hypochondroplasia may be allelic (13).

More than 80 percent of recorded cases of achondroplasia are sporadic, representing point mutations. Less than 20 percent of reported cases are familial, showing an autosomal dominant mode of transmission (17). Increased paternal age at time of conception is associated with sporadic cases (17, 18).

The gene frequency of achondroplasia has been estimated to range between 0.00004 and 0.00014 in various populations (3, 15, 16, 19, 24, 27, 31). These are probably gross overestimates because various chondrodystrophies are undoubtedly included in these surveys (17, 29).

Affected individuals are heterozygous for the achondroplasia gene. Presumed homozygosity has been reported in a few instances in which both parents were achondroplastic. Homozygous achondroplastic infants are more severely affected, clinically and radiologically. The homozygous state resembles thanatophoric dwarfism in many respects, and the condition is lethal during infancy (9).

The possible existence of an autosomal recessive mode of transmission in achondroplasia has been the subject of numerous discussions. Most examples cited in support of this thesis either represent various recessively inherited chondrodystrophies or are insufficiently documented to establish diagnosis with certainty (14). The one known instance of affected sibs with normal parents (4) can probably be explained by gonadal mosaicism, since one sib has subsequently produced an affected child (J. Hall, personal communication, 1975).

Cases of achondroplasia within the same kindred which seemingly do not show complete penetrance have been reported on rare occasion (20, 35). Such pedigrees may be explained by the inheritance of an unstable premutation (20), which could also explain instances of mosaic achondroplasia, such as the case reported by Rimoin and McKusick (25).

The basic defect is unknown. Early histologic studies, which suggested gross disorganization of endochondral ossification, were misleading because they described patients with thanatophoric dwarfism, metatropic dwarfism, or achondrogenesis (Parenti-Fraccaro type), rather than true achondroplasia (26). Achondroplasia appears to be associated with a quantitative decrease in endochondral ossification but a normal rate of membranous ossification (24a).

Rimoin and his associates found well-organized endochondral ossification with longitudinal columns of cartilage cells in chondroosseous rib junctions. Iliac crest cartilage was found to be normal. These findings suggested that the abnormality in achondroplasia might be quantitative, affecting the rate of cartilage growth (26). Different findings have been reported by Ponseti (23) and Stanescu (30).

Histologic, histochemical, ultrastructural, and biochemical studies of growth plates from different anatomic locations (including both weight-bearing and non-weight-bearing areas) in different age groups are necessary to resolve further the pathogenesis of achondroplasia.

Defective oxidative energy formation with decreased phosphorylation at the NADH dehydrogenase region of the terminal respiratory system has been demonstrated in achondroplastic muscle (13a). A defect in peripheral glucose utilization has also been shown (6).

SYSTEMIC MANIFESTATIONS

Mean birth lengths are 47.7 cm for males and 47.2 cm for females. Mean birth weights are 3,500 g for males and 3,150 g for females. Both lengths and weights are somewhat less for achondroplastic offspring of dwarfed mothers.

Motor milestones are slow. Head control may not occur until 3 to 4 months and affected children may not walk until 24 to 36 months. Ultimately, however, development is normal.

Final height attainment is 130 cm for males and 123 cm for females. Mean adult weights are 55 kg for males and 46 kg for females. There is a predilection for obesity.

Reproductive fitness is considerably reduced among achondroplastics, because of social difficulties in finding mates and because of the obstetrical problems of achondroplastic women (prematurity and caesarean deliveries).

Facies. The head is enlarged, with frontal bossing and depression of the nasal bridge. These features occasionally may not be present at birth, but disproportionate growth of the head occurs during the first year of life and then parallels the normal curve (5, 12) (Fig. 4-1).

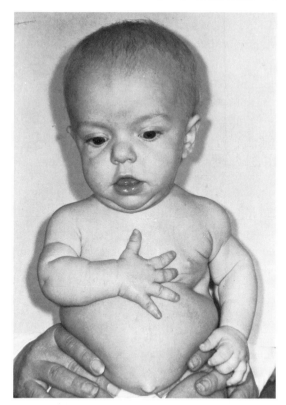

Figure 4-1. *Achondroplasia.* Note enlarged head with frontal bossing and depressed nasal bridge. Rhizomelia and short hands with trident deformity are evident.

Central nervous system. Intelligence is almost always normal, although the acquisition of motor skills may be somewhat delayed because of the large head and short extremities (5). Enlargement of the head in achondroplasia may be due to true megalencephaly (7). Mild ventricular dilatation has been demonstrated by pneumoencephalographic studies (5, 7, 37). However, gross mechanical block caused by obliteration of the basal cisterns, by obliteration at the level of the foramen magnum, or by kinking of the cerebral aqueduct has not been demonstrated in most cases (11). Significant hydrocephaly (stepwise increase in the head-growth slope) with neurologic signs and symptoms has occurred in a few instances (5, 7) and is probably caused by cerebrospinal fluid obstruction at the level of the foramen magnum. Cohen and associates (5) demonstrated poor filling of the basal cisterns in two cases of achondroplasia with significant hydrocephaly. Communicating hydrocephaly without ventricular stasis was demonstrated by James et al. (10).

The narrow spinal canal predisposes to neurologic complications with age. Compression of the spinal cord and nerve rootlets results from osteophytes, prolapsed intervertebral disks, or deformed vertebral bodies (1, 8, 33, 34).

Skeletal system. Enlarged calvaria with shortening of the cranial base and basilar kyphosis are constant features. The foramen magnum is small. The maxilla is hypoplastic resulting in midface deficiency and relative mandibular prognathism. The frontal and occipital bones and, in some cases, the temporal bones may be prominent (11, 12). Partial occipitalization of the first cervical vertebra occurs in most cases.

The interpediculate distances in the upper to the lower lumbar spine are progressively narrowed, the pedicles are shortened in anteroposterior diameter, the posterior aspect of the vertebral bodies is concave, and the bony spinal canal diameters are decreased, especially in the lumbar region. Anterior wedging of the vertebral bodies (particularly in the region of the thoracolumbar junction) with resultant kyphosis may be prominent (11, 12).

The lumbar spine appears to articulate low in relationship to the crests of the iliac bone. The sacrum is narrow and horizontally oriented. The pelvis is broad and short. Narrowing of the pelvic inlet prevents vaginal delivery in pregnant achondroplastic females. The superior acetabular margins are oriented horizontally, and the sacrosciatic notch is acute. The thoracic cage is relatively small in anteroposterior diameter (2, 11, 12). The legs are frequently bowed because of lax knee ligaments.

Limb bones are shortened in a rhizomelic pattern, which is more prominent in the upper extremities. There is incomplete extension at the elbows. The metacarpals and phalanges, although shortened, are disproportionately large in relation to the humerus, radius, and ulna (11, 12). The fibula is overlong at the ankle compared to the tibia, leading in some cases to varus foot deformity. There is limitation of elbow extension.

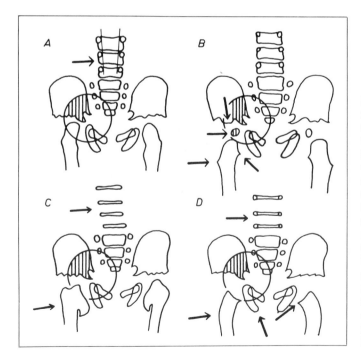

Figure 4-2. Schematic drawings of pelvic features of (*A*) achondroplasia, (*B*) chondroectodermal dysplasia, (*C*) metatropic dwarfism, and (*D*) thanatophoric dwarfism. Deformity of acetabulum is nearly the same in the four conditions. In achondroplasia, interpediculate distances diminish downward. In chondroectodermal dysplasia, ossification centers of femur and spikelike exostoses at the trochanters are present. In metatropic dwarfism, reduced height of vertebral bodies, halberd form of femur, and, occasionally, scoliosis are seen. In thanatophoric dwarfism, vertebral bodies are flat, spikelike exostoses are present at the os pubics and at the femur, and the femur is bowed. (*From K. Gefferth*, Prog. Pediatr. Radiol. **4**:137, 1973.)

Other findings. Otitis media is common during the first 6 years of life, and if untreated, may lead to hearing loss.

Oral manifestations. Malocclusion is commonly observed. Anterior crowding, anterior overjet, and various crossbites have been noted (M. M. C., unpublished data, 1972).

DIFFERENTIAL DIAGNOSIS

Achondroplasia should be distinguished from *achondrogenesis, thanatophoric dwarfism, Ellis-van Creveld syndrome, metatropic dwarfism, diastrophic dwarfism,* asphyxiating thoracic dystrophy, hypochondroplasia, pseudoachondroplasia, *Nance-Sweeney chondrodysplasia,* and other types of short-limbed dwarfism (11–14, 18, 28, 36) (Fig. 4-2).

LABORATORY AIDS

Roentgenographic studies permit differentiation from other forms of dwarfism that simulate achondroplasia (29).

REFERENCES

1 Alexander, E., Jr., Significance of the Small Lumbar Spinal Canal: Cauda Equina Compression Syndromes Due to Spondylosis. Part 5: Achondroplasia. *J. Neurosurg.* **31:**513–519, 1969.

2 Bailey, J. A., Orthopedic Aspects of Achondroplasia. *J. Bone Joint Surg.* **52A:**1285–1301, 1970.

3 Böök, J. A., The Incidence of Congenital Diseases and Defects in a South Swedish Population. *Acta Genet.* (*Basel*) **2:**289–311, 1951.

4 Bowen, P., Two Achondroplasts from Normal Parents. *Birth Defects,* in press.

5 Cohen, M. E., et al., Neurological Abnormalities in Achondroplastic Children. *J. Pediatr.* **71:**367–376, 1967.

6 Collipp, P. J., et al., Abnormal Glucose Tolerance in Children with Achondroplasia. *Am. J. Dis. Child.* **124:**682–689, 1972.

7 Dennis, J. P., et al., Megencephaly, Internal Hydrocephalus and Other Neurological Aspects of Achondroplasia. *Brain* **84:**427–445, 1961.

8 Duvoisin, R. C., and Yahr, M., Compressive Spinal Cord and Root Syndromes in Achondroplastic Dwarfs. *Neurology* (*Minneap.*) **12:**202–207, 1962.

9 Hall, J. G., et al., Two Probable Cases of Homozygosity for the Achondroplasia Gene. *Birth Defects* **5**(4):24–34, 1969.

10 James, A. E., et al., Hydrocephalus in Achondroplasia Studied by Cisternography. *Pediatrics* **49:**46–49, 1972.

11 Langer, L. O., et al., Achondroplasia. *Am. J. Roentgenol.* **100:**12–26, 1967.

12 Langer, L. O., et al., Achondroplasia: Clinical Radiologic Features with Comment on Genetic Implications. *Clin. Pediatr.* **7:**474–485, 1968.

13 McKusick, V. A., et al., Observations Suggesting Allelism of the Achondroplasia and Hypochondroplasia Genes. *J. Med. Genet.* **10:**11–16, 1973.

13a Mackler, B., et al., Oxidative Energy Deficiency. II. Human Achondroplasia. *Arch. Biochem. Biophysics* **159:**885–888, 1973.

14 Maroteaux, P., and Lamy, M., Achondroplasia in Man and Animals. *Clin. Orthop.* **33:**91–103, 1964.

15 Master-Notani, P., et al., Congenital Malformations in the Newborn in Bombay. *Acta Genet.* (*Basel*) **18:**193–205, 1968.

16 Mørch, E. T., *Chondrodystrophic Dwarfs in Denmark.* Munksgaard, Copenhagen, 1941.

17 Murdoch, J. L., et al., Achondroplasia—a Genetic and Statistical Survey. *Ann. Hum. Genet.* **33:**227–244, 1970.

18 Nance, W. E., and Sweeney, A., A Recessively Inherited Chondrodystrophy. *Birth Defects* **6**(4):25–27, 1970.

19 Neel, J. V., A Study of Major Congenital Defects in Japanese Infants. *Am. J. Hum. Genet.* **10:**398–445, 1958.

20 Opitz, J. M., Delayed Mutation in Achondroplasia? *Birth Defects* **5**(4):20–23, 1969.

21 Parrot, J. M., Sur les malformations achondroplasiques et le dieu Ptah. *Bull. Soc. Antropol.* (*Paris*) **1:**296, 1878.

22 Penrose, L. S., Parental Age in Achondroplasia and Mongolism. *Am. J. Hum. Genet.* **9:**167–169, 1957.

23 Ponseti, I. V., Skeletal Growth in Achondroplasia. *J. Bone Joint Surg.* **52-A:**701–716, 1970.

24 Potter, E. L., and Coverstone, V., Chondrodystrophy fetalis. *Am. J. Obstet. Gynecol.* **65:**790–793, 1948.

24a Rimoin, D. L., Histopathology and Ultrastructure of Cartilage in the Chondrodystrophies. *Birth Defects* **10**(9):1–18, 1974.

25 Rimoin, D. L., et al., Somatic Mosaicism in an Achondroplastic Dwarf. *Birth Defects* **5**(4):17–19, 1969.

26 Rimoin, D. L., et al., Endochondral Ossification in Achondroplastic Dwarfism. *N. Engl. J. Med.* **283:**728–735, 1970.

27 Schull, W. J., Consanguinity and the Etiology of Congenital Malformations. *Pediatrics* **23:**195–201, 1959.

28 Silverman, F. N., A Differential Diagnosis of Achondroplasia. *Radiol. Clin. North Am.* **6:**223–237, 1968.

29 Spranger, J., et al., *Bone Dysplasias.* Gustav Fischer-Verlag, Stuttgart, 1974.

30 Stanescu, V., Study of Bone Growth. *N. Engl. J. Med.* **284:**110–111, 1971.

31 Stevenson, A. C., Achondroplasia: An Account of the Condition in Northern Ireland. *Am. J. Hum. Genet.* **9**:81–91, 1957.

32 Tyson, J. E., et al., Obstetric and Gynecologic Considerations of Dwarfism. *Am. J. Obstet. Gynecol.* **108**:688–704, 1970.

33 Vogl, A., The Fate of the Achondroplastic Dwarf (Neurological Complications of Achondroplasia). *Exp. Med. Surg.* **20**:108–117, 1962.

34 Vogl, A., and Osborne, R. L., Lesions of the Spinal Cord (Transverse Myelopathy) in Achondroplasia. *Arch. Neurol. Psychiatr. (Chic.)* **61**:644–662, 1949.

35 Wadia, R., Achondroplasia in Two First Cousins. *Birth Defects* **5**(4):227–229, 1969.

36 Walker, B. A., et al., Hypochondroplasia. *Am. J. Dis. Child.* **122**:95–104, 1971.

37 Wise, B. L. et al., Achondroplasia und Hydrocephalus. *Neuropädiatrie* **3**:106–113, 1971.

5

Acrodermatitis Enteropathica

(*Danbolt-Closs Syndrome*)

Acrodermatitis enteropathica is a rare familial disorder, occurring in childhood, the primary signs of which are (*a*) skin lesions, (*b*) hair loss, (*c*) nail changes, and (*d*) gastrointestinal disturbances. Before 1942, when Danbolt and Closs (6) presented the first comprehensive description of the syndrome and suggested the name "acrodermatitis enteropathica," the condition was mentioned in the literature under such varying diagnoses as systemic thrush, moniliasis, and "dermatitis in children with disturbances in the general condition and the absorption of food elements" (2). Comprehensive reviews of the literature have been made by Dillaha et al. (7), Wells and Winkelmann (21), and Heite and Ody (9). About 200 cases have been reported (9).

Etiology is still obscure but theories have abounded (1, 3, 7, 8). Most have suggested deficiency of an unknown food element. The onset of the syndrome often coincides with the time of weaning. In 1953, Dillaha et al. (7) reported dramatic improvement of the condition after oral administration of diiodohydroxyquin. The beneficial effect of the compound, a local disinfectant absorbed in negligible quantities, is not understood. On the basis of histochemical studies, Moynahan et al. (13) suggested a possible intestinal enzyme deficiency. Barnes and Moynahan (2) demonstrated a zinc deficiency. Low serum zinc levels have been demonstrated by others (15, 19) who effected dramatic improvement of their patients given zinc therapy. Possibly the efficacy of

diiodohydroxyquin is based on its possible role in transporting the zinc ion across the intestinal barrier.

In 65 percent of reported cases, there is a history of familial occurrence (21). A recessive mode of transmission appears evident (1, 6). The disease is evenly distributed over the world (9).

SYSTEMIC MANIFESTATIONS

Acrodermatitis begins early in life, usually between the ages of three weeks and ten years, with an average age at onset of nine months in reported cases (20). Many patients, however, exhibit the full syndrome at about the age of one year (4). A review of reported cases shows females to be affected only slightly more frequently than males (21). Rarely has the syndrome been reported in adults (18, 23). The disorder seems to improve by puberty (21). The onset is insidious and follows an intermittent course, often with spontaneous, partial remissions, succeeded by increasingly severe exacerbations. The majority of cases have ended fatally.

Body growth is retarded in 80 percent of the patients, and 40 percent present mental changes (21), often in the form of schizoid features (6) associated with the exacerbations.

Facies. Children suffering from acrodermatitis enteropathica exhibit a striking uniformity of appearance, mainly because of the alopecia and

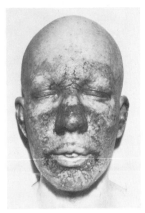

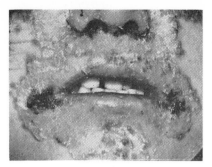

Figure 5-3. Circumoral changes.

Figure 5-1. Acrodermatitis enteropathica in a 20-year-old male.

the orificial location of lesions (Fig. 5-1). Dillaha et al. (7) pointed out that the affected child holds his head at an angle, with his face downward.

Skin. The syndrome usually starts with small erythematous, moist skin eruptions localized around the natural orifices and symmetrically on the buttocks, elbows, knees, hands, and feet, especially between the fingers and toes and around the nails (Fig. 5-2). The trunk is only slightly affected. The rash, in most cases, is of a vesiculo-bullous type, but vesicles or bullae are not always present. After a short period of time, the

vesicular lesions begin to dry and crust, subsequently turning into sharply marginated lesions, sometimes with a psoriasiform appearance (7). When the lesions heal, they leave no scars.

Gastrointestinal tract. The gastrointestinal tract disturbances consist of bouts of diarrhea, with increased excretion of fat (6). Lombeck et al. (12) described inclusions in Paneth cells. A large number of children with the syndrome suffer from thrush. The buccal mucosa (less often the palate, gingiva, and tonsils) presents red and white spots (17, 20) or edema with erosions, ulcerations, and desquamation (4, 10). The white coating of the oral mucosa is reported to be rather firmly attached to underlying structures (11, 23). On the buccal mucosa and borders of the tongue, there may be numerous small papillomas with a whitish, thickened epithelial covering (6) (Figs. 5-3, 5-4). Severe halitosis is often present. Wells and Kierland (20) noted delayed eruption of the deciduous teeth.

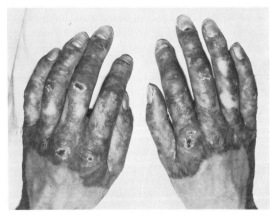

Figure 5-2. Hand changes in acrodermatitis enteropathica in the same patient. (*From N. Thyresson,* Acta Derm. Venereol **54**:383, 1974.)

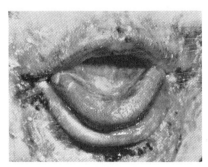

Figure 5-4. Circumoral changes and white coating of tongue.

PATHOLOGY

Biopsy of skin lesions has not revealed any specific changes. The findings comprise hyperkeratosis, acanthosis, and mild chronic inflammation in corium (21). Lodin and Gentele (11) found intraepithelial cutaneous vesicles. Autopsies have been performed by Danbolt (4) and by Wells and Winkelmann (21). Although Danbolt found erosions in the large intestines, Wells and Winkelmann were unable to demonstrate abnormalities. Histochemical studies (13) of duodenal and jejunal biopsies have revealed a decrease in leucine aminopeptidase and succinic dehydrogenase activity. Electron microscopy failed to reveal a consistent abnormality.

DIFFERENTIAL DIAGNOSIS

Differential diagnosis should include generalized moniliasis; the likelihood of confusing this condition with acrodermatitis enteropathica is increased by the fact that *Candida albicans* has been found in over 50 percent of reported cases of acrodermatitis enteropathica. The monilial infection, however, does not have an intermittent course, and there is no total alopecia or familial background. The celiac syndrome also has some features in common with acrodermatitis enteropathica, but skin lesions, nail changes, and total alopecia are rarely seen in celiac disease. Furthermore, there is a rather high incidence of enamel hypoplasia in patients with celiac syndrome, which has not been observed in acrodermatitis enteropathica. Other conditions with signs similar to acrodermatitis enteropathica are *dystrophic epidermolysis bullosa* and acrodermatitis continua Hallopeau. Moniliasis may also be seen in association with the *endocrine cardidosis syndrome*.

LABORATORY AIDS

None is known.

REFERENCES

1 Bloom, D., Acrodermatitis Enteropathica: Another Inborn Error of Metabolism? Follow-up Case Reported in 1955 and Review of Recent Literature. *N.Y. State J. Med.* **60:**3609–3616, 1960.
2 Barnes, P. M., and Moynahan, E. J., Zinc deficiency in acrodermatitis enteropathica. *Proc. R. Soc. Med.* **66:** 327–329, 1973.
3 Cash, R., and Berger, C. K., Acrodermatitis Enteropathica: Defective Metabolism of Unsaturated Fatty Acids. *J. Pediatr.* **74:**717–729, 1969.
4 Danbolt, N., Acrodermatitis Enteropathica. *Acta Derm. Venereol.* (*Stockh.*) **36:**257–271, 1956.
5 Danbolt, N., Acrodermatitis Enteropathica. *Hautarzt* **15:**27–29, 1964.
6 Danbolt, N., and Closs, K., Akrodermatitis Enteropathica. *Acta Derm. Venereol.* (*Stockh.*) **23:**127–169, 1943.
7 Dillaha, C. J., et al., Acrodermatitis Enteropathica: Review of Literature and Report of a Case Successfully Treated with Diodoquin. *J.A.M.A.* **152:**509–512, 1953.
8 Hansson, O., Acrodermatitis Enteropathica: Report of 2 Cases with a Hypothesis Concerning the Pathogenesis of the Disease. *Acta Derm. Venereol.* (*Stockh.*) **43:**465–571, 1963.
9 Heite, H. J., and Ody, R., Die Acrodermatitis enteropathica im Lichte der Häufigkeitsanalyse. *Hautarzt* **16:**529–534, 1965, and **17:**1–7, 1966.
10 Hodgson-Jones, I. S., Acrodermatitis Enteropathica. *Br. J. Dermatol.* **67:**222–224, 1955.
11 Lodin, A., and Gentele, H., *One Hundred Clinical Cases; Presented at the Eleventh International Congress of Dermatology, Stockholm, 1957.* Lund, 1958, pp. 10–15.
12 Lombeck, I., et al., Ultrastructural Findings in Acrodermatitis Enteropathica, *Pediatr. Res.* **8:**82–88, 1974.
13 Moynahan, E. J., et al., Demonstration of Possible Intestinal Enzyme Defect. *Proc. R. Soc. Med.* **56:**300–301, 1963.
14 Nowak, T., Acrodermatitis enteropathica bei zwei Brüdern. *Arch. Kinderheilkd.* **174:**44–53, 1966.
15 Portnoy, B., and Molokhia, M., Acrodermatitis Enteropathica Treated by Zinc. *Brit. J. Dermatol.* **91:**701–703, 1974.
16 Schulze, R. R., and Winkelmann, R. K., Acrodermatitis enteropathica. *Mayo Clin. Proc.* **41:**331–341, 1966.
17 Sundal, A., Enteropathica Acrodermatitis (Danbolt-Closs) and Diodoquin Treatment. *Ann. Paediatr. Fenn.* **3:**486–493, 1957.
18 Tompkins, R. R., and Livingood, C. S., Acrodermatitis Enteropathica Persisting into Adulthood. *Arch. Dermatol.* **99:**190–195, 1969.
19 Thyresson, N., Acrodermatitis Enteropathica Report of a Case Treated with Zinc Therapy. *Acta Derm. Venereol.* (*Stockh.*) **54:**383–385, 1974.
20 Wells, B. T., and Kierland, R. R., Acrodermatitis En-

teropathica: Report of a Case. *Acta Derm. Venereol. (Stockh.)* **41**:227–234, 1961.

21 Wells, B. T., and Winkelmann, R. K., Acrodermatitis Enteropathica. *Arch. Dermatol.* **84**:40–52, 1961.

22 Wirsching, L., Eye Symptoms in Acrodermatitis En-

teropathica. *Acta Ophthalmol.* (*Kbh.*) **40**:567–574, 1962.

23 Wittels, W., Akrodermatitis enteropathica beim Erwachsenen (Danbolt u. Closs). *Dermatol. Wochenschr.* **144**:765–772, 1961.

6

Acrodynia

Acrodynia is a syndrome described in children that is characterized by (a) profound changes in temperament, (b) skin alterations, (c) neurologic symptoms, (d) tachycardia, and (e) stomatitis. The term "acrodynia" was introduced in 1830 by Chardon (6), who presented the first description of the syndrome. Under the name "trophodermatoneurose," Selter (19), in 1903, reported eight children, all between one and three years of age, exhibiting the characteristic picture. Thorough descriptions were given by Swift (23) in Australia in 1914, and by Feer (12) in Switzerland in 1923, both emphasizing the neurologic aspects. A comprehensive review is that of Warkany (25).

Mercury was shown to be the etiologic agent in this condition (10, 20, 25, 26), the evidence being based on (a) increased excretion of mercury in the urine, (b) a frequent history of contact with mercury before the onset of the syndrome, and (c) similarity between symptoms in adults with mercury poisoning and in children with acrodynia. Prominent among mercury-containing medicaments are teething powders, ointments for skin rashes, and calomel for worm infestations.

The syndrome was seen most often in children between five months and two years of age (13), both sexes being equally affected. The disorder was reported occasionally as locally epidemic (6) and among members of the same family (4, 21). It had an average duration of 4 months (13). The mortality rate was reported to be about 5 percent.

The incidence and mortality rate of acrodynia have fallen dramatically since mercury-containing teething powders were withdrawn from the market in 1954 (8). Supporting the theory of metal intoxication is the sensitivity of the condition to treatment with BAL (dimercaprol) (1) and with N-acetyl D,L-penicillamine (15). It is likely that mercury potentiates sympathetic activity in acrodynia (11, 15).

A survey, carried out in England for the 5-year period 1961–1965 among 220 pediatricians, revealed an incidence of 52 cases (14). In half these cases there was established association with mercury.

SYSTEMIC MANIFESTATIONS

Acrodynia has a vague febrile onset, often accompanied by an upper respiratory infection and gastrointestinal disturbance. The children become fretful and suffer from muscular hypotonia. They lie in a characteristic attitude with the knees drawn up to the abdomen and the head buried in the pillow (salaam position) (Fig. 6-1).

Skin. The cutaneous symptoms, which vary considerably as to time of onset, intensity, and duration, are seen mainly on the hands, feet, and nose. These parts become cold, swollen, and pink and start to peel. Because of pruritus, the children chew on the hands and feet, which assume a "raw-beef" appearance. Other parts of

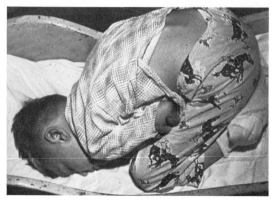

Figure 6-1. *Acrodynia.* Salaam position. (*Courtesy of M. Feingold, Boston, Massachusetts.*)

the body may be affected. There is profuse sweating, sometimes giving rise to a "sweat rash." The nails and hair may be shed.

Nervous system. A varied picture of superficial sensory loss, generalized hypotonia, and tremor is present (12). Increased blood pressure and tachycardia are usually noted. Paresthesia occurs over the entire cutaneous surface.

Other findings. The individual usually exhibits photophobia. The stools may be loose and have an especially offensive odor. Electrolyte changes in acrodynia include chloride and sodium loss from the vascular space (7).

Oral manifestations. The onset of the syndrome seems to coincide with the eruption of the primary teeth, the mother often ascribing the state of the child to teething. In 1947, Sundvall-Haggland (22) presented a comprehensive review of oral signs.

The changes in the oral cavity that cause the children considerable discomfort may be divided into three categories: (*a*) alterations in the oral mucosa, (*b*) changes of the teeth and gingiva, and (*c*) neurologic signs.

The oral mucosa is often the seat of generalized stomatitis. The mucosa, initially red and swollen, subsequently becomes covered by a whitish-gray exudate or membrane. Localized, deep ulcerations may simulate necrotic ulcerative stomatitis. Histologically, the buccal epithelium shows increased thickness, with intra- and

intercellular edema and deposits of small, round bodies within the cells (3).

The gingiva is spongy and red, and pocket formation occurs around the teeth (17, 22) (Fig. 6-2). At times, periodontal abscesses are seen. Destruction of the supporting tissue progresses rapidly, the teeth becoming loose and finally exfoliated. The incisors are attacked first. During the exfoliative process, the permanent tooth follicles may also be shed (16, 21, 24). In rare cases, portions of the alveolar bones are also exfoliated, the condition simulating osteomyelitis. Premature eruption of single permanent teeth has been reported by several authors (4). Histologic examination of teeth in acrodynia has shown broadening of the predentin, very irregular wavy dentin apically, and extensive hemorrhage in the pulp (22).

Follow-up examination of six children ($3\frac{1}{2}$ to $12\frac{1}{2}$ years after recovery from acrodynia) has shown occlusal irregularities in four children as a result of damage to buds of permanent teeth during the acute phase of the illness (2).

The changes in the nervous system causing a hyperkinetic state may also explain the excessive bruxism from which these patients suffer. The continuous grinding of the teeth accelerates shedding. The children also chew the buccal

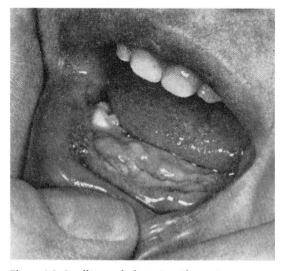

Figure 6-2. Swelling and ulceration of anterior mandibular gingiva. (*From A. M. Nussey, Br. Dent. J.* **96:**266, 1954.)

mucosa and tongue, producing a deep, beefy appearance. Increased salivation has been mentioned by several authors (12, 18).

PATHOLOGY

Microscopic examination of the nervous system reveals peripheral neuritis and chronic inflammatory changes in the spinal cord and nerve roots. The histologic changes in the affected skin are said to be specific for acrodynia (3). They consist of acanthosis in connection with papillomatosis, causing anastomosing epithelial strands, marked parakeratosis, widening of the granular cell layer, and necrobiotic changes in the spinous and basal cell layers. In the connective tissue, a diffuse polymorphic infiltrate with disappearance of elastic fibers may be noted.

DIFFERENTIAL DIAGNOSIS

The differential diagnosis may be difficult. Acrocyanosis may be seen in several conditions, such as dermatomyositis and acrosclerosis. Intoxication with substances other than mercury may produce a similar complex of symptoms, e.g., arsenic intoxication.

An acrodynia-like syndrome has been described in African infants who apparently had no contact with mercury (9).

Premature loss of teeth may also be seen in osteomyelitis, histiocytosis X, hypophosphatasia, *Papillon-Lefèvre syndrome*, acatalasia, various neutropenias, and leukemia.

LABORATORY AIDS

Urinary mercury levels should be determined.

REFERENCES

1 Alexander, I. F., and Rosario, R., A Case of Mercury Poisoning: Acrodynia in a Child of 8. *Canad. Med. Assoc. J.* **104**:929–930, 1971.
2 Barbacki, M., Follow-up Examination of 6 Children after Acrodynia. *J. Pediatr.* **76**:981–982, 1970.
3 Bode, H.-G., Die Feersche Krankheit im Lichte der Dermatologie. *Arch. Dermatol. Syph. (Berl.)* **167**:15–46, 1933.
4 Boisrame, R., Manifestations bucco-dentaires d'acrodynie infantile chez deux soeurs. *Inform. Dent. (Madr.)* **30**:935–961, 1948.
5 Braithwaite, J. V., On the Aetiology and Treatment of Pink Disease. *Arch. Dis. Child.* **8**:1–16, 1933.
6 Chardon, Fils, De l'acrodynie. *Rev. Méd. Franç.* **3**:51–74, 1830.
7 Cheek, D. B., Pink Disease (Infantile Acrodynia). *J. Pediatr.* **42**:239–260, 1953.
8 Dathan, J. G., and Harvey, C. C., Pink Disease—Ten Years After (the Epilogue). *Br. Med. J.* **1**:1181–1182, 1965.
9 Davies, P., African Pink Disease. *East Afr. Med. J.* **39**:52–54, 1962.
10 Fanconi, G., and Botztejn, A., Die Feersche Krankheit (Akrodynie) und Quecksilbermedikation. *Helv. Paediatr. Acta* **3**:264–271, 1948.
11 Farquhar, J. W., et al., Urinary Sympathin Excretion of Normal Infants and of Infants with Pink Disease. *Br. Med. J.* **2**:276–281, 1956.
12 Feer, E., Eine eigenartige Neurose des vegatativen Systems beim Kleinkinde. *Ergeb. Inn. Med. Kinderheilkd.* **24**:100–122, 1923.
13 Fisher, T. N., Pink Disease: A Review of 65 Cases. *Br. Med. J.* **1**:251–253, 1947.
14 Granger, C. D., Pink Disease. *Br. Med. J.* **2**:1657–1658, 1966.
15 Hirschman, S. Z., et al., Mercury in House Paint as a Cause of Acrodynia. *N. Engl. J. Med.* **269**:889–893, 1963.
16 Nussey, A. M., Pink Disease. *Br. Dent. J.* **96**:266–268, 1954.
17 Obura, C. W., Pink Disease: Report of a Case. *Br. Dent. J.* **119**:273–274, 1965.
18 Rachet, M., *Les manifestations bucco-dentaires de l'acrodynie infantile*. Vigne, Paris, 1935.
19 Selter, P., Über Trophodermatoneurose. *Verh. Ges. Kinderheilkd.* 20 Versammlung:45–50, 1903.
20 Stelgens, P., Zur Ätiologie, Pathogenese und Therapie der Feerschen Krankheit. *Dtsch. Med. Wochenschr.* **82**:378–381, 1957.
21 Stones, H. H., et al., *Oral and Dental Diseases*, 4th ed., E. & S. Livingstone, Ltd., Edinburgh, 1962, pp. 114–115.
22 Sundvall-Haggland, I., Swift-Feer's Disease (Akrodyni). *Sven. Tandläk. Tidskr.* **40**:243–326, 1947.
23 Swift, H., Erythroedema, in *Australian Medical Congress Transactions*, 10th Session, New Zealand, 1914, p. 575 [quoted in Cheek (7)].
24 Townsend, B. R., Pink Disease: Report of a Case in Which Extensive Exfoliation of Deciduous and Permanent Teeth Occurred. *Br. Dent. J.* **68**:514–517, 1940.
25 Warkany, J., Acrodynia—Postmortem of a Disease. *Am. J. Dis. Child.* **112**:146–156, 1966.
26 Warkany, J., and Hubbard, D. M., Acrodynia and Mercury. *J. Pediatr.* **42**:365–386, 1953.

7

Acrodysostosis

(Peripheral Dysostosis, Nasal Hypoplasia, and Mental Retardation)

Described initially by Singleton (13) in 1960, the syndrome of (a) peripheral dysostosis, (b) nasal and midface hypoplasia, (c) mental retardation, and (d) growth failure was termed "acrodysostosis" by Maroteaux and Malamut (8) in 1968. A complete review of the syndrome is that of Robinow et al. (12). More than 25 cases have been described.

All cases reported to date have been sporadic. Paternal age at time of conception has been increased in several cases. It may possibly have dominant inheritance, all cases representing point mutations.

SYSTEMIC MANIFESTATIONS

Facies. Most common is marked hypoplasia of the nose (Fig. 7-1*A, B*). The bridge is low, and in some cases the bony framework may be missing (3, 13). The entire nose is flat and short, with a broad, sometimes dimpled tip and anteverted nostrils. The center of the nasal tip is more severely reduced than the sides, so that the alae extend below the columella. The philtrum is usually unduly long. In other cases, the bridge is depressed but the nose is not especially short (2, 12). Apparent hypertelorism has been noted by several authors (8, 12). Epicanthus is often present (2, 8, 12), probably because of the low nasal bridge.

Skeletal abnormalities. The short stubby fingers, resembling those of cartilage hair hypo-

plasia, is a cardinal feature. The feet are similarly affected (Fig. 7-2*A*). The deformities may be obvious at birth, may become apparent during the first year (2, 4, 14) or not until some years later (12). Skin and subcutaneous tissues gradually outgrow the skeleton, forming bulges and folds over the dorsal aspects of the hands and fingers. The fingernails are broad and very short. Mesomelic brachymelia of the upper extremities is less conspicuous.

Intrauterine growth retardation and short stature are almost constant findings. Birth weight at normal term has ranged from 1,800 to 3,000 g, and birth length from 44 to 48 cm. Growth failure is progressive. Apparently inadequate growth and/or epiphyseal closure occur not only at the deformed epiphyses but also in bones that appear radiographically uninvolved.

Because of the premature arrest of metacarpal and phalangeal growth, the relative shortness of the fingers becomes more pronounced with age, resulting in difficulties with manual skills. Arthritic changes supervene early in hands and feet and may be generalized. In addition, range of motion is usually limited in the elbows and may be considerably restricted in the spine (1, 6, 13). Some children start to walk unduly late,

Radiographically, the most striking abnormalities are found in the hands and feet, with severe shortening of metacarpals and phalanges. In most cases, involvement is general, but rarely, some proximal phalanges are spared (2, 10). Often the growth disturbance is most severe in metacarpals. Their epiphyses are deformed and

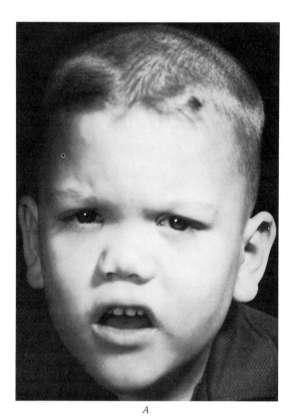
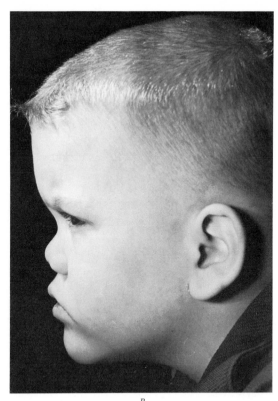

A   *B*

Figure 7-1. (*A* and *B*). *Acrodysostosis.* Marked hypoplasia of nose and midface. (*From M. Robinow et al.,* Am. J. Dis. Child. **121**:195, 1971.)

fuse prematurely. The phalanges have cone-shaped epiphyses, usually with a λ-base (Giedion, type 35), which also fuse prematurely (5). Continued remodeling broadens and deforms the bones into even more grotesque shapes. Carpal maturation is usually advanced (12) (Fig. 7-2*B*).

Forearm shortening seems to become more severe with age. In standing adults, the hands barely reach the trochanters. Epiphyses of the elbow region appear and fuse prematurely (8, 12). The distal radius and ulna are often malformed. Hypoplastic ulna with a poorly developed or absent styloid process is common.

The foot changes are comparable to those in the hands but somewhat less striking. The metatarsal and phalanges of the hallux are usually large and broad, sometimes accompanied by hallux valgus. The first cuneiform and navicular participate in relative hyperplasia of the first ray. The remaining metatarsals and phalanges are disproportionately small.

Partially collapsed vertebral bodies and irregularly deformed end plates in the thoracic and lumbar spines with resultant dorsolumbar kyphosis has suggested juvenile spondylitis in several cases (1, 6, 8, 12, 13). Brachycephaly and occasionally mild microcephaly are evident. Nasal bones are hypoplastic or even missing.

Mental retardation. Most patients have presented intellectual deficit, intelligence quotients ranging from 35 to 85. Associated neurologic defects have included internal hydrocephalus, optic atrophy (8), seizures (6, 10), choreoathetosis (10), and strabismus (8, 12). Hearing loss has been noted by several observers (3, 4, 8).

Hypogonadism. Delayed puberty has been seen occasionally (4, 10, 12).

Skin. A few patients have had numerous pigmented nevi (1, 6, 13).

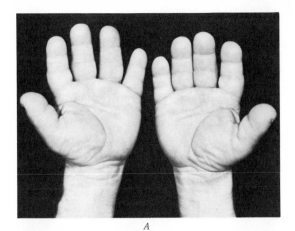

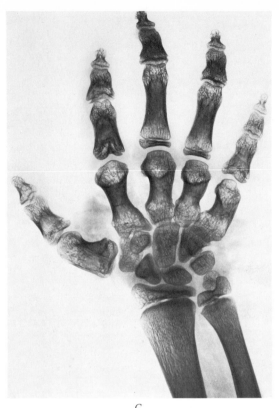

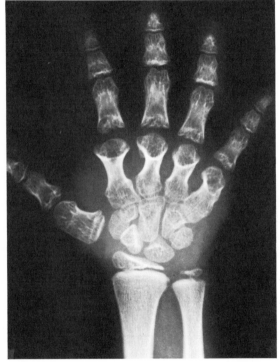

Figure 7-2. (*A*). Hands are short and stubby. Feet are similarly deformed. (*B*). Radiograph showing shortened metacarpals and phalanges. (*C*). Similar radiographic alterations in another patient. (*From A. Giedion*, Fortschr. Roentgenstr. **110**:507, 1969.)

while the ramus is long and slender. Tooth formation is occasionally delayed (4, 8, 12), but erupted teeth show no defects.

Oral manifestations. Frequently associated with the hypoplastic nose is maxillary hypoplasia, producing a peculiar flattening of the cheeks. In contrast, the upper alveolar process is usually prominent. Open bite is common, and relative mandibular prognathism may be conspicuous (10, 12). The mandibular angle is often increased. In some patients, the mandibular body is short

DIFFERENTIAL DIAGNOSIS

A striking feature of the syndrome is the severe, generalized peripheral dysostosis. The term implies shortening of the tubular bones of the hands and feet, associated with cone-shaped epiphyses, and exhibiting only minor changes in the remaining skeleton. Peripheral dysostosis may occur as an isolated finding (9). It should be emphasized, however, that cone-shaped epiphyses can be found in numerous bone disorders (*trichorhinophalangeal syn-*

dromes, pseudohypoparathyroidism, etc.) and, in fact, can be seen in the hand in about 7 percent of normal males and in 4 percent of normal females.

None of the features of acrodysostosis is, by itself, diagnostic. Hyperplasia of the first ray of the foot with hypoplasia of the second to fifth rays have been observed in other, unrelated disorders, such as *the Morquio syndrome* and *diastrophic dwarfism*. Short forearms, restricted elbow extension, increased mandibular angle, and cranial hyperostosis all occur in other conditions. Nasal hypoplasia and mental retardation are neither specific nor invariably present in the syndrome. The facies is reminiscent of that seen in the *fetal face syndrome* (11).

One should also exclude "snub-nose dwarfism," acromesomelic dwarfism, and pseudo-achondroplasia.

LABORATORY AIDS

None is known.

REFERENCES

1 Arkless, R., and Graham, C. B., An Unusual Case of Brachydactyly. *Am. J. Roentgenol.* **99:**724–735, 1967.
2 Cohen, P., and van Creveld, S., Peripheral Dysostosis. *Br. J. Radiol.* **36:**761–765, 1963.
3 Evans, P. R., Sotos' syndrome (cerebral gigantism) with peripheral dysostosis. *Amer. J. Dis. Child.* 46:199–202, 1971.
4 Garces, L. Y., et al., Peripheral Dysostosis: Investigation of Metabolic and Endocrine Function. *J. Pediatr.* **74:**730–737, 1969.
5 Giedion, A., Zapfenepiphysen. Naturgeschichte und diagnostische Bedeutung des enchondralen Wachstums. *Ergeb. Med. Radiol.* **1:**59–124, 1968.
6 Giedion, A., Die periphere Dysostose (PD)–ein Sammelbegriff. *Fortschr. Roentgenstr.* **110:**507–524, 1969.
7 Jewelewicz, R., and Nachtigall, L. E., Pseudo-pseudohypoparathyroidism and Pregnancy. *Obstet. Gynecol.* **37:**396–401, 1971.
8 Maroteaux, P., and Malamut, G., L'acrodysostose. *Presse Méd.* **76:**2189–2192, 1968.
9 Newcombe, D. S., and Keats, T. E., Roentgenographic Manifestations of Hereditary Peripheral Dysostoses. *Am. J. Roentgenol.* **106:**178–189, 1969.
10 Ortolani, M., and Cremonese, M., Su di un caso di acromicria vera. *Clin. Orthop.* **15:**193–203, 1963.
11 Pfeiffer, R. A., and Müller, H., Ein Komplex multipler Missbildungen bei zwei nicht verwandten Kindern. *Pädiatr. Pädol.* **6:**262–267, 1971.
12 Robinow, M., et al., Acrodysostosis. A Syndrome of Peripheral Dysostosis, Nasal Hypoplasia and Mental Retardation. *Am. J. Dis. Child.* **121:**195–203, 1971.
13 Singleton, E. B., et al., Peripheral Dysostosis. *Am. J. Roentgenol.* **84:**499–505, 1960.
14 Steinbach, H., and Young, D. A., The Roentgen Appearance of Pseudohypoparathyroidism (PH) and Pseudopseudohypoparathyroidism (PPH). *Am. J. Roentgenol.* **97:**49–66, 1966.

8

Acroosteolysis

A croosteolysis consists of (*a*) dissolution of the terminal phalanges, (*b*) short stature, (*c*) bizarrely shaped skull, and (*d*) premature loss of teeth. Several excellent reviews are those of Chawla (1), Cheney (2), Jänner et al. (8), and Herrmann et al. (7).

The syndrome is inherited as an autosomal dominant trait (2, 11, 15). Cheney (2) indicated that the disorder was less severe in females, but this does not seem to be supported in other families.

SYSTEMIC MANIFESTATIONS

Facies. Several patients seen by one of the authors (R. J. G.) have had remarkably long noses. This was also evident in the patient illustrated by Hajdu and Kauntze (6). Abnormal facies was noted by Shaw (14) and by Matisonn and Zaidy (11) (Fig. 8-1). Among patients personally examined, the scalp hair was coarse and abundant.

Skeletal alterations. Most striking are shortening and clubbing of the distal portion of fingers and toes, primarily the former. The terminal portion of the thumb is especially short (2, 12) (Fig. 8-4*A*). The interphalangeal joints are often hyperflexible (1, 5, 14, 15). Pain or paresthesia may be experienced in the joints, especially on motion.

Basilar impression of the skull is noted, together with dolichocephaly and unusual protu-berance of the squamous portion of the occipital bone (bathrocephaly), with widening of the metopic, coronal, and lambdoidal sutures with associated Wormian bones. There may be depression at the anterior fontanel (1, 2, 6). The frontal sinuses are absent. The sella turcica is enlarged, with slender clinoids (Fig. 8-3).

Adult height is seldom greater than 157 cm and decreases with age. This is in part because of severe kyphosis, marked osteoporosis, and compression of thoracic vertebras. The superior and inferior surfaces of the vertebras are concave, assuming a so-called "fish-bone" shape. Toglia (15) noted straightening of the cervical spine. Intervertebral disks may appear denser than the vertebral bodies. The kyphosis becomes progressive and is associated with pain (1, 2, 6). Multiple fractures have involved the spine (2, 6), long bones (2), and hands or feet (5,12). Some patients have exhibited fusion of the dorsal processes of the third to fifth cervical vertebras. Valgus deformity of the elbows and knees has also been observed (Fig. 8-2*A*, *B*).

Narrowing of the metacarpophalangeal and/or metatarsophalangeal spaces has been noted (2, 5, 6, 14). Striking is lysis of terminal phalanges (Fig. 8-4*B*). Looser's zones, or possible fracture of the metatarsals or metacarpals, have been reported by a number of authors (5, 9, 12).

Other manifestations. Conductive deafness, blurred vision, headache, and sixth nerve palsy have been noted (6), as well as hypogonadism (11).

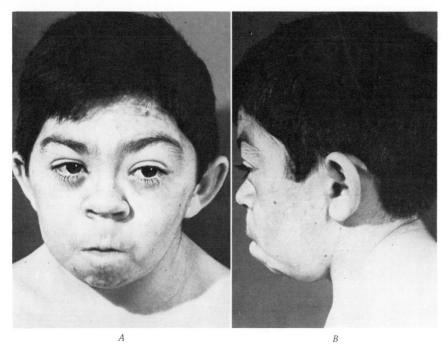

Figure 8-1. *Acroosteolysis.* (*A* and *B*). Unusual facies marked by midfacial hypoplasia, fullness of outer supraorbital ridges, mild ocular hypertelorism, small mouth, and receding chin. (*From A. Matisonn and F. Zaidy*, S. Afr. Med. J. **47**:2060, 1973.)

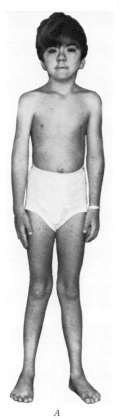

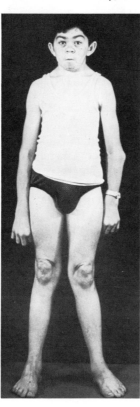

Figure 8-2. (*A*). Ten-year-old boy exhibiting shortness of stature, hirsutism, genua valga, unusual facial appearance. (*From J. Hermann et al.*, Z. Kinderheilkd. **114**:93, 1973.) (*B*). Compare with 18-year-old boy. Note similar facies, genu valgum, subluxation of radial head. (*From Matisonn and Zaidy, op. cit.*)

A

B

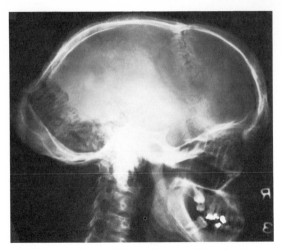

Figure 8-3. Bathrocephaly with many Wormian bones in suture lines, depressed anterior fontanel, and basilar impression, (*From W. D. Cheney*, Am. J. Roentgenol. **94:**595, 1965.)

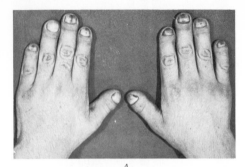

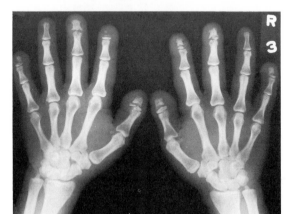

Figure 8-4. (*A*). Observe abbreviation of terminal phalanges. (*From A. Matisonn and F. Zaidy*, S. Afr. Med. J. **47:**2060, 1973.) (*B*). Radiograph showing lysis of terminal phalanges. (*From W. D. Cheney*, Am. J. Roentgenol. **94:**595, 1965.)

Oral manifestations. Early loss of teeth with marked atrophy of the alveolar processes of the maxilla and mandible is an almost constant feature (1, 2, 5, 6, 12). The molar roots have been found to be resorbed (12). Some patients have been prognathic (6, 15). Others have had a very small mandible.

DIFFERENTIAL DIAGNOSIS

Acroosteolysis may also be seen in *pyknodysostosis, progeria, epidermolysis bullosa,* scleroderma, syringomyelia, leprosy, syphilis, psoriasis, trauma, neurogenic ulcerative acropathy (3, 10), and polyvinyl chloride intoxication.

Young et al. (17) described acroosteolysis in association with severe mandibular and clavicular hypoplasia, stiff joints, and cutaneous atrophy in two unrelated males. They called the disorder "mandibuloacral dysplasia."

LABORATORY AIDS

Matisonn and Zaidy (11) described elevated levels of serum alkaline phosphatase and lactic dehydrogenase.

REFERENCES

1 Chawla, S., Cranio-skeletal Dysplasia with Acro-osteolysis. *Br. J. Radiol.* **37:**702–705, 1964.

2 Cheney, W. D., Acro-osteolysis. *Am. J. Roentgenol.* **94:**595–607, 1965.

3 Crecelius, W., Ein Beitrag zum Krankheitsbild der Osteopathia dysplastica familiaris. *Fortschr. Roentgenstrahl.* **76:**196–202, 1952.

4 Giaccai, L., Familial and Sporadic Neurogenic Acro-osteolysis. *Acta Radiol. (Stockh.)* **38:**17–29, 1952.

5 Greenberg, B. D., and Street, D., Idiopathic Nonfamilial Acro-osteolysis. *Radiology* **69:**259, 1957.

6 Hajdu, N., and Kauntze, R., Cranio-skeletal Dysplasia. *Br. J. Radiol.* **21:**42–48, 1948.

7 Herrmann, J., et al., Arthro dento-osteo Dysplasia

(Hajdu-Cheney Syndrome) *Z. Kinderheilkd.* **114**:93–110, 1973.

8 Jänner, M., et al., Zum Krankheitsbild der familiärer Akroosteolyse. *Z. Haut Geschlechtskr.* **34**:65–73, 1963.

9 Kleinsorge, H., Akroosteolystische Erscheinungen der Osteomalacie. *Fortschr. Roentgenstr.* **73**:471–475, 1950.

10 Kozlowski, K., et al., Neurogene ulcerierende Akropathie. Akroosteolyse-Syndrom. *Monatsschr. Kinderheilkd.* **119**: 169–175, 1971.

11 Matisonn, A., and Zaidy, F., Familial Acro-osteolysis. *S. Afr. Med. J.* **47**:2060–2063, 1973.

12 Papavasiliou, C., et al., Idiopathic Nonfamilial Acro-osteolysis Associated with Other Bone Abnormalities. *Am. J. Roentgenol.* **83**:687–691, 1960.

13 Schulze, R., and Gulbin, O., Beitrag zum Problem der Akroosteolyse (gleichzeitig ein Beitrag zur Kenntnis der Patella profunda). *Fortschr. Roentgenstr.* **109**:209–216, 1968.

14 Shaw, D. G., Acro-osteolysis and Bone Fragility. *Br. J. Radiol.* **42**:934–936, 1969.

15 Toglia, J. V., Hereditary Dysostosis. *Tex. State J. Med.* **62**:36–41, 1966.

16 Wieland, H., Ein Beitrag zur Kenntnis der Akroosteolyse. *Fortschr. Roentgenstr.* **77**:193–198, 1952.

17 Young, L. W., et al., New Syndrome Manifested by Mandibular Hypoplasia, Acroosteolysis, Stiff Joints, and Cutaneous Atrophy (Mandibuloacral Dysplasia) in Two Unrelated Boys. *Birth Defects* **7**(7):291–297, 1971.

9

Apert Syndrome

(*Acrocephalosyndactyly*)

Apert-type acrocephalosyndactyly is a rare developmental deformity syndrome characterized by (*a*) craniosynostosis leading to turribrachycephaly and (*b*) syndactyly of hands and feet. Other features include (*c*) various ankyloses and (*d*) progressive synostoses of the hands, feet, and cervical spine. Apert (1) was credited with the discovery of the disorder, although the condition was reported earlier by Baumgartner (2) and others. Park and Powers (17), Valentin (25), Blank (4), and Schauerte and St-Aubin (20) have made significant contributions to our understanding of Apert-type acrocephalosyndactyly. Over 200 cases have been reported to date.

In the Anglo-American literature prior to 1960, all acrocephalosyndactylies were thought to constitute a single syndrome. In 1960, Blank (4), in examining 54 cases, divided acrocephalosyndactyly into typical and atypical forms. Typical, or Apert-type, acrocephalosyndactyly included only those cases in which there was a mid-digital hand mass consisting of osseous and soft-tissue syndactyly of digits 2 through 4.

Park and Powers (17) suggested that acrocephalosyndactyly was caused by a hereditary defect in the tissues which separates the various bone anlagen from one another before the fifth to sixth week of embryonic life. This theory provides a uniform explanation of premature synostoses, syndactylies, and ankyloses observed in the Apert syndrome.

Most cases are sporadic (4, 11). On a few occasions, a female with the Apert syndrome has given birth to an affected child (3, 15, 19, 26, 28). Increased paternal age at the time of conception was found by Blank (4) and confirmed by Erickson and Cohen (12a). The few familial cases, lack of sex predilection, the increased paternal age at conception, and the large number of sporadic cases suggest autosomal dominant transmission, with most cases representing fresh mutations. In most instances karyotypes have been normal, but chromosomal alterations have been reported in a few cases (12, 13), probably having aleatory association.

The mutation rate was estimated to be 3×10^{-6} per gene per generation by Blank (4) and 4×10^{-6} per gene per generation by Tünte et al. (24). The Apert syndrome occurs once in 160,000 births and, because of the high mortality rate in the neonatal period, occurs once in 2,000,000 in the general population (4).

SYSTEMIC MANIFESTATIONS

Facies. Facial variability is more pronounced than isolated medical reports indicate (10). The forehead is high and steep and, during infancy, a horizontal groove may be present above the supraorbital ridges. The occiput is flattened. Hypertelorism is commonly observed. Proptosis and antimongoloid obliquity of the palpebral fissures are variable in degree (Fig. 9-1*A, B*). Strabismus is present in some cases. When the nasal bridge is severely depressed, the nose may have a parrot-beaked appearance but, in general, nasal structure is quite variable. The middle

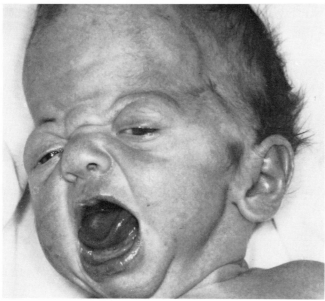
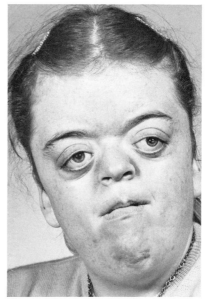

A   B

Figure 9-1. (*A*). *Apert syndrome.* Note turribrachycephaly, proptosis, and horizontal grooves above supraorbital ridges. (*B*). Note turribrachycephaly, ocular hypertelorism, antimongoloid slant of palpebrial fissures, beaked nose, midface hypoplasia, and relative mandibular prognathism. (*From A. Kahn, Jr., and J. Fulmer,* N. Engl. J. Med. **252:**379, 1955.)

third of the face is underdeveloped, lending prominence to the mandible. Facial asymmetry is often present and may be very pronounced in some cases (10, 17).

Skeletal system. The skull is turribrachycephalic. The frontal and occipital bones are flattened, and the apex of the cranium is located near or anterior to the bregma. There is irregular, early obliteration of cranial sutures, especially of the coronal, but frequently of other sutures as well. An accentuation of digital markings is usually observed. The anterior fontanel may remain open longer than normal. The orbits are hyperteloric, and the maxilla is hypoplastic (11, 17).

Deformities of the hands and feet are symmetric. A mid-digital hand mass with osseous and soft-tissue syndactyly of digits 2, 3, and 4 is always found (Fig. 9-2*A, B*). Digits 1 and 5 may be joined to digits 2 and 4, respectively, or may be separate. In the feet, toes 2, 3, and 4 are joined by soft-tissue syndactyly (Fig. 9-2*D*). Toes 1 and 5 are sometimes free; at times they are joined by

soft tissue to the second and fourth toes, respectively (4, 15). In several cases, six metatarsals have been observed (11, 16). The interphalangeal joints of the fingers are stiff. Fingernails of the mid-digital hand mass may be continuous or partially continuous, and toenails may be partially continuous with some segmentation. The thumb usually deviates radially at the metacarpophalangeal joint (15).

The upper extremities are shortened. Aplasia or ankylosis of several joints, especially elbow, shoulder, and hip, is commonly observed (1, 4, 11, 18, 20). Progressive synostosis of the bones of the hands, feet, and cervical portion of the spine has been reported (15, 20) (Fig. 9-2*C*). Not uncommonly there is a delay in the appearance of the epiphyses of long bones and carpal and tarsal bones (18). Epiphyseal dysplasia is also frequently noted. The thumb may have but a single phalanx.

Central nervous system. Some degree of mental retardation is found in most patients, although normal intelligence has been observed in some

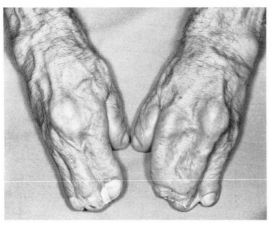

A

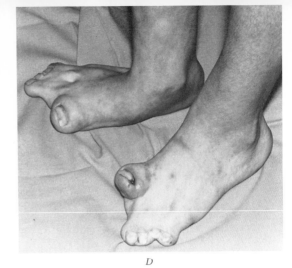

D

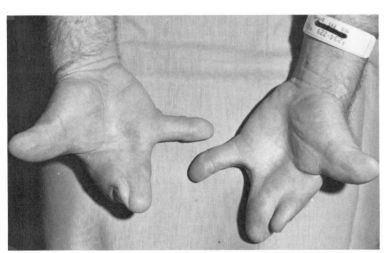

B

Figure 9-2. (*A*). Syndactyly of second to fourth fingers. Note broad, radially deviated thumbs. (*B*). Mid-digital hand mass with first and fifth digits free. (*C*). Radiograph showing bony synostoses. (*B* and *C* from J. Opitz, Madison, Wisconsin.) (*D*). Syndactyly of second to fourth toes. Note broad, proximally placed halluces. (*Courtesy of R. Bauer, Innsbruck, Austria.*)

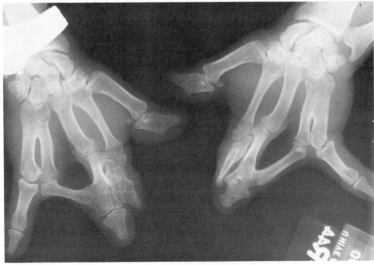

C

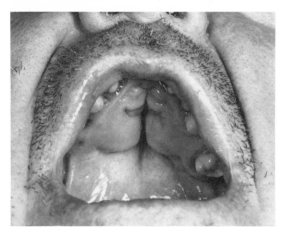

Figure 9-3. Note Byzantine arch-shaped palate.

The palate is highly arched, is constricted, and may have a marked median furrow (Fig. 9-3). Cleft soft palate is observed in approximately 30 percent of the cases. Bifid uvula may also occur. The soft palate is excessively long in over half the cases (17a). The maxillary dental arch may be V-shaped, with severely crowded teeth and bulging alveolar ridges. Class III malocclusion is usually present, with anterior open bite or cross bite and unilateral or bilateral posterior cross bite. Retarded dental eruption is a common finding (2, 11, 21, 25).

DIFFERENTIAL DIAGNOSIS

Differential diagnosis includes the *Pfeiffer syndrome, Crouzon syndrome, Carpenter syndrome, Summitt syndrome,* and various other craniosynostosis syndromes. Marked syndactyly resembling that in the Apert syndrome may be seen in *cryptophthalmos syndrome.* A bizarre form of total syndactyly of the hands and distal radioulnar synostosis in brothers was described by Cenani and Lenz (8).

LABORATORY AIDS

None is known.

cases. Various forms of encephalopathy may be present (5, 6, 27).

Other findings. Fixation of the stapes has been frequently observed (3). Acne vulgaris is commonly noted with unusual extension to the forearms (22). A variety of cardiovascular and other internal anomalies (4, 9, 11) has been reported.

Oral manifestations. In the relaxed state, the lips frequently form a trapezoidal configuration.

REFERENCES

1 Apert, E., De l'acrocéphalosyndactylie. *Bull. Soc. Méd. (Paris)* **23**:1310–1330, 1906.

2 Baumgartner, K. H., *Kranken-Physiognomik,* 2d ed., L. F. Rieger & Co., Stuttgart, 1842, p. 189 and Fig. 60.

3 Bergstrom, L., et al., Otologic Manifestations of Acrocephalosyndactyly. *Arch. Otolaryngol.* **96**:117–123, 1972.

4 Blank, C. E., Apert's Syndrome (a Type of Acrocephalosyndactyly): Observations on a British Series of Thirty-nine Cases. *Ann. Hum. Genet.* **24**:151–164, 1960.

5 Böök, J. A., and Hesselvik, L., Acrocephalosyndactyly. *Acta Paediatr. Scand.* **42**:359–364, 1953.

6 Born, E., Beobachtungen am Zwischenhirn-Hypophysensystem bei einer Akrocephalosyndaktylie. *Psychiatr. Neurol. (Basel)* **141**:26–37, 1961.

7 Buchanan, R. C., Acrocephalosyndactyly, or Apert's Syndrome. *Br. J. Plast. Surg.* **21**:406–418, 1968.

8 Cenani, A., and Lenz, W., Totale Syndaktylie und totale radioulnare Synostose bei zwei Brüdern. *Z. Kinderheilkd.* **101**:181–190, 1967.

9 Cohen, M. M., Jr., Cardiovascular Anomalies in Apert Type Acrocephalosyndactyly. *Birth Defects* **8**(5):132–133, 1972.

10 Cohen, M. M., Jr., et al., Facial Variability in Apert Type Acrocephalosyndactyly. *Birth Defects* **7**(7):143–152, 1971.

11 Cohen, M. M., Jr., An Etiologic and Nosologic Overview of Craniosynostosis Syndromes. *Birth Defects* **11**(2):137–189, 1975.

12 Dodson, W. E., et al., Acrocéphalosyndactylia Associated with a Chromosomal Translocation. *Am. J. Dis. Child.* **120**:360–362, 1970.

12a Erickson, J. D., and Cohen, M. M., Jr., A Study of Parental Age Effects on the Occurrence of Fresh Mutations for the Apert Syndrome. *Ann. Hum. Genet.* **38**:89–96, 1974.

13 Genest, P., et al., Le syndrome d'Apert (acrocephalosyndactylie). *Arch. Fr. Pédiatr.* **23**:887–897, 1966.

14 Herrmann, J., et al., Craniosynostosis and Craniosynostosis Syndromes. *Rocky Mt. Med. J.* **66**:45–56, 1969.

15 Hoover, G. H., et al., The Hand in Apert's Syndrome. *J.*

Bone Joint Surg. **52A:**878–895, 1970.

16 Matucci-Cerinic, L., Un caso di acrocefalosindattilia *Riv. Clin. Pediatr.* **71:**104–114, 1963.

17 Park, E. A., and Powers, G. F., Acrocephaly and Scaphocephaly with Symmetrically Distributed Malformations of the Extremities. *Am. J. Dis. Child.* **20:**235–315, 1920.

17a Peterson, S. J., and Pruzansky, S., Palatal Anomalies in the Syndromes of Apert and Crouzon. *Cleft Palate J.* **11:**394–403, 1974.

18 Pillay, V. K., Acrocephalosyndactyly in Singapore. *J. Bone Joint Surg.* **46B:**94–101, 1964.

19 Roberts, K. B., and Hall, J. G., Apert's Acrocephalosyndactyly in Mother and Daughter: Cleft Palate in the Mother. *Birth Defects* **7**(7):262–263, 1971.

20 Schauerte, E. W., and St-Aubin, P. M., Progressive Synosteosis in Apert's Syndrome (Acrocephalosyndactyly). *Am. J. Roentgenol.* **97:**67–73, 1966.

21 Schwarzweller, F., Die Akrocephalosyndaktylie. *Z. Menschl. Vererb.-u. Konstit. Lehre* **20:**341–349, 1937.

22 Solomon, L. M., et al., Pilosebaceous Abnormalities in Apert's Syndrome. *Arch. Dermatol.* **102:**381–385, 1970.

23 Solomon, L. M., et al., Apert Syndrome and Palatal Mucopolysaccharides. *Teratology* **8:**287–292, 1973.

24 Tünte, W., and Lenz, W., Zur Häufigkeit und Mutationsrate des Apert-Syndroms. *Humangenetik* **4:**104–111, 1967.

25 Valentin, B., Die Korrelation (Koppelung) von Missbildungen, erläutert am Beispiel der Akrocephalosyndaktylie. *Acta Orthop. Scand.* **9:**235–316, 1938.

26 van den Bosch, J., cited in C. E. Blank, Apert's Syndrome (a Type of Acrocephalosyndactyly): Observations on a British Series of Thirty-nine Cases. *Ann. Hum. Genet.* **24:**151–164, 1960.

27 Verger, P., et al., L'acrocéphalo-syndactylie (syndrome d'Apert). *Arch. Fr. Pédiatr.* **29:**91–106, 1962.

28 Weech, A. A., Combined Acrocephaly and Syndactylism Occurring in Mother and Daughter. *Bull. Johns Hopkins Hosp.* **40:**73–76, 1927.

10

Ataxia-telangiectasia

(*Louis-Bar Syndrome*)

Delineation of the syndrome of (*a*) ataxia, (*b*) oculocutaneous telangiectasia, and (*c*) sinopulmonary infections is usually credited to Mme. Louis-Bar (4) in 1941, although earlier examples were reported by Syllaba and Henner (24). Boder and Sedgwick (4), who coined the name "ataxia-telangiectasia" and clearly defined the syndrome, subsequently published an exhaustive review in 1975 (3). Over 200 cases have been described.

The syndrome is inherited as an autosomal recessive trait. The parental consanguinity rate of 3 to 4.5 percent suggests that the gene is far more frequent in the population than heretofore supposed (25).

Rarely does an affected person live past twenty years of age. There appears to be heightened sensitivity to radiation and to radiomimetic drugs (6).

SYSTEMIC MANIFESTATIONS

Facies and appearance. The face is described as thin, and the expression as relaxed, dull, or sad (Fig. 10-1). The patient often stoops, with the shoulders drooped and the head held to one side. Mild athetoid movements may be noted around the shoulders. Growth is markedly diminished in over 65 percent of patients (21).

Nervous system. The ataxia is of the cerebellar type and usually becomes apparent when the child begins to walk. The truncal ataxia is slowly progressive. Eventually there may be dyssynergia and intention tremor of the upper extremities. Hypotonia and diminished tendon reflexes are noted. Speech is slow, slurred, and often scanning.

Mental deficiency is usually not apparent until the child reaches the age of nine years, when mental development begins to taper off. This has been noted in about 30 percent of cases.

Pneumoencephalographic study shows there is cerebellar atrophy, and, on necropsy, thinning of the granular layer of the cerebellum, with diminished numbers of Purkinje cells (27).

Eyes. Usually at four to six years of age, fine, symmetric, bright-red streaks are noted in the temporal and nasal areas of the conjunctiva. The telangiectasia has been shown to be venous (11) (Fig. 10-2).

Ataxia of the eyes due to atrophy of the cerebellar cortex, strabismus, poor convergence, and nystagmus are commonly found. Movement of the eyes is slow and interrupted, halting midway on lateral and upward gaze. This movement is often accompanied by rapid blinking. Fixation nystagmus is present in over 80 percent of patients (21).

Skin. The cutaneous telangiectasia is first noted on the ears, butterfly area of face, bridge of nose, and periorbitally, i.e., in areas receiving the greatest sun exposure (Fig. 10-3). With time it extends to the neck, antecubital and popliteal areas, and the dorsum of hands and feet.

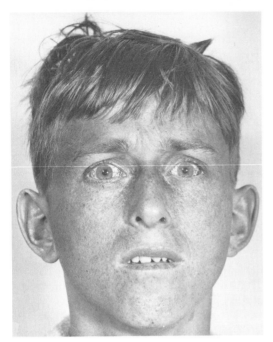

Figure 10-1. *Ataxia-telangiectasia.* Note rigid facies marked by staring expression and prominent bulbar conjunctival vessels. (*From S. J. Miller and W. Gooddy,* Brain **87:**581, 1964.)

With continued sun exposure and/or aging, the skin tends to become sclerodermatous in appearance (5, 19), with a mottled pattern of hyperpigmentation and hypopigmentation (poi-

kiloderma). Diffuse graying of the scalp hair is frequent, even in young patients. Seborrheic dermatitis, follicular keratosis, and hirsutism of the arms and legs are constant features (3, 4, 19, 21).

Respiratory system. Recurrent sinopulmonary infections have occurred in 75 to 80 percent of affected patients (4, 20). These may vary in severity from acute rhinitis with infections of the ears to chronic bronchitis, recurrent pneumonia, and bronchiectasis.

Neoplasia. A number of authors (1, 6, 7, 11, 15, 17) have pointed out the high frequency (about 10 percent) of lymphoreticular malignancy (lymphosarcoma, Hodgkin's disease, reticular cell sarcoma, leukemia) which eventuates. An increased number of chromosome breaks (15) and mutant clones with translocation chromo-

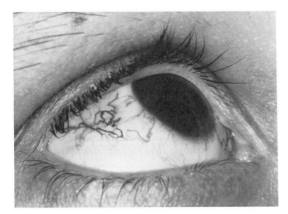

Figure 10-2. Telangiectasia of bulbar conjunctiva. (*From G. Karapati et al.,* Am. J. Dis. Child. **110:**51, 1965.)

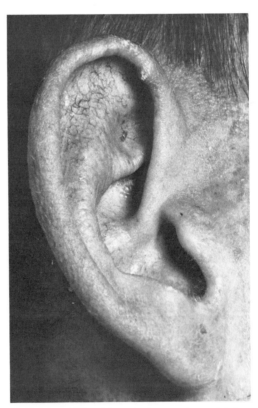

Figure 10-3. Telangiectasia of pinna. (*From M. Ruiter,* Hautarzt **15:**667, 1964.)

Table 10-1. Genetic cutaneous disorders with similarities to ataxia-telangiectasia

Disease	Skin changes	Ataxia	Mental retardation	Growth	Aminoaciduria	Inheritance
Ataxia-telangiectasia	Telangiectasia, atrophy, pigmentation sometimes, sclerodermatitis	Primary cerebellar	Sometimes	Retarded	Reported but unconfirmed	Autosomal recessive
Hartnup disease	Pellagra-like, pigment changes in hair	Cerebellar	Sometimes	Sometimes retarded	Characteristic	Autosomal recessive
Cockayne syndrome	Sunlight sensitivity, aging of skin	Cerebellar	Always	Retarded	Not reported	Autosomal recessive
Bloom syndrome	Sunlight sensitivity, aging of skin		Sometimes	Retarded	Not reported	Autosomal recessive
Werner syndrome	Premature aging, sclerodermatitis		Sometimes	Retarded	Not reported	Autosomal recessive
De Sanctis-Cacchione syndrome (xerodermic iodicy)	Xeroderma pigmentosum in sun-exposed areas, sun sensitivity	Reported to be like Friedreich's ataxia	Retarded	Retarded	Reported	Autosomal recessive
Rothmund-Thomson syndrome	Poikiloderma, more so in sun-exposed areas, cutaneous malignancy		Sometimes	Retarded	Not reported	Autosomal recessive

somes (12) have been found on lymphocyte culture. Other types of cancer have been reported, including ovarian dysgerminoma, medulloblastoma, glioma, and adenocarcinoma (1, 5, 10).

Oral manifestations. Telangiectasia of the hard and soft palate has also been reported (3, 4, 20, 28). Nasal mucosal involvement with telangiectasia may be inferred from recurrent episodes of epistaxis (20). Drooling has been noted in the vast majority of patients (4, 21), but its cause has not been established (3). Speech, as noted above, is often of the bulbar type. Oropharyngeal lymphatic tissue is diminished or absent. Lymphosarcoma of the palate has been noted in several cases (8, 22).

DIFFERENTIAL DIAGNOSIS

Ordinarily considered in differential diagnosis are cerebral palsy, structural anomaly or neoplasm of the posterior fossa or foramen magnum, or any of several degenerative or metabolic disorders such as Friedreich's ataxia, hepatolenticular degeneration, Pelizaeus-Merzbacher disease, and Hallevorden-Spatz disease.

Various other genetic cutaneous disorders are reviewed in Table 10-1.

LABORATORY AIDS

Many patients have exhibited a deficiency in immunoglobulin formation. This has been characterized as a decreased production of gammaglobulin, particularly IgA and IgE (2, 3, 18, 26), in over 60 percent of patients. Rarely IgG (8) is decreased. Alpha-fetoprotein is elevated (29).

The thymus is absent or hypoplastic without Hassall's corpuscles, and there is a defect in cellular immunity. The patient characteristically exhibits delayed homograft rejection and poor-to-absent response to the monilia skin test. There is also an inability to sensitize to dinitrochlorobenzene, absent follicles in lymph nodes or other lymphatic tissues, and decreased in vitro lymphocyte transformation (3, 8, 15, 17).

Of interest have been the absence of ovarian follicles (16) and bizarre nuclear changes or cytomegaly in the pituitary gland (23).

Over 50 percent of patients with ataxia-telangiectasia have abnormal glucose tolerance, but rarely with glycosuria and never with ketosis, implying insulin resistance (15).

REFERENCES

1 Aguilar, M. J., et al., Pathologic Observations in Ataxia-telangiectasia. *J. Neuropathol. Exp. Neurol.* **27:**659–676, 1968.

2 Ammann, A. J., et al., Immunoglobulin E Deficiency in Ataxia-telangiectasia. *N. Engl. J. Med.* **281:**469–472, 1969.

3 Boder, E., Ataxia-telangiectasia: Some Historic, Clinical, and Pathologic Observations. *Birth Defects* **11**(1):255–270, 1975.

4 Boder, E., and Sedgwick, R. P., Ataxia-telangiectasia: A Familial Syndrome of Progressive Cerebellar Ataxia, Oculocutaneous Telangiectasia and Frequent Pulmonary Infection. *Pediatrics* **21:**526–554, 1958.

5 Dunn, H. G., Ataxia-telangiectasia. *J. Can. Med. Assoc.* **91:**1106–1118, 1964.

6 Feigin, R. D., et al., Ataxia-telangiectasia with Granulocytopenia. *J. Pediatr.* **77:**431–438, 1970.

7 Gatti, R. A., and Good, R. A., Occurrence of Malignancy in Immunodeficiency Disease. *Cancer* **28:**89–98, 1971.

8 Gimeno, A., et al., Ataxia-telangiectasia with Absence of IgG. *J. Neurol. Sci.* **8:**545–554, 1969.

9 Gotoff, S. P., et al., Ataxia-telangiectasia, Neoplasia, Untoward Response to X-irradiation and Tuberous Sclerosis. *Am. J. Dis. Child.* **114:**617–625, 1967.

10 Haerer, A., et al., Ataxia-telangiectasia with Gastric Adenocarcinoma. *J.A.M.A.* **210:**1884–1887, 1970.

11 Harris, V. J., and Seeler, R. A., Ataxia-telangiectasia and Hodgkin's Disease. *Cancer* **32:**1415–1420, 1973.

12 Hecht, F., et al., Ataxia-telangiectasia—Clonal Growth of Translocation Lymphocytes. *N. Engl. J. Med.* **289:**286–291, 1973.

13 Hyams, S. W., et al., The Eye Signs in Ataxia-telangiectasia. *Am. J. Ophthalmol.* **62:**1118–1124, 1966.

14 Louis-Bar (Mme.), Sur un syndrome progressif comprenant des telangiectasies capillaires cutanées et conjonctivales symetriques, à disposition naevoide et des troubles cerebelleux. *Confin. Neurol.* **4:**32–42, 1941.

15 McFarlin, D. E. et al., Ataxia-telangiectasia. *Medicine* **51:** 281–305, 1972.

16 Miller, M. E., and Chatten, J., Ovarian Changes in Ataxia-telangiectasia. *Acta Paediatr. Scand.* **56:**559–561, 1967.

17 Peterson, R. D. A., et al., Lymphoid Tissue Abnormalities Associated with Ataxia-telangiectasia. *Am. J. Med.* **41:**342–359, 1966.

18 Polmar, S. H., et al., Immunoglobulin E in Immunologic Deficiency Diseases. *J. Clin. Invest.* **51:**326–330, 1972.

19 Reed, W. B., et al., Cutaneous Manifestations of Ataxia-

telangiectasia. J.A.M.A. **195:**746–753, 1966.

20 Reye, C., Ataxia-telangiectasia. *Am. J. Dis. Child.* **99:**238–241, 1960.

21 Sedgwick, R. P., and Boder, E., Progressive Ataxia in Childhood with Particular Reference to Ataxia-telangiectasia. *Neurology* **10:**705–715, 1960.

22 Smeby, B., Ataxia-telangiectasia. *Acta Paediatr. Scand.* **55:**239–243, 1966.

23 Solitare, G. B., Louis-Bar's Syndrome (Ataxia-telangiectasia). *Neurology* **18:**1180–1186, 1968.

24 Syllaba, L., and Henner, K., Contribution à l'independence de l'athétose double idiopathique et congénital atteinte familiale, syndrome dystrophique, signe du reseau vasculaire conjunctival intégrité psychique. *Rev. Neurol.* **15:**541–562, 1926.

25 Tadjoedin, M. K., and Fraser, F. C., Heredity of Ataxia-telangiectasia (Louis-Bar Syndrome). *Am. J. Dis. Child.* **110:**64–68, 1965.

26 Terhaggen, H. G., et al., Ataxia-telangiectasia (Louis-Bar Syndrome). Bericht über sieben Fälle. *Z. Kinderheilkd.* **107:**324–342, 1970.

27 Terplan, K. L., and Krauss, R. F., Histopathologic Brain Changes in Association with Ataxia-telangiectasia. *Neurology* **19:**446–454, 1969.

28 Utian, H. L., and Plit, J., Ataxia-telangiectasia. *J. Neurol. Neurosurg. Psychiatry* **27:**38–40, 1964.

29 Waldman, T. A., and McIntire, K. R., Serum Alpha-fetoprotein Levels in Patients with Ataxia-telangiectasia. *Lancet* **2:**1112–1115, 1972.

11

Beckwith-Wiedemann Syndrome

(*Macroglossia-Omphalocele Syndrome, EMG Syndrome*)

In 1963, Beckwith (2) reported three cases of a newly recognized syndrome consisting of (*a*) macroglossia, (*b*) omphalocele, (*c*) cytomegaly of the adrenal cortex, (*d*) hyperplasia of the gonadal interstitial cells, (*e*) renal medullary dysplasia, and (*f*) hyperplastic visceromegaly. Subsequently, Beckwith (3) enlarged his series of patients, noting (*g*) postnatal somatic gigantism, (*h*) mild microcephaly, and (*i*) severe hypoglycemia. In 1964, Wiedemann (29) independently reported the syndrome in three sibs and observed a further component—(*j*) a dome-shaped defect of the diaphragm. Other important contributions have been made by several investigators (10–12, 15–20, 25, 33). An early report of the syndrome is that of Helbing (16) in 1896.

Most cases of the Beckwith-Wiedemann syndrome are sporadic. Affected sibs have been reported occasionally (5–7, 29) and consanguinity was established in one case (10). Several have occurred in more than one sibship in the same family (12a, 18, 19, 19a, 20a). Based on familial cases, autosomal recessive (3, 12, 19), autosomal dominant (12a, 19a), polygenic (13), and autosomal dominant, sex-dependent (20a) inheritance have been proposed. Etiologic heterogeneity is possible.

Thorburn et al. (28) estimated the frequency of the syndrome as 1 per 13,700 births; and they suggested that it occurs in perhaps more than 15 percent of infants with omphalocele (27).

Wiedemann et al. (32, 33) regarded congenital generalized lipodystrophy, the Beckwith-Wiedemann syndrome, cerebral gigantism, and the Russell-Silver syndrome as examples of "congenital diencephalic syndromes of childhood."

Because of the endocrine cytomegaly present in the syndrome, Beckwith (3) suggested that the fetal adrenal cortex is either overactive or underactive, with excessive stimulation caused by a feedback mechanism similar to that found in the adrenogenital syndrome. He further noted that abnormalities observed in the hypophysis, gonads, islets of Langerhans, and paraganglia should be considered in evaluating the abnormal growth in this syndrome, and that altered placental endocrine physiology could conceivably play a role in producing many of the features found during the neonatal period.

Hydramnios has been noted in about 60 percent of cases, and some infants have been premature. Placentas have also been large (18, 19).

SYSTEMIC MANIFESTATIONS

Symptomatic neonatal hypoglycemia may be present in one-third to one-half of the patients (3). Some later become prediabetic (17, 29).

Facies. Macroglossia, evident at birth, is discussed below (Figs. 11-1 and 11-2). Maxillary hypoplasia and relative mandibular prognathism were regular features of Irving's series (18). The occiput may be prominent. Mild microcephaly

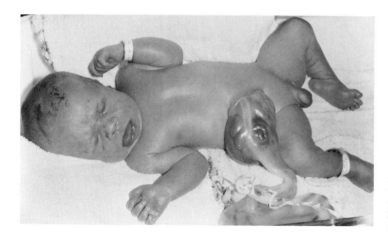

Figure 11-1. *Beckwith-Wiedemann syndrome.* Note large tongue and omphalocele. (*From M. W. Moncrieff et al.*, Postgrad. Med. J. **46**:162, 1970.)

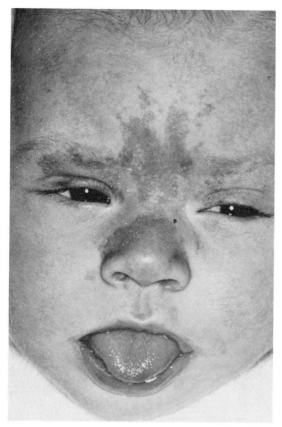

Figure 11-2. Glabellar nevus flammeus and macroglossia. (*From H. R. Wiedemann,* Z. Kinderheilkd. **106**:171, 1969.)

has been noted in about half the cases (28). Asymmetric earlobe grooves and pits (Fig. 11-3*A, B*) have been observed in about 60 percent of patients (28). Circular depressions on the posterior rim of the helices have been noted in about 50 percent (31). Facial nevus flammeus, a finding seen in over 90 percent of patients, tends to become less prominent during the first year of life (18, 19). It occurs principally in the glabellar area and over the upper eyelids (Fig. 11-2).

Gastrointestinal system. Omphalocele, or umbilical hernia, is a common feature (Fig. 11-1). Malrotation anomalies are present in most cases (18, 28). Several patients have had diastasis recti (3). Hepatomegaly is common (9, 10).

Skeletal system. Gigantism is not necessarily present at birth, but mean birth weight is about 3,900 g (range, 2,775 to 6,235 g) (20). Growth may even be subnormal for a few months, but somatic gigantism eventually results. Height and weight are often above the 90th percentile. Advanced bone age is present in the majority (28) of cases, and widening of the metaphyses and cortical thickening of long bones have been reported. Hemihypertrophy has been noted in about 15 percent (3, 21, 22, 32, 34).

Central nervous system. Mental retardation, which occurs in some cases, is probably due, in

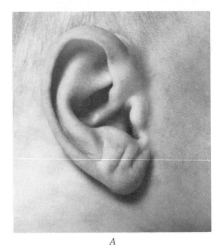

A

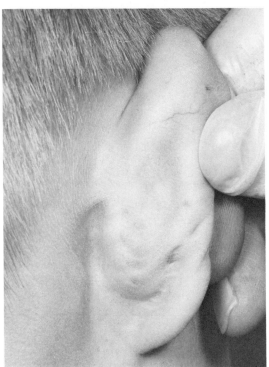

B

Figure 11-3. (*A*). Linear grooves on earlobe. (*From H. R. Wiedemann,* Z. Kinderheilkd. **106:**171, 1969.) (*B*). Punched-out depressions of posterior pinna.

part, to undetected hypoglycemia during infancy (34). Intelligence has been normal in many cases (18), although mild to moderate retardation was a regular feature in Beckwith's series (3). Hydro-

cephalus has been observed in two instances (10, 19).

Neoplasia. Wilms tumor and adrenal cortical carcinoma occur with a frequency of about 5 percent (3, 23, 26, 32, 34). Hepatoblastoma, glioma, embryonal rhabdomyosarcoma, carcinoid tumor, myxoma, and fibroma have also been noted (19, 27a). The presence of hemihypertrophy does not increase the risk for malignancy (32).

Other findings. Diaphragmatic eventration (Fig. 11-4) in about 30 percent of patients (3, 10, 18, 20, 29) and clitoromegaly (3, 18, 19, 20a, 29) have been noted. Various other abnormalities, such as genitourinary tract anomalies, have been described (19, 27, 28).

Oral manifestations. Macroglossia is a very common but not essential feature (Figs. 11-1, 11-2, 11-5). Tongue biopsies have been normal (3, 10, 11, 17–19, 25, 28, 29). Class III malocclusion, anterior open bite, and retroclined mandibular incisors were features emphasized in Irving's series (18). The dentofacial characteristics of the syndrome received further comment

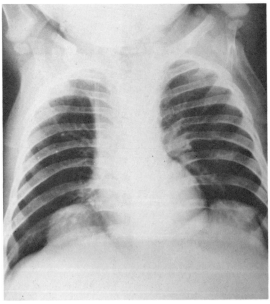

Figure 11-4. Bilateral diaphragmatic eventration. (*From I. Irving,* J. Pediatr. Surg. **2:**499, 1967.)

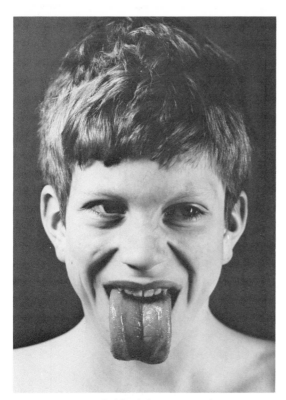

Figure 11-5. Remarkable ability to extend tongue. (*Courtesy of H. R. Wiedemann, Kiel, Germany.*)

by Cohen (8). Some patients have Class II malocclusion. Cleft palate was noted in a few cases (4, 5, 27) and the Robin anomalad has also been observed (10).

PATHOLOGY

Nephromegaly is common, and pancreatomegaly may also occur (19, 27). Hyperplasia of the bladder, uterus, liver, and thymus has also been reported (2, 37). In Beckwith's autopsy series (3), increased renal lobulation was noted. Each lobule was capped by a wide, persistent nephrogenic activity zone. Medullary dysplasia was evident, with most pyramids showing an increased amount of stroma. The collecting tubules were immature. Hyperplasia of acini, islets, and ducts was evident in the pancreas. Cytomegaly of the fetal adrenal cortex was a constant feature—the cells containing sudano-

philic droplets (19, 27) (Fig. 11-6). The adrenal cortex was cystic, and the medulla was hyperplastic. An increased number of amphophils was present in the pituitary gland. The gonadal interstitial cells were hyperplastic. The paraganglia were also hyperplastic.

DIFFERENTIAL DIAGNOSIS

The facial features of patients with the Beckwith-Wiedemann syndrome may, at times, suggest hypothyroidism or a *mucopolysaccharidosis.* Infants of diabetic or prediabetic mothers resemble infants with the Beckwith-Wiedemann syndrome in being gigantic and hypoglycemic. However, the duration of hypoglycemia is different, and, furthermore,

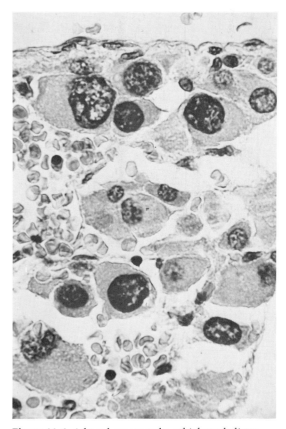

Figure 11-6. Adrenal cytomegaly, which we believe represents polyploidy. (*From K. Bech,* Acta Pathol. Microbiol. Scand. **79A:**279, 1971.)

congenital anomalies occur rarely in infants born to diabetic mothers. A distinct entity consisting of macroglossia, transient neonatal diabetes mellitus, and intrauterine growth failure was reported (11a). Earlobe grooves can be inherited as an isolated autosomal dominant trait (31).

Other possible considerations in differential diagnosis include the *Down syndrome, hemihypertrophy,* the *mucolipidoses, lipoatrophic diabetes,* and *cerebral gigantism.*

Adrenal cytomegaly is not rare in stillborn infants (1).

LABORATORY AIDS

Blood glucose determinations should be utilized to screen patients for possible hypoglycemia during the neonatal period (23a). Hyperlipemia, hypercholesterolemia, and hypocalcemia have been occasionally reported (3, 15, 25, 31). Neonatal polycythemia has also been described (3, 11, 27). Hyperinsulinemia and insulin hyperresponsiveness to glucose has been reported (24). Greene et al. (13) discussed associated immunodeficiency.

REFERENCES

1 Bech, K., Cytomegaly of the Fetal Adrenal Cortex. *Acta Pathol. Microbiol. Scand.* **79A:**279–286, 1971.

2 Beckwith, J. B., Extreme Cytomegaly of the Adrenal Fetal Cortex, Omphalocele, Hyperplasia of Kidneys and Pancreas, and Leydig-cell Hyperplasia: Another Syndrome? Presented at Annual Meeting of Western Society for Pediatric Research, Los Angeles, Calif., Nov. 11, 1963.

3 Beckwith, J. B., Macroglossia, Omphalocele, Adrenal Cytomegaly, Gigantism, and Hyperplastic Visceromegaly. *Birth Defects* **5**(2):188–196, 1969.

4 Beckwith, J. B., Personal communication, 1969.

5 Bohlmann, H. G., and Havers, W., Exomphalos-Makroglossie-Gigantismus-Syndrom (Wiedemann-Beckwith-Syndrom) bei drei Geschwistern. *Arch. Kinderheilkd.* **183:**175–182, 1971.

6 Borit, A., and Kosek, J., Cytomegaly of the Adrenal Cortex: Electron Microscopy in Beckwith's Syndrome. *Arch. Pathol.* **88:**58–64, 1969.

7 Chambionnat, D., *A propos de deux nouveaux cas d'un syndrome associant une omphalocèle, une macroglossie, une macrosomie, et plusieurs anomalies mineures.* Thesis, Faculté de Médicine, Paris, 1969.

8 Cohen, M. M., Jr., Comments on the Macroglossia-Omphalocele Syndrome. *Birth Defects* **5**(2):197, 1969.

9 Cohen, M. M., Jr., Macroglossia, Omphalocele, Visceromegaly, Cytomegaly of the Adrenal Cortex and Neonatal Hypoglycemia. *Birth Defects* **7**(7):226–232, 1971.

10 Cohen, M. M., Jr., et al., The Beckwith-Wiedemann Syndrome: Seven New Cases. *Am. J. Dis. Child.* **122:**515–520, 1971.

11 Combs, J. T., et al., New Syndrome of Neonatal Hypoglycemia. *N. Engl. J. Med.* **275:**236–243, 1966.

11a Dakou-Voutetakis, C., et al., Macroglossia, Transient Neonatal Diabetes Mellitus and Intrauterine Growth Failure: A New Distinct Entity. *Pediatrics* **55:**127–131, 1975.

12 Filippi, G., and McKusick, V. A., Beckwith-Wiedemann Syndrome (Exomphalos-Macroglossia-Gigantism Syndrome): Report of Two Cases and Review of the Literature. *Medicine* **49:**279–298, 1970.

12a Forrester, R. M., Wiedemann-Beckwith Syndrome. *Lancet* **2:**47, 1973.

13 Greene, R. J., Immunodeficiency Associated with Exomphalos-Macroglossia-Gigantism Syndrome. *J. Pediatr.* **82:**814–820, 1973.

14 Gustavson, K. H., et al., A 4-5/21-22 Chromosomal Translocation Associated with Multiple Congenital Anomalies. *Acta Paediatr. Scand.* **53:**172–181, 1964.

15 Harris, F., and Zachary, R. B., Exomphalos and Macroglossia (Beckwith's Syndrome). *Proc. R. Soc. Med.* **62:**905–906, 1969.

16 Helbing, C., Zur Casuistik der muskulären Makroglossie. *Jb. Kinderheilkd.* **41:**442–454, 1896.

17 Hooft, C., et al., Le syndrome de Wiedemann et Beckwith (omphalocèle-macroglossie-gigantisme). *Ann. Pédiatr.* **16:**49–56, 1969.

18 Irving, I., Exomphalos with Macroglossia: A Study of 11 Cases. *J. Pediatr. Surg.* **2:**499–507, 1967.

19 Irving, I., The E.M.G. Syndrome (Exomphalos, Macroglossia, Gigantism) in P. P. Rickham, W. Ch. Hacker and J. Prevolt (eds.), *Progress in Pediatrics,* vol. 1. Urban & Schwarzenberg, Munich, 1970, pp. 1–61.

19a Kosseff, A. L., et al., The Wiedemann-Beckwith Syndrome: Genetic Considerations and a Diagnostic Sign. *Lancet* **1:**844, 1972.

20 Lee, F. A., Radiology of the Beckwith-Wiedemann Syndrome. *Radiol. Clin. North Am.* **10:**261–276, 1972.

20a Lubinsky, M., et al., Autosomal Dominant Sex-Dependent Transmission of the Wiedemann-Beckwith Syndrome. *Lancet* **1:**932, 1974.

21 Mangold, B. L., et al., Exomphalos-Macroglossie-Gigantismus-Syndrome. *Pädiat. Pädol.* **9:**365–372, 1974.

22 Mucke, J., Zum Exomphalos-Makroglossie-Gigantismus-Syndrom. *Kinderärztl. Prax.* **40:**10–14, 1972.

23 Reddy, J. K., et al., Beckwith-Wiedemann Syndrome. *Arch. Pathol.* **94:**523–532, 1972.

23a Roe, T. F., et al., Beckwith's Syndrome with Extreme Organ Hyperplasia. *Pediatrics* **52:**372–381, 1973.

24 Schiff, D., et al., Metabolic Aspects of the Beckwith-Wiedemann Syndrome. *J. Pediatr.* **82:**258–262, 1973.

25 Shafer, A. D., Primary Macroglossia. *Clin. Pediatr.* **7:**357–363, 1968.

26 Sherman, F. E., et al., Congenital Metastasizing Adrenal

Cortical Carcinoma Associated with Cytomegaly of the Fetal Adrenal Cortex. *Am. J. Clin. Pathol.* **30:**439–446, 1958.

27 Sotelo-Avila, C., and Singer, D. B., Syndrome of Hyperplastic Fetal Visceromegaly and Neonatal Hypoglycemia (Beckwith's Syndrome): A Report of Seven Cases. *Pediatrics* **46:**240–251, 1970.

27a Sotelo-Avila, C., personal communication, 1975.

28 Thorburn, M. J., et al., Exomphalos-Macroglossia-Gigantism Syndrome in Jamaican Infants. *Am. J. Dis. Child.* **119:**316–321, 1970.

29 Wiedemann, H. R., Complexe malformatif familial avec hernie ombilicale et macroglossie-un syndrome nouveau? *J. Génét. Hum.* **13:**223–232, 1964.

30 Wiedemann, H. R., Das EMG Syndrom: Exomphalos, Makroglossie, Gigantismus und Kohlenhydratstoffwechselstörung. *Z. Kinderheilkd.* **102:**1–36, 1968.

31 Wiedemann, H. R., Über das "Kerbenohr" beim Exomphalos-Makroglossie-Gigantismus Syndrom, über Ohrläppchen-Fisteln und über das Vorkommen entsprechender Erscheinungen bei anderweitigen Syndromen sowie bei Gesunden. *Z. Kinderheilkd.* **115:**95–110, 1973.

32 Wiedemann, H. R., Exomphalos-Makroglossie-Gigantismus-Syndrom, Berardinelli-Seip-Syndrom und Sotos-Syndrom-ein vergleichende Betrachtung unter ausgewählten Aspekten. *Z. Kinderheilkd.* **115:**193–207, 1973.

33 Wiedemann, H. R., et al., Über das Syndrom Exomphalos-Makroglossie-Gigantismus, über generalisierte Muskelhypertrophie, progressive Lipodystrophie und Miescher-Syndrom im Sinne diencephaler Syndrome. *Z. Kinderheilkd.* **102:**1–36, 1968.

34 Wilson, F. C., and Orlin, H., Crossed Congenital Hemihypertrophy Associated with Wilms' Tumor. *J. Bone Joint Surg.* **47A:**1609–1614, 1965.

12

Behçet Syndrome

(Recurrent Genitooral Aphthosis and Uveitis with Hypopyon)

The syndrome presently carrying Behçet's name was probably described by Hippocrates in his third book of endemic disease (10). Blüthe (5) in 1908 and Adamantiades (1) in 1931 mentioned the simultaneous occurrence of iritis, hypopyon, and lesions of the mouth and genitals. However, it was not until the Turkish dermatologist Hulusi Behçet published his classic paper (3) that the disease was recognized as a clinical entity, comprising the triad of aphthous stomatitis, genital ulcers, and recurring uveitis (hypopyon). Touraine (26) considered the affection of the eyes, mouth, and genitals in the Behçet syndrome to be part of what he called "l'aphtose," a systemic disease with potential manifestations in many organs. An excellent historic and clinical review is that of Monacelli and Nazzaro (19).

Theories of etiology abound. The syndrome has been thought to be the result of an allergic reaction, a concept to some extent supported by the rather frequent association with erythema nodosum. In recent years, support has been found for an autoimmune etiology. Oshima et al. (20) showed the presence of autoantibodies against oral mucosa and a rise in immunoglobulins in the oral mucosa and blood of patients with the Behçet syndrome. In 1969, Lehner (16) described an intense lymphomonocytic infiltration of the epithelium and concluded that the changes were consistent with those of a delayed hypersensitivity reaction. Saito et al. (22) demonstrated a constant association of macrophages with degenerated cells in the prickle cell layer of the oral mucosa adjacent to the ulcerations. Because of this association they suggested an autoimmune basis.

SYSTEMIC MANIFESTATIONS

The Behçet syndrome occurs between the ages of ten and forty-five years, with a marked predilection (between 3:1 and 5:1) for males (9, 18). Many of the cases have been reported from the Middle East, especially in the eastern Mediterranean area. Perhaps a disproportionate number of cases have been described in patients of Jewish extraction (4). Relatively few examples have been reported in the United States.

The syndrome has a tendency to recur. Relapses of varying duration may be seen several times yearly, often accompanied by fever and poor general health (18, 25). Malaise, weakness, mild fever, bouts of sore throat and tonsillitis, and muscular pain and joint stiffness, especially involving the lower extremities, may appear 6 months to 5 years before the appearance of the major triad.

Eyes. The ocular signs, occurring in about 80 percent of cases, usually begin in one eye and spread to the other. Various types of lesions have been reported (conjunctivitis, keratitis, retinitis, etc.), the most common being chronic recurrent uveitis with hypopyon, which eventually leads to severe visual damage or blindness (4, 9). The frequency of ocular signs varies considerably in different surveys (12). Recurrent conjunctivitis may precede the appearance of uveitis by years. Usually the patient experiences intense periorbital pain and photophobia. Histopathologic studies have demonstrated that the primary defect is an obliterative vasculitis which results secondarily in hemorrhagic infarcts, retinal detachment, and iridocyclitis (11).

Genitalia. The genital lesions, noted in about 85 percent of patients, consist of recurrent aphthae, larger than those involving the oral mucosa, which in males appear on the penis, the inner thigh, and, particularly, on the scrotum (Fig. 12-1). In women, the ulcers occur on the vulva, where they may lead to fenestration of the labia minora (Fig. 12-2). Healing of these ulcerations may lead to severe scarring. The perineum may be involved in both sexes.

Skin. The lesions may present a varied picture. Pyoderma is seen in about 30 percent of cases, being manifested in one of the following types:

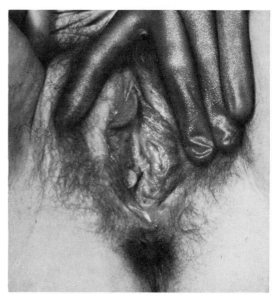

Figure 12-2. Deep ulcer of labia. (*From D. L. Phillips, Glasgow, Scotland.*)

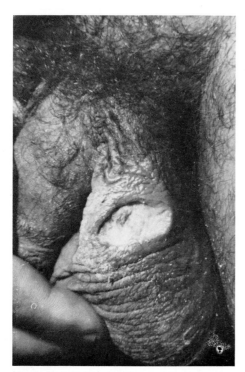

Figure 12-1. *Behçet syndrome.* Large ulcer on scrotum. (*From A. Mortada, Cairo, Egypt.*)

pustules, impetigo, folliculitis, furuncles, or simple ulcerations (9). Erythema nodosum is found in about 30 percent (9). The nodules occur predominantly on the lower extremities and are, at times, accompanied by fever. The skin exhibits an increased sensitivity. Rashes of the erythema multiforme type have also been described.

Other findings. Other signs in the Behçet syndrome include recurrent thrombophlebitis of superficial veins of the legs in about 45 percent of the patients (13), arthralgia in about 35 percent (9), and epididymitis in about 5 percent (10, 14, 15). Several reports note involvement of the central nervous system in 20 to 50 percent, with meningitis, spastic weakness, external ophthalmoplegia, and other features of midbrain disease and acute confusional states or progressive dementia being the more common manifestations (9, 14, 23, 27). The prognosis for patients having neurologic symptoms is more grave, and in about 65 percent of the cases the patient dies within a year of the appearance of central nervous system involvement (23).

Visceral involvement, particularly of the pulmonary system and of the gastrointestinal tract, may also be seen (7, 14). Cardiac involvement has also been described (17).

Oral manifestations. Oral lesions are an almost constant feature of the Behçet syndrome and are the initial manifestation of the syndrome in about 60 percent of cases. The ulcers may be located anywhere on the oral mucosa and tend to appear in crops. Morphologically they resemble aphthae, being well demarcated and varying in size from a few millimeters to a centimeter in diameter. The ulcer base is covered with a yellowish-gray exudate, and the margin is surrounded by a red halo (Fig. 12-3*A–C*). The ulcers, which are extremely painful, at times extend into the pharynx and esophagus, resulting in dysphagia (2). Involvement of the central nervous system may cause slurred speech and difficulty in swallowing (23). Absence or scantiness of lingual fungiform papillae has been described as characteristic for the Behçet syndrome (8).

PATHOLOGY

Few cases of the Behçet syndrome with autopsy reports have been recorded (19). Sulheim et al. (25) described extensive pulmonary and splenic fibrosis, atrophic esophagogastroenteritis, subchronic panophthalmitis, and disseminated atrophic-degenerative lesions in the brain. Certain features suggested a relationship with collagen diseases.

DIFFERENTIAL DIAGNOSIS

Some authors regard the Behçet syndrome as a variant of *erythema multiforme*. The present authors feel that a separation between the two syndromes should be maintained, since the oral and ocular lesions in the two conditions are completely different in appearance. In the syndrome of Behçet, the oral manifestations are aphthae; in erythema multiforme the oral lesions are much more extensive, producing superficial sloughing of the mucosa, often combined with crust formation of the lips.

It has been observed that the three major clinical signs need not occur simultaneously; at

times only two are present and years may elapse before the third appears (6). It has also been maintained that patients exhibiting only two

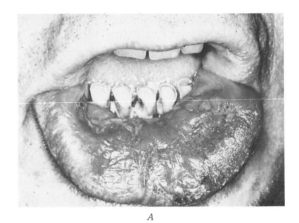

A

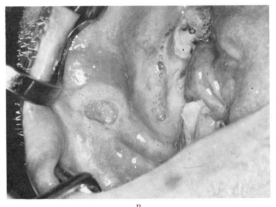

B

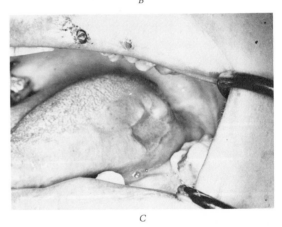

C

Figure 12-3. (*A, B, and C*). Deep scarifying oral ulcers. (*From H. Mathis and D. Herrmann*, Dtsch. Zahnärztl. Z. **25**:1154, 1970.)

signs, for example, ocular-oral or genital-oral involvement, should be considered as having abortive forms of the Behçet syndrome. This concept immediately raises the question of whether all cases of recurrent oral and genital aphthae are abortive cases of this syndrome. At the present time, this question cannot be answered.

The Reiter syndrome is also similar to the Behçet syndrome insofar as it occurs mainly in men and the prominent symptoms are limited to the eyes, mouth, genitals, and skin. However, the clincial appearance of the lesions is different. In the Reiter syndrome, the genital involvement consists usually of urethritis. The oral lesions are not a constant finding; when occurring, they have a whitish, circinate, nonaphthous-like appearance, similar to that of lesions on the penis.

DIAGNOSTIC AIDS

According to Katzenellenbogen (15) and Sobel (24), patients with the Behçet syndrome may show a characteristic erythematous reaction when given an intracutaneous injection of saline solution. Even a prick with a sterile needle may result in a pustule. Berlin (4) gave an intradermal injection of 0.1 ml saline solution to 10 patients and found eight positive reactions. Moderate leukocytosis and slight elevation of the sedimentation rate may be observed during episodes of the disease (19).

REFERENCES

1 Adamantiades, B., Sur un cas d'iritis à hypopyon recidivant. *Ann. Ocul. (Paris)* **168:**271–278, 1931.

2 Arma, S., et al., Dysphagia in Behçet's Syndrome. *Thorax* **26:**155–158, 1971.

3 Behçet, H., Über rezidiverende Aphthöse, durch ein Virus verursachte Geschwüre am Mund, am Auge und an den Genitalien. *Dermatol. Wochenschr.* **105:**1152–1157, 1937.

4 Berlin, C., Behçet's Disease as a Multiple Symptom Complex: Report of Ten Cases. *Arch. Dermatol.* **82:**73–79, 1960.

5 Blüthe, L., *Zur Kenntnis des recidivierenden Hypopyons.* D. Straus, Heidelberg, 1908.

6 Curth, H. O., Recurrent Genito-oral Aphthosis and Uveitis with Hypopyon (Behçet's Syndrome). *Arch. Dermatol. Syph.* **54:**179–196, 1946; and *Mod. Med. (Minneap.)* **16:**131–137, 1955.

7 Davies, J. D., Behçet's Syndrome with Haemoptysis and Pulmonary Lesions. *J. Pathol.* **109:**351–356, 1973.

8 Davis, E., and Melzer, E., A New Sign in Behçet's Syndrome: Scanty Fungiform Papillae in Tongue. *Arch. Intern. Med.* **124:**720–721, 1969.

9 Dowling, G. B., et al., Behçet's Disease. *Proc. R. Soc. Med.* **54:**101–107, 1961.

10 Feigenbaum, A., Description of Behçet's Syndrome in the Hippocratic Third Book of Endemic Diseases. *Br. J. Ophthalmol.* **40:**355–357, 1956.

11 Fenton, R. H., and Eason, H. A., Behçet's Syndrome: A Histopathologic Study of the Eye. *Arch. Ophthalmol.* **72:**71–81, 1964.

12 Haim, S., Contribution of Ocular Symptoms in the Diagnosis of Behçet's Disease. *Arch. Dermatol.* **98:**478–480, 1968.

13 Haim, S., et al., Involvement of Veins in Behçet's Syndrome. *Br. J. Dermatol.* **84:**238–241, 1971.

13a Hamza, M., et al. La maladie de Behçet. Etude de 22 cas. *Nouv. Presse Méd.* **4:**563–566, 1975.

14 Kalbian, V. V., and Challis, M. T., Behçet's Disease. *Am. J. Med.* **49:**823–829, 1970.

15 Katzenellenbogen, I., and Feurman, E. J., Beitrag zur Morbus Behçet: Die Bedeutung der spezifischen Hauthyperaktivität und der Behçetinreaktion. *Hautarzt* **16:**13–18, 1965.

16 Lehner, T., Characterization of Mucosal Antibodies in Recurrent Aphthous Ulceration and Behçet's Syndrome. *Arch. Oral Biol.* **14:**843–853, 1969.

17 Lewis, P. S., Behçet Disease and Carditis. *Br. Med. J.* **1:**1026–1027, 1964.

18 Mamo, J. G., and Baghdassarian, A., Behçet's Disease: A Report of 28 Cases. *Arch. Ophthalmol.* **71:**4–14, 1964.

19 Monacelli, M., and Nazzaro, P. (eds.), *Behçet's Disease,* S. Karger, Basel, 1966.

20 Oshima, Y., et al., Clinical Studies on Behçet's Syndrome. *Ann. Rheum. Dis.* **22:**36–45, 1963.

21 Rogers, R. S., et al., Lymphocytotoxicity in Recurrent Aphthous Stomatitis. *Arch. Dermatol.* **109:**361–363, 1974.

22 Saito, T., et al., Auto-immune Mechanisms as a Probable Aetiology of Behçet's Syndrome, an Electron Microscopic Study of the Oral Mucosa. *Virchows Arch. (Pathol. Anat.) (Abt. A)* **353:**261–272, 1971.

23 Schotland, D. L., et al., Neurologic Aspects of Behçet's Disease. *Am. J. Med.* **34:**544–553, 1963.

24 Sobel, J. D., et al., Cutaneous Hyperreactivity in Behçet's Disease. *Dermatologica* **146:**350–356, 1973.

25 Sulheim, O., et al., Behçet's Syndrome: Report of a Case with Complete Autopsy Performed. *Acta Pathol. Microbiol. Scand.* **45:**145–158, 1959.

26 Touraine, A., L'aphtose. Donnees récentes et synthése. *Presse Méd.* **63:**1493–1494, 1955.

27 Winter, F. C., and Yukins, R. E., Ocular Pathology of Behçet's Disease. *Am. J. Ophthalmol.* **62:**257–262, 1966.

13

Bloom Syndrome

(Congenital Telangiectatic Erythema with Growth Retardation)

A syndrome consisting of (*a*) growth retardation and (*b*) telangiectatic erythema was first described by Bloom (1) and Torre and Cramer (16) in 1954. Since then about 50 other patients have been recognized.

German (5, 6) was the first to point out the tendency of these children to have chromosome breaks and to develop malignancies. Several patients have exhibited immunologic deficiency as expressed by multiple infections (5, 7).

The syndrome exhibits autosomal recessive inheritance. About half the reported patients have been of eastern European Jewish origin (5), and two-thirds have been male. Parental consanguinity (4–6) has been higher among non-Jews, indicating the rarity of the gene in this group. A family history of rheumatoid arthritis is not uncommon (13).

SYSTEMIC MANIFESTATIONS

Facies. There is disproportionate microcephaly, accentuated by the delicacy and narrowness of the face (2, 4, 7–9, 16). The head is dolichocephalic. Some patients have a prominent nose and ears, with slightly receding mandible (15) (Fig. 13-1*A, B*).

Dwarfism. Growth retardation of prenatal onset is a prominent clinical feature (Fig. 13-2). Mild mental retardation has been noted in a few patients (3, 5, 8, 15, 16). Birth weight is low, rarely exceeding 2,300 g at normal term. Mean birth length is 44 cm (mean normal, 50 cm). Maximal adult height rarely exceeds 145 cm for men and 130 cm for women (8).

Skin. Sensitivity to light is noticed early in infancy and leads to the development of telangiectatic erythema, which may first appear any time between early infancy and two years of age (1–3, 7, 9, 12). The erythema involves light-exposed areas of the face; superficially it resembles lupus erythematosus because of the butterfly arrangement across the nose (1). The eyelashes are commonly lost. The forearms and dorsa of the hands, nape, and ears may become involved, but rarely does the erythema extend to the trunk. Exposure to sunlight may cause bullae and vesicles (1, 15). Milia may be noted in the scarred areas (2).

Café-au-lait spots have been noted in about 60 percent of the patients for whom this information is available (4, 5), and keratosis follicularis in about 20 percent. Acanthosis nigricans was noted in one patient who developed diabetes mellitus during puberty (2). Pilonidal cyst or sacral dimpling has also been observed (5).

Eyes. Conjunctivitis and telangiectasia of the conjunctival vessels may be seen (15). Colloid bodylike spots in Bruch's membrane have been reported in two patients (10).

Malignancies. There is a high incidence of leukemia, lymphoma, and "solid tumors." About

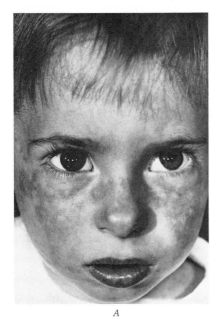

A

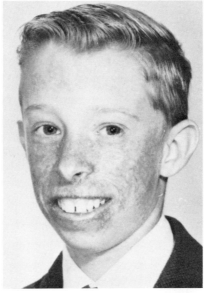

B

Figure 13-1. (*A*). Bloom syndrome. Telangiectatic erythema of face. (*B*). Extensive facial telangiectasia in fourteen-year-old male. (*From J. German,* Am. J. Hum. Genet. **21:**196, 1969.)

15 percent of patients have subsequently died of malignant neoplasia (3, 4, 5).

Other findings. Patients have been reported with skeletal abnormalities, including syndactyly, clinodactyly, supernumerary digits, absence of the toe and its corresponding metatarsal, dislocation of hips, and pes equinus (2, 5, 9).

The testes may be small and soft and have been undescended in several patients. Urethral stricture or meatal narrowing has been observed (5, 7).

Oral manifestations. Chronic cheilitis is a prominent feature of the Bloom syndrome (15). The voice may be high-pitched (2, 7, 8). One author commented on the absence of maxillary lateral incisors (16), but it is doubtful whether this is a significant finding. One patient developed squamous cell carcinoma of the tongue (12).

DIFFERENTIAL DIAGNOSIS

Bloom syndrome has been grouped with *ataxia-telangiectasia,* the *Cockayne syndrome, Rothmund-Thomson syndrome, Werner syndrome,*

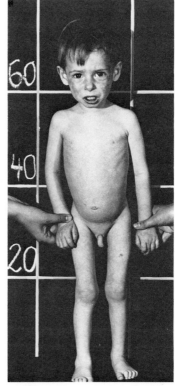

Figure 13-2. Four-year-old boy, far below 3d percentile in height, with telangiectatic erythema of face. (*From J. Keutel et al.,* Z. Kinderheilkd. **101:**165, 1967.)

dyskeratosis congenita, Fanconi anemia, and *xerodermic idiocy* (5, 9, 11). Nearly all these disorders are characterized by growth retardation, increased incidence of neoplasia (both lymphoreticular and carcinomatous), immunologic deficiency, late-onset diabetes, and premature senility of the skin and conjunctiva (11).

Sunlight sensitivity is also a feature of the Cockayne syndrome, Rothmund-Thomson syndrome, and xeroderma pigmentosum. Pigmentary skin changes are seen in sun-exposed areas of patients with ataxia-telangiectasia, the Werner syndrome, dyskeratosis congenita, and Fanconi anemia.

Increased chromosomal breaks have also been reported in Fanconi anemia, Cockayne syndrome, ataxia-telangiectasia, and dyskeratosis congenita (5, 9). However, they are unlike the changes seen in Bloom syndrome (14).

LABORATORY AIDS

Cytogenetic studies have demonstrated a proclivity for chromosomal breakage and rearrangement in cells cultured in vitro and. consequently a high incidence of aneuploidy (5, 6, 8, 14). Homologous sites on homologous chromosomes form sister chromatid exchanges (6, 14).

Low levels of serum immunoglobulins (IgG, IgA, and IgM) have been a rather consistent finding (5, 7–9, 13).

REFERENCES

1 Bloom, D., Congenital Telangiectatic Erythema in a Levi-Lorain Dwarf. *Arch. Dermatol.* **69:**526, 1954.

2 Bloom, D., The Syndrome of Congenital Telangiectatic Erythema and Stunted Growth. *J. Pediatr.* **68:**103–113, 1966.

3 Braun-Falco, O., and Marghescu, S., Kongenitales telangiektatisches Erythem (Bloom-Syndrom) mit Diabetes insipidus. *Hautarzt* **17:**155–161, 1966.

4 Braun-Falco, O., and Marghescu, S., Bloom-Syndrom. Eine Krankheit mit relativ hoher Leukämie-Morbidität. *Münch. Med. Wochenschr.* **111:**65–69, 1969.

5 German, J., Bloom's Syndrome, Genetic and Clinical Observations in the First 27 Patients. *Am. J. Hum. Genet.* **21:**196–227, 1969.

6 German, J., et al., Bloom's Syndrome. III. Analysis of the Chromosome Aberration Characteristic of this Disorder. *Chromosoma (Berlin)* **48:**361–366, 1974.

7 Katzenellenbogen, I., and Laron, Z., A Contribution to Bloom's Syndrome. *Arch. Dermatol.* **82:**609–616, 1960.

8 Keutel, J., et al., Bloom-Syndrom. *Z. Kinderheilkd.* **101:**165–180, 1967.

9 Landau, J. W., et al., Bloom's Syndrome. *Arch. Dermatol.* **94:**687–694, 1966.

10 Landau, J., et al., Eye Findings in Congenital Telangiectatic Erythema and Growth Retardation. *Am. J. Ophthalmol.* **62:**753–754, 1966.

11 Reed, W. B., et al., Cutaneous Manifestations of Ataxia-Telangiectasia. *J.A.M.A.* **195:**746–753, 1966.

12 Sawitsky, A., et al., Chromosomal Breakage and Acute Leukemia in Congenital Telangiectatic Erythema and Stunted Growth. *Ann. Intern. Med.* **65:**487–495, 1966.

13 Schoen, E. J., and Shearn, M. A., Immunoglobulin Deficiency in Bloom's Syndrome. *Am. J. Dis. Child.* **113:**594–596, 1967.

14 Schroeder, T. M., and German, J., Bloom's Syndrome and Fanconi's Anemia. Demonstration of Two Distinctive Patterns of Chromosome Disruption and Rearrangement. *Humangenetik* **25:**299–306, 1974.

15 Szalay, G. C., Dwarfism with Skin Manifestations. *J. Pediatr.* **62:**686–695, 1963.

16 Torre, D. P., and Cramer, J., Primordial Dwarfism. Discoid Lupus Erythematosus. *Arch. Dermatol.* **69:**511–513, 1954.

14

Carpenter Syndrome

(*Acrocephalopolysyndactyly*)

The syndrome consists of (*a*) acrocephaly, (*b*) soft-tissue syndactyly, especially involving the third and fourth fingers, and brachymesophalangy, (*c*) preaxial polydactyly and syndactyly of the toes, (*d*) coxa valga and pes varus, (*e*) congenital heart disease, (*f*) mental retardation, (*g*) hypogenitalism, (*h*) mild obesity, and (*i*) hernia. Less commonly there is (*j*) postminimal polydactyly of the hands.

Originally described by Carpenter (1, 2) in 1901, this syndrome was not recognized as a distinct entity until Temtamy's report in 1966 (11). Several cases have been erroneously classified as Apert syndrome or as examples of Bardet-Biedl syndrome.

Less than 20 cases have been reported to date. The syndrome is clearly inherited as an autosomal recessive trait. Affected siblings have been described by Carpenter (1, 2), Nørvig (5), Rudert (7), Schönenberg and Scheidhauer (9), and Eaton et al. (3a). Consanguinity was noted by Der Kaloustian et al. (3), and may have been present in the case of Rudert (7). The child described by Warkany et al. (13) was Afro-American.

SYSTEMIC MANIFESTATIONS

Height is usually below the 25th percentile, but weight is often above average. The obesity mainly involves the trunk, proximal portion of the limbs, face, and nape.

Skull and facies. The distortion of the skull and peculiar facies are quite distinctive. The skull is usually tower-shaped. Though there may be premature synostosis of all cranial sutures, this often occurs asymmetrically, producing distorted calvaria. Flat nasal bridge and dystopia canthorum add to this distinctive quality (Fig. 14-1*A–C*).

Radiologically, the sagittal and lambdoidal sutures often fuse first, the coronal being the last to close. Wormian bones can be found in the anterior fontanel (6).

Skeletal alterations. The hands are short, the fingers being somewhat stubby. Marked soft-tissue syndactyly may be present between the third and fourth fingers, with less marked syndactyly between other fingers. Several fingers have but a single flexion crease.

Radiologically, the proximal phalanx of the thumb has two ossification centers. A tongue-shaped projection may extend from the radial side of the epiphysis for the proximal phalanx of the index finger (11, 13). Often there is brachymesophalangy of all digits or agenesis of some middle phalanges of the second to fifth digits.

Usually there are bilateral varus deformities of the feet and preaxial polydactyly with duplication of first or second toe. In many cases, toes exhibit soft-tissue syndactyly (Fig. 14-2). Radiographically, metatarsus varus and replication of the second toe are seen, and, to a lesser extent, replication of the second metatarsal. The first

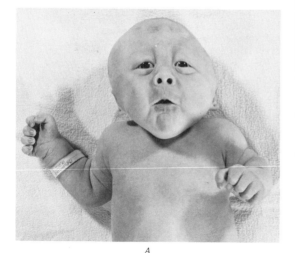

A

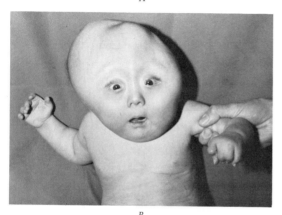

B

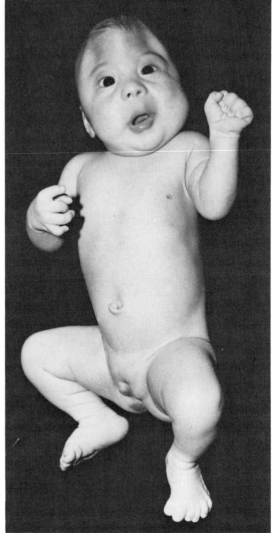

C

Figure 14-1. *Carpenter syndrome.* (*A*). Asymmetric tower-shaped skull, low-set ears, and short neck. (*From E. Sunderhaus and J. R. Wolter,* J. Pediatr. Ophthalmol. **5**:118, 1968.) (*B*). Asymmetric malformation of skull and soft-tissue syndactyly of third and fourth digits. (*C*). Compare with *A* and *B*. (*From V. Der Kaloustian et al.,* Am. J. Dis. Child. **124**:716, 1972.)

metatarsal is short and remarkably broad. Only two phalanges are present in each toe. The proximal phalanx of the hallux has two rounded ossification centers and a triangular distal one (Fig. 14-3*A*, *B*).

In nearly all cases, there has been genu valgum with lateral displacement of the patellas. Hip joint mobility may be reduced (9).

Miscellaneous findings include spina bifida occulta (5, 11), absent coccyx (11), iliac flaring with poor acetabular development (5, 9, 11), coxa valga (11), postminimus digits of the hands (9, 10), scoliosis (5), and vertically oriented orbits (9).

Ears and eyes. Dystopia canthorum (primary telecanthus) is nearly a constant feature, i.e., the medial intercanthal distance is increased but the interpupillary and bony interorbital distances are normal. Often this is combined with epicanthal folds and depressed nasal bridge, giving the eyes a "downthrust" appearance (11, 13).

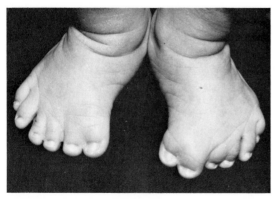

Figure 14-2. General webbing as well as bilateral poly-syndactyly of halluces. (*From V. Der Kaloustian et al.,* Am. J. Dis. Child. **124**:716, 1972.)

Maldeveloped cornea or microcornea (1, 2, 4) and corneal opacity (1, 2) have been noted, as well as slight optic atrophy and blurring of disk margins (11). The ears are usually low-set (3a, 10, 11), and the neck is short. Preauricular fistulas have been noted (13).

Heart. Congenital heart disease has been reported in several cases (1, 2, 4, 6, 10, 11). Various types have included ventricular septal defect (6, 10), atrial septal defect (6), patent ductus arteriosus (11), pulmonic stenosis (6), and tetralogy of Fallot (4).

Abdominal organs. Omphalocele (1, 2, 4, 9, 10), accessory spleen (4), hydronephrosis and/or hy-

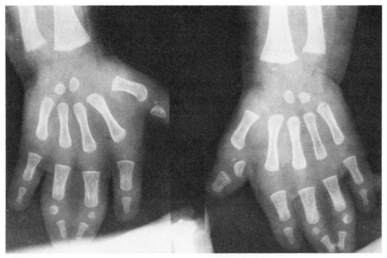

A

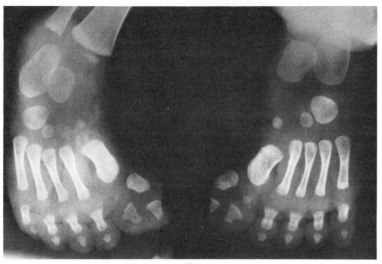

B

Figure 14-3. (*A* and *B*). Note especially brachymesophalangy and agenesis of middle phalanges together with soft-tissue syndactyly and clinodactyly of the third and fourth digits; also polysyndactyly of halluces, varus deformity, broadening of the first metatarsal, and absent middle phalanges. (*From H. Schönenberg and E. Scheidhauer,* Monatsschr. Kinderheilkd. **114**:322, 1966.)

Table 14-1. Main differences and overlap between the Apert, Carpenter, and Bardet-Biedl syndromes

Syndrome	Skull		Mental retardation	Obesity and hypo-genitalism	Retinitis pigmentosa
	Acrocephaly	Mild deformity			
Apert	+	−	±	−	−
Carpenter	+	−	+	+	−
Bardet-Biedl	−	+	+	+	+

Syndrome	Hands			Feet			Inheritance	
	Complete syndactyly with bone fusion	Partial syndactyly with brachymeso-phalangy	Postaxial poly-dactyly	Complete syndactyly	Preaxial polydactyly and syndactyly	Postaxial poly-dactyly	Domi-nant	Reces-sive
Apert	+	−	−	+	−	−	+	
Carpenter	−	+	−*	+	+	−		+
Bardet-Biedl	−	−	+	−	−	+		+

Note: +, present; −, absent; ± variable.
* Turner's patient had pedunculated postminimi on both hands, a frequent finding in patients with preaxial polydactyly.

droureter (4, 16), and inguinal hernia (6) have been noted.

Genitalia. Undescended testes (3a, 13) have been described.

Mental retardation. A relatively low level of intelligence is usually achieved by those who do not succumb to congenital heart disease. The intelligence quotient of Warkany's patient was estimated at 70 (13) and we have heard of one patient with normal intelligence (B. D. Hall, personal communication, 1975).

Oral manifestations. The mandible is somewhat smaller than normal, and the palate is narrow and highly arched, but otherwise there are no remarkable oral changes.

DIFFERENTIAL DIAGNOSIS

The *Apert syndrome* and the Bardet-Biedl syndromes are most often confused with the Carpenter syndrome (Table 14-1). Also to be excluded is the condition described by Sakati et al. (8) (see Chap. 40).

LABORATORY AIDS

Generalized aminoaciduria with especially elevated glycine levels has been noted (11).

REFERENCES

1 Carpenter, G., Two Sisters Showing Malformations of the Skull and Other Congenital Abnormalities. *Rep. Soc. Study Dis. Child. (London)* **1**:110, 1901.
2 Carpenter, G., Case of Acrocephaly with Other Congenital Malformations. *Proc. R. Soc. Med.* **II**, part I:45–53, 199–201, 1909.
3 Der Kaloustian, V., et al., Acrocephalopolysyndactyly, Type II—Carpenter's Syndrome. *Am. J. Dis. Child.* **124**:716–718, 1972.
3a Eaton, A. P., et al., Carpenter Syndrome—Acrocephalopolysyndactyly Type II. *Birth Defects* **10**:(9):249–260, 1974.
3b Kapras, J., et al., Acrocephalopolysyndactylia *Cs. Pediatr.* **29**:279–282, 1974.

4 McLoughlin, T. G., et al., Heart Disease in the Laurence-Moon-Biedl-Bardet Syndrome: A Review and Report of Three Brothers. *J. Pediatr.* **65:**388–399, 1964.

5 Nørvig, J., To tilfaelde af akrocephalosyndaktyli hos søskende. *Hospitalstidende* **72:**165–178, 1929.

6 Owen, R. H., Acrocephalosyndactyly: A Case with Congenital Cardiac Abnormalities. *Br. J. Radiol.* **25:**103–106, 1952.

7 Rudert, I., Über die Vererblichkeit der präaxialen Polydaktylie, *Z. Menschl. Vererb. Konstit. Lehre.* **21:**545–557 (case 2), 1938.

8 Sakati, N., et al., A New Syndrome with Acrocephalopolysyndactyly, Cardiac Disease and Distinctive Defects of the Ear, Skin and Lower Limbs. *J. Pediatr.* **79:**104–109, 1971.

9 Schönenberg, H., and Scheidhauer, E., Über zwei ungewöhnliche Dyscranio-Dysphalangien bei Geschwistern (atypische Akrocephalosyndaktylie) und fragliche Dysencephalia splanchnocystica. *Monatsschr. Kinderheilkd.* **114:**322–327, 1966.

10 Sunderhaus, E., and Wolter, J. R., Acrocephalosyndactylism. *J. Pediatr. Ophthalmol.* **5:**118–120, 1968.

11 Temtamy, S. A., Carpenter's Syndrome: Acrocephalopolysyndactyly. An Autosomal Recessive Syndrome. *J. Pediatr.* **69:**111–120, 1966.

12 Turner, H., Endocrine Clinic; Diabetes Insipidus, Laurence-Moon-Biedl Syndrome. *J. Oklahoma Med. Assoc.* **24:**148–419, 1931.

13 Warkany, J., et al., The Laurence-Moon-Biedl Syndrome. *Am. J. Dis. Child.* **53:**455–470 (case 1), 1937.

15

Cartilage-Hair Hypoplasia

(Metaphyseal Chondrodysplasia, Type McKusick)

McKusick (21, 22) first described a new syndrome characterized by (a) short-limbed dwarfism and (b) fine, sparse, light-colored hair in the old-order Amish. Subsequently, other non-Amish cases have been reported (1, 10, 17–19). We have seen the disorder in sibs of Finnish extraction and an increased incidence has been reported in Finland (25). Fewer than 100 cases have been reported to date.

Autosomal recessive inheritance is definitely established (21, 22), but there appears to be reduced penetrance. Heterogeneity probably exists with a typical form, a mild form, and a severe type with an immune defect (J. G. Hall, personal communication, 1975).

SYSTEMIC MANIFESTATIONS

Cesarean section is necessary for childbirth.

Facies and hair. The head is of normal size. The hair is very blond, brittle, fine, silky, and sparse on the scalp and elsewhere on the body. The eyebrows, eyelashes, and beard are deficient (Fig. 15-1). Microscopically, the caliber of the hair shaft is reduced to 50 to 65 percent of normal diameter and there is no central pigment core (7, 8, 14a, 18, 21, 22, 28).

Skeletal alterations. Affected individuals have short stature, with an adult height of 110 to 150 cm (21, 22). The legs are relatively short,

with mild bowing of the femurs (Fig. 15-2). The hands are short and pudgy, and the fingernails and toenails are small (19) (Fig. 15-3). Some patients have marked hyperextensibility of joints, particularly of the hands, wrists, and feet. However, most of them are unable to extend their elbows. Several patients were noted to have been "floppy" babies (1, 22).

Radiologically, irregularly scalloped metaphyses with sclerotic margins are noted. Small cystic radiolucencies may be scattered throughout the metaphyses. The epiphyses tend to be flattened. There is often some narrowing of interpediculate distances, and about one-third of patients have mild hypoplasia of the odontoid. There is mild flaring of the lower rib cage, with prominent proximal sternum and normal or increased vertebral height with mild lumbar lordosis. The tibia is characteristically shorter than the fibula.

Microscopically, hypoplasia of cartilage is seen, as well as failure of the cartilage cells to form orderly columns.

Infections. An important clinical feature of the severe type is the unexplained susceptibility to severe varicella and other infections (otitis media, pneumonia) (1, 14, 16–19, 21, 22). Malabsorption and megacolon have been noted in a few patients (2, 3, 14, 17, 21, 22). Chronic noncyclic neutropenia with maturation arrest has also been noted occasionally (1, 18, 22). Immunologic investigation in two children re-

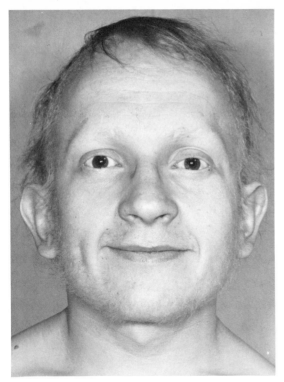

Figure 15-1. *Cartilage-hair hypoplasia.* Note sparse blond hair and deficiency of eyebrows and eyelashes.

vealed persistent lymphopenia, diminished skin hypersensitivity, diminished responsiveness of their lymphocytes to phytohemagglutinin *in vitro*, and, in one, delayed rejection of a skin allograft. Serum immunoglobulin levels were normal or elevated (18). Patients have been able to synthesize antibodies to a variety of viral and bacterial antigens. It has been suggested that these persons have a distinct form of cellular immune defect that is responsible for their unusual susceptibility to varicella infection. One child has been vaccinated with vaccinia without serious complications, but cellular immunity appears to decrease with increased age. Smallpox vaccination should probably be avoided (18).

Other findings. Renal proximal and distal tubular function may be altered.

DIFFERENTIAL DIAGNOSIS

Fine blond hair may be seen in *hypohidrotic ectodermal dysplasia* and in Marinesco-Sjögren syndrome.

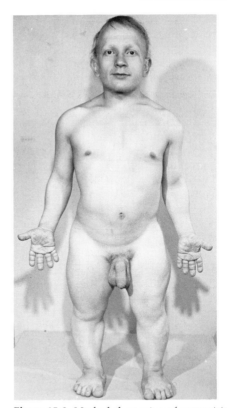

Figure 15-2. Marked shortening of extremities.

Three other somewhat similar disorders, commonly referred to as metaphyseal dysostosis, must be distinguished: The Jansen type is a rare syndrome associated with mental and motor retardation, decreased muscle mass, abnormally shaped skull, ocular hypertelorism, flexion deformities of many joints, beading at

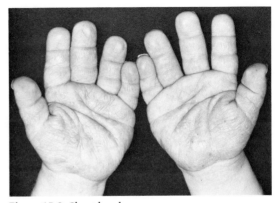

Figure 15-3. Short hands.

the costochondral junction, and gross enlargement of the metaphyses (13). Inheritance is possibly autosomal dominant. The Schmidt type of metaphyseal dysostosis is characterized by mild growth retardation, normal intelligence, normal facies, and autosomal dominant inheritance (27). Transient abnormalities are seen at the growth plate, mostly slight widening and irregularity. The Spahr type is similar to the Schmidt type, except that it apparently has an autosomal recessive pattern of inheritance.

Patients with cartilage-hair hypoplasia are easily distinguished from those with other lymphopenic immunologic deficiency diseases (hereditary thymic dysplasia, *ataxia-telangiectasia*, and Wiskott-Aldrich syndrome) (18). There are defects of thymic function with abnormal cellular immunity and normal serum immunoglobulin levels. These are DiGeorge syndrome (thymus-parathyroid aplasia) (9, 15) and Nezelof syndrome (24). The course of Nezelof syndrome is variable. Some patients die in infancy; others survive but are prone to severe infections with varicella and vaccinia (23).

Gatti and associates (11) reported a brother and sister with lymphopenic agammaglobulinemia associated with short-limbed dwarfism, cutis laxa, alopecia of the scalp, and an ichthyosiform dermatosis (metaphyseal chondrodysplasia with thymolymphopenia). The disorder is probably inherited as an autosomal recessive trait. Similar patients were reported by McKusick and Cross (20) in an old-order Amish family with both ataxia-telangiectasia and Swiss-type agammaglobulinemia. There are other reported cases of various combinations of metaphyseal dysostosis, fine hair, susceptibility to varicella, neutropenia, and malabsorption (21–24, 26, 27).

Also to be excluded in differential diagnosis are *achondroplasia*, hypophosphatasia, and vitamin D–resistant rickets. Radiologically the first two may be easily ruled out. The metaphyseal irregularities in cartilage-hair hypoplasia are sharp, in contrast to the frayed and indistinct metaphyses in vitamin D–resistant rickets.

L. S. Levin (personal communication, 1975) reported sibs with a possible allelic variant form of cartilage-hair hypoplasia. The incisors were notched at the incisal edge. The premolars were small, the lower premolars exhibiting doubling of the lingual cusps.

The reader is referred to a checklist of conditions associated with retarded longitudinal growth (16).

LABORATORY AIDS

None is known.

REFERENCES

1 Ammann, A. J., et al., Antibody-mediated Immunodeficiency in Short-limbed Dwarfism. *J. Pediatr.* **84:**200–203, 1974.

2 Beals, R. K., Cartilage-hair Hypoplasia. *J. Bone Joint Surg.* **50A:**1245–1249, 1968.

3 Boothby, C. B., and Bower, B. C., Cartilage-hair Hypoplasia. *Arch. Dis. Child.* 48:919–921, 1973.

4 Burgert, E. O., Jr., et al., A New Syndrome – Aregenerative Anemia, Malabsorption (Celiac), Dyschondroplasia and Hyperphosphatemia. *J. Pediatr.* 67:711–712, 1965.

5 Burke, V., et al., Association of Pancreatic Insufficiency and Chronic Neutropenia in Childhood. *Arch. Dis. Child.* 42:147–157, 1967.

6 Clinicopathological Conference, A Case of Swiss-type Agammaglobulinemia and Achondroplasia, Demonstrated at the Royal Postgraduate Medical School. *Br. Med. J.* 2:1371–1374, 1966.

7 Coupe, R. L., and Lowry, R. B., Abnormality of the Hair in Cartilage-hair Hypoplasia. *Dermatologica* 141:329–334, 1970.

8 D'Apuzzo, V., and Joss, E., Metaphysäre Dysostose und Hypoplasie der Haare: Knorpel-Haar-Hypoplasie. *Helv. Paediatr. Acta* 27:241–252, 1972.

9 DiGeorge, A. M., Congenital Absence of the Thymus and Its Immunologic Consequences: Concurrence with Congenital Hypoparathyroidism, Immunologic Deficiency Diseases in Man. The National Foundation–March of Dimes, New York City, 1968, pp. 116–123.

10 Fauchier, C., Nanisme diastrophique ou "dysostose métaphysaire." *Ann. Pédiatr.* (Paris) 17:876–881, 1970.

11 Gatti, R. A., et al., Hereditary Lymphopenic Agammaglobulinemia Associated with a Distinctive Form of Short-limbed Dwarfism and Ectodermal Dysplasia. *J. Pediatr.* 75:675–684, 1969.

12 Goldstein, R., Congenital Lipomatosis of the Pancreas: Malabsorption, Dwarfism, Leukopenia with Relative Granulocytopenia and Thrombocytopenia. *Clin. Pediatr.* 7: 419–422, 1908.

13 Gram, P. B., et al., Metaphyseal Chondrodysplasia of Jansen. *J. Bone Joint Surg.* 41A:951–959, 1959.

14 Irwin, G. A., Cartilage-hair Hypoplasia (HCH), Variant of Familial Metaphyseal Dysostosis. *Radiology* **86**:920–928, 1966.

14a Kelling, C., et al., Biophysical and Biochemical Studies of the Hair in Cartilage-Hair Hypoplasia. *Clin. Genet.* **4**:500–506, 1973.

15 Kretschmer, R., et al., Congenital Aplasia of the Thymus Gland (DiGeorge's Syndrome). *N. Engl. J. Med.* **279**:1295–1301, 1968.

16 Langer, L. O., Short Stature. Check List of Conditions Associated with Retarded Longitudinal Growth. *Clin. Pediatr.* **8**:142–153, 1969.

17 Lowry, R. B., et al., Cartilage-hair Hypoplasia: A Rare and Recessive Cause of Dwarfism. *Clin. Pediatr.* **9**:44–46, 1970.

18 Lux, S. E., et al., Chronic Neutropenia and Abnormal Cellular Immunity in Cartilage-hair Hypoplasia. *N. Engl. J. Med.* **282**:231–236, 1970.

19 McKusick, V. A., *Heritable Disorders of Connective Tissue.* 4th ed., Mosby, St. Louis, 1972.

20 McKusick, V. A., and Cross, H. E., Ataxia-telangiectasia and Swiss-type Agammaglobulinemia: Two Genetic Disorders of the Immune Mechanism in Related Amish Sibships. *J.A.M.A.* **195**:739–745, 1966.

21 McKusick, V. A., et al., Dwarfism in the Amish. *Trans. Assoc. Am. Physicians* **77**:151–168, 1964.

22 McKusick, V. A., et al., Dwarfism in the Amish. II. Cartilage-hair Hypoplasia. *Bull. Johns Hopkins Hosp.* **116**:285–326, 1965.

23 Meuwissen, H. J., et al., Combined Immunodeficiency Disease Associated with Adenosine Deaminase Deficiency. *J. Pediatr.* **86**:169–181, 1975.

24 Nezelof, C., Thymic Dysplasia with Normal Immunoglobulins and Immunologic Deficiency: Pure Alymphocytosis, Immunologic Deficiency Diseases in Man. The National Foundation–March of Dimes, New York City, 1968, pp. 104–115.

25 Norio, R., et al., Hereditary Diseases in Finland. *Ann. Clin. Res.* **5**:109–141, 1973.

26 Ray, H. C., and Dorst, J. P., Cartilage-hair Hypoplasia. *Prog. Pediatr. Radiol.* **4**:270–298, 1973.

27 Rosenbloom, A. L., and Smith, W. D., The Natural History of Metaphyseal Dysostosis. *J. Pediatr.* **66**:857–868, 1965.

28 Wiedemann, H. R., et al., Knorpel-Haar Hypoplasie. *Arch. Kinderheilkd.* **176**:74–85, 1967.

16

Cerebral Gigantism

(*Sotos Syndrome*)

In 1964, Sotos et al. (14) defined a syndrome of (*a*) advanced height and bone maturation, dating from infancy, (*b*) mental deficiency, and (*c*) unusual craniofacial appearance. Occurrence is sporadic, but it has been noted in two generations (D. Rimoin, J. Sotos, personal communication, 1975) and has been concordant in monozygotic twins (4). There is no sex predilection. Over 75 cases have been reported, about two-thirds in males (12, 13).

SYSTEMIC MANIFESTATIONS

Facies. The facies is characterized by macrocrania with dolichocephaly and ocular hypertelorism, with antimongoloid obliquity of palpebral fissures (10). The frontal hairline is often receded (1) (Fig. 16-1).

Nervous system. Most patients have had a nonprogressive neurologic dysfunction, manifested by unusual clumsiness, dull intelligence (mean intelligence quotient of 60), and, at times, aggressive behavior (1, 6, 10). Over 80 percent have had dilatation of the cerebral ventricles (10, 12). Convulsions and respiratory and feeding problems have been noted in at least 40 percent of cases (5). Delay in walking until after fifteen months of age, and delay in speech development until after two and one-half years are usual.

Skeletal alterations. Many patients are large at birth, the mean being about 4,250 g and 55 cm (1, 12). Bone age is usually 2 to 3 years in advance of chronologic age in the absence of obvious endocrine dysfunction in about 75 percent (12, 13). Hands and feet are disproportionately large in over 80 percent (1, 2, 5, 6). Head circumference and height are well above the 97th percentile for age, and frontal bossing is marked (6) (Fig. 16-2). The span is greater than the height in about 90 percent of cases (5, 6). Kyphoscoliosis has been present in about 30 percent.

Oral manifestations. Highly arched palate (in over 90 percent of patients) and precocious dentition (in over 50 percent) have been described (5, 8, 10). Mandibular prognathism has been noted in over 80 percent (5).

DIFFERENTIAL DIAGNOSIS

Diagnosis can be difficult in adults. Generalized lipodystrophy, gigantism due to hypophyseal tumor, and the XYY syndrome should be excluded.

The so-called autosomal recessive form of cerebral gigantism (10a) probably represents another disorder (3a).

LABORATORY AIDS

Growth hormone levels have been normal (15). Dermatoglyphic alterations have been described (2, 10).

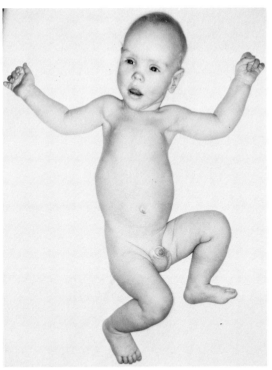

Figure 16-1. *Cerebral gigantism.* Eighteen-month-old male, showing typical facies. Note receding hairline and small nose. (*From M. M. Steiner, Chicago, Illinois.*)

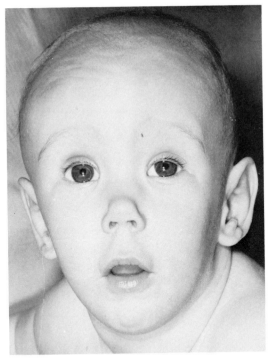

Figure 16-2. Six-month-old female. Note facies similar to that in Fig. 16-1.

Branched-chain essential amino acids in plasma have been found at higher levels than normal, the glycine:valine ratio being especially altered (2). This finding has not been confirmed, however. Levels of 17-ketosteroids and gonadotropins have been elevated in several patients (6, 15).

Pneumoencephalography usually shows dilated ventricles. About 40 percent of patients have had abnormal electroencephalographic studies (17).

REFERENCES

1 Abraham, J. M., and Snodgrass, G., Sotos' Syndrome of Cerebral Gigantism. *Arch. Dis. Child.* **44**:203–210, 1969.

2 Bejar, R. L., et al., Cerebral Gigantism: Concentrations of Amino Acids in Plasma and Muscle. *J. Pediatr.* **76**:105–111, 1970.

3 Cohen, M. I., Cerebral Gigantism in Childhood. *N. Engl. J. Med.* **271**:635, 1964.

3a Cohen, M. M. Jr., Diagnostic Problems in Cerebral Gigantism *J. Med. Genet.*, in press.

4 Hook, E. B., and Reynolds, J. W., Cerebral Gigantism. *J. Pediatr.* **70**:900–914, 1967.

5 Jaeken, J., et al., Cerebral Gigantism Syndrome. *Z. Kinderheilkd.* **112**:332–346, 1972.

6 Kjellman, B., Cerebral Gigantism. *Acta Paediatr. Scand.* **54**:603–609, 1965.

7 Kowlessar, M., Cerebral Gigantism. Abnormal Urinary Corticoid Excretion. *Minn. Med.* **48**:1610–1614, 1965.

8 Ludwig, G. D., et al., Cerebral Gigantism with Intermittent Fractional Hypopituitarism and Normal Sella Turcica. *Ann. Intern. Med.* **67**:123–131, 1967.

9 Marie, J., et al., Gigantism avec encéphalopathie et dysmorphie cranio-faciale. *Ann. Pédiatr.* **12**:682–691, 1965.

10 Milunsky, A., et al., Cerebral Gigantism in Childhood. *Pediatrics* **40**:395–402, 1967.

10a Nevo, S., et al., Evidence for Autosomal Recessive Inheritance in Cerebral Gigantism. *J. Med. Genet.* **11**:158–165, 1974.

11 Poznanski, A. K., and Stephenson, J. M., Radiographic Findings in Hypothalamic Acceleration of Growth Associated with Cerebral Atrophy and Mental Retardation

(Cerebral Gigantism). *Radiology* **88**:446–456, 1967.

12 Schelling-Dürst, V., Makrozephaler Grosswuchs. *Klin. Pädiatr.* **186**:97–106, 1974.

13 Schneider, H., and Vasella, F., Zerebraler Gigantismus. *Helv. Paediatr. Acta* **26**:2–13, 1971.

14 Sotos, J. F., et al., Cerebral Gigantism in Childhood. *N. Engl. J. Med.* **271**:109–116, 1964.

15 Stephenson, J. N., et al., Cerebral Gigantism. *Pediatrics* **41**:130–138, 1968.

16 Turner, E. K., and Sloan, L. E. G., Cerebral Gigantism in Childhood. *Aust. Paediatr. J.* **1**:243–251, 1965.

17 Zappella, M., and Boscherini, B., Considerations à propos de sept cas de gigantisme cérébral. *Pédiatrie* **28**:419–428, 1973.

17

Cerebrohepatorenal Syndrome

(*Zellweger Syndrome*)

Bowen and associates (1) in 1964 and, independently, Smith and coworkers in 1965 (9) described a syndrome consisting of (*a*) hypotonia, (*b*) high forehead and other craniofacial anomalies, (*c*) flexion contractures, (*d*) hypoprothrombinemia, (*e*) hepatomegaly, (*f*) renal cortical cysts, and (*g*) developmental abnormalities of the brain. Over 20 cases have been reported to date, an excess of females being noted (1–18).

Affected sibs (1, 6–8, 12–14) and three instances of parental consanguinity (7, 10, 12, 18) indicate autosomal recessive inheritance.

The frequency of the disorder has been estimated to be one per 100,000 live births (2).

SYSTEMIC MANIFESTATIONS

Failure to thrive and early demise (neonatal to six months of age) are characteristic.

Facies. The forehead is high. The skull may be pear-shaped or may show some degree of turribrachycephaly. The occiput is flattened in about half the cases (9). The facies and especially the supraorbital ridges are flat (Fig. 17-1*A, B*). Puffy eyelids, ocular hypertelorism, mild mongoloid obliquity of the palpebral fissures, epicanthal folds, Brushfield spots, cataracts, and nystagmus may be observed, as well as full cheeks, anteverted nostrils, micrognathia, and redundant skin on the neck (9). The ears may be posteriorly rotated (7, 12).

Central nervous system. Severe hypotonia (Fig. 17-2), seizures, abnormal electroencephalographic findings, dilated ventricles, a tendency toward megalencephaly, polymicrogyria, macrogyria, pachygyria (Fig. 17-3), lissencephaly, olfactory hypoplasia, absent corpus callosum, histologic leukoencephalomyelopathic changes, and disorganized neuronal migration have been reported (3, 7–10, 17).

Skeletal system. Camptodactyly of one or more fingers, simian or transitional simian creases, ulnar deviation of hands, cubitus valgus, flexion at knees and hips, talipes equinovarus, metatarsus adductus, rocker bottom feet, and dorsiflexion of fourth toes have been reported (7, 9, 10, 12).

Fontanels and sutures are widely patent. Bone age may be retarded, and hypomineralization and Wormian bones have been noted (9, 10, 18).

Calcific stippling has been observed, especially in the acetabular cartilages and along the inferior medial margin of the patellas (Fig. 17-4). Stippled epiphyses may be present in long bones in about half the cases (9). Calcification of the hyoid bone and thyroid cartilage has also been noted. Metaphyseal radiolucencies have also been described (2, 6, 9, 10, 18).

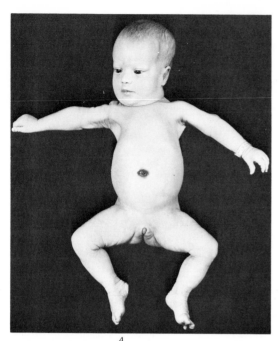
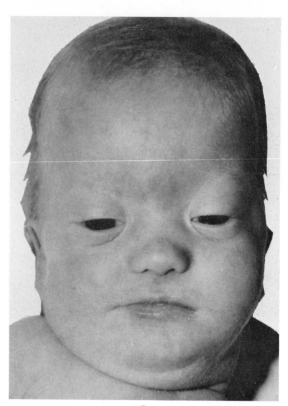

A   *B*

Figure 17-1. (*A*). *Cerebrohepatorenal syndrome of Zellweger.* High forehead, mongoloid slant to palpebral fissures in severely hypotonic female infant. (*From J. E. Jan et al.,* Am. J. Dis. Child. **119**:274, 1970.) (*B*). Compare with facies shown in *A*. (*From E. Passarge and A. J. McAdams,* J. Pediatr. **71**:691, 1967.)

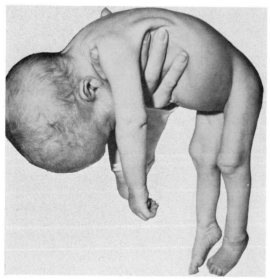

Figure 17-2. Extreme hypotonia. (*From E. Passarge and A. J. McAdams.* J. Pediatr. **71**:691, 1967.)

Liver. Hepatomegaly, intrahepatic biliary dysgenesis, small cysts, and progressive parenchymal damage to the liver with disturbances of lobular architecture, diffuse fibrosis, and iron pigment deposition have been documented (2, 7).

Kidneys. The kidneys may be normal or slightly decreased in size. Renal cortical cysts and, less frequently, foci of renal dysgenesis may be found (7, 15) (Fig. 17-5).

Other findings. Cardiac anomalies include patent ductus arteriosus and patent foramen ovale. Widely spaced nipples, deep sacral dimple, hypoplastic dermal ridges, small penis, hypospadias, cryptorchism, prominent clitoris, umbilical hernia, diastasis recti, hypertrophied pylorus, partial malrotation of colon, splenomegaly, extramedullary hematopoiesis, pancreatic islet cell

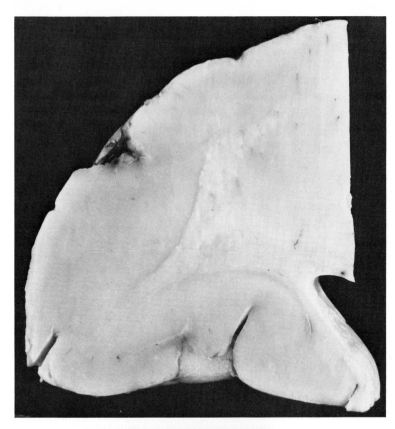

Figure 17-3. Cross section of cerebrum showing macrogyria, flattening of cortical surface, and thickened cortical gray matter. (*From A. Poznanski et al.*, Am. J. Roentgenol. **109:**313, 1970.)

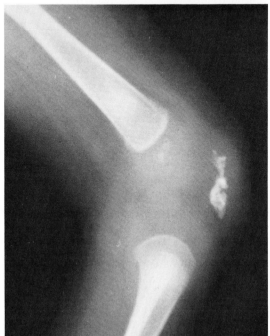

Figure 17-4. Extensive calcification of patella. (*From A. Poznanski et al.*, Am. J. Roentgenol. **109:**313, 1970.)

hyperplasia, absent thoracic lobes, and generalized hypoplasia of the thymus gland have also been described (1, 7, 9, 10, 12).

Oral manifestations. Narrow, highly arched palate and protruding tongue have been noted (7).

DIFFERENTIAL DIAGNOSIS

The Zellweger syndrome may occasionally be confused with *trisomy 21 syndrome,* since flat facies, epicanthal folds, Brushfield spots, and hypotonia may occur in both conditions. However, the overall pattern of anomalies in each syndrome allows differentiation. The syndrome also shares several features in common with *chondrodysplasia punctata,* including calcific stippling, cataracts, highly arched palate, contractures, and foot abnormalities. The presence of high forehead, severe hypotonia, and hepatomegaly in the former should aid in distinguishing the two disorders.

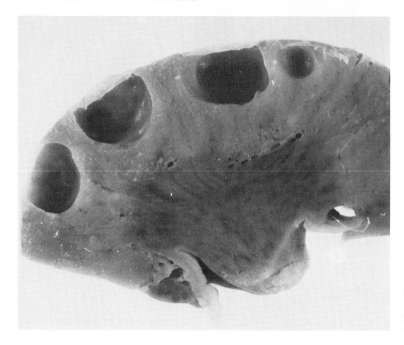

Figure 17-5. Kidney showing large cortical cysts. (*From A. Poznanski et al.*, Am. J. Roentgenol. **109**:313, 1970.)

LABORATORY AIDS

Neonatal determination of serum iron concentration may aid in diagnosis (7, 16). However, it should be noted that the serum iron level is not always increased (9). Excess hepatic iron has been implicated as being responsible for the cirrhotic changes and alterations in liver function (7, 16). However, it has been impossible to establish a pathogenetic relationship between the iron storage defect and the various morphologic abnormalities observed in the Zellweger syndrome. That iron overload plays an important role in pathogenesis has been denied. It has been stated that the apparent increase in iron observed in some patients may not represent a congenital tissue overload, but redistribution or deficient utilization of iron (9).

Hyperbilirubinemia with jaundice, hypoprothrombinemia with gastrointestinal bleeding, proteinuria, decreased immunoglobulins, and hypoglycemia have been reported in some cases (1–10, 12–18). The present authors regard the aminoaciduria noted in several instances (7, 10) as being secondary to failure to thrive.

Danks et al. (2) reported elevated serum levels of pipecolic acid. Goldfischer et al. (5) found abnormal peroxisomes and mitochondria.

REFERENCES

1 Bowen, P., et al., A Familial Syndrome of Multiple Congenital Defects. *Johns Hopkins Med. J.* **114**:402–414, 1964.

2 Danks, D. M., et al., Cerebrohepato-renal Syndrome of Zellweger. *J. Pediatr.* **86**:382–387, 1975.

3 Garzuly, F., et al., Neuronale Migrations störung bei cerebro-hepato-renal Syndrom "Zellweger." *Neuropädiatrie* **5**:319–328, 1974.

4 Gilchrist, K. W., et al., Immunodeficiency in Cerebrohepato-renal Syndrome. *Lancet* **1**:164–165, 1974.

5 Goldfischer, S., et al., Peroxisomal and Mitochondrial Defects in the Cerebrohepatorenal Syndrome. *Science* **182**:62–64, 1973.

6 Jan, J. E., et al., Cerebro-hepato-renal Syndrome of Zellweger. *Am. J. Dis. Child.* **119**:274–277, 1970.

7 Opitz, J. M., et al., The Zellweger Syndrome. *Birth Defects* **5**(2):143–158, 1969.

8 Passarge, E., and McAdams, A. J., Cerebro-hepato-renal Syndrome. *J. Pediatr.* **71**:691–702, 1967.

9 Patton, R. G., et al., Cerebro-hepato-renal Syndrome of Zellweger: Two Cases with Islet Cell Hyperplasia, Hypo-

glycemia, and Thymic Anomalies, and Comments on Iron Metabolism. *Am. J. Dis. Child.* **124:**840–844, 1972.

10 Poznanski, A. K., et al., The Cerebro-hepato-renal Syndrome (CHRS): Zellweger's Syndrome. *Am. J. Roentgenol.* **109:**313–322, 1970.

11 Punnett, H. H., and Kirkpatrick, J. A., A Syndrome of Ocular Abnormalities, Calcification of Cartilage and Failure to Thrive. *J. Pediatr.* **73:**602–606, 1968.

12 Smith, D. W., et al., A Syndrome of Multiple Developmental Defects Including Polycystic Kidneys and Intrahepatic Biliary Dysgenesis in 2 Siblings. *J. Pediatr.* **67:**617–624, 1965.

13 Sommer, A., et al., The Cerebro-hepato-renal Syndrome (Zellweger's Syndrome). *Biol. Neonate* **25:**219–230, 1974.

14 Taylor, J. C., et al., A New Case of the Zellweger Syndrome. *Birth Defects* **5**(2):159–160, 1969.

15 Vincens, A., et al., A propos d'un cas de syndrome de Zellweger (syndrome hépato-cérébro-rénal). *Ann. Pédiat.* **20:**553–560, 1972.

16 Vitale, L., et al., Congenital and Familial Iron Overload. *N. Engl. J. Med.* **280:**642–645, 1969.

17 Volpe, J. J., and Adams, R. D., Cerebro-hepato-renal Syndrome of Zellweger. An Inherited Disorder of Neuronal Migration. *Acta Neuropath.* **20:**175–198, 1972.

18 Williams, J. P., et al., Roentgenographic Features of the Cerebrohepatorenal Syndrome of Zellweger. *Am. J. Roentgenol.* **115:**607–610, 1972.

18

Chédiak-Higashi Syndrome

The Chédiak-Higashi syndrome is a rare genetic disease manifested clinically by (a) defective pigmentation, (b) abnormal granulation of leukocytes, and (c) increased susceptibility to infection. Although it was discussed earlier by Beguez Cesar (1) in 1943 and Steinbrinck (21) in 1948, Chédiak (5), in 1952, and Higashi (9), in 1954, defined the syndrome and emphasized the leukocyte anomaly. About 60 patients have since been described.

The syndrome is inherited as an autosomal recessive trait. Parental consanguinity has been noted in over 45 percent of patients (3, 22).

Most patients die in early childhood of overwhelming infection, over 50 percent succumbing before the end of the first decade of life (3, 26); occasionally some survive into adulthood (19). This disorder occurs in other species — the Aleutian mink, the beige mouse, and cattle (14, 18, 23, 30).

Chédiak-Higashi syndrome is a disorder of giant lysosomal inclusion bodies found in all circulating granulocytes and in many other cells of the body. The large size of the inclusion bodies reflects a functional abnormality leading to the improper handling or distribution of normal lysosomal enzymes (11, 27–31). There is normal phagocytosis but failure of postphagocytic degranulation and diminished intracellular bactericidal capacity, reflecting the ineffective delivery of lysosomal products to the phagocytic vacuole (30). Kanfer et al. (11) suggested accelerated turnover of sphingolipids in leukocytes.

SYSTEMIC MANIFESTATIONS

Skin. Most patients have lighter hair, skin, and eyes than their unaffected sibs (20, 26), but the degree of pigmentary dilution is variable. Comparison with sibs and parents is important. The hair has a frosted-gray sheen (2, 3, 12, 23, 25) (Fig. 18-1). Large melanin granules are visible by light microscopy, and large melanosomes by electron microscopy (20). The structural defect in the melanin granules probably accounts for the dilution of the pigment. Heterozygotes exhibit the same microscopic pigmentary alterations but to a lesser degree (2).

The patients exhibit cutaneous stigmata of albinism, including a marked pallor and absent pigmentation of the areolas and genitals. They may show scattered pigmented nevi or numerous ephelides on exposed areas and an unusual slate-gray coloration of the skin (2, 3, 12, 24, 25).

Several reports have mentioned hyperhidrosis, heat rash, and marked photosensitivity (3, 8, 20, 24, 25). Severe and extensive pyoderma may be seen (25, 26) (Fig. 18-2).

Hematologic features. Some peripheral circulatory granulocytes as well as their marrow precursors have giant granules — some up to 10 times normal size (5, 12, 17, 19). In Giemsa preparations, they are slate-gray. However, there may be normal-appearing granules in the same cell with one or more giant granules. Anemia has

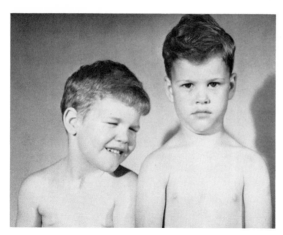

Figure 18-1. *Chédiak-Higashi syndrome.* Frosted-gray sheen of hair in affected boy (left) as compared with unaffected brother. (*Courtesy of O. C. Stegmaier, Fort Wayne, Indiana.*)

been noted in 80 percent of cases, thrombocytopenia in 50 percent, and leukopenia in 40 percent.

The characteristic lymphocytic inclusions have also been found in normal relatives of patients with the Chédiak-Higashi syndrome (6, 12, 16).

Eye. The ocular albinism is more definite than the cutaneous "partial" albinism. Pale lavender irides and pale fundi, photophobia, and coarse horizontal nystagmus are usually readily apparent (3, 15, 22, 24, 25). A definite pink coloration is visible upon transillumination of the ocular globe (25).

Pathologic examination of the eye confirms the diminution of the melanin pigment in the iris, ciliary epithelium, choroid, and pigment epithelium of the retina (4, 10). There may be invasion of the eye structures by inflammatory cells, some with cytoplasmic inclusions, and, at times, associated papilledema.

Nervous system. Progressive cranial and peripheral neuropathy as well as muscle weakness, foot drop, and decreased muscle stretch reflexes are sometimes part of Chédiak-Higashi syndrome, resembling spinocerebellar degeneration (12, 13, 19). Headache, transitory paresis, tremor, emotional lability, and EEG abnormalities have also been noted (8, 25).

Lymphohistiocytic infiltration of central and peripheral nervous systems has been reported. Characteristic cytoplasmic inclusions resembling lysosomes are seen within nerve cells, astrocytes, Schwann cells, etc. Within the neurons of the substantia nigra, the melanin pigment granules are especially large and irregular (22).

Recurrent infections. Respiratory (3, 8, 12, 20, 24) and skin (8, 12, 20, 23, 25) infections are most frequent. The bouts of infection are repeated, the most common offending organisms being *Staphylococcus aureus*, *Streptococcus pyogenes*, and *Pneumococci* (31). The neutropenia is thought to be due to the intramedullary destruction of granulocytes.

The terminal "accelerated" phase of the disorder is lymphoma-like, being characterized by generalized lymphohistiocytic infiltrates of the bone marrow, lymphoid tissues, and nervous

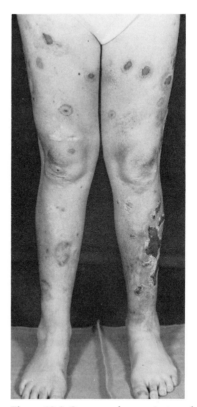

Figure 18-2. Severe and extensive pyoderma. (*Courtesy of P. Weary, Charlottesville, Virginia.*)

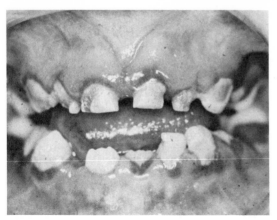

Figure 18-3. Marked gingivitis. (*From J. Gilly, Dayton, Ohio.*)

system that preserve the integrity of the involved organ (3, 7, 23). The patient clinically presents adenopathy, hepatosplenomegaly, peripheral neuropathy, and hemorrhage prior to death. However, Hodgkin's disease has been described in a child with the disorder (23).

ORAL MANIFESTATIONS

Aphthae and/or gingivitis are present in most cases (8) (Fig. 18-3). Rapid breakdown of the periodontium has also been observed (3, 25). This may be a reflection of the neutropenia or defective leukocyte function (15, 16, 22). Cervical adenopathy, though not a constant feature, is especially frequent (8, 12, 15, 17).

DIFFERENTIAL DIAGNOSIS

Oculocutaneous albinism has been suggested in several cases (20), but should be readily excluded.

LABORATORY AIDS

See Hematologic features. The abnormal granules in the leukocytes are striking. Those in the neutrophils are large (up to 4 μ in diameter) and stain a greenish-gray with Romanowsky stain. They are peroxidase-positive and stain with Sudan black B, but not with PAS. The lymphocytes contain abnormal azurophilic granules which are PAS-positive but Sudan black B- and peroxidase-negative (16).

REFERENCES

1 Beguez Cesar, A., Neutropenia crónica maligna familiar con granulaciones atípicas de los leucocítos. *Bol. Soc. Cuba Pediatr.* **15:**900–922, 1943.

2 Beyoda, U., Pigmentary Changes in Chédiak-Higashi Syndrome: Microscopic Study of 12 Homozygous and Heterozygous Subjects. *Br. J. Dermatol.* **85:**336–347, 1971.

3 Blume, R. S., and Wolff, S. M., The Chédiak-Higashi Syndrome: Studies in Four Patients and Review of the Literature. *Medicine* (*Baltimore*) **51:**247–280, 1972.

4 Bregeat, P., et al., Manifestations oculaires du syndrome de Chédiak-Higashi. *Arch. Ophtalmol.* (*Paris*) **26:**611–676, 1966.

5 Chédiak, M., Nouvelle anomalie leucocytaire de caractère constitutionnel et familial. *Rev. Hematol.* **7:**362–367, 1952.

6 Danes, B. S., and Bearn, A. G., Cell Culture and the Chédiak-Higashi Syndrome. *Lancet* **2:**65–67, 1967.

7 Dent, P. B., et al., Chédiak-Higashi Syndrome, Observations on the Nature of the Associated Malignancy. *Lab. Invest.* **15:**1634–1642, 1966.

8 Donohue, W. L., and Bain, H. W., Chédiak-Higashi Syndrome: A Lethal Familial Disease with Anomalous Inclusions in the Leukocytes and Constitutional Stigmata. *Pediatrics* **20:**416–430, 1957.

8a Hamilton, R. E., Jr., et al., The Chédiak-Higashi Syndrome. *Oral Surg.* **37:**754–761, 1974.

9 Higashi, O., Congenital Gigantism of Peroxidase Granules. *Tohoku J. Exp. Med.* **59:**315–332, 1954.

10 Johnson, D. L., et al., Histopathology of Eyes in Chédiak-Higashi Syndrome. *Arch. Ophthalmol.* **75:**84–88, 1966.

11 Kanfer, J. W., et al., Alteration of Sphingolipid Metabolism in Leukocytes from Patients with the Chédiak-Higashi Syndrome. *N. Engl. J. Med.* **279:**410–413, 1968.

12 Kritzler, R. A., et al., Chédiak-Higashi Syndrome. Cytologic and Serum Lipid Observations in a Case and Family. *Am. J. Med.* **36:**583–594, 1964.

13 Lockman, L. A., et al., The Chédiak-Higashi Syndrome: Electrophysiological and Electron Microscopic Observations on the Peripheral Neuropathy. *J. Pediatr.* **70:**942–951, 1967.

14 Lutzner, M. A., et al., Giant Granules and Widespread Cytoplasmic Inclusions in a Genetic Syndrome of Aleutian Mink. *Lab. Invest.* **14:**2063–2079, 1965.

15 McLelland, R., and Estevez, J. M., The Chédiak-Higashi Syndrome. *J. Can. Assoc. Radiol.* **19,** 78–82, 1968.

16 Millis, R. R., et al., The Chédiak-Higashi Anomaly. *Arch. Dis. Child.* **42:**100–105, 1967.

17 Moran, T. J., and Estevez, J. M., Chédiak-Higashi Disease. *Arch. Pathol.* **88:**329–339, 1969.

18 Padgett, G. A., et al., Comparative Studies of the Chédiak-Higashi Syndrome. *Am. J. Pathol.* **51:**553–572, 1967.

19 Sheramata, W., et al., The Chédiak-Higashi-Steinbrinck Syndrome. *Arch. Neurol.* **25:**289–294, 1971.

20 Stegmaier, O. C., and Schneider, L. A., Chédiak-Higashi Syndrome, Dermatologic Manifestations. *Arch. Dermatol.* **91:**1–9, 1965.

21 Steinbrinck, W., Über eine neue Granulationsanomalie der Leukocyten. *Dtsch. Arch. Klin. Med.* **193:**577–581, 1948.

22 Sung, J. H., et al., Neuropathological Changes in Chediak-Higashi Disease. *J. Neuropathol. Exp. Neurol.* **28:**86–118, 1969.

23 Tan, C., et al., Chédiak-Higashi Syndrome in a Child with Hodgkin's Disease. *Am. J. Dis. Child.* **121:**135–139, 1971.

24 Tay, C. H., et al., Chédiak-Higashi Syndrome. *Med. J. Aust.* **2:**1024–1029, 1970.

25 Weary, P. E., and Bender, A. S., Chédiak-Higashi Syndrome with Severe Cutaneous Involvement. *Arch. Intern. Med.* **119:**381–386, 1967.

26 Wegelius, R., et al., Chédiak-Steinbrinck-Higashi's Anomaly. *Acta Med. Scand.* **181:**367–372, 1967.

27 White, J. G., The Chédiak-Higashi Syndrome. *Blood* **28:**143–156, 1966.

28 White, J. G., Chédiak-Higashi Syndrome. *Am. J. Pathol.* **72:**503–519, 1973.

29 Windhorst, D. B., et al., A Human Pigmentary Dilution Based on a Heritable Subcellular Structural Defect—the Chédiak-Higashi Syndrome. *J. Invest. Dermatol.* **50:**9–18, 1968.

30 Wolff, S. M., et al., The Chédiak-Higashi Syndrome: Studies of Host Defenses. *Ann. Intern. Med.* **76:**293–306, 1972.

31 Zelickson, A. S., et al., The Chédiak-Higashi Syndrome: Formation of Giant Melanosomes and the Basis of Hypopigmentation. *J. Invest. Dermatol.* **49:**575–581, 1967.

19

Chondrodysplasia Punctata

(Chondrodystrophia Calcificans Congenita, Conradi-Hünermann Syndrome, Stippled Epiphyses)

Described initially by Conradi (5) in 1914, chondrodysplasia punctata consists of (*a*) punctate or stippled alterations most marked in the epiphyses of long bones, (*b*) congenital cataract, (*c*) joint contractures, and other skeletal alterations.

Chondrodysplasia punctata is extremely rare, the frequency being estimated at two to three cases per million births (18, 28). It has genetic heterogeneity, being inherited as an autosomal dominant and as an autosomal recessive trait (25). The former is known as the *Conradi-Hünermann type.* Cases probably exhibiting direct transmission are those of Curth (8), Kremens and Orloff (14), and Lischi and Menichini (16). Paternal age at conception in sporadic cases is elevated. Parental consanguinity was, however, noted in the cases of Melnik (17) and Mosekilde (19). Heterogeneity within this "dominant" group is probable (J. G. Hall, personal communication, 1975). The *rhizomelic type,* which is autosomal recessive, is so called because of marked shortening of the humerus, femur, or both. Parental consanguinity has been found in about 8 percent of rhizomelic cases.

SYSTEMIC MANIFESTATIONS

At least 65 percent of affected children with the rhizomelic type die before the end of the first year of life; few if any survive to puberty. In contrast, only a few infants with the Conradi-Hünermann type die in early infancy. If they survive the first few months of life, prognosis is good.

Facies. The face in both types is flat, because of hypoplasia of the malar bones. The forehead is prominent, with ocular hypertelorism. The palpebral fissures have a mongoloid slant. The bridge of the nose is flat, with the nostrils rather anteverted. Only about 50 percent, of either type, however, exhibit the typical facies (Figs. 19-1*B*, 19-2*A, B*).

Eyes. In the Conradi-Hünermann type, cataracts have been found in about 20 percent of the cases at birth. In contrast, cataracts have been noted in at least 70 percent of the rhizomelic cases (25).

Skin. The skin is dry, scaly, and atrophic (follicular atrophoderma). These changes are seen in about 25 percent of both forms of chondrodysplasia punctata (8).

Musculoskeletal alterations. In the *Conradi-Hünermann type,* height is reduced but head circumference is normal (3). Punctate calcifications are seen in the vertebral column, epiphyses, flat and round bones, and in some extraskeletal tissues such as the larynx and tracheal rings. There is mild or asymmetric shortening of tubular bones (Fig. 19-1*A*). Multiple, often asymmetric, dysplastic alterations in the epiphyses with flattening or irregular outlines are noted.

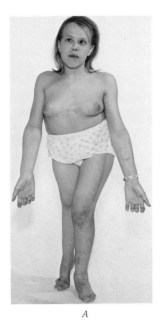

A

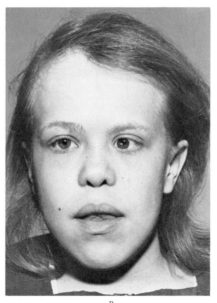

B

Figure 19-1. *Chondrodysplasia punctata. (A). (Conradi-Hüner-mann type.)* Height is reduced. Note disproportionate limb length and scoliosis. *(B).* Sparse hair, flat midface, anteverted nostrils, and cataract. *(From D. Comings et al.,* J. Pediat. **72**:63, 1968.)

The metaphyses are intact. The vertebral bodies are usually deformed, and scoliosis often develops after the first year of life (26). Contractures, particularly of large joints, have been noted in about 25 percent of the cases. Foot deformities, primarily talipes calcaneovalgus, have been present in about 20 percent (25) (Table 19-1).

In the *rhizomelic type,* in contrast to the Conradi-Hünermann type, there is severe congenital rhizomelic shortening of the extremities. Small head circumference tends to be present at birth and is a constant finding in older infants and children. Radiologically, severe shortening, metaphyseal cupping, splaying, and disturbed ossification of the humerus and/or femur are

Table 19-1. Differentiation of the Conradi-Hünermann and rhizomelic types of chondrodysplasia punctata

Findings	Conradi-Hünermann type	Rhizomelic type
Radiologic		
Severe bilateral shortening of femur and/or humerus	Absent	Present
Severe metaphyseal changes of femur and/or humerus	Absent	Present
Distribution of lesions	Frequently asymmetric	Mostly symmetric
Clinical		
Cataracts	About 17% of cases	At least 72% of cases
Head circumference	Normal for age	Small for age
Psychomotor retardation	Rare	Frequent
Prognosis	Good after neonatal period	Death usually in the first year of life
Histologic	Normal or mildly affected endochondral bone formation	Severely disturbed endochondral bone formation
Inheritance	Autosomal dominant	Autosomal recessive

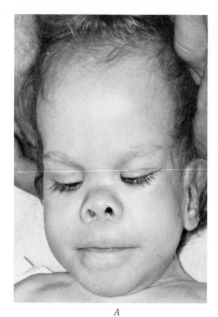
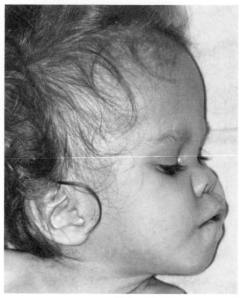

A
B

Figure 19-2. *Chondrodysplasia punctata.* (*A*). *Rhizomelic type.* Flat midface and small upturned nose. (*B*). Depressed midface and posteriorly rotated ears. (*C*). Severe shortening, metaphyseal cupping, splaying, and disturbed ossification of humerus and femur. Note marked stippling of epiphyses.

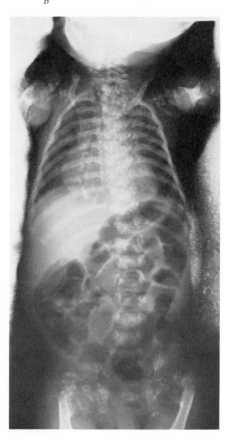

C

observed (Fig. 19-2*C*). Epiphyseal and extraepiphyseal calcifications are usually severe. Lateral views of the spine show a universal coronal cleft of the vertebral bodies (27). Contractures have been noted in over 60 percent of patients, and foot deformities in about 10 percent.

Histopathologic study of bones has shown focal disruption of the growth plate by fibrous tissue (D. Rimoin, personal communication, 1973).

Oral manifestations. Cleft palate (2, 4, 6, 7, 11, 12, 16a, 21) and submucous palatal cleft (1) have been noted in the rhizomelic type.

DIFFERENTIAL DIAGNOSIS

Punctate intra- and extracartilaginous calcifications in infants are nonspecific, may be seen in a number of hereditary and nonhereditary conditions, and may lead to erroneous diagnosis. These include calcifying arthritis and chondritis secondary to bacteremia, *cerebrohepatorenal syndrome of Zellweger* (20), and multiple epiphyseal dysplasia (25), and other disorders. A phenocopy may be produced by maternal ingestion of dicoumaral or Warfarin in early gestation (23).

LABORATORY AIDS

In the rhizomelic type, enchondral bone formation is grossly abnormal (29), with severely disturbed maturation of cartilage cells. Tongues of cartilage extend deep into the osseous shaft; cancellous bone is found directly on resting cartilage (7).

REFERENCES

1 Armaly, M. F., Ocular Involvement in Chondrodystrophia Calcificans Congenita Punctata. *Arch. Ophthalmol.* **57**:491–502, 1957.

2 Brogdon, B. G., and Crow, N. E., Chondrodystrophia Calcificans Congenita. *Am. J. Roentgenol.* **80**:443–448, 1958.

3 Comings, D., et al., Conradi's Disease. *J. Pediatr.* **72**:63–69, 1968.

4 Condron, C. J., Conradi's Disease: A Case without Cutaneous Manifestations. *Birth Defects* **7**(8):214–215, 1971.

5 Conradi, E., Vorzeitiges Auftreten von Knochen- und eigenartigen Verkalkungskernen bei Chondrodystrophia foetalis hypoplastica. *Jb. Kinderheilkd.* **80**:86–97, 1914.

6 Coté, P. E., Observations sur la chondrodysplasie épiphysaire. *Laval Méd.* **20**:481–489, 1955.

7 Coughlin, E. J., et al., Chondrodystrophia Calcificans Congenita. *J. Bone Joint Surg.* **32A**:938–942, 1950.

8 Curth, H. O., Follicular Atrophoderma and Pseudopelade Associated with Chondrodystrophia Calcificans Congenita. *J. Invest. Dermatol.* **13**:233–247, 1949.

9 Fraser, F. C., and Scriver, J. B., A Hereditary Factor in Chondrodystrophia Calcificans Congenita. *N. Engl. J. Med.* **250**:272–277, 1954.

10 Fritsch, H., and Manzke, H., Beitrag zur Chondrodystrophia calcificans connata (Conradi-Hünermann-Syndrom. *Arch. Kinderheilkd.* **169**:235–254, 1963.

11 Hammond, A., Dysplasia Epiphysalis Punctata with Ocular Anomalies. *Br. J. Ophthalmol.* **54**:755–758, 1970.

12 Hewitt, H. L., and van Bochove, W., Chondrodystrophia Calcificans Congenita (Case 1). *Radiol. Clin. Biol.* **40**:175–183, 1971.

13 Josephson, B. M., and Oriatti, M. D., Chondrodystrophia Calcificans Congenita. *Pediatrics* **28**:425–435, 1961.

14 Kremens, V., and Orloff, T. L., Congenital Calcific Chondrodystrophy. *J. Einstein Med. Cent.* **3**:137–139, 1955.

15 Lightwood, R. C., Congenital Deformities with Stippled Epiphyses and Congenital Cataract. *Proc. R. Soc. Med.* **24**:564–566, 1930.

16 Lischi, G., and Menichini, G., L'évolution clinique et radiologique de la chondropathie calcifiante congénitale. *Helv. paediatr. Acta* **22**:289–301, 1967.

16a Louvar, R. D., et al., Conradi-Hünermann Syndrome. *Clin. Pediatr.* **13**:680–685, 1974.

17 Melnik, J. C., Chondrodystrophia Calcificans Congenita. *Am. J. Dis. Child.* **110**:218–225, 1965.

18 Mørch, E. T., *Chondrodystrophic Dwarfs in Denmark.* E. Munksgaard, Copenhagen, 1941.

19 Mosekilde, E., Stippled Epiphyses in the Newborn and in Infants. *Acta Radiol. Scand.* **37**:291–307, 1958.

20 Opitz, J. M., et al., The Zellweger Syndrome (Cerebro-Hepato-Renal Syndrome). *Birth Defects* **5**(2):144–148, 1969.

21 Phillips, L. I., Chondrodystrophia Calcificans Congenita (Case 1), *N.Z. Med. J.* **56**:22–27, 1957.

22 Selakovich, W. G., and White, J. W., Chondrodystrophia Calcificans Congenita. *J. Bone Joint Surg.* **37A**:1271–1277, 1955.

23 Shaul, W. L., et al., Chondrodysplasia Punctata and Maternal Warfarin Use During Pregnancy. *Am. J. Dis. Child.* **129**:360–362, 1975.

24 Silverman, F., Dysplasias épiphysaires. Entité protéiforme. *Ann. Radiol.* **4**:833–867, 1961.

25 Spranger, J. W., et al., Heterogeneity of Chondrodysplasia punctata. *Humangenetik* **11**:190–212, 1971.

26 Spranger, J. W., et al., Chondrodysplasia punctata (Chondrodystrophia Calcificans). I. Typ Conradi-Hünermann. *Fortschr. Roentgenstr.* **113**:717–726, 1970.

27 Spranger, J., et al., Chondrodysplasia punctata (Chondrodystrophia calcificans). II. Der rhizomelic Typ. *Fortschr. Roentgenstr.* **114**:327–335, 1971.

28 Verschuer, O. F., von, Die Häufigkeit krankhafter Erbmerkmale im Berzirk Münster. *Z. Menschl. Vererb. Konstit. Lehre* **36**:383–412, 1962.

29 Yakovac, W. C., Calcareous Chondropathies in the Newborn Infant. *Arch. Pathol.* **57**:62–79, 1957.

20

Chondroectodermal Dysplasia

(Ellis-van Creveld Syndrome)

Although the syndrome was described in part by several authors (14, 18, 21, 32) prior to the classic paper of Ellis and van Creveld (8) in 1940, credit is given the latter authors for describing the complete syndrome and coining the name "chondroectodermal dysplasia." The syndrome consists of (*a*) bilateral manual postaxial polydactyly, (*b*) chondrodysplasia of long bones resulting in acromelic dwarfism, (*c*) hidrotic ectodermal dysplasia affecting principally the nails and teeth, and less often, (*d*) congenital heart malformations. More than 100 cases have been reported to date.

The syndrome manifests autosomal recessive inheritance (16, 17, 22), with parental consanguinity in about 30 percent of cases (6, 8, 9, 16, 19, 22).

This condition is the most common type of dwarfism among the Amish. McKusick et al. (16) found 52 cases distributed in 30 sibships among the Amish isolate of Lancaster County, Pennsylvania.

SYSTEMIC MANIFESTATIONS

Facies. The facies is not especially characteristic except for a mild defect in the middle of the upper lip, which, although often present, is not striking.

Skeletal anomalies. The extremities are often plump and markedly shortened progressively distalward, i.e., from the trunk to the phalanges (Fig. 20-1). Bilateral manual hexadactyly is frequent, the extra digit being on the ulnar side (Fig. 20-2). Heptadactyly has also been noted (7, 12). Frequently the patient cannot make a tight fist. Only rarely are there extra toes (9, 12, 16, 17). A widened space frequently is present between the hallux and the rest of the toes (23). Genu valgum (5, 19), curvature of the humerus, talipes equinovarus (25, 28), talipes calcaneovalgus (6), and pigeon breast with thoracic constriction (7, 16, 23) have also been reported.

Radiographically, the tubular bones are seen to be short and thickened. The diaphyseal ends of the humerus and the femur are plump. Shortening of the radius and ulna is even more marked than that of the humerus. The proximal end of the ulna and the distal end of the radius are unusually large, and the proximal end of the radius and the distal end of the ulna are unusually small. The widened end of the tibial shaft is irregular, and the ossification centers in the proximal epiphysis are hypoplastic (Fig. 20-3*A*, *B*). There is peaking of the proximal tibia, with a long lateral and a short medial slope, resulting in genu valgum (16) after the age of six years (5). The fibula is most severely shortened, being only about 50 percent of normal length (7). Phalangeal bones are often missing (22), and syncarpalism (hamate and capitate), synmetacarpalism, and polymetacarpalism are frequent (5, 12, 16, 19). Cone-shaped epiphyses of the hands (type 37 of Giedion) are pathognomonic for the syndrome (10) (Fig. 20-3*A*, *B*, *C*).

In infancy the pelvis is dysplastic with low

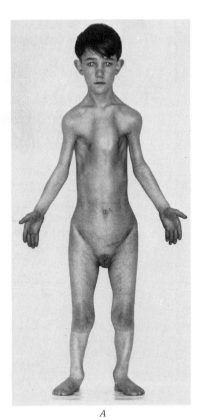
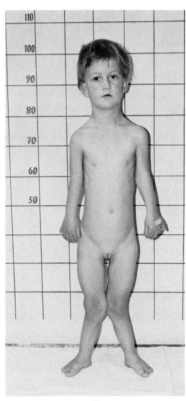

A   *B*

Figure 20-1. *(A). Chondroec-todermal dysplasia* (Ellis-van Cre-veld syndrome). Long appearing thorax with pectus carinatum; mesomelia of lower extremities. *(From G. B. Winter and M. Geddes,* Br. Dent. J. **122:**103, 1967.) *(B).* Compare phenotype with *A*. *(From H. O. Bützler et al.* Fortschr. Roentgenstr. **118:**537, 1973.)

iliac wings and hooklike downward projection of the medial acetabulum. The capital femoral epiphysis may ossify prematurely. In childhood, the pelvic shape normalizes (5).

Heart. Congenital heart defect has been seen in 40 to 50 percent of the cases reported to date (14). It is the most serious feature, being largely responsible for frequent neonatal deaths. Most patients with the heart defect have demonstrated single atrium and endocardial cushion defect (9, 14). Some patients have had cor triloculare (19) or even cor biloculare (23). Lynch et al. (14) have presented a comprehensive review of the heart anomalies.

Hair and nails. The hair, especially the eyebrows and pubic hair, has been stated to be thin and sparse (8, 12, 16, 19, 29). However, we have not been impressed by this feature in patients that we have seen. Nearly all patients have severe dystrophy of the fingernails (Fig. 20-2). They are markedly hypoplastic, thin, and often wrinkled or spoon-shaped. The skin is normal, and there is no alteration in sweating.

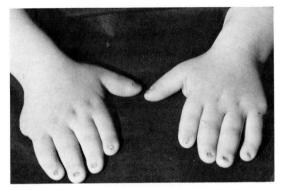

Figure 20-2. Digits abbreviated, with hypoplastic nails. Note that digits have been amputated on ulnar side. *(From D. H. Altman, Miami, Florida.)*

Eyes. The eyes are usually normal, but internal strabismus (19) and congenital cataract (12, 17) have been observed.

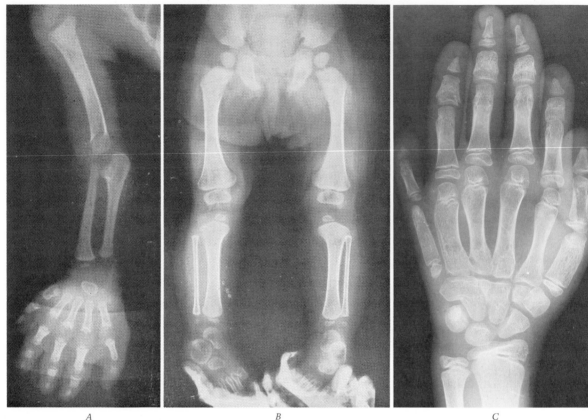

A   *B*   *C*

Figure 20-3. (*A* and *B*). Radiographs demonstrating unusually large proximal end of ulna and distal end of radius, and unusually small proximal end of radius, as well as progressive shortening. Extra digit had been amputated shortly after birth. Also note peaking of proximal tibia. (*Courtesy of D. Gutman and A. Jungmann, Hadera, Israel.*) (*C*). Malformed middle phalanges with cone-shaped epiphysis of middle phalanx of fifth finger. Note extra finger on ulnar side, malformed fifth metacarpal, capitate-hamate fusion.

Genitalia. About one-third of patients have genital anomalies. All these patients have been male. These anomalies have included cryptorchism (8), mild epispadias (17), and hypospadias (16, 27).

Mental status. Some patients were noted to be mentally retarded, but McKusick (16) suggests that mental retardation is not an integral part of the disorder. Hydrocephalus has been reported in several instances (3, 10).

Oral manifestations. The most striking oral finding is fusion of the middle portion of the upper lip to the maxillary gingival margin so that no mucobuccal fold or sulcus exists anteriorly. This is a constant finding and has been reported in all cases in which this change has been sought (2, 6, 8–12, 17, 19, 22, 29). Because of this fusion, the middle portion of the upper lip appears hypoplastic, resembling a lip that has undergone cheiloplasty (Fig. 20-4*A*–*C*).

Natal teeth have been observed in at least 25 percent of infants, and it is possible that this condition may be even more frequent than reported. Oligodontia is also a constant finding, especially in the mandibular anterior region (2, 6, 8, 9, 17, 18, 27). In this area, the alveolar ridge is often serrated (2, 6, 8, 23, 25) (Fig. 20-4*C*). The present authors believe that the notching of the

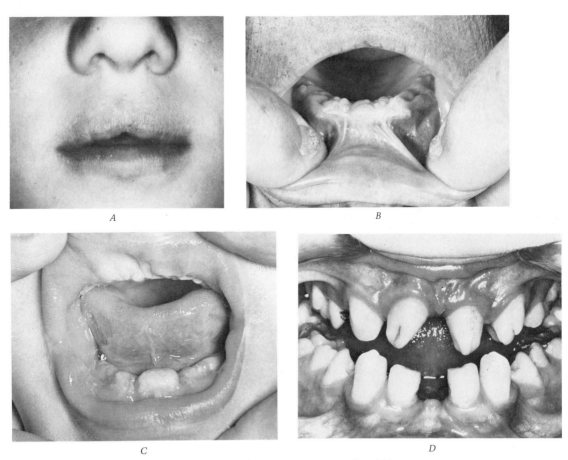

Figure 20-4. (*A*). Mild midline defect of upper lip. (*From R. H. Biggerstaff and M. Mazaheri,* J. Am. Dent. Assoc. **77**:1090, 1968.) (*B*). Attachment of upper lip to gingival margin. (*From V. A. McKusick, Baltimore, Maryland.*) (*C*). In infant, note absence of superior mucobuccal fold, serrated lower anterior alveolar process. (*D*). Malformed and absent incisors. (*From G. B. Winter and M. Geddes,* Br. Dent. J. **122**:103, 1967.)

lower alveolar process may represent the continuation of the normal serrated condition of the gingiva from the third to the seventh month *in utero* (30). The teeth which erupt are usually small (2, 17), conically crowned (2, 7, 8, 18, 33), and irregularly spaced (2, 8, 9, 18). The crown form of many of the teeth is distinctive. Those that are not conical are somewhat bicuspid in form, with accentuated cuspal height and deep, steep fissures (Fig. 20-4*D*). The enamel has been noted to be hypoplastic in about half the cases. A comprehensive review of the oral findings has been presented by Biggerstaff and Mazaheri (2).

DIFFERENTIAL DIAGNOSIS

It may be almost impossible to differentiate radiographically the Ellis-van Creveld syndrome from asphyxiating thoracic dystrophy (13). Both syndromes may present identical changes in hands, pelvis, and long bones. Differential diagnosis is based upon the following clinical changes present in the Ellis-van Creveld syndrome: cardiac anomalies, nail hypoplasia, fusion of upper lip and gingiva and, when they are present, the neonatal teeth. Later in life, the presence of genu valgum in chondroectodermal dysplasia and renal failure with hypertension in thoracic asphyxiating dystrophy will help to establish a more positive diagnosis.

The Ellis-van Creveld syndrome is differentiated from other chondrodystrophies such as *achondroplasia, chondrodysplasia punctata,* the *Morquio syndrome,* and *cartilage-hair hypoplasia* by its distinctive radiographic features, discussed above.

Polydactyly and hypodontia or other dental anomalies have been seen in several generations without other apparent stigmata (24) and in association with *acrofacial dysostosis of Weyers* and *trisomy 13.*

Polydactyly is also seen as a component of the Bardet-Biedl syndrome (adiposity, retinitis pigmentosa, and genital hypoplasia).

Partial fusion of the upper lip due to hyperplastic frenula is seen in *OFD syndrome.* Natal teeth are observed in *pachyonychia congenita (Type II), oculomandibulodyscephaly, and cyclopia.*

LABORATORY AIDS

Maroteaux and Lamy (15) found increased urinary excretion of chondroitin sulfate A in some patients with chondroectodermal dysplasia, a finding denied by Spranger (personal communication, 1972).

REFERENCES

1 Baisch, A., Anonychia congenita, kombiniert mit Polydaktylie und verzögertem abnormen Zahndurchbruch. *Dtsch. Z. Chir.* **232:**450–457, 1931.

2 Biggerstaff, R. H., and Mazaheri, M., Oral Manifestations of the Ellis-van Creveld Syndrome. *J. Am. Dent. Assoc.* **77:**1090–1095, 1968.

3 Blackburn, M. G., and Belliveau, R. E., Ellis-van Creveld Syndrome: A Report of Previously Undescribed Anomalies in Two Siblings. *Am. J. Dis. Child.* **122:**267–270, 1971.

4 Bode,-, *Entwicklung des Zahnsystems gekoppelt mit Polydaktylie und Anonychia congenita.* Thesis, Göttingen, 1935.

5 Bützler, H. O., et al., Die Röntgendiagnose der Skelettveränderungen des Ellis-van Creveld-Syndroms im Wachstumsalter. *Fortschr. Roentgenstr.* **118:**538–552, 1973.

6 Douglas, W. F., et al., Chondroectodermal Dysplasia (Ellis-van Creveld Syndrome): Report of Two Cases in Sibship and Review of Literature. *Am. J. Dis. Child.* **97:**472–478, 1959.

7 Ellis, R. W. B., and Andrew, J. D., Chondroectodermal Dysplasia. *J. Bone Joint Surg.* **44-B:**626–636, 1962.

8 Ellis, R. W. B., and van Creveld, S., A Syndrome Characterized by Ectodermal Dysplasia, Polydactyly, Chondrodysplasia and Congenital Morbus Cordis. *Arch. Dis. Child.* **15:**65–84, 1940.

9 Engle, M. A., and Ehlers, K. H., Ellis-van Creveld Syndrome with Asymmetric Polydactyly and Successful Surgical Correction of Common Atrium. *Birth Defects* **5**(4):65–67, 1969.

10 Giedion, A., Cone-shaped Epiphyses of the Hands and Their Diagnostic Value: The Tricho-rhino-phalangeal Syndrome. *Ann. Radiol.* **10:**322–329, 1967.

11 Guastini, M. R. et al., Considerazioni clinico-radiologiche su un caso di sindrome di Ellis-van Creveld. *Minerva Pediatr.* **23:**525–531, 1971.

12 Hartwein, L., Zur Kasuistik des Ellis-van Creveld Syndroms. *Kinderärztl. Prax.* **27:**229–233, 1959.

13 Langer, L. O., The Thoracic-pelvic-phalangeal Dystrophy. *Birth Defects* **5**(4):55–64, 1969.

14 Lynch, J. I., et al., Congenital Heart Disease and Chondroectodermal Dysplasia. *Am. J. Dis. Child.* **115:**80–87, 1968.

15 Maroteaux, P., and Lamy, H., Hurler's Disease. Morquio's Disease and Related Mucopolysaccharidoses. *J. Pediatr.* **67:**312–323, 1965.

16 McKusick, V. A., et al., Dwarfism in the Amish. I. The Ellis-van Creveld Syndrome. *Bull. Johns Hopkins Hosp.* **115:**306–336, 1964.

17 Metrakos, J. D., and Fraser, F. C., Evidence for a Hereditary Factor in Chondroectodermal Dysplasia (Ellis-van Creveld Syndrome). *Am. J. Hum. Genet.* **6:**260–269, 1954.

18 Miller, H. A., Dental Abnormalities in a Patient with Achondroplasia. *Int. J. Orthodont.* **23:**296–299, 1937.

19 Mitchell, F. N., and Waddell, W. W., Jr., Ellis-van Creveld Syndrome: Report of 2 Cases in Siblings. *Acta Paediatr.* **47:**142–151, 1958.

20 Neiman, N., et al., Maladie d' Ellis-van Creveld. *Sem. Hop. Paris* **29:**1702–1704, 1953.

21 Pires de Lima, J. A., Dents à la naissance. *Bull. Mem. Soc. Anthropol. Paris* **4:**71–74, 1923.

22 Rössler, H., Beitrag zum Ellis-van Creveld Syndrom. *Neue Oest. Z. Kinderheilkd.* **3:**301–312, 1958.

23 Smith, H. L., and Hand, A. M., Chondroectodermal Dysplasia (Ellis-van Creveld Syndrome). *Pediatrics* **21:**298–307, 1958.

24 Thomas,-, Uber einen Fall von hereditären Polydaktylie mit Anomalien der Zahne. *Dtsch. Monatsschr. Zahnheilkd.* **6:**407–408, 1888.

25 Turner, E. K., The Ellis-van Creveld Syndrome: Report of a Case. *Med. J. Aust.* **1:**366–367, 1956.

26 Uehlinger, E., Pathologische Anatomie der chondroektodermalen Dysplasie Ellis-van Creveld. *Schweiz. Z. Allg. Pathol.* **20:**754–766, 1957.

27 Walls, W. L., et al., Chondroectodermal Dysplasia (Ellis-van Creveld Syndrome): Report of a Case and Review of

the Literature. *Am. J. Dis. Child.* **98:**242–248, 1959.

28 Weiss, H., and Crosett, A., Jr., Chondroectodermal Dysplasia. *J. Pediatr.* **46:**268–275, 1955.

29 Weller, S. D. V., Chondroectodermal Dysplasia (Ellis-van Creveld Syndrome). *Proc. R. Soc. Med.* **44:**731–732, 1951.

30 West, C. M., The Development of the Gums and Their Relationship to the Deciduous Teeth in the Human Foetus. *Carnegie Inst. Contrib. Embryol.* **16:**23–46, 1925.

31 Weyers, H., Zur Kenntnis der Chondroektodermaldysplasie (Ellis-van Creveld): Bericht über 2 Beobachtungen. *Z. Kinderheilkd.* **78:**111–129.

32 Willner, H., Ektodermale Missbildungen. Kasuistischer Beitrag zur Unterzahl von Zähnen. *Dtsch. Zahn Mund Kieferheilkd.* **3:**279–285, 1936.

33 Winter, G. B., and Geddes, M., Oral Manifestations of Chondroectodermal Dysplasia (Ellis-van Creveld Syndrome). *Br. Dent. J.* **122:**103–107, 1967.

21

Chromosomal Syndromes
and Orofacial Anomalies

Since the discovery that man has 46 chromosomes in each somatic cell, interest in human chromosomes and the conditions that arise from their abnormalities has mushroomed. The reader is referred to several excellent reviews of the present status of the knowledge of human chromosomes (1–10).

Several surveys have shown that many of these syndromes are relatively common. In newborns, the XXY Klinefelter syndrome is present in 0.3 percent of males; the XO chromatin-negative Turner syndrome, in 0.03 percent; and the XXX syndrome, in 0.13 percent of females. In institutionalized patients, the incidence is 1.0 percent, 0.05 percent, and 0.4 percent, respectively (4). Trisomy 21 (Down syndrome) accounts for at least 15 percent of institutionalized individuals. However, for some of the rarer autosomal disorders, such as trisomy 13 or 18, the incidence is not precisely known but has been estimated to be about 1 per 6,000 births. For many of the syndromes, orofacial changes have not been extensively studied—or if studied, have been sparsely documented, with the exception of trisomy 21. For purposes of presenting the orofacial anomalies, they will be considered under two categories: (a) autosomal chromosome syndromes and (b) sex chromosome syndromes.*

---

*The following symbols will be employed: p for short arm, q for long arm, r for ring, + for trisomy, and − for deletion. For example, 6p− means deletion of the short arm of chromosome 6 and 8+ means trisomy for chromosome 8. The symbol 7q+ means partial trisomy for the long arm of chromosome 7.

AUTOSOMAL CHROMOSOME SYNDROMES

1q+ SYNDROME

Two patients had common features of beaked nose, large outstanding pinnas, micrognathia, long tapered fingers, congenital heart disease, and involution or absence of the thymus (1, 2). One had cleft lip-palate (3).

3p+ SYNDROME

Common features include microbrachycephaly with frontal bossing, high forehead, hypertelorism, epicanthus, large mouth, short neck, congenital heart disease, and large numbers of digital whorls. Half the patients had cleft palate (1, 2).

4p− SYNDROME (WOLF-HIRSCHHORN SYNDROME)

The syndrome described independently in 1965 by Wolf et al. (11) and Hirschhorn et al. (3) results from deletion of the short arm of a No. 4 chromosome. It is characterized by severe psychomotor and growth retardation. Birth weight is usually less than 2,000 g in spite of prolonged gestation. Fetal activity is diminished. Most infants are hypotonic. Seizures have occurred in 70 percent of the patients. Males commonly exhibit cryptorchism and, especially, hypospadias. Congenital heart malformations, most often atrial or ventricular septal defects, have been noted in about 60 percent of cases (12).

In several patients there has been dimpling of the skin over the sacrum and elsewhere, as over shoulders, elbows, or knuckles (4, 5, 10, 11). The

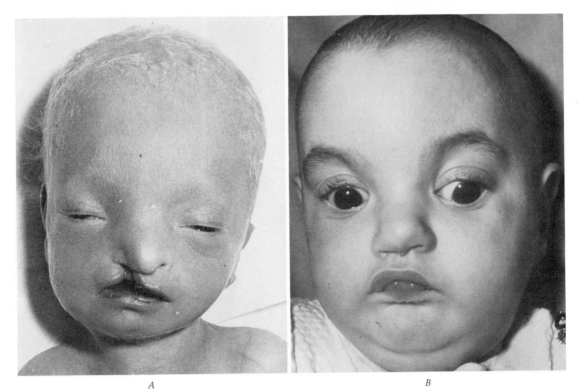

A   B

Figure 21-1. 4p— (*Wolf-Hirschhorn*) *syndrome*. (*A*). Small head, ocular hypertelorism,
flattened nose, cleft lip with short philtrum, down-turned mouth. (*From A. I. Taylor*, J.
Med. Genet. **5**:227, 1968.) (*B*). Microcephaly with cranial asymmetry, wide-spaced eyes,
strabismus, broad-based nose with asymmetric nares, short philtrum, down-turned
mouth. (*From D. Arias et al.*, J. Pediatr. **76**:82, 1970.)

pelvic and carpal bones are late in ossification.
Pseudoepiphyses are seen in the phalanges and
at the base of each metacarpal. Simian creases
have been present in about 20 percent of cases.
The dermal ridges tend to be underdeveloped,
and the finger ridge count tends to be low because of increased numbers of arches. About 35
cases have been described to date.

Oral and facial manifestations. The skull is microcephalic, and often there is cranial asymmetry. In a few cases, midline scalp defects have
been noted (2, 3, 9, 11). Hemangioma on the
brow is frequent (2) (Fig. 21-1*A*, *B*).

A prominent glabella and ocular hypertelorism are almost constant features. Strabismus
epicanthal folds, and antimongoloid obliquity of
the palpebral fissures have been noted in over 50
percent of cases. Iris coloboma has been found
occasionally.

The ears have narrow external canals and are
low set and simplified in form. A preauricular
dimple or sinus has been present in 50 percent of
patients. The nose is misshapen or beaked with
a broad base. The philtrum is short with a down-
turned mouth. Cleft lip or, especially, cleft palate has been noted in two-thirds of the cases.
The mandible is micrognathic in about 70 percent of cases.

4p+ SYNDROME

Characteristics included marked growth and
psychomotor retardation, microcephaly with
prominent glabella, bulbous nasal tip, low-set
ears with broad concha and helix and protruding
anthelix, hypertelorism, large mouth, prominent
chin, short neck, hypoplastic ribs, abnormal vertebras, limb anomalies, membranous anal
atresia, distal palmar axial triradius, and increased numbers of finger-tip whorls (1–3).

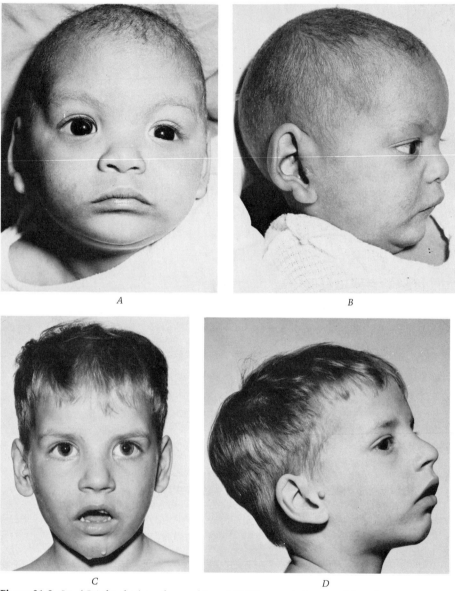

A   *B*

C   *D*

Figure 21-2. *5p−* (*Cri-du-chat*) syndrome. (*A and B*). Microcephaly, round face, hyperte-lorism with broad nasal bridge, malformed pinnas. (*From C. Weinkove and R. Mc-Donald,* S. Afr. Med. J. **43**:218, 1969.) (*C* and *D*). As child ages round face disappears. Note preauricular tag. (*From H. B. Dyggve and M. Mikkelsen,* Arch. Dis. Child. **40**:82, 1965.)

5p− (CRI-DU-CHAT) SYNDROME

This disorder was described initially in 1963 by Lejeune et al.; over 150 examples have been documented to date. The syndrome is present in about 1 percent of institutionalized individuals who have intelligence quotients less than 35.

The syndrome results from deletion of 35 to 55 percent of the short arm of a chromosome No. 5. About 10 to 15 percent of cases result from translocation.

As the name implies, the syndrome is characterized by a catlike, weak, shrill cry in infancy which is due to hypoplasia of the larynx. However, the cry disappears with time, even within a few weeks of age (1, 3).

There are severe mental retardation (I.Q. less than 25), failure to thrive, and hypotonia in infancy. Adult height usually ranges from 124 to 168 cm (49 to 66 in.). Various musculoskeletal anomalies have included hypotonia, flatfoot, scoliosis, small ilia, and short metacarpals and metatarsals. Simian creases are seen in about 35 percent of patients (4, 5) and eight or more whorls in about 30 percent.

There is considerable overlap of the clinical signs in the 5p− and 4p− syndromes. However, in the latter, one finds no catlike cry, a lower birth weight, more severe mental retardation, and a more frequent association with cleft palate, seizures, hypospadias, skin dimples, and midline scalp defects.

Oral and facial manifestations. The infant facies is characterized by microcephaly, round form, hypertelorism, antimongoloid obliquity of palpebral fissures, bilateral alternating strabismus, broad nasal bones, and low-set ears (Fig. 21-2A–D). The frontal sinuses are usually enlarged. Preauricular tags are occasionally noted. Most patients have mild micrognathia. However, the roundness of the face and the ocular hypertelorism disappear with age. The face becomes thin and the philtrum short. Premature graying of the hair has been noted in about 30 percent of patients. Dental malocclusion is common.

GROUP C DELETION, TRISOMY, TRISOMY MOSAICISM, AND PARTIAL TRISOMY

There are seven pairs of C-group chromosomes and hence many possible types of trisomy, partial trisomy, or deletion involving the 6–12 group. Many of these states have only recently been clinically recognized by use of newer banding techniques.

6r SYNDROME
Moore et al. (14) described a mentally retarded child with microcephaly, microphthalmia, microstomia, large pinnas, stiff ankles, and hyperkeratosis of the soles.

7q+ SYNDROME
Several reports indicate that common features are low birth weight, mental retardation, fuzzy hair, wide anterior fontanel, small palpebral fissures, hypertelorism, small nose, cleft palate, large tongue, low-set abnormal pinnas, kyphoscoliosis, dislocated hips, abnormal ribs, and pes cavus (2, 24).

8+ SYNDROME
The most striking aspects of trisomy 8 or trisomy 8 mosaicism syndrome are mild to moderate mental retardation, asymmetric skull or scaphocephaly, strabismus, dysplastic pinnas, long slender trunk with sloping shoulders, slender pelvis, vertebral and rib anomalies, reduced joint mobility, absent patellas, and deep linear grooves of the palms and soles. A few have exhibited agenesis of the corpus callosum (3, 5, 11, 12, 22) (Fig. 21-3A to D).

9p+ SYNDROME
The syndrome is characterized by mental retardation, mild microcephaly, brachycephaly, flat forehead, enophthalmos, iris coloboma, prominent nose with broad root and bridge and globular tip, short upper lip, carp mouth, protuberant ears, hypoplasia of phalanges and nails, clinodactyly, simian crease, decreased whorls, and absence of B or C triradius. Sexual maturation is delayed (13, 15, 16, 20, 23, 27). Cleft lip-palate has also been found.

9p− SYNDROME
Common clinical features include mental retardation, hypertonia, trigonocephaly with frontal bossing, biparietal flattening, flat occiput, flat nasal bridge, anteverted nostrils, long philtrum, exophthalmos, short neck, abnormal pinnas with small external canals, short neck, congenital heart disease, and excessive whorls (1). 9r syndrome has similar features (9).

9+ SYNDROME
This lethal condition is characterized by mild microcephaly, hypotonia, small mongoloid palpebral fissures, prominent nose, low-set ears, micrognathia, long flexed fingers, multiple joint dislocations, small penis, cryptorchism, and severe congenital heart disease (4, 8, 10).

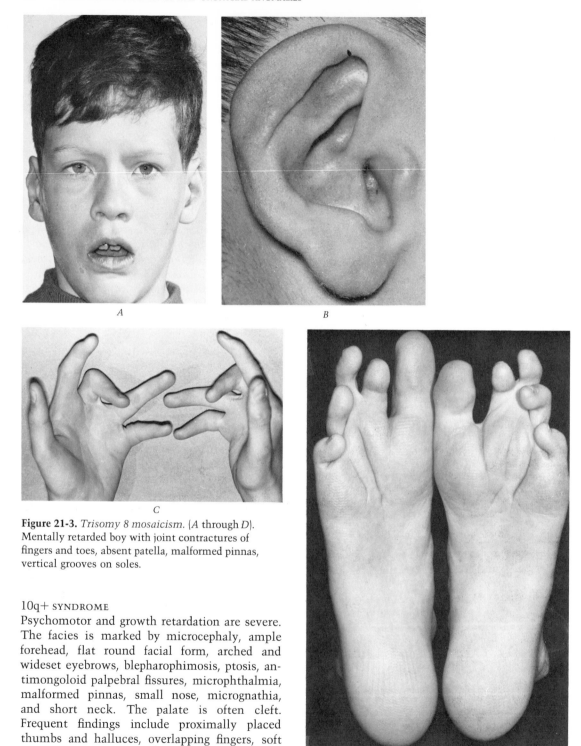

Figure 21-3. *Trisomy 8 mosaicism. (A through D).* Mentally retarded boy with joint contractures of fingers and toes, absent patella, malformed pinnas, vertical grooves on soles.

10q+ SYNDROME

Psychomotor and growth retardation are severe. The facies is marked by microcephaly, ample forehead, flat round facial form, arched and wideset eyebrows, blepharophimosis, ptosis, antimongoloid palpebral fissures, microphthalmia, malformed pinnas, small nose, micrognathia, and short neck. The palate is often cleft. Frequent findings include proximally placed thumbs and halluces, overlapping fingers, soft tissue syndactyly, camptodactyly, deep plantar furrows, and reduced renal function (13, 18, 21, 26).

11p+ SYNDROME

Characteristic are mental retardation, hypotonia, marked frontal bossing, strabismus, nystagmus, enophthalmos, antimongoloid obliquity of palpebral fissures, broad fingers and toes, and cleft palate (7, 19).

11q+ SYNDROME

Features include mental retardation, low birth weight, broad flat nose, micrognathia with retracted lower lip, congenital heart disease, renal anomalies, and dysplastic dermal ridges. Death occurred in all cases prior to the ninth extrauterine month (17, 25).

TRISOMY 13 SYNDROME (TRISOMY D₁)

The phenotype is so striking that diagnosis is usually made on clinical grounds before the karyotype has been studied. The incidence has been estimated to be about 1 per 6,000 births (1, 6, 8, 10). There is no sex predilection.

Holoprosencephaly, apneic spells, seizures, feeding difficulties, severe mental retardation, and apparent deafness are characteristic. Musculoskeletal abnormalities include postaxial polydactyly of the hands or feet with overlapping flexed fingers (about 75 percent) (2, 3). At least 80 percent have congenital heart defects (ventricular septal defect, patent ductus arteriosus, atrial septal defect, dextroposition) (8). Genital anomalies include cryptorchism, abnormal scrotum in males, and bicornuate uterus and hypoplastic ovaries in females (8, 9). Dermatoglyphic alterations include simian crease and distal palmar axial triradius. The reader is referred to several excellent sources for associated anomalies (6, 8).

Mean birth weight is about 2,500 g, and often there is a single umbilical artery. About 45 percent of patients die within the first month, 70 percent by the sixth month, and less than 5 percent survive more than 3 years (4). The mean maternal age at birth of an affected child is about 31 years. As with 21 and 18 trisomies, most cases result from nondisjunction.

Different forms of incomplete trisomy 13 have been reviewed by Schinzel et al. (5) and Escobar et al. (1a).

Oral and facial manifestations. Moderate microcephaly with sloping forehead and wide sagittal suture and large fontanels have been noted in over 60 percent of patients. Microphthalmia or iris coloboma with retinal dysplasia and ocular hypertelorism occur in about 80 percent. The pinnas are usually malformed. Capillary hemangiomas in the glabellar region and localized scalp defects in the parieto-occipital area are common (6) (Fig. 21-4A–C).

Cleft lip with or without cleft palate or isolated cleft palate occurs in 60 to 70 percent of patients (8), and micrognathia is present in over 80 percent. The tongue tip has been noted to be bifid in several cases, and ankyloglossia may occur (6). Tooth crown structure has been somewhat bizarre in cases we have personally examined.

13q− AND 13r SYNDROMES

There are reports on over 60 cases in which part of the long arm of a D chromosome has been missing or in which a D-group chromosome was replaced by a ring. Although these cases may represent a heterogeneity, there is good evidence to suggest that the chromosome involved is number 13. Mean survival is 39 months for 13q− cases and 89 months for 13r survivors (8).

All patients have exhibited mental and somatic retardation, and many have been hypotonic. Thumbs have been absent or hypoplastic in about 70 percent of the 13q− cases but in less than 30 percent of the 13r cases. Congenital cardiovascular anomalies (ventricular septal defect or malformation of the aorta) have been reported in about 50 percent of both groups.

Genitourinary anomalies have included hypospadias, cryptorchism, cleft or hypoplastic scrotum, small penis, and pelvic kidney (7, 10). Anal atresia has been occasionally found (3).

Musculoskeletal abnormalities have included bilateral hip dislocation, focal lumbar vertebral agenesis, inguinal hernia, coxa valga, and synostosis of the fourth and fifth metacarpals. Simian creases are commonly noted. Niebuhr and Ottosen (6) have discussed the phenotypic alterations associated with different degrees of deletion.

Oral and facial manifestations. Microcephaly has been present in 60 to 80 percent of the cases.

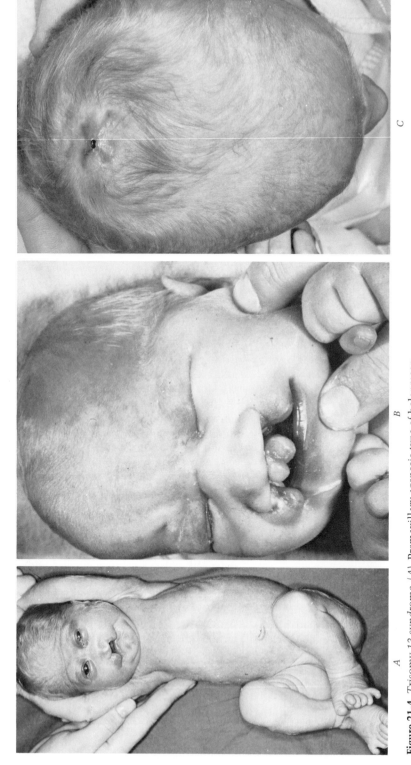

Figure 21-4. *Trisomy 13 syndrome.* (*A*). Premaxillary agenesis type of holoprosencephaly with trisomy 13. Note ocular hypotelorism, lack of nasal bones, extra digits. (*From P. E. Conen,* Am. J. Dis. Child. **111:**236, 1966.) (*B*). Bilateral cleft lip-palate, microphthalmia, ulnar hexadactyly, superficial angioma over brow. (*C*). Skin defect at vertex of skull.

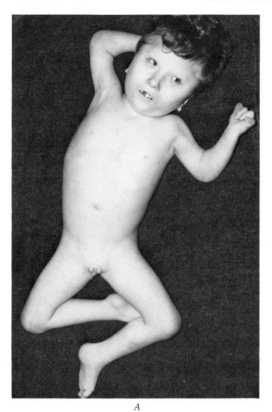 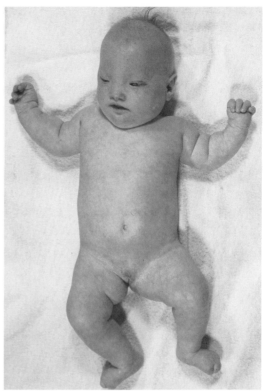

A *B*

Figure 21-5. *13q— syndrome.* (*A*). Absence of thumbs, micropenis, cleft scrotum in severely retarded child. (*From R. S. Sparkes et al.,* Am. J. Hum. Genet. **19**:644, 1967.) (*B*). Broad-based nose, ptosis of lids, absence of thumbs. (*From R. C. Juberg et al.,* J. Med. Genet. **6**:314, 1969.)

Some have exhibited various degrees of holo-prosencephaly.

Most striking has been unilateral or bilateral retinoblastoma, which has been documented in over half the 13q— cases (8) but in only one of the 13r examples (3). Other eye defects, seen in almost 50 percent of patients, have included microphthalmia, iris and/or retinal coloboma, and apparent ocular hypertelorism. The earlobes are often large (Fig. 21-5).

Several of the children have had protrusion of the maxillary incisors (2, 4). Cleft palate has been described in several cases of 13q— syndrome (1, 5, 9, 11).

TRISOMY 18 SYNDROME

These patients present a clinical picture that is readily recognizable. The incidence is about 1 per 7,000 newborn babies, and there is an over 3 : 1 female sex predilection. Although due to

nondisjunction in almost all cases, this syndrome, like trisomy 21, may rarely be caused by translocation. The mean maternal age at birth of an affected child is 32 years. The reader is referred to several comprehensive reviews of over 130 abnormalities which have been associated (1, 3–5).

The most common features are polyhydramnios, small placenta, single umbilical artery, mental retardation, weak cry, hypertonicity, feeding difficulty, failure to thrive, flexion of fingers with the index overlapping the third finger and the fifth overlapping the fourth, cryptorchism, dorsiflexion of halluces, interventricular septal defect, patent ductus arteriosus, inguinal and/or umbilical hernia, and short sternum. Less commonly seen are epicanthus, talipes calcaneovalgus, "rocker-bottom" feet, soft-tissue syndactyly of the second and third toes, Meckel's diverticulum, heterotopic pan-

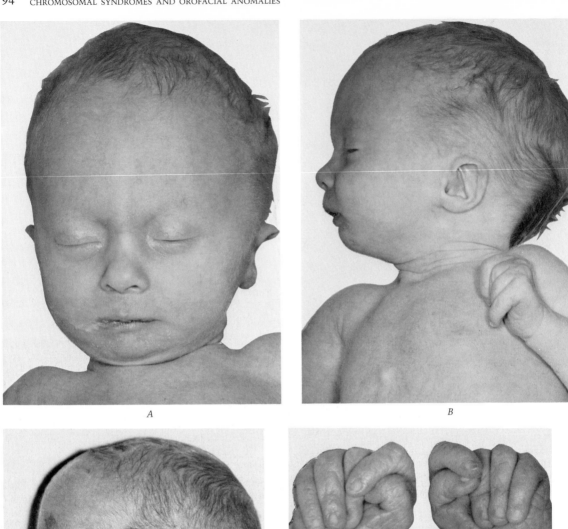

A

B

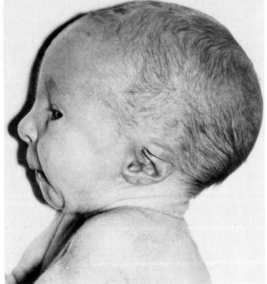

C

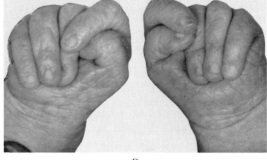

D

Fig. 21-6. *Trisomy 18 syndrome.* (*A*). Narrow bifrontal diameter, small lower jaw. (*B*). Prominent occiput, eyelid ptosis, malformed low-set pinna, micrognathia. (*C*). Compare facies with that in *B*. (*From P. Paerregård*, Acta Pathol. Microbiol. Scand. **67**:479, 1966.) (*D*). Overlapping fingers.

creatic tissue, and thin diaphragm with eventration.

A combination of trisomy 18 with XXX or XXY syndrome occurs in about 7.5 percent of cases. The fingerprints usually manifest six or more arches, and dermal ridges may be dysplastic. Mean birth weight is less than 2,300 g. Thirty percent of patients fail to survive more than 1 month, 50 percent live 2 months, and fewer than 10 percent live more than 1 year. Mean survival is about 70 days.

Oral and facial anomalies. Most commonly seen are prominent occiput, narrow bifrontal diameter, mild hirsutism of forehead, low-set malformed pinnas, and micrognathia. Less commonly noted are microcephaly, corneal opacity, and ptosis of eyelids. Cleft lip and/or palate have been tabulated in 15 percent of the cases (2) (Fig. 21-6A–C).

18p− SYNDROME

Deletion of the short arms of a chromosome 18 is associated with a variable phenotype (2, 5, 7, 13). Heterogeneity is likely due to interstitial or terminal deletions, unequal interchromatid exchanges, and reciprocal translocation. Maternal age is elevated. There is a 2:1 female sex predilection. Mental retardation, of variable degree, is a constant feature. Birth weight is low, and somatic growth retarded. Over half the patients have pectus excavatum, incurved fifth fingers, and muscular hypotonia (13). Serum IgA has been absent in several cases (2).

Oral and facial manifestations. There is usually variable facial dysmorphia. Common are hypertelorism, epicanthal folds, strabismus, and ptosis of lids. The ears are low-set, large, floppy, and poorly formed. The nose is short and broad based and the mouth is wide. The mandible is

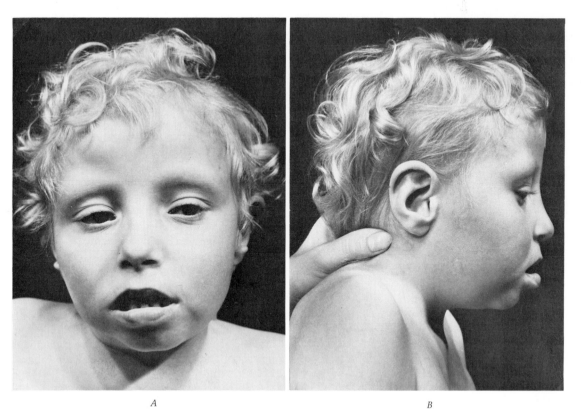

A   B

Figure 21-7. *18q− syndrome.* (*A* and *B*). Midface hypoplasia, deep-set eyes, and prominent antihelix and antitragus in patient with 18r syndrome. (*From J. D. Mürken et al.,* Z. Kinderheilkd. **109:**1, 1970.)

generally small. The neck is short with a low hairline. Dental caries is usually marked.

Among 18p— cases, there is a distinct group exhibiting various degrees of holoprosencephaly (1, 3, 8, 13, 14). Possibly these cases arise from deletion of the normal allele in the heterozygote allowing expression of a recessive holoprosencephalic gene.

18q— SYNDROME

The phenotype is rather distinct (5, 9). Birth weight is generally below 2,700 g. Mental retardation is variable, a few patients having an I.Q. less than 30, others being only mildly retarded. Somatic growth is also retarded. Hypotonia and seizures are frequent. Skin dimples are present over the subacromial area, epitrochlear area, lateral to the patella, and over the knuckles. The fingers are long and tapering. Skeletal anomalies are limited to supernumerary ribs. Congenital heart anomalies are present in over 65 percent of cases. The genitalia are hypoplastic in both sexes, the labia, clitoris, and penis being small. Fingerprint whorls characteristically exceed five in number (6, 7, 15).

Oral and facial manifestations. Most characteristic are midfacial hypoplasia and mild microcephaly. The eyes are deeply set, and there are frequent ocular defects: glaucoma, strabismus, nystagmus, tapetoretinal degeneration, atrophy of optic nerve. The nose is short. A small subcutaneous nodule may be present at the site of cheek dimples. The mouth is carp-shaped. The pinnas are somewhat unusual, the antitragus and antihelix being especially prominent (Fig. 21-7A, B). The ear canals are often atretic. In several cases cleft lip and/or cleft palate have been noted (4). The voice is often husky.

18r SYNDROME

This syndrome exhibits features of both 18p— and 18q— syndrome. Of the approximately 20 described patients, all are mentally retarded and nearly all are microcephalic and hypotonic. Birth weight has been low in about 50 percent. These cases have been reviewed by de Grouchy (5).

Oral and facial manifestations. As in the above-mentioned syndromes, facial alterations have included hypertelorism, epicanthus, carp-shaped mouth, and low-set ears. Cleft palate has been seen in several cases (4).

TRISOMY 21 SYNDROME (DOWN SYNDROME, G₁ TRISOMY SYNDROME)

Trisomy 21 is the most common and well known of all malformation syndromes. More than 100 different signs have been presented in several reviews (6, 38, 43). The reader is referred to the following sources for comprehensive coverage: Penrose and Smith (43) and Benda (7) for general coverage; Hall (28) for pediatric aspects; Cowie (21) for performance; Carter (12) for causes of death; several authors for genetic considerations (42–45); Lilienfeld and Benesch (39) for epidemiology; Kisling (32) for craniofacial aspects; Cohen and Cohen (14) for oral manifestations; and Smith and Wilson (51) for a presentation suitable for the layman, especially for parents of an affected child.

The incidence is reported to vary from approximately one in 600 to one in 700 births. Fifteen percent of patients institutionalized for mental deficiency have trisomy 21 syndrome. Most cases result from nondisjunction associated with increased maternal age at the time of conception. Approximately 4 percent result from reciprocal translocation (D/G, G/G), and fewer than 3 percent are mosaics (12, 43, 44). Frequent causes of death include cardiac anomalies (20 percent), lower respiratory infections, gastrointestinal malformations (8 percent), and acute leukemia (1 percent) (12, 20, 34, 43).

Hall (28) noted 10 common signs in the newborn period, including hypotonia, poor Moro reflex, hyperextensibility of joints, loose skin on nape, flat facial profile, mongoloid obliquity of palpebral fissures, ear anomalies, dysplastic pelvis, clinodactyly of the fifth fingers, and simian creases. At least four of these abnormalities were present in all cases, and six or more were present in 89 percent.

Other common signs include mental deficiency, short stature, brachycephaly, flat occiput, epicanthic folds, Brushfield spots, fine lens opacities, short neck, short broad hands, distal axial triradius, wide gap between the first and second toes, and tibial arch pattern (6, 38, 43).

Cardiovascular anomalies occur in 40 percent of cases (43). Especially common are atrioventricular communis, ventricular septal defect, patent ductus arteriosus, atrial septal defect, and aberrant subclavian artery. Gastrointestinal mal-formations occur in 10 to 18 percent (12, 34). Findings have included tracheoesophageal fistula, pyloric stenosis, duodenal atresia, annular pancreas, Hirschsprung's disease, and imperforate anus (34).

Craniofacial and oral manifestations. Brachycephaly and flat occiput result in a cephalic index which is usually greater than 0.80 and may exceed 1.00 (normal, 0.75 to 0.80) (47). Fontanels are large, and closure is late (43). In the study of Chemke and Robinson (13), a "third fontanel" was noted in all affected patients. Persistent metopic suture is found in 67 percent of males (normal, 8.8 percent) and in 42 percent of females (normal, 12.3 percent) (47). Frontal and sphenoidal sinuses are absent and maxillary sinuses are hypoplastic in over 90 percent of cases (8, 29, 47, 48, 52). Bony midface hypoplasia produces ocular hypotelorism, small nose with flattening of the nasal bridge, and relative mandibular prognathism (9, 25, 27). The nasion-sella-basion angle is increased (10) (Fig. 21-8).

Upward slanting of palpebral fissures and epicanthic folds are common. Other ocular findings include Brushfield spots (85 percent) (Fig. 21-8C), fine lens opacities (50 percent), convergent strabismus (33 percent), nystagmus (15 percent), keratoconus (6 percent), and cataract (1.3 percent) (43).

The ears tend to be small (1). Overlapping of the superior rim of the helix and small or absent lobes are common (28, 43).

The lips are broad, irregular, fissured, and dry in about 65 percent of cases (11). Open mouth with the tongue protruding beyond the lips is observed in over 65 percent. The tongue appears relatively large because of the small oral cavity. That the "large tongue" is relative was demonstrated by Ardran et al. (3). Occasionally, true macroglossia may be present. Fissured tongue is common (about 30 percent). Lingual papillae have been noted to be large even during infancy (14).

The palate is narrower and shorter but not higher than average (49). Radiographically, palatal length averages about 25 mm (normal, 31 ± 3 mm) in the newborn (4). Cleft of the lip and/or palate is present in 0.5 percent (26).

Parotid salivary flow rate is decreased. A significant rise in pH, sodium, calcium, bicar-bonate, uric acid, and nonspecific esterase in pure parotid saliva has been reported (14, 22, 56, 57).

Periodontal disease has been observed in over 90 percent of cases. Severe involvement even below the age of six years is especially common in the mandibular anterior and maxillary molar regions. Exfoliation of lower central incisors from periodontal bone loss occurs frequently. However, calculus formation is neither common nor severe. Necrotizing ulcerative gingivitis has been reported to occur in about 30 percent of patients (9, 16, 30, 33, 53).

The incidence of dental caries has been stated to be low by several authors (9, 14, 41, 55), although these findings have recently been challenged (36).

Eruption of both deciduous and permanent teeth is delayed in 75 percent of cases. An irregular sequence of eruption is common, deciduous first molars sometimes preceding incisors (6, 29, 37, 46, 53).

Missing teeth have been reported in 23 to 47 percent of patients. Third molars, second premolars, and lateral incisors are most frequently absent in the permanent dentition. In 12 to 17 percent of patients, deciduous lateral incisors are absent. Extreme hypodontia and anodontia have been noted occasionally (5, 14, 40, 54).

Microdontia in permanent (24) and macrodontia in deciduous (2) dentitions have been found. Crown-size asymmetry (23) and a gradient of reduction along a mesial to distal axis (17) have been reported. Fusion of a deciduous mandibular lateral incisor with a canine or, less commonly, with a central incisor is a low-frequency finding (6, 11, 14).

Morphologic crown alterations have been reported (14, 18, 35). Almost 50 percent of patients have three or more dental irregularities (35). Peg-shaped maxillary lateral incisors have been observed in 10 percent (5, 14, 15, 18). Enamel hypocalcification has been noted (14, 15).

Irregular alignment of teeth is common. Posterior crossbite, mandibular overjet, mesiocclusion, anterior open bite, crowded teeth, and widely spaced teeth have been discussed by several authors (9, 14, 19, 32).

NONMONGOLOID TRISOMY G

Some of these examples have been designated as trisomy 22, as distinguished from trisomy 21

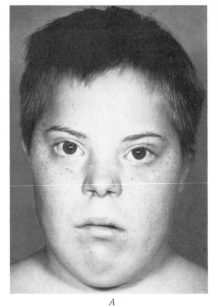

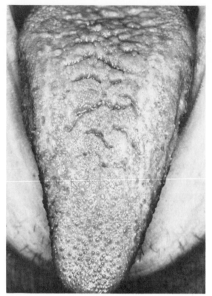

A

B

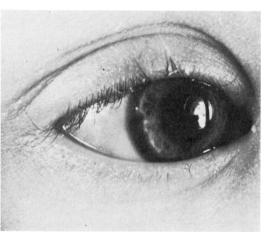

C

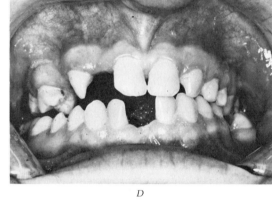

D

Figure 21-8. *Trisomy 21 (Down) syndrome. (A).* Typical facies of child with Down syndrome. *(B).* Fissured tongue present in over 30 percent of Down syndrome patients. *(C).* Brushfield spots. *(D).* Oligodontia. *(E).* Extensive periodontal destruction in 12-year-old Down syndrome patient. *(From M. Bessermann-Nielsen, Copenhagen, Denmark.)*

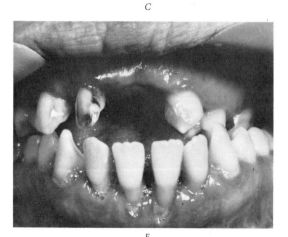

E

(Down syndrome). At this time, within this group, with two possible exceptions, there seems to be no characteristic phenotype, and it would appear likely that some cases may represent centric fragments from several different chromosomes (5–7).

The so-called "cat's-eye syndrome" represents a distinct entity representing 22q+ (2, 8). Several examples have been reported (2–4, 8–11). In addition to anal atresia, rectovaginal fistula,

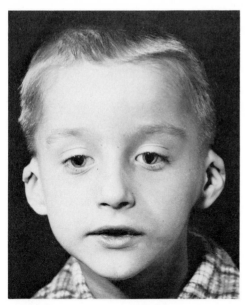

Figure 21-9. *Trisomy 22 syndrome.* Boy with "cat's-eye syndrome." Note iris coloboma and deformed pinnas in mentally retarded child. *(From A. Dollmann and W. Jaeger,* Monatsschr. Kinderheilkd. **116**:144, 1968.)

and coloboma of the iris and choroid, there has been found a wide variety of other anomalies: antimongoloid palpebral fissures, ocular hypertelorism, preauricular fistulas, and various cardiac, genitourinary, and skeletal anomalies (Fig. 21-9). Partial trisomy 22 may be associated with cleft palate (1, 3, 8).

G-DELETION SYNDROMES (21q− and 22q−)
There are at least two relatively distinct phenotypes presumably representing monosomy or deletion of the two different G-group chromosomes. G_1-*deletion syndrome* (antimongolism or 21q− syndrome) consists of mental and somatic retardation, hypertonia, nail anomalies, skeletal malformations, cryptorchism, hypospadias, inguinal hernia, pyloric stenosis, thrombocytopenia, eosinophilia, and hypogammaglobulinemia. Facial and oral manifestations include microcephaly, large low-set ears, antimongoloid obliquity of palpebral fissures, highly arched or cleft palate, cleft lip-palate, and micrognathia. (1–9, 11). There is a marked increase in radial loops (12) (Fig. 21-10A). G_2-*deletion syndrome* or 22q− syndrome has less distinc-

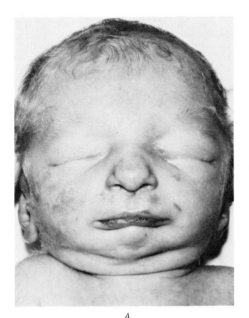

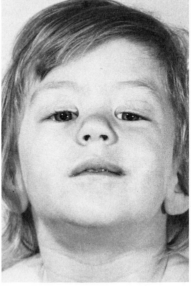

A   B

Figure 21-10. *G-deletion syndromes.* (*A*). *Type I.* In addition to severe mental retardation, child had antimongoloid obliquity of palpebral fissures and broad-based nose. *(From L. E. Reisman et al.,* Lancet **1**:394, 1966.) (*B*). *Type II.* Hypotonia, low-set ears, eyelid ptosis, epicanthal folds. *(From R. G. Weleber et al.* Am. J. Dis. Child. **115**:489, 1968.)

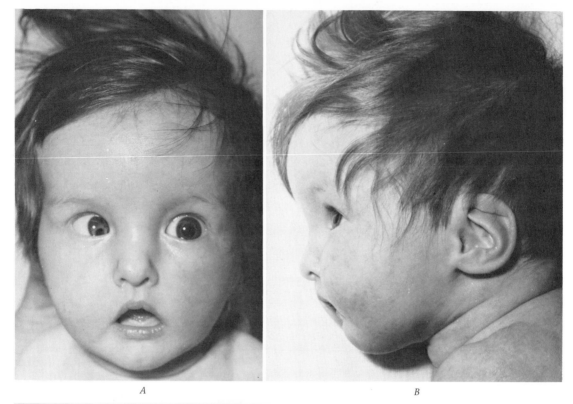

A

B

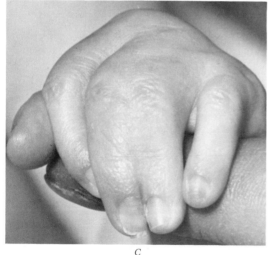

C

Figure 21-11. *Triploidy.* (*A* and *B*). Frontal bossing, coloboma of iris, strabismus, malformed pinna. (*C*). Soft-tissue syndactyly of the third and fourth fingers. (*From W. Schmid and D. Vischer,* Cytogenetics **6**:145, 1967.)

lids, highly arched palate, and bifid uvula (2a, 6, 10, 11, 13, 14, 16). There is a marked increase in whorls and in distal axial triradiuses (12) (Fig. 21-10*B*).

TRIPLOIDY

Triploidy is a frequent cause of fetal wastage prior to the eighth week of intrauterine development (8). Polyploidy is markedly increased in abortuses from pregnancies following discontinuation of oral contraceptives (7). Over 30 cases of triploidy (3, 4, 6, 9, 12, 13, 16, 20–23, 25, 26, 29–34) and diploid/triploid mosaicism (2, 5, 10, 11, 14, 15, 18, 19, 24, 27) have been reported to date. In general, the latter condition is less severe, more compatible with life, and harder to diagnose clinically.

Only two cases of tetraploid mosaicism have

tive features: severe mental retardation, hypotonia, soft-tissue syndactyly of the second and third toes, and clinodactyly of the fifth fingers. Facial and oral manifestations include large, low-set ears, epicanthal folds, ptosis of eye-

been noted. In one instance of tetraploid/diploid mosaicism, microcephaly, closed fontanels, overriding sutures, iris coloboma, aphakia, retinal detachment, two phalanges in each finger, and oligosyndactyly of toes were reported (17). Triple mosaicism for tetraploidy, trisomy 18, and a normal cell line has also been recorded in a six-year-old boy (1).

In triploidy, at birth, the placenta is nearly always large, with hydatidiform degeneration.

Most patients with triploidy or diploid/triploid mosaicism have exhibited low birth weight. Pronounced asymmetry has been observed in diploid/triploid mosaicism and in pure triploidy (10, 11, 14, 15, 20). Hypotonia has been documented in about 60 percent of the cases. Syndactyly of the third and fourth fingers (Fig. 21-11), simian creases, and clubfoot have been noted in at least 60 percent. Camptodactyly of the fifth finger and an increased number of digital whorls have been reported.

Mental deficiency has been noted in most patients. Hydrocephalus, absent corpus callosum, dilated ventricles, large posterior fontanel, lumbosacral meningomyelocele, and less frequently Arnold-Chiari malformation have been reported. Holoprosencephaly has also been noted (34).

The genitalia are frequently small and incompletely formed. Hypospadias, bifid scrotum, cryptorchism, and Leydig cell hyperplasia have been documented frequently. Hydronephrosis, glomerular abnormalities, and adrenal hypoplasia have also been noted. Congenital heart defects, especially ventricular septal defects and atrial septal defects, are common. A variety of other low-frequency findings has been reported.

Craniofacial abnormalities. The posterior fontanel is always large at birth. Asymmetry was restricted to the head in one case of diploid/triploid mosaicism (2). Microphthalmia, iris and choroid colobomas, and mild hypertelorism are seen in 60 to 70 percent of patients. The ears are usually dysplastic and/or low set (Fig. 21-11).

Micrognathia is frequently observed. Isolated cleft palate (12, 16, 18, 24, 28, 33) or cleft lip with or without cleft palate has been noted (22, 28, 31, 33) in about 30 percent of the cases. Oral asymmetry and short tooth crowns have been described (19). Macroglossia has been documented in one instance (25).

SEX CHROMOSOMAL SYNDROMES

XO SYNDROME (TURNER SYNDROME, GONADAL DYSGENESIS)

The syndrome consists of short stature (usually 127 to 147 cm), primary amenorrhea, infantile uterus, infantile vagina and breasts, ovarian agenesis, pterygium colli, cubitus valgus, and low posterior hairline (1–3, 5, 6, 8, 11). The frequency is about 1 per 2,500 female births. Other changes often present include peripheral lymphedema in infancy which usually disappears by the second year, spadelike chest, hypoplastic, at times, inverted nipples, short fourth metacarpals, renal anomalies, coarctation of the aorta, hypoplastic nails, and multiple pigmented nevi (Fig. 21-12A–B). The palmar axial triradius may be distally displaced. Most patients exhibit a neurocognitional defect in space for perception and orientation (10).

Buccal smear reveals a chromatin-negative pattern in most patients. Usually only 45 chromosomes are present, because of loss of one of the X chromosomes. Several variants have been described (2, 3, 9).

Oral and/or facial manifestations. Epicanthal folds, ptosis of the eyelids, prominent ears, and micrognathia are common facial features. Two of the most constant oral findings appear to be a higher than normal bulgy palatal vault which becomes more pronounced with age (6a, 7), and hypoplastic mandible. The corners of the mouth are pulled down by the pterygium colli, producing a characteristic sphinxlike visage. The pterygium of the neck appears in the embryo as neck blisters or hygromas (12). Chronic suppurative otitis with resultant deafness is not uncommon (13).

There is retarded development of the skull in both appositional and sutural growth. This is manifested in the condylar cartilage and in the sphenooccipital synchondrosis.

The teeth may erupt prematurely, the first permanent molars appearing between one and one-half and four years of age (4, 11). The mesial-distal width of the permanent teeth is smaller than normal, and the roots may undergo idiopathic resorption (11). Cleft palate may occur with a somewhat higher than normal frequency (13).

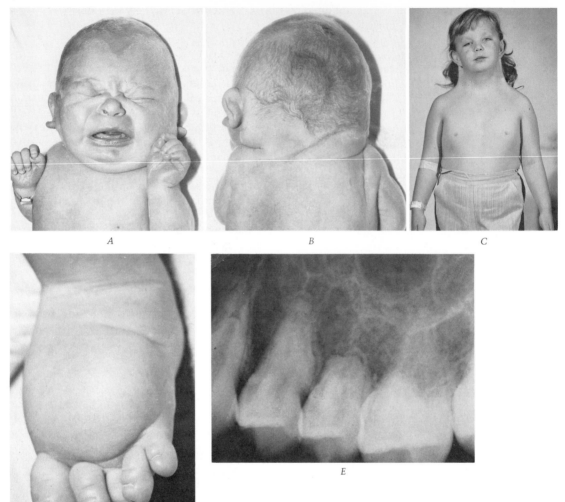

A *B* *C*

D *E*

Figure 21-12. *Turner (XO) syndrome. (A and B).* At birth, excess skin is present at nape rather than pterygium, which develops later. Note protruding pinnas, widely spaced nipples. (*From R. R. Gordon,* Br. Med. J. **1**:483, 1969.) (*C*). Pterygium colli, protruding ears, broad shieldlike chest with small nipples. (*D*). Lymphedema of foot with hypoplastic toenails. (*E*). Hypoplasia and/or resorption of dental roots.

KLINEFELTER SYNDROME AND ITS VARIANTS

Klinefelter syndrome has been found in about 1 percent of mentally retarded institutionalized males, in about 2 per 1,000 males in the general population, and in approximately 10 percent of males manifesting sterility.

The clinical picture may vary, but patients with the XXY syndrome have small testes and, after the age of puberty, aspermatogenesis, eunuchoid build with female pubic escutcheon, variable gynecomastia, and elevated urinary gonadotropin levels. Social, especially sexual, behavior is often deviant. Biopsy of the postpubertal testes demonstrates characteristic tubular hyalinization. Orofacial anomalies, apart from diminished facial hair, have not been associated with the XXY syndrome.

Other variants, including the XXXY and XXXXY syndromes, have been observed, arising from nondisjunction in both the first and second

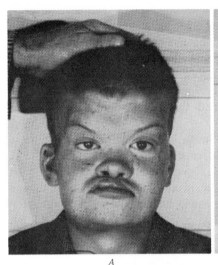
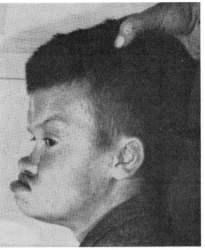

A   *B*

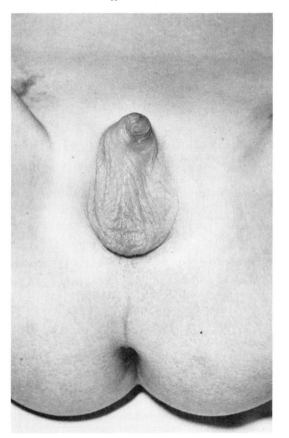

C

Figure 21-13. *Klinefelter (XXXXY) syndrome.* (*A* and *B*). Facies of patient with XXXXY syndrome. Some patients with this syndrome have cleft palate. Marked mandibular growth occurs after puberty. (*Courtesy of H. Schade, Münster.*) (*C*). Micropenis. (*From M. C. Joseph et al.,* J. Med. Genet. **1**:95, 1964.)

meiotic divisions. Individuals with the **XXXXY** syndrome have exhibited the most severe anomalies. These include severe mental retardation, hypotonia, small penis, cryptorchism, very small testes, radioulnar synostosis with reduced ability to pronate the forearm, cubitus valgus, retarded bone age, coxa valga, genu valgum, elongation of distal ulna and proximal radius, hypoplasia of the middle phalanx of the fifth digit, wide proximal ulna, malformed cervical vertebras, pseudo-epiphyses of metacarpals and metatarsals, and pes planus (4, 6, 7a, 9).

Patients with the XXYY variant tend to be taller and more aggressive than those with the XXY type of Klinefelter syndrome (7).

Craniofacial abnormalities. In XXXXY Klinefelter's syndrome there are mild microcephaly, ocular hypertelorism, myopia, strabismus, mild mongoloid obliquity of palpebral fissures, epicanthus, and short neck with redundant skin on the posterior part of the neck. About 5 percent of patients have cleft palate (6) (Fig. 21-13*A–C*). Somewhat similar changes are seen in females with the XXXXX syndrome (3). In infancy the face is often rounded. This, however, disappears with age and midfacial growth is retarded, resulting in a dish face, with relative mandibular prognathism, especially after puberty. We have been impressed by the high frequency of tauro-dontism in the XXXXY syndrome. Some patients with the XXY and XXYY syndrome exhibit mandibular prognathism [7], taurodontism, and shovel-shaped incisors [5].

REFERENCES

1 Bartalos, M., and Baramki, T. A., *Medical Cytogenetics.* Williams & Wilkins, Baltimore, 1967.
2 Bergsma, D. (ed.), Phenotype Aspects of Chromosomal Aberrations. *Birth Defects* **5**(5):1–210, 1969.
3 Gardner, L. I. (ed.), *Endocrine and Genetic Disease of Childhood.* Saunders, Philadelphia, 1969.
4 Gorlin, R. J., Clinical Manifestations of Chromosome Disorders, in J. Yunis (ed.), *Human Chromosome Methodology.* Academic, New York, 1974.
5 Hamerton, J., *Human Cytogenetics.* Academic, New York, 1973.
6 Pfeiffer, R. A., *The Karyotype and the Phenotype of Autosomal Aberrations in Man.* Gustav Fischer Verlag, Stuttgart, 1968.
7 Reisman, L. E., and Matheny, A. P., *Genetics and Counseling in Medical Practice.* Mosby, St. Louis, 1969.
8 Smith, D. W., Autosomal Abnormalities. *Am. J. Obstet. Gynecol.* **90**:1005–1077, 1964.
9 Turpin, R., and Lejeune, J., *Human Afflictions and Chromosomal Aberrations.* Pergamon, Oxford, 1969.
10 Valentine, G. H., *The Chromosome Disorders.* 2d ed., Lippincott, Philadelphia, 1970.

1q+ SYNDROME

1 Berghe, H. van den, et al., Partial Trisomy 1. *Humangenetik* **18**:225–230, 1973.
2 Neu, R. L., and Gardner, L. I., A Partial Trisomy of Chromosome 1 in a Family with a t(1q−; 4p+) Translocation. *Clin. Genet.* **9**:914–918, 1973.
3 Norwood, T. H., and Hoehn, H., Trisomy for the Long Arm of Human Chromosome 1. *Humangenetik* **25**:79–82, 1974.

3p+ SYNDROME

1 Ballesta, F., and Behi, L., Trisomie partielle pour la partie distale du bras court du chromosome 3. *Ann. Génét.* **17**:287–290, 1974.
2 Sachdeva, S., et al., An Unusual Chromosomal Segregation in a Family with a Translocation Between Chromosomes 3 and 12. *J. Med. Genet.* **11**:303–306, 1974.

4p− SYNDROME (WOLF-HIRSCHHORN SYNDROME)

1 Arias, D., et al., Human Chromosomal Deletion—Two Patients with the 4p− Syndrome. *J. Pediatr.* **76**:82–88, 1970.
2 Fryns, J. P., et al., The 4p− Syndrome, with a Report on Two New Cases. *Humangenetik* **19**:99–109, 1973.
3 Hirschhorn, K., et al., Deletion of Short Arms of Chromosome 4–5 in a Child with Defects of Midline Fusion. *Humangenetik* **1**:479–482, 1965.
4 Leão, J. C., et al., New Syndrome Associated with Partial Deletion of Short Arms of Chromosome No. 4. *J.A.M.A.* **202**:434–437, 1967.

5 Miller, O. J., et al., Partial Deletion of the Short Arm of Chromosome No. 5 (5p-): Clinical Studies in Five Unrelated Patients. *J. Pediatr.* **77**:792–801, 1970.
6 Passarge, E., et al., Human Chromosomal Deficiency: The 4p− Syndrome. *Humangenetik* **10**:51–57, 1970.
7 Pfeiffer, R. A., Neue Dokumentation zur Abgrenzung eines Syndroms der Deletion des kurzen Arms eines Chromosoms Nr. 4. *Z. Kinderheilkd.* **102**:49–61, 1968.
8 Taylor, A. I., et al., Short Arm Deletion, Chromosome 4, (4p−), a Syndrome? *Ann. Hum. Genet.* **34**:137–144, 1970.
9 Wilcock, A. R., et al., Deletion of Short Arm of No. 4 (4p−). *J. Med. Genet.* **7**:171–176, 1970.
10 Wilson, M. G., et al., Wolf-Hirschhorn Syndrome Associated with an Unusual Abnormality of Chromosome No. 4. *J. Med. Genet.* **7**:164–170, 1970.
11 Wolf, V., et al., Defizienz an den kurzen Armen eines Chromosoms Nr. 4. *Humangenetik* **1**:397–413, 1965.
12 Zellweger, H., et al., The Short Arm Deletion Syndrome of Chromosome 4 (4p− Syndrome). *Arch. Otolaryngol.* **101**:29–32, 1975.

4p+ SYNDROME

1 Owen, L., Multiple Congenital Defects Associated with Trisomy for the Short Arm of Chromosome 4. *J. Med. Genet.* **11**:291–296, 1974.
2 Rethoré, M. O., et al., La trisomie 4p. *Ann. Génét.* **17**:125–128, 1974.
3 Sartori, A., et al., Familial 4/22 Translocation with Partial Trisomy for the Short Arm of Chromosome 4 in Two Sibs. *Acta Paediatr. Scand.* **63**:631–635, 1974.

5p− (CRI-DU-CHAT) SYNDROME

1 Breg, W. R., et al., The Cri du Chat Syndrome in Adolescents and Adults: Clinical Findings in 13 Older Patients with Partial Deletion of the Short Arms of Chromosome No. 5 (5p−). *J. Pediatr.* **77**:782–791, 1970.
2 de Capoa, A., et al., Translocation Heterozygosis: A Cause of Five Cases of Cri du Chat Syndrome and Two Cases with a Duplication of Chromosome Number Five in Three Families. *Am. J. Hum. Genet.* **19**:586–603, 1967.
3 Gordon, R. R., and Cooke, P., Facial Appearance in Cri-du-Chat Syndrome. *Dev. Med. Child. Neurol.* **10**:69–76, 1968.
4 Mennicken, U., et al., Klinische und cytogenetische Befunde von 7 Patienten mit Cri-du-Chat Syndrom. *Z. Kinderheilkd.* **104**:230–256, 1968.
5 Neuhäuser, G., and Lother, K., Das Katzenschrei Syndrom. *Monatsschr. Kinderheilkd.* **114**:278–280, 1966.
6 Taylor, A. I., Patau's, Edwards' and Cri-du-Chat Syndromes: A Tabulated Summary of Current Findings. *Dev. Med. Child. Neurol.* **9**:76–86, 1967.
7 Warburton, D., and Miller, O. J., Dermatoglyphic Features

of Patients with a Partial Short Arm Deletion of a B Group Chromosome. *Ann. Hum. Genet.* **31**:189–208, 1967.

8 Ward, P. H., et al., The Larynx in the Cri-du-chat (Cat Cry) Syndrome. *Trans. Am. Acad. Ophthalmol. Otolaryngol.* **72**:90–102, 1968.

GROUP C DELETION, TRISOMY, TRISOMY MOSAICISM, AND PARTIAL TRISOMY

1 Alfi, O. S., et al., 46, del (9) (22): A New Deletion Syndrome. *Birth Defects* **10**:27–34, 1974.

2 Bass, H. N., et al., Two Different Chromosome Abnormalities Resulting from a Translocation Carrier Father. *J. Pediatr.* **83**:1034–1038, 1973.

3 Bijlsma, J. B., et al., C8 Trisomy Mosaicism Syndrome. *Helv. Paediat. Acta* **27**:281–288, 1972.

4 Bowen, P., et al., Trisomy 9 Mosaicism in a Newborn Infant with Multiple Malformations. *J. Pediatr.* **85**:95–97, 1974.

5 Caspersson, T., et al., Four Patients with Trisomy 8 Identified by the Fluorescence and Giemsa Banding Techniques. *J. Med. Genet.* **9**:1–7, 1972.

6 Crandall, B. F., et al., The Trisomy 8 Syndrome. *J. Med. Genet.* **11**:393–397, 1974.

7 Falk, R. E., et al., Partial Trisomy of Chromosome 11. *Am. J. Ment. Defic.* **77**:383–388, 1973.

8 Feingold, M., and Atkins, L., A Case of Trisomy 9. *J. Med. Genet.* **10**:184–187, 1973.

9 Fraisse, J., et al., A propos d'un cas de chromosome 9 en anneau. *Ann. Génét.* **17**:175–180, 1974.

10 Haslam, R. H. A., et al., Trisomy 9 Mosaicism with Multiple Congenital Anomalies. *J. Med. Genet.* **10**:180–184, 1973.

11 Jacobsen, P., et al., The Trisomy 8 Syndrome. *Ann. Génét.* **17**:87–94, 1974.

12 Kakati, S., et al., An Attempt to Establish Trisomy 8 Syndrome. *Humangenetik* **19**:293–300. 1973.

13 Lewandowski, R. C., Jr., and Yunis, J. J., New Chromosomal Syndromes. *Am. J. Dis. Child.* **129**:515–529, 1975.

14 Moore, C. M., et al., Developmental Abnormalities Associated with a Ring Chromosome 6. *J. Med. Genet.* **10**:299–303, 1973.

15 Podruch, P. E., and Weisskopf, B., Trisomy for the Short Arms of Chromosome 9 in Two Generations, with Balanced Translocations t(15p+; 9q−) in Three Generations. *J. Pediatr.* **85**:92–95, 1974.

16 Rethoré, M. O., et al., Analyse de la trisomie 9p par denaturation menagée. *Humangenetik* **18**:129–138, 1973.

17 Rott, H. D., et al., C11/D13 Translocation in Four Generations. *Humangenetik* **14**:300–305, 1972.

18 Roux, C., et al., Trisomie partielle 10q par translocation familiale t(10q−; 22p+). *Ann. Génét.* **16**:59–62, 1974.

19 Sanchez, O., et al., Partial Trisomy 11 in a Child Resulting from a Complex Maternal Rearrangement of Chromosomes 11, 12, and 13. *Humangenetik* **22**:59–65, 1974.

20 Schwanitz, G., et al., Partial Trisomy 9 in the Case of Familial Translocation 8/9 mat. *Ann. Génét.* **17**:163–166, 1974.

21 Talvik, T., et al., Inherited Translocation in Two Families: t(14q+; 10q−) and t(13q−; 21q+). *Humangenetik* **19**:215–226, 1973.

22 Tuncbilek, E., et al., Trisomy 8 Syndrome. *Humangenetik* **23**:23–30, 1974.

23 Turleau, C., et al., Trisomie 9p: deux nouvelles observations. *Ann. Génét.* **17**:167–174, 1974.

24 Vogel, W., et al., Partial Trisomy 7q. *Ann. Génét.* **16**:227–230, 1973.

25 Wright, Y. M., et al., Craniorachischisis in a Partially Trisomic 11 Fetus in a Family with Reproductive Failure and a Reciprocal Translocation t(6p+; 11q−). *J. Med. Genet.* **11**:69–75, 1974.

26 Zaremba, J., et al., Four Cases of 9p Trisomy Resulting from a Balanced Familial Translocation (9; 15) (q13; q11). *J. Ment. Defic. Res.* **18**:153–190, 1974.

TRISOMY 13 SYNDROME

1 Conen, P. E., and Erkman, B., Frequency and Occurrence of Chromosomal Syndromes. I. D-Trisomy. *Am. J. Hum. Genet.* **18**:374–386, 1966.

1a Escobar, J. I., et al., Trisomy for the Distal Segment of Chromosome 13: a New Syndrome. *Am. J. Dis. Child.* **128**:217–220, 1974.

2 Fujimoto, A., et al., Trisomy 13 in Two Infants with Cyclops. *J. Med. Genet.* **10**:294–296, 1973.

3 James, A. E., et al., Trisomy 13–15. *Radiology* **92**:44–49, 1969.

4 Magenis, R. E., et al., Trisomy 13 (D₁) Syndrome: Studies on Parental Age, Sex Ratio and Survival. *J. Pediatr.* **73**:222–228, 1968.

5 Schinzel, A., et al., Different Forms of Incomplete Trisomy 13 Mosaicism and Partial Trisomy for the Proximal and Distal Long Arm. *Humangenetik* **22**:287–298, 1974.

6 Smith, D. W., The 18 Trisomy and 13 Trisomy Syndromes. *Birth Defects* **5**(5):67–71, 1969.

7 Snodgrass, G., et al., The D (13–15) Trisomy Syndrome. *Arch. Dis. Child.* **41**:250–261, 1966.

8 Taylor, A. I., Autosomal Trisomy Syndromes. *J. Med. Genet.* **5**:227–252, 1968.

9 Warkany, J., et al., Congenital Malformations in Autosomal Trisomy Syndromes. *Am. J. Dis. Child.* **112**:502–517, 1966.

10 Yu, F., Trisomy 13 in Chinese Children: Clinical Findings and Incidence. *J. Med. Genet.* **7**:132–137, 1970.

13q− AND 13r SYNDROMES

1 Cagianut, B., and Theiler, K., Bilateral Coloboma of Iris and Choroid, Association with Partial Deletion of a Chromosome of Group D. *Arch. Ophthalmol.* **83**:141–144, 1970.

2 Coffin, G. S., and Wilson, M. G., Ring Chromosome D (13). *Am. J. Dis. Child.* **119**:370–373, 1970.

3 Grace, E., et al., The 13 q− Deletion Syndrome. *J. Med. Genet.* **8**:351–357, 1971.

4 Lejeune, J., et al., Le phenotype Dr. Etude de trois cas de chromosomes D en anneau. *Ann. Génét.* **11**:79–87, 1968.

5 Masterson, J. G., A Malformation Syndrome with Ring D Chromosome. *J. Irish Med. Assoc.* **61**:398–399, 1968.

6 Niebuhr, E., and Ottosen, J., Ring Chromosome D (13) Associated with Multiple Congenital Malformations. *Ann. Génét.* **16**:157–166, 1973.

7 Sparkes, R. S., et al., Absent Thumbs with a Ring D₂ Chromosome: A New Deletion Syndrome. *Am. J. Hum. Genet.* **19**:644–659, 1967.

8 Taylor, A. I., Dq—, Dr and Retinoblastoma. *Humangenetik* **10:**209–217, 1970.

9 Thompson, H., and Lyons, R. B., Retinoblastoma and Multiple Congenital Anomalies Associated with Complex Mosaicism with Deletion of D— Chromosome and Probably D/C Translocation. *Hum. Chrom. Newsl.* **15:**21, 1965.

10 Tolksdorf, M., et al., Die Symptomatik von Ringchromosomen der D— Gruppe. *Arch. Kinderheilkd.* **181:**282–295, 1970.

11 Wilson, M. G., et al., Retinoblastoma and Deletion D (14) Syndrome. *J. Med. Genet.* **6:**322–324, 1969.

TRISOMY 18 SYNDROME

1 Butler, L. J., et al., No. E (16–18) Trisomy Syndrome: Analysis of 13 Cases. *Arch. Dis. Child.* **40:**600–611, 1965.

2 Gorlin, R. J., et al., Facial Clefting and Its Syndromes. *Birth Defects* 7(7):3–49, 1971.

3 Smith, D. W., Autosomal Abnormalities. *Am. J. Obstet. Gynecol.* **90:**1055–1077, 1964.

4 Taylor, A. I., Autosomal Trisomy Syndromes: A Detailed Study of 27 Cases of Edwards' Syndrome and 27 Cases of Patau's Syndrome. *J. Med. Genet.* **5:**227–252, 1968.

5 Warkany, J., et al., Congenital Malformations in Autosomal Trisomy Syndromes. *Am. J. Dis. Child.* **112:**502–517, 1966.

18p—, 18q—, 18r SYNDROMES

1 Dumars, K. W., et al., Median Facial Cleft Associated with Ring E Chromosome. *J. Med. Genet.* **7:**86–90, 1970.

2 Fischer, P., et al., Autosomal Deletion Syndrome: 46, XX, 18p—: A New Case Report with Absence of IgA in Serum. *J. Med. Genet.* **7:**91–98, 1970.

3 Gorlin, R. J., et al., Short Arm Deletion of Chromosome 18 in Cebocephaly. *Am. J. Dis. Child.* **115:**453–476, 1968.

4 Gorlin, R. J., et al., Facial Clefting and Its Syndromes. *Birth Defects* 7(7):3–49, 1971.

5 Grouchy, J. de., The 18p—, 18q—, and 18r Syndromes. *Birth Defects* 5(5):74–87, 1969.

6 Law, E. M., and Masterson, J. G., Familial 18q— Syndromes. *Ann. Génét.* 215–222, 1969.

7 Lurie, I., and Lazjuk, G., Partial Monosomies 18. *Humangenetik* **15:**203–222, 1972.

8 McDermott, A., et al., Arrhinencephaly Associated with a Deficiency Involving Chromosome 18. *J. Med. Genet.* **5:**60–67, 1968.

9 Parker, C. E., et al., The Syndrome Associated with Partial Deletion of the Long Arms of Chromosome 18 (18q—). *Calif. Med.* **117**(4):65–71, 1972.

10 Parker, C. E., et al., A Short Retarded Child with Deletion of the Short Arm of Chromosome 18 (18p—). *Clin. Pediatr.* **12:**42–46, 1973.

11 Nitowsky, H. M., et al., Partial 18 Monosomy in the Cyclops Malformation. *Pediatrics* **37:**260–269, 1966.

12 Pfeiffer, R. A., Deletion der kurzen Arme des Chromosoms Nr. 18. *Humangenetik* **2:**178–185, 1966.

13 Schinzel, A., et al., Structural Aberrations of Chromosome 18. I. The 18p— Syndrome. *Arch. Genet.* **47:**1–15, 1974.

14 Uchida, I. A., Familial Short Arm Deficiency of Chromosome 18 Concomitant with Arrhinencephaly and Alopecia Congenita. *Am. J. Hum. Genet.* **17:**410–419, 1965.

15 Wolf, U., et al., Deletion on Long Arm of Chromosome 18 (46, XX, 18q—). *Humangenetik* **5:**70–72, 1967.

TRISOMY 21 SYNDROME

1 Aase, J. M., et al., Small Ears in Down's Syndrome: A Helpful Diagnostic Aid. *J. Pediatr.* **82:**845–847, 1973.

2 Alexandersen, V., *The Odontometrical Variation of the Deciduous and Permanent Teeth in Down's Syndrome.* Thesis, Wisconsin, Madison, 1970.

3 Ardran, G. M., et al., Tongue Size in Down's Syndrome. *J. Ment. Defic. Res.* **16:**160–166, 1972.

4 Austin, J. H. M., et al., Short Hard Palate in Newborn: Roentgen Sign of Mongolism. *Radiology* **92:**775–776, 1969.

5 Barkla, D. H., Congenital Absence of Permanent Teeth in Mongols. *J. Ment. Defic. Res.* **10:**198–203, 1966.

6 Barkla, D. H., Eruption of Permanent Teeth in Mongols. *J. Ment. Defic. Res.* **10:**190–197, 1966.

7 Benda, C. E., *Down's Syndrome. Mongolism and Its Management.* Grune & Stratton, New York, 1969.

8 Betlejewski, S., et al., Radiologische Untersuchungen der Entwicklung der Nasennebenhölen im Down-Syndrom. *Ann. Paediatr. (Basel)* **203:**355–362, 1964.

9 Brown, R. H., and Cunningham, W. M., Some Dental Manifestations of Mongolism. *Oral Surg.* **14:**664–676, 1961.

10 Burwood, R. J., et al., The Skull in Mongolism. *Clin. Radiol.* **24:**475–480, 1973.

11 Butterworth, T., et al., Cheilitis of Mongolism. *J. Invest. Dermatol.* **35:**347–351, 1960.

12 Carter, C. O., A Life-Table for Mongols with the Causes of Death. *J. Ment. Defic. Res.* **2:**64–74, 1958.

13 Chemke, J., and Robinson, A., The Third Fontanelle. *J. Pediatr.* **75:**617–622, 1969.

14 Cohen, M. M., Sr., and Cohen, M. M., Jr., The Oral Manifestations of Trisomy G$_1$ (Down's Syndrome). *Birth Defects* 7(7):241–251, 1971.

15 Cohen, M. M., and Winer, R. A., Dental and Facial Characteristics in Down's Syndrome (Mongolism). *J. Dent. Res.* **44:**197–208, 1965.

16 Cohen, M. M., et al., Oral Aspects of Mongolism. Periodontal Disease in Mongolism. *Oral Surg.* **14:**92–107, 1961.

17 Cohen, M. M., et al., Crown-size Profile Pattern in Trisomy G. *J. Dent. Res.* **49:**460, 1970.

18 Cohen, M. M., et al., Abnormalities of the Permanent Dentition in Trisomy G. *J. Dent. Res.* **49:**1386–1393, 1970.

19 Cohen, M. M., et al., Occlusal Disharmonies in Trisomy G (Down's Syndrome, Mongolism). *Am. J. Orthodont.* **58:**367–372, 1970.

20 Conen, P. E., and Erkman, B., Combined Mongolism and Leukemia. *Am. J. Dis. Child.* **112:**429–443, 1966.

21 Cowie, V. A., *A Study of the Early Development of Mongols.* Pergamon, Oxford, 1970.

22 Cutress, T. W., Composition, Flow-rate and pH of Mixed and Parotid Saliva from Trisomic and Other Mentally Retarded Subjects. *Arch. Oral Biol.* **17:**1081–1094, 1972.

23 Garn, S. M., et al., Increased Crown-size Asymmetry in Trisomy G. *J. Dent. Res.* **49:**465, 1970.

24 Geciauskas, M. A., and Cohen, M. M., Mesiodistal Crown Diameters of Permanent Teeth in Down's Syndrome (Mongolism). *Am. J. Ment. Defic.* **74:**563–567, 1970.

25 Gerald, B. E., and Silverman, F. N., Normal and Abnormal Interorbital Distances with Special Reference to Mongolism. *Am. J. Roentgenol.* **95:**154–161, 1965.

26 Gorlin, R. J., et al., Facial Clefting and Its Syndromes. *Birth Defects* 7(7):3–49, 1971.

27 Gosman, S. D., Facial Development in Mongolism. *Am. J. Orthodont.* **37:**332–349, 1951.

28 Hall, B., Mongolism in Newborns: A Clinical and Cytogenetic Study. *Acta Paediatr. Scand.*, suppl. **154:**1–95, 1964.

29 Jensen, G. M., Dentoalveolar Morphology and Developmental Changes in Down's Syndrome. *Am. J. Orthodont.* **64:**607–618, 1973.

30 Johnson, N. P., and Young, M. A., Periodontal Disease in Mongols *J. Periodont.* **34:**41–47, 1963.

31 Johnson, N. P., et al., Tooth Ring Analysis in Mongolism. *Aust. Dent. J.* **10:**282–286, 1965.

32 Kisling, E., *Cranial Morphology in Down's Syndrome: A Roentgenocephalometric Study in Adult Males.* Munksgaard, Copenhagen, 1966.

33 Kisling, E., and Krebs, G., Periodontal Conditions in Adult Patients with Mongolism (Down's Syndrome). *Acta Odontol. Scand.* **21:**391–405, 1963.

34 Knox, G. E., and ten Bensel, R. W., Gastrointestinal Malformations in Down's Syndrome. *Minn. Med.* **55:**542–544, 1972.

35 Kraus, B. S., et al., Mental Retardation and Abnormalities of the Dentition. *Am. J. Ment. Defic.* **72:**905–917, 1968.

36 Kroll, R. G., et al., Incidence of Dental Caries and Periodontal Disease in Down's Syndrome. *N.Y. State Dent. J.* **36:**151–156, 1970.

37 Kučera, J., Age at Walking, Age at Eruption of Deciduous Teeth and Response to Ephedrine in Children with Down's Syndrome. *J. Ment. Defic. Res.* **13:**143–148, 1969.

38 Levinson, A., et al., Variability of Mongolism. *Pediatrics* **16:**43–54, 1955.

39 Lilienfeld, A. M., and Benesch, C. H., *Epidemiology of Mongolism.* Johns Hopkins, Baltimore, 1969.

40 MacGillivrary, R. C., Anodontia in Mongolism. *Br. Med. J.* **2:**282, 1966.

41 McMillan, R. S., Relation of Human Abnormalities of Structure and Function to Abnormalities of the Dentition. II. Mongolism. *J. Am. Dent. Assoc.* **63:**368–373, 1961.

42 Mikkelsen, M., and Stene, J., Genetic Counselling in Down's Syndrome. *Hum. Hered.* **20:**457–464, 1970.

43 Penrose, L. S., and Smith, L. S., *Down's Anomaly.* Little, Brown, Boston, 1966.

44 Pergament, E., Inheritance of Down's Syndrome: Fact and Theory. *Lancet* **1:**93, 1970.

45 Richards, B. W., et al., Cytogenetic Survey of 225 Patients Diagnosed Clinically as Mongols. *J. Ment. Defic. Res.* **9:**245–259, 1965.

46 Roche, A. F., and Barkla, D. H., The Eruption of Deciduous Teeth in Mongols. *J. Ment. Defic. Res.* **8:**54–65, 1964.

47 Roche, A. F., et al., Growth Changes in the Mongoloid Head. *Acta Paediatr. Scand.* **50:**133–140, 1961.

48 Roche, A. F., et al., Non-metrical Observations on Cranial Roentgenogram in Mongolism. *Am. J. Roentgenol.* **85:**659–662, 1961.

49 Shapiro, B. L., et al., The Palate and Down's Syndrome. *N. Engl. J. Med.* **276:**1460–1463, 1967.

50 Shapiro, B. L., Prenatal Dental Anomalies in Mongolism: Comments on the Basis and Implications of Variability. *Ann. N.Y. Acad. Sci.* **171:**562–577, 1970.

51 Smith, D. W., and Wilson, A. A., *The Child with Down's Syndrome (Mongolism).* Saunders, Philadelphia, 1973.

52 Spitzer, R., et al., A Study of the Abnormalities of the Skull, Teeth, and Lenses in Mongolism. *Can. Med. Assoc. J.* **84:**567–572, 1961.

53 Swallow, J. N., Dental Diseases in Children with Down's Syndrome. *J. Ment. Defic. Res.* **8:**102–118, 1964.

54 Thomas, D., Anodontia in Mongolism. *Br. J. Psychiatr.* 566–568, 1939.

55 Winer, R. A., and Cohen, M. M., Dental Caries in Mongolism. *Dent. Prog.* **2:**217–219, 1962.

56 Winer, R. A., and Feller, R. P., Composition of Parotid and Submandibular Saliva and Serum in Down's Syndrome. *J. Dent. Res.* **51:**449–454, 1972.

57 Winer, R. A., et al., Composition of Human Saliva, Parotid Gland Secretory Rate, and Electrolyte Concentration in Mentally Retarded Persons. *J. Dent. Res.* **44:**632–634, 1965.

NONMONGOLOID TRISOMY G

1 Bass, H., et al., Probable Trisomy 22 Identified by Fluorescent and Trypsin-Giemsa Banding. *Ann. Génét.* **16:**189–192, 1973.

2 Bühler, E., et al., Cat's Eye Syndrome, a Partial Trisomy 22. *Humangenetik* **15:**150–162, 1972.

3 Freedom, R. M., and Gerald, P. S., Congenital Cardiac Disease and the "Cat's Eye" Syndrome. *Am. J. Dis. Child.* **126:**16–18, 1973.

4 Gerald, P. S., et al., A Novel Syndrome Basis for Imperforate Anus (the "Cat's Eye Syndrome"). *Pediatr. Res.* **2:**297, 1968.

5 Goodman, R. M., et al., The Question of Trisomy 22 Syndrome. *J. Pediatr.* **79:**174–175, 1971.

6 Gustavson, K., et al., Three Non-Mongoloid Patients of Similar Phenotype with an Extra G-like Chromosome. *Clin. Genet.* **3:**135–146, 1972.

7 Hsu, L., et al., Trisomy 22, a Clinical Entity. *J. Pediatr.* **79:**12–19, 1971.

8 Peterson, R. A., Schmid-Fraccaro Syndrome (Cat's Eye Syndrome). *Arch. Ophthalmol.* **90:**287–291, 1973.

9 Schachenmann, G., et al., Chromosomes in Coloboma and Anal Atresia. *Lancet* **2:**290, 1965.

10 Thomas, C., Un syndrome rare, atteinte colobomateuse du globe oculaire, atrésie anale, anomalies congénitales multiples et presence d'un chromosome surnumeraire. *Ann. Ocul. (Paris)* **202:**1021–1031, 1969.

11 Weber, F. M., et al., Anal Atresia, Eye Anomalies and an Additional Small Abnormal Acrocentric Chromosome (47,XX, mar+). *J. Pediatr.* **76:**594–597, 1970.

G-DELETION SYNDROMES

1 Böhm, R., and Fuhrmann, W., Lebensfähigkeit bei Monosomie G. *Monatsschr. Kinderheilkd.* **117:**184–187, 1969.

2 Crandall, B. F., et al., Identification of 21r and 22r Chromosomes by Quinacrine Fluorescence. *Clin. Genet.* **3:**264–270, 1972.

2a De Cicco, F., et al., Monosomy of Chromosome 22. *J. Pediatr.* **83:**836–838, 1973.

3 Emberger, J. M., et al., Monosomie 21 avec mosaique 45, XX, 21/46, XX, 21 pi. *Arch. Fr. Pédiatr.* **27:**1069–1080, 1970.

4 Endo, A., et al., Antimongolism Syndrome. *Br. Med. J.* **4:**148–149, 1969.

5 Hall, B., et al., A Case of Monosomy G? *Hereditas* **57:**356–366, 1967.

6 Kelch, R. P., et al., Group G Deletion Syndromes. *J. Med. Genet.* **8:**341–345, 1971.

7 Lejeune, J., et al., Monosomie partielle pour un petit acrocentrique. *C. R. Acad. Sci. (D) (Paris)* **259:**4187–4190, 1964.

8 Mikkelsen, M., and Vestermark, S., Karyotype 45, XX, −21/46, XX, 21q− in an Infant with Symptoms of G-deletion Syndrome I. *J. Med. Genet.* **11**:389–393, 1974.

9 Reisman, L. E., et al., Anti-mongolism: Studies in an Infant with a Partial Monosomy of the 21 Chromosome, *Lancet* **1**:394–397, 1966.

10 Reisman, L. E., et al., A Child with Partial Deletion of a G-group Autosome, *Am. J. Dis. Child.* **114**:336–339, 1967.

11 Schulz, J., and Krmpotic, E., Monosomy G Mosaicism in Two Unrelated Children (Case 1 — Type 1, Case 2 — Type II). *J. Ment. Defic. Res.* **12**:255–268, 1968.

12 Schindeler, J. D., and Warren, R. J., Dermatoglyphics in the G-deletion Syndromes. *J. Ment. Defic. Res.* **17**:149–156, 1973.

13 Stoll, C., et al., Chromosome 22 en anneau r (22): identification par denaturation thermique ménagés. *Ann. Génét.* **16**:193–198, 1973.

14 Warren, R. J., and Rimoin, D. L., The G Deletion Syndromes. *J. Pediatr.* **77**:658–663, 1970.

15 Weber, F. M., et al., Anal Atresia, Eye Anomalies and an Additional Small Abnormal Acrocentric Chromosome (47, XX, mar+). *J. Pediatr.* **76**:594–597, 1970.

16 Weleber, R. G., et al., Ring-G Chromosome, a New G-Deletion Syndrome? *Am. J. Dis. Child.* **115**:489–493, 1968.

17 Zellweger, H., et al., Two Cases of Multiple Malformations with an Autosomal Chromosomal Aberration — Partial Trisomy D? *Helv. Paediatr. Acta* **17**:290–300, 1962.

TRIPLOIDY

1 Atnip, R. L., and Summitt, R. L., Tetraploidy and 18-trisomy in a Six-year-old Triple Mosaic Boy. *Cytogenetics* **10**:305–317, 1971.

2 Berghe, H. van den, Triploid-diploid Mosaicism in the Lymphocytes of a Liveborn Child with Multiple Malformations. *Humangenetik* **11**:16–21, 1970.

3 Bernard, R., et al., Triploidie chromosomique chez un nouveau-né "polymalforme." *Ann. Génét.* **10**:70–74, 1965.

4 Bernard, R., et al., Polymalformation chez un nouveau-né presentant une triploidie chromosomique. *Pédiatrie* **22**:721–722, 1967.

5 Böök, J. D., and Santesson, B., Malformation Syndrome in Man Associated with Triploidy (69 Chromosomes). *Lancet* **1**:858, 1960.

6 Butler, L. J., et al., A Liveborn Infant with Complete Triploidy (69,XXX). *J. Med. Genet.* **6**:413–421, 1969.

7 Carr, D. H., Chromosome Studies in Selected Spontaneous Abortions. I. Conception after Oral Contraceptives. *Can. Med. Assoc. J.* **103**:343–348, 1970.

8 Carr, D. H., et al., Chromosome Studies in Selected Spontaneous Abortion: Polyploidy in Man. *J. Med. Genet.* **8**:164–174, 1971.

9 Edwards, J. H., et al., Three Cases of Triploidy in Man. *Cytogenetics* **6**:81–104, 1967.

10 Ellis, J. R., et al., A Girl with Triploid Cells. *Nature* **198**:411, 1963.

11 Ferrier, P., et al., Congenital Asymmetry Associated with Diploid-triploid Mosaicism and Large Satellites. *Lancet* **1**:80, 1964.

12 Finley, W. H., et al., Triploidy in a Liveborn Male Infant. *J. Pediatr.* **81**:855–856, 1972.

13 Henriksson, P., et al., A Liveborn Triploid Infant. *Acta Paediatr. Scand.* **63**:447–449, 1974.

14 Jenkins, M. E., et al., Congenital Asymmetry and Diploid-Triploid Mosaicism. *Am. J. Dis. Child.* **122**:80–84, 1971.

15 Johnston, A. W., and Penrose, L. S., Congenital Asymmetry. *J. Med. Genet.* **3**:77–85, 1966.

16 Keutel, J., et al., Triploidie (69,XXY) bei einem lebend geborenen Kind. *Z. Kinderheilkd.* **109**:104–117, 1970.

17 Kohn, G., et al., Tetraploid-diploid Mosaicism in a Surviving Infant. *Pediatr. Res.* **1**:461–469, 1967.

18 Lejeune, J., et al., Chimere 46, XX/69, XXY. *Ann. Génét.* **10**:188–192, 1967.

19 Nicolas, G., Myxodiploidia in a Young Child: Its Effect on Orodental Anatomy. *Rev. Fr. Odontostomatol.* **16**:97–108, 1969.

20 Niebuhr, E., et al., Triploidy in Man: Cytogenetical and Clinical Aspects. *Humangenetik* **21**:103–126, 1974.

21 Papiernik-Berkhauser, E., Enfant triploide à terme et thérapeutique hormonale. *Bull. Féd. Soc. Gynecol. Obstet. Lang. Fr.* **20**:248, 1968.

22 Paterson, W. G., et al., Two Cases of Hydatidiform Degeneration of the Placenta with Fetal Abnormality and Triploidy Chromosome Constitution. *J. Obstet. Gynaecol. Br. Commonw.* **78**:136–142, 1971.

23 Prats, J., et al., Triploid Live Full-term Infant. *Helv. Paediatr. Acta* **26**:164, 1971.

24 Sacrez, R., et al., La triploidie chez l'enfant. *Pédiatrie* **22**:267–275, 1967.

25 Schindler, A. M., and Mikamo, K., Triploidy in Man: Report of a Case and a Discussion on Etiology. *Cytogenetics* **9**:116–130, 1970.

26 Schmickel, R. D., et al., A Live Born Infant with 69 Chromosomes. *J. Pediatr.* **79**:97–103, 1971.

27 Schmid, W., and Vischer, D., A Malformed Boy with Double Aneuploidy and Diploid-triploid Mosaicism 48, XXYY/71, XXXYY. *Cytogenetics* **6**:145–155, 1967.

28 Shepard, T. H., et al., Chromosomal Aberrations in Two Embryos from the Same Mother. *Am. J. Obstet. Gynecol.* **102**:48–52, 1968.

29 Simpson, J. L., et al., Triploidy (69, XXY) in a Liveborn Infant. *Ann. Génét.* **15**:103, 1972.

30 Sparrevohn, S., et al., A Case of Live Born Triploidy. *Nord. Med.* **85**:90–91, 1971.

31 Tarkkanen, A., Ocular Pathology in Triploidy (69, XXY). *Ophthalmologica* **163**:90–97, 1971.

32 Uchida, I. A., et al., Identification of Triploid Genome by Fluorescence Microscopy. *Science* **176**:304–305, 1972.

33 Walker, S., et al., Three Further Cases of Triploidy in Man Surviving to Birth. *J. Med. Genet.* **10**:135–141, 1973.

34 Zergollern, L., et al., A Liveborn Infant with Triploidy (69, XXX). *Z. Kinderheilkd.* **112**:293–300, 1972.

TURNER'S SYNDROME

1 Baker, D. H., et al., Turner's Syndrome and Pseudo-Turner's Syndrome. *Am. J. Roentgenol.* **100**:40–47, 1967.

2 Engel, E., and Forbes, A. P., Cytogenetic and Clinical Findings in 48 Patients with Congenitally Defective or Absent Ovaries. *Medicine* **44**:135–164, 1965.

3 Ferguson-Smith, M. A., Karyotype-Phenotype Correlations in Gonadal Dysgenesis and Their Bearing on the Pathogenesis of Malformations. *J. Med. Genet.* **2**:142–155, 1965.

4 Filipsson, R., et al., Time of Eruption of the Permanent Teeth, Cephalometric and Tooth Measurement and Sul-

phation Factor Activity in 45 Patients with Turner's Syndrome with Different Types of X Chromosome Aberrations. *Acta Endocrinol. (Kbh.)* **48:**91–113, 1965.

5 Gordon, R. R., Turner's Infantile Phenotype. *Br. Med. J.* **1:**483–485, 1969.

6 Greenblatt, R. B., et al., The Spectrum of Gonadal Dysgenesis. *Am. J. Obstet. Gynecol.* **98:**151–172, 1967.

6a Horowitz, S. L., and Morishima, A., Palatal Abnormalities in the Syndrome of Gonadal Dysgenesis and its Variants and in Noonan's Syndrome. *Oral Surg.* **38:**839–844, 1974.

7 Johnson, R., and Baghdady, V. S., Maximum Palatal Height in Patients with Turner's Syndrome. *J. Dent. Res.* **48:**472–476, 1969.

8 Lemli, L., and Smith, D. W., The XO Syndrome. A Study of the Differentiated Phenotype in 25 Patients. *J. Pediatr.* **63:**577–588, 1963.

9 Lindsten, J., *The Nature of Origin of X Chromosome Aberrations in Turner's Syndrome: A Cytogenetical and Clinical Study of 57 Patients.* Almquist and Wiksells Press, Uppsala, 1963.

10 Money, J., et al., Visual-Constructional Deficit in Turner's Syndrome. *J. Pediatr.* **69:**126–127, 1966.

11 Silver, H., and Dodd, S. G., Gonadal Dysgenesis. *Am. J. Dis. Child.* **94:**702–707, 1957.

12 Singh, R. P., Hygroma of the Neck in XO Abortuses. *Am. J. Clin. Pathol.* **53:**104–107, 1970.

13 Szpunar, J., and Rybak, M., Middle Ear Disease in Turner's Syndrome. *Arch. Otolaryngol.* **87:**34–40, 1968.

KLINEFELTER SYNDROME AND ITS VARIANTS

1 Becker, K. L., et al., Klinefelter's Syndrome: Clinical and Lab Findings in 50 Patients. *Arch. Intern. Med.* **118:**314–321, 1966.

2 Christensen, M. F., and Therkelsen, A. J., A Case of the XXXXY Chromosome Anomaly with 4 Maternal X Chromosomes and Diabetic Glucose Tolerance. *Acta Paediatr. Scand.* **59:**706–710, 1970.

3 Dallapiccola, B., and Pistocchi, G., Alterazioni scheletriche in un caso di rara aberrazione cromosomica. *Radiol. Med.* **54:**737–750, 1968.

4 Houston, C. S., Roentgen Findings in the XXXXY Chromosome Anomaly. *J. Can. Assoc. Radiol.* **18:**258–267, 1967.

5 Keeler, C., Taurodont Molars and Shovel Incisors in Klinefelter's Syndrome. *J. Hered.* **64:**234–236, 1973.

6 Sacrez, R., et al., Dysgénesie gonadosomatique. XXXXY. *Arch. Fr. Pédiatr.* **22:**41–52, 1965.

7 Schlegel, R. J., et al., A Boy with XXYY Chromosome Constitution. *Pediatrics* **36:**113–119, 1965.

7a Simpson, J. L., et al., Abnormalities of Human Sex Chromosomes. *Humangenetik* **21:**301–308, 1974.

8 Terheggen, H. G., et al., Das XXXXY Syndrom. Bericht über 7 neue Fälle und Literaturübersicht. *Z. Kinderheilkd.* **115:**209–234, 1973.

9 Zaleski, W. A., et al., The XXXXY Chromosome Anomaly: Report of Three New Cases and Review of 30 Cases from the Literature. *Can. Med. Assoc. J.* **94:**1143–1154, 1966.

10 Zollinger, H., Das XXXY Syndrom. *Helv. Paediatr. Acta* **24:**589–599, 1969.

22

Facial Clefts and Associated Anomalies

Before cleft-palate syndromes are considered, the epidemiologic and genetic aspects of isolated cleft lip and cleft palate will be reviewed. Readers who wish to examine the subject in greater detail should consult the papers of Drillien et al. (7), Fraser (10), and Gorlin et al. (12).

Clefts of the primary and/or secondary palates are included among the more common congenital anomalies. Clinically, there is great variability in the degree of cleft formation. The minimal degrees of involvement include such anomalies as bifid uvula, linear lip indentations or so-called "intrauterine healed clefts," and submucous cleft of the soft palate.

A cleft may involve only the upper lip or may extend to involve the nostril and the hard and soft palates. Isolated palatal clefts may be limited to the uvula (bifid uvula) or they may be more extensive, cleaving the soft palate or both the soft and hard palates.

A combination of cleft lip and cleft palate is most common. The breakdown according to type has differed somewhat in several large surveys. Roughly, however, cleft lip-cleft palate comprises about 50 percent of the cases, with cleft lip and isolated cleft palate constituting about 25 percent each.

CLEFT LIP WITH OR WITHOUT CLEFT PALATE

Cleft lip with or without cleft palate would appear to occur in about 1 per 1,000 Caucasian births (range 0.6 to 1.3), although data differ somewhat from study to study. Fogh-Andersen (8) indicated that the incidence appears to be increasing in Denmark, probably because of declining postnatal mortality, decreasing operative mortality, steadily improving operative results, and attendant increase in marriage and child-bearing.

The prevalence is higher in Orientals (about 1.7 per 1,000 births) (25, 29) and lower among Afro-Americans (approximately 1 per 2,500 births) (1, 4). The frequency of cleft lip and/or palate in Amerindians must surely be the highest of any group in the world (over 3.6 per 1,000 live births). In general, the more severe the defect, the greater the proportion of males affected (i.e., cleft lip-cleft palate greater than cleft lip and bilateral cleft greater than unilateral cleft) (8, 14). However, not all races have similar sex predilections. Kobayashi (18) analyzed Japanese data on facial clefts and pointed out that for isolated cleft lip the Japanese differ significantly from Caucasians by demonstrating a slight female excess. However, for cleft lip with cleft palate and isolated cleft palate, the same sex predominance noted in Caucasians was also observed in Japanese. These findings have been confirmed by Sanui (31) and Kurozumi (19).

Among Afro-Americans, if all forms of facial clefts are considered, more clefts of all types are found in the female (14, 30). This is in direct contrast to other races, in which summation of total clefts indicates a male predominance.

Isolated cleft lip may be unilateral or bilateral

(approximately 20 percent). When unilateral, the cleft is more common on the left side (about 70 percent), although no more extensive (38). Lips are somewhat more frequently cleft bilaterally (approximately 25 percent) when combined with cleft palate. Cleft lip-palate is more common in males (about 2:1). About 85 percent of cases of bilateral cleft lip and 70 percent of unilateral cleft lip are associated with cleft palate.

Cleft lip is not always complete (i.e., extending into the nostril). In about 10 percent of the cases, the cleft is associated with skin bridges (Simonart's bands).

ISOLATED CLEFT PALATE

Isolated cleft palate appears to be a separate entity from cleft lip with or without cleft palate. This has been demonstrated by several authors (7a, 8, 37). Sibs of patients with cleft lip with or without cleft palate have an increased frequency of the same anomaly but not of isolated cleft palate, and vice versa.

The incidence of isolated cleft palate among Caucasians and Afro-Americans (4, 11) would appear to be between 1 per 2,000 and 1 per 2,500 births (7). Gordon et al. (11) found a relative excess of cleft palate in the so-called Cape Colored of South Africa. It may be somewhat more frequent in Orientals (26, 27). Lowry and Renwick (21), however, studying British Columbia Indians, found a relatively infrequent occurrence of isolated cleft palate (14 percent) versus cleft lip-palate (78 percent). Isolated cleft palate is more common in females.

When the number of cases of cleft palate is broken down according to extent, a 2:1 female predilection for complete clefts of the hard and soft palates is clearly indicated, while the ratio approaches 1:1 for clefts of the soft palate only (8, 17, 23, 24).

Cleft uvula appears to be an incomplete form of cleft palate (33). However, the incidence of cleft uvula (1 per 80 Caucasian individuals) is much higher than that for cleft palate (1 per 2,500 births). Like cleft of the soft palate, cleft uvula approaches a 1:1 sex ratio (22).

The frequency of cleft uvula among various Amerindian and Inuit groups is high, ranging from 1 per 9 to 1 per 14 individuals (3, 15a, 16, 16a). In Afro-Americans, it is extremely rare (1 per 300) (30, 32).

Congenital pharyngeal incompetence, in which the patient has cleft-palate speech without an overt cleft, is associated with bifid or absent uvula or a short soft palate in over 80 percent of the patients. The remainder have a thin soft palate or increased depth of the nasopharynx.

Submucous palatal cleft refers to the condition in which there is an imperfect muscle union across the velum but an intact mucosal surface. The palate is usually short and velopharyngeal closure is incompetent, resulting in hypernasal speech. However, great variation occurs (5). There is usually a deficiency or notch in the bone at the posterior edge of the hard palate, and often there is a bifid uvula.

Approximately 30 percent of the patients with submucous palatal cleft described by Gylling and Soivio (15) had bifid uvula, and over 60 percent had palates considered to be short, with poor mobility demonstrated in 20 percent.

Among the collective cases of submucous palatal cleft presented by Calnan (2) and Gylling and Soivio (15), over 50 percent occurred in males, an unusual finding since isolated cleft palate is decidedly more common in females. Stewart et al. (36), studying 10,000 school children in Denver, Colorado, found an incidence of 1 per 1,200.

RISK

The risk for the occurrence of clefts of the lip and/or palate in a child ranges from 1 in 2,500 for isolated cleft palate in the random population to somewhat less than 1 in 2 for cleft lip and/or cleft palate in association with congenital pits or fistulas of the lower lip.

In the vast majority of cases, the cleft is either isolated or associated with a constellation of anomalies that do not form a recognizable syndromal pattern. Well-defined cleft syndromes perhaps contribute only a small percentage of the cases. However, all efforts must be made to recognize a cleft syndrome, since the pattern of inheritance may be a simple one and the genetic risk for future affected children may then be quite predictable.

However, in the event of failure to recognize such a pattern, we must resort to risk figures based on pooled data. These have been calculated by several authors (6, 37, 38) and are summarized in Tables 22-1 to 22-6. In the use of such tables, it should be borne in mind that the data apply only to risks for similar anomalies (i.e., a parent with isolated cleft palate has no greater risk of having a child with cleft lip-cleft palate than anyone else, and vice versa). The parents and relatives of an affected individual should also be examined carefully for even such

Table 22-1. Frequency of cleft lip and/or palate in sibs of propositi with and without associated anomalies

Propositi	Total no. of sibs	% affected
Females without associated anomalies	503	5.17
Females with associated anomalies	75	1.33
Males without associated anomalies	849	4.00
Males with associated anomalies	147	1.36
Total without associated anomalies	1,352	4.44
Total with associated anomalies	222	1.35

SOURCE: Courtesy of C. M. Woolf, modified from *J. Med. Genet.* **8**:65–83, 1971.

Table 22-2. Frequency of CL(P) (cleft lip and/or palate) with bilateral and unilateral CL(P)

Propositi	Total no. of sibs	% affected
Female–bilateral	128	8.59
Female–unilateral	195	4.10
Male–bilateral	200	5.50
Male–unilateral	405	3.70
Total–bilateral	328	6.71
Total–unilateral	600	3.83

SOURCE: Courtesy of C. M. Woolf, modified from *J. Med. Genet.* **8**:65–83, 1971.

Table 22-3. Frequency of cleft lip and/or palate in sibs of male and female propositi

Propositi	Total no. of sibs	% affected
Females	578	4.67
Males	996	3.61

SOURCE: Courtesy of C. M. Woolf, modified from *J. Med. Genet.* **8**:65–83, 1971.

Table 22-4. Influence of family history of CL(P) (cleft lip and/or palate) on frequency of CL(P) in sibs of propositi

Family history	Total no. of sibs	% affected
None	848	2.24
Occurrence of CL(P) in fourth-degree relative	298	3.69
Occurrence of CL(P) in third-degree relative	87	6.90
Occurrence of CL(P) in second-degree relative	111	9.91
Occurrence of CL(P) in parent	45	15.55

SOURCE: Courtesy of C. M. Woolf, modified from *J. Med. Genet.* **8**:65–83, 1971.

Table 22-5. Frequency of isolated cleft palate (CP) in families of patients with this anomaly

Relatives	Frequency, %
Sibs when neither parent has CP	1.96
Sibs when one parent has CP	13.64
Parents	1.48
Children	8.70
Grandparents	0.18
Aunts and uncles	0.32
First cousins	0.09

SOURCE: Courtesy of C. M. Woolf, modified from *J. Med. Genet.* **8**:65–83, 1971.

minor stigmata as bifid uvula, submucous cleft, or velo-pharyngeal insufficiency.

Woolf et al. (37, 38) have demonstrated that the risk of transmission to the offspring is en-

Table 22-6. Recurrence risk for clefts

		CL(P), %	CP, %
Normal parents:			
Affected sibs	Normal sibs		
1	0	4.0	3.5
1	1	4.0	3.0
2	0	14.0	13.0
One parent affected:			
Affected sibs	Normal sibs		
0	0	4.0	3.5
1	0	12.0	10.0
1	1	10.0	9.0
2	0	25.0	24.0
Both parents affected:			
Affected sibs	Normal sibs		
0	0	35.0	25.0
1	0	45.0	40.0
1	1	40.0	35.0
2	0	50.0	45.0

SOURCE: Derived from M. Tolarová, Empirical recurrence risk figures for genetic counseling of clefts. *Acta Chir. Plast.* (Praha) **14**:234–235, 1972.

hanced if the affected parent is the mother. Furthermore, the risk of having a second affected child is increased also if the first affected sib is female and/or if a close relative has a similar anomaly (39).

Within recent years there has been increasing evidence that facial clefting is multifactorial (i.e., caused by many factors, both genetic and environmental) (3, 10, 12, 39). The rates of closure of the primary and secondary palates are quasi-continuous variables, and a threshold exists beyond which an individual is, by definition, affected. Rarely, X-linked inheritance has been demonstrated (20).

Twin studies have indicated the role of genetic and nongenetic influences in cleft production. Especially comprehensive reviews on clefting in twins are those of Metrakos et al. (25) and Gorlin et al. (12).

In twins with cleft lip-palate, concordance is far greater in monozygotic twins (35 percent) than in dizygotic twins (7 percent). In twins with isolated cleft palate, concordance is less different in the two groups (monozygotic, 28 percent; dizygotic, 10 percent), a fact that would suggest a somewhat greater genetic basis for cleft lip-cleft palate than for isolated cleft palate.

ASSOCIATED ANOMALIES

Many investigators have tabulated the frequency and types of anomalies that accompany facial clefts (12). Data secured at birth differ from those on patients who have undergone surgery, since those with more serious defects often succumb prior to surgery. When the data are broken down according to subtype, there is general agreement that isolated cleft palate (13 to 50 percent) is far more often associated with other congenital defects than either isolated cleft lip (7 to 13 percent) or cleft lip with cleft palate (2 to 11 percent) (3, 10, 13, 14, 17, 35).

More malformations have been found in infants with bilateral cleft lip, with or without cleft palate, than in those with unilateral cleft lip. The more malformations a child had, the lighter the birth weight (13). Associated anomalies are more frequently noted in patients without a familial history of clefts than in patients with affected relatives. Congenital palatopharyngeal incompetence has been noted to be frequently associated with cervical spine anomalies (28).

REFERENCES

1 Altemus, L. A., The Incidence of Cleft Lip and Palate among North American Negroes. *Cleft Palate J.* **3**: 357–361, 1966.

2 Calnan, J., Submucous Cleft Palate. *Br. J. Plast. Surg.* **6**: 264–282, 1954.

3 Červenka, J., and Shapiro, B., Cleft Uvula in Chippewa Indians: Prevalence and Genetics. *Hum. Biol.* **42**:47–52, 1970.

4 Chung, C. E., and Myrianthopoulos, N. C., Racial and Prenatal Factors in Major Congenital Malformations. *Am. J. Hum. Genet.* **20**:44–60, 1968.

5 Crickelair, G. F., et al., The Surgical Treatment of Submucous Cleft Palate. *Plast. Reconstr. Surg.* **45**:58–65, 1970.

6 Curtis, E. J., et al., Congenital Cleft Lip and Palate. *Am. J. Dis. Child.* **102**:853–857, 1961.

6a Dahl, E., Craniofacial Morphology in Congenital Clefts of the Lip and Palate. *Acta Odontol. Scand.* **28,** suppl. **57:**1–167, 1970.

7 Drillien, C. M., et al., *The Causes and Natural History of Cleft Lip and Palate.* E. & S. Livingstone, Edinburgh, 1966.

7a Emanuel, I., et al., The Further Differentiation of Cleft Lip and Palate: A Population Study of Clefts in King County, Washington, 1956–1965. *Teratology* **7:**231–282, 1973.

8 Fogh-Andersen, P., *Inheritance of Harelip and Cleft Palate.* Nyt Nordisk Forlag, Copenhagen, 1942.

9 Fogh-Andersen, P., Incidence of Cleft Lip and Palate Constant or Increasing? *Acta Chir. Scand.* **122:**106–111, 1961.

10 Fraser, F. C., The Genetics of Cleft Lip and Cleft Palate. *Am. J. Hum. Genet.* **22:**336–352, 1970.

11 Gordon, H., et al., Cleft Lip and Palate in Cape Town. *S. Afr. Med. J.* **43:**1267–1268, 1969.

12 Gorlin, R. J., et al., Facial Clefting and Its Syndromes. *Birth Defects* **7**(7):3–49, 1971.

13 Greene, J. C., et al., Epidemiologic Study of Cleft Lip and Cleft Palate in Four States. *J. Am. Dent. Assoc.* **68:**387–404, 1964.

14 Greene, J. C., et al., Utilization of Birth Certificates in Epidemiologic Studies of Cleft Lip and Palate. *Cleft Palate J.* **2:**141–156, 1965.

15 Gylling, U., and Soivio, A. I., Submucous Cleft Palate; Surgical Treatment and Results. *Acta Chir. Scand.* **129:**282–287, 1965.

15a Heathcote, G. M., The Prevalence of Cleft Uvula in an Inuit Population. *Am. J. Phys. Anthropol.* **41:**433–437, 1974.

16 Jaffe, B. F., and De Blanc, G. B., Cleft Palate, Cleft Lip and Cleft Uvula in Navajo Indians. *Cleft Palate J.* **7:**301–305, 1970.

16a Jarvis, A., and Gorlin, R. J., Minor Facial Abnormalities in an Eskimo Population. *Oral Surg.* **33:**417–427, 1972.

17 Knox, F., and Braithwaite, F., Cleft Lips and Palates in Northumberland and Durham. *Arch. Dis. Child.* **38:**66–70, 1963.

18 Kobayashi, Y., A Genetic Study of Harelip and Cleft Palate. *Jap. J. Hum. Genet.* **3:**73–107, 1958.

19 Kurozumi, S., et al., A Genetic Study of Harelip and Cleft Palate. *Jap. J. Hum. Genet.* **8:**120–127, 1963.

20 Lowry, R. B., X-linked Cleft Palate. *Birth Defects* **7**(7):76–79, 1971.

21 Lowry, R. B., and Renwick, D. H. G., Incidence of Cleft Lip and Palate in British Columbia Indians. *J. Med. Genet.* **6:**67–69, 1969.

22 Meskin, L. H., et al., Abnormal Morphology of the Soft Palate. I. The Prevalence of Cleft Uvula. *Cleft Palate J.* **1:**324–346, 1964.

23 Meskin, L. H., et al., An Epidemiologic Investigation of Factors Related to the Extent of Facial Clefts. *Cleft Palate J.* **5:**23–29, 1968.

24 Meskin, L. H., and Pruzansky, S., Epidemiologic Relationship of Age of Parents to Type and Extent of Facial Clefts. *Acta Chir. Plast.* **10:**249–259, 1968.

25 Metrakos, J. D., et al., Clefts of the Lip and Palate in Twins. *Plast. Reconstr. Surg.* **22:**109–122, 1958.

26 Neel, J. V., A Study of Major Congenital Defects in Japanese Infants. *Am. J. Hum. Genet.* **10:**398–445, 1958.

27 Niswander, J., and Adams, M. S., Oral Clefts in the American Indians. *Public Rep. (Wash.)* **82:**807–812, 1967.

28 Osborne, G. S., et al., Upper Cervical Spine Anomalies and Osseous Nasopharyngeal Depth. *J. Speech Disord.* **14:**14–22, 1971.

29 Rank, B. K., and Thomson, J. A., Cleft Lip and Palate in Tasmania. *Med. J. Aust.* **47**(2):681–689, 1960.

30 Richardson, E. R., Cleft Uvula: Incidence in Negroes. *Cleft Palate J.* **7:**669–672, 1970.

31 Sanui, Y., Clinical Statistics and Genetics on the Cleft Lip and Cleft Palate. *Jap. J. Hum. Genet.* **7:**194–233, 1962.

32 Schaumann, B. F., et al., Minor Craniofacial Anomalies among a Negro Population. *Oral Surg.* **29:**566–575, 1970.

33 Shapiro, B., et al., Cleft Uvula, a Microform of Facial Clefts and Its Genetic Basis. *Birth Defects* **7**(7):80–82, 1971.

34 Shields, E. D., et al., A Study of Facial Clefts in Danish Twins, *Proc. 2d Int. Cong. Cleft Palate, 1973,* Copenhagen, p. 200.

35 Spriestersbach, D. C., et al., Incidence of Clefts of the Lip and Palate in Families with Children with Clefts and Families with Children without Clefts. *Plast. Reconstr. Surg.* **29:**392–401, 1962.

36 Stewart, J., et al., Submucous Cleft Palate. *Birth Defects* **7**(7):64–66, 1971.

37 Woolf, C. M., et al., A Genetic Study of Cleft Lip and Palate in Utah. *Am. J. Hum. Genet.* **15:**209–215, 1963.

38 Woolf, C. M., et al., Cleft Lip and Heredity, *Plast. Reconstr. Surg.* **34:**11–14, 1964.

39 Woolf, C. M., Congenital Cleft Lip: A Genetic Study of 496 Propositi. *J. Med. Genet.* **8:**65–83, 1971.

23

Cleft Lip-Palate and Congenital Lip Fistulas

The first report of congenital fistulas of the lower lip appears to be that of Demarquay (4) in 1845. Since that time over 450 cases have been reported. A large percentage of these patients have also manifested cleft lip or palate, or both. Hilgenreiner (7) in 1924, Ludy and Shirazy (9) in 1938, and Watanabe et al. (23) in 1951 carried out extensive reviews and analyses of the published cases.

The hereditary pattern seems to be that of an autosomal dominant gene with penetrance estimated to be that of about 80 percent (2, 20, 22). Červenka et al. (2), in their genetic analysis of cases published prior to 1966, could find no evidence of sex predilection. The reader is referred to their article for purposes of genetic counseling.

SYSTEMIC MANIFESTATIONS

Manifestations of the syndrome, apart from the oral or facial areas, are unusual.

Extremities. Bilateral talipes equinovarus, or clubfoot (5, 14, 18, 19), and syndactyly (3, 11, 14) have been reported, as well as popliteal pterygia (19) (see Chap. 25).

Other findings. Ankyloblepharon and symblepharon have been described in association with this condition (12, 13). These patients, however, may have had mild expression of the *pop-liteal pterygium syndrome.* Accessory nipples were observed by Pohl (14).

Oral manifestations. Usually, bilateral, symmetrically placed depressions are observed on the vermilion portion of the lower lip, one on each side of the midline. These dimples are circular, or they may be transverse slits (Fig. 23-1). Upon occasion, they may be located at the apex of nipple-like elevations. Rarely, these elevations may fuse in the midline, producing a snoutlike structure (13). The depressions represent blind sinuses that descend through the orbicularis oris muscle to a depth of 0.5 to 2.5 cm and communicate with the underlying minor salivary glands through their excretory ducts. These fistulas often transport a viscid saliva to the surface, either spontaneously or upon pressure.

The fistulas may be so small as barely to permit a hair probe, or they may be as large as 3 mm or more. Nipple-like processes occasionally occur without demonstrable fistulas (8, 21, 24).

Although usually bilateral and symmetrically placed, variations may be seen, such as an asymmetric single pit (8, 10, 15, 21, 23), central single pit (15, 16, 21), or pits of the upper lip and frenum (9).

Sicher and Pohl (17) and Warbrick et al. (22) suggested that the congenital fistulas arise from arrested development, i.e., persistence of a median and/or lateral sulcus or sulci which normally are evanescent structures. These median

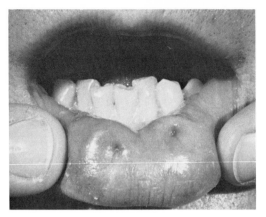

Figure 23-1. *Cleft lip-palate and congenital lip fistulas.* Paramedian pits of lower lip may occur as an isolated finding or combined with cleft lip and/or cleft palate.

and lateral grooves appear in the 5- to 6-mm embryo and disappear at the 10- to 16-mm stage (Fig. 23-2). It should be pointed out that the grooves disappear at about the same time that fusion occurs between several facial processes. This probably accounts for the simultaneous occurrence of pits and facial clefts. An extremely rare but, in the opinion of the authors, related anomaly consists of the bilateral lower-lip clefts observed by Abramson (1). In his patient, epi-palatus was also found.

About 70 percent of patients with lower-lip pits have associated cleft lip, cleft palate, or both. Červenka et al. (2) estimated the frequency of the syndrome to be 1:75,000 to 1:100,000 in the white population.

Adhesions between maxilla and mandible (syngnathia) have been described (12).

Schneider (16a) reported associated absence of maxillary and mandibular second premolars.

DIFFERENTIAL DIAGNOSIS

Because of the variable expressivity, affected family members may exhibit only pits, clefts without pits or a combination of pits and clefts.

The chances of transmitting cleft lip-palate differ drastically according to whether this stigma is associated with lip pits or is an isolated phenomenon. Lip pits may occur in the *popliteal pterygium syndrome.*

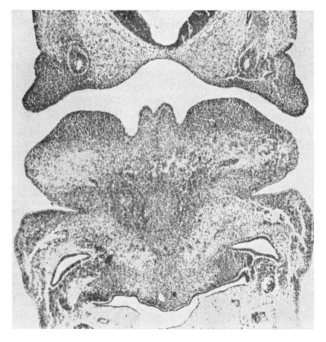

Figure 23-2. Photomicrograph of 7.5-mm embryo demonstrating three invaginations in mandibular process. These disappear by the 14-mm stage. (*From J. G. Warbrick et al.,* Br. J. Plast. Surg. **4**:254, 1952.)

LABORATORY AIDS

None is known.

REFERENCES

1 Abramson, P. D., Bilateral Congenital Clefts of the Lower Lip. *Surgery* **31**:761-764, 1952.
2 Červenka, J., et al., The Syndrome of Pits of the Lower Lip and Cleft Lip and/or Palate: Genetic Considerations. *Am. J. Hum. Genet.* **19**:416-432, 1967.
3 Colman, J., Congenital Double Lip: Record of a Case with a Note on the Embryology. *Br. J. Plast. Surg.* **5**:197-202, 1952-1953.
4 Demarquay, J. N., Quelques considérations sur le bec-de-lièvre. *Gaz. Med. (Paris)* **13**:52-53, 1845.
5 Hamilton, E., Congenital Deformity of the Lower Lip. *Dublin J. Med. Sci.* **72**:1-2, 1881.
6 Heiner, H., and Leutert, G., Zur Klinik und Genese der kongenitalen Unterlippenfisteln. *Arch. Klin. Chir.* **299**:775-788, 1962.
7 Hilgenreiner, H., Die angeborenen Fisteln bzw: Schleimhauttaschen der Unterlippe. *Dtsch. Z. Chir.* **188**:273-309, 1924.
8 Koberg, W., Zur Kenntnis der kongenitalen Unterlippenfisteln. *Oest. Z. Stomatol.* **63**:60-74, 1966.
9 Ludy, J. B., and Shirazy, E., Concerning Congenital Fistulae of the Lips; Their Mooted Significance; Review of the Literature; and Report of a Family with Congenital Fistulae of the Lower Lip. *N. Int. Clin.* **3**:75-88, 1938.
10 Madelung, Zwei seltene Missbildung des Gesichtes. *Arch. Klin. Chir.* **37**:271-277, 1888.
11 Murray, J., cited by Hilgenreiner (7), *Br. Foreign Med. Chir. Rev.* **26**:502-523, 1860.
12 Neuman, Z., and Shulman, J., Congenital Sinuses of the Lower Lip. *Oral Surg.* **14**:1415-1420, 1961.
13 Oberst, –, Über die angeborenen Unterlippenfisteln. *Beitr. Klin. Chir.* **68**:795-801, 1910.
14 Pohl, L., Letter to the Editor. *Dent. Pract. Dent. Rec.* **7**:112, 1956.
15 Ruppe, C., and Magdelaine, J., Fistules muqueuse congénitales des lèvres. *Rev. Stomatol. (Paris)* **29**:1-8, 1927.
16 Sato, K., Three Cases of Congenital Fistulas of the Lower Lip. *Jap. J. Orthop.* **13**:581-584, 1938.
16a Schneider, E. L., Lip Pits and Congenital Absence of Second Premolars. Varied Expression of the Lip Pits Syndrome. *J. Med. Genet.* **10**:346-349, 1973.
17 Sicher, H., and Pohl, L., Zur Entstehung des menschlichen Unterkiefers (ein Beitrag zur Entstehung des Unterlippenfisteln). *Oest. Z. Stomatol.* **32**:552-560, 1934.
18 Taylor, W. B., and Lane, D. K., Congenital Fistulas of the Lower Lip: Associations with Cleft Lip-Palate and Anomalies of the Extremities. *Arch. Dermatol.* **94**:421-424, 1966.
19 Trélat, U., Sur un vice conformation très rare de la lèvre-inférieure. *J. Méd. Chir. Prat.* **40**:442-445, 1869.
20 Van der Woude, A., Fistula Labii Inferioris Congenita and Its Association with Cleft Lip and Palate. *Am. J. Hum. Genet.* **6**:244-256, 1954.
21 Wange, M. K. H., and Macomber, W. B., Congenital Lip Sinuses. *Plast. Reconstr. Surg.* **18**:319-328, 1956.
22 Warbrick, J. G., et al., Remarks on the Etiology of Congenital Bilateral Fistulae of Lower Lip. *Br. J. Plast. Surg.* **4**:254-262, 1952.
23 Watanabe, Y., et al., Congenital Fistulas of the Lower Lip. *Oral Surg.* **4**:709-722, 1951.
24 Zeller, O., cited by Ludy and Shirazy (9).

Cleft Lip-Palate, Lobster-Claw Deformity, and Nasolacrimal Duct Obstruction

(Ectrodactyly-Ectodermal Dysplasia-Clefting (EEC) Syndrome)

The syndrome of (a) lobster-claw deformity of the hands and feet, (b) nasolacrimal duct obstruction, and (c) cleft lip-palate was possibly first described by Eckoldt and Martens (10) in 1804. Another early case is that of Cruveilhier (9).

Although most cases have been isolated examples, there have been affected sibs (1, 20, 23, 33) with normal parents, and several cases in which the disorder has been transmitted from a parent to one or more children (37). The syndrome appears to have autosomal dominant inheritance with incomplete penetrance and variable expressivity (8, 24, 35), although we cannot rule out a recessive form. Some evidence suggests genetic heterogeneity (26).

SYSTEMIC MANIFESTATIONS

Facies. The facies is characterized by cleft lip, dacrocystitis, keratoconjunctivitis, tearing, and photophobia. The scalp hair, lashes, and eyebrows may be sparse.

Extremities. The lobster-claw deformity (ectrodactyly) usually involves all four extremities, but there have been exceptions (8) (Fig. 24-1A). Occasionally there has been some degree of soft-tissue syndactyly (1), especially of the toes. Among 19 patients with lobster-claw deformity, Barsky (2) found three with cleft lip-palate.

Eyes. Absent lacrimal punctas have been noted in most cases (Fig. 24-1B). This is associated with tearing, blepharitis, dacrocystitis, keratoconjunctivitis, and photophobia (8, 18, 22, 28, 31–37). Primary telecanthus has been observed (5). There is a reduction in the number of meibomian orifices (23).

Skin. An albinoid alteration in the skin and hair has been noted by Pashayan et al. (23) and in a few other cases (1, 5, 27). The scalp hair, eyebrows, and lashes have been sparse (28). The nails may be hypoplastic and brittle (5). Skin biopsy has shown an absence of sebaceous glands (23). Several patients have had numerous pigmented nevi.

Central nervous system. Microcephaly and mental retardation were described in several cases (1, 3, 5, 12, 14, 19, 23, 31). Conduction deafness was noted by Hillman and Fraser (16), Pashayan et al. (23), and others (5, 7a, 18, 23, 24a, 26a).

Other findings. Inguinal hernia (17) and kidney and ureter malformations (absent kidney, hydronephrosis, hydroureter) (1, 6, 14, 18, 21, 22, 27, 33) have been described. Gehler and Grosse (14) and we have noted cryptorchism.

Oral manifestations. Cleft lip-palate, more often bilateral, has been described in many cases but has been absent in others (15, 23, 37). Lack

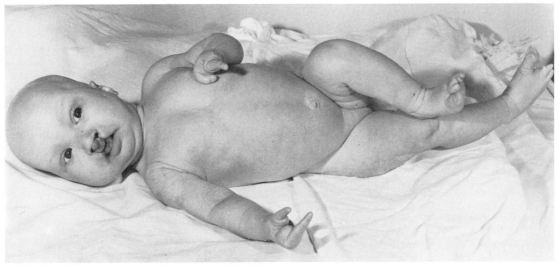

A

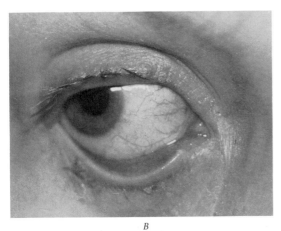

B

Figure 24-1. *Cleft lip-palate, lobster-claw deformity, and nasolacrimal duct obstruction. (A), Bilateral cleft lip-palate and ectrodactyly. (From R. A. Rüdiger et al., Am. J. Dis. Child. 120:160, 1970.) (B), Absence of lacrimal point.*

of permanent incisors was described (3, 7a, 31, 33), as well as anodontia, severe oligodontia, or enamel hypoplasia (5, 7, 12, 15, 32, 34, 35). Xerostomia and deeply furrowed tongue have also been noted. The mucous membranes are predisposed to cardidosis (23).

DIFFERENTIAL DIAGNOSIS

Isolated ectrodactyly has been observed to follow autosomal dominant transmission. The syndrome of *cleft lip-palate, hypohidrosis, thin wiry hair,* and *dystrophic nails* also has autosomal dominant inheritance. The syndrome of *cleft lip-palate, tetraperomelia, deformed pinnas, and ectodermal dysplasia* appears to follow an autosomal recessive mode of inheritance. Finally, the syndrome of *craniosynostosis, symmetrically malformed extremities, and cleft lip-palate* bears some resemblance to the EEC syndrome.

Though lacrimal duct obstruction occurs in 1 to 6 percent of the general childhood population, it has been found with an increased frequency–of about 10 percent–in the cleft lip-palate population (36).

Reed et al. (26) described a mother and daughter with ectrodactyly, lacrimal duct obstruction, early graying of the hair with pili torti, subtotal alopecia, and atrophic pigmented macules on the extensor surfaces of the body.

LABORATORY AIDS

None is known.

REFERENCES

1 Ahrens, K., Chromosomale Untersuchungen bei craniofacialen Missbildungen (Cases 3A, B). *H.N.O.* **15**:106–109, 1967.

2 Barsky, A. J., Cleft Hand: Classification, Incidence and Treatment. *J. Bone Joint Surg.* **46A**:1707–1720, 1961.

3 Berendt, H., Case Report of Partial Anodontia Connected with Missing and Stunted Phalanges of Hands and Feet. *Oral Surg.* **1**:283–290, 1948.

4 Berndorfer, A., Gesichtsspalten gemeinsam mit Hand- und Fussspalten. *Z. Orthop.* **107**:344–354, 1970.

5 Bixler, D., et al., The Ectrodactyly-Ectodermal Dysplasia–Clefting (EEC) Syndrome. *Clin. Genet.* **3**:43–51, 1971.

6 Brill, C. B., et al., The Syndrome of Ectrodactyly, Ectodermal Dysplasia and Cleft Lip and Palate. *Clin. Genet.* **3**:293–302, 1972.

7 Brunn, C., Et tilfaelde af dysplasia acro-dentalis. *Tandlaegebladet* **72**:162–167, 1968.

7a Bystrom, E. B., et al., The Syndrome of Ectrodactyl Ectodermal Dysplasia and Clefting (EEC). *J. Oral Surg.* **33**:192–198, 1975.

8 Cockayne, E. A., Cleft Palate, Hare Lip, Dacrocystitis and Cleft Hand and Feet. *Biometrika* **28**:60–63, 1936.

9 Cruveilhier, J., *Anatomie pathologique du corps humaine. Maladies des extremites.* Vol. II, part 38. S. Bailliere, Paris, 1829–1842.

10 Eckoldt, J. G., and Martens, F. H., *Über eine sehr komplicierte Hasenscharte.* Steinacker, Leipzig, 1804.

11 Fraser, F. C., Congenital Clefts of the Face. *De Genet. Med.* **3**:289–295, 1961.

12 Freuenthaller, P., Kephalometrische Untersuchungen und Berichte über Fälle von Anodontie und Oligodontie. *Schweiz. Monatsschr. Zahnheilkd.* **76**:484–489, 1966.

12a Fried, K. Ectrodactyly-Ectodermal Dysplasia-Clefting (EEC) Syndrome. *Clin. Genet.* **3**:396–400, 1972.

13 Fuss, H., Über die Hasenscharten und ihre Behandlung (Case 4). *Arch. Klin. Chir.* **182**:252–272, 1935.

14 Gehler, J., and Grosse, R., Fehlbildungs-Retardierungs-Syndrom mit Spalthänden-Spaltfüssen, Iriskolobom, Nierenagenesie und Ventrikelseptumdefekt. *Klin. Pädiatr.* **184**:389–392, 1972.

15 Gorcznski, H., Congenital Edentulous Condition and the Accompanying Developmental Disorders of the Upper and Lower Extremities. *Čs. Stomatol.* **9**:439–444, 1956.

16 Hillman, D. A., and Fraser, F. C., Artificial Sweeteners and Fetal Malformations: A Rumored Relationship. *Pediatrics* **44**:299–300, 1969.

17 Jaworska, M., and Popiolek, J., Genetic Counselling in Lobster Claw Anomaly: Discussion of Variability of Genetic Influence in Different Families. *Clin. Pediatr.* **7**:396–399, 1968.

18 Kaiser-Kupfer, M., Ectrodactyly, Ectodermal Dysplasia and Clefting Syndrome. *Am. J. Ophthalmol.* **76**:992–998, 1973.

19 Kellner, A. W., Über Spalthand und -Fuss mit Oligodaktylie. *Klin. Wochenschr.* **13**:1507–1509, 1934.

20 Kompe, K., Kasuistische Beiträge zur Lehre von den Missbildungen. *Münch. Med. Wochenschr.* **50**:165–166, 1903.

21 Levy, W. J., Mesoectodermal Dysplasia: A New Combination of Anomalies. *Am. J. Ophthalmol.* **63**:978–982, 1967.

22 Maisels, D. O., Lobster-claw Deformity of the Hands and Feet. *Br. J. Plast. Surg.* **23**:269–282, 1970.

23 Pashayan, H. M., et al., The EEC Syndrome. *Birth Defects* **10**(7):105–127, 1974.

24 Pfeiffer, R. A., and Verbeck, C., Spalthand und Spaltfuss, ektodermale Dysplasie und Lippen-Kiefer-Gaumen-Spalte: ein autosomal dominant vererbtes Syndrom. *Z. Kinderheilkd.* **115**:235–244, 1973.

24a Pries, C., et al., The EEC Syndrome. *Am. J. Dis. Child.* **127**:840–844, 1974.

25 Preus, M., and Fraser, F. C., The Lobster Claw Defect with Ectodermal Defects, Cleft Lip-Palate, Tear Duct Anomaly and Renal Anomalies. *Clin. Genet.* **4**:369–375, 1973.

26 Reed, W. B., et al., The REEDS Syndrome. *Birth Defects* **10**(8):61–73, 1974.

26a Robinson, G. C., et al., Ectrodactyly, Ectodermal Dysplasia and Cleft Lip-Palate Syndrome. *J. Pediatr.* **82**:107–109, 1973.

27 Rosselli, D., and Gulienetti, R., Ectodermal Dysplasia (Case 1). *Br. J. Plast. Surg.* **14**:190–204, 1961.

28 Rüdiger, R. A., et al., Association of Ectrodactyly, Ectodermal Dysplasia and Cleft Lip-Palate: The EEC Syndrome. *Am. J. Dis. Child.* **120**:160–163, 1970.

29 Schönenberg, H., Über die Kombination von Lippen-Kiefer-Gaumen-Spalten mit Extremitatenmissbildungen (Cases 3 and 4). *Z. Kinderheilkd.* **76**:79–90, 1955.

30 Schönenberg, H., Über Missbildungen der Extremitäten. *Bibl. Paediatr.* **80**:80–82, 1962.

31 Strouzer, W., Aplasies congénitales multiples hémimélies transverses symétriques des extrémités. Edentation. *J. Radiol. Électrol.* **23**:169–170, 1939–1940.

31a Swallow, J. N., et al., Ectrodactyly, Ectodermal Dysplasia and Cleft Lip and Cleft Palate (EEC Syndrome). *Br. J. Derm.* **89**:suppl. 9:54–56, 1973.

32 Temtamy, S., and McKusick, V. A., Synopsis of Hand Malformations with Particular Emphasis on Genetic Factors. *Birth Defects* **5**(3):125–184, 1969.

33 Walker, J. C., and Clodius, L., The Syndromes of Cleft Lip, Cleft Palate and Lobster-Claw Deformities of Hands and Feet. *Plast. Reconstr. Surg.* **32**:627–636, 1963.

34 Walker, J. C., et al., Ectodermal Dysplasia. *Trans. 4th Int. Cong. Plast. Reconstr. Surg.*, Rome, 1967, pp. 122–128.

35 Wegner, H., Über Hypodontia vera der Milch- und Ersatzzähne bei vererbter Ekto- und Mesoderm Dysplasie. *Dtsch. Zahnärztl. Z.* **13**:1019–1026, 1958.

36 Whitaker, L., et al., The Lacrimal Apparatus in Patients with Cleft Lip and Palate. *Proc. 2d Int. Cong. Cleft Palate*, Copenhagen, 1973, p. 167.

37 Wiegmann, O. A., and Walker, F. A., The Syndrome of Lobster Claw Deformity and Nasolacrimal Obstruction. *J. Pediatr. Ophthalmol.* **7**:79–85, 1970.

25

Cleft Lip-Palate, Popliteal Pterygium, Digital and Genital Anomalies

(Popliteal Pterygium Syndrome)

This syndrome is quite rare, fewer than 30 cases having been described to date. The first recorded case would appear to be that of Trèlat (28) in 1869. Extensive reviews of the popliteal pterygium syndrome have been those of Gorlin et al. (11), Pfeiffer et al. (22), and Bixler et al. (5). Rintala and Lahti (23) suggested the term "faciogenitopopliteal syndrome."

Although most cases have been isolated, probably because of hypoplastic genitalia, the condition has been transmitted from affected parents to one or more children (13–15, 18, 22). In a few other cases, several sibs have been affected but the parents have been ostensibly normal (6, 16, 24). Thus, the evidence suggests autosomal dominant inheritance with variable expressivity and incomplete penetrance (11, 13, 22). X-linkage has been ruled out on the basis of male-to-male transmission (18, 22).

SYSTEMIC MANIFESTATIONS

Facies. The most obvious facial alterations are cleft lip, with or without cleft palate, and filiform adhesions between the eyelids.

Cutaneous and musculoskeletal anomalies. Certainly the most striking component, the pterygium or skin web (Flughaut), extends from the heel to the ischial tuberosity, limiting extension and abduction as well as rotation of the leg (Fig. 25 1A–C). In all but a few cases (10, 15, 22, 25, 27, 30), these webs have been bilateral. Along the free edge of the pterygium runs a hard, inelastic, subcutaneous cord or fibrous band. The sciatic nerve lies free within the pterygium, deep to the fibrous band about halfway between the free edge and the apex, being covered by a fibromuscular septum. Special caution must thus be taken in repair of the skin fold. The popliteal vessels are normally situated deep in the popliteal space. In many cases, muscle groups are absent or muscle insertions are abnormal.

Patients with this syndrome may also have hypoplasia or agenesis of digits (6, 12, 13, 24, 30), varus or valgus deformities of the foot (4, 10, 12, 13, 16, 27, 28), variable soft-tissue syndactyly of the second to fifth toes (2, 4–8, 12, 16, 19, 20, 22, 25, 27, 30), spina bifida occulta (12, 15, 19, 24, 30), and scoliosis or lordosis (12, 15, 20, 30). Bipartite or absent patella has also been noted (12, 22, 30).

The skin over the hallux has a somewhat pyramidal form, one vertex extending over the nail. Occasionally the hallucal or other toenails (most often the second) are hypoplastic (11–13, 15, 19, 22, 23, 24, 28). Congenital filiform adhesions (ankyloblepharon filiforme) between the upper and lower lids also have been noted (2, 4, 11, 14, 22, 23, 24).

Genitourinary system. Anomalies in the male have included cryptorchism (1, 8, 11, 16, 20, 24, 27); absent, cleft, or ectopic scrotum (2, 4, 11, 19,

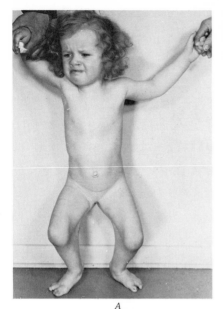

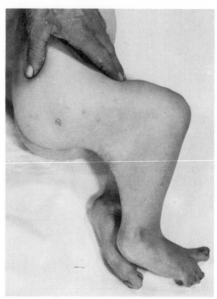

A

B

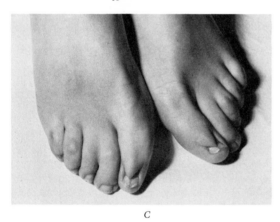

C

Figure 25-1. *Cleft lip-palate, popliteal pterygium, digital and genital anomalies.* (A). Child with repaired bilateral cleft lip-palate, bilateral popliteal pterygia, and hypoplasia of external genitalia. (*From G. Dahmen*, Z. Orthop. **95**:112, 1962.) (B). Side view showing popliteal pterygium. Sciatic nerve is located in web under free margin. (*From G. Dahmen*, Z. Orthop. **95**:112, 1962.) (C). Pyramidal skin folds extending to free edge of hallucal nails. (*From D. Klein*, J. Génét. Hum. **11**:65, 1962.)

threads of mucous membrane extending between the jaws (syngnathia) have been reported (2, 4, 22, 23, 24) (Fig. 25-3A, B).

23, 25, 29); and inguinal hernia (11, 19, 25, 27) (Fig. 25-2B). In the female, absence or displacement of the labia majora (1, 10, 12, 13, 14, 22, 24, 25) and enlarged clitoris (12, 13, 14, 24, 26) have been noted (Fig. 24-2A). Hypoplastic uterus was also described (12).

There also may be a crural pterygium extending between the thighs ventral to the anus (6, 8, 11, 19, 24).

Oral manifestations. Cleft lip with or without cleft palate has been described in nearly all cases. Pits or fistulas of the lower lip (6, 8, 11–15, 22, 24, 28) and congenital bands or

DIFFERENTIAL DIAGNOSIS

The popliteal pterygia make this syndrome rather distinctive. It is possible that the case described by Neuman and Shulman (21) with cleft palate, lip pits, oral mucosal adhesions, and ankyloblepharon is an incomplete form of the syndrome. Lip pits may occur as an isolated phenomenon or in combination with cleft lip and/or cleft palate. Pterygia of the axilla, neck, and antecubital and popliteal areas constitute the *multiple pterygrium syndrome.* Pterygia-like alterations of the lower extremities occur as a

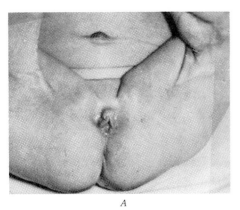

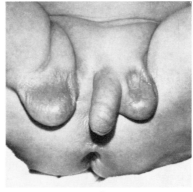

A   B

Figure 25-2. (*A*). Agenesis of labia majora and enlarged clitoris. (*From R. Champion and J. C. F. Cregan,* J. Bone Joint Surg. **41B:**355, 1959.) (*B*). Testicle displaced to upper right thigh. (*From A. Rintala and A. Lahti,* Scand. J. Plast. Reconstr. Surg. **4:**67, 1970.)

part of the so-called "caudal regression syndrome" (16).

Bartsocas and Papas (3) described an autosomal recessive syndrome which included mental retardation, microcephaly, filiform eyelid adhesions, corneal aplasia, hypoplastic nose, microstomia, cleft lip-palate, soft-tissue syngnathia, micrognathia, aplastic labia majora, and bicornuate uterus. Anomalies of the extremities comprised popliteal pterygia, thumb aplasia, syndactyly of fingers and toes, and progressive distal reduction of metacarpals, metatarsals, and phalanges.

LABORATORY AIDS

None is known.

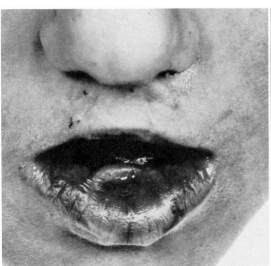

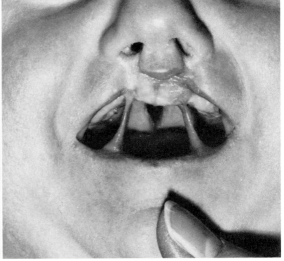

A   B

Figure 25-3. (*A*). Repaired bilateral cleft lip, lower lip pits. (*B*). Bilateral synechiae connecting upper and lower jaws. (*From A. Rintala and A. Lahti,* Scand. J. Plast. Reconstr. Surg. **4:**67, 1970.)

REFERENCES

1 Aberle-Horstenegg, A., Flughautbildung zwischen Ober- und Unterschenkel mit abnormer Muskelbildung (M. ischiosuralis). *Z. Orthop.* **67:**21–29, 1937.

2 Bajaj, P. S., and Bailey, B. M., Ectopic Scrotum: A Case Report. *Br. J. Plast. Surg.* **22:**87–89, 1969.

3 Bartsocas, C. S., and Papas, C. V., Popliteal Pterygium Syndrome: Evidence for a Severe Autosomal Recessive Form. *J. Med. Genet.* **9:**222–226, 1972.

4 Basch, K., Ein weiterer Fall von sog. Flughautbildung. *Prag. Med. Wochenschr.* **16:**572–573, 1891; and **17:**287–291, 1892.

5 Bixler, D., et al., Phenotypic Variation in the Popliteal Pterygium Syndrome. *Clin. Genet.* **4:**220–228, 1973.

6 Champion, R., and Cregan, J. C. F., Congenital Popliteal Webbing in Siblings: Report of Two Cases. *J. Bone Joint Surg.* **41B:**355–359, 1959.

7 Dahmen, G., Über die Versorgung einer doppelseitigen Kniestreckhemmung wegen Flügelfell mit einem provisorischen Knie-Ruhebein. *Z. Orthop.* **95:**112–113, 1962.

8 Fèvre, M., and Languepin, A., Les brides cruro-jambières contenant le nerf sciatique: Le syndrome bride poplitée et malformations multiples (division palatine, fistules de la lèvre inférieure, syndactylie des orteils). *Presse Méd.* **70:**615–618, 1962.

9 Fèvre, M., and Languepin, S., Brides poplitées simples et brides poplitées avec quadruple syndrome. *Ann. Chir. Plast.* **11:**124, 1966.

10 Fisher, H., Ein Fall von sogenannter Flughautbildung zwischen Ober- und Unterschenkel. *Prag. Med. Wochenschr.* **18:**579, 1893.

11 Gorlin, R. J., et al., Popliteal Pterygium Syndrome: A Syndrome Comprising Cleft Lip-Palate, Popliteal and Intercrural Pterygia, Digital and Genital Anomalies. *Pediatrics* **41:**503–509, 1968.

12 Hackenbroch, M., Über einen Fall von kongenitaler Kontraktur der Kniegelenke mit Flughautbildung. *Z. Orthop.* **43:**508–524, 1923.

13 Hecht, F., and Jarvinen, J. M., Heritable Dysmorphic Syndrome with Normal Intelligence. *J. Pediatr.* **70:**927–935, 1967.

14 Kind, H. P., Popliteales Pterygiumsyndrom. *Helv. Paediatr. Acta* **25:**508–516, 1970.

15 Klein, D., Un curieux syndrome héréditaire: cheilo-palatoschizis avec fistules de la lèvre inférieure associé a une syndactylie, une onychodysplasie particulière, un ptérygion poplité unilatérale et des pieds varus équins. *J. Génèt. Hum.* **11:**65–71, 1962.

16 Kopits, E., Die als ''Flughaut'' bezeichneten Missbildung und deren operative Behandlung. *Arch. Orthop. Unfallchir.* **37:**539–549, 1937.

17 Kučera, J., Exposure to Fat Solvents: a Possible Cause of Sacral Agenesis in Man. *J. Pediatr.* **72:**857–859, 1968.

18 Lewis, E., Congenital Webbing of the Lower Limbs. *Proc. R. Soc. Med.* **41:**864, 1948.

19 Marquardt, W., Die angeborene Flughautbildung und ihre konservative Behandlung. *Z. Orthop.* **67:**379–386, 1937.

20 Matolcsy, T., Über die chirurgische Behandlung der angeborene Flughaut. *Arch. Klin. Chir.* **185:**675–681, 1936.

21 Neuman, Z., and Shulman, J., Congenital Sinuses of the Lower Lip. *Oral Surg.* **14:**1415–1420, 1961.

22 Pfeiffer, R. A., et al., Das Kniepterygium-Syndrom. Ein autosomal dominant vererbtes Missbildungssyndrom. *Z. Kinderheilkd.* **108:**103–116, 1970.

23 Rintala, A., and Lahti, A., The Facio-Genito-Popliteal Syndrome. *Scand. J. Plast. Reconstr. Surg.* **4:**67–71, 1970.

24 Rosselli, D., and Gulienetti, R., Ectodermal Dysplasia. *Br. J. Plast. Surg.* **14:**190–204, 1961.

25 Rydgier, L., Demonstration von Abbildungen seltener Fälle von Missbildungen. *Arch. Klin. Chir.* **42:**769, 1891.

26 Schönenberg, H., Über die Kombination von Lippen-Kiefer-Gaumen-Spalten mit Extremitätenmissbildung. *Z. Kinderheilkd.* **76:**79–90, 1955.

27 Schramm, G., Über die angeborene Flughautbildung. *Z. Orthop.* **70:**189–195, 1940.

28 Trèlat, U., Sur un vice conformation très-rare de la lèvre-inférieure. *J. Méd. Chir. Prat.* **40:**442–445, 1869.

29 Williams, D. W., Anomaly of Scrotum and Testes: Simple Plastic Repair. *J. Urol.* **89:**860–863, 1963.

30 Wolff, J., Über einen Fall von angeborener Flughautbildung. *Arch. Klin. Chir.* **38:**66–73, 1889.

26

Cleft Lip-Palate and Tetraphocomelia

(*Appelt-Gerken-Lenz Syndrome, Roberts Syndrome*)

There have been several examples of a syndrome consisting of (*a*) bilateral cleft lip-palate, (*b*) tetraphocomelia with a reduction in digit number, (*c*) ocular proptosis with hypertelorism, and (*d*) growth deficiency. Although it was described earlier by Roberts (9) and others, Appelt et al. (1) should be credited for clear recognition of this syndrome entity. Several other examples have been reported (2–14), including a description as early as 1671 (see 8).

The syndrome follows an autosomal recessive mode of transmission. Parental consanguinity and occurrence in sibs have been noted (4, 9, 11, 12).

SYSTEMIC MANIFESTATIONS

Facies. The facies is characterized by ocular hypertelorism, proptosis, and bilateral cleft lip-palate.

Skeletal alterations. The birth weight is nearly always less than 2,200 g. There are reduction deformities in the bones of all four extremities (4), although variability may occur from case to case. For example, the femur, radius, and ulna were essentially spared in the cases of Roberts (9), while the tibia, fibula, and humerus were severely hypoplastic. In nearly all cases, the number of digits has been reduced more frequently in the hands than in the feet. Soft-tissue syndactyly has been noted in 70 percent of cases (Fig. 26-1).

Genitalia. Although enlarged phallus has been noted (4, 5, 9), it is possible that the striking growth deficiency in this syndrome is responsible for making a normal-sized phallus appear enlarged. Cryptorchism has been described in nearly all affected males (4). Enlargement of the clitoris has been reported (1, 4, 10). The labia minora have been enlarged or cleft (1), and vaginal septum has been observed (4).

Eyes and ears. The pinnas may be somewhat bizarre (9) or even rudimentary (5), and nearly all patients have exhibited ocular proptosis with shallow orbits and hypertelorism (Fig. 26-1*B, C*). Cataracts, corneal opacity, and colobomas of the eyelids have been noted (4).

Other findings. Hydrocephalus, frontal encephalocele, spina bifida, atrial septal defect, patent ductus arteriosus, polycystic kidneys, horseshoe kidney, and bicornuate uterus have been reported (4).

Oral manifestations. Bilateral cleft lip with or without cleft palate has been present in almost all cases (1–14).

DIFFERENTIAL DIAGNOSIS

A relationship between this syndrome and the *pseudothalidomide syndrome* has been postulated. See Differential Diagnosis in Chap. 122, *Pseudothalidomide Syndrome*, for discussion of

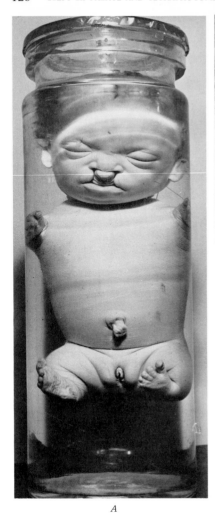

A

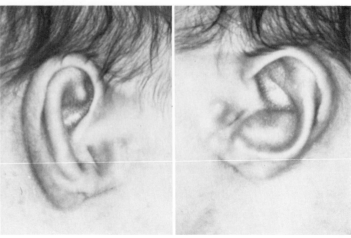

B   *C*

Figure 26-1. *Cleft lip-palate and tetraphocomelia.* (*A*). Ocular hypertelorism, reduction in digits, clitoral enlargement, bizarre pinnas. (*From J. Appelt et al.,* Pädiatr. Pädol. **2:**119, 1966.) (*B, C*). Close-up of ears in similarly affected child. (*Courtesy of S. Pruzansky, Chicago, Ill.*)

this problem. Phocomelia-like deformities may be observed in a variety of other conditions. In thalidomide embryopathy, limbs are usually asymmetrically malformed.

LABORATORY AIDS

None is known.

REFERENCES

1 Appelt, J., et al., Tetraphokomelie mit Lippen-Kiefer-Gaumenspalte und Clitorishypertrophie–ein Syndrom. *Pädiatr. Pädol.* **2:**119–124, 1966.

2 Doerffer, C., Ein Fall von Phokomelie. *Monatsschr. Geburtsh. Gynäk.* **72:**195–198, 1926.

3 Engelhart, E., and Pischinger, A., Über eine durch Röntgenstrahlen verursachte menschliche Missbildung. *Münch. Med. Wochenschr.* **86:**1315–1316, 1939.

4 Freeman, M. V. R., et al., The Roberts Syndrome. *Clin. Genet.,* **5:**1–16, 1974.

5 Grillo, R. A., Über einen Fall von Phokomelie. *Dtsch. Med. Wochenschr.* **62:**1332–1333, 1936.

6 Gruber, G., Die Entwicklungsstörungen der menschlichen Gliedmassen, in E. Schwalbe and G. Gruber (eds.), *Die Morphologie der Missbildungen der Menschen und der Tiere.* III, G. Fischer, Jena, 1937, p. 310.

7 Kaul, A., Über eine besondere Form der Phokomelie verbunden mit Hasenscharte und Wolfsrachen nebst Bemerkungen über die Ätiologie dieser Missbildung. *Thesis,* Würzburg, 1899.

8 Krueger, R., *Die Phocomelie und ihre Übergänge.* (Case 87). August Hirschwald, Berlin, 1906, p. 92.

9 Roberts, J. B., A Child with Double Cleft of Lip and Palate, Protrusion of the Intermaxillary Portion of the Upper Jaw

and Imperfect Development of the Bones of the Four Extremities. *Ann. Surg.* **70:**252, 1919.

10 Slingenberg, B., Missbildungen von Extremitäten (Case 11). *Virchows Arch. Pathol. Anat.* **193:**1–92, 1908.

11 Stroer, W. F. H., Über das Zusammentreffen von Hasenscharte mit ernsten Extremitätenmissbildungen. *Erbarzt* **7:**101–107, 1939.

12 Temtamy, S. A., and Loutfi, A. H., Some Genetic and Surgical Aspects of Cleft Lip/Cleft Palate Problem in Egypt. *Cleft Palate J.* **7:**578–594, 1970.

13 Virchow, R., Die Phokomelien und das Bärenweib. *Z. Ethnol.* **30:**55–61, 1898.

14 Werthemann, A., Die Entwicklungsstörungen der Extremitaten, in O. Lubarsch et al. (eds.), *Handbuch der speziellen pathologischen Anatomie und Histologie,* Vol. IX. Springer-Verlag, Berlin, 1952.

27

Cleft Palate, Flattened Facies, and Multiple Congenital Dislocations

(Larsen Syndrome)

The syndrome first recognized as a distinct entity by Larsen (8), in 1950, includes (a) flattened facies, (b) multiple congenital dislocations, (c) foot deformities, and frequently, (d) cleft palate. Several authors have reported similar cases (1, 2, 4, 7, 11, 12, 14a, 19). Other examples are less certain (14, 15, 18).

The syndrome has been noted in sibs (1, 2, 19). Most cases are consistent with autosomal recessive transmission (4), but others have manifested dominant inheritance (1, 5, 10, 19a). There is an apparent female sex predilection.

SYSTEMIC MANIFESTATIONS

Facies. The face is typically flattened, because of a depressed nasal bridge. The eyes appear widely spaced. Frontal bossing may be marked, with arrested hydrocephaly (Fig. 27-1).

Skeletal system. Bony alterations include bilateral anterior dislocation of the tibia on the femur, with displaced patella, subluxation of humeral head, dislocation of radial head, hip dislocation, and talipes equinovarus or equinovalgus. Adult height is reduced, the patient usually being less than 168 cm tall (Fig. 27-2A, B). The fingers are long and cylindric, with extra creases (Fig. 27-3). The thumb is spatulate, without normal taper.

Radiographically, the terminal phalanx of the thumb is triangular. The metacarpals are rela-tively shortened, and numerous additional carpal bones are noted (4, 7) (Fig. 27-4A). The carpal tunnel syndrome has been described in several

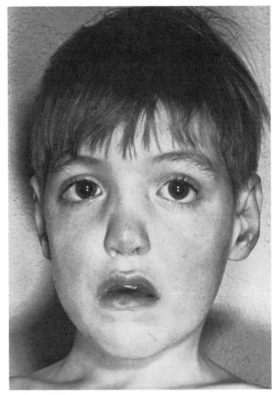

Figure 27-1. *Larsen syndrome.* Flattened midface with broad nasal bridge.

128

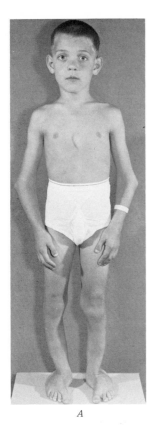

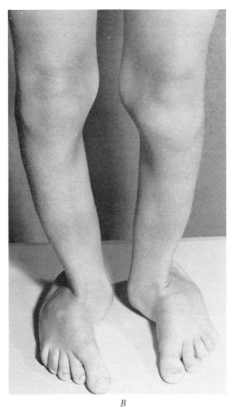

A   *B*

Figure 27-2. (*A, B*). Note similar facies in boy shown in Fig. 27-1, subluxation of radial heads, sternal anomaly, dislocated knees, "windmill" feet, spatulate thumbs.

patients. Abnormal segmentation of one or more vertebras has been seen (3, 7, 8, 19, 20). Latta et al. (9), Steel and Kohl (19), and Szabó and Perjés (20) described a juxtacalcaneal accessory bone, or bifid calcaneus (Fig. 27-4*B*). We have also noted this alteration in our cases.

Cardiovascular anomalies. Anomalies of the heart were observed by McFarland (11). These were probably of the interventricular septal type.

Oral manifestations. Oral changes seem to be essentially limited to cleft palate, which occurs in about 50 percent of cases (3, 12). This may be limited to the soft palate and/or uvula and apparently is never combined with cleft lip.

Some patients have laryngotracheomalacia (20).

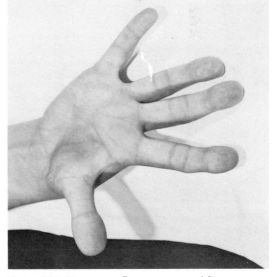

Figure 27-3. Note extra flexion creases of fingers, spatulate thumb.

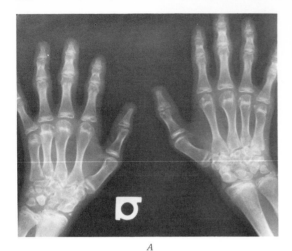

A

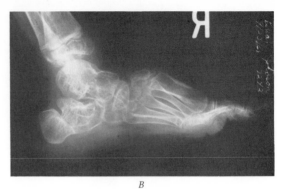

B

Figure 27-4. (*A*). The carpal bones, late to appear, are supernumerary. (*B*). Juxtacalcaneal bone fuses with calcaneus just prior to puberty. Also note unusual relationship of metatarsals to tarsal bones.

DIFFERENTIAL DIAGNOSIS

The X-linked *otopalatodigital syndrome* is most often mistaken for Larsen syndrome. In contrast, these patients exhibit paddle-shaped metacarpal and metatarsal bones, do not have a juxtacalcaneal bone, and do not have supernumerary carpal bones.

Schröder (16) described a syndrome in five sibs consisting of bizarre pinnas and bilateral luxation of the radius, radiohumeral ankylosis, bilateral dislocation of the hips, shoulders, and knees, genu valgum, and camptodactyly.

Multiple congenital dislocations may occur as an isolated finding (6, 13).

Larsen syndrome differs sufficiently enough from arthrogryposis that the disorders should be easily separated (20).

REFERENCES

1 Bartsocas, C. S., and Dimitriou, J. K., Multiple Joint Dislocation in Mother and Child. *J. Pediatr.* **80:**299–301, 1972.

2 Block, C., and Peck, H. M., Bilateral Congenital Dislocation of the Knees. *J. Mt. Sinai Hosp.* **32:**607–608, 1965.

3 Curtis, B. H., and Fisher, R. L., Heritable Congenital Tibiofemoral Subluxation: Clinical Features and Surgical Treatment (Case 5). *J. Bone Joint Surg.* **52A:**1104–1114, 1970.

4 Hackenbroch, M., Multiple kongenitale Gelenkmissbildungen. *Z. Orthop. Chir.* **45:**467–476, 1924.

5 Harris, R., and Cullen, C. H., Autosomal Dominant Inheritance in Larsen's Syndrome. *Clin. Genet.* **2:**87–90, 1971.

6 Hayashi, K., and Matsuoko, M., Angeborene Missbildungen kombiniert mit der kongenitalen Huftverrenkung. *Z. Orthop. Chir.* **31:**369–399, 1913.

7 Kaijser, R., Über kongenitale Kniegelenksluxationen. (Case 6). *Acta Orthop. Scand.* **6:**1–20, 1935.

8 Larsen, L. J., et al., Multiple Congenital Dislocations Associated with Characteristic Facial Abnormality. *J. Pediatr.* **37:**574–581, 1950.

9 Latta, R. J., et al., Larsen's Syndrome: A Skeletal Dysplasia with Multiple Joint Dislocations and Unusual Facies. *J. Pediatr.* **78:**291–298, 1971.

10 McFarlane, A. L., A Report in Four Cases of Congenital Genu Recurvatum Occurring in One Family. *Br. J. Surg.* **34:**388–391, 1947.

11 McFarland, B. L., Congenital Dislocation of the Knee. *J. Bone Joint Surg.* **11:**281–285, 1929.

12 Niebauer, J. J., and King, D. E., Congenital Dislocation of the Knee. (Case 2). *J. Bone Joint Surg.* **42A:**207–225, 1960.

13 Provenzano, R. W., Congenital Dislocation of the Knee. *N. Engl. J. Med.* **236:**360–362, 1947.

14 Reiner, M., Über einen blutig reponirten Fall von angeborener Kniegelenksluxationen. *Z. Orthop. Chir.* **13:**442–450, 1904.

14a Robertson, F. W., et al., Larsen's Syndrome. *Clin. Pediat.* **14:**53–60, 1975.

15 Rotter, W., and Erb, W., Über eine Systemerkrankung des Mesenchyms mit multiplen Luxationen aus angeborener Gelenkschlaffheit und über Wirbelbogenspalten. *Virchows Arch. Pathol. Anat.* **316:**233–263, 1949.

16 Schröder, C. H., Familiäre kongenitale Luxationen. *Z. Orthop. Chir.* **57:**580–596, 1932.

17 Silverman, F. N., Larsen's Syndrome: Congenital Dislocation of the Knees and Other Joints, Distinctive Facies and

Frequently, Cleft Palate. *Ann. Radiol.* **15:**297–328, 1972.

18 Stause, M., Zur Kenntnis der multiplen kongenitalen Gelenkdeformitäten. *Z. Orthop. Chir.* **16:**322–327, 1906.

19 Steel, H. H., and Kohl, E. J., Multiple Congenital Dislocations Associated with Other Skeletal Anomalies (Larsen's Syndrome) in Three Siblings. *J. Bone Joint Surg.* **54A:**75–82, 1972.

19a Sugarman, G. I., The Larsen Syndrome, Autosomal Dominant Form. *Birth Defects* **11**(2):121–129, 1975.

20 Szabó, L., and Perjés, K., Über die Differenzierung der Arthrogyrposis multiplex congenita und des Larsen-Syndroms. *Z. Orthop.* **112:**1275–1281, 1974.

28

Cleft Palate, Micrognathia, and Glossoptosis

(Robin Anomalad)

The well-recognized combination of micrognathia, glossoptosis, and cleft palate, ordinarily known as the Pierre Robin syndrome (often incorrectly hyphenated), was described earlier by St. Hilaire in 1822 (20), Fairbairn (7) in 1846, and Shukowsky (22) in 1910. Smith and Stowe (23) reported on the ocular findings in 39 cases. Historic development is thoroughly discussed by Dennison (4), Grimm et al. (8), and Randall et al. (16). We prefer to think of the disorder as a nonspecific anomalad which may occur as an isolated defect or as part of a broader pattern of malformations.

Various conditions known to be associated with the Robin anomalad are listed in Table 28-1. Preeminent among these is the Stickler syndrome, which may often present with the Robin anomalad. Active detection of myopia should be sought because blindness, a consequence of retinal detachment, can probably be prevented in this syndrome. Since there is further ill-defined heterogeneity with respect to the Robin anomalad, the reader may expect to find this complex with other unrecognized or ill-defined syndromes not listed in Table 28-1, some of which may be hereditary (2). A variety of associated anomalies is listed below. In general, anomalies that are part of a known pattern of malformation listed in the table have been omitted to avoid redundancy. There may be others that we have not recorded.

The pathogenesis of the Robin anomalad is probably based on arrested development. The primary defect lies in hypoplasia of the mandible, preventing the normal descent of the tongue between the palatal shelves (10). In this connection, the palate in the Robin anomalad has been found to be U-shaped (caused by tongue interference) in contrast to the more frequent V-shaped cleft palate (8a). During embryologic development, because the upper jaw grows markedly during the 10- to 12-week period, the disparity becomes quite apparent by the fourth or fifth month, the embryo being micrognathic during this stage. As additional evidence of intrauterine insult, several investigators have produced the anomalad experimentally (3).

SYSTEMIC MANIFESTATIONS

Difficulty in the inspiratory phase of respiration is apparent, with periodic cyanotic attacks, labored breathing, and recession of the sternum and ribs. This becomes especially apparent when the child is in the supine position. The respiratory difficulty is usually evident at birth, although it may not be severe for the first week. Only rarely is its initiation delayed until the first month.

Facies. The facies is striking at birth. The mandible is small and symmetrically receded, producing an "Andy Gump" appearance. Commonly the base of the nose is flattened (Fig. 28-1A).

Table 28-1. Conditions associated with the Robin anomalad

Condition	Frequency of Robin anomalad in given condition	References for details
Stickler syndrome	Common	Chapter 29
Cerebrocostomandibular syndrome	Common; micrognathia in all patients	Chapter 29
Campomelic syndrome	Common	Chapter 29
Persistent left superior vena cava syndrome	Common	Chapter 29
Spondyloepiphyseal dysplasia congenita	Uncommon	Chapter 29
Severe congenital myotonic dystrophy		J. M. Opitz, personal communication
Diastrophic dwarfism	Uncommon; isolated cleft palate common	Chapter 44
Beckwith—Wiedemann syndrome	Uncommon; isolated cleft palate also observed uncommonly	Chapter 11
Femoral hypoplasia—unusual facies syndrome	Micrognathia and cleft palate common; glossoptosis uncommon	Chapter 29
Radiohumeral synostosis syndrome	? Too few cases known	J. Hanson, personal communication
Fetal alcohol syndrome	Uncommon	Chapter 144
Fetal hydantoin syndrome	Uncommon	Chapter 144
Fetal trimethadione syndrome	Uncommon	Chapter 144
Cleft palate—Accessory second-finger metacarpal syndrome	? Too few cases known	Chapter 29
Cleft palate and amelia	? Too few cases known	Chapter 29

The association of various congenital heart defects and the Robin anomalad is discussed in Chap. 29.

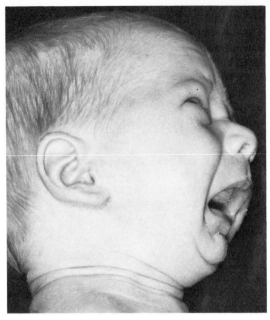

A

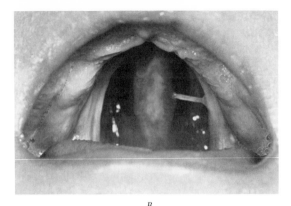

B

Figure 28-1. *Robin anomalad.* (*A*). Severe micrognathia. (*B*). U-shaped cleft palate.

Heart and blood vessels. Congenital murmurs and/or heart disease have been observed in about 15 to 25 percent of the patients who die in early infancy (21). Necropsy has revealed patent ductus arteriosus and foramen ovale, atrial and/or ventricular septal defect, ventricular hypertrophy, cor triloculare with coarctation of the aorta, biventricular aorta, and dextrocardia (4, 5, 6, 18, 20, 21, 23).

Skeletal system. Congenital amputations, bilateral talipes equinovarus, hip dislocation, syndactyly, and rib and sternal anomalies have been described (8, 18, 23).

Eyes and ears. Ocular findings are apparently common. Smith and Stowe (23) found 13 major lesions in nine patients, including esotropia, congenital glaucoma, and microphthalmia. Ortlepp and Brandt (13) also described congenital glaucoma.

Less frequently, there are ear anomalies: low-set ears, deformed pinna (8, 23).

Nervous system. About 20 percent of patients have exhibited major mental retardation. In ad-

dition, hydrocephaly, microcephaly, and the Moebius syndrome have been associated (23).

Oral manifestations. Although there is no complete agreement concerning the exact mechanism by which the respiratory and feeding difficulties are produced, the classic explanation suggests that the micrognathia makes for little support of the tongue musculature. This allows the tongue to fall downward and backward (glossoptosis) into the lower postpharyngeal space, obstructing the epiglottis. In this position the tongue permits egress of air but prevents inhalation, acting much as a ball valve, causing periodic cyanosis and sternal retraction. Feeding problems are thought to be due to inadequate control of the tongue. Nursing, even when performed in a favorable position, is an ordeal (5, 6).

Routledge (18), on the other hand, suggested that the respiratory difficulty might be due, in large part, to impaction of the tongue tip in the palatal cleft, from which it is not easily disengaged. The violent muscular contractions resulting from the efforts to free it cause the tongue to bulge into the nasopharynx, resulting in asphyxia. The resultant anoxia would cause the tongue to become limp and flaccid, dropping out of the nasopharynx and restoring the airway. Routledge realized that this theory did not account for those cases in which plastic correction of the palate did not correct the situation, or for those cases associated with ankyloglossia which did not permit upward movement of the tongue

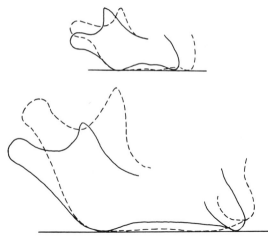

Figure 28-2. Superimposed tracings from normal (broken line) and Robin (solid line) mandibles. Note differences in height of ramus, length of body, gonial angle, and inclination of condyle to ramus. (*From S. Pruzansky,* Birth Defects **5**(2):120, 1969.)

tip. He stated that some cases are truly due to "having too large a tongue too far back in too small a mouth."

It has been shown, most notably by Pruzansky and coworkers (2, 14, 15) and Stellmach and Schettler (24), that the growth of the jaws will progress so that an essentially normal profile is achieved by four to six years of age. Pruzansky (14) described the mandible as having a foreshortened body with a characteristic ratio of ramus to mandibular body length (Fig. 28-2).

The tongue has been stated by some investigators to be small, by others, normal, and by still others, large. It has been suggested that the cases showing delayed appearance of the anomaly are due to disproportionate growth of the tongue during this period (18). Pruzansky and Richmond (15) concluded from cephalometric studies that the micrognathia, of itself, was insufficient to produce respiratory embarrassment unless the tongue is normal or enlarged. Ankyloglossia is a commonly associated complication.

The palatal defect may vary widely from cleft uvula to clefting which involves two-thirds of the hard palate and is horseshoe in shape. The majority of patients have a defect of intermediate degree (Fig. 28-1B). Cleft lip does not occur in combination with cleft palate in this anomalad.

DIFFERENTIAL DIAGNOSIS

Micrognathia and cleft palate are seen in a wide variety of disorders (see Chap. 29). Some examples of the *Stickler syndrome* have been erroneously called "Robin syndrome" (19, 26).

The difficulty in nursing, the choking fits, and the cyanotic bouts may also suggest tracheoesophageal fistula, but the "bird facies" of the infant with the Robin anomalad is so distinctive that even the inexperienced clinician should have little difficulty in recognizing it.

DIAGNOSTIC AIDS

None is known.

REFERENCES

1 Beers, M. D., and Pruzansky, S., The Growth of the Head of an Infant with Mandibular Micrognathia: Glossoptosis and Cleft Palate Following the Beverly Douglas Operation. *Plast. Reconstr. Surg.* **16**:189–193, 1955.

2 Carroll, D. B., et al., Hereditary Factors in the Pierre Robin Syndrome. *Br. J. Plast. Surg.* **24**:43–47, 1971.

3 Cocke, W. J., Experimental Production of Micrognathia and Glossoptosis Associated with Cleft Palate (Pierre Robin Syndrome). *Plast. Reconstr. Surg.* **38**:395–403, 1966.

4 Dennison, W. M., The Pierre Robin Syndrome. *Pediatrics* **36**:336–341, 1965.

5 Douglas, B., The Treatment of Micrognathia Associated with Obstruction by a Plastic Procedure. *Plast. Reconstr. Surg.* **1**:300, 1946.

6 Douglas, B., The Treatment of Micrognathia with Obstruction by a Plastic Operation. *Lyon Chir.* **52**:420–431, 1956.

7 Fairbairn, P., Suffocation in an Infant from Retraction of the Base of the Tongue, Connected with Defect of the Frenum. *Month. J. Med. Sci.* **6**:280–281, 1846.

8 Grimm, G., et al., Die klinische Bedeutung des Pierre Robin Syndroms und seine Behandlung. *Dtsch. Zahn Mund Kieferheilkd.* **43**:385–416, 1964.

8a Hanson, J., and Smith, D. W., U-shaped Palatal Defect in the Robin Anomaly: Developmental and Clinical Relevance. *J. Pediatr.* **87:**30–33, 1975.

9 Jersty, R. M., et al., Pierre Robin Syndrome. *Am. J. Dis. Child.* **117:**710–716, 1969.

10 Latham, R. A., The Pathogenesis of Cleft Palate Associated with the Pierre Robin Syndrome. *Br. J. Plast. Surg.* **19:**205–214, 1966.

11 Lenstrup, E., Hypoplasia Mandibulae as Cause of Choking Fits in Infants. *Acta Paediatr.* **5:**154–165, 1925.

12 Opitz, J., Familial Anomalies in the Pierre Robin Syndrome. *Birth Defects* **5**(2):119, 1969.

13 Ortlepp, J., and Brandt, H. P., Hydrophthalmos bei Pierre Robin Syndrom. *Klin. Monatsbl. Augenheilkd.* **148:**46–49, 1966.

14 Pruzansky, S., Not All Dwarfed Mandibles Are Alike. *Birth Defects* **5**(2):120–129, 1969.

15 Pruzansky, S., and Richmond, J. B., Growth of the Mandible in Infants with Micrognathia. *Am. J. Dis. Child.* **88:**29–42, 1954.

16 Randall, P., et al., Pierre Robin and the Syndrome that Bears His Name. *Cleft Palate J.* **2:**237–246, 1965.

17 Robin, P., La chute de la base de la langue considerée comme une nouvelle cause de gène dans la respiration naso-pharyngienne. *Bull. Acad. Méd.* (Paris) **89:**37–41, 1923.

18 Routledge, R. T., The Pierre-Robin (sic) Syndrome: A Surgical Emergency in the Neo-natal Period. *Br. J. Plast. Surg.* **13:**204–218, 1960.

19 Schreiner, R. L., et al., Stickler Syndrome in a Pedigree of the Pierre Robin Syndrome. *Am. J. Dis. Child.* **126:**86–91, 1973.

20 Schönenberg, H., and Lautermann, R., Das Robin Syndrom. *Z. Kinderheilkd.* **97:**326–346, 1966.

21 Shah, C. V., et al., Cardiac Malformations with Facial Clefts. *Am. J. Dis. Child.* **119:**238–244, 1970.

22 Shukowsky, W. P., Zur Ätiologie des Stridor inspiratorius congenitus. *Jb. Kinderheilkd.* **73:**459, 1911.

23 Smith, J. L., and Stowe, F. R., The Pierre Robin Syndrome (Glossoptosis, Micrognathia, Cleft Palate): A Review of 39 Cases with Emphasis on Associated Ocular Lesions. *Pediatrics* **27:**128–133, 1961.

24 Stellmach, R., and Schettler, D., Beobachtungen zum Robin-Syndrom und kephalometrische Untersuchungen bei 12 Behandlungsfällen. *Dtsch. Zahn Mund Kieferheilkd.* **49:**137–149, 1967.

25 Stern, L. M., Management of Pierre Robin Syndrome in Infancy by Prolonged Nasoesophageal Intubation. *Am. J. Dis. Child.* **124:**78–80, 1972.

26 Turner, G., The Stickler Syndrome in a Family with the Pierre Robin Syndrome and Severe Myopia. *Aust. Paediat. J.* **10:**103–108, 1974.

29

Miscellaneous Cleft Syndromes

CLEFT LIP-PALATE AND CONGENITAL FILIFORM FUSION OF THE EYELIDS

The association of cleft lip and/or cleft palate and congenital filiform fusion of the eyelids (ankyloblepharon filiforme adnatum) appears to be inherited as an autosomal dominant trait (1–5, 7, 9).

Multiple connective tissue bands, 0.3 to 5.0 mm in width, extend from the white line of one lid to that of the other lid, posterior to the cilia and anterior to the Meibomian orifices. No associated anomalies are found in the eyeballs. Filiform adhesions of the eyelids may occur in combination with lip pits (1, 6, 10) and in the popliteal pterygium syndrome (Fig. 29-1).

CLEFT LIP-PALATE, CLEFT LARYNX, AND LARYNGEAL WEB

Cleft lip-palate has been associated with cleft larynx in two patients described by Cameron and Williams (2). One patient had associated esophageal atresia, tracheoesophageal fistula, ventricular septal defect, coarctation of the aorta, and hypoplasia of penis and testes. The other child had an arachnoidal cyst of the brain and fenestration of the foramen ovale. In both patients the laryngeal cleft extended from the interarytenoid fold to the cricoid cartilage; it was associated with laryngeal stridor, respiratory obstruction, and aspiration of food with resultant pneumonia. Clefts may also be associated with laryngeal web (2–4). Both combinations have been sporadic to date.

CLEFTING AND THORACOPAGOUS TWINS

Thoracopagous twins, i.e., conjoined twins having part of the thoracic wall in common and having various abnormalities of the mediastinum and the viscera of the upper part of the abdomen, would appear to have a higher rate of facial clefting than might be expected by chance (4).

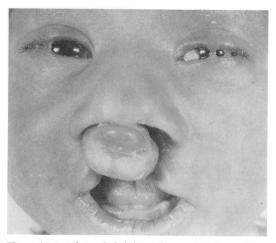

Figure 29-1. *Bilateral cleft lip-palate and filiform adhesions of eyelids. (From J. C. Long and S. E. Blandford, Am. J. Ophthalmol. 53:126, 1962.)*

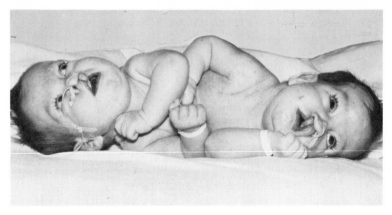

Figure 29-2. *Conjoined twins with mirror image clefts. (From R. Stellmach and G. Frenkel,* Dtsch. Zahnärztl. Z. **25**:28, 1970.)

Among 42 cases of thoracopagous twins, Nichols et al. (7) noted four cases of cleft lip and two cases of cleft palate in one of the twin pair and a mirror image cleft lip in both conjoined twins. Robertson and McKenzie (8) noted discordance for cleft lip in thoracopagous twins, and Stellmach and Frenkel (9) described mirror image concordance (Fig. 29-2).

Bartlett (2) described cleft palate, and Herbst and Apffelstaedt (5) cleft lip and palate in cephalothoracopagus. Ayer and Mariappa (1) observed unilateral cleft lip and palate in both thoracopagous twins and bilateral cleft lip and palate in both faces of a diprosopic child. Ivy (6) described a two-headed fetus, one with cleft lip-palate, the other normal. Buchta (3) described anencephaly in thoracopagous twins with facial clefting. Cleft palate has been reported in craniopagus (11).

FACIAL CLEFTS AND CONGENITAL "RING" CONSTRICTIONS (STREETER BANDS) OR AMPUTATIONS

Several cases of congenital ring constrictions of one or more limbs have been reported in association with facial clefts (Fig. 29-3A, B). Other cases have exhibited congenital amputation of one or more digits or even limbs (5) and distal syndactyly. The most complete discussions of the anomaly are those of Patterson (7), Torpin (9), and Baker and Rudolph (1), who estimated the incidence of ring constrictions to be about 1 per 15,000 births. Associated malformations are common, the more frequent being talipes equin-

ovarus (20 to 40 percent) and syndactyly (10 to 35 percent). Among 50 cases of ring constriction, Patterson (7) noted four with cleft lip and palate and one with lateral facial cleft. A similar frequency was noted by Baker and Rudolph (1). Other patients with this combination have been recorded (1–6, 8, 18), and all known instances have been sporadic. The condition may result from premature rupture of the amnion with subsequent encirclement of fetal extremities (1, 3a, 9).

Jones et al. (5a) and Kubaček and Pěnkava (5b) reported several patients with a variety of severe craniofacial anomalies in association with intrauterine amputation or constriction of limbs and/or pseudosyndactyly of digits. Survival beyond the neonatal period occurred in most cases. Frequency is one per 10,000 births and all have been sporadic.

The craniofacial anomalies included severe microcephaly with deficiencies of anterior calvaria, asymmetric usually anteriorly located occasionally multiple encephaloceles, microphthalmia with distortion of palpebral fissures, nasal deformities, bizarre facial clefts and various bands about the face (29-3C, D). Less frequent findings were unilateral proboscis, gastroschisis and talipes equinovarus.

CLEFT PALATE AND ORAL SYNECHIAE

Mathis (8) described syngnathism resulting from a membrane which joined the jaws from the canine region to the angle of the jaws. It is not

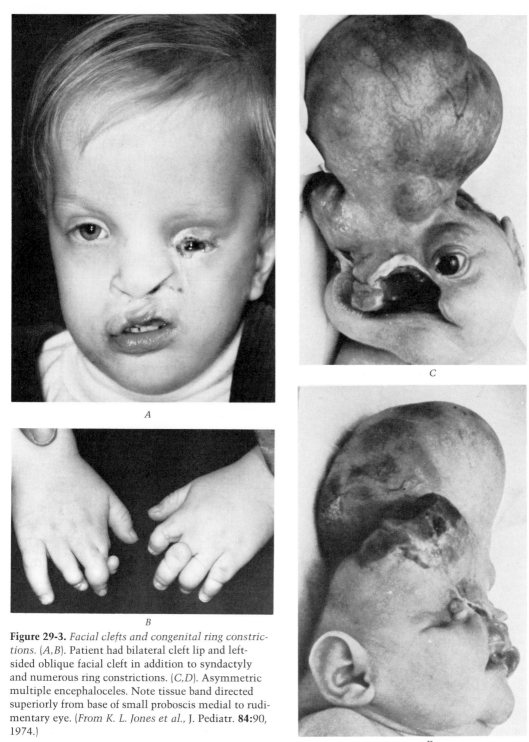

A

B

C

D

Figure 29-3. *Facial clefts and congenital ring constrictions.* (*A,B*). Patient had bilateral cleft lip and left-sided oblique facial cleft in addition to syndactyly and numerous ring constrictions. (*C,D*). Asymmetric multiple encephaloceles. Note tissue band directed superiorly from base of small proboscis medial to rudimentary eye. (*From K. L. Jones et al., J. Pediatr.* **84:**90, 1974.)

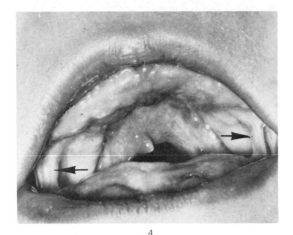

A

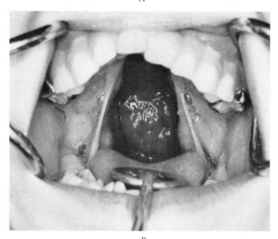

B

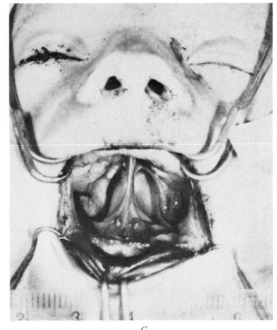

C

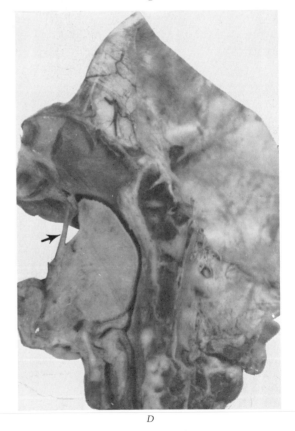

D

Figure 29-4. *Cleft palate and oral synechiae. (A).* Syngnathia; arrows point to fibrous bands joining upper and lower gingiva. *(Courtesy of H. Weyers, Cuxhaven, Germany.) (B).* Autosomal dominantly inherited synechiae. *(Courtesy of M. Mazaheri, Lancaster, Pa.) (C,D).* Cleft palate and persistence of buccopharyngeal membrane. *(From M. Hub and J. Jirásek,* Čas. Lék Čes. **99:** 1297, 1960.)

certain that these synechiae represent remnants of the buccopharyngeal membrane. Longacre (7) described extension of the soft palate to the base of the tongue in the region of the foramen cecum. The velum was cleft. Palatal cleft in association with various synechiae has been noted by Wassermann (9), Lamothe (6), Kouyoumdjian and McDonald (5), Hayward and Avery (3), Hub and Jirasek (4), Berendes (1), Fuhrmann et al. (2), and C. S. Bartsocas (personal communication, 1974) (Figs. 29-4A–D).

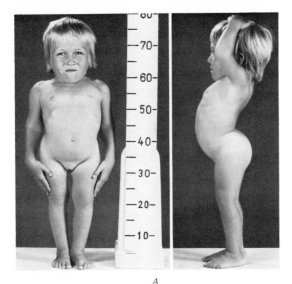

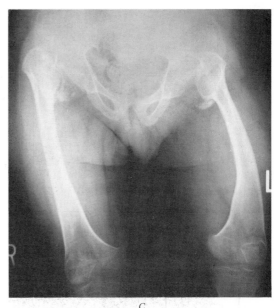

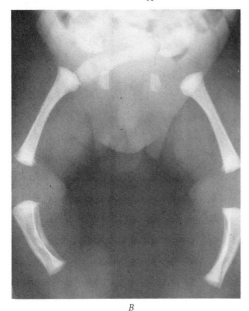

Figure 29-5. *Cleft palate and spondyloepiphyseal dysplasia congenita.* (*A*). Markedly reduced stature, shortened neck and trunk, severe myopia, and retinal detachment. Cleft palate occurs in about 35 percent of cases. Note marked lumbar lordosis. (*Courtesy of J. Spranger, Kiel, Germany.*) (*B*). Note retardation in ossification of pubic bones. (*From W. Holthusen,* Ann. Radiol. (Paris) **15**:253, 1972.) (*C*). The femoral epiphyses are deformed, late in development, and in severe coxa vara position.

ably either X-linked or autosomal recessive inheritance (1).

The hearing defect proved to be a conduction deficit in all but one child. The digital anomaly consisted of shortening and broadening of the distal portion of the thumbs and great toes. Roentgenographic examination revealed that the distal phalanges were rudimentary, with bifid ends. The urinary tract anomalies were bandlike constrictions of the ureter and replication of the renal pelvis and ureter.

The uvula was bifid in two of five affected males. This appears to be statistically significant, since the incidence of bifid uvula in Caucasians is about 1 in 70 (2).

It is conceivable that this represents a heterogeneous group of disorders. At least one example suggests trisomy 13 (5), while others represent an autosomal dominant syndrome (1, 2).

CLEFT UVULA, DEAFNESS, NEPHROSIS, CONGENITAL URINARY TRACT AND DIGITAL ANOMALIES

The syndrome was found in five of seven boys and in none of five girls in a sibship. It was the authors' contention that the syndrome had prob-

CLEFT PALATE AND CONGENITAL SPONDYLOEPIPHYSEAL DYSPLASIA

Defined first by Spranger and Wiedemann in 1966 (5), this autosomal dominantly inherited disorder appears to be as frequent as the Morquio syndrome. It is associated with congenitally reduced stature, which is largely due to disproportionate shortness of the neck and trunk. The extremities are proportionately shortened. Myopia is noted in about 50 percent of the cases (2), and detached retina has been occasionally observed (Fig. 29-5A).

Roentgenographically, there is reduction in the height of the vertebral bodies, which, during infancy, appear ovoid in lateral view. There are mild to moderate metaphyseal alterations in long tubular bones and retardation in ossification of the pubic bones, knee epiphyses, and talus and calcaneus. The long bones are slightly squat. The upper femoral epiphysis is deformed, late in development, and in coxa vara position (Fig. 29-5B, C).

Cleft palate has been observed in about 35 percent of cases (1–6). Lymphocytic granulations are characteristic, but urinary mucopolysaccharides are normal.

CLEFT LIP-PALATE AND LATERAL PROBOSCIS

Lateral proboscis usually occurs in association with unilateral absence of the nose on the same side, but it may result from an accessory nasal placode (2). The blind-ended tubular structure usually arises above the inner canthus, the eye being laterally displaced (5). There is unilateral absence of the olfactory bulb and cribriform plate on the side of the proboscis, i.e., unilateral arhinencephaly (Fig. 29-6).

Cleft lip-palate has been present in most cases. It is unilateral and occurs on the same side. The cleft, however, may be incomplete (1, 4). Bilateral cleft lip and cleft palate were seen in association with anencephaly and lateral proboscis in the case of Rating (3).

CLEFT LIP-PALATE, OCULAR HYPERTELORISM, AND MICROTIA

This syndrome was described in 1969 by Bixler et al. (1) in two sisters. Ocular hypertelorism was observed (Fig. 29-7A). The pinnas were markedly hypoplastic (Fig. 29-7B). Tomographic examination revealed hypoplasia of the auditory ossicles and canals. Mild microcephaly was

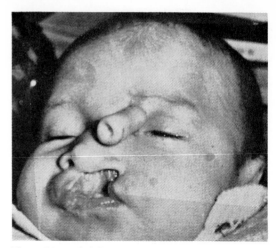

Figure 29-6. *Cleft lip and palate* with lateral nasal proboscis. (*Courtesy of L. R. McLaren*, Br. J. Plast. Surg. **8:**57, 1955.)

present, as well as ectopic kidneys and congenital heart defects. Growth was below the 3d percentile. The parents were normal, suggesting autosomal recessive inheritance.

CLEFT PALATE, MICROGNATHIA, TALIPES EQUINOVARUS, ATRIAL SEPTAL DEFECT, AND PERSISTENT LEFT SUPERIOR VENA CAVA

Gorlin et al. (1) presented a kindred exhibiting cleft palate, micrognathia, talipes equinovarus, atrial septal defect, persistence of the left superior vena cava, and a cardiac conduction anomaly. The occurrence of the syndrome in several male children of sisters suggested X-linked recessive inheritance.

CLEFT LIP-PALATE, MICROCEPHALY, AND HYPOPLASIA OF RADIUS AND THUMB

Juberg and Hayward (1) noted cleft lip-palate, microcephaly, hypoplastic and distally positioned thumbs, and shortened radii (Fig. 29-8). This constellation was present in three of six siblings. The parents were normal and nonconsanguineous. Somewhat similar findings were described by Murphy and Lubin (2).

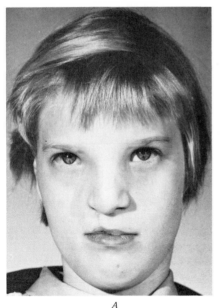

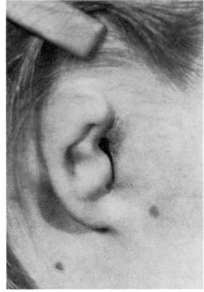

A   *B*

Figure 29-7. *Cleft lip-palate, ocular hypertelorism, and microtia. (A).* Note hypertelorism, repaired cleft lip. Sister has similar anomalies. *(B).* Dysplastic pinna, narrowing of ear canal. *(From D. Bixler, et al.,* Birth Defects **5**(2):77, 1969.)

CLEFT LIP-PALATE AND HYPOPHYSEAL DWARFISM

Francés et al. (1) described clefts in two female hypophyseal dwarfs. The first cleft involved both the lip and palate. The second cleft was stated to be median, involving the lip but not the palate. The photographs and description suggest premaxillary agenesis in this latter case. Congenital hip dysplasia was also present in the second child. Other examples are those of Laron et al. (2), Zimmermann et al. (3), and Zuppinger et al. (4). The association may be one of chance.

CLEFT LIP-PALATE AND SACRAL AGENESIS

There are a few examples of partial or complete sacral agenesis combined with clefts of the lip and/or palate (1, 2). The most commonly associated anomalies have been talipes equinovarus, dislocated hips, and hernia.

CLEFT PALATE AND ANIRIDIA

Lindberg (1) reported the combination of cleft palate and aniridia in two members of a family.

CLEFT PALATE AND AMELIA

Centa and Rovei (1) noted amelia, micrognathia, and cleft palate in a child described as having the Robin anomalad. A child reported by Holthusen (2) was less severely affected. The arms, femurs, and fibulas were absent. Perhaps this case should be classified with cleft palate and absent femurs (see below).

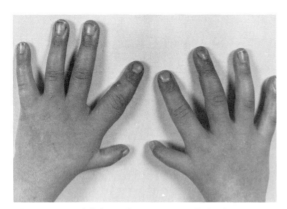

Figure 29-8. *Cleft lip-palate, microcephaly, hypoplasia of radius and thumb.* Severe hypoplasia of thumbs. *(From R. C. Juberg and J. R. Hayward, J. Pediatr.* **74**:755, 1969.)

CLEFT PALATE AND APLASIA OF THE TROCHLEA

Mead and Martin (1) described cleft palate in a patient who also had aplasia of the trochlea. Conceivably the association is one of chance. However, because of the rarity of aplasia of the trochlea, the finding may be significant.

CLEFT PALATE AND ACCESSORY METACARPAL OF INDEX FINGER

Manzke (3) reported a female child with cleft palate, micrognathia, glossoptosis, pectus carinatum, and an accessory metacarpal at the base of the index finger bilaterally, producing clinodactyly. Similar cases were reported by Farnsworth and Pacik (1) and Holthusen (2). All cases to date are sporadic (Fig. 29-9A, B).

CLEFT PALATE, CUTIS GYRATUM, AND ACANTHOSIS NIGRICANS

Beare et al. (1) described a patient exhibiting an apparently unique syndrome of cutis gyratum of the facial skin, acanthosis nigricans, ocular hypertelorism, neonatal teeth, hypodontia, bifid nipples, hypogonadism, and cleft palate (Fig. 29-10A–C).

CLEFT LIP-PALATE, HYPOHIDROSIS, THIN WIRY HAIR, AND DYSTROPHIC NAILS

Rapp and Hodgkins (4) and Wannarachue et al. (6) noted the combination of hypohidrosis, sparse, wiry scalp hair, nail dystrophy, short stature, and clefting of the lip and/or palate in a mother and in her son and daughter. Summitt and Hiatt (5)

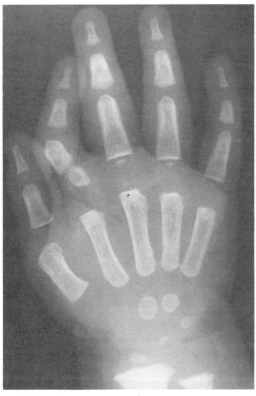
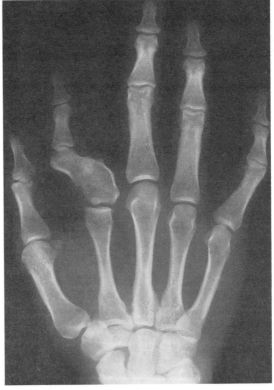

A   B

Figure 29-9. *Cleft palate and accessory metacarpal of index finger. (A).* Note separate bone at base of proximal phalanx of index finger. *(B).* Same anomaly in older patient, but fusion has taken place. *(From W. Holthusen,* Ann. Radiol. *(Paris)* **15**:253, 1972.)

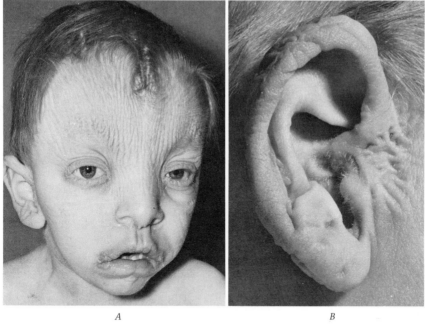

A   *B*

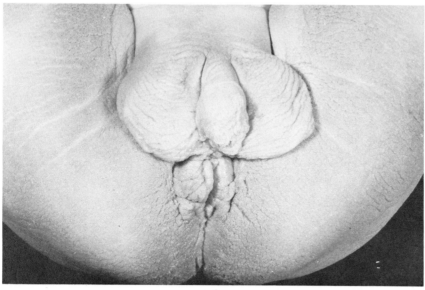

C

Figure 29-10. *Cleft palate, cutis gyratum, and acanthosis nigricans.* (*A*). Cutis gyratum of facial skin, broad nasal bridge, acanthosis nigricans around mouth. Patient had cleft palate and natal teeth. Note unusual hairline. (*B*). Malformed pinna showing "forceps-mark" indentations in tragal area. (*C*). Marked acanthosis nigricans in anogenital area. (*From J. M. Beare et al.,* Br. J. Dermatol. **81**:241, 1969.)

described a white male child with bilateral cleft lip-palate, hypospadias, chordee, sparse and wiry scalp hair, hypohidrosis, nail dysplasia, deficiency of Meibomian glands, few lashes, corneal opacities, photophobia, ectropion of lower lids, slow growth, and slitlike ear canals. An affected mother and similarly affected children have been observed by P. Spaulding (personal communication, 1975). A female infant with blond wiry hair, nail dysplasia, frontal bossing, hypohidrosis, and cleft palate was seen by W. F. Schorr (personal communication, 1974). This disorder is probably inherited as an autosomal dominant trait (Fig. 29-11).

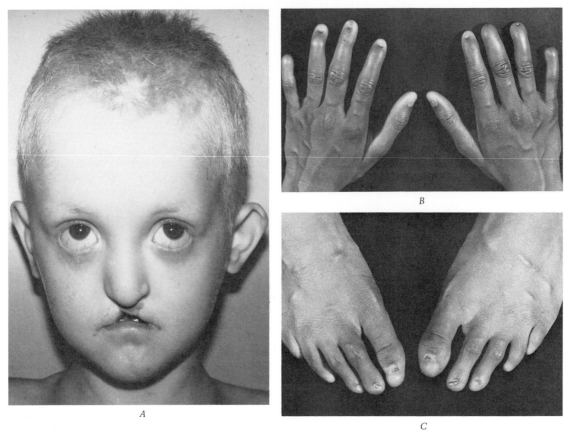

Figure 29-11. *Cleft lip-palate, hypohidrosis, thin wiry hair, and dystrophic nails. (A).* Sparse wiry hair, absent lashes and lacrimal puncta, ectropion of lower lids, hypoplasia of nasal alae, abnormal pinnas, bilateral cleft lip-palate. *(From R. L. Summitt and R. L. Hiatt,* Birth Defects **7**(8):121, 1971.) *(B,C).* Hypoplastic nails of fingers and toes. *(From R. M. Watson and C. E. Hardwick,* Br. Dent. J. **130**:77, 1971.)

Moynahan (3) described what he called the XTE syndrome in sibs who were the product of a consanguineous union. The syndrome consisted of cleft palate, hypohidrosis and dry skin, nail deformities, dry coarse hair, evanescent cutaneous bullae, absence of lashes on lower lids, small lacrimal punctae, and defective enamel. The relationship of this disorder to those cases described above is unknown.

Fára (1) and Massengill et al. (2) each described a female with sparse hair, severe hypodontia, and cleft lip-palate. Watson and Hardwick (7) described a girl with bilateral cleft lip-palate, hypoplastic pinnas, anodontia, and dystrophic nails. A sib who died soon after birth had cleft lip-palate and congenital heart defect. The parents were consanguineous. Perhaps there is genetic heterogeneity.

Possibly some of these cases are incomplete forms of the EEC syndrome.

CLEFT LIP-PALATE, TETRAPEROMELIA, DEFORMED PINNAS, AND ECTODERMAL DYSPLASIA

Freire-Maia and coworkers (1, 2) described a unique disorder in four of eight Brazilian sibs which they have called "odontotrichomelic hypohidrotic dysplasia." The parents were normal and apparently not consanguineous but were from a highly inbred region. Rather extensive bone deficiencies involved all four extremities. There was marked reduction in the amount of body hair. The ears were large, thin, outstanding, and deformed. Oligodontia and conical crown form were noted. The nipples and areolas were hypoplastic, and hypogonadism was found, as well as mental retardation. Two of four affected sibs died in infancy. Cleft lip occurred in only one boy (Fig. 29-12).

Herrmann et al. (3) described a mentally re-

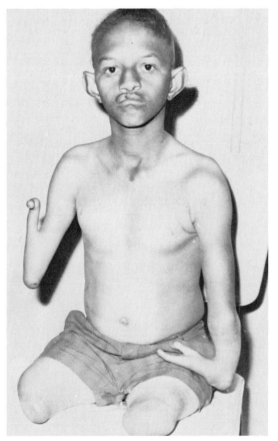

Figure 29-12. *Cleft lip-palate, tetraperomelia, deformed pinnas, and ectodermal dysplasia.* Sparsity of hair, deformed ears, hypoplastic nipples, deficient teeth, and cleft lip-palate. Sister was similarly affected. (*From N. Freire-Maia,* Am. J. Hum. Genet. **22:**370, 1970.)

tarded Amerindian boy with some of the stigmata seen in the syndrome noted above. However, their case probably represents another syndrome and is considered in Chap. 40 which discusses *unusual craniosynostosis syndromes.*

CLEFT PALATE, CAMPTODACTYLY, AND CLUBFOOT

Gordon et al. (1) reported a syndrome having autosomal dominant inheritance and variable expressivity and comprising camptodactyly, talipes equinovarus, and cleft palate.

CLEFT PALATE, STAPES FIXATION, AND OLIGODONTIA

We have seen two sisters, the offspring of a consanguineous marriage, who had stapes fixation, cleft soft palate, and marked reduction in the number of teeth (1). Neither girl had ever had more than three or four deciduous teeth, and those had conical crown form. No permanent teeth were ever present, and alveolar ridges were absent.

There was coalition of all cuneiform bones, as well as coalition of the navicular and talus, the talus and calcaneus, and the first cuneiform with the first metatarsal. The talus was malformed, having a superior and medial lump. The carpal navicular was sharply wedge-shaped, lacking its normal convexity (Fig. 29-13).

CLEFT PALATE AND ORAL DUPLICATION

There is a group of perhaps a dozen cases of oral duplication, which have been thoroughly reviewed by Gorlin (4). Among them are several infants with a rather complex set of anomalies which include cleft palate (2, 7, 8). The child described by Avery and Hayward (1) had not only two cleft palates but a double set of maxillary teeth and a bilaterally grooved or trifurcated tongue. Virtually identical examples were noted by Koblin (5) and Robertson (8). Other apparent cases are those of Kohnz (6) and Bell (3). Another possibly related example without cleft palate is that of Steinhilber (9) (Fig. 29-14).

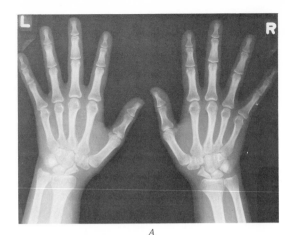

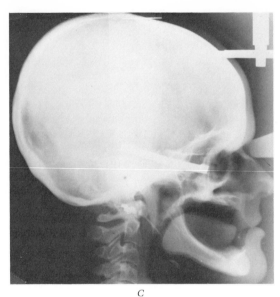

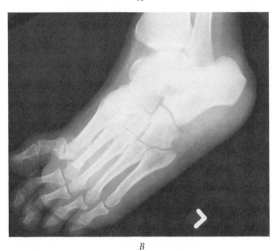

Figure 29-13. *Cleft palate, stapes fixation, and oligodontia.* (*A*). Hypoplasia of navicular bones. (*B*). Talocalcaneal fusion with unusual tibiotalar articulation and talar hump. (*C*). Absence of alveolar processes due to severe oligodontia. (*From R. J. Gorlin et al.*, Birth Defects **7**(7):87, 1971.)

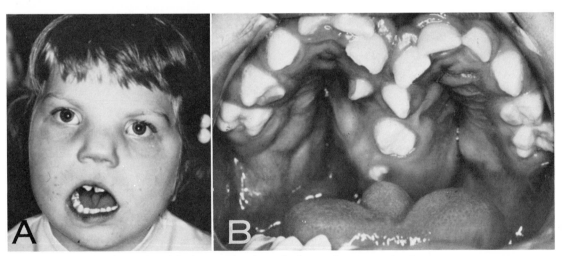

Figure 29-14. *Cleft palate and oral duplication.* (*A,B*). Ocular hypertelorism, two hard palates, and two dental arches. Note two cleft palates and partial duplication of the tongue. (*From J. Avery and J. R. Hayward*, Cleft Palate J. **6**:505, 1969.)

CLEFT PALATE AND CEREBROCOSTOMANDIBULAR SYNDROME

Doyle (1) and McNicholl et al. (4) described a syndrome in three children of nonconsanguineous parents. Similar cases have been reported by a number of authors (2, 3, 5–7). Each had microcephaly and a Robin-like complex associated with thoracic deformity, marked by rib gaps, hypoplastic or absent ribs and bizarre vertebral anomalies. Most infants died during the neonatal period. The disorder presumably has autosomal recessive inheritance (Fig. 29-15).

CLEFT PALATE, RETINAL DETACHMENT, AND HEREDITARY ARTHROOPHTHALMOPATHY (STICKLER SYNDROME)

The Stickler syndrome is an autosomal dominant disorder with markedly variable expressivity. It has been considered to be a connective tissue dysplasia with pleiotropic manifestations. First recognized by Strickler (16, 17), the condition has been described under a variety of different names (1–8, 10–15). The most extensive discussion of the Stickler syndrome was presented by Herrmann et al. (7). Although genetic

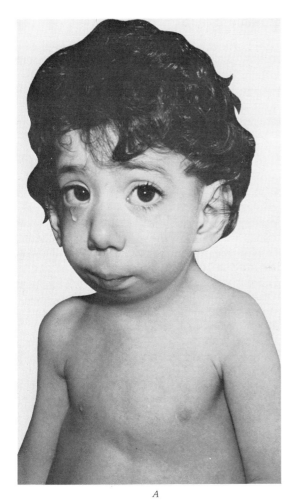

A

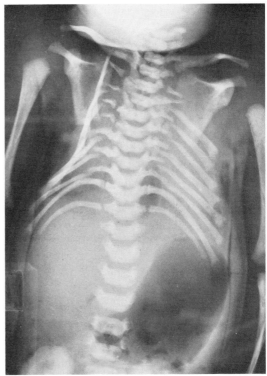

B

Figure 29-15. *Cleft palate and cerebrocostomandibular syndrome.* (A). One of three sibs with microcephaly, thoracic deformity with rib gaps, and vertebral anomalies. (B). Roentgenogram showing severely narrowed upper part of the thorax and bizarre vertebral and rib anomalies. (*From B. McNicholl et al.*, Arch. Dis. Child. **45**:421, 1970.)

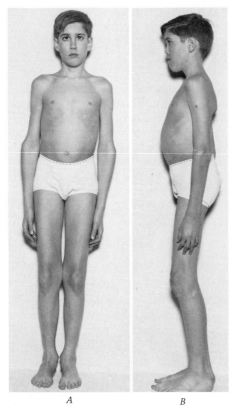

A   B

Figure 29-16. *Cleft palate, retinal detachment, and arthroophthalmopathy (Stickler syndrome).* (A, B). Severe myopia, retinal detachment, and bony changes (flattened vertebral bodies, thinned diaphyses of long bones, hypoplastic pelvic bones). (*From G. B. Stickler and D. G. Pugh,* Mayo Clin. Proc. **42:**495, 1967.)

heterogeneity may exist at a more basic level, Herrmann et al. (7) indicated that there was no good reason to justify nosologic splitting on the clinical level at the present time.

The joints are enlarged, often hyperextensible, and sometimes painful with use, becoming stiff with rest. Rarely, they are reddened and warm.

Roentgenographically, there are multiple epiphyseal ossification disturbances, moderate flattening of vertebral bodies, and diminution of the width of the shaft in tubular bones. The very thin diaphysis contrasts with the normally broad metaphysis. The pelvic bones are hypoplastic,

the femoral neck being poorly modeled and plump (15) (Fig. 29-16). The skeletal features observed radiographically and the clinical joint involvement are not always present in every case of the Stickler syndrome (7).

Congenital myopia, as great as 18 diopters, is characteristic. Before the tenth year of life, broad zones of retinal detachment may be experienced, which, if untreated, lead to blindness and ultimately to cataract, keratopathy, and glaucoma. Eye findings have been more extensively discussed by Herrmann et al. (7).

The craniofacial spectrum has varied from a reasonably normal face to midfacial flattening and the Robin anomalad. Cleft palate has been noted by several authors (6, 15, 17) and submucous cleft palate and abnormal palatal mobility have also been described (1, 7). Herrmann et al. (7) indicated that a sizable proportion of newborns with the Robin anomalad may have the Stickler syndrome. Epicanthal folds have been observed in many cases that we have personally examined. Sensorineural deafness was reported by Stickler and Pugh (18). Hearing deficit has also been noted by other authors (7). Dental abnormalities have been described (7) (Fig. 29-17).

Various other findings have been discussed by Herrmann et al. (7).

Wagner's autosomal dominant hyaloideoretinal degeneration bears great resemblance to the ophthalmologic findings in the Stickler syndrome, but since no other features of the latter are observed, it probably represents a distinct nosologic entity.

The Marshall syndrome (9) has many features in common with the Stickler syndrome. However, because of differences discussed in Chapter 144, it appears to be a distinct entity.

CLEFT LIP-PALATE AND ENCEPHALOMENINGOCELE

Cleft lip with or without cleft palate has been described in association with glioma or encephalomeningocele which herniates through the sphenoid bone to present in the mouth (Fig. 29-18). The encephalocele may also present as a bulge on the frontal bone (5) and may be as-

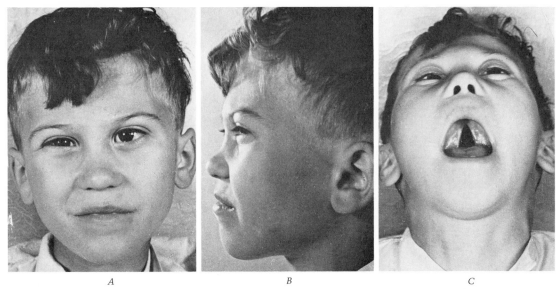

A   *B*   *C*

Figure 29-17. *Cleft palate, retinal detachment, and myopia features of the Stickler syndrome. (A–C).* Note midfacial flattening and cleft palate. Patients sometimes present during infancy with the Robin anomalad.

sociated with ocular hypertelorism. The condition should be differentiated from oral teratoma.

The cleft in most cases has involved both lip and palate (3, 5, 7, 8). Low et al. (6) described isolated cleft palate, and Exner (2) illustrated a most unusual midline cleft of the upper lip and a separate cleft of the hard and soft palates.

CLEFT PALATE AND CONGENITAL ORAL TERATOMA

Epignathus is a term used to describe a teratoma arising in the region of the Rathke pouch and projecting into and filling the pharynx or oral cavity between the palatal halves and protruding from the mouth (1–8). Erich (4), reviewing 22 cases, noted that 11 of the teratomas were attached to the sphenoid bone, six to the lateral wall of the epipharynx near the opening of the eustachian tube, two to the soft palate, and one to the hard palate (Fig. 29-19). The term "epignathus" is thus ill chosen and should be abandoned. Congenital oral teratomas appear to be far more common in females. In most cases, the

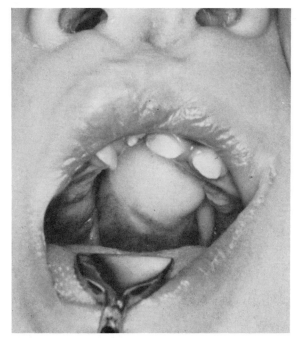

Figure 29-18. *Cleft palate and encephalomeningocele.* Repaired cleft lip, unrepaired cleft palate.

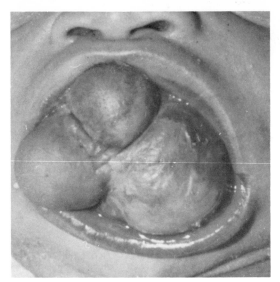

Figure 29-19. Cleft palate and congenital oral teratoma. (*Courtesy of C. O. Dummett, Los Angeles, Calif.*)

infant seldom lives beyond the neonatal period. At times, the skull base is intact, but in some cases the skull is separated, the teratoma being hourglass in shape, with intra- and extracranial portions. Still others have had no connection with the sphenoid bone.

CLEFT PALATE AND BILATERAL FEMORAL AND FIBULAR DYSGENESIS

Bailey and Beighton (1), Daentl et al. (2), and others (3, 5, 6) described patients with femoral and fibular dysgenesis, with consequent short stature, several of whom had cleft palate. The facies was characterized by mongoloid obliquity of palpebral fissures, short nose with alar hypoplasia, long philtrum, and thin upper lip and micrognathia. In addition, they had dislocated and hypoplastic patellas, hypoplastic pelvis, talipes equinovarus, derangement of elbow joints, and lower spine abnormalities. The genetic nature of the syndrome, if it exists, is not known. Patients described by Holthusen (4) may have the same disorder (Fig. 29-20A–C).

CLEFT PALATE, VENTRICULAR SEPTAL DEFECT, TRUNCUS ARTERIOSUS, AND INTRAUTERINE DEATH

Lowry and Miller (1) noted sibs with cleft palate, truncus arteriosus, and abnormal right pulmonary artery. The left pulmonary artery came off the truncus. Presumably the syndrome has autosomal recessive inheritance.

CLEFT LIP AND/OR PALATE AND ENLARGED PARIETAL FORAMENS

It would appear likely that enlarged parietal foramens, commonly inherited as an isolated autosomal dominant trait, may be associated with clefting of the lip or palate with a greater-than-chance frequency.

The nature of these odd cranial defects has been discussed by numerous authors (5, 6, 8). The frequency of parietal foramens would appear to be less than 1 in 25,000 individuals. Over 250 cases of their isolated occurrence have been described. Warkany and Weaver (7) and Lother (5) discussed other malformations associated with enlarged parietal foramens. Cases in which clefting has been noted are those of Irvine and Taylor (3), Hässler (1), James (4), and Hollender (2).

CLEFT LIP AND/OR PALATE AND CONGENITAL NEUROBLASTOMA

There are at least four published reports on the combination of congenital neuroblastoma with cleft lip-palate or isolated cleft palate. To date, this combination represents a loose association, although various anomaly combinations are described below.

Mittelbach and Szekely (4) described an infant with congenital neuroblastoma, cleft lip-palate, patent ductus arteriosus, microcephaly, agenesis of the corpus callosum, and hypertonia. Kouyoumdjian and McDonald (3) noted the following anomalies in an infant: congenital neuroblastoma, imperforate buccopharyngeal

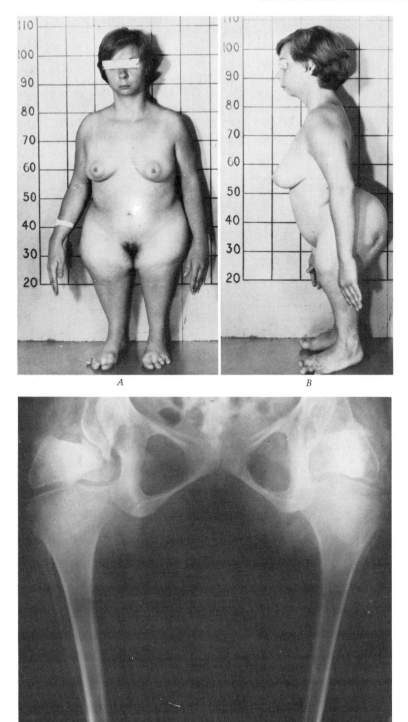

Figure 29-20. *Cleft palate and bilateral femoral dysgenesis.* (A,B). Severe abbreviation of lower limbs. Patients had dislocated and hypoplastic patellas, abnormal toes. (C). Roentgenogram showing minuscule femurs, absent acetabula, hypoplastic pelvis. (*From J. A. Bailey and P. Beighton,* Clin. Pediatr. **9:**668, 1970.)

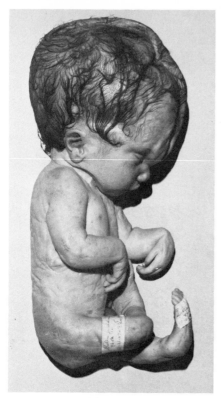

Figure 29-21. *Cleft palate and congenital neuroblastoma.* Hydrocephalus, cleft palate, malformed pinnas, joint contractures, hip dislocation. *(From J. A. Aase and D. W. Smith,* J. Pediatr. **73:**606, 1968.)

membrane, congenital cataract, polydactyly, tracheoesophageal fistula, patent foramen ovale, ureteral atresia, and Meckel diverticulum. Beckwith and Perrin (2) described a newborn with congenital neuroblastoma, cleft palate, hydrocephalus, microphthalmia, and cataracts. The resemblance to alterations seen in trisomy 13 is probably not accidental (5).

Aase and Smith (1) described two sibs and their father. Both sibs had cleft palate, hydrocephalus, Dandy-Walker malformation, hip dislocation, and malformed pinna. One child had congenital neuroblastoma. The other had multiple ventricular septal defects and a single sternal ossification center. The father exhibited oculomotor palsy, joint contractures, dislocated hip, and malformed pinnas. This same syndrome was probably described in the case of Potter and Parrish (6) (Fig. 29-21).

CLEFT PALATE, SHORT HUMERUS AND FEMUR, LONG RADIUS AND TIBIA

Walden et al. (1) described an infant with cleft palate who had extremities of normal length but the humerus and femur were short and the radius and tibia were longer than normal.

CLEFT PALATE AND SHORT STATURE

Gareis and Smith (1) described a kindred in which several affected members had stature below the 3d percentile because of relative shortness of the extremities. All affected males and about half the affected females had cleft palate or submucous cleft palate and bifid uvula. Micrognathia was also present in about half of those affected. The condition is dominantly inherited, possibly X-linked.

CLEFT LIP-PALATE AND CONGENITAL HEART DISEASE

Forming a rather ill-defined group are cases of clefting and congenital heart disease. Some of these are considered toward the end of this chapter, under Cleft Lip-palate and Forearm Bone Aplasia or Hypoplasia.

Clefting can be associated with a wide spectrum of congenital heart defects. Boeson et al. (1) noted 11 cases of cleft lip and/or cleft palate among 516 patients with congenital heart disease. The cardiac anomalies were of various types, the most common being atrial and ventricular septal defects. An equally diverse group was described by Holt and Oram (3). Rabl and Schulz (5) noted the association of cleft lip-palate and pulmonary valvular atresia and septal defect in twins. They also described two sibs with clefts.

Shah et al. (6), in an extensive review of congenital cardiac malformations in children with facial clefts, found no consistent pattern of heart abnormalities. Of 32 children with cleft lip or cleft palate who died, cardiac anomalies were present in 21 (66 percent). Seventeen of these had cleft palate. Six of the 21 had the Robin anomalad. Four had tetralogy of Fallot; four, tricuspid stenosis; three, coarctation of the aorta; and three, atrial septal defect of the secundum type. Of interest was the fact that there were no cases of transposition of the great vessels or examples of a single ventricle among the group. Similar observations were made by Okada et al. (4). They noted that the Robin anomalad was associated with coarctation of the aorta and tetralogy of Fallot.

Didier et al. (2a) described a child with cleft lip-palate and extrathoracic heart.

CLEFT LIP-PALATE AND ANENCEPHALY

Anencephaly is characterized by absence of cranial vault, brain, and pituitary gland. Associated with the condition are protruding eyeballs and tongue, aquiline nose, malformations of the cranial base, and changes secondary to absence of the pituitary, such as hypoplasia of the adrenal

glands and gonads (1). The protruding eyeballs presumably result from the presence of abnormally large retroorbital fat pads. The protruding tongue may be due to an abnormally small oral cavity.

The incidence varies considerably in different parts of the world, but roughly is about 15 to 18 per 10,000 live births.

The concurrence of clefting and anencephaly is certainly higher than chance would dictate. Among 114 infants with isolated cleft palate, MacMahon and McKeown (8) found one anencephalic, but three with this condition were enumerated among 105 infants with cleft lip with or without cleft palate. Neel (10) found one infant with cleft palate and three with cleft lip and palate among 34 Japanese anencephalics. Fogh-Andersen (4) also noted the association. Gleeson and Stovin (5) described an anencephalic child with cleft palate, a Klippel-Feil-like alteration, and a neuroenteric cyst. Heintel (6) stated

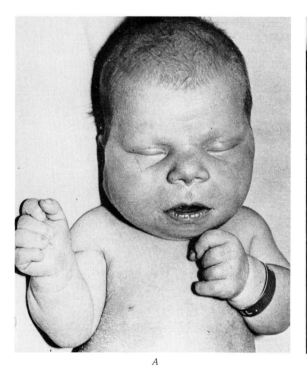
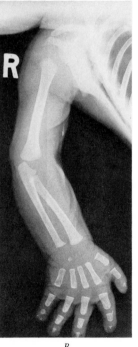

A   *B*

Figure 29-22. *Cleft palate and Rüdiger syndrome.* (*A*). Coarse facies, finger contractures. (*B*). Small middle phalanges and small triangular terminal phalanges. (*From R. A. Rüdiger et al.,* J. Pediatr. **79**:977, 1971.)

that every anencephalic he examined had a sub-mucous palatal cleft. Both Deppe (3) and Roches (11) described a high correlation between anen-cephaly and facial clefting. Christakos and Simpson (2) noted cleft lip in one of three sibs with anencephaly. Mufarrij and Kilejian (9) de-scribed an anencephalic with cleft palate. Smithells et al. (12) noted two with cleft lip, one with cleft lip and palate, and one with cleft pal-ate among 180 anencephalics. Jones (7) described 12 with cleft palate and one with cleft lip among 67 anencephalics.

CLEFT PALATE AND RÜDIGER SYNDROME

Rüdiger et al. (1) described a lethal, probably au-tosomal recessive syndrome in sibs, the infants succumbing within the first year of life. The disorder is characterized by somatic retardation, flexion contracture of hands with thick palmar creases, simian lines, small fingers and nails, and ureteral stenosis. Arches were noted on all fingers. The facies was coarse, and the soft palate was cleft (Fig. 29-22).

CLEFT PALATE AND NANCE-SWEENEY CHONDRODYSPLASIA

Nance and Sweeney (1) noted a unique chondro-dysplasia having autosomal recessive inheri-tance. Cousins were similarly affected, and there was parental consanguinity. Clinically, the cases superficially resembled achondroplasia. In addi-tion, thick leathery skin, soft-tissue calcifica-tions, and dysplastic ears were noted. Cleft pal-ate was present in at least two of four affected sibs (Fig. 29-23A–D).

CLEFT PALATE, UNUSUAL FACIES, MENTAL RETARDATION, AND LIMB ABNORMALITIES

Palant et al. (1) described sisters with mild mi-crocephaly, short stature, mental retardation, almond-shaped deep-set eyes, bulbous nasal tip, cleft palate, clinodactyly of toes, and firm non-bony prominence of the anteromedial aspect of the wrists. The syndrome probably has autosomal recessive inheritance (Fig. 29-24).

CLEFT PALATE AND RARE LETHAL DWARFISM

Distinct from achondrogenesis and thana-tophoric dwarfism is a condition described in sibs by de la Chapelle et al. (1). This micromelic dwarfism is characterized by cleft palate, short curved bones (especially the radius and ulna), tri-angular fibula and ulna, double phalanges, various vertebral anomalies (small vertebral bodies, hemivertebras), and anomalies of the scapula and pelvis.

Inheritance is autosomal recessive.

CLEFT PALATE AND CAMPOMELIC DWARFISM

Spranger et al. (10) called attention to a syndrome consisting of prominent forehead with flat face, ocular hypertelorism, cleft palate, and micro-gnathia. Death has occurred in 90 percent of the cases before six months of age. At least 75 per-cent of these patients have exhibited respiratory distress.

Roentgenographically, there is anterior bow-ing of the femurs and tibias, which, if se-vere, is associated with skin dimpling. The fibu-las are hypoplastic. There are reduced numbers of ribs, hypoplasia of scapulas, vertebral ossifica-tion defects, vertical pelvis, and talipes cal-caneovalgus. Engel et al. (4) and Gardner et al. (5) described the disorder in phenotypic females with XY sex chromosomes. Stüve and Wiede-mann (12) and Cremin et al. (3) described af-fected female sibs. Thurman and Kityakara (13) reported the syndrome in half-sibs. The disorder is probably heterogeneous, some having au-tosomal recessive inheritance (Fig. 29-25A–C). In some cases, the long bones are abbreviated. Poly-hydramnios has been noted in 25 percent of cases. Good reviews are those of Schmickel et al. (9), Opitz et al. (8), and Storer and Grossman (11).

CLEFT LIP-PALATE AND HYPOGONADOTROPIC HYPOGONADISM

There have been a few reports of individuals, both male and female, with cleft lip-palate and low urinary gonadotropin levels and oligomen-orrhea or infantile testes with aspermia and ab-

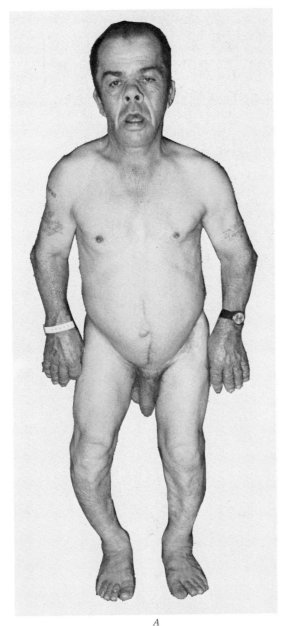

A

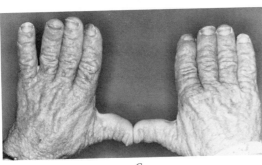

C

Figure 29-23. *Cleft palate and Nance-Sweeney chondro-dysplasia.* (*A*). Short male with bowed legs, short nose with anteverted nostrils, limited elbow extension. (*B*). Dysplastic pinna. (*C*). Fingers of same length, thick leathery skin. (*D*). Squat bones of hand. (*From W. E. Nance and A. Sweeney,* Birth Defects **6**(4):25, 1970.)

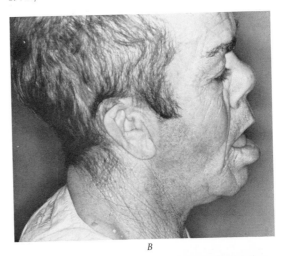

B

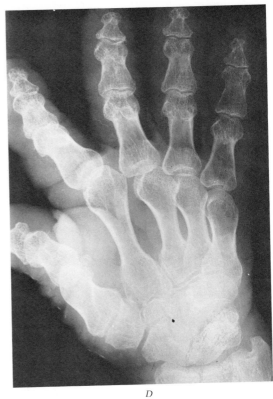

D

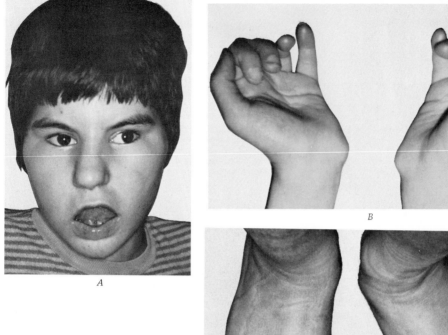

Figure 29-24. *Cleft palate, unusual facies, mental retardation, and limb abnormalities. (A). One of the two female sibs with cleft palate, short stature, bulbous nasal tip. (B). Firm nonbony prominences of anteromedial aspects of wrists. (C). Short halluces with space between hallux and second toe. (From D. Palant et al., J. Pediatr. **78**:686, 1971.)*

sent Leydig cells. Some have the Kallmann syndrome, i.e., associated anosmia (1–3).

Rosen (2) suggested autosomal recessive inheritance, although this is not likely in the family reported by Sparkes et al. (3).

CLEFT PALATE AND KNIEST SYNDROME

The disorder described by Kniest (1) in 1952 is a rare form of disproportionate dwarfism, often confused with the Morquio syndrome or metatropic dwarfism. At this writing, nearly all cases have been sporadic (1–6). Maroteaux and Spranger (2) observed the syndrome in a mother and daughter.

The face is round, with the midface flat and the nasal bridge depressed, giving the eyes an exophthalmic appearance. The neck is short, and the head appears to sit upon the thorax (Fig. 29-26A, B). At birth, the patient is frequently noted to have cleft palate, clubfoot, and prominent knees. Lordosis and/or kyphoscoliosis and tibial bowing usually develop within the first few years of life. The child may not sit and walk until two and three years of age, respectively. By that time, most joints become progressively enlarged, stiff, and painful. Movement at the metacarpophalangeal joint is normal, but the child cannot make a fist. The fifth fingers are generally not involved. The elbows and wrists become especially enlarged, and flexion and extension of

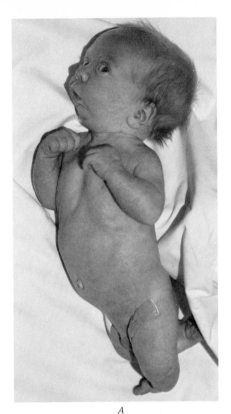

A

most joints become progressively reduced. Gait is markedly altered. Adult height ranges between 105 and 145 cm.

Severe myopia and lattice degeneration with or without retinal detachment and/or cataract formation have been present in less than half of reported cases, as has cleft palate. Conduction and/or sensorineural deafness may develop before puberty. Recurrent respiratory infections are common.

Roentgenographically, the neurocranium is large in comparison with the facial skeleton. Platyspondyly, especially of the upper thoracic part of the spine, is severe. The interpediculate distances in the lumbar portion of the spine narrow sacrally. The bones of the upper limbs are

Figure 29-25. *Cleft palate and campomelic dwarfism.* (*A*). Child with bent femurs and tibias, micrognathia, cleft palate. (*B*). Roentgenogram showing camptomelia (bent bones). (*From J. Opitz, Madison, Wis.*) (*C*). Similar stigmata in another child with same syndrome. (*From R. D. Schmickel,* J. Pediatr. **82**:299, 1973.)

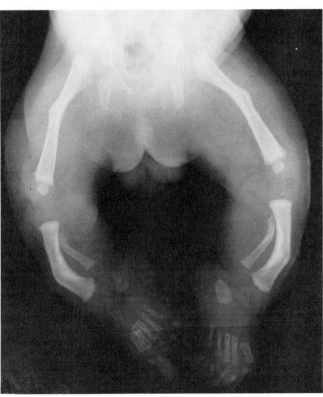

B

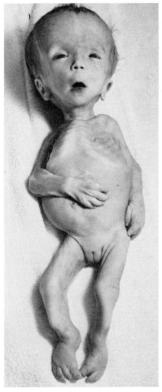

C

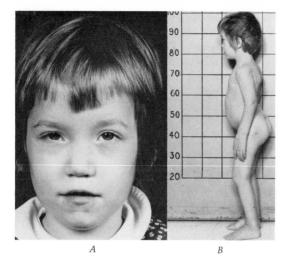

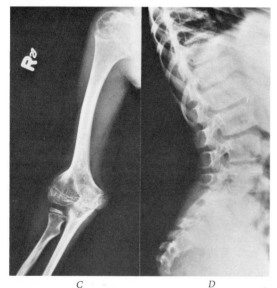

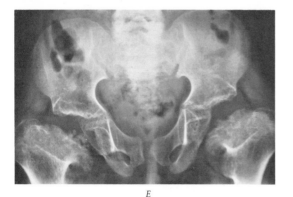

short. The metaphyses of long bones flare, and the epiphyses are large, irregular, and punctate.

The proximal row of carpal bones is small, but bone age is normal or advanced. The pelvic bones are markedly small, especially in relation to the large capital femoral epiphysis and proximal femoral metaphysis. The femoral capital epiphysis forms late, the neck is wide and short with a poorly ossified central area, and there may be coxa vara. The trochanter is prominent (Fig. 29-26C, E).

Histopathologic examination of the bones has shown that the cartilage contains large chondrocytes which lie in a very loosely woven matrix containing numerous empty spaces ("Swiss cheese cartilage") (3).

CLEFT PALATE AND MEGEPIPHYSEAL DWARFISM

Gorlin et al. (1973) described a male with cleft palate, dislocated lenses, deafness, somatic and mental retardation, epicanthal folds, and snub nose. Striking were enlarged joints (shoulders, elbows, hips, knees, ankles). Roentgenographic study showed marked shortening of long bones, with flared metaphyses and extremely large proximal and distal epiphyses. The carpal bones were large (Fig. 29-27A–E).

Homocystinuria, found on biochemical study, would account for the dislocated lenses and the mental retardation, but the skeletal alterations were unique. The child was the product of father-daughter incest.

Figure 29-26. *Cleft palate and Kniest syndrome. (A, B).* Five-year-old girl with flat midface, myopia, cleft palate. At birth, legs were noted to be abnormally short and hips were stiff. Umbilical and inguinal hernia were repaired. During early childhood, joints became enlarged, painful, and stiff. Note flexion deformities. *(C).* Roentgenograms showing irregularity of epiphyses and flared metaphyses of shortened humerus. *(D).* Platyspondyly with irregularity of anterior margins of vertebral bodies. *(E).* Coxa vara with irregular mineralization of femoral capital epiphyses, wide femoral heads and trochanters. Irregularity of acetabular roofs.

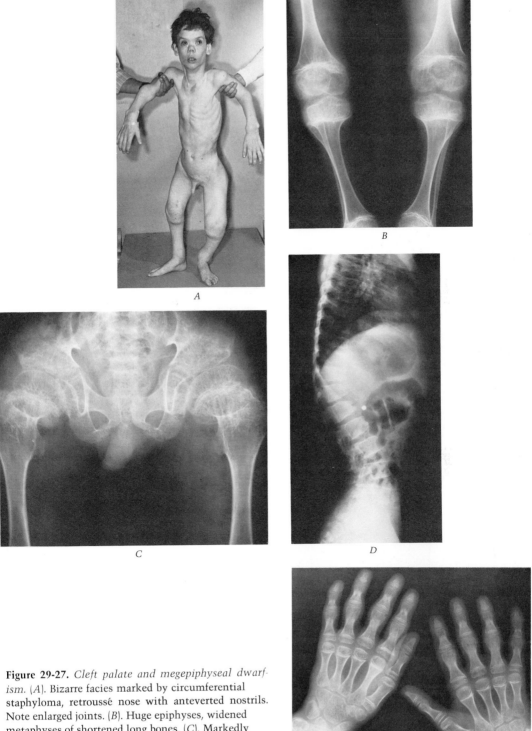

Figure 29-27. *Cleft palate and megepiphyseal dwarfism.* (*A*). Bizarre facies marked by circumferential staphyloma, retroussé nose with anteverted nostrils. Note enlarged joints. (*B*). Huge epiphyses, widened metaphyses of shortened long bones. (*C*). Markedly enlarged femoral heads, trochanters. (*D*). Anterior wedging of several lumbar vertebras. (*E*). Note flattened epiphyses of metacarpals, large carpal bones.

CLEFT PALATE, MACULAR COLOBOMA, AND SKELETAL ABNORMALITY

Phillips and Griffiths (1) reported male and female sibs with bilateral macular colobomas, cleft palate, hallux valgus, somatic retardation, and flexion deformities of distal interphalangeal joints of the little fingers. The male sib was mentally retarded, with dislocation of the patella, coxa valga, and genu valgum.

CLEFT LIP-PALATE AND FOREARM BONE APLASIA OR HYPOPLASIA

The association of aplasia of the ulna, antecubital pterygia, reduction of ulnar marginal

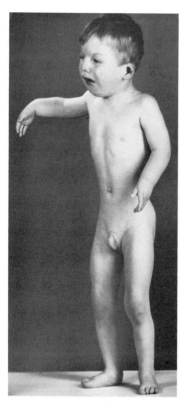

Figure 29-28. *Cleft palate, bilateral absence of fifth rays of hands and feet, and mental retardation.* Patient also had hypoplasia of ulnas, malformed ears and eyelids, and congenital heart disease. (*From H. R. Wiedemann,* Klin. Pediätr. **185:**181, 1973.

radiation and sternal segments, malformation of spleen and kidney, and premaxillary anomalies, such as mesiodens and cleft lip-palate, was described by Weyers (9). Its inheritance pattern, if any, is not known.

Wiedemann (10) defined a mental retardation syndrome characterized by bilateral absence of the fifth rays in both hands and feet, hypoplasia of the ulnas, cleft palate, malformed ears and eyelids, and congenital heart disease (Fig. 29-28). He suggested autosomal recessive inheritance and cited "similar" cases. We are not convinced that the cases cited are, in fact, the same disorder.

Birch-Jensen (1) found nine cases of cleft lip and palate among 625 cases of congenital deformities or absence of the upper limbs.

Radial aplasia has been noted to occur in association with cleft lip and palate by a number of investigators (1–4, 6, 7, 8). Kato (6) and Birch-Jensen (1) found facial clefts present in 2 to 7 percent of patients with aplasia of the radius. The early literature was especially well reviewed by Kummel (8).

Immeyer (5), in an exhaustive study, documented 16 cases of radius defects and facial clefts. In 14 cases, there was bilateral cleft lip and palate. Other commonly associated anomalies include horseshoe kidney, interventricular septal defects, and hydrocephalus (6).

CLEFT LIP-PALATE, LID ECTROPION, AND OCULAR HYPERTELORISM

A possible syndrome involving cleft lip and/or cleft palate, ectropion of the lower eyelids, and digital and/or limb reduction has been noted in several case reports (1–5). Zellweger (5) found the condition in a mother and her son. Whether they represent variants of mandibulofacial dysostosis or of Nager syndrome cannot be stated at this time.

The patient described by Genée (2) had cleft palate, mild microtia, supernumerary vertebras, 13 ribs, and only four digits on each extremity. The boy reported by Piper (3) had cleft lip-palate but no other anomalies. Warburg's patient (4) had ventricular septal defect and coloboma of the optic nerve and choroid but no limb abnor-

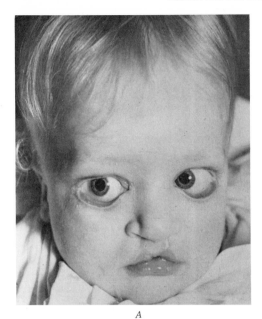
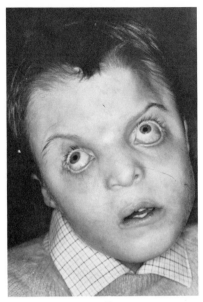

A   *B*

Figure 29-29. (*A*, *B*). Compare facies of two unrelated children. Note ectropion of lower eyelids, repaired cleft lip, and ocular hypertelorism. (*From. H. F. Piper*, Monatsschr. Kinderheilkd. **105:**107, 1957, and M. Warburg, Copenhagen, Denmark.)

malities (Fig. 29-29*A*, *B*). Several patients have exhibited rudimentary nipples and cryptorchism (1).

CLEFT PALATE AND MICROGNATHIC DWARFISM

Maroteaux et al. (1) and others (2, 3) have described a micromelic type of dwarfism characterized by a small mandible and marked widening of the metaphyses of long bones. Cleft vertebras are often visible in the lumbar region, and a slight median fissure of the bony plates is observed in anteroposterior views (Fig. 29-30*A–C*). Later, the development of the epiphyses is insufficient, particularly in the femoral heads, and growth is slow. The disorder appears to have autosomal recessive inheritance. Cleft palate has been present in all those affected.

Weissenbacher (personal communication, 1974) has reported that, with time, the long bones exhibit normal length and almost normal form. Thoracic platyspondyly is evident, and the second lumbar vertebra is kyphotic. The child

that he described, now is about ten years old, and has marked sensori neural deafness.

MEDIAN CLEFT LIP-PALATE AND SHORT RIB–POLYDACTYLY SYNDROME (MAJEWSKI TYPE)

There are several examples of a lethal condition in which short-ribbed dwarfs have polydactyly. These conditions have been described by Spranger et al. (6). In the so-called "Majewski type," the infant is hydropic with thoracic dystrophy characterized by a short and narrow thorax and short ribs, pre- and postaxial polydactyly of the hands and feet, short extremities due to short tibia, and protuberant abdomen (Fig. 29-31*A*, *B*). Hypoplasia of epiglottis, larynx, and lungs, persistent left superior vena cava, patent ductus arteriosus, various genital anomalies, and polycystic kidney have been found on autopsy.

Polyhydramnios is common. After a brief period, the infant dies because of severe respiratory distress.

Oral anomalies have included median cleft of

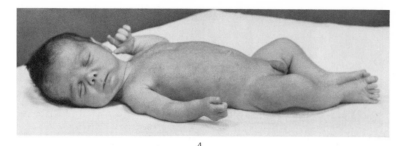

A

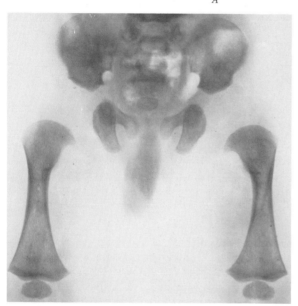

B

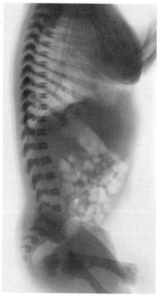

C

Figure 29-30. *Cleft palate and micrognathic dwarfism.* (*A*). Three-week-old infant showing sunken nasal root, small nose with anteverted nostrils, and micrognathia. Proximal upper and lower extremities are shortened. (*B*). Roentgenogram of child at three months of age showing small pelvis, widened femoral metaphyses. (*C*). Note widened intervertebral spaces, unusual form of second to fourth lumbar vertebras, cleft lumbar vertebral bodies. (*Fig.* 29-30A–C, *from G. Weissenbacher and E. Zweymuller*, Monatsschr. Kinderheilkd. **112**:315, 1964.)

the upper lip and/or cleft palate (2–6), ankyloglossia (2, 3, 5), tongue hamartoma (3), bifid tongue tip (3), and natal teeth (1).

CLEFT PALATE AND LETHAL MICROMELIC DWARFISM WITH MARKED SHORTNESS OF THE RADIUS AND FIBULA

De la Chapelle et al. (1) reported a unique form of lethal micromelic dwarfism in a brother and sister whose parents were consanguineous. The disorder probably has autosomal recessive inheritance.

Extension of the elbows and knees was limited. The joints were somewhat enlarged, and there was talipes equinovarus. The fingers and toes, although normal in number, were very short. The trunk length was reduced, and the belly was large. The root of the nose was rather flat, with associated ocular hypertelorism. The ears were low set. Both children had cleft-palate.

Roentgenographically, the radius and the fibula were particularly affected, being wide, short, and somewhat triangular. A certain degree of campomelia was present in the femurs and tibias. The proximal portion of the humerus was

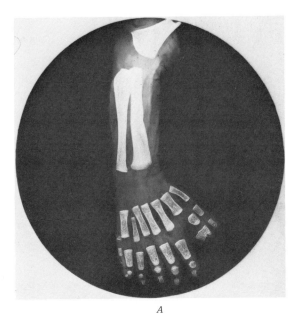
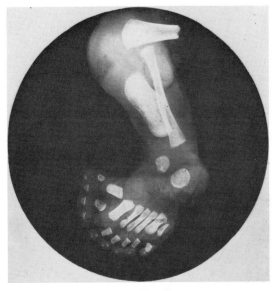

A   B

Figure 29-31. *Median cleft lip-palate and short rib–polydactyly syndrome (Majewski type).* (A,B). Roentgenograms showing preaxial and postaxial polydactyly, shortened tibia. *(From E. Pitschi, Thesis, Zurich, 1904–1905.)*

widened. The bones of the hand were inadequately ossified. The proximal phalanges were not visible, and in the boy the middle phalanges were doubled. The form of the scapula was abnormal. The iliac wings were small. The vertebral bodies were small and unequal, and numerous hemivertebras were present.

Hepatosplenomegaly was present in both children, but only the boy had multiple heterotopic hyperplastic adenomas of the parathyroid and adrenal glands and hyperplasia of endocrine pancreatic tissue. In addition, both children had patent foramen ovale and ductus arteriosus.

PSEUDODIASTROPHIC DWARFISM AND CLEFT PALATE

Burgio et al. (1) reported two sisters who were found to be short at birth. The facies were characterized by flat nose, ocular hypertelorism, micrognathia, and full cheeks. The pinnas were malformed with large lobes. Micromelia was noted as well as talipes equinovarus and anomalies of the toes. The hands were externally rotated. The proximal phalanges were hyperextended. The second phalanges were deviated and flexed. Movement at the metatarsophalangeal and metacarpophalangeal joints was very limited as was that at the elbow. Limitation was less severe at the knees, hips, and shoulders. The thorax was bell-shaped and there was progressive scoliosis and marked kyphosis at the thoracolumbar junction and lordosis at the lumbosacral junction. Platyspondyly was severely marked. The fifth lumbar vertebra was particularly small, rounded, and subluxated. Interpediculate distances diminished from L1 to L5. The ribs were delicate and somewhat sinuous. The long bones were short and massive and their distal and proximal epiphyses were spatulate. Luxation of the radius was noted. The elbow was enlarged. The first metacarpal was enlarged.

Microscopically, the changes in the cartilage were not similar to those reported in diastrophic dwarfism. The vertebral anomalies and histochemical alterations in the cartilage separate this entity from diastrophic dwarfism.

MICROCEPHALY, LARGE EARS, SHORT STATURE, AND CLEFT PALATE

Say et al. (1) reported a dominantly inherited syndrome in which cleft palate was associated with small head size, large ears, and short stature.

The mother and her sister had distally tapering fingers with hypoplastic distal phalanges involving the second to fourth digits bilaterally, ulnar deviation of the middle fingers, low set thumbs, and bilateral acromial dimples.

RECURRENT BRACHIAL PLEXUS NEURITIS AND CLEFT PALATE

Erikson (1) reported a syndrome in a father and his two daughters. The syndrome was characterized by sudden attacks of pain in the shoulder which radiated to the arms and hands. The pain gradually disappeared, but paresthesia and weakness in the upper extremity were noted. There was also limitation of extension at the elbow and winging of the scapulas. Sensory loss over the hand and forearm was also evident. An electromyogram revealed partial denervation of several muscles of the arm and hand, the distribution being compatible with a lesion of the brachial plexus. The neuritis initially appeared around the age of 3 or 4 years.

In all three individuals the facies appeared unusual. There was facial asymmetry and mild mongoloid obliquity of the palpebral fissures and

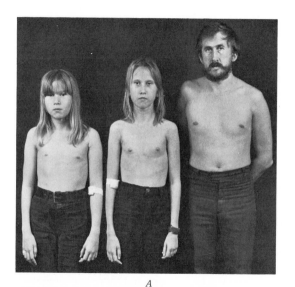

A

Figure 29-32. *Recurrent brachial plexus neuritis and cleft palate.* (A) Father and two daughters. Note deeply set eyes, ocular hypotelorism and mongoloid obliquity of palpebral fissures. (B). Patient exhibiting wrist drop during attack of recurrent brachial neuritis. (C). Winged scapulas are clearly evident. (Figures A to C from A. Erikson, *Acta Paediatr. Scand.* **63**:885, 1974.) (D). Typical facies. Note deep set hypoteloric eyes. (*Courtesy of J. C. Jacob, St. John's, Newfoundland.*)

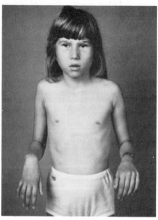

B

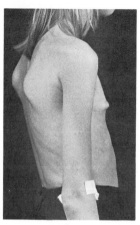

C

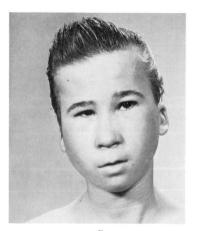

D

the eyes appeared deeply set and hypoteloric. All three patients had cleft palate. Other patients exhibiting brachial neuritis, similar facies, and cleft palate were reported by Jacob et al. (2). Similar facies was evident in the cases of Poffenbarger (4) and Gardner and Maloney (3). The syndrome has autosomal dominant inheritance.

REFERENCES

CLEFT LIP-PALATE AND CONGENITAL FILIFORM ADHESIONS OF THE EYELIDS

1 Ehlers, N., and Jensen, I. K., Ankyloblepharon Filiforme Congenitum Associated with Hare-lip and Cleft Palate. *Acta Ophthalmol. (Kbh.)* **48**:465–467, 1970.

2 Gupta, S. P., and Saxena, R. C., Ankyloblepharon Filiforme Adnatum. *J. All-India Ophthalmol. Soc.* **10**:19–21, 1962.

3 Khanna, V. D., Ankyloblepharon Filiforme Adnatum. *Am. J. Ophthalmol.* **43**:774–777, 1957.

4 Lemtis, H., and Neubauer, H., Ankyloblepharon Filiforme et Membraniforme Adnatum. *Klin. Monatsbl. Augenheilkd.* **135**:510–516, 1959.

5 Long, J. C., and Blandford, S. E., Ankyloblepharon Filiforme Adnatum with Cleft Lip and Palate. *Am. J. Ophthalmol.* **53**:126–129, 1962.

6 Neuman, A., and Shulman, J., Congenital Sinuses of the Lower Lip. *Oral Surg.* **14**:1415–1420, 1961.

7 Pahwa, J. M., and Sud, S. D., Ankyloblepharon Filiforme Adnatum. *Orient. Arch. Ophthalmol.* **4**:170–172, 1966.

8 Rogers, J. W., Ankyloblepharon Filiforme Adnatum. *Arch. Ophthalmol.* **65**:114–117, 1961.

9 Sood, N. M., et al., Ankyloblepharon Filiforme Adnatum with Cleft Lip and Palate. *J. Pediatr. Ophthalmol.* **5**:30–32, 1968.

10 Van der Woude, A., Fistula Labii Inferioris Congenita and Its Association with Cleft Lip and Palate. *Am. J. Hum. Genet.* **6**:244–256, 1954.

CLEFT LIP-PALATE, CLEFT LARYNX, AND LARYNGEAL WEB

1 Bhatia, M. L., et al., Congenital Laryngeal Web (Case 3). *Indian J. Otolaryngol.* **20**:107–111, 1968.

2 Cameron, A. H., and Williams, T. C., Cleft Larynx: A Case of Laryngeal Obstruction and Incompetence. *J. Laryngol.* **76**:381–387, 1962.

3 Cavanagh, F., Congenital Laryngeal Web. *Proc. R. Soc. Med.* **58**:272–277, 1965.

4 McHugh, H. E., and Lock, W. E., Congenital Webs of the Larynx. *Laryngoscope* **52**:43–65, 1942.

5 Phelan, P. D., et al., Familial Occurrence of Congenital Laryngeal Clefts. *Arch. Dis. Child.* **48**:275–278, 1973.

CLEFTING AND THORACOPAGOUS TWINS

1 Ayer, A. A., and Mariappa, D., Hare-lip and Cleft Palate in Double Monsters. *Indian Acad. Sci.* **38**:153–156, 1953.

2 Bartlett, R. C., Cephalothoracopagus. *Arch. Pathol.* **68**:292–298, 1959.

3 Buchta, R. M., Anencephaly in Female Thoracopagous Conjoined Twins. *Clin. Pediatr.* **12**:598–599, 1973.

4 Guttmacher, A. F., and Nichols, B. L., Teratology of Conjoined Twins. *Birth Defects* **3**:2–9, 1967.

5 Herbst, E., and Apffelstaedt, M., *Atlas und Grundriss der Missbildungen der Kiefer und Zähne.* J. F. Lehmann, 1928.

6 Ivy, R. J., A Curiosity in the Area of Cleft Lip-Cleft Palate. *Plast. Reconstr. Surg.* **42**:160, 1968.

7 Nichols, B. L., et al., General Clinical Management of Thoracopagous Twins. *Birth Defects* **3**:38–51, 1967.

8 Robertson, G. S., and McKenzie, J., Thoracopagous Twins with Different First Arch Defects. *Br. J. Surg.* **51**:362–363, 1964.

9 Stellmach, R., and Frenkel, G., Über das Vorkommen von spiegelbildlich konkordanten vollständigen einseitigen Lippen-Kiefer-Gaumenspalten bei einem siamesischen Zwillingspaar. *Dtsch. Zahnärztl. Z.* **25**:28–31, 1970.

10 Vestergaard, P., Triplets Pregnancy with a Normal Foetus and a Dicephalus Dibrachius Sirenomelus. *Acta Obstet. Gynecol. Scand.* **51**:93–94, 1972.

11 Wieczorkiewicz, B., and Komraus-Gatniejewski, M., Craniopagus. *Z. Kinderchir.* **14**:207–209, 1974.

FACIAL CLEFTS AND CONGENITAL RING CONSTRICTIONS [STREETER BANDS]

1 Baker, C. J., and Rudolph, A. J., Congenital Ring Constrictions and Intrauterine Amputations. *Am. J. Dis. Child.* **121**:393–400, 1971.

2 Custer, E. M., *Über das Wesen der schrägen Gesichtsspalten.* Thesis, Zürich, 1943.

3 Emmett, A. J. J., Syndactylism of the Hand: A Review of 60 Cases. *Br. J. Plast. Surg.* **16**:357–375, 1963.

3a Field, J. H., and Krag, D. O., Congenital Constricting Bands and Congenital Amputation of the Fingers: Placental Studies. *J. Bone Joint Surg.* **55A**:1035–1041, 1973.

4 Heinrich, R., and Vavuras, E., Zum Problem der Syndaktylie der Kinderhand. *Z. Kinderheilkd.* **6**:216–228, 1968.

5 Huffstadt, A. J. C., Aangeboren snoerringen aan de ledematen en daarmee samenhangende afwijkingen. *Ned. Tijdschr. Geneeskd.* **109**:2077–2082, 1965.

5a Jones, K. L., et al., A Pattern of Craniofacial and Limb Defects Secondary to Aberrant Tissue Bands. *J. Pediatr.* **84**:90–95, 1974.

5b Kubaček, V., and Pěnkava, J., Oblique Clefts of the Face. *Acta Chir. Plast.* **16**:152–163, 1974.

6 Maisels, D. O., Acrosyndactyly. *Br. J. Plast. Surg.* **15**:166–172, 1962.

7 Patterson, T. J. S., Congenital Ring Constrictions. *Br. J. Plast. Surg.* **14**:1–13, 1961.

8 Pfeiffer, R. A., Associated Deformities of the Head and Hands. *Birth Defects* **5**(3):18–34, 1969.

9 Torpin, R., *Fetal Malformations Caused by Amnion Rupture During Gestation.* Charles C Thomas, Springfield, 1968.

CLEFT PALATE AND ORAL SYNECHIAE

1 Berendes, J., Angeborene Synechie zwischen der Mundbodenschleimhaut und der Oberkieferfortsätzen am Rande einer Gaumenspalte. *H.N.O.* **9:**180–182, 1961.

2 Fuhrmann, W., Autosomal dominante Vererbung von Gaumenspalte und Synechien zwischen Gaumen und Mundboden oder Zunge. *Humangenetik* **14:**196–203, 1972.

3 Hayward, J. R., and Avery, J. K., A Variation in Cleft Palate. *J. Oral Surg.* **15:**320–324, 1957.

4 Hub, M., and Jirásek, J. E., Persistence of the Middle Portion of the Buccopharyngeal Membrane. *Čas. Lék. Česk.* **99:**1297–1300, 1960.

5 Kouyoumdjian, A. O., and McDonald, J. J., Association of Congenital Adrenal Neuroblastoma with Multiple Anomalies, Including an Unusual Oropharyngeal Cavity (Imperforate Buccopharyngeal Membrane?). *Cancer* **4:**784–788, 1951.

6 Lamothe, D. de, Un cas d'absence congénitale de la langue avec persistance de la membrane orale. *Ann. Mal. Oreil Larynx* **49:**717–719, 1930.

7 Longacre, J. J., Congenital Atresia of the Oropharynx. *Plast. Reconstr. Surg.* **8:**341–348, 1951.

8 Mathis, H., Über einen Fall von Ernährungsschwierigkeit bei connataler Syngnathie. *Dtsch. Zahnärztl. Z.* **17:**1167–1171, 1962.

9 Wassermann, M., Ein kongenitales Diaphragma pharyngopalatinum. *Arch. Laryngol. Rhinol.* **15:**611–612, 1904.

CLEFT UVULA, DEAFNESS, NEPHROSIS, CONGENITAL URINARY TRACT, AND DIGITAL ANOMALIES

1 Braun, F. C., Jr., and Bayer, J. F., Familial Nephrosis Associated with Deafness and Congenital Urinary Tract Anomalies in Siblings. *J. Pediatr.* **60:**33–41, 1962.

2 Meskin, L. H., and Gorlin, R. J., Abnormal Morphology of the Soft Palate: I. The Prevalence of Cleft Uvula. *Cleft Palate J.* **1:**342–344, 1964.

CLEFT PALATE AND CONGENITAL SPONDYLOEPIPHYSEAL DYSPLASIA

1 Bach, C., et al., Dysplasie spondylo-épiphysaire congénitale avec anomalies multiples. *Arch. Fr. Pédiatr.* **24:**23–33, 1967.

2 Fraser, G. R., Dysplasia Spondyloepiphysaria Congenita and Related Generalized Skeletal Dysplasia among Children with Severe Visual Handicaps. *Arch. Dis. Child.* **44:**490–498, 1969.

2a Ginter, D. N., and Lee, S. O., Spondyloepiphyseal Dysplasia Congenita. *Birth Defects* **10**(12):379–382, 1974.

3 Holthusen, W., The Pierre Robin Syndrome: Unusual Associated Developmental Defects. *Ann. Radiol. (Paris)* **15:**253–262, 1972.

4 Rupprecht, E., Dysplasia Spondylo-epiphysaria Congenita. *Kinderärztl. Prax* **37:**161–166, 1969

5 Spranger, J., and Wiedemann, H. R., Dysplasia spondyloepiphysaria congenita. *Helv. Paediatr. Acta* **21:**598–611, 1966.

6 Spranger, J. W., and Langer, L. O., Spondyloepiphyseal Dysplasia Congenita. *Radiology* **94:**313–322, 1970.

CLEFT LIP-PALATE AND LATERAL PROBOSCIS

1 Meeker, L. H., and Aebli, R., Cyclopian Eye and Lateral Proboscis with Normal One-half Face. *Arch. Ophthalmol.* **38:**159–173, 1947.

2 McLaren, L. R., A Case of Cleft Lip and Palate with Polypoid Nasal Tubercle. *Br. J. Plast. Surg.* **8:**57–59, 1955–1956.

3 Rating, B., Über eine ungewöhnliche Gesichtsmissbildung bei Anencephalie. *Virchows Arch. Pathol. Anat.* **288:**223–242, 1933.

4 Tendlau, A., Ein Fall von Proboszis lateralis. *Albrecht von Graefes Arch. Klin. Ophthalmol.* **95:**135–144, 1918.

5 Young, F., The Surgical Repair of Nasal Deformities. *Plast. Reconstr. Surg.* **4:**59–91, 1949 (Fig. 22).

CLEFT LIP-PALATE, OCULAR HYPERTELORISM, AND MICROTIA

1 Bixler, D., et al., Hypertelorism, Microtia and Facial Clefting: A Newly Described Inherited Syndrome. *Am. J. Dis. Child.* **118:**495–498, 1969; and *Birth Defects* **5**(2):77–81, 1969.

CLEFT PALATE, MICROGNATHIA, TALIPES EQUINOVARUS, ATRIAL SEPTAL DEFECT, AND PERSISTENCE OF LEFT SUPERIOR VENA CAVA

1 Gorlin, R. J., et al., Robin's Syndrome: A Probably X-linked Subvariety Exhibiting Persistence of Left Superior Vena Cava and Atrial Septal Defect. *Am. J. Dis. Child.* **119:**176–179, 1970.

CLEFT LIP-PALATE, MICROCEPHALY, AND HYPOPLASIA OF RADIUS AND THUMB

1 Juberg, R. C., and Hayward, J. R., A New Familial Syndrome of Oral, Cranial and Digital Anomalies. *J. Pediatr.* **74:**755–762, 1969.

2 Murphy, S., and Lubin, B., Triphalangeal Thumbs and Congenital Erythroid Hypoplasia. *J. Pediatr.* **81:**987–989, 1972.

CLEFT LIP-PALATE AND HYPOPHYSEAL DWARFISM

1 Francés, J. M., et al., Hypophysärer Zwergwuchs bei Lippen-Kiefer-Spalte. *Helv. Paediatr. Acta* **21:**315–322, 1966.

2 Laron, Z., et al., Pituitary Growth Hormone Insufficiency Associated with Cleft Lip and Palate. *Helv. Paediatr. Acta* **24:**576–581, 1969.

3 Zimmerman, T. S., et al., Hypopituitarism with Normal or Increased Height. *Am. J. Med.* **42:**146–150, 1967.

4 Zuppinger, K. A., et al., Cleft Lip and Choroidal Coloboma Associated with Multiple Hypothalmo-pituitary Dysfunction. *J. Clin. Endocrinol.* **33:**934–939, 1971.

CLEFT LIP-PALATE AND SACRAL AGENESIS

1 Blummel, J., et al., Partial and Complete Agenesis or Malformation of the Sacrum with Associated Anomalies. *J. Bone Joint Surg.* **41A:**497–518, 1959.
2 Feller, A., and Sternberg, H., Zur Kenntnis der Fehlbildungen der Wirbelsäule (Case 3). *Virchows Arch. Pathol. Anat.* **280:**649–692, 1931.
3 Holthusen, W., The Pierre Robin Syndrome. *Ann. Radiol. (Paris)* **15:**253–262, 1972.

CLEFT PALATE AND ANIRIDIA

1 Lindberg, J. G., Beitrag zur Kenntnis der kongenitalen sog. Aniridia. *Klin. Monatsbl. Augenheilkd.* **70:**133–138, 1923.

CLEFT PALATE AND AMELIA

1 Centa, A., and Rovei, S., Dismelia grave non talidomidica associata a sindrome di Pierre Robin. *Pathologica* **57:**245–250, 1965.
2 Holthusen, W., The Pierre Robin Syndrome: Unusual Associated Developmental Defects. *Ann. Radiol. (Paris)* **15:**253–262, 1972.

CLEFT PALATE AND APLASIA OF THE TROCHEA

1 Mead, C. A., and Martin, M., Aplasia of the Trochea in an Original Mutation. *J. Bone Joint Surg.* **45A:**379–383, 1963.

CLEFT PALATE AND ACCESSORY METACARPAL OF INDEX FINGER

1 Farnsworth, P. B., and Pacik, P. T., Glossoptotic Hypoxia and Micrognathia: The Pierre Robin Syndrome Reviewed. *Clin. Pediatr.* **10:**600–606, 1971.
2 Holthusen, W., The Pierre Robin Syndrome: Unusual Associated Developmental Defects. *Ann. Radiol. (Paris)* **15:**253–262, 1972.
3 Manzke, H., Symmetrische Hyperphalangie des zweiten Fingers durch ein akzesorisches Metacarpale. *Fortschr. Roentgenstr.* **105:**425–427, 1966.

CLEFT PALATE, CUTIS GYRATUM, AND ACANTHOSIS NIGRICANS

1 Beare, J. M., et al., Cutis Gyratum, Acanthosis Nigricans and Other Congenital Anomalies: A New Syndrome. *Br. J. Dermatol.* **81:**241–247, 1969.

CLEFT LIP-PALATE, HYPOHIDROSIS, THIN WIRY HAIR, AND DYSTROPHIC NAILS

1 Fára, M., Regional Ectodermal Dysplasia with Total Bilateral Cleft. *Acta Chir. Plast.* **13:**100–105, 1971.
2 Massengill, R., et al., An Abnormal Speech Pattern Associated with an Orofacial Anomaly. *Acta Oto-laryngol. (Stockh.)* **68:**537–542, 1969.
3 Moynahan, E., XTE (Xeroderma, Talipes and Enamel Defect): A New Heredo-familial Syndrome. Two Cases. Homozygous Inheritance of a Dominant Gene. *Proc. R. Soc. Med.* **63:**447–448, 1970.
4 Rapp, R. S., and Hodgkins, W. E., Anhidrotic Ectodermal Dysplasia: Autosomal Dominant Inheritance with Palate and Lip Anomalies. *J. Med. Genet.* **5:**269–272, 1968.

5 Summitt, R. L., and Hiatt, R. L., Hypohidrotic Ectodermal Dysplasia with Multiple Associated Anomalies. *Birth Defects* **7**(8):121–124, 1971.
6 Wannarachue, N., et al., Ectodermal Dysplasia and Multiple Defects (Rapp-Hodgkins Type). *J. Pediatr.* **81:** 1217–1218, 1972.
7 Watson, R. M., and Hardwick, C. E., Hypodontia Associated with Cleft Palate. *Br. Dent. J.* **130:**77–80, 1971.

CLEFT LIP-PALATE, TETRAPEROMELIA, DEFORMED PINNA, AND ECTODERMAL DYSPLASIA

1 Cat, I., et al., Odontotrichomelic Hypohidrotic Dysplasia: A Clinical Reappraisal. *Hum. Hered.* **22:**91–95, 1972.
2 Freire-Maia, N., A Newly Recognized Genetic Syndrome of Tetramelic Deficiencies, Ectodermal Dysplasias, Deformed Ears, and Other Anomalies. *Am. J. Hum. Genet.* **22:**370–377, 1970.
3 Herrmann, J., et al., Craniosynostosis and Craniosynostosis Syndromes. *Rocky Mt. Med. J.* (May) 45–56, 1969.

CLEFT PALATE, CAMPTODACTYLY, AND CLUBFOOT

1 Gordon, H., et al., Camptodactyly, Cleft Palate and Club Foot: A Syndrome Showing the Autosomal Dominant Pattern of Inheritance. *J. Med. Genet.* **6:**266–274, 1969.

CLEFT PALATE, STAPES FIXATION, AND OLIGODONTIA

1 Gorlin, R. J., et al., Cleft Palate, Stapes Fixation and Oligodontia—A New Autosomal Recessively Inherited Syndrome. *Birth Defects* **7**(7):87–88, 1971.

CLEFT PALATE AND ORAL DUPLICATION

1 Avery, J. K., and Hayward, J. R., Duplication of Oral Structures with Cleft Palate. *Cleft Palate J.* **6:**505–516, 1969.
2 Bacsich, P., et al., A Rare Case of Duplicitas Anterior: A Female Infant with Two Mouths and Two Pituitaries. *J. Anat.* **98:**292–293, 1964.
3 Bell, R. C., A Child with Two Tongues (Oral-Facial-Digital Syndrome). *Br. J. Plast. Surg.* **24:**193–196, 1971.
4 Gorlin, R. J., Developmental Anomalies of the Face and Oral Structures, in R. J. Gorlin and H. M. Goldman (eds.), *Thoma's Oral Pathology*, 6th ed., Mosby, St. Louis, 1970.
4a Hausamen, J. E., and Scheunemann, H., Partielle Doppelanlage des Oberkiefers mit multiplen Spaltbildungen Gesicht, in press.
5 Koblin, I., Zwischenkieferverdoppelung mit normotoper und heterotoper Zahnüberzahl sowie Gaumenspalte. *Dtsch. Zahn Mund Kieferheilkd.* **54:**204–210, 1970.
6 Kohnz, R., Erstbeobachtung einer Zwischenkieferverdoppelung beim Menschen mit Epignathus, Zungenkörper- und Gaumenspalte. *Dtsch. Zahn Mund Kieferheilkd.* **35:**18–32, 1961.
7 Morton, W. R. M., Duplication of the Pituitary and Stomatodaeal Structures in a 38-week Male Infant. *Arch. Dis. Child.* **32:**135–141, 1957.

8 Robertson, N. R. E., Apparent Duplication of the Upper Alveolar Process and Dentition. *Br. Dent. J.* **129**:333–334, 1970.

9 Steinhilber, W., Partielle Doppelanlage des Unterkiefers mit Epignathus, Zwischenkieferbürzel und Zungenspalte. *Z. Kinderheilkd.* **112**:171–176, 1972.

CLEFT PALATE AND CEREBROCOSTOMANDIBULAR SYNDROME

1 Doyle, J. F., The Skeletal Defects of the Cerebro-costo-mandibular Syndrome. *Irish J. Med. Sci.* (7 ser.) **2**:595–603, 1969.

2 Kuhn, J. P., et al., Cerebro-costo-mandibular Syndrome: A Case with Cardiac Anomaly. *J. Pediatr.* **86**:243–244, 1975.

3 Langer, L. O., and Herrmann, J., The Cerebrocostomandibular Syndrome. *Birth Defects* **10**(7):167–170, 1974.

4 McNicholl, B., et al., Cerebro-costo-mandibular Syndrome: A New Familial Developmental Disorder. *Arch. Dis. Child.* **45**:421–424, 1970.

5 Miller, K. E., et al., Rib Gap Defects with Micrognathia: The Cerebro-costo-mandibular Syndrome: A Pierre Robin-like Syndrome with Rib Dysplasia. *Am. J. Roentgenol.* **114**:253–256, 1972.

6 Nicholls, S. J., and Fletcher, E., Congenital Rib Defects with the Pierre Robin Syndrome. *Pediatr. Radiol.* **1**:246–247, 1973.

7 Smith, D. N., et al., Rib-gap Defect with Micrognathia, Malformed Tracheal Cartilages and Redundant Skin: A New Pattern of Defective Development. *J. Pediatr.* **69**:799–803, 1966.

CLEFT PALATE, RETINAL DETACHMENT, AND PROGRESSIVE ARTHROOPHTHALMOPATHY

1 Cohen, M. M., et al., A Dominantly Inherited Syndrome of Hyaloideoretinal Detachment, Cleft Palate and Maxillary Hypoplasia. *Birth Defects* **7**(7):83–86, 1971.

2 Daniel, R., et al., Hyalo-retinopathy in the Clefting Syndrome. *Br. J. Ophthalmol.* **58**:96–102, 1974.

3 Delaney, W. V., et al., Inherited Retinal Detachment. *Arch. Ophthalmol.* **69**:44–50, 1963.

4 Falger, E. L. F., et al., Hereditary Hyaloideo-retinal Degeneration and Palatoschisis. *Ophthalmologica* **160**:384, 1970.

5 Frandsen, E., Hereditary Hyaloideo-retinal Degeneration (Wagner) in a Danish Family. *Acta Ophthalmol. (Kbh.)* **44**:223–232, 1966.

6 Hall, J., Stickler Syndrome Presenting as a Syndrome of Cleft Palate, Myopia and Blindness Inherited as a Dominant Trait. *Birth Defects* **10**(8):157–171, 1974.

7 Herrmann, J., et al., The Stickler Syndrome (Hereditary Ophthalmopathy). *Birth Defects* **11**(2):76–103, 1975.

8 Hirose, T., et al., Wagner's Hereditary Vitreoretinal Degeneration and Retinal Detachment. *Arch. Ophthalmol.* **89**:176–185, 1973.

9 Marshall, D., Ectodermal Dysplasia. Report of a Kindred with Ocular Abnormalities and Hearing Defects. *Am. J. Ophthal.*, Suppl. **45**:143–156, 1958.

10 Opitz, J. M., Ocular Anomalies in Malformation Syndromes. *Trans. Am. Acad. Ophthalmol. Otolaryngol.* **76**:1193–1202, 1972.

11 Herrmann, J., et al., The Stickler Syndrome. *Birth Defects* **11**(2):76–103, 1975.

12 Perkins, J., Pierre Robin Syndrome. *Trans. Ophthalmol. Soc. U.K.* **40**:179–180, 1970.

13 Popkin, J. S., and Polomino, R. C., Stickler's Syndrome (Hereditary Progressive Arthro-ophthalmopathy). *Can. Med. Assoc. J.* **111**:1071–1076, 1974.

14 Schreiner, R. L., et al., Stickler Syndrome in a Pedigree of Pierre Robin Syndrome. *Am. J. Dis. Child.* **126**:86–90, 1973.

15 Smith, W. K., Pierre Robin Syndrome in Brothers. *Birth Defects* **5**(2):220–221, 1969.

16 Spranger, J., Arthro-ophthalmopathia hereditaria. *Ann. Radiol. (Paris)* **11**:359–364, 1968.

17 Stickler, G. B., et al., Hereditary Progressive Arthro-ophthalmopathy. *Mayo Clin. Proc.* **40**:433–455, 1965.

18 Stickler, G. B., and Pugh, D. G., Hereditary Progressive Arthro-Ophthalmopathy. II. Additional Observation on Vertebral Anomalies, a Hearing Defect and a Report of a Similar Case. *Mayo Clin. Proc.* **42**:495–500, 1967.

CLEFT LIP-PALATE AND ENCEPHALOMENINGOCELE

1 Crockford, D. A., et al., Some Observations on Congenital Teratomata and Ectopic Cerebromata. *Plast. Reconstr. Surg.* **24**:31–42, 1971.

2 Exner, A., Über basale Cephalocele. *Dtsch. Z. Chir.* **90**:23–41, 1907.

3 Fogh-Andersen, P., *Inheritance of Harelip and Cleft Palate.* Nyt Nordisk Forlag, Copenhagen, 1942, pp. 26–38.

4 Ingraham, F. D., and Matson, D. D., Spina Bifida and Cranium Bifidum. IV. An Unusual Nasopharyngeal Encephalocele. *N. Engl. J. Med.* **228**:815–820, 1943.

5 Lewin, M. L., and Shuster, M. M., Transpalatal Correction of Basilar Meningocoele with Cleft Palate. *Arch. Surg.* **90**:687–693, 1965.

6 Low, N. L., et al., Brain Tissue in the Nose and Throat (Case 3). *Pediatrics* **18**:254–259, 1956.

7 Neumann, H., and Peters, U. H., Frontale Cephalocele kombiniert mit Kiefergaumenlippenspalte und psychomotorischen Anfällen. *Arch. Psychiatr. Nervenkr.* **200**:531–540, 1960.

8 Pruzansky, S., and Lis, E. P., Cephalometric Roentgenography of Infants: Sedation, Instrumentation and Research. *Am. J. Orthod.* **44**:156–186, 1958.

9 Stuart, E. A., An Otolaryngologic Aspect of Frontal Meningocoele. *Arch. Otolaryngol.* **40**:171–174, 1944.

10 Vistnes, L. M., et al., Nasal Glioma: Case Report. *Plast. Reconstr. Surg.* **43**:195–197, 1969.

11 Zarem, H. A., et al., Heterotopic Brain in the Nasopharynx and Soft Palate. *Surgery* **61**:483–486, 1967.

CLEFT PALATE AND CONGENITAL ORAL TERATOMA

1 Arnold, J., Über behaarte Polyposen der Rachen-Mundhöhle und deren Stellung zur den Teratomen. *Virchows Arch. Pathol. Anat.* **111**:176–210, 1888 (reviews early literature).

2 Dohlman, G., and Sjövall, A., Large Epignathous Teratoma Successfully Operated upon Immediately after Birth. *Glasgow Med. J.* **34**:122–126, 1953.

3 Dummett, C. O., et al., Epignathoid Teratoma. *J. Can. Dent. Assoc.* **29**:788–791, 1963.

4 Erich, W. E., Teratoid Parasites of the Mouth (Episphenoids, Epipalati, Epignathia). *Am. J. Orthod.* **31**:650–659, 1945.

5 Hoyek, H., von, Über die Beziehungen des Epignathus zum Diprosopus. *Zentralbl. Allg. Pathol.* **85:**171–175, 1949.

6 Kraus, E. J., Über ein epignathisches Teratom der Hypophysengegend. *Virchows Arch. Pathol. Anat.* **271:** 546–555, 1929.

7 Miller, A. P., and Owens, J. B., Teratoma of the Tongue. *Cancer* **19:**1583–1586, 1966.

8 Wynn, S. K., et al., Epignathus. *Am. J. Dis. Child.* **91:**495–497, 1956.

CLEFT PALATE AND BILATERAL FEMORAL AND FIBULAR DYSGENESIS

1 Bailey, J. A., and Beighton, P., Bilateral Femoral Dysgenesis. *Clin. Pediatr.* **9:**668–674, 1970.

2 Daentl, D. L., et al., Femoral Hypoplasia – Unusual Facies Syndrome. *J. Pediatr.* **86:**107–111, 1975.

3 Frantz, C. H., and O'Rahilly, R., Congenital Skeletal Limb Deficiencies. *J. Bone Joint Surg.* **43A:**1218–1224, 1961.

4 Holthusen, W., The Pierre Robin Syndrome: Unusual Associated Developmental Defects. *Ann. Radiol. (Paris)* **15:**253–262, 1972.

5 Kučera, J., et al., Missbildungen der Beine und der kaudalen Wirbelsäule bei Kindern diabetischer Mütter. *Dtsch. Med. Wochenschr.* **90:**901–905, 1965.

6 Passarge, E., Congenital Malformation and Maternal Diabetes. *Lancet* **1:**324–325, 1965.

CLEFT PALATE, VENTRICULAR SEPTAL DEFECT, TRUNCUS ARTERIOSUS, AND INTRAUTERINE DEATH

1 Lowry, R. B., and Miller, J. R., Cleft Palate and Congenital Heart Disease. *Lancet* **1:**1302–1303, 1971.

CLEFT LIP AND/OR PALATE AND ENLARGED PARIETAL FORAMENS

1 Hässler, E., Fenestrae parietalis symmetrica. *Monatsschr. Kinderheilkd.* **64:**337–340, 1936.

2 Hollender, L., Enlarged Parietal Foramina. *Oral Surg.* **23:**447–453, 1967.

3 Irvine, E. D., and Taylor, F. W., Hereditary and Congenital Large Parietal Foramina. *Br. J. Radiol.* **9:**456–462, 1936.

4 James, F. E., Hypertelorism Associated with Poor Frontal Development of Skull and Bilateral Sprengel's Shoulders. *Br. Med. J.* **1:**1019–1020, 1959.

5 Lother, K., Familiäres Vorkommen von Foramina parietalia permagna. *Arch. Kinderheilkd.* **160:**156–168, 1959.

6 Pepper, O. H. P., and Pendergrass, E. P., Hereditary Occurrence of Enlarged Parietal Foramina. *Am. J. Roentgenol.* **35:**1–8, 1936.

7 Warkany, J., and Weaver, T. A., Heredofamilial Deviations. II. Enlarged Parietal Foramens Combined with Obesity, Hypogenitalism, Microphthalmos and Mental Retardation. *Am. J. Dis. Child.* **60:**1147–1154, 1940.

8 Zarfl, M., Fenestrae parietales symmetricae. *Z. Kinderheilkd.* **57:**54–66, 1934.

CLEFT LIP AND/OR PALATE AND CONGENITAL NEUROBLASTOMA

1 Aase, J. M., and Smith, D. W., Dysmorphogenesis of Joints, Brain and Palate: A New Dominantly Inherited Syndrome. *J. Pediatr.* **73:**606–609, 1968.

2 Beckwith, J. B., and Perrin, E. V., In Situ Neuroblastoma: A Contribution to the Natural History of Neural Crest Tumors. *Am. J. Pathol.* **43:**1089–1104, 1963.

3 Kouyoumdjian, A. O., and McDonald, H., Association of Congenital Adrenal Neuroblastoma with Multiple Anomalies Including an Unusual Oropharyngeal Cavity (Imperforate Buccopharyngeal Membrane?). *Cancer* **4:**784–788, 1951.

4 Mittelbach, M., and Szekely, P., Ein Fall von Neuroblastom des Nebennieresmarkes mit mehreren Missbildungen. *Frankfurt Z. Pathol.* **47:**517–521, 1934.

5 Nevin, N. C., et al., Two Cases of Trisomy D Associated with Adrenal Tumors. *J. Med. Genet.* **9:**119–121, 1972.

6 Potter, E. L., and Parrish, J. M., Neuroblastoma, Ganglioneuroma and Fibroneuroma in a Stillborn Fetus. *Am. J. Pathol.* **18:**141–152, 1942.

CLEFT PALATE, SHORT HUMERUS AND FEMUR, LONG RADIUS AND TIBIA

1 Walden, R. H., et al., Pierre Robin Syndrome in Association with Combined Lengthening and Shortening of the Long Bones. *Plast. Reconstr. Surg.* **48:**80–82, 1971.

CLEFT PALATE AND SHORT STATURE

1 Gareis, F. J., and Smith, D. W., Diminished Stature-Defective Palate Syndrome: A Dominantly Inherited Disorder. *J. Pediatr.* **79:**470–472, 1971.

CLEFT LIP-PALATE AND CONGENITAL HEART DISEASE

1 Boeson, I., et al., Extracardiac Congenital Malformations in Children with Congenital Heart Diseases. *Acta Paediatr. Scand. (Suppl.)* **146:**28–33, 1963.

2 Brans, Y. W., and Lintermans, J. P., The Upper Limb-Cardiovascular Syndrome. *Am. J. Dis. Child.* **124:**779–783, 1972.

2a Didier, F., et al., Un cas d'ectopie cardiaque extra-thoracique. *Z. Kinderchir.* **14:**252–259, 1974.

3 Holt, M., and Oram, S., Familial Heart Disease with Skeletal Malformations. *Br. Heart J.* **22:**236–242, 1960.

4 Okada, R., et al., Extracardiac Malformations Associated with Congenital Heart Disease. *Arch. Pathol.* **85:**649–657, 1968.

5 Rabl, R., and Schulz, F., Angeborene Herzfehler und Lippen-Kiefer-Gaumenspalten bei Zwillingen. *Virchows Arch. Pathol. Anat.* **305:**505–520, 1939.

6 Shah, C. V., et al., Cardiac Malformations with Facial Clefts: with Observation on the Pierre Robin Syndrome. *Am. J. Dis. Child.* **119:**238–244, 1970.

CLEFT LIP-PALATE AND ANENCEPHALY

1 Brown, F. J., The Anencephalic Syndrome in Its Relation to Apituitarism. *Edinburgh Med. J.* **25:**296–307, 1920.

2 Christakos, A. C., and Simpson, J. L., Anencephaly in Three Siblings. *Obstet. Gynecol.* **33:**267–270, 1969.

3 Deppe, B., *Beitrag zum anatomischen Wesen der Anencephalie, Amyelie und Craniorhachischisis.* Thesis, Göttingen, 1935.

4 Fogh-Andersen, P., *Inheritance of Harelip and Cleft Palate.* Nyt Nordisk Forlag, Copenhagen, 1942.

5 Gleeson, J. A., and Stovin, P. G. I., Mediastinal Enterogenous Cysts Associated with Vertebral Anomalies. *Clin. Radiol.* **12:**41–48, 1961.
6 Heintel, H., Die Palatoschisis und ihre Beziehung zum Anencephalie-Syndrom. *Stoma (Heidelb.)* **9:**204–211, 1956.
7 Jones, W. R., Anencephalus, A 23-year Survey in a Sydney Hospital. *Med. J. Aust.* **1:**104–105, 1967.
8 MacMahon, B., and McKeown, T., Incidence of Harelip and Cleft Palate. Related to Birth Rank and Maternal Age. *Am. J. Hum. Genet.* **5:**176–183, 1953.
9 Mufarrij, I. K., and Kilejian, V. O., An Analysis of Anencephalic Births and Report of a Case of Repeated Anencephaly. *Obstet. Gynecol.* **22:**657–661, 1963.
10 Neel, J. V., A Study of Major Congenital Defects in Japanese Infants. *Am. J. Hum. Genet.* **10:**398–445, 1958.
11 Roches, P., *Zur Frage der Anenkephalie.* Thesis, Basel, 1951.
12 Smithells, R. W., et al., Anencephaly in Liverpool. *Dev. Med. Child. Neurol.* **6:**231–240, 1964.

CLEFT PALATE AND RÜDIGER SYNDROME
1 Rüdiger, R. A., et al., Severe Developmental Failure with Coarse Facial Features, Distal Limb Hypoplasia, Thickened Palmar Creases, Bifid Uvula and Ureteral Stenosis: A Previously Undescribed Familial Disorder with Lethal Outcome. *J. Pediatr.* **79:**977–981, 1971.

CLEFT PALATE AND NANCE-SWEENEY CHONDRODYSPLASIA
1 Nance, W. E., and Sweeney, A., A Recessively Inherited Chondrodysplasia. *Birth Defects* **6**(4):25–27, 1970.

CLEFT PALATE, UNUSUAL FACIES, MENTAL RETARDATION, AND LIMB ABNORMALITIES
1 Palant, D. I., et al., Unusual Facies, Cleft Palate, Mental Retardation and Limb Abnormalities in Siblings—a New Syndrome. *J. Pediatr.* **78:**686–689, 1971.

CLEFT PALATE AND RARE LETHAL DWARFISM
1 de la Chapelle, A., et al., Une rare dysplasie osseuse léthale de transmission recessive autosomique. *Arch. Fr. Pédiatr.* **29:**759–770, 1972.

CLEFT PALATE AND CAMPTOMELIC DWARFISM
1 Bain, A. D., and Barrett, H. S., Congenital Bowing of the Long Bones. *Arch. Dis. Child.* **34:**516–524, 1959.
2 Bianchine, J., et al., Camptomelic Dwarfism. *Lancet* **1:**1017–1018, 1971.
3 Cremin, B. J., et al., Autosomal Recessive Inheritance in Camptomelic Dwarfism. *Lancet* **1:**488–489, 1973.
4 Engel, W., et al., Multiple Missbildungen bei einem Mädchen mit dem Karyotypus 46, XY, 17q⁻. *Humangenetik* **6:**311–325, 1968.
5 Gardner, L. T., et al., Syndrome of Multiple Osseous Defects with Pretibial Dimples. *Lancet* **2:**98, 1971.
6 Hoefnagel, D., et al., Camptomelic Dwarfism. *Lancet* **1:**1068, 1972.
7 Lee, F. A., et al., The "Camptomelic" Syndrome. *Am. J. Dis. Child.* **124:**485–496, 1972.

8 Opitz, J. M., et al., The Campomelic Syndrome—Comments. *Birth Defects* **10**(9):97–99, 1974.
9 Schmickel, R. D., et al., The Camptomelique Syndrome. *J. Pediatr.* **82:**299–302, 1973.
10 Spranger, J., et al., Increasing Frequency of a Syndrome of Multiple Osseous Defects? *Lancet* **2:**716, 1970.
11 Storer, J., and Grossman, H., The Campomelic Syndrome. *Radiology* **111:**673–681, 1974.
12 Stüve, A., and Wiedemann, H. R., Angeborene Verbiegungen langer Röhrenknochen-eine Geschwisterbeobachtung. *Z. Kinderheilkd.* **111:**184–192, 1971.
13 Thurmon, T. F., and Kityakara, A., Camptomelic Dwarfism. *Birth Defects* **10**(9):89–95, 1974.

CLEFT LIP-PALATE AND HYPOGONADOTROPIC HYPOGONADISM
1 Christian, J. C., et al., Hypogonadotropic Hypogonadism with Anosmia. The Kallmann Syndrome (Case 4). *Birth Defects* **7**(6):166–171, 1971.
2 Rosen, S. W., The Syndrome of Hypogonadism, Anosmia, and Midline Cranial Anomalies. *Proc. 47th Meet. Endocr. Soc.,* New York, 1965.
3 Sparkes, R. S., et al., Familial Hypogonadotropic Hypogonadism with Anosmia. *Arch. Intern. Med.* **121:**534–538, 1968.

CLEFT PALATE AND KNIEST DISEASE
1 Kniest, W., Zur Abgrenzung der Dysostosis enchondralis von der Chondrodystrophie. *Z. Kinderheilkd.* **70:**633–640, 1952.
2 Maroteaux, P., and Spranger, J., La maladie de Kniest. *Arch. Fr. Pédiatr.* **30:**735–750, 1973.
3 Rimoin, D., Histopathology and Ultrastructure of Cartilage in the Chondrodystrophies. *Birth Defects* **10**(9):1–18, 1974.
4 Roaf, R., et al., A Childhood Syndrome of Bone Dysplasia, Retinal Detachment and Deafness (Case 2). *Dev. Med. Child. Neurol.* **9:**463–473, 1967.
5 Rolland, J. C., et al., Nanisme chondrodystrophique et division palatine chez un nouveau-né. *Ann. Pédiatr.* **19:**139–143, 1972.
6 Siggers, D. C., et al., The Kniest Syndrome. *Birth Defects,* **10**(9):193–208, 1974, and **10**(12):432–442, 1974.
7 Spranger, J., and Maroteaux, P., Kniest Disease. *Birth Defects* **10**(12):50–56, 1974.

CLEFT PALATE AND MEGEPIPHYSEAL DWARFISM
1 Gorlin, R. J., et al., Megepiphyseal Dwarfism. *J. Pediatr.* **83:**633–635, 1973.

CLEFT PALATE, MACULAR COLOBOMA, AND SKELETAL ABNORMALITIES
1 Phillips, C. I., and Griffiths, D. L., Macular Coloboma and Skeletal Abnormality. *Br. J. Ophthalmol.* **53:**346–349, 1969.

CLEFT LIP-PALATE AND FOREARM BONE APLASIA OR HYPOPLASIA
1 Birch-Jensen, A., *Congenital Deformities of the Upper Extremities.* Munksgaard, Copenhagen, 1949.
2 Drinnenberg, A., Klumphandbildung infolge angeborener

Radiusdefekte und ihre Behandlung (Case 1). *Z. Orthop. Chir.* **63:**297–307, 1936.

3 Gruber, W., Über congenitalen unvollständigen Radiusmangel. *Virchows Arch. Pathol. Anat.* **40:**427–435, 1867.

4 Heikel, H. V. A., Aplasia and Hypoplasia of the Radius: Studies on 64 Cases and an Epiphyseal Transplantation in Rabbits with the Imitated Defect. *Acta Orthop. Scand.* Suppl. **39:**1–155, 1959.

5 Immeyer, F., Lippen-Kiefer-Gaumenspalten bei Thalidomidgeschädigten Kindern. *Acta Genet. Med. (Roma)* **16:**244–274, 1967.

6 Kato, K., Congenital Absence of the Radius. *J. Bone Joint Surg.* **6:**589–626, 1924.

7 Kruckemeyer, K., *Talipomanus. Ein Beitrag zur Kenntnis des sogen. kongenitalen Radiusdefektes.* Thesis, Göttingen, 1938.

8 Kummel, W., *Die Missbildungen der Extremitäten durch Defekt, Verwachsung und Überzahl.* T. G. Fischer, Cassel, 1895.

9 Weyers, H., Das Oligodactylie-Syndrom des Menschen und seine Parallelmutation bei der Hausmaus. *Ann. Paediatr.* **189:**351–370, 1957.

10 Wiedemann, H. R., Missbildungs-Retardierungs-Syndrom mit Fehlen des 5 Strahl an Händen und Füssen, Gaumenspalte, dysplastischen Ohren und Augenlidern und radioulnarer Synostose. *Klin. Pädiatr.* **185:**181–186, 1973.

CLEFT LIP-PALATE, LID ECTOPION, AND OCULAR HYPERTELORISM

1 Bergsma, D., Case 28. *Syndrome Identification* 3(1):7–13, 1975.

2 Genée, E., Une forme extensive de dysostose mandibulofaciale. *J. Génét. Hum.* **17:**45–52, 1969.

3 Piper, H. F., Augenärztliche Befunde bei frühkindlicher Entwicklungsstörungen. *Monatsschr. Kinderheilkd.* **105:** 170–176, 1957.

4 Warburg, M., Personal communication, 1974.

5 Zellweger, H., Personal communication, 1975.

CLEFT PALATE AND MICROGNATHIC DWARFISM

1 Maroteaux, P., et al., Le nanisme micrognathe. *Presse Med.* **78:**2371–2374, 1970.

2 Rolland, J. C., et al., Un nanisme chondrodystrophique avec division palatine. *Arch. Fr. Pédiatr.* **27:**331, 1970.

3 Weissenbacher, G., and Zweymüller, E., Gleichzeitiges Vorkommen eines Syndroms von Pierre Robin und einer fetalen Chondrodysplasie. *Monatsschr. Kinderheilkd.* **112:**315–317, 1964.

MEDIAN CLEFT LIP-PALATE AND SHORT RIB–POLYDACTYLY SYNDROME [MAJEWSKI TYPE]

1 Casper, J. L., Ein Missgeburt seltenster Art. *Berl. Klin. Wochenschr.* **1:**9–10, 1864.

2 Dreibholz, E., *Beschreibung einer sogenannten Phokomelie.* Thesis, Berlin, 1873.

3 Majewski, F., et al., Polysyndaktylie, verkürzte Gliedmassen und Genitalfehlbildungen: Kennzeichen eines selbständigen Syndroms? *Z. Kinderheilkd.* **111:**118–138, 1971.

4 Otto, A. W., *Seltene Beobachtung zur Anatomie, Physiologie und Pathologie gehörig.* Breslau, Holäufer, 1816.

5 Pitschi, E., Zur Kasuistik der Poly- und Syndaktylie aller Extremitäten nebst beiderseitigem partiellem Tibiadefekt und anderen Missbildungen (doppelte Anlage des Unterkiefers). Thesis, Zürich, 1904–1905.

6 Spranger, J., et al., Short Rib-Polydaktyly (SRP) Syndromes, Typus Majewski and Saldino-Noonan. *Z. Kinderheilkd.* **116:**73–94, 1974.

CLEFT PALATE AND LETHAL MICROMELIC DWARFISM WITH MARKED SHORTNESS OF THE RADIUS AND FIBULA

1 de la Chapelle, A., et al., Une rare dysplasie osseuse léthale de transmission recessive autosomique. *Arch. Fr. Pédiatr.* **29:**759–770, 1972.

PSEUDODIASTROPHIC DWARFISM AND CLEFT PALATE

1 Burgio, G. R., et al., Nanisme pseudodiastrophique. Etude de deux soeurs nouveau-nées. *Arch. Fr. Pédiatr.* **31:** 681–696, 1974.

MICROCEPHALY, LARGE EARS, SHORT STATURE, AND CLEFT PALATE

1 Say, B., et al., A New Dominantly Inherited Syndrome of Cleft Palate. *Humangenetik* **26:**1–3, 1975.

RECURRENT BRACHIAL PLEXUS NEURITIS AND CLEFT PALATE

1 Erikson, A., Hereditary Syndrome Consisting in Recurrent Attacks Resembling Brachial Plexus Neuritis, Special Facial Features and Cleft Palate. *Acta Paediat. Scand.* **63:**885–888, 1974.

2 Jacob, J. C., et al., Heredofamilial Neuritis with Brachial Predilection. *Neurology (Minneap.)* **11:**1025–1033, 1961.

3 Gardner, J. H., and Maloney, W., Hereditary Brachial and Cranial Neuritis. Genetically Linked with Ocular Hypotelorism and Syndactyly. *Neurology (Minneap.)* **18:**278, 1968.

4 Poffenbarger, A. L., Heredofamilial Neuritis with Brachial Predilection. *W. Virginia Med. J.* **64:**425–429, 1968.

30

Lateral Facial Cleft and Associated Anomalies

Occasionally, lateral cleft (marcrostomia) is associated with anomalies of the ear, lower-lid coloboma, malar bone hypoplasia, etc. (see Chap. 90, Mandibulofacial Dysostosis). Other cases of lateral cleft may be found in association with unilateral microphthalmia, cystic eye, supernumerary ear tags, absence of mandibular ramus and condyle, and mastoid process (5, 10, 12) (see Chap. 104, Oculoauriculovertebral Dysplasia).

It may also occur as an isolated phenomenon (Fig. 30-1*A–D*). Like the oblique facial cleft, the isolated lateral facial cleft does not appear to have a genetic basis. Blackfield and Wilde (4), Boo-Chai (5), and Ogo et al. (10a) suggested that there is one lateral facial cleft for every 100 cases of cleft lip, while Fogh-Andersen (8) indicated that he found about 1 case per 350 cases of facial cleft. Lateral facial cleft appears to be more common in males and, when unilateral, is more common on the left side.

The lateral facial cleft may represent failure of penetration of ectomesenchyme between the developing maxillary and mandibular processes and may be unilateral or bilateral, partial or (rarely) complete, extending from the angle of the mouth to the ear. It probably more often represents postfusion tears, since there is considerable clinical variability. It may be associated with anomalies of the extremities, such as polydactyly, syndactyly, or absence of digits (4), with

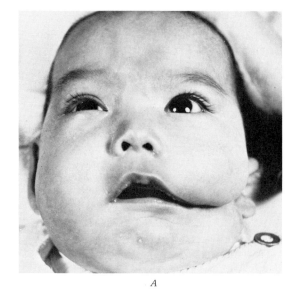

A

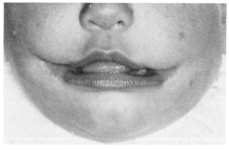

B

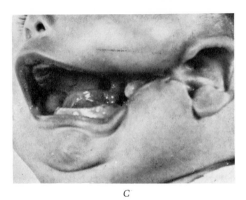 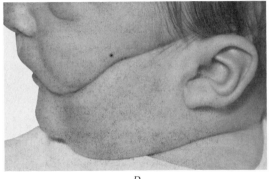

C D

Figure 30-1. *Lateral facial cleft.* (*A*). Unilateral lateral facial cleft. (*B*). Bilateral lateral facial cleft. (*C*). Unilateral lateral facial cleft extending to tragus. (*D*). Lateral facial cleft extending above helix of low-set, posteriorly rotated ear. (1*B, courtesy of K. Schuchardt, Hamburg, Germany; 1A and C, from P. Fogh-Andersen,* Acta Chir. Scand. **129:**275, 1964; 1D, from H. M. Blackfield and N. J. Wilde, Plast. Reconstr. Surg. **6:**62, 1950.)

micrognathia (3), amniotic bands (14), supernumerary teeth (13), ear tags (2), nasal dermoid (4), rib and vertebral defects (6), congenital heart defects (6), other facial clefts (7), or epignathus (1).

REFERENCES

1 Ahlfeld, F., Beiträge zur Lehre von der Zwillingen. *Arch. Gynäkol.* **7:**210–286, 1875.

2 Ballantyne, J. W., Preauricular Appendages. *Teratologia* **2:**18–36, 1895.

3 Benavent, W. J., and Ramos-Oller, A., Micrognathia: Report of Twelve Cases. *Plast. Reconstr. Surg.* **22:**486–490, 1958.

4 Blackfield, H. M., and Wilde, N. J., Lateral Facial Clefts. *Plast. Reconstr. Surg.* **6:**62–78, 1950.

5 Boo-Chai, K., The Transverse Facial Cleft: Its Repair. *Br. J. Plast. Surg.* **22:**119–124, 1969.

6 Davies, J., Two Cases of Macrostomia Described with Some Observations on the Incidence of Defective Development of the Mandibular Arch in the Sheep. *Br. Dent. J.* **86:**217–225, 1949.

7 Edington, G. H., Macrostomia Associated with Clefts of Soft Palate. *Glasgow Med. J.* **71:**338–341, 1909.

8 Fogh-Andersen, P., Rare Clefts of the Face. *Acta Chir. Scand.* **129:**275–281, 1965.

9 Keith, A., Concerning the Origin and Nature of Certain Malformations of the Face, Head and Foot. *Br. J. Surg.* **28:**173–192, 1940.

10 May, H., Transverse Facial Clefts and Their Repair. *Plast. Reconstr. Surg.* **29:**240–249, 1962.

10a Ogo, K., et al., Ten Year Survey of Macrostoma. *Jap. J. Plast. Reconstr. Surg.* **16:**431–438, 1973.

11 Padgett, E. C., *Plastic and Reconstructive Surgery.* Charles C Thomas, Springfield, Ill., 1948.

12 Powell, W. J., and Jenkins, H. P., Transverse Facial Clefts. *Plast. Reconstr. Surg.* **42:**454–459, 1968.

13 Rushton, M. A., and Walder, F. A., Unilateral Secondary Facial Cleft with Excess Tooth and Bone Formation. *Proc. R. Soc. Med.* **30:**79–82, 1936.

14 Van der Hoeve, J., Eye and Amnion Bands. *Tr. Ophthalmol. Soc. U.K.* **50:**237–243, 1930.

31

Oblique Facial Cleft and Associated Anomalies

Oblique facial cleft (meloschisis) is exceedingly rare and variable in extent. From the approximately 75 published cases, the cleft appears to be bilateral in about 20 percent of the cases and more often on the right side when unilateral (1). It is nearly always associated with cleft lip, cleft palate, or lateral facial cleft. Fogh-Andersen (8) found one case of oblique cleft per 1,300 cases of facial cleft, while Gunter (11) noted four among 900 cases of facial clefts.

There is no sex predilection (1). For historic discussion, see Morian (13) and Boo-Chai (1).

This type of cleft may extend through the upper lip to the nose (as a typical lip cleft) and

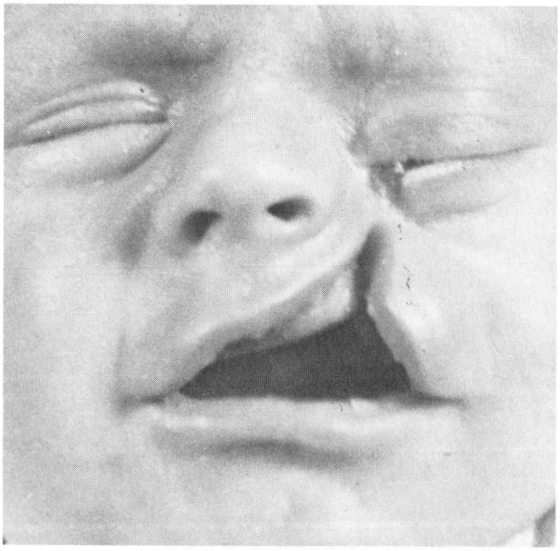

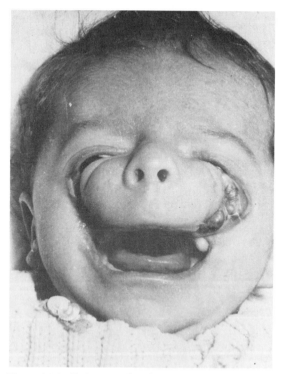

Figure 31-1. *Oblique facial cleft.* Cleft which bypasses nostril and extends roughly along line of closure of nasolacrimal canal. (*From P. Fogh-Andersen,* Acta Chir. Scand. **129**:275, 1965.)

Figure 31-2. Clefts extending from angles of mouth to outer canthi of eyes, following no line of embryonic fusion of facial processes. (*From I. Pitanguy and T. Franco,* Plast. Reconstr. Surg. **39**:569, 1967.)

involve the eye, at times even reaching the brow or temple (1, 16), or it may arise lateral to the philtrum and extend to the eye without involving the nose (Figs. 31-1, 31-2). The more severe types are, not uncommonly, incompatible with life. An attempt has been made to divide the oblique cleft into two types: (a) nasoocular cleft—extending from nostril to lower eyelid border with possible extension to temporal region, i.e., along the line of closure of the naso-lacrimal groove, and (b) oroocular cleft—extending from eye to lip. This last form is further subdivided into (a) oromedial canthal type and (b) orolateral canthal type (1, 3, 12). Our own view is that this classification is rather arbitrary and does not fit all cases (see further on). It has been stated to represent failure of penetration of ecto-mesenchyme between the lateral nasal and maxillary processes and failure of coverage of the nasolacrimal groove. Not uncommonly the oblique facial cleft fails to follow the line of fusion of the globular and maxillary processes and/or the nasolacrimal or other facial groove and may represent tears in ectomesenchyme. To date, all known cases are sporadic.

The oblique facial cleft may also be associated with encephalocele (12, 12a), hydro-cephaly (13), intrauterine amputation of digits (1, 2, 17, 19), hernia (15), absence of lacrimal puncta or involvement of the nasolacrimal duct and/or upper- or lower-lid colobomas (4), choroid colo-bomas (5, 10, 14, 16), exophthalmos (11), lateral facial cleft (1, 4, 19), anomalies of the extremities, such as syndactyly, polydactyly, adactyly, or ring constrictions (16, 17), frontonasal dysplasia (6), genitourinary abnormalities (11), and spinal and costal defects (4).

REFERENCES

1 Boo-Chai, K., The Oblique Facial Cleft: A Report of 2 Cases and a Review of 41 Cases. *Br. J. Plast. Surg.* **23:**352–359, 1970.

2 Davies, J., Two Cases of Macrostomia Described with Some Observations on the Incidence of Defective Development of the Mandibular Arch in the Sheep. *Br. Dent. J.* **86:**217–225, 1949.

3 Dey, D. L., Oblique Facial Clefts. *Plast. Reconstr. Surg.* **52:**258–263, 1973.

4 Dodds, G. E., A Case Showing Partial Deficient Fusion of a Maxillary Process with Lateral Nasal Process on One Side. *Br. J. Ophthalmol.* **27:**414–415, 1943.

5 Ecker, H. A., An Unusual Bilateral Oblique Facial Cleft. *J. Oral Surg.* **8:**618–619, 1970.

6 Ergin, N. O., Naso-ocular Cleft. *Plast. Reconstr. Surg.* **38:**573–575, 1966.

7 Fleischer, K., Die schräge Gesichtsspalte. *H.N.O.* **9:**280–281, 1961.

8 Fogh-Andersen, P., Rare Clefts of the Face. *Acta Chir. Scand.* **129:**275–281, 1965.

9 Gorlin, R. J., Developmental Anomalies of Face and Oral Structures, in R. J. Gorlin and H. M. Goldman, (eds.), *Thoma's Oral Pathology,* 6th ed., Mosby, St. Louis, 1970.

10 Grob, M., *Lehrbuch der Kinderchirurgie.* Georg Thieme Verlag, Stuttgart, 1957, pp. 101–104.

11 Gunter, G. S., Nasomaxillary Cleft. *Plast. Reconstr. Surg.* **32:**637–645, 1963.

12 Harkins, C. S., et al., A Classification of Cleft Lip and Cleft Palate. *Plast. Reconstr. Surg.* **29:**31–39, 1962.

12a Kubaček, V., and Pěnkava, J., Oblique Clefts of the Face. *Acta Chir. Plast.* **16:**152–163, 1974.

13 Morian, R., Über die schräge Gesichtsspalte. *Arch. Klin. Chir.* **35:**245–288, 1887.

14 Ortega, J., and Flor, E., Incomplete Naso-ocular Cleft. *Plast. Reconstr. Surg.* **43:**630–632, 1969.

15 Potter, J., A Case of Bilateral Cleft of the Face. *Br. J. Plast. Surg.* **3:**209–213, 1951.

16 Sakurai, E. H., et al., Bilateral Oblique Facial Clefts and Amniotic Bands. *Cleft Palate J.* **3:**181–185, 1966.

17 Schwalbe, E., *Die Morphologie der Missbildungen des Menschen und der Tiere.,* part 3, Gustav Fischer Verlag, Jena, 1913, pp. 113–204.

18 Tange, I., and Murofushi, H., Six Cases with Oblique Facial Cleft. *Jap. J. Plast. Surg.* **9:**114–119, 1966.

19 Tower, P., Coloboma of Lower Lid and Choroid with Facial Defects and Deformity of Hand and Forearm. *Arch. Ophthalmol.* **50:**333–343, 1953.

32

Median Cleft of Lower Lip, Mandible, and Tongue

Cleft tongue is usually associated with the oral-facial-digital syndrome (Chap. 107), but may be an isolated phenomenon (8) or associated with the Robin anomalad (12).

Of special interest is the association of bifid tongue and median cleft of the lower lip and mandible. Some cases are mild, involving only the soft tissues of the lower lip and sparing the bone (3, 11). Some patients have had cleft lower jaw without tongue involvement (15, 18). Most other patients have associated complete cleavage of the mandible, tongue, and structures of the midneck down to the hyoid bone (4, 5, 21, 25) (Figs. 32-1, 32-2). Some patients have a midline cervical cord (5a).

This anomaly results either from failure of development of the unpaired copula which normally arises between the primary paired mandibular processes and gives rise to the mandibular arch, or from persistence of the central of three evanescent grooves which appear in the mandibular process of the 5- to 6-mm embryo and normally disappear by the 10- to 16-mm stage (22).

Such a cleft has been found in association with oblique cleft (14). The patient described by

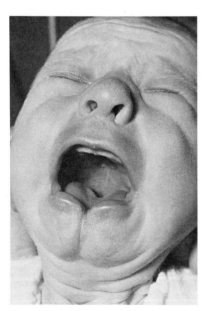

Figure 32-1. *Cleft mandible.* Incomplete cleft of lower lip and chin with complete cleft of mandible. (*From C. C. Knowles et al.,* Br. Dent. J. **127:**337, 1969.)

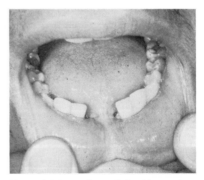

Figure 32-2. *Median cleft of lower lip.* Tongue tip attached to mandible. (*From H. A. Ecker,* Am. J. Surg. **96:**815, 1958.)

Ashley and Richardson (1) had associated cleft palate, absence of parotid glands, anophthalmia, and anencephaly. Davis (4) noted associated strabismus and heart murmur. A heart anomaly was also noted by Stewart (21). In another case, the lower jaw was involved in a symphyseal cystic process (26). The infant described by Petit and Psaume (16) had bizarre pinnas and bilateral colobomas of the iris.

The disorder is not hereditary. Its precise incidence is unknown. Petit and Psaume (16) estimated it to be about 1 per 600 cases of cleft upper lip with or without cleft palate. Recent reviews are those of Monroe (13) and Gorlin (6).

Malfusion of the mandibular symphysis that does not give rise to a clinical cleft has been described in association with hypodontia, microdontia, polydactyly, synostosis, and absence of carpals, metacarpals, tarsals, and metatarsals by Weyers (23, 24) as *acrofacial dysostosis*.

True doubling or replication of the tongue has also been described (7, 19).

REFERENCES

1 Ashley, L. M., and Richardson, G. E., Multiple Congenital Anomalies in a Stillborn Infant. *Anat. Rec.* **86:**457–473, 1943.

2 Ballesti, J., *Le bec-de-lièvre inférieure médian*. Thesis, Paris, 1909.

3 Braithwaite, F., and Watson, J., A Report of Three Unusual Cleft Lips. *Br. J. Plast. Surg.* **2:**38–49, 1949.

4 Davis, A. D., Median Cleft of the Lower Lip and Mandible. *Plast. Reconstr. Surg.* **6:**62–67, 1950.

5 Ecker, H. A., Median Clefts of the Lip. *Am. J. Surg.* **96:**815–819, 1958.

5a Fujino, H., et al., Median Cleft of the Lower Lip Mandible and Tongue with Midline Cervical Cord. *Cleft Palate J.* **7:**679–684, 1970.

6 Gorlin, R. J., Developmental Anomalies of Face and Oral Structures, in R. J. Gorlin and H. Goldman (eds.), *Thoma's Oral Pathology*, 6th ed., Mosby, St. Louis, 1970.

7 Greig, D. M., Schistoglossum and Double Tongue. *Edinburgh Med. J.*, **32:**1–16, 1925.

8 Hubinger, H. L., Bifid Tongue: Report of a Case. *J. Oral Surg.* **10:**64, 1952.

9 Knowles, C. C., et al., Incomplete Cleft of the Lower Lip and Chin with Complete Cleft of the Mandible. *Br. Dent. J.* **127:**337–339, 1969.

10 Lagrot, F., et al., Bifidité mandibulo-glosso-labiale. *Ann. Chir. Infant.* **3:**88–90, 1962.

11 Magrinos Torres, C., et al., Cheiloschisis e cheilognathoschisis inferior. *Mem. Inst. Oswaldo Cruz*, **54:**409–412, 1956.

12 Mathis, H., Exzessive Unterentwicklung des Unterkiefers als Todesursache. *Dtsch. Zahnärztl. Z.*, **4:**482–487, 1949.

13 Monroe, C. W., Midline Cleft of the Lower Lip, Mandible and Tongue with Flexion Contracture of the Neck. *Plast. Reconstr. Surg.* **38:**312–319, 1966.

14 Morian, R., Über schräge Gesichtsspalte. *Arch. Klin. Chir.* **35:**245–288, 1887.

15 Morton, C. B., and Jordan, H. E., Median Cleft of Lower Lip and Mandible, Cleft Sternum and Absence of Basihyoid. *Arch. Surg.* **30:**647–656, 1935.

16 Petit, P., and Psaume, J., Fente médiane de la lèvre inférieure. *Ann. Chir. Plast.* **10:**91–96, 1965.

17 Rea, E., Median Cleft of Lower Lip. *Cent. Afr. J. Med.* **13:**209–210, 1967.

18 Redard, P., and Michel, F., Sillon médian profond de la lèvre inférieure et du menton. *Presse Méd.* **7:**191–193, 1899.

19 Seitz, A., A Case of Double Tongue. *N.Y. Med. Rec.* **61:**474–475, 1902.

20 Silas, V., Réparation du bec-de-lièvre inférieure avec bifidité de l'arc mandibulaire. *Ann. Chir. Infant.* **8:**233–236, 1967.

21 Stewart, W. J., Congenital Median Cleft of the Chin. *Arch. Surg.* **31:**813–815, 1935.

22 Warbrick, J. G., et al., Remarks on the Etiology of Congenital Bilateral Fistulas of Lower Lip. *Br. J. Plast. Surg.* **4:**254–262, 1952.

23 Weyers, H., Hexadactylie, Unterkieferspalt und Oligodontia, ein neuer Symptomenkomplex: Dysostosis acrofacialis. *Ann. Paediatr. (Basel)* **181:**45–60, 1953.

24 Weyers, H., Über Wachstums- und Entwicklungsstörungen der Unterkiefersymphyse und ihre Begleitmissbildungen. *Stoma (Heidelb.)* **8:**86–102, 1955.

25 Wolfler, A., Zur Casuistik der medianen Gesichtsspalte. *Arch. Klin. Chir.* **40:**795–805, 1890.

26 Wynn-Williams, D., Congenital Midline Cervical Cleft and Web. *Br. J. Plast. Surg.* **5:**87–93, 1952–1953.

33

Cleidocranial Dysplasia

(Cleidocranial Dysostosis)

Over 700 cases of cleidocranial dysplasia have been documented in the medical literature from the time of Martin (17) and Meckel (18). Scheuthauer (24) described the syndrome quite accurately in 1871. Marie and Sainton (16), in 1897, independently reported the combination of (*a*) aplasia or hypoplasia of one or both clavicles, (*b*) exaggerated development of the transverse diameter of the cranium, and (*c*) delayed ossification of fontanels. They coined the name "cleidocranial dysostosis."

Since that time, many extensive reviews and analyses of the syndrome have been carried out and over 100 associated anomalies have been recorded (5, 6, 7, 19). Perhaps the most classic anatomic study is that of Hultkrantz (13). A good review is that of Schuch and Fleischer-Peters (25).

The syndrome has autosomal dominant inheritance (3, 6, 7, 19, 25).

SYSTEMIC MANIFESTATIONS

Facies and general appearance. The appearance is usually so marked as to be pathognomonic. The individual is usually short, males averaging 156.6 cm and females, 144.6 cm. The neck appears long, and the shoulders are narrow and droop markedly. The skull is brachycephalic, with pronounced frontal and parietal bossing, causing the face to appear small. The nose is broad at the base, with the bridge depressed (Fig. 33-1).

Cranium. The skull is large and short, the cephalic index being usually in excess of 80. Usually a groove, overlying the metopic suture, extends from the nasion to the sagittal suture.

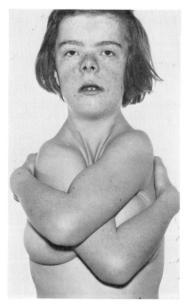

Figure 33-1. *Cleidocranial dysplasia.* Frontal and parietal bossing, glabellar groove in thirteen-year-old girl attempting to approximate shoulders. (*From M. Fons,* Acta Otolaryngol. (Stockh.) **67**:483, 1969.)

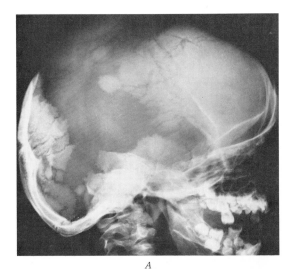

A

B

Figure 33-2. (*A*). Numerous Wormian bones found in lambdoidal sutures, delayed cranial bone formation. (*Courtesy of F. Silverman, Cincinnati, Ohio.*) (*B*). Wormian bones in lambdoidal sutures.

Because of the failure of various bones to unite, closure of the fontanels and sutures is delayed, often for life. Secondary centers of ossification appear in the suture lines, and many Wormian bones are formed (Fig. 33-2*A, B*). There is short sagittal diameter to the cranial base. The accessory sinuses are often underdeveloped or absent (3, 11). The mastoids are usually not pneumatized, because of altered function of the sternocleidomastoid muscles.

Eyes. The orbital height may be great compared with the width, and the orbital ridges may overhang the sockets. Mild exophthalmos associated with a depressed orbital roof may be seen.

Clavicle. The clavicle may be unilaterally (more often on the right side) or bilaterally totally aplastic but more frequently is defective at the acromial end. Some patients have manifested a central gap (pseudoarthrosis), with bone replacement by fibrous connective tissue (7) (Fig. 33-3).

The deficiency of the clavicle is reponsible for the long appearance of the neck and the narrow shoulders. The range of shoulder movements permitted by this bony defect is often remarkable, frequently allowing the individual to approximate his shoulders in front of his chest. This ability is not always recognized by the patient, nor are the parents of an affected child necessarily aware of it (Fig. 33-1).

In this syndrome, there are variations in size, origin, and insertion of muscles related to the clavicles, especially the sternocleidomastoid, trapezius, deltoid, and pectoralis major; yet function is noted to be remarkably good (4).

Other skeletal deformities. Although cleidocranial dysplasia was originally believed to involve only bones of membranous origin, involvement of bones of both intramembranous and intracartilaginous origin has been recognized from the time of Fitchet's writings (6). The most frequent deformities include delayed closure of the pubic symphysis, coxa vara or (less often) coxa valga with lateral notching of the capital femoral epiphysis (14), spina bifida occulta of the cervical, thoracic, or lumbar regions of the spine, pseudoepiphyses at the base of one

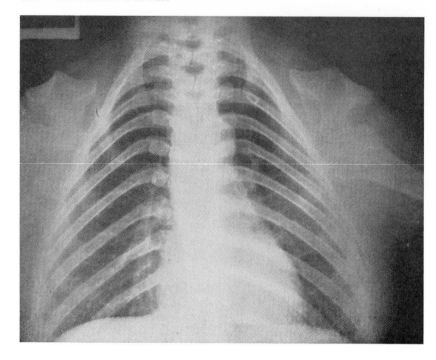

Figure 33-3.
Roentgenogram of chest demonstrating complete bilateral aplasia of clavicles.

or more metacarpals, abnormally pointed terminal phalangeal tufts of the hands and feet, and cone-shaped epiphyses of the distal phalanges.

Other findings. Conduction deafness (9, 10) has been described in several patients. A number of patients have experienced dystocia (14).

Oral manifestations. The palate is highly arched and may have submucous cleft or even complete palatal cleft involving both the hard and soft tissues (30). Nonunion at the mandibular symphysis has also been noted. Development of the premaxilla is poor, and since growth of the mandible is usually normal, relative prognathism results.

Though "lack of teeth" was recognized by many early authors, it was not until 1925 that Hesse (12) undertook extensive roentgenographic study of the jaws in cleidocranial dysplasia, which seemed to stimulate a number of similar investigations during the next two decades in both Germany and England (11, 12, 21, 22, 31).

The delayed eruption or failure of eruption of the deciduous and permanent teeth, which in some cases is total, results in pseudoanodontia. Fleischer-Peters (8) suggested that the jaw bones have increased density, which may inhibit tooth eruption. Cyst formation around these impacted, often inverted or displaced, teeth is not unusual and has been described by several authors (11, 12, 21, 22, 31). There is also a tendency for nonexfoliation of deciduous teeth. Winter (30) observed that those teeth without deciduous predecessors have a greater chance to erupt. Extraction of deciduous teeth does not seem to promote eruption of the permanent teeth (30). Gemination and dilaceration of roots are also common (11, 12, 21, 22, 30, 31).

One of the most remarkable oral aspects is the number of supernumerary teeth (Fig. 33-4). The crown form of many of these teeth is similar to that of a premolar, although somewhat more flattened. Fröhlich (11) suggested that the number of molars formed is less than normal. Extracted teeth have been found to be severely deformed (11, 21, 22, 30) and to have hypoplastic enamel.

Rushton (23) studied the teeth microscopically and noted that their roots lacked a

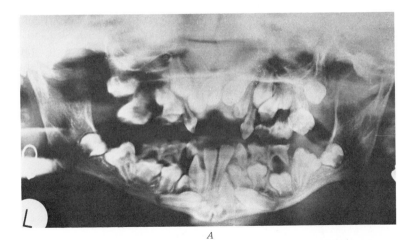

A

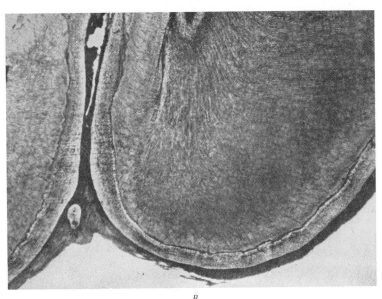

B

Figure 33-4. (*A*). Panorex showing multiple supernumerary, unerupted teeth. (*From A. Fleischer-Peters*, Stoma (Heidelb.) **23**:212, 1970.) (*B*). Tooth roots, exhibiting complete absence of cellular cementum. (*Courtesy of M. Rushton*, Br. Dent. J. **100**:81, 1956.)

layer of cellular cementum (Fig. 33-4*B*), a finding confirmed by several others (1, 26). This most interesting observation certainly merits further investigation.

DIFFERENTIAL DIAGNOSIS

Though the appearance is quite characteristic, the brachycephaly and frontal bossing may suggest rickets, prenatal syphilis, *achondroplasia*, hydrocephaly, and *pyknodysosto-*

sis. A deficient premaxilla may also be seen in *Apert syndrome* and in *craniofacial dysostosis*. Depressed nasal bridge is seen in *hypohidrotic ectodermal dysplasia* and in prenatal syphilis. A similar appearance of the shoulders may be seen in intrauterine or natal fracture. True widening of the pubic symphysis is seen most often with extrophy of the bladder and epispadias (20).

A peculiar variant, in which there were dolichocephaly, severe lordosis, generalized joint hypermobility, and dystrophic toenails, was described by Winkler (29). Also to be excluded is *mandibuloacral dysplasia.* The right clavicle may be hypoplastic in *focal dermal hypoplasia.* Bilateral absence of the clavicles was described in a syndrome called *cleidofacial dysplasia* (15). Associated were microbrachycephaly, exophthalmos with hypoplasia of lids, and mental retardation. Inheritance is autosomal recessive.

We have had occasion to see a girl with congenital absence of both clavicles and the sternum. She also had contractures of the fingers.

Failure of eruption of all permanent teeth has been reported as a dominant disorder (25a).

REFERENCES

1 Alderson, C. G. P., Hereditary Cleidocranial Dysostosis. *Br. Dent. J.* **108:**157–159, 1960.
2 Bjorn, H., and Grahnén, H., Cleido-cranial Dysostosis. *Odontol. Revy* **17:**67–74, 1966.
3 Chemin, J. P., et al., Une nouvelle observation de dysostose cleidocranienne. *Rev. Stomatol.* (*Paris*) **61:**900–905, 1960.
4 Eckstein, H. B., and Hoare, R. D., Congenital Parietal "Foramina" Associated with Faulty Ossification of the Clavicles. *Br. J. Radiol.* **36:**220–221, 1963.
5 Eldridge, W. W., et al., Cleidocranial Dysostosis. *Am. J. Roentgenol.* **34:**41–49, 1935.
6 Fitchet, S. M., Cleidocranial Dysostosis: Hereditary and Familial. *J. Bone Joint Surg.* **11:**838–866, 1929.
7 Fitzwilliams, D. C. L., Hereditary Cranio-cleido-dysostosis; with a Review of all the Published Cases of This Disease: Theories of the Development of the Clavicle Suggested by this Condition. *Lancet* **2:**1466–1475, 1910.
8 Fleischer-Peters, A., Zur Pathohistologie des Alveolarknochens bei Dysostosis cleidocranialis. *Stoma* (*Heidelb.*) **23:**212–215, 1970.
9 Föns, M., Ear Malformations in Cleidocranial Dysostosis. *Acta Oto-laryngol.* (*Stockh.*) **67:**483–489, 1969.
10 Forland, M., Cleidocranial Dysostosis. *Am. J. Med.* **33:**792–799, 1962.
11 Fröhlich, E., Die Erblichkeit der Dysostosis cleidocranialis. *Dtsch. Zahn Mund Kieferheilkd.* **41:**157–168, 1937.
12 Hesse, G., Dysotosis cleidocranialis unter besonderer Berücksichtigung des Gebisses. *Vjschr. Zahnheilkd.* **41:**162–177, 1925.
13 Hultkrantz, J. W., Über Dysostosis cleidocranialis. *Z. Morphol. Anthropol.* **11:**385–528, 1908.
14 Jarvis, J. L., and Keats, T. E., Cleidocranial Dysostosis: A Review of 40 New Cases. *Am. J. Roentgenol.* **121:**5–16, 1974.
15 Kozlowski, K., et al., Dysplasia cleidofacialis. *Z. Kinderheilkd.* **108:**331–338, 1970.
16 Marie, P., and Sainton, P., Observation d'hydrocéphalie héréditaire (père et fils) par vice de développement du crâne et du cerveau. *Bull. Soc. Méd. Hôp. Paris* **14:**706–712, 1897.
17 Martin, –, Sur un déplacement natural de la clavicule. *J. Méd. Chir. Pharmacol.* **23:**456–460, 1765.
18 Meckel (1760), cited by Terry, R. J., Rudimentary Clavicles and Other Abnormalities of the Skeleton of a White Woman. *J. Anat. Physiol.* (*Lond.*) **33:**413–422, 1899.
19 Miles, P. W., Cleidocranial Dysostosis: A Survey of Six New Cases and 126 from the Literature. *J. Kansas Med. Soc.* **41:**462–468, 1940.
20 Muecke, E. C., and Currarino, G., Congenital Widening of the Pubic Symphysis. *Am. J. Roentgenol.* **103:**178–185, 1968.
21 Rushton, M. A., The Dental Condition in Cleidocranial Dysostosis. *Guy's Hosp. Rep.* **87:**354–361, 1937.
22 Rushton, M. A., The Failure of Eruption in Cleidocranial Dysostosis. *Br. Dent. J.* **63:**641–645, 1937.
23 Rushton, M. A., An Anomaly of Cementum in Cleidocranial Dysostosis. *Br. Dent. J.* **100:**81–83, 1956.
24 Scheuthauer, G., Kombination rudimentärer Schlüsselbeine mit Anomalien des Schädels beim erwachsenen Menschen. *Allg. Wien Med. Ztg.* **16:**293–295, 1871.
25 Schuch, P., and Fleischer-Peters, A., Zur Klinik der Dysostosis cleidocranialis. *Z. Kinderheilkd.* **98:**107–132, 1967.
25a Shokeir, M. H. K., Complete Failure of Eruption of All Permanent Teeth: An Autosomal Dominant Disorder. *Clin. Genet.* **5:**322–326, 1974.
26 Smith, N. H., A Histological Study of Cementum in a Case of Cleidocranial Dysostosis. *Oral Surg.* **25:**470–478, 1968.
27 Soule, A. B., Jr., Mutational Dysostosis. *J. Bone Joint Surg.* **28:**81–102, 1946.
28 Wee, L. K., and Pillay, V. K., Hereditary Cleido-cranial Dysostosis with a Note on the Anomaly of Cementum. *Singapore Med. J.* **5:**3–9, 1964.
29 Winkler, H., Ein eigenartiger Fall von Dysostosis cleidocranialis bei einem siebenjährigen Kinde. *Jb. Kinderheilkd.* **149:**238–260, 1937.
30 Winter, G. R., Dental Conditions in Cleidocranial Dysostosis. *Am. J. Orthod.* **29:**61–89, 1943.
31 Zilkens, –, Zahnbefunde bei zwei Fällen von Dysostosis cleidocranialis. *Dtsch. Monatsschr. Zahnheilkd.* **45:**477–482, 1927.

34

Cockayne Syndrome

The Cockayne syndrome is characterized by (a) cachectic dwarfism, (b) premature aging, (c) mental deficiency, (d) microcephaly, (e) intracranial calcifications, (f) neurologic deficits, (g) retinal pigmentary abnormalities, (h) sensorineural deafness, and (i) photosensitivity.

Cockayne in 1936 described dwarfism with retinal atrophy and deafness in two sibs, and 10 years later published a brief review of their progress (4, 5). About 30 patients have been described in the literature, and autosomal recessive inheritance has been established (10, 20). However, a 3:1 male sex predilection has been observed.

SYSTEMIC MANIFESTATIONS

Facies. Lack of subcutaneous facial fat, particularly of the cheeks, gives prominence to the facial bones. This feature, combined with microcephaly, sunken eyes, thin, often beaklike nose, and large ears, gives the patient a birdlike appearance (24) (Fig. 34-1).

Musculoskeletal alterations. Dwarfism is the most prominent feature of the disorder. Growth retardation becomes evident during the second year of life after a normal gestation, birth weight, and infancy. Kyphosis and ankylosis are frequent (10, 15, 20, 21, 25). The limbs are disproportionately long, and the hands and feet dis-

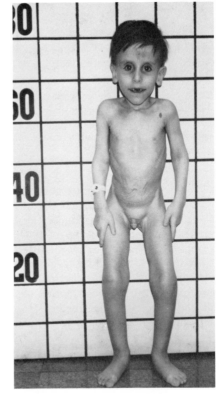

Figure 34-1. *Cockayne syndrome.* Note marked enophthalmos and horse-riding stance. (*From R. L. Summitt, Nashville, Tenn.*)

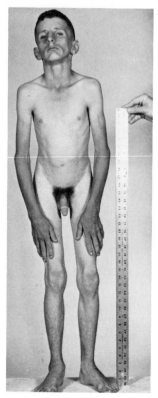

Figure 34-2. Sixteen-year-old male who experienced marked mental and somatic retardation, eye difficulties, deafness. Note wizened appearance, photodermatitis of sun-exposed areas, horse-riding stance. (*From R. M. Paddison, New Orleans, La.*)

proportionately large (14, 23). Flexion contractures may involve the ankles, knees, and elbows. The interphalangeal joints of the hands and feet may show periarticular thickening (Fig. 34-2).

Roentgenographic studies show abnormalities in the skull, extremities, and spine. There is increased thickening of the bones, particularly the skull base and calvaria, most noticeable in the frontal and parietooccipital regions (15, 21, 23). Often there is an associated osteoporosis (21).

Skin. Photosensitivity is a prominent feature. Dermatitis appears on the sun-exposed parts of the body by the second year of life, with a butterfly arrangement on the face (14, 25). The forehead is spared, but the pinnas and chin are involved. The photodermatitis may result in

scarring and pigmentary changes in older patients (15). Seborrheic dermatitis may also be present. The scalp hair and sometimes the eyebrows are diminished (10). Subcutaneous fat appears to be decreased throughout the body except for the suprapubic area (10).

Eyes. In nearly all patients there is enophthalmos. The retina is studded with fine, speckled pigment of the salt-and-pepper type, with the greatest concentration in the macular area. Also present are optic atrophy and arteriolar narrowing (3, 5, 15, 16, 25). Cataracts develop by adolescence (5, 6, 11, 20). A poor response to mydriasis with homatropine or Neo-synephrine has been noted (6). Corneal dystrophy with recurrent epithelial erosions, nystagmus, and photophobia are less frequently observed (2, 16).

Nervous system. Progressive neurologic signs include cerebellar ataxia, choreoathetosis, moderate to severe mental deficiency, sensorineural deafness, and blindness. Neuropathologic studies of the brain have shown microcephaly; widespread mineralization in the cortex, basal ganglia, and cerebellum; and patchy demyelinization, often severe, in the subcortical white matter (9, 18, 22). Normal intelligence has been reported in one patient (13).

Oral manifestations. An increase in dental caries has been noted by most authors (5, 11, 14, 16, 22). In some patients, numerous permanent teeth were congenitally absent (10, 22, 23). Atrophy of alveolar processes (10, 23) and condylar hypoplasia (8) have also been observed.

DIFFERENTIAL DIAGNOSIS

The Cockayne syndrome is one of a group of disorders which has certain common characteristics. The photosensitivity may suggest *Bloom syndrome*, Hartnup disease, *xerodermic idiocy*, or erythropoietic porphyria. Bloom syndrome has many of the features of the Cockayne syndrome except for the neurologic and ophthalmologic findings. Both have reduced IgA levels (4). No patient with the Cockayne syndrome has been reported with leukemia or lymphoma, and chromosomal breakage is absent (20, 25).

Rothmund-Thomson syndrome is not a neurologic disease, and although cataracts are seen in about half the patients, there are no retinal changes. *Xerodermic idiocy* is characterized by multiple cutaneous malignancies in light-exposed areas. Skin cancers have not been reported thus far in the photosensitive areas in patients with the Cockayne syndrome.

Progeria does not feature photosensitivity, neurologic disease, or retinal changes, and the phenotype is quite different from that of the Cockayne syndrome.

LABORATORY AIDS

Hyperinsulinemia and hyperlipoproteinemia but normal growth hormone levels have been noted in several patients (7, 8, 10).

REFERENCES

1 Bender, S. W., et al., Das Cockayne-Syndrom, eine Minderwuchsform mit vermehrter Wachstumhormonausshüttung. *Acta Endocrinol. [Suppl.] (Kbh.)* **152:**9, 1971.

2 Brodrick, J. D., and Dark, A. J., Corneal Dystrophy in Cockayne's Syndrome. *Br. J. Ophthalmol.* **57:**391–399, 1973.

3 Civantos, F., Human Chromosomal Abnormalities. *Bull. Tulane Med. Fac.* **20:**241–253, 1961.

4 Cockayne, E. A., Dwarfism with Retinal Atrophy and Deafness. *Arch. Dis. Child.* **11:**1–8, 1936.

5 Cockayne, E. A., Dwarfism with Retinal Atrophy and Deafness. *Arch. Dis. Child.* **21:**52–54, 1946.

6 Coles, W. H., Ocular Manifestations of Cockayne's Syndrome. *Am. J. Ophthalmol.* **67:**762–764, 1969.

7 Conly, P. W., et al., Hyperinsulinemia in Cockayne's Syndrome. *South. Med. J.* **63:**1491–1495, 1970.

8 Cotton, R. B., et al., Abnormal Blood Glucose Regulation in Cockayne's Syndrome. *Pediatrics* **46:**54–60, 1970.

9 Crome, L., and Kanjilal, G. C., Cockayne's Syndrome. *J. Neurol. Neurosurg. Psychiatr.* **34:**171–178, 1971.

10 Fujimoto, W. Y., et al., Cockayne's Syndrome, Report of a Case with Hyperlipoproteinemia, Hyperinsulinemia, Renal Disease and Normal Growth Hormone. *J. Pediatr.* **75:**881–884, 1969.

11 Guzetta, F., La sindrome di Cockayne. *Minerva Pediatr.* **19:**891–895, 1967.

12 Land, V. J., and Nogrady, M. B., Cockayne's Syndrome. *J. Can. Assoc. Radiol.* **20:**194–203, 1970.

13 Lanning, M., and Simila, S., Cockayne's Syndrome: Report of a Case with Normal Intelligence. *Z. Kinderheilkd.* **109:**70–75, 1970.

14 Lieberman, W. J., et al., Cockayne's Disease. *Am. J. Ophthalmol.* **52:**116–118, 1961.

15 Macdonald, W. B., et al., Cockayne's Syndrome. *Pediatrics* **25:**997–1007, 1960.

16 Marie, J., et al., Nanisme avec surdi-mutité et rétinite pigmentaire: Syndrome de Cockayne. *Arch. Fr. Pédiatr.* **15:**1101–1103, 1958.

17 Moosa, A., and Dubowitz, V., Peripheral Neuropathy in Cockayne's Syndrome. *Arch. Dis. Child.* **45:**674–677, 1970.

18 Moossy, J., The Neuropathology of Cockayne's Syndrome. *J. Neuropathol. Exp. Neurol.* **26:**654–660, 1967.

19 Neill, C. A., and Dingwall, M. M., A Syndrome Resembling Progeria. *Arch. Dis. Child.* **25:**213–221, 1950.

20 Paddison, R. M., et al., Cockayne's Syndrome. *Dermatol. Trop.* **2:**196–203, 1963.

21 Riggs, W. Jr., and Seibert, J., Cockayne's Syndrome. Roentgen Findings. *Am. J. Roentgenol.* **116:**623–633, 1972.

22 Rowlatt, V., Cockayne's Syndrome: Report of a Case with Necropsy Findings. *Acta Neuropathol.* **14:**52–61, 1969.

23 Schönenberg, H., and Frohn, K., Das Cockayne-Syndrom. *Monatsschr. Kinderheilkd.* **117:**103–108, 1969.

24 Tympner, K. D., et al., Cockaynes Syndrom. *Z. Kinderheilkd.* **104:**298–307, 1968.

25 Windmiller, J., et al., Cockayne Syndrome with Chromosomal Analysis. *Am. J. Dis. Child.* **105:**204–208, 1963.

35

Congenital Indifference to Pain

(Congenital Insensitivity to Pain)

Dearborn (7), in 1931, described a syndrome in which there was congenital complete indifference to pain, resulting in injury to both soft and hard tissues with subsequent severe scarring. Trauma to bones caused aseptic necrosis, osteomyelitis, or fractures. His patient worked in a sideshow as a "human pincushion."

Over 90 cases have been reported to date. Parental consanguinity (8, 10, 11, 17, 22) and affected sibs (1, 9, 12, 15) indicate autosomal recessive inheritance (21).

SYSTEMIC MANIFESTATIONS

Facies and general appearance. Frequent scarring of the face, with mutilation of the lips, arms, and legs, as well as phalangeal amputation

due to self-mutilation have been noted (1, 7–23) (Figs. 35-1, 35-2).

Nervous system. There is total absence of reaction to painful stimuli over the entire body. Deep-tendon reflexes are intact. The corneal reflex is often absent or diminished (1, 7, 9, 12, 13, 15, 23); taste, touch, temperature sensation, joint position sense, tickling, itching, and vibration are generally normal (1, 4, 9, 11, 14–17). Anosmia has been occasionally observed (23). Thrush (23) noted a reduction in large myelinated fibers but abundant normal unmyelinated fibers.

Intelligence has ranged from dull to normal (1). Patients with severe mental retardation represent examples of other syndromes (see Table 35-1).

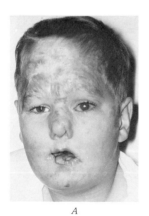

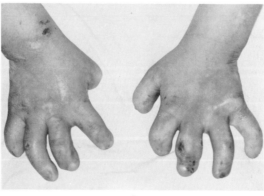

A

B

Figure 35-1. *Congenital indifference to pain.* (*A*). Five-year-old male chewed off anterior tongue and lower lip. Repeatedly traumatized nose, eye, forehead. Parents were first cousins. (*B*). Hands of same child.

Table 35-1. Comparison of major clinical features in childhood sensory syndromes.

Condition	Inheritance	Manifestations in infancy	Touch appreciation	Temperature appreciation	Tears	Sweat	Mental retardation	Abnormal histology
Congenital indifference to pain	Autosomal recessive	+	+	+	+	+	±	−
Congenital sensory neuropathy	Mostly sporadic	+	−	−	+	+	±	+
Congenital sensory neuropathy with anhidrosis	Autosomal recessive	+	+	−	+	−	+	±
Familial dysautonomia	Autosomal recessive	+	+	±	−	+	±	−
Lesch-Nyhan syndrome	X-linked recessive	+	+	+	+	+	+	−
Hereditary sensory radicular neuropathy	Autosomal dominant	−	±	±	+	+	±	+

Musculoskeletal system. Osteomyelitis, aseptic necrosis, fracture, Charcot joint, and distal necrosis with spontaneous resorption of toes and fingers are virtually constant features (1–4, 9, 11, 13, 15–18, 20). These complications have been ascribed to lack of pain sensation, the patient being unable to recognize trauma. Several patients have exhibited loose joints. Haaxma et al. (12) have shown insufficient calcium absorption in the digestive tract with an excess of osteoid tissue formation, a finding which merits further evaluation.

Oral manifestations. Lack of pain sensation results in severe oral mutilation (1, 9, 10, 12, 13, 15, 17, 23). The tongue and lips are especially subject to injury, with resultant scarring (4, 9, 10, 13, 19, 20). This becomes apparent as soon as the teeth appear and may lead to early diagnosis (9). Extensive decay is not accompanied by toothache, and teeth may be lost early on this account (10). In many cases, the patient has painlessly extracted his own teeth. Thrush (23) described a fibrous cord buccal to the teeth in each of his patients.

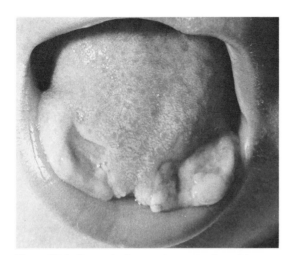

Figure 35-2. *Congenital sensory neuropathy with anhidrosis.* Extensive mutilation of anterior tongue. (*From F. Vassella et al.,* Arch. Dis. Child. **43**:124, 1968.)

DIFFERENTIAL DIAGNOSIS

Indifference to pain also occurs in leprosy, oligophrenia, hysteria, multiple sclerosis, postleukotomy state, and asymbolia (23). Indifference to pain may also be seen in syringobulbia and syringomyelia, but in these conditions temperature sense is also lost. *Familial dysautonomia,* radicular sensory neuropathy, sensory neuropathy with anhidrosis, and congenital sensory neuropathy should also be considered (Table 35-1).

In familial dysautonomia there is a great reduction in unmyelinated fibers and an absence of myelinated fibers greater than 12 μm in diameter. In insensitivity to pain with anhidrosis there is an absence of Lissauer's tract and of small dorsal root ganglion cells and axons. In hereditary sensory radicular neuropathy there is primary degeneration of dorsal root ganglion cells (1). Asymbolia for pain is a form of aplasia associated with lesions of the supramarginal gyrus of the parietal lobe, usually due to trauma, tumor, or infection.

The sisters described by Appenzeller and Kornfeld (1) demonstrated marked loss of large myelinated fibers and virtual absence of small myelinated fibers. Mosaic Schwann cells and an increase in endoneural and perineural collagen were also noted.

Patients with *Lesch-Nyhan* syndrome also show signs of self-mutilation, especially of lips and hands, but they have severe mental retardation, choreoathetosis, and hyperuricemia. Critchley et al. (5), in 1968, described an autosomal recessively inherited syndrome characterized by acanthocytosis and neurologic disorder without beta-lipoproteinemia. Tongue, lip, and buccal mucosal biting leading to severe mutilation was present because of uncontrollable, jerky movements which generally occurred at night. Patients responded normally to pain stimulation, but deep-tendon reflexes were absent.

LABORATORY AIDS

Da Costa Maia et al. (6) reported an unidentified metabolite in the urine of several patients with congenital indifference to pain. The metabolite was described as having an aromatic nucleus with carboxylic and primary aromatic amine groups. Normal controls failed to show this metabolite. This finding has not been further substantiated.

REFERENCES

1 Appenzeller, O., and Kornfeld, M., Indifference to Pain: A Chronic Peripheral Neuropathy with Mosaic Schwann Cells. *Arch. Neurol.* **27**:322–339, 1972.

2 Arbuse, D., Congenital Indifference to Pain. *J. Pediatr.* **35**:221–226, 1951.

3 Baxter, D. W., and Olszewski, J., Congenital Universal Insensitivity to Pain. *Brain* **83**:381–393, 1960.

4 Boyd, D. H., Jr., and Nie, L. W., Congenital Universal Indifference to Pain. *Arch. Neurol. Psychiatr.* **61**:402–412, 1949.

5 Critchley, E. M. R., et al., Acanthocytosis and Neurological Disorder without Betalipoproteinemia. *Arch. Neurol.* **18**:134–140, 1968.

6 Da Costa Maia, J. C., et al., Isolation of a New Urine Metabolite Excreted in Generalized Congenital Analgesia. *Clin. Chim. Acta* **12**:122–124, 1965.

7 Dearborn, G., A Case of Congenital General Pure Analgesia. *J. Nerv. Ment. Dis.* **75**:612–615, 1931.

8 Fanconi, G., and Ferrazzini, F., Kongenitale Analgie (kongenitale generalisierte Schmerzindifferenz). *Helv. Paediatr. Acta* **12**:79–115, 1957.

9 Gaudier, B., et al., L'indifférance congénitale à la douleur. A propos de deux nouvelles observations. *Arch. Fr. Pédiatr.* **26**:1027–1040, 1969.

10 Guillermo, A., and Grinspan, G. A., Indifférance congéni-

tale à la douleur, à propos d'un cas avec antécédents de consanguinité. *Rev. Neurol. (Paris)* **123**:434–435, 1970.

11 Gwinn, J. L., and Barnes, G. R., Radiological Case of the Month: Congenital Indifference to Pain. *Am. J. Dis. Child.* **112**:583–584, 1966.

12 Haaxma, R., et al., Congenital Indifference to Pain Associated with a Defect in Calcium Metabolism. *Acta Neurol. Scand.* **47**:194–208, 1971.

13 Ingwersen, O. S., Congenital Indifference to Pain: Report of a Case. *J. Bone Joint Surg.* **49B**:704–709, 1967.

14 Jewsbury, E. C. O., Insensitivity to Pain. *Brain* **74**:336–353, 1951.

15 Khan, S. A., and Peterkin, G. A. G., Congenital Indifference to Pain. *St. Johns Hosp. Dermatol. Soc. Trans.* **56**:122–130, 1970.

16 Lamy, et al., L'analgésie généralisée congénitale. *Arch. Fr. Pédiatr.* **15**:433–448, 1958.

17 Lievre, J. A., et al., Analgésie généralisée congénitale (indifferance congénitale à la douleur) chez deux frères issu de cousins germains. *Soc. Méd. Hôp. Paris* **119**:447–456, 1968.

18 Murray, R. O., Congenital Indifference to Pain with Special Reference to Skeletal Changes. *Br. J. Radiol.* **30**:2–6, 1957.

19 Nissler, K., and Parnitzke, K. H., Fehlen der Schmerzemp-

findung bei einem Kinde. *Dtsch. Med. Wochenschr.* **76:**861–863, 1951.

20 Petrie, J. G., A Case of Progressive Joint Disorders Caused by Insensitivity to Pain. *J. Bone Joint Surg.* **35B:**399–401, 1953.

21 Saldanha, P. H., et al., A Genetical Investigation of Congenital Analgesia. *Acta Genet. (Basel)* **14:**143–158, 1964.

22 Thiemann, H. H., Analgesia congenita (angeborene universelle Schmerzindifferenz). *Arch. Kinderheilkd.* **164:**255–262, 1961.

23 Thrush, D. C., Congenital Insensitivity to Pain. *Brain* **96:**369–386, 1973.

36

CRST Syndrome

(Calcinosis, Raynaud Phenomenon, Sclerodactyly, and Telangiectasia)

Although calcinosis occurring in association with scleroderma was described early in this century (5), the more benign complex of (a) calcinosis, (b) sclerodactyly, (c) Raynaud phenomenon, and (d) telangiectasia was probably first recorded by Thomas (11) in 1942. The name "CRST syndrome" was coined by Winterbauer (12).

The disorder is not hereditary. There is a marked (possibly 6:1) female predilection. Fewer than 50 cases have been reported to date.

SYSTEMIC MANIFESTATIONS

The several aspects of the syndrome characteristically appear at various times in a patient's life. Only rarely does the disorder present prior to puberty; in these cases, the Raynaud phenomenon first becomes evident.

Facies. As noted below, the facies is marked by telangiectases (Fig. 36-1).

Calcinosis. The calcinosis is subcutaneous or in the dermis, being usually but not always limited to areas of sclerodactyly. Rarely, calcinosis is absent (3) (Fig. 36-2A, B).

Raynaud phenomenon. Paresthesia and blueness of the extremities is usually the primary complaint, often appearing 20 to 30 years prior to the onset of other signs of the syndrome.

It often is associated with frank ischemic changes in the fingertips.

Sclerodactyly. The alterations in the fingers in no way differ from those found in ordinary

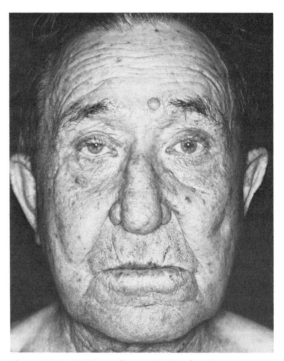

Figure 36-1. *CRST syndrome.* Facies showing numerous telangiectases. (*From R. H. Winterbauer,* Johns Hopkins Hosp. Bull. **114**:361, 1964.)

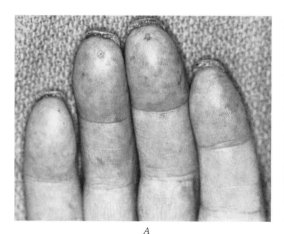

A

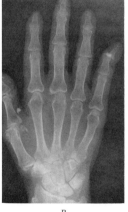

B

Figure 36-2. (*A*). Sclerodactyly of terminal phalanges. Note extrusion of particulate calcium salts. (From Berris et al., Can. Med. Assoc. J. **96:**1528.) (*B*). Joint degeneration and numerous calcium deposits. (*From R. H. Winterbauer,* Bull. Johns Hopkins Hosp. **114:**361, 1964.)

scleroderma. Sclerodermatous alterations may be present elsewhere in the body, but they are usually mild and often atypical (4) (Fig. 36-2*A*). The face is free of sclerodermatous changes, but the esophagus is often involved, and most patients exhibit gastrointestinal tract dysfunction (3, 10).

Telangiectasia. The face (especially the cheeks, nose, and lips), oral mucosa, hands, and upper trunk are the most common sites of involvement with punctate telangiectases (Fig. 36-1). Retiform and linear telangiectases may also be scattered among the punctate lesions. The nasal mucosa is characteristically spared.

Telangiectases occurring on mucosal surfaces are not likely to hemorrhage, although there have been a few exceptions (2, 5, 9).

Hepatic and other changes. Primary biliary cirrhosis has been described in several patients (5, 9). Various collagen disorders, such as lupus erythematosus, dermatomyositis, rheumatoid arthritis, etc., have been associated with the CRST syndrome (3, 10).

Oral manifestations. In our survey of the literature, the oral sites most often involved with telangiectasia, in decreasing order, are the lips, buccal mucosa, tongue, and palate (Fig. 36-3*A*, *B*).

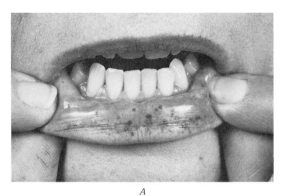

A

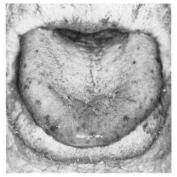

B

Figure 36-3. (*A*, *B*). Telangiectasia of oral mucosa resembling that of hereditary hemorrhagic telangiectasia. (*A from Berris et al.,* Can. Med. Assoc. J. **96:**1528, 1967; *B from R. H. Winterbauer,* Johns Hopkins Hosp. Bull. **114:**361, 1964.)

DIFFERENTIAL DIAGNOSIS

Although the telangiectases may result in the erroneous diagnosis of *hereditary hemorrhagic telangiectasia* (HHT) (6), calcinosis cutis, Raynaud phenomenon, and scleroderma are not found in that disorder. Moreover, HHT is inherited as an autosomal dominant trait, and epistaxis and melena are common, being unusual in the CRST syndrome.

LABORATORY AIDS

Calcium metabolism is normal. Alteration of the skin of the involved extremities is typical for scleroderma. Roentgenographic study of the extremities usually demonstrates calcinosis cutis (5). Esophageal changes of scleroderma have also been observed roentgenographically. Cryoglobulin levels are normal in this syndrome.

REFERENCES

1 Berris, B., et al., Telangiectases Simulating Hereditary Hemorrhagic Telangiectasia in Scleroderma. *Can. Med. Assoc. J.* **96:**1528–1531, 1967.

2 Binford, R. T., CRST Syndrome with Gastrointestinal Bleeding. *Arch. Dermatol.* **97:**603–604, 1968.

3 Carr, R. D., and Heisel, E. B., CRST Syndrome and Variant. *Acta Derm. Venereol. (Stockh.)* **47:**345–349, 1967.

4 Carr, R. D., et al., CRST Syndrome: A Benign Variant of Scleroderma. *Arch. Dermatol.* **92:**519–525, 1965.

5 Dellipiani, A. W., and George, M., Syndrome of Sclerodactyly, Calcinosis, Raynaud's Phenomenon and Telangiectasia. *Br. Med. J.* **4:**334–335, 1967.

6 Gottron, H. A., and Korting, G. W., Über Ablagerung körpereigener Stoffe (Amyloidosis, Calcinosis) bei Morbus Osler. *Arch. Klin. Exp. Dermatol.* **207:**177–201, 1958.

7 McAndrew, G. M., and Barnes, E. G., Familial Sclero-

derma. *Ann. Phys. Med.* **8:**128–131, 1965.

8 Ohm, O. J., The CRST Syndrome. *Nord. Med.* **83:**268–269, 1970.

9 Reynolds, T. B., et al., Primary Biliary Cirrhosis with Scleroderma, Raynaud's Phenomenon and Telangiectasia. *Am. J. Med.* **50:**302–312, 1971.

10 Schimke, R. N., et al., Calcinosis, Raynaud's Phenomenon, Sclerodactyly, and Telangiectasia. *Arch. Intern. Med.* **119:**365–370, 1967.

11 Thomas, E. W. P., Calcinosis Cutis and Scleroderma: Thibierge-Weissenbach Syndrome. *Lancet* **2:**389–392, 1942.

12 Winterbauer, R. H., Multiple Telangiectasia, Raynaud's Phenomenon, Sclerodactyly, and Subcutaneous Calcinosis: A Syndrome Mimicking Hereditary Hemorrhagic Telangiectasia. *Bull. Johns Hopkins Hosp.* **114:**361–383, 1964.

37

Cranial Nerve Syndromes
with Orofacial Manifestations

Because of the large number of possible combinations of involvement of cranial nerves, both within and outside the cranial cavity, a considerable number of eponymic syndromes have been created to describe these conditions. Many of these syndromes overlap, and some of them have been given several eponyms. They will be considered under three general sections: (*a*) those involving the trigeminal nerve, (*b*) those largely involving the other cranial nerves that may have oral manifestations, and (*c*) a group of miscellaneous cranial nerve syndromes.

SYNDROMES OF THE TRIGEMINAL NERVE

Pain, temperature, and tactile sensation for the lips, teeth, and oral mucosa is mediated largely through the second and third divisions of the *trigeminal nerve.* From the gasserian ganglion, which lies in a cavity in the dura mater near the petrous tip of the temporal bone, the three divisions pass forward:

1. The *ophthalmic* branch passes through the cavernous sinus, where it is intimately associated with the third, fourth, and sixth cranial nerves.

2. The *maxillary* division leaves the skull through the foramen rotundum, crosses the pterygopalatine fossa, where it supplies branches to the sphenopalatine ganglion and the upper posterior teeth and alveolar process, enters the orbit through the inferior orbital fissure, runs through the infraorbital canal, sending off branches to the rest of the upper teeth and alveoli, and supplies the skin and mucous membrane of the lower eyelid, upper part of the cheek, and upper lip. In addition, the maxillary division supplies the maxillary and most of the sphenoid and ethmoid sinuses, hard palate, soft palate (except for its posterior border), and uvula. In the sphenopalatine ganglion, there is communication with the geniculate ganglion of the seventh nerve and the sympathetic nervous system via the lesser and greater superficial and deep petrosal nerves.

3. The *mandibular* division leaves the skull through the foramen ovale with the motor root, after which they unite and then divide into small anterior (mostly motor) and large posterior (chiefly sensory) branches. The sensory portion of the anterior division is the buccinator nerve. The posterior division divides into three branches, two of which, the lingual and auriculotemporal, are entirely sensory. The inferior branch supplies sensation to the lower teeth and alveolar process and carries motor fibers to the mylohyoid and anterior belly of the digastric muscles. The mandibular division also supplies the skin of the posterior and lower cheek, chin, and temporal area, and the mucous membrane of the lower lip and cheek, tongue, and oral floor, as well as the temporomandibular joint. It also sends branches to the otic and submandibular ganglions.

Several syndromes involving the trigeminal

nerve merit interest because of pain or dysfunction of one or more oral structures supplied by this nerve. Again, it must be emphasized that rarely is a single cranial nerve involved in a pathologic process. Because of the intimate association of the trigeminal nerve with the third, fourth, and sixth nerves in the cavernous sinus, a host of eponymic syndromes exists. Diffuse processes, such as primary basal brain tumors or tumors that invade the cranium from the nasopharynx, may involve the last four cranial nerves in combination with the fifth, but this is less common.

Trigeminal neuralgia (tic douloureux). This syndrome is characterized by extremely severe, recurrent episodic attacks of unilateral pain distributed over a branch, or more than one branch, of the fifth cranial nerve. The pain may occur spontaneously or may be initiated by stimulation of a trigger zone, most often extending from the lateral border of the nose to the angle of the mouth (Fig. 37-1A, B). It occurs suddenly, without warning, and lasts from 10 to 30 seconds, producing a jabbing sensation. In the later stages of the condition, secondary trigger zones develop which may be "tripped" by mastication, talking, shaving, or even a draft of air on the face. The syndrome appears to occur more often on the right side. Trigeminal neuralgia is about twice as common in women as in men and is far more often seen in persons over fifty years of age (9, 12). About 2 percent of the cases of trigeminal neuralgia have been associated with multiple sclerosis (11, 19).

Facial pain of nondental origin may, however, be due to a number of causes: periodic migrainous neuralgia, temporomandibular joint syndrome, giant-cell arteritis, atypical facial pain with personality changes, and postherpetic neuralgia (4, 7, 10).

Trotter syndrome (sinus of Morgagni syndrome). First described by Trotter (22) in 1911, this syndrome consists of (a) unilateral deafness, (b) pain over the area supplied by the mandibular division, (c) ipsilateral defective mobility of the palate, and (d) subsequent trismus. The syndrome results from invasion of the lateral wall of the nasopharynx (sinus of Morgagni) by a tumor, usually anaplastic carcinoma. Immediately below the sinus is the attachment of the levator

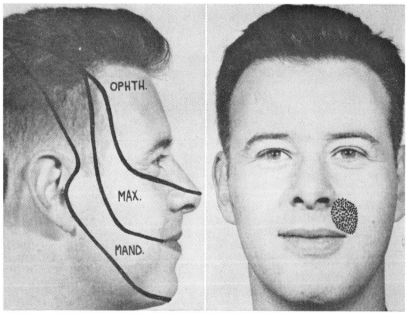

A   *B*

Figure 37-1. (*A*). *Trigeminal nerve.* Areas supplied by the three sensory branches of the trigeminal nerve. (*B*). *Trigeminal neuralgia.* Most common "trigger zone" area.

veli palatini muscle; just laterally is the foramen ovale; posteriorly is the opening to the eustachian canal or tube. As the tumor extends, it compresses the tube (causing deafness) and invades the palatal musculature (decreasing soft palate mobility) and the mandibular nerve (producing pain in the temporal area, ear, lower jaw, teeth, and tongue, and anesthesia over the mental area). Trismus results from extension of the tumor into the pterygoids. The syndrome is seen most often in males during the third and fourth decades. There are usually no symptoms due to nasopharyngeal obstruction (1, 8, 16, 22).

Trigeminal sensory neuropathy. This term refers to sensory disturbances of the trigeminal nerve, principally the second and third divisions, characterized by tingling, numbness, and impaired taste. The corneal reflex is intact (2).

Pterygopalatine fossa syndrome. This syndrome resembles that of Trotter. It is due to tumor metastatic to the pterygopalatine fossa. The fossa, located behind the maxillary sinus and below the inferior surface of the sphenoid, contains the maxillary division, sphenopalatine ganglion, and internal maxillary artery. There are several apertures through which a tumor may spread: the foramen rotundum, pterygoid canal, sphenopalatine foramen, pterygopalatine canal, pharyngeal canal, etc. In its extension the tumor involves the maxillary division and adjacent structures, producing (a) pain in the *upper* teeth, (b) anesthesia of the infraorbital area, (c) blindness, (d) anesthesia of the palate, and (e) motor nerve paralysis of the pterygoids. For contrast with the Trotter syndrome, see Table 37-1.

Jacod syndrome (petrosphenoidal space syndrome). This syndrome combines most of the features of the two syndromes already described in this chapter. However, it differs from them in that it refers to the signs and symptoms resulting from an *intracranial* lesion arising on the floor of the middle cranial fossa and involving the nerves that pass through the foramen ovale, foramen rotundum, and sphenoidal fissure. The tumor may extend along any of these paths or intracranially to produce ophthalmoplegia by involvement of the third, fourth, and sixth nerves and blindness by spread to the optic nerve (amaurosis) (15, 18).

Godtfredsen syndrome (cavernous sinus–nasopharyngeal tumor syndrome). Tumors arising in the nasopharynx, in addition to extending into the skull, thereby producing ophthalmoplegia and trigeminal neuralgia, may also be associated with paralysis of the tongue (hypoglossal paralysis). This is produced by compression of the hypoglossal nerve by enlarged, involved, retropharyngeal lymph nodes, because

Table 37-1. Trotter syndrome and pterygopalatine fossa syndrome

Manifestation or area affected	Trotter syndrome	Pterygopalatine fossa syndrome
Tumor	Primary	Metastatic
Location	Sinus of Morgagni	Pterygopalatine fossa
Pain	First, third division of trigeminal nerve (mandible, ear, tongue, lower teeth); later, second division of trigeminal	First, second division of trigeminal nerve (maxilla, upper teeth); later, third division of trigeminal
Anesthesia	Over mental foramen	Over infraorbital foramen
Deafness	Early	Late
Blindness	No	Yes
Palate	Infiltration, asymmetric at rest	Anesthesia
Pterygoids	Infiltration, trismus	Motor paralysis, deviation to affected side, no trismus

Source: Modified from Asherton (1).

of their proximity to the hypoglossal canal (8). The syndrome may also be caused by trauma or vascular disease.

Foix syndrome (cavernous sinus–lateral wall syndrome). This syndrome is due to tumors (rarely pituitary), intracranial aneurysms, or thrombosis involving the cavernous and/or lateral sinuses. Ophthalmoplegia results from involvement of the third, fourth, and sixth nerves. The ophthalmic and, often, the maxillary divisions of the fifth nerve are affected, producing a trigeminal neuralgia (5).

Sluder syndrome (sphenopalatine neuralgia). The existence of this syndrome, supposedly consisting of pain in the palate, upper jaw and teeth, cheek, root of nose, orbit, etc., has been denied by many outstanding investigators (20).

Horner syndrome (enophthalmos, miosis, partial ptosis, ipsilateral vascular dilation, and anhidrosis of the face, neck, and arms). The syndrome may also be seen in association with fifth and tenth nerve involvement in the *Wallenberg syndrome* (see Syndromes of Other Cranial Nerves, further on in this chapter).

Raeder syndrome (paratrigeminal syndrome). This syndrome is a combination of a Horner-like syndrome (no facial sweating) with ipsilateral motor and sensory fifth nerve dysfunction due to a neoplasm of the middle cranial fossa or a primary tumor of the gasserian ganglion. It is essentially limited to men in the fourth to sixth decades (3, 6, 13, 14, 17, 21).

SYNDROMES OF OTHER CRANIAL NERVES

The lips receive their motor supply from the facial, or seventh, cranial nerve via its zygomatic, buccal, and mandibular branches. Sensation is received by the second and third divisions of the trigeminal nerve.

Melkersson-Rosenthal syndrome and the Duchenne syndrome (progressive bulbar palsy or labioglossolaryngeal paralysis) are among the very few cranial nerve syndromes associated with labial paralysis.

The soft palate and superior and middle con-

strictors of the pharynx receive their motor supply largely from the vagus, or tenth cranial nerve. The glossopalatine, pharyngopalatine, uvular, and levator veli palatini muscles are supplied by the vagus (and possibly the accessory nerve) via the pharyngeal plexus. The tensor veli palatini is supplied by the fifth nerve via a branch to the medial pterygoids. The sensory supply to the posterior soft palate is furnished by the glossopharyngeal, or ninth, cranial nerve. The uvula is supplied by the lesser palatine nerves (3). The anterior part of the soft palate receives branches from the fifth nerve via its middle and posterior palatine nerves.

The sensory and motor supply of the pharynx and fauces comes from the ninth and tenth nerves via the pharyngeal plexus. The soft palate may be paralyzed in the following syndromes: Avellis, Cestan-Chenais, Collet-Sicard, Duchenne, Garcin, Jackson, Moebius, Schmidt, Vernet, Villaret, and Wallenberg. Paralysis of the soft palate may also be seen in the *Heerfordt syndrome* and in an inordinate number of other conditions (3). All the muscles of the tongue (the intrinsic, genioglossus, and hyoglossus) are supplied by the hypoglossal, or twelfth cranial nerve, with the exception of the glossopalatine (see above) and the geniohyoid (ansa hypoglossi).

General sensation to the anterior two-thirds of the tongue is carried by the lingual branch of the fifth nerve. Taste to the same area is supplied by the chorda tympani branch of the seventh nerve. In the posterior third, both general sensation and taste are carried by the glossopharyngeal nerve. The tongue is paralyzed completely or in part in the following syndromes: Collet-Sicard, Dejerine, Duchenne, Garcin, Jackson, Moebius, Tapia, and Villaret (Fig. 37-2).

The syndromes of interest, therefore, in this section are those involving the motor branch of the fifth, the seventh, and the ninth through the twelfth cranial nerves (20, 29).

The nuclei of several of these nerves lie in close proximity in the floor of the fourth ventricle or in the medulla, and several exit from the skull together and enter the retroparotid space. Hence, the reader can see the reason for combined involvement, whether vascular, inflammatory, neoplastic, or traumatic. It is rare for a single nucleus or nerve trunk to be affected.

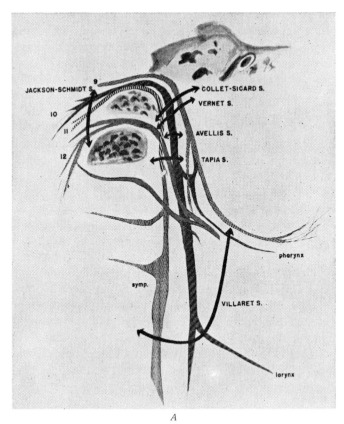

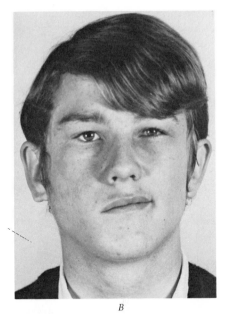

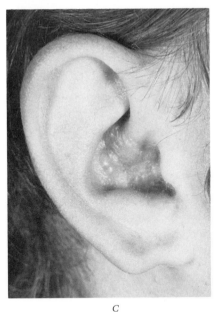

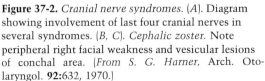

Figure 37-2. *Cranial nerve syndromes.* (*A*). Diagram showing involvement of last four cranial nerves in several syndromes. (*B, C*). *Cephalic zoster.* Note peripheral right facial weakness and vesicular lesions of conchal area. (*From S. G. Harner,* Arch. Otolaryngol. **92:**632, 1970.)

In the case of both nuclear and infranuclear lesions, simultaneous involvement of the ninth, tenth, and eleventh nerves is common. The association of these three cranial nerves in various combinations with the twelfth, the cervical sympathetic chain, and, rarely, the spinothalamic tracts has led to a plethora of eponymic syndromes, only a few of which are discussed below. They may be roughly divided into *central medullary lesions* (about 10 percent) and *peripheral lesions* (about 90 percent). The central lesions may be vascular in origin (Avellis syndrome, Cestan-Chenais syndrome, Wallenberg syndrome, and Dejerine syndrome), or they may be due to other causes, such as syringobulbia, multiple sclerosis, poliomyelitis, neoplasms, or trauma, resulting in such syndromes as those of Jackson, Schmidt, and Tapia.

The peripheral lesions may be located close to the base of the skull at the jugular foramen (Vernet syndrome) or in a lateral pharyngeal or retroparotid space where tumors of the nasopharynx, fractures, or aneurysms of the internal carotid artery may affect the last four cranial nerves with (Villaret syndrome) or without (Collet-Sicard) the cervical sympathetic trunk.

Avellis syndrome. This syndrome is usually due to occlusion of the vertebral artery and is characterized by combined involvement of the nucleus ambiguus and spinothalamic tracts, with (*a*) ipsilateral paralysis and anesthesia of the soft palate, pharynx, and larynx, (*b*) contralateral loss of pain and temperature sensation of the trunk and extremities, (*c*) frequently contralateral body loss of proprioception and tactile senses, and (*d*) rarely, ipsilateral Horner syndrome (2, 5, 7, 16, 43).

Wallenberg syndrome. Arteriosclerotic thrombosis of the posterior inferior cerebellar artery results in degeneration of the nucleus ambiguus, nuclei and descending tracts of the fifth nerve, descending sympathetic pathways, afferent spinocerebellar and lateral spinothalamic tracts, producing (*a*) ipsilateral paralysis and anesthesia of the soft palate, pharynx, and larynx, (*b*) ipsilateral loss of the corneal reflex and anesthesia of the face for pain and temperature, (*c*) ipsilateral Horner syndrome, (*d*) ipsilateral coarse ataxia, (*e*) contralateral loss of temperature and pain sensation of the trunk and extremities, and (*f*) rarely, involvement of the sixth to eighth nerves (24, 50).

Cestan-Chenais syndrome. This syndrome is caused by thrombosis of the vertebral artery below the point of origin of the posterior inferior cerebellar artery. It differs from the Wallenberg syndrome by the presence of pyramidal tract signs, medial lemniscus involvement (causing hemiplegia and contralateral body diminution of touch and proprioceptive senses), and absence of changes in pain and temperature sensation (6).

Dejerine syndrome (anterior bulbar syndrome, pyramid-hypoglossal syndrome, alternating hypoglossal hemiplegia syndrome). Hemorrhage or thrombosis of the anterior spinal artery (which supplies the pyramids, medial lemniscus, and emerging hypoglossal fibers) produces ipsilateral paralysis of the tongue, contralateral pyramidal paralysis of the arm and leg, and, occasionally,

contralateral loss of proprioceptive and tactile senses.

Jackson-Mackenzie syndrome (vago-accessory-hypoglossal syndrome). Characterized by unilateral involvement of the last three cranial nerves, it results in unilateral paralysis of the soft palate, pharynx, larynx, sternocleidomastoid muscle, and tongue and partial paralysis of the trapezius muscle (8, 27, 32, 33, 37).

Schmidt syndrome (vago-accessory syndrome). Involving the radicular fibers of the tenth and eleventh cranial nerves, it is similar to the Jackson syndrome but without lingual paralysis (39, 41).

Tapia syndrome (vagohypoglossal syndrome). This is another variant of the Jackson syndrome in which the sternocleidomastoid and trapezius muscles are spared (43, 44).

Vernet syndrome (jugular foramen syndrome). Vernet syndrome is characterized by (*a*) ipsilateral paralysis of the ninth, tenth, and eleventh cranial nerves with resultant paralysis of the soft palate, larynx, pharynx, sternocleidomastoid muscle, and part of the trapezius muscle; (*b*) anesthesia of the posterior soft palate; and (*c*) loss of sensation and taste over the posterior third of the tongue (30, 33, 46, 47). About one-half of the cases have been due to brain tumors (43).

Villaret syndrome (retroparotid space syndrome). Ipsilateral paralysis of the last four cranial nerves and the cervical sympathetic chain produces the *Horner* syndrome (enophthalmos, ptosis, miosis). Occasionally, the seventh nerve is also involved. The syndrome is due to a lesion in the retroparotid space, which is bounded posteriorly by the cervical vertebras, medially by the pharynx, anteriorly by the parotid gland, laterally by the sternocleidomastoid muscle, and superiorly by the skull near the jugular foramen (30, 33, 48).

Collet-Sicard syndrome. It is similar to the Villaret syndrome except for the absence of the Horner syndrome (32, 41).

Garcin syndrome (half-base syndrome). Occasionally in cases of tumors of the nasopharynx, all or nearly all cranial nerves on one side become involved without signs of motor or sensory disturbances of the extremities and without evidence of increased intracranial pressure (papilledema, spinal fluid changes). Often roentgenographic changes are apparent in the skull base. The Garcin syndrome has been reported to occur frequently in Chinese.

It is distinguished by a peculiar spread of the tumor via the foramen lacerum in the epidural cavity and by the tendency, late in its course, to infiltrate the dura. In addition to the nasopharynx, the tumor may invade the skull base from the maxillary or sphenoid sinus, or it may, on occasion, represent metastasis from the breast or bronchus or even extension of a glomus tumor from the middle ear (18, 19, 25, 30, 32, 38, 41, 49).

It is interesting to note that in spite of destruction of the pituitary gland by the tumor there are seldom signs of hypophyseal cachexia.

Duchenne syndrome (progressive bulbar palsy; glossopharyngolabial paralysis). Principally seen in individuals in their sixth and seventh decades, the syndrome is characterized by a slowly ascending process that involves the motor nuclei of the medulla and often the pons and midbrain. The twelfth nerve is usually involved first. Early signs are bilateral atrophy, fasciculations, and atrophy of the tongue. The tenth nerve is then affected, with resultant dysphagia of both liquids and solids, pseudosialorrhea, dysarthria, and thickened nasal speech. Atrophy and fasciculations of the palatal and pharyngeal musculature may be seen. Involvement of the nuclei of the seventh and fifth nerves causes paralysis and wasting of the muscles of facial expression and mastication. The nucleus of the accessory nerve is less often affected. This syndrome may represent the first manifestation of amyotrophic lateral sclerosis (11, 28).

In *pseudobulbar palsy,* usually due to arteriosclerosis, the syndrome is caused by interruption of the supranuclear cortical fibers. Essentially the same symptoms are experienced. However, in spite of paralysis of the tongue, this condition involves neither atrophy nor fasciculations and the palatal and pharyngeal musculature is less severely affected. This condition differs from true bulbar palsy in that pyramidal tract signs are present and sensory alterations are common (20, 29).

Moebius syndrome. This syndrome is discussed in Chap. 109.

Glossopharyngeal neuralgia syndrome. This syndrome is characterized by unilateral paroxysmal stabbing pain (lasting from 20 to 30 seconds) followed by a burning sensation (2 to 5 minutes) in the posterior tongue, pharynx, and soft palate that extends to the ear. The pain is associated, as is trigeminal neuralgia, with a "trigger zone." This area is usually located on the lateral wall of the pharynx, at the base of the tongue, or in the external ear area posterior to the mandibular ramus. Swallowing and talking, i.e., moving the tongue, usually trip the trigger, although it may also be tripped by yawning or coughing (23, 31, 34, 42, 45). The syndrome seems to occur with equal frequency in both sexes (45).

The pain is usually of an intense, severe quality and occurs most often at night (3). It is followed by homolateral tearing and salivation caused by neuronal bombardment of the lacrimal and parotid glands. Between attacks, tinnitus, partial deafness, and facial tics may be experienced. Cocainization of the lateral pharyngeal wall is ordinarily performed to ascertain whether one is dealing with true glossopharyngeal neuralgia, for this brings about immediate but temporary relief in this condition. Associated with the neuralgia may be bradycardia, hypotension, syncope and cardiac arrest.

In the idiopathic, or essential, type, the majority of cases occurs after the fifth decade. However, organically caused cases usually are seen in a younger age group, in whom the syndrome may be due to anomalous arteries at the cerebellopontine angle, arachnoiditis, perineural fibrosis, elongation of the styloid process (1, 10, 12), or a viral infection (15).

The glossopharyngeal neuralgia syndrome may be seen in association with the Hunt (geniculate ganglion) syndrome (14). Pain in the region of the trigeminal nerve may occur occasionally with glossopharyngeal neuralgia.

DIAGNOSTIC AIDS

The sensory function of the *trigeminal nerve* is ordinarily tested with cotton wisp, pinprick, cold, and heat. Care must be taken to distinguish the three divisions of cutaneous supply. A portion of the lower part of the face below the ear and over the angle of the mandible is supplied by cervical nerves, and the clinician should not attribute abnormalities in this area to the mandibular division.

The muscles of mastication are tested in several ways. With firm closure of the jaws, the masseters and temporal muscles are palpated bilaterally and differences in weakness and/or atrophy are noted. The patient is then asked to open his mouth. Deviation of the chin to one side may indicate weakness of the muscles on the same side, though it may also signify abnormalities in the temporomandibular joint of the same or contralateral side. Facial weakness or paralysis may sometimes be misinterpreted as jaw deviation. The jaw should also be moved laterally in both directions to test pterygoid function.

The jaw reflex is tested by tapping the chin horizontally with the mouth held half open. The reflex may be exaggerated in such syndromes as pseudobulbar palsy, being demonstrated by brisk closure.

The degree of function of the several components of the *facial nerve* may be determined as follows:

1. *Motor.* The muscles of facial expression may be examined by asking patient to frown, raise eyebrows, wrinkle forehead, close eyes (singly and bilaterally, lightly and tightly), expose teeth, blow out cheeks, whistle, and retract chin.

2. *Gustatory.* To detect alteration of taste sensation, solutions of 4 percent glucose, 2.5 percent sodium chloride, 1 percent citric acid, and 0.075 percent quinine hydrochloride are ordinarily applied to the anterior two-thirds of the protruded tongue with an applicator. The patient should not be allowed to speak during the test but should point to the correct answer on a printed form. These same solutions may be applied to the posterior third of the tongue to test glossopharyngeal function but are usually not so satisfactory because of physical difficulties. Galvanic stimulation which may be accurately measured and recorded is gaining wider use (21, 26).

3. *Secretory.* This function is less often tested. Increased lacrimation is usually apparent, and decreased lacrimation may be determined from the history. Submandibular and sublingual function may be determined by placing a highly flavored substance on the tongue and noting the subsequent salivary flow from the salivary ducts beneath the tongue.

Since the *glossopharyngeal nerve* supplies tactile sensation to the pharyngeal vault, nasopharynx, posterior soft palate, and posterior third of the tongue, the degree of dysfunction of this nerve can easily be tested with a swabbed applicator. The motor and secretory functions of this nerve are not ordinarily tested.

The amount of *vagal* impairment can be ascertained by determining the degree of paralysis of the soft palate, pharynx, and larynx. The pharyngeal, or gag, reflex may be tested by stimulating the posterior pharyngeal wall with a tongue blade, and the palatal or uvular reflex may be tested by stimulating the undersurface of the uvula. With palatal paralysis, the affected side of the soft palate is flattened and does not elevate on phonation of "ah"; the uvula deviates to the normal side. With vagus nerve dysfunction, difficulty is experienced in swallowing solids and the larynx fails to elevate on swallowing. Nasal regurgitation of fluids is common, and a brassy or hoarse sound is detected in the voice. With unilateral vagal paralysis, only minimal change in the voice may be noted. One should observe the palatal and pharyngeal musculature for a fibrillary tremor which may accompany nuclear degeneration, as in progressive bulbar palsy, syringomyelia, etc.

Examination of the *eleventh nerve* is usually limited to evaluation of function of the sternocleidomastoid and trapezius muscles. The former is inspected and palpated when the head is rotated against resistance applied by the examiner's hand. The paralyzed muscle is flat and does not tense when attempts are made to turn the head toward the opposite shoulder. Trapezius function is tested by having the patient elevate each shoulder against resistance. With loss of function, the shoulder cannot be elevated, the arm cannot be raised above the horizontal, and the head cannot be tilted toward the side of the paralysis. The shoulder contour is depressed.

Hypoglossal dysfunction is determined by

noting atrophy or loss of function of tongue musculature. If the nerve is affected bilaterally, the tongue cannot be protruded. With unilateral involvement, the protruded tongue will deviate to the paralyzed side because of the unopposed action of the normal side when the geniohyoglossal muscles pull the base forward. The paralyzed side becomes wrinkled, furrowed, and wasted. If nuclear degeneration is slow, as in progressive bulbar palsy, fine or coarse fasciculations are seen on the surface of the tongue (9).

ASYMMETRIC CRYING FACIES (CARDIOFACIAL SYNDROME)

Asymmetric crying facies, caused by unilateral weakness of the lower-lip depressors, is a valuable index of congenital anomalies, especially of the cardiovascular, genitourinary, and respiratory systems. The sign was described as being without significance by several authors (6, 8). However, Cayler and others (1–5, 7, 10, 12) subsequently reported many examples associated with congenital heart disease. Cayler et al. (2–4) referred to the condition as the cardiofacial syndrome and suggested that over 5 percent of in-

fants with cardiac defects had this syndrome. An extensive analysis of associated anomalies was provided by Pape and Pickering (10). Papadatos et al. (9) found congenital heart disease in 3 of 37 affected. Perlman and Reisner (11) found associated anomalies in only 5 percent of cases. They found asymmetric crying facies in 1 per 150 children. In their series, there was a 5:1 left-sided predilection. Similar findings were noted by Papadatos et al. (9).

The present authors regard asymmetric crying facies as a nonspecific sign which may occur with a variety of anomalies in most cases. Although cardiovascular defects predominated in the large series of Pape and Pickering (9), 10 of 44 had anomalies other than cardiac defects and 10 of 44 had only minor anomalies or were normal.

Papadatos et al. (9) reported familial occurrence and suggested multifactorial inheritance. The defect results from unilateral partial paralysis of the seventh nerve, specifically the ramus marginalis mandibulare, which supplies the mentalis and quadratus labii inferior muscles of the lower lip. Parity and delivery histories indicate that neither intrauterine molding nor

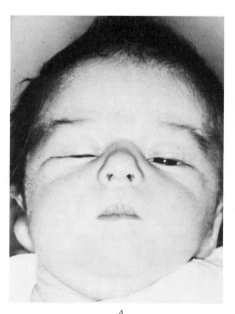
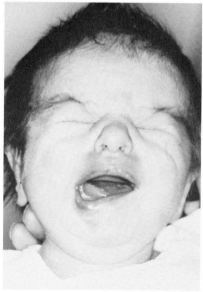

A   B

Figure 37-3. *Asymmetric crying facies.* (*A*). Face at rest. (*B*). Asymmetry during crying. (*From G. Cayler, Sacramento, Calif.*)

forceps injury during delivery is responsible for the condition. Because the muscles involved act only to depress the lower-lip margin, the defect does not interfere with sucking or smiling and does not foster drooling. The lips are symmetric at rest, the sign becoming apparent only during crying (Fig. 37-3). In most cases lower facial weakness persists, but occasionally it may diminish to some degree. Pape and Pickering (10), however, found no side predilection and, furthermore, that the side on which the defect occurs was unrelated to the sex of the child. However, associated defects expressed on one side of the body tended to occur on the same side as the partial lower facial palsy.

Cardiovascular anomalies have included ventricular septal defect, patent ductus arteriosus, tetralogy of Fallot, right aortic arch, double aortic arch, pulmonic stenosis, coarctation of the aorta, atrial septal defect, atrioventricular communis, tricuspid atresia, single ventricle, hypoplastic right ventricle, hypoplastic pulmonary arteries, and bicuspid aortic valve (1–5, 9).

Hemivertebra, fused vertebras, sternal and rib anomalies, hypoplastic or absent radius and thumb, and various other skeletal defects have been reported (10).

Genitourinary anomalies have included absent kidney, hypoplastic kidney, ectopic kidney, bifid kidney, polycystic kidneys, bifid scrotum, hypogonadism, cryptorchism, and hypospadias (10).

Tracheoesophageal atresia or fistula, laryngomalacia, bronchial stenosis, absent bronchus, absent lung lobe, anal stenosis, imperforate anus, absent thymus, and a variety of other defects have been discussed by Pape and Pickering (10).

A number of cases have been associated with ear anomalies. Of 44 patients in the study of Pape and Pickering (10), three had cleft lip-palate, one had isolated cleft palate, and three had highly arched palate.

GENICULATE GANGLION SYNDROME (HUNT SYNDROME, HERPES ZOSTER SYNDROME, CEPHALIC ZOSTER SYNDROME)

Infection of the geniculate, or sensory, ganglion of the facial nerve with the virus of herpes zoster results in (a) zoster lesions of the external ear and oral mucosa, (b) facial palsy which is usually complete (Fig. 37-2B, C), and (c) severe pain in the external auditory canal and pinna. The syndrome, named after Hunt (7) (often listed as Ramsay Hunt), who described and classified the condition in 1907, was noted earlier by others (5). It comprises about 3 to 9 percent of cases of facial palsy (5). The peripheral ganglions of the eighth, ninth, and tenth cranial nerves may also be affected (8), though some authors have restricted the syndrome to involvement of the ganglions of the seventh or seventh and eighth nerves (5). Tschiassny (10) limits the syndrome to those cases in which the "geniculate zone" (concha, external meatus, root of helix, crura of antihelix, intercrural fossa, antitragus, and external surface of the upper part of the lobe) is involved. Denny-Brown et al. (3) and others (1, 2) established that cases of so-called Hunt syndrome were not due to involvement of the geniculate ganglion. Nevertheless the term "geniculate herpes" has persisted. Round-cell infiltration of the facial nerve has been demonstrated repeatedly.

Ear. The pain is severe and paroxysmal, and, as in zoster infection of other areas, it often precedes and survives the cutaneous and mucosal lesions. The ear becomes red and swollen; this is followed by vesicular eruption of the auditory meatus and tympanic membrane. The concha, tragus, antitragus, antihelix, and lobule may also be involved. Associated signs and symptoms may include diminished lacrimation, tinnitus, diminished hearing, vertigo, nystagmus, hoarseness, and loss of superficial and deep sensation of the face (5). Rarely, there is no auricular eruption (9).

Oral manifestations. Oral signs and symptoms include vesicles or eroded areas in the peritonsillar region, oral pharynx, and posterolateral third of the tongue. Pain in the same areas and occasional loss of taste, diminished salivation, and palatal paralysis may also be present (5, 10). Occasionally, these changes may precede the auricular signs (4).

DIMINISHED AND PERVERTED TASTE AND SMELL

Henkin et al. (2) described a syndrome consisting of (a) decreased taste acuity (hypogeusia), (b) unpleasant or perverted taste (dysgeusia), (c) decreased olfactory acuity (hyposmia), and (d) perverted or unpleasant perception of odors (dysosmia). Other symptoms included persistent salty, sweet, sour, bitter, or metallic taste, a sensation of foul odor in the nasopharynx, and, less often, vertigo, hearing loss, decreased libido, and unexplained hypertension.

In about half the patients, an upper respiratory illness preceded the onset of hypogeusia, and onset was abrupt in about 75 percent. Not all components were present in every patient: hypogeusia (100 percent), hyposomia (80 percent), dysgeusia (65 percent), and dysosmia (50 percent).

The disorder is not inherited (1, 2).

GUSTATORY LACRIMATION (PAROXYSMAL LACRIMATION, CROCODILE TEARS SYNDROME, BOGORAD SYNDROME, GUSTOLACRIMAL REFLEX)

The syndrome of lacrimation that accompanies eating was described by Berg (see 1) in 1924, and, in far more detail, by Bogorad (2) in 1928. The last author called it the "syndrome of crocodile tears," referring to the tale that the crocodile weeps hypocritical tears while devouring his victims (4). Since the original report, over 100 cases have been recorded. Ford (7, 8) wrote the first report in English and linked the syndrome with gustatory sweating and flushing (auriculotemporal or Frey syndrome), both conditions being caused by misdirected regrowth of nerve fibers. Ford used the term "paroxysmal lacrimation" to describe the condition. To parallel the use of the term "gustatory sweating and flushing," the present authors suggest the use of "gustatory lacrimation." Axelsson and Laage-Hellman (1) have employed "gustolacrimal reflex."

In many cases, the syndrome has followed facial palsy (1). By the time motor function is becoming restored, the patient usually notices that when eating, tears flow from the eye on the affected side. Ford (7) noted that the syndrome is not associated with the common form of Bell palsy, in which the lesion is distal to the geniculate ganglion, but occurs only when the lesion is proximal to the ganglion. Rarely, the syndrome is bilateral and/or congenital (10–12,

15). The congenital cases have usually been associated with lateral rectus palsy. Obviously aberrant regeneration cannot explain congenital examples of this disorder, which in these cases, is probably supranuclear (13).

The facial nerve has several components: a motor component supplying the muscles of facial expression; a sensory component, which carries gustatory impulses from the anterior two-thirds of the tongue and proprioceptive impulses from the face; and an autonomic-parasympathetic component. These latter fibers arise in the superior salivary nucleus and provide secretory and vasodilatory function to the submandibular and sublingual glands via the nerve of Wrisberg, the chorda tympani, and the lingual nerve, as well as to the lacrimal gland via the nerve of Wrisberg, the greater superficial petrosal nerve, the vidian nerve, the sphenopalatine ganglion, and the zygomaticotemporal nerve. Proximal to the geniculate ganglion, all these components are in contiguity.

If a lesion occurs proximal to the geniculate ganglion, then during regeneration, fibers destined for the submandibular and sublingual glands may become partially interchanged with those destined for the lacrimal gland. Thus, when the gustatory stimulus is evoked, lacrimation is produced (Fig. 37-4).

In the exceptional cases cited by Boyer and Gardner (3), the syndrome appeared after surgery on the greater superficial petrosal nerve for relief of headache. During the course of surgery, the lesser superficial petrosal nerve was injured, as it runs only 2 mm lateral to the greater superficial petrosal nerve in the middle cranial fossa. In regeneration, the fibers of the two nerves became interchanged, producing the syndrome. This was proved by resection of the glossopharyngeal nerve, which abolished the syndrome.

The syndrome has also been seen in association with neurosyphilis, acoustic neuroma, vascular disease, and facial palsy in association with herpes zoster of the ear (the Hunt syndrome discussed above).

Facial contracture or diffuse facial muscle response is often associated with the tearing. If, for example, the teeth are shown, the forehead may wrinkle and the eyelid close. Conversely, wrinkling the forehead or closing the eye may cause the corner of the mouth to be retracted and the nasolabial fold to deepen. This indicates

The Gusto-lacrimal Reflex

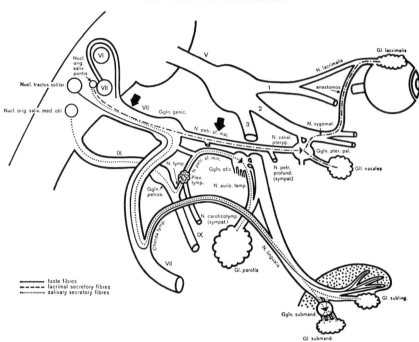

taste fibres
----- lacrimal secretory fibres
··········· salivary secretory fibres

Figure 37-4. *Gustatory lacrimation.* Diagram shows two possible mechanisms for production of the syndrome. Most often, lesion is proximal to geniculate ganglion and in regeneration, fibers destined for the submandibular and sublingual salivary glands may become interchanged with those for the lacrimal gland. The lesion may also be distal to the geniculate ganglion and involve interchange of fibers of the greater and lesser superficial petrosal nerves. (*Courtesy of A. Axelsson and J. E. Laage-Hellman,* Acta Oto-laryngol. (Stockh.) **54:**239, 1962.)

that impulses formerly directed toward isolated muscle groups are diffusely distributed over the face, thus bolstering the concept of misdirected fiber regeneration. This has been called "the Marin Amat phenomenon."

DIFFERENTIAL DIAGNOSIS

This syndrome should not be confused with lacrimation seen in association with facial paralysis, in which the tearing is due to ectropion which permits tears to flow out of the conjunctival sac. The latter is not associated with hypersecretion of the lacrimal gland and is unaffected by eating.

LABORATORY AIDS

None is known.

GUSTATORY SWEATING AND FLUSHING—AURICULOTEMPORAL AND CHORDA TYMPANI SYNDROMES (FREY SYNDROME)

The earliest references to the syndrome of gustatory sweating and flushing appear to be those of Duphenix (5) in 1757, Dupuy (6) in 1816, and

Baillarger (2) in 1853. In 1897, Weber (35) described the syndrome and recognized that it was related in some manner to the auriculotemporal nerve. However, credit for bringing the syndrome to the attention of the medical public goes to Frey (8), who, in 1923, described a case following an infected bullet wound in the parotid region. The syndrome is often referred to under her name. Although several hundred cases have been published subsequently, possibly the greatest contributions have been made by the studies of Freedberg et al. (7), Glaister et al. (12), Gardner and McCubbin (11), Hogeman (16), Spiro and Martin (30), and especially, Laage-Hellman (18–21), who showed that the syndrome, far from being rare, is a constant complication of conservative parotidectomy. For an excellent historical survey, see Hogeman (16).

It should be pointed out that the term "auriculotemporal syndrome" is misleading, since the skin innervated by the greater auricular nerve, the lesser occipital nerve, or any cutaneous branch of the cervical plexus may be involved.

SYSTEMIC MANIFESTATIONS

The syndrome is clinically manifested by sweating, flushing, a sense of warmth and, sometimes, pain in the preauricular and temporal areas during eating of foods that produce a strong salivary stimulus. The syndrome has been noted to follow suppurative parotitis (2, 6, 7–9, 17, 22), septicemia (17), direct trauma to the parotid region (26), mandibular resection (16), and, most frequently, conservative parotidectomy (18). It has even been noted to follow exercise in cold weather (28).

The etiologic factor in most cases is damage to the auriculotemporal nerve. This nerve, in addition to supplying sensory fibers to the preauricular and temporal areas, carries parasympathetic fibers to the parotid gland and sympathetic vasomotor and sudomotor fibers to the skin of the same area.

The parasympathetic fibers arise in the inferior salivary nucleus of the midbrain and leave in the glossopharyngeal nerve. This nerve enters the middle ear as the Jacobson nerve and emerges as the lesser superficial petrosal nerve from the roof of the petrous pyramid. It then passes through the foramen ovale medial to the mandibular nerve to the otic ganglion, the postganglionic fibers passing to the parotid gland via the auriculotemporal nerve. The sympathetic vasomotor and sudomotor fibers of the auriculotemporal nerve are derived from the superior cervical ganglion via the carotid plexus.

Injury to the auriculotemporal nerve denervates the sweat glands and vessels of the skin over its distribution, in addition to producing sensory disturbances. This is demonstrated by the failure of applied heat to induce sweating in the area prior to the advent of the syndrome.

Both the parasympathetic and sympathetic nerves of the face are cholinergic, and in the process of regeneration, parasympathetic fibers become misdirected and grow along sympathetic pathways (3, 11, 18–21). Thus, a gustatory stimulus produces sweating and flushing.

Other theories have been proposed, among them denervation hypersensitivity, i.e., hypersensitivity of the skin of the affected area to acetylcholine released from the salivary gland (7, 22). However, Gardner and McCubbin (11) demonstrated the failure of hypersensitivity to occur after sympathectomy, and Laage-Hellman (20) further pointed out that if denervation hypersensitivity were the cause, it should develop suddenly, not gradually as is the case.

That the syndrome is caused by misdirection of parasympathetic fibers is shown by the ability of procaine, injected over the auriculotemporal nerve, to abolish the syndrome. Severing of the auriculotemporal, glossopharyngeal (11), or Jacobson (15) nerve, local atropine injection, blockage of the otic ganglion (12, 16), or local application of 3 percent scopolamine hydrobromide cream (19) have all been shown to inhibit or abolish the reaction. Conversely, acetylcholine injection increases the reaction (7, 12). Procaine blockage of the superior cervical ganglion has no effect.

Misdirected regrowth of fibers cannot be the explanation of the few cases in which the syndrome has appeared a few days postoperatively (9, 26, 29); the alternate possibility of transaxonal excitation exists. Laage-Hellman (18–21) has shown, however, that it was present in 100 percent of his cases, though in approximately 50 percent it was essentially subclinical (30). In only 10 to 15 percent were the signs and symptoms of sufficient degree to cause embarrassment or distress (18, 33).

Some patients exhibit only sweating or flushing, the former being more common in men, the latter in women (16, 18).

Pain over the involved area is usually mild and probably does not cause sufficient discomfort in most cases to be recorded. However, Turner (33) noted that 4 of his 11 patients experienced pain. Hypo- or hyperesthesia is far more common (9, 28). It is of interest that parotid pain also occurs following superior cervical ganglionectomy in over half the cases, probably as a result of vasodilation (10).

The time of the first appearance of the fully developed syndrome varies considerably. Though most observers have noted its occurrence within 2 months to 2 years (average, 9 months) postoperatively (12, 18, 30, 33), there are cases in which the syndrome has appeared in a few days (9, 26, 30) or as much as 17 years after surgery (30). The very careful laboratory studies of Laage-Hellman (18–21) have indicated, however, that in reality the first signs are seen after the fifth postoperative week.

The initial appearance of the flushing does not necessarily occur at the same time as the sweating. In one case (28), though flushing was noted 2 years postoperatively, sweating did not appear for another 3 years. When the full syndrome appears, a sense of warmth usually pre-

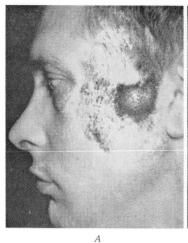 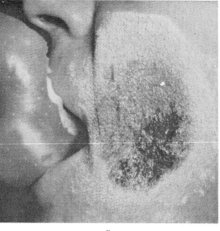

A   B

Figure 37-5. (*A*). *Gustatory sweating and flushing* (*Frey syndrome*). Following meals there is profuse sweating immediately in front of ear. This is demonstrated by starch-iodine test. (*B*). Patient drove scissors into cheek as child. Severe sweating and flushing are noted at mealtime.

cedes the flushing and sweating, but this is by no means constantly observed. Skin temperature measurements have revealed an increase in temperature of 1 to 2°C (28).

As a rule, once the syndrome appears, the area of skin involved increases (20) and remains increased for life (1, 16). However, about 5 percent of patients (18) experience regression and disappearance of the symptoms. The area involved varies both in degree and in extent, in some persons being seen at the corner of the mouth or extending down to the angle of the mandible, an area supplied by the greater auricular nerve (18) (Fig. 37-5A).

Related to the auriculotemporal syndrome is the *chorda tympani syndrome* described by Urprus et al. (34) and Young (36). In this syndrome, the sweating and flushing are limited to the skin of the chin and submental region. This syndrome, apparently rare, may accompany operation or injury to the submandibular gland (18). It has been shown to be abolished by blockage of the lingual nerve proximal to the chorda tympani.

Also related is *gustatory lacrimation,* previously described.

One of the authors (R. J. G.) saw a patient whose sole area of gustatory sweating was a half-dollar-sized area near the corner of his mouth where he had driven a scissor blade many years prior to development of the syndrome. Presumably the parasympathetic fibers came from those supplying the minor salivary glands of the cheek (Fig. 37-5B). Another example was reported by Storrs (31).

Oral manifestations. The degree of parotid salivary secretory inhibition during the syndrome has not been studied quantitatively. Freedberg et al. (7) indicated that it was not possible to express saliva from the duct on the involved side during eating. The overall inhibition is not severe enough, however, to produce an increase in dental caries on the involved side.

DIFFERENTIAL DIAGNOSIS
This syndrome should not be confused with excessive sweating sometimes seen as a possibly hereditary trait in persons who have just eaten spicy or sour foods (23, 27). In this case, the sweating appears limited to the forehead, tip of nose, and upper lip. Neither should it be confused with signs or symptoms of hysteria or postsympathectomy sweating.

LABORATORY AIDS
To detect sweating, the simplest method is application of the Minor starch-iodine test (15 ml of 1.0 percent iodine, 5 ml castor oil, 80 ml of 95 percent alcohol) (18, 24). A more quantitative estimate can be made by using plastic tape (12, 32).

HEREDITARY QUIVERING OF THE CHIN

Hereditary chin quivering, a transient, fine, oscillating tremor of the mentalis muscle, was probably first described by Frey (1) in 1930. Since then, numerous kindreds have demonstrated autosomal dominant inheritance with complete penetrance (3, 4).

The trait is precipitated by emotional disturbances and/or specific activities, both pleasant and otherwise, and disappears during sleep. The quivering may interfere with speech. It is present at birth and decreases in frequency with age. In some cases, there has been associated nystagmus (1, 3).

Nocturnal myoclonus and tongue biting were noted by Johnson et al. (2) in dizygous twins with hereditary chin trembling.

JAW-WINKING AND WINKING-JAW SYNDROMES (MARCUS GUNN AND INVERSE MARCUS GUNN SYNDROMES)

The short communication by Marcus Gunn (11) (often erroneously hyphenated) in 1883, describing the syndrome of (a) unilateral congenital ptosis and (b) rapid exaggerated elevation of the ptotic lid on moving the lower jaw to the contralateral side, stimulated immediate interest in this problem. By 1895, 33 cases had been reviewed by Sinclair (19), and since then at least another 100 cases have been published. The most comprehensive studies have been those of Villard (21), Cooper (2), Spaeth (20), Wartenberg (22, 23), and Simpson (18). The syndrome is seen in about 2 percent of all cases of congenital ptosis of the eyelid.

The name "jaw-wink" syndrome is not well chosen, for the symptom is not a wink but an exaggerated opening of the eye. However, the term has been used so long and extensively that

until the cause is clarified, its use will probably be continued.

There appears to be some hereditary pattern, though a history of familial involvement is rarely obtained. The cases of a number of investigators reveal an irregular dominance (2, 5, 10, 15) (Fig. 37-6A–D). Though the syndrome has been stated to be more common in males (10), the survey by the present authors would suggest that there is no sex predilection.

The cause is unknown, but it was originally assumed that the syndrome was based on aberrant innervation of the levator palpebrae superioris from the motor branch of the trigeminal because of the close approximation of the nuclei of the third and fifth cranial nerves. However, a supranuclear, or at least a combined supranuclear-nuclear, involvement has been suggested, and the view has gained support (3, 6, 22). A good review of theories of etiology has been compiled by Simpson (18).

SYSTEMIC MANIFESTATIONS

Facies. The only abnormality usually apparent is ptosis of one eyelid.

Eyes. The ptosis is congenital in over 90 percent of the reported cases. It may, however, arise spontaneously in older persons (10, 15, 18). Ordinarily the lid cannot be raised to any significant degree. The left eye has been stated to be more frequently affected (10, 15), though there is some doubt that this is statistically significant. Seven percent of patients have experienced the syn-

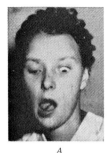 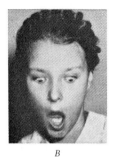 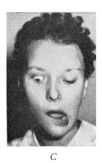 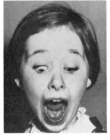

| A | B | C | D |

Figure 37-6. (A–C). *Jaw-winking syndrome.* Note exaggerated opening of eye. This patient demonstrated opening of left lid when jaw was opened and deviated to the right, and vice versa. There was exaggerated lid opening of both eyes when jaw was opened wide without deviation. (D). Similar phenomenon in daughter of patient in A to C. (*Courtesy of D. Kanter,* Klin. Monatsbl. Augenheilkd. **126**:50, 1955.)

drome without having ptosis, and 3 percent have had bilateral ptosis (10).

Occasionally, associated paresis of the extraorbital eye muscles is seen (10, 15, 18–20). The pupillary and corneal reflexes are normal. The pupil in the ptotic eye may be smaller, but true Horner syndrome is not present (11, 22).

Jaws. About 40 percent of these patients manifest the syndrome both on depressing the mandible and on moving it to the side opposite the ptotic eye. Another 40 percent only need the jaw to be depressed (19). However, in some individuals the syndrome may be produced by movement of the lips, whistling, clenching the teeth, puffing out the cheeks, protrusion of the tongue, etc. (18, 22). It may even be precipitated by swallowing or, rarely, by moving the jaw to the ipsilateral side (7) or to both sides (8). The syndrome has also been triggered by closing the other eye (8). It may even temporarily disappear (18). Several muscles and cranial nerves come into play during these acts; the most important appears to be the external pterygoid (trigeminal). That the masseter and temporal muscles play no significant role was demonstrated by Dupuy-Dutemps (4). A comprehensive review of critical jaw movements was made by Simpson (18).

Other anomalies. Schultz and Burian (17) reported a patient with associated anomalies including ectrodactyly, bilateral pes cavus with ankle varus and forefoot adduction, cryptorchism, and duplication of incisor teeth.

The so-called *winking-jaw* syndrome (inverse Marcus Gunn syndrome, corneomandibular reflex, pterygocoroneal reflex) is manifested by a brisk movement of the mandible to the contralateral side when the cornea is touched. The jaw may also be thrust forward (9, 22, 23). Both the jaw-winking and winking-jaw syndromes are considered to be release phenomena due to a supranuclear lesion (caused either by malformation or by severe cerebral or brainstem lesions) that reunites the orbicularis oculi and external pterygoid muscles, which phylogenetically belong together (22, 23).

The so-called *Marin Amat syndrome or phenomenon* appears to be an intrafacial reaction on the part of a regenerating facial nerve after a facial palsy (1, 13, 22, 23). A partially ptosed

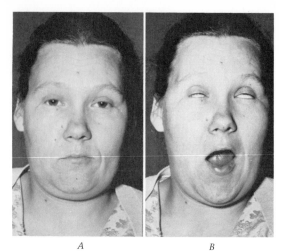

A   *B*

Figure 37-7. *Inverse jaw-winking.* (*A*). Note slight ptosis of single eyelid. (*B*). On opening jaw, there is drooping of eyelids with conjugate upward deviation of eyes. (*From J. Jancar,* Ophthalmologica **151:** 548, 1966.)

eyelid droops further when the mandible moves from side to side (Fig. 37-7*A, B*). Also see Gustatory Lacrimation, earlier in this chapter.

PALATAL MYOCLONUS

Palatal myoclonus (palatal nystagmus, rhythmic myoclonus) is a relatively rare disorder, less than 200 cases having been recorded (7). The soft palatal and uvular musculature undergo continuous, rhythmic (usually 100 to 240 per minute) contractions of small amplitude. Not uncommonly, there are associated movements of the pharynx, larynx, tongue, and oral floor, as well as of the eyelid and/or eyeball (3). The clonus is usually bilateral and accompanied in over 50 percent of cases by a clicking sound in the ear which can be heard by others. The sound is thought to arise from the opening of the cartilaginous eustachian tube. Talking, swallowing, deep inspiration, expiration, or other pharyngeal activities interrupt the involuntary movements, and the clicking sound ceases during these actions (4).

Palatal myoclonus appears more often in older individuals, and its complications are usually more severe in this group. The causative factor in most cases is thought to be cerebral arteriosclerosis, but other causes, such as tumors of the corpora quadrigemina or cerebellum, multiple sclerosis, trauma, encephalitis, or syphilis, have also been indicated as involving the central tegmental tract and inferior olivary nucleus in demyelinating processes (1, 2, 3, 5). The phenomenon has been experimentally produced (2).

SUBMANDIBULAR, RECTAL, AND OCULAR PAIN AND FLUSHING

This syndrome, first described in 1959 by Hayden and Grossman (2), consists of very brief, excruciating pain of the submandibular, rectal, and ocular areas, as well as flushing of the surrounding skin accompanying bowel movement.

Genetic study of the affected family suggested that the condition was inherited as an autosomal dominant trait with variable penetrance of the components (1, 2, 4). The submandibular and ocular pain occurs with greater frequency than the rectal pain.

The pathogenesis is unknown, but the condition is thought to be a dysautonomia.

SYSTEMIC MANIFESTATIONS

Rectum. The episodes of pain begin in infancy and last for 10 to 60 seconds, then culminate in a normal bowel movement. The pain may occur about once a week or once a day for 5 to 10 days,

followed by remission for several weeks. Subsequently, there is flushing of the buttocks and legs extending to the toes. This gradually fades within 10 to 20 minutes. The pain may radiate to the feet.

Eyes. The orbital pain is nonradiating and burning but poorly localized. It is associated with profuse tearing, squint, and blurred vision. The pain may last for 10 seconds and is usually experienced every 1 or 2 days.

ORAL MANIFESTATIONS

The submandibular or parotid pain is dull and nonradiating. It seems to be brought about by sight of food. It lasts for about 30 seconds and is followed by profuse salivation.

DIFFERENTIAL DIAGNOSIS

Proctalgia fugax must be excluded. The differences are discussed by Hayden and Grossman (2). Pain is not seen in the *chorda tympani syndrome* (see Gustatory Sweating and Flushing—Auriculotemporal and Chorda Tympani Syndromes, earlier in this chapter).

Painful ophthalmoplegia has been described by a number of investigators (3, 5, 6). It is unilateral and accompanied or preceded by pain behind the eye. The paresis involves the third, fourth, and sixth cranial nerves, with paresthesia of the first branch of the trigeminal nerve. Its cause is inflammation of the carotid sinus.

REFERENCES

SYNDROMES OF THE TRIGEMINAL NERVE

1 Asherton, N., Trotter's Syndrome and Associated Lesions. *J. Laryngol.* **65:**349–366, 1951.

2 Blau, J. N., Trigeminal Sensory Neuropathy. *N. Engl. J. Med.* **281:**873–876, 1969.

3 Cohen, D. N., et al. Paratrigeminal Syndrome. *Am. J. Ophthalmol.* **79:**1044–1049, 1975.

4 Eggleston, D. J., Periodic Migrainous Neuralgia. *Oral Surg.* **29:**524–529, 1970.

5 Foix, C., Syndrome de la paroi externe du sinus caverneux. *Rev. Neurol. (Paris)* **38:**827–832, 1922.

6 Ford, F. R., and Walsh, F. B., Raeder's Paratrigeminal Syndrome: A Benign Disorder, Possibly a Complication of Migraine. *Bull. Johns Hopkins Hosp.* **103:**296–298, 1958.

7 Foster, J. B., Facial Pain. *Br. Med. J.* **4:**667–669, 1969.

8 Godtfredsen, E., Studies on the Cavernous Sinus Syndrome. *Acta Neurol. Scand.* **40:**69–75, 1964.

9 Graham, J. G., Trigeminal Neuralgia. *Practitioner* **198:**497–504, 1967.

10 Hurwitz, L. J., Facial Pain of Non-dental Origin. *Br. Dent. J.* **124:**167–171, 1968.

11 Kahana, E., et al., Brainstem and Cranial Nerve Involvement in Multiple Sclerosis. *Acta Neurol. Scand.* **49:**269–279, 1973.

12 Kerr, F. W., and Miller, R. H., The Pathology of Trigeminal Neuralgia. *Arch. Neurol.* **15:**308–319, 1966.

13 Klingon, G. H., and Smith, W. M., Raeder's Paratrigeminal Syndrome. *Neurology* **6:**750–753, 1956.

14 Minton, L. R., and Bounds, G. W., Raeder's Paratrigeminal Syndrome. *Am. J. Ophthalmol.* **58:**271–275, 1964.

15 Moses, L., Superior Orbital Fissure Syndrome. *Am. J. Ophthalmol.* **62:**163–164, 1966.

16 Olivier, R. M., Trotter's Syndrome. *Oral Surg.* **15:**527–530, 1962.

17 Raeder, J. G., "Paratrigeminal" Paralysis of the Oculopupillary Sympathetic. *Brain* **47:**149–158, 1924.

18 Robinson, B. C., and Jarrett, W. J., Superior Orbital Fissure

Syndrome with Bell's Palsy. *J. Oral Surg.* **31**:203–206, 1973.

19 Rushton, J. G., and Olafson, R. A., Trigeminal Neuralgia Associated with Multiple Sclerosis. *Arch. Neurol.* **13**:383–386, 1965.

20 Sluder, G., Etiology, Diagnosis and Prognosis and Treatment of Sphenopalatine Ganglion Neuralgia. *J.A.M.A.* **61**:1261–1266, 1913.

21 Smith, J. L., Raeders's Paratrigeminal Syndrome. *Am. J. Ophthalmol.* **46**:194–199, 1958.

22 Trotter, W., On Clinically Obscure Malignant Tumors of the Nasopharyngeal Wall. *Br. Med. J.* **2**:1057–1059, 1911.

SYNDROMES OF OTHER CRANIAL NERVES

1 Asherton, N., Glossopharyngeal Neuralgia (Otalgia) and the Elongated Styloid Process: A Record of Five Cases. *J. Laryngol.* **71**:453–470, 1957.

2 Avellis, G., Klinische Beiträge zur halbseitigen Kehlkopflähmung. *Berl. Klin.* **41**:1–26, 1891.

3 Böhme G., Zur Klinik organischer Gaumensegellähmungen. *Z. Laryngol. Rhinol. Otol.* **47**:104–110, 1968.

4 Bohn, E., and Strang, R., Glossopharyngeal Neuralgia. *Brain* **85**:371–388, 1962.

5 Burger, H., Classification and Nomenclature of Associated Paralysis of Vocal Cords. *Acta Oto-laryngol. (Stockh.)* **19**:389–403, 1934.

6 Cestan, R., and Chenais, L., Du myosis dans certaines lésions bulbaires en foyer (hemiplégie du type Avellis associée au syndrome oculaire sympathique). *Gaz. Hôp. (Paris)* **76**:1229–1233, 1903.

7 Cody, C. C., Jr., Associated Paralyses of the Larynx. *Ann. Otol. Rhinol. Laryngol.* **55**:549–561, 1946.

8 Crue, B. L., et al., Syndrome of the Jugular Foramen: A Syndrome Resulting from Neoplasms of the Posterior Fossa. *Arch. Otolaryngol.* **63**:384–391, 1956.

9 De Jong, R. N., *The Neurologic Examination.* 3d ed., Hoeber, New York, 1967.

10 Donahue, W. B., Styloid Syndrome. *Can. Dent. Assoc. J.* **25**:283–286, 1959.

11 Duchenne, G. B. A., Glosso-labial-laryngeal Paralysis: Selections from the Clinical Works of Dr. Duchenne (edited by G. V. Poore). *New Sydenham Soc.* **105**:143–172, 1883.

12 Eagle, W. W., Symptomatic Elongated Styloid Process: Report of Two Cases of Styloid Process – Carotid Artery Syndrome with Operation. *Arch. Otolaryngol.* **49**:490–503, 1949.

13 Elkin, D. C., and Woodhall, B., Combined Vascular and Nerve Injuries of Warfare. *Ann. Surg.* **119**:411–413, 1944.

14 Engstrom, H., and Wohlfart, G., Herpes Zoster of the Seventh, Eighth, Ninth and Tenth Cranial Nerves. *Arch. Neurol. Psychiatr.* **62**:638–652, 1949.

15 Font, J. H., The Jugular Foramen Syndrome. *Arch. Otolaryngol.* **56**:134–141, 1952.

16 Fox, S. L., and West, G. B., Jr., Syndrome of Avellis: A Review of the Literature and Report of One Case. *Arch. Otolaryngol.* **46**:773–778, 1947.

17 Furstenberg, A. C., and Magielski, J. E., A Motor Function of the Nucleus Ambiguus: Its Clinical Significance. *Ann. Otol. Rhinol. Laryngol.* **64**:788–793, 1955.

18 Garcin, R., Le syndrome paralytique unilatérale globale des nerfs crâniens. Thesis, Paris, 1927.

19 Gelin, G., and Saulnier, G., La paralysie unilatérale globale des nerfs crâniens (syndrome de Garcin). *Ann. Méd.* **52**:518–538, 1951.

20 Globus, J. H., Neurological Disorders of Interest to the Oral Surgeon. *Oral Surg.* **4**:1410–1419, 1951.

21 Harbert, F., et al., The Quantitative Measurement of Taste Function. *Arch. Otolaryngol.* **75**:138–143, 1962.

22 Herceg, S. J., and Harding, R. L., Gradenigo's Syndrome Following Correction of Posterior Choanal Atresia. *Plast. Reconstr. Surg.* **48**:181–183, 1971.

23 Holt, G. W., Clinical Syndromes of the Glossopharyngeus: Practical Neurologic Concepts. *Am. J. Med. Sci.* **238**:85–96, 1959.

24 Hörnsten, G., Wallenberg's Syndrome. *Acta Neurol. Scand.* **50**:434–468, 1974.

25 Kono, C., A Case of Garcin's Syndrome Associated with Carcinoma of the Middle Ear. *Nagoya J. Med. Sci.* **33**:47–54, 1970.

26 Krarup, B., Taste Reactions of Patients with Bell's Palsy. *Acta Oto-laryngol. (Stockh.)* **49**:389–399, 1958.

27 Mackenzie, S., Case of Intracranial Disease Involving the Medulla Oblongata. *Br. Med. J.* **1**:408–410, 1883.

28 Madsen, E., Dysphagia in Bulbar and Pseudobulbar Lesions and Its Similarity to Esophageal Carcinoma. *Acta Radiol. (Stockh.)* **41**:517–524, 1954.

29 Meyers, C. E., Diagnosis of Neurological Disease. *Oral Surg.* **1**:481–484, 1948.

30 New, G. B., Laryngeal Paralysis Associated with the Jugular Foramen Syndrome and Other Syndromes. *Am. J. Med. Sci.* **165**:727–737, 1923.

31 Orton, C. J., Glossopharyngeal Neuralgia. *Br. J. Oral Surg.* **9**:228–232, 1972.

32 Pisi, E., Contributo anatomo-clinico alla conoscenza della sindrome di Garcin. *Arch. Patol. Clin. Med.* **30**:1–39, 1952.

33 Pollack, L. J., Case of Multiple Cranial Nerve Palsies Due to Extracranial Disease. *J.A.M.A.* **78**:502–503, 1922.

34 Reichert, F. L., Neuralgias of the Glossopharyngeal Nerve with Particular Reference to the Sensory, Gustatory and Secretory Functions of the Nerves. *Arch. Neurol. Psychiatr.* **32**:1032–1037, 1934.

35 Robinson, B. C., and Jarret, W. J., Superior Orbital Fissure Syndrome with Bell's Palsy. *J. Oral Surg.* **31**:203–206, 1973.

36 Rosenbaum, H. E., and Seaman, W. B., Neurologic Manifestations of Nasopharyngeal Tumors. *Neurology* **5**:868–874, 1955.

37 Rullan, A., Associated Laryngeal Paralysis. *Arch. Otolaryngol.* **64**:207–212, 1956.

38 Schiffer, K. H., Das Halbbasissyndrom (Garcin), seine Diagnostik und seine Genese. *Arch. Psychiatr.* **186**:298–326, 1951.

39 Schmidt, A., Casuistische Beiträgezur Nervenpathologie: II: Doppelseitige Accessoriuslähmung bei Syringomyelie. *Dtsch. Med. Wochenschr.* **18**:606–608, 1892.

40 Sherman, I. C., and Tentler, R. L., Subacute Ascending Paralysis of Duchenne. *J. Neuropathol. Clin. Neurol.* **1**:285–290, 1961.

41 Spiegel, L. A., Garcin Syndrome: Unilateral Total Involvement of the Cranial Nerves with Report of One Case. *Ann. Otol. Rhinol. Laryngol.* **52**:706–712, 1943.

42 Spurling, R. G., and Grantham, E. G., Glossopharyngeal Neuralgia. *South. Med. J.* **35**:509–512, 1942.

43 Svien, H. J., et al., Jugular Foramen Syndrome and Allied Syndromes. *Neurology* **13**:797–809, 1963.

44 Tapia, —, Un nouveau syndrome: Quelques cas d'hemiplégia du larynx et de la langue avec ou sans paralysie du sterno-cléïdo-mastoïden et du trapèze. *Arch. Int. Laryngol.* **22**:780–785, 1906.

45 Uhlein, A., et al., Intracranial Section of the Glossopharyngeal Nerve. *Arch. Neurol. Psychiatr.*, **74**:320–324, 1955.

46 Vernet, M., Sur le syndrome des quatre dernières paires crâniennes d'après une observation personelle chez un blessé de guerre. *Bull. Soc. Med. Paris* **40**, Ser. 3:210–223, 1916.

47 Vernet, M., The Classification of the Syndromes of Associated Laryngeal Paralysis. *J. Laryngol.* **33**:354–365, 1918.

48 Villaret, M., Sur le syndrome du trou déchiré postérieur. *Paris Méd.* **23**:78–81, 1917.

49 Weiss, H., Halbbasissyndrom (Syndrom Garcin) bei Glomustumoren. *Nervenarzt* **26**:289–291, 1955.

50 Wilkins, R. H., and Brody, L. A., Wallenberg's Syndrome. *Arch. Neurol.* **22**:379–382, 1970.

ASYMMETRIC CRYING FACIES

1 Caylor, G. G., An "Epidemic" of Congenital Facial Paresis and Heart Disease. *Pediatrics* **40**:666–668, 1967.

2 Cayler, G. G., Additional Cases of the Cardiofacial Syndrome. *J. Pediatr.* **73**:953–954, 1968.

3 Cayler, G. G., Cardiofacial Syndrome: Congenital Heart Disease and Facial Weakness, a Hitherto Unrecognized Association. *Arch. Dis. Child.* **44**:69–75, 1969.

4 Cayler, G. G., et al., Further Studies of Patients with the Cardiofacial Syndrome. *Chest* **60**:161–165, 1971.

5 Chantler, C., and McEnery, G., Cardiofacial Syndrome. *Proc. R. Soc. Med.* **64**:20, 1971.

6 Clark, D. N., Diseases of the Autonomic Nervous System, in W. E. Nelson, C. V. Vaughan III, and R. J. McKay (eds.), *Textbook of Pediatrics.* 9th ed., Saunders, Philadelphia, 1969, p. 1309.

7 Hepner, W. R., Some Observations on Facial Paresis in the Newborn Infant: Etiology and Incidence. *Pediatrics* **8**:494–497, 1951.

8 Hoefnagel, D., and Penry, J. K., Partial Facial Paralysis in Young Children. *N. Engl. J. Med.* **262**:1126–1128, 1960.

9 Papadatos, C., et al., Congenital Hypoplasia of Depressor Anguli Oris Muscle. A Genetically Determined Condition? *Arch. Dis. Child.* **49**:927–931, 1974.

10 Pape, K. E., and Pickering, D., Asymmetric Crying Facies: An Index of Other Congenital Anomalies. *J. Pediatr.* **81**:21–30, 1972.

11 Perlman, M., and Reisner, S. H., Asymmetric Crying Facies and Congenital Anomalies. *Am. J. Dis. Child.* **48**:627–629, 1973.

12 Strong, W. B., and Silbert, D. R., Paralysis of the Facial Nerve and Congenital Heart Defects. *Am. Heart J.* **78**:279–280, 1969.

CEPHALIC ZOSTER SYNDROME

1 Blackley, B., et al., Herpes Zoster Auris Associated with Facial Nerve Palsy and Auditory Nerve Syndrome. *Acta Oto-laryngol. (Stockh).* **63**:533–550, 1967.

2 Crabtree, J. A., Herpes Zoster Oticus. *Laryngoscope* **78**:1853–1878, 1968.

3 Denny-Brown, D., et al., Pathologic Features of Herpes Zoster: A Note on "Geniculate" Herpes. *Arch. Neurol. Psychiatr.* **51**:216–231, 1944.

4 Dworkin, H., and Imburgia, R., Ramsay Hunt Syndrome Presenting Symptoms of Acute Pharyngitis. *N.Y. State J. Med.* **62**:3976–3977, 1962.

5 Engstrom, H., and Wohlfart, G., Herpes Zoster of the Seventh, Eighth, Ninth and Tenth Cranial Nerves. *Arch. Neurol. Psychiatr.* **62**:638–652, 1949.

6 Harbert, F., and Young, I. M., Audiologic Findings in Ramsay Hunt Syndrome. *Arch. Otolaryngol.* **85**:632–639, 1967.

7 Hunt, J. R., On Herpetic Inflammation of the Geniculate Ganglion: A New Syndrome and Its Complications. *J. Nerv. Ment. Dis.* **34**:73–96, 1907.

8 McGovern, F. H., and Fitz-Hugh, G. S., Herpes Zoster of the Cephalic Extremity. *Arch. Otolaryngol.* **55**:307–320, 1952.

9 Phillips, B. L. D., Auditory Herpes Zoster without Auricular Eruption. *Br. J. Clin. Pract.* **17**:715–719, 1963.

10 Shevick, I. M., Mandibular Herpes Zoster. *Calif. Med.* **79**:444–448, 1953.

11 Tschiassny, K., Herpes Zoster Oticus (Ramsay Hunt's Syndrome). *Arch. Otolaryngol.* **51**:73–82, 1950.

12 Wilson, A. A., Geniculate Neuralgia. *J. Neurosurg.* **7**:473–481, 1950.

DIMINISHED AND PERVERTED TASTE AND SMELL

1 Henkin, R. I., and Bradley, D. F., Hypogeusia Corrected by Na^{++} and Zn^{++}. *Life Sci.* **9**:701–709, 1970.

2 Henkin, R. I., et al., Idiopathic Hypogeusia with Dysgeusia, Hyposomia, and Dysosmia: A New Syndrome. *J.A.M.A.* **217**:434–440, 1971.

GUSTATORY LACRIMATION

1 Axelsson, A., and Laage-Hellman, J. E., The Gustolachrymal Reflex: The Syndrome of Crocodile Tears. *Acta Oto-laryngol. (Stockh.)* **54**:239–254, 1962.

2 Bogorad, F. A., Symptom of Crocodile Tears. *Vraču. Delo* **11**:1328–1330, 1928.

3 Boyer, F. C., and Gardner, W. J., Paroxysmal Lacrimation (Syndrome of Crocodile Tears) and Its Surgical Treatment: Relation to Auriculotemporal Syndrome. *Arch. Neurol. Psychiatr. (Chic.)* **61**:56–64, 1949.

4 Chorobski, J., Syndrome of Crocodile Tears. *Arch. Neurol. Psychiatr. (Chic.)* **65**:299–318, 1951.

5 Cricchi, M., Su di un nuovo caso di sindrome di lacrime di coccodrillo di natura congenita associata alla sindrome di Stilling-Türk-Duane. *Boll. Ocul.* **41**:587–594, 1962.

6 Dereux, J., Sur le larmoiement prandial homolatérale post paralytique: Syndrome des larmes de crocodile. *Rev. Neurol. (Paris)* **88**:120, 1953.

7 Ford, F. R., Paroxysmal Lacrimation during Eating as Sequel of Facial Palsy: Syndrome of Crocodile Tears. *Arch. Neurol. Psychiatr.* **29**:1279–1288, 1933.

8 Ford, F. R., and Woodhall, B., Phenomena Due to Misdirection of Regenerating Fibers of Cranial, Spinal and Autonomic Nerves: Clinical Observations. *Arch. Surg.* **36**:480–496, 1938.

9 Golding-Wood, P. H., Crocodile Tears. *Br. Med. J.* **1**:1518–1521, 1963.

10 Jacklin, H. N., The Gusto-lacrimal Reflex (Syndrome of Crocodile Tears). *Arch. Ophthalmol.* **61**:1521–1526, 1966.

11 Jampel, R. S., and Titone, C., Congenital Paradoxical Gustatory Lacrimal Reflex and Lateral Rectus Paralyses. *Arch. Ophthalmol.* **67**:123–126, 1962.

12 Lutman, F. C., Paroxysmal Lacrimation When Eating. *Am. J. Ophthalmol.* **30**:1583–1585, 1947.

13 Regenbogen, L., and Stein, R., Crocodile Tears Associated with Homolateral Duane's Syndrome. *Ophthalmologica* **156**:353–360, 1968.

14 Sarda, R. P., et al., Congenital Neuro-lacrimal Syndrome. *Ophthalmologica* **153**:353–360, 1968.

15 Spiers, A. S. D., Syndrome of "Crocodile Tears": Pharmacological Study of a Bilateral Case. *Br. J. Ophthalmol.* **54**:330–334, 1970.

GUSTATORY SWEATING AND FLUSHING

1 Adie, R., Gustatory Sweating. *Aust. N.Z. J. Surg.* **38**:98–103, 1968.

2 Baillarger, –, Mémoire sur l'obliteration du canal de sténon. *Gaz. Méd.* (*Paris*) **23**:194–197, 1853.

3 Bloor, K., Gustatory Sweating and Other Responses after Cervicothoracic Sympathectomy. *Brain* **92**:137–146, 1969.

4 Daly, R. F., New Observations Regarding the Auriculotemporal Syndrome. *Neurology* (*Minneap.*) **17**:1159–1168, 1967.

5 Duphenix, –, Sur une playe compliqué à la joue ou le canal salivaire fut déchiré. *Mém. Acad. Chir.* **3**:431–437, 1757.

6 Dupuy, –, Sur l'enlèvement des ganglions gutturaux des nerfs tresplanchniques sur des chevaux. *J. Méd. Chir. Pharmacol.* **37**:340–350, 1816.

7 Freedberg, A. S., et al., The Auriculotemporal Syndrome – a Clinical and Pharmacologic Study. *J. Clin. Invest.* **27**:669–676, 1948.

8 Frey, L., Le syndrome du nerf auriculo-temporal. *Rev. Neurol.* (*Paris*) **2**:97–104, 1923.

9 Fridberg, R., Das auriculo-temporale Syndrom. *Dtsch. Z. Nervenheilkd.* **121**:225–239, 1931.

10 Gardner, W. J., and Abdullah, A. F., Parotid Pain Following Superior Cervical Ganglionectomy: A Clinical Example of the Antagonistic Action of the Parasympathetic and Sympathetic Systems. *Am. J. Med. Sci.* **230**:65–69, 1955.

11 Gardner, W. J., and McCubbin, J. W., Auriculotemporal Syndrome: Gustatory Sweating Due to Misdirection of Regenerating Nerve Fibers. *J.A.M.A.* **160**:272–277, 1956.

12 Glaister, D. H., et al., The Mechanism of Post-parotidectomy Gustatory Sweating (the Auriculo-temporal Syndrome). *Br. Med. J.* **2**:942–946, 1958.

13 Goatcher, P. D., The Auriculo-temporal Syndrome. *Br. Med. J.* **1**:1233–1234, 1954.

14 Gorlin, R. J., personal observations, 1961.

15 Hemenway, W. G., Gustatory Sweating and Flushing: The Auriculo-Temporal Syndrome: Frey's Syndrome. *Laryngoscope* **70**:84–90, 1960.

16 Hogeman, K. E., Surgical-orthopedic Correction of Mandibular Protrusion. *Acta Chir. Scand.* (*Suppl.*) **159**:94–111, 1951.

17 Karnosh, L. J., The Syndrome of the Auriculo-temporal Nerve. *Cleveland Clin. Quart.* **13**:194–198, 1946.

18 Laage-Hellman, J. E., Gustatory Sweating and Flushing after Conservative Parotidectomy. *Acta Oto-laryngol.* (*Stockh.*) **48**:234–252, 1957.

19 Laage-Hellman, J. E., Treatment of Gustatory Sweating and Flushing. *Acta Oto-laryngol.* (*Stockh.*) **49**:132–143, 1958.

20 Laage-Hellman, J. E., Aetiologic Implications of Latent Period and Mode of Development after Parotidectomy. *Acta Oto-laryngol.* (*Stockh.*) **49**:306–314, 1958.

21 Laage-Hellman, J. E., Aetiologic Implications of Response of Separate Sweat Glands to Various Stimuli. *Acta Oto-laryngol.* (*Stockh.*) **49**:363–374, 1958.

22 Langenskiöld, A., Gustatory Local Hyperhidrosis Following Injuries in the Parotid Region. *Acta Chir. Scand.* **93**:294–306, 1946.

23 Mailander, J. C., Hereditary Gustatory Sweating. *J.A.M.A.* **201**:203–204, 1967.

24 Minor, V., Ein neues Verfahren zu der klinischen Untersuchung der Schweissabsonderung. *Dtsch. Z. Nervenheilkd.* **101**:302–308, 1928.

25 Morfit, H. M., and Kramish, D., Auriculotemporal Syndrome (Frey's Syndrome) Following Surgery of Parotid Tumors. *Am. J. Surg.* **102**:777–780, 1961.

26 New, G. B., and Bozer, H. E., Hyperhidrosis of the Cheek Associated with Injury to the Parotid Region. *Minn. Med.* **5**:652–657, 1922.

27 Payne, R. T., Pneumococcal Parotitis and Antecedent Auriculotemporal Syndrome. *Lancet* **1**:634–636, 1940.

28 Pfeffer, W., Jr., and Gellis, S. S., Auriculotemporal Syndrome: Report of a Case Developing in Early Childhood with a Review of the Literature. *Pediatrics* **7**:670–678, 1951.

29 Smith, R. O., et al., Jacobson's Neurectomy for Frey's Syndrome. *Am. J. Surg.* **120**:478–480, 1970.

30 Spiro, R. H., and Martin, H., Gustatory Sweating Following Parotid Surgery and Radical Neck Dissection. *Ann. Surg.* **165**:118–127, 1967.

31 Storrs, T. J., A Variation of the Auriculotemporal Syndrome. *Br. J. Oral Surg.* **11**:236–242, 1974.

32 Thomson, M. L., and Sutarman, –, The Identification and Enumeration of Active Sweat Glands in Man from Plastic Impressions of the Skin. *Trans. R. Soc. Trop. Med.* **47**:412–417, 1953.

33 Turner, J. C., Jr., et al., The Auriculotemporal (Frey) Syndrome Occurring after Parotid Surgery. *Surg. Gynecol. Obstet.* **111**:564–568, 1960.

34 Urprus, V., et al., Localized Abnormal Flushing and Sweating on Eating. *Brain* **57**:443–453, 1934.

35 Weber, F., A Case of Localized Sweating and Blushing on Eating, Possibly Due to Temporary Compression of Vasomotor Fibers. *Trans. Chir. Soc. London* **31**:277–280, 1897–1898.

36 Young, A. G., Unilateral Sweating of the Submental Region after Eating (Chorda Tympani Syndrome). *Br. Med. J.* **2**:976–979, 1956.

HEREDITARY QUIVERING OF THE CHIN

1 Frey, E., Ein streng dominant erbliches Kinnmuskelzittern. *Dtsch. Z. Nervenheilkd.* **115**:9–26, 1930.

2 Johnson, L. F., et al., Hereditary Chin-trembling with Nocturnal Myoclonus and Tongue-biting in Dizygous Twins. *Dev. Med. Child. Neurol.* **13**:726–729, 1971.

3 Laurance, B. M., et al., Hereditary Quivering of the Chin. *Arch. Dis. Child.* **43:**249–251, 1968.
4 Wadlington, W. B., Familial Trembling of the Chin. *J. Pediatr.* **53:**316–321, 1958.

JAW-WINKING AND WINKING-JAW SYNDROMES

1 Abraham, J. E., and Selvam, E. T., Inverse Marcus Gunn Phenomenon. *Br. J. Ophthalmol.* **46:**186–187, 1962.
2 Cooper, E. L., The Jaw-winking Phenomenon. Report of a Case. *Arch. Ophthalmol.* **18:**198–203, 1937.
3 Domke, H., and Habild, D., Zur Kiefer-Lidsynkinese im Kindesalter (Marcus Gunn Phänomen). *Monatsschr. Kinderheilkd.* **116:**517–522, 1968.
4 Dupuy-Dutemps, L., Ptosis congénital et phénomène de Marcus Gunn. *Bull. Soc. Ophthalmol. (Paris)* **41:**136–140, 1929.
5 Falls, H. F., et al., Three Cases of Marcus Gunn Phenomenon in Two Generations. *Am. J. Ophthalmol.* **32**(2):53–59, 1949.
6 Feric-Seiwerth, F., et al., Marcus-Gunn Syndrom. *Klin. Monatsbl. Augenheilkd.* **154:**519–524, 1969.
7 Friedenwald, H., On Movements of the Eyelids Associated with Movements of the Jaws with Lateral Movements of the Eyeballs. *Bull. Johns Hopkins Hosp.* **7:**134–136, 1896.
8 Fromaget, C., and Brun, C., Phénomène de Marcus Gunn, compliqué. *Bull. Soc. Ophthalmol. (Paris)* **38:**153–158, 1926.
9 Gordon, R. M., and Binder, M. B., The Corneomandibular Reflex. *J. Neurol. Neurosurg. Psychiatr.* **34:**236–242, 1971.
10 Grant, F. C., The Marcus Gunn Phenomenon: Report of a Case with Suggestions as to Relief. *Arch. Neurol. Psychiatr.* **35:**487–500, 1936.
11 Gunn, R. M., Congenital Ptosis with Peculiar Associated Movements of the Affected Lid. *Trans. Ophthalmol. Soc. U.K.* **3:**283–287, 1883.
12 Howe, G. L., Hereditary Opalescent Dentine Associated with the Marcus Gunn Phenomenon. *Br. J. Oral Surg.* **1:**119–123, 1963.
13 Jancar, J., Inverse Jaw-winking with Exaggerated Bell's Phenomenon. *Ophthalmologica* **151:**548–554, 1966.
14 Kirkham, T. H., Familial Marcus Gunn Phenomenon. *Br. J. Ophthalmol.* **53:**282–283, 1969.
15 Lutz, A., Jaw-winking Phenomenon and Its Explanation. *Arch. Ophthalmol.* **48:**144–158, 1919.
16 Marin Amat, M., Sur le syndrome ou phénomène de Marcus Gunn. *Ann. Ocul. (Paris)* **156:**513–528, 1919.
17 Schultz, R. O., and Burian, H. M., Bilateral Jaw Winking: Reflex in Association with Multiple Congenital Anomalies. *Arch. Ophthalmol.* **64:**946–949, 1960.
18 Simpson, D. G., Marcus Gunn Phenomenon Following Squint and Ptosis Surgery. Definition and Review. *Arch. Ophthalmol.* **56:**743–748, 1956.
19 Sinclair, W. W., Abnormal Associated Movements of the Eyelids. *Ophthalmol. Rev.* **14:**307–319, 1895.
20 Spaeth, E. B., The Marcus Gunn Phenomenon: Discussion, Presentation of Four Instances and Consideration of Its Surgical Correction. *Am. J. Ophthalmol.* **30:**143–158, 1947.
21 Villard, H., Le phénomène de Marcus Gunn. *Bull. Soc. Fr. Ophthalmol.* **38:**725–753, 1925.
22 Wartenberg, R., Winking-jaw Phenomenon. *Arch. Neurol. Psychiatr.* **59:**734–753, 1948.
23 Wartenberg, R., Inverted Marcus Gunn Phenomenon (So-called Marin Amat Syndrome). *Arch. Neurol. Psychiatr.* **60:**584–596, 1948.

PALATAL MYOCLONUS

1 Ablin, G., and Schwartz, A. W., Myoclonus of the Palate. *Br. J. Plast. Surg.* **16:**264–267, 1963.
2 Bender, M. B., et al., Myoclonus of Muscles of the Eye, Face and Throat. *Arch. Neurol. Psychiatr.* **67:**44–58, 1952.
3 Chokroverty, S., and Barron, K. D., Palatal Myoclonus and Rhythmic Ocular Movements: A Polygraphic Study. *Neurology* **19:**975–982, 1969.
4 Heller, M. F., Vibratory Tinnitus and Palatal Myoclonus. *Acta Oto-laryngol. (Stockh.)* **55:**292–298, 1962.
5 Herrmann, C., and Brown, J. W., Palatal Myoclonus. *J. Neurol. Sci.* **5:**473–492, 1967.
6 McCarty, W., Ocular and Palatal Myoclonus. *Am. J. Ophthalmol.* **43:**121–124, 1957.
7 Pulec, J. L., and Siminton, K. M., Palatal Myoclonus: A Report of Two Cases. *Laryngoscope* **71:**668–671, 1961.
8 Tyler, R., Palato-pharyngeal Myoclonus. *J. Nerv. Ment. Dis.* **117:**267–269, 1953.
9 Yap, C. B., et al., "Ocular Bobbing" in Palatal Myoclonus. *Arch. Neurol.* **18:**304–310, 1968.

SUBMANDIBULAR, RECTAL, AND OCULAR PAIN AND FLUSHING

1 Dugan, R. E., Familial Rectal Pain. *Lancet* **1:**854, 1972.
2 Hayden, R., and Grossman, M., Rectal, Ocular, and Submaxillary Pain: A Familial Autonomic Disorder Related to Proctalgia Fugax. Report of a Family. *Am. J. Dis. Child.* **97:**479–482, 1959.
3 Hunt, W. E., et al., Painful Ophthalmoplegia. *Neurology (Minneap.)* **11:**56–58, 1961.
4 Mann, T. P., and Cree, J. E., Familial Rectal Pain. *Lancet* **1:**1016–1017, 1972.
5 Other, A., Painful Ophthalmoplegia. *Acta Ophthalmol. (Kbh.)* **45:**371–373, 1967.
6 Smith, J. L., and Taxdal, D., Painful Ophthalmoplegia: The Tolosa-Hunt Syndrome. *Am. J. Ophthalmol.* **61:**1466–1472, 1966.

38

Craniocarpotarsal Dysplasia

(Whistling Face Syndrome, Freeman-Sheldon Syndrome)

In 1938, Freeman and Sheldon (5) described a syndrome characterized by (*a*) microstomia and flat midface, (*b*) talipes equinovarus, and (*c*) ulnar deviation of the fingers. Unaware of this report, Burian (1), in 1963, described the same complex, utilizing the term "whistling face syndrome." Weinstein and Gorlin (15) in 1969 reviewed all published cases employing the term "craniocarpotarsal dysplasia."

Although most cases are sporadic, there are several examples of the syndrome in two generations (4, 6, 9, 11), and, in view of the male-to-male transmission, it would appear to be inherited as an autosomal dominant trait. Less certain are the cases of Pitanguy and Bisaggio (10).

Sauk et al. (11a) pointed out the possible depiction of the condition in a pre-Columbian vase.

SYSTEMIC MANIFESTATIONS

Facies. The stiff, immobile, flat midface, long philtrum and puckered mouth are characteristic. The eyes appear deeply sunken (Fig. 38-1).

Eyes. Convergent strabismus, epicanthus, and ocular hypertelorism have been noted in several cases (5, 7, 8, 11, 13). Several patients have exhibited antimongoloid obliquity and ptosis of the upper lids (3, 13, 15) (Fig. 38-2).

Nose. The nose is small and the philtrum long. The nostrils are narrow, the alae often being bent, thus simulating nostril colobomas. Near the tip, the alae are of normal thickness, but they thin dorsally to be inserted close to the columella. The nasolabial folds are evident only near the sides of the nose.

Musculoskeletal system. Growth has been retarded below the 3d percentile in about half the cases (7). Flexion contractures of the fingers are a constant feature, the thumbs being especially involved at the metacarpophalangeal joints. There is ulnar deviation of the fingers without bony abnormalities (Fig. 38-1).

Talipes equinovarus has been an almost constant feature. Occasionally this is unilateral (7). Other less frequently found anomalies include moderate to severe scoliosis, spina bifida occulta (8, 15), and inguinal hernia (11).

The facial skeleton is small. The anteroposterior length of both face and cranium is short, while the height is relatively great. Most patients have shown a steep cranial base (11, 15).

Other findings. Hashemi (6a) noted atrophy of one kidney and hydronephrosis of the other.

Oral manifestations. There is marked microstomia, the interangular or intercommissural distance being about two-thirds of that for a child of the same age (2). The lips are pursed or held as in whistling (Fig. 38-3*A, B*). The palate

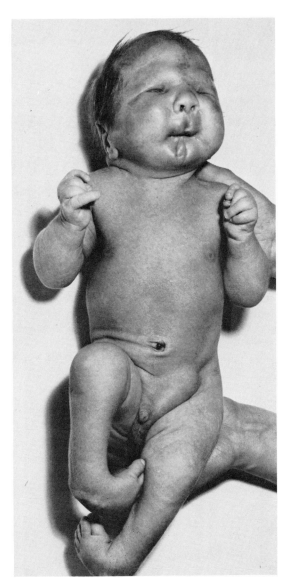

Figure 38-1. *Craniocarpotarsal dysplasia.* Sunken eyes, chin grooves, overlapping fingers, talipes equinovarus, and inguinal hernia. (*From A. E. Rintala,* Acta Paediatr. Scand. **57**:553, 1968.)

is highly arched and the mandible and tongue tend to be small.

Extending from the middle of the lower lip to the chin is a fibrous band or elevation which is demarcated by two paramedian grooves, forming an H- or V-shaped scarlike structure (Fig. 38-2).

Biopsy of buccinator muscles has shown fibrous connective tissue replacement of muscle bundles (11a).

DIFFERENTIAL DIAGNOSIS

The constellation of anomalies is sufficiently characteristic to cause little confusion with other entities.

LABORATORY AIDS

Electromyography has shown hypoplasia of facial musculature (11a).

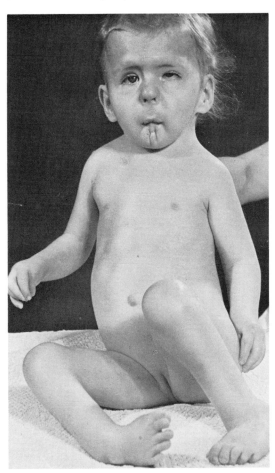

Figure 38-2. Deep-set eyes, lid ptosis, convergent strabismus, H-shaped chin grooves, overlapping fingers, and talipes. (*From J. Külz, Rostock, East Germany.*)

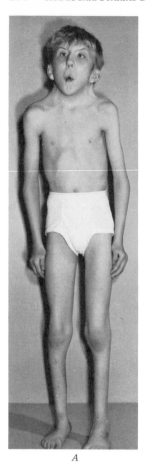
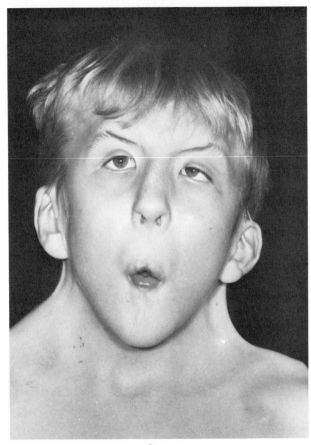

A   *B*

Figure 38-3. (*A, B*). Whistling facies is produced by small puckered mouth. Note pterygium colli and notched nostrils.

REFERENCES

1 Burian, F., The "Whistling Face" Characteristic in a Compound Cranio-facio-corporal Syndrome. *Br. J. Plast. Surg.* **16:**140–163, 1963.

2 Cervenka, J., et al., Cranio-carpo-tarsal Dysplasia or the Whistling Face Syndrome. II. Oral Intercommissural Distance in Children. *Am. J. Dis. Child.* **117:**434–435, 1969.

3 Cervenka, J., et al., Craniocarpotarsal Dysplasia or Whistling Face Syndrome. *Arch. Otolaryngol.* **91:**183–187, 1970.

4 Fraser, F. C., et al., Cranio-carpo-tarsal Dysplasia. *J.A.M.A.* **211:**1374–1376, 1970.

5 Freeman, E. A., and Sheldon, J. H., Cranio-carpo-tarsal Dystrophy — an Undescribed Congenital Malformation. *Arch. Dis. Child.* **13:**277–283, 1938.

6 Gross-Kieselstein, E., et al., Familial Occurrence of the Freeman-Sheldon Syndrome; Cranio-carpo-tarsal Dysplasia. *Pediatrics* **47:**1064–1067, 1971.

6a Hashemi, G., The Whistling Face Syndrome. *Indian J. Pediatr.* **40:**23–24, 1973.

7 MacLeod, P., and Patriquin, H., The Whistling Face Syndrome — Cranio-carpo-tarsal Dysplasia. *Clin. Pediatr.* **13:**184–189, 1974.

8 Otto, F. M. G., Die "Cranio-carpo-tarsal Dystrophie" (Freeman and Sheldon): Ein kasuistischer Beitrag. *Z. Kinderheilkd.* **73:**240–250, 1953.

9 Pfeiffer, R. A., et al., Das Syndrom von Freeman und Sheldon. *Z. Kinderheilkd.* **112:**43–53, 1972.

10 Pitanguy, I., and Bisaggio, S., A Chiro-cheilo-podalic Syndrome. *Br. J. Plast. Surg.* **22:**79–85, 1969.

11 Rintala, A. E., Freeman-Sheldon's Syndrome: Cranio-carpo-tarsal Dystrophy. *Acta Paediatr. Scand.* 57:553–556, 1968.

11a Sauk, J. J., Jr., et al., Electromyography or Oral-Facial Musculature in Craniocarpaltarsal Dysplasia (Freeman-Sheldon Syndrome). *Clin. Genet.* **6:**132–137, 1974.

12 Sharma, R. N., and Tandon, S. N., "Whistling Face" Deformity in Cranio-facio-corporal Syndrome. *Br. Med. J.* **4:**33, 1970.

13 Temtamy, S. A., *Genetic Factors in Hand Malformations.* Thesis, Johns Hopkins, Baltimore, 1966.

14 Walbaum, R., et al., Le syndrome de Freeman-Sheldon (syndrome du siffleur). *Ann. Pédiatr.* **20:**357–364, 1973.

15 Weinstein, S., and Gorlin, R. J., Cranio-carpo-tarsal Dysplasia or the Whistling Face Syndrome. I. Clinical Considerations. *Am. J. Dis. Child.* **117:**427–433, 1969.

39

Craniofacial Dysostosis

(*Crouzon Syndrome*)

Craniofacial dysostosis is characterized by (*a*) premature craniosynostosis, (*b*) midface hypoplasia with shallow orbits, and (*c*) ocular proptosis.

The condition clearly has autosomal dominant transmission. Impressive pedigrees have been reported by various authors (3, 10–12, 21, 23, 24, 28). In almost every affected family reported to date, penetrance has been complete. This has also been the experience of the authors. However, seemingly incomplete penetrance was noted by Crouzon (8, 9). The possibility of an autosomal recessive form of Crouzon syndrome was first raised by Cross and Opitz (6). We cannot accept the recessive examples published by Juberg and Chambers (17) for the reasons stated by Jones and Cohen (16). However, heterogeneity for the Crouzon syndrome may yet be demonstrated.

Sporadic cases, representing fresh mutations, have also been observed (20, 29) and amount to almost one-third of the cases (1). A large number of sporadic cases should be studied to determine if increased paternal age at time of conception is a significant factor in producing fresh mutations.

Cranial deformity in the Crouzon syndrome depends upon the order and rate of progression of sutural involvement. Bertelsen (3), employing detailed cranial measurements on 15 patients, concluded that there was no characteristic calvaria in craniofacial dysostosis. Thus, variability of expression characterizes the disorder. Nowhere is this more apparent than in the pedigree reported by Schiller (24). The proband, the most severely affected member of the family, presented with the Kleeblattschädel anomalad (14), a nonspecific deformity which may be observed in several disorders. Several sibs manifested classical craniofacial dysostosis. The affected mother and various other members of the family exhibited proptosis and ocular hypertelorism but without evidence of craniosynostosis.

SYSTEMIC MANIFESTATIONS

Face. Midface hypoplasia is characteristically observed. Relative mandibular prognathism, with drooping lower lip and short upper lip, are frequent findings. The nose may be parrot-beaked (3, 7) (Fig. 39-1*A*, *B*).

Eyes. Proptosis is secondary to shallow orbits. Divergent strabismus and nystagmus as well as hypertelorism are commonly found. Bertelsen (3) noted that 80 percent of patients with craniofacial dysostosis had optic nerve involvement. Spontaneous luxation of the globes has been reported (2). Megalocornea, ectopia lentis, iris coloboma, and corectopia have been noted occasionally (5).

Cranium. The shape of the cranium depends upon which sutures are involved. Brachycephaly, scaphocephaly, trigonocephaly, and, rarely, the Kleeblattschädel anomalad have been observed.

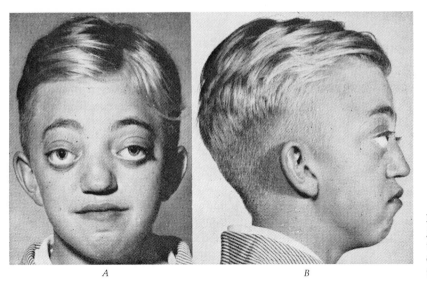

A   *B*

Figure 39-1. (*A, B*). *Cranio-facial dysostosis* in fourteen-year-old boy. Note exophthalmos, hypertelorism, and short upper lip.

Palpable ridging is usually evident. A prominent bulge may be present at the bregma (3).

Premature craniosynostosis is variable in onset but frequently commences during the first year of life and is usually complete by two to three years of age. In some cases, synostosis may not be evident until ten years of age. In a few instances, no craniosynostosis may be present (24). Roentgenographically, the coronal, sagittal, and lambdoidal sutures are most frequently involved. Other findings may include digital impressions, basilar kyphosis, widening of the hypophyseal fossa, and small paranasal sinuses (3) (Fig. 39-2*A, B*).

Central nervous system. Increased intracranial pressure and mental deficiency may be observed in some cases. Epilepsy was noted by Crouzon (7).

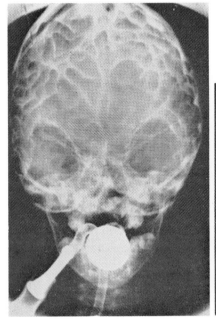

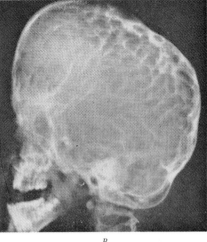

A   *B*

Figure 39-2. (*A, B*). Roentgenograms of patient with Crouzon syndrome. Note shortening of anteroposterior diameter of skull and the marked digital impressions.

Ears. Bilateral atresia of the auditory meatus have been reported in some instances (4, 18, 22, 29). About one-third of patients with the Crouzon syndrome have hearing loss, mostly conductive (2, 4, 25).

Other findings. Ankylosis at the elbows and subluxation of the head of the radius have been described by several investigators (3).

Oral manifestations. Crowding of the upper teeth, V-shaped dental arch, class III malocclusion, and open bite have been reported (1, 3, 26). The palate may be narrow and highly arched. Bifid uvula has been reported by Kelln et al. (18). Oligodontia, macrodontia, peg-shaped teeth, and widely spaced teeth have been described occasionally (10, 15, 18).

DIFFERENTIAL DIAGNOSIS

Craniofacial dysostosis should be distinguished from simple craniosynostosis, the *Apert syndrome,* the *Pfeiffer syndrome,* and *Saethre-Chotzen syndrome.*

Franceschetti (13) used the term pseudo-Crouzon syndrome to designate those cases which simulate craniofacial dysotosis, but which do not have relative mandibular prognathism, parrot-beaked nose, strabismus, or familial occurrence. This distinction is meaningless since these findings are not obligatory and none is essential in making a diagnosis of craniofacial dysostosis. These cases, in our opinion, are examples of the *Saethre-Chotzen syndrome.*

Cases of so-called "Vogt cephalosyndactyly" (27), a condition in which the Crouzon syndrome is said to be combined with the Apert syndrome, are simply cases of Apert-type acrocephalosyndactyly.

LABORATORY AIDS

None is known.

REFERENCES

1 Atkinson, F. R. B., Hereditary Cranio-facial Dysostosis, or Crouzon's Disease. *Presse Med.* **195**:118–121, 1937.
2 Baldwin, J. L., Dysostosis Craniofacialis of Crouzon. *Laryngoscope* **78**:1660–1676, 1968.
3 Bertelsen, T. I., *The Premature Synostosis of the Cranial Sutures.* Munksgaard, Copenhagen, 1958.
4 Boedts, D., La surdité dans la dysostose crâniofaciale ou maladie de Crouzon. *Acta Oto-rhino-laryng. Belg.* **21**:143–155, 1967.
5 Cohen, M. M., Jr., An Etiologic and Nosologic Overview of Craniosynostosis Syndromes. *Birth Defects,* **11**(2):137–189, 1975.
6 Cross, H. E., and Opitz, J. M., Craniosynostosis in the Amish. *J. Pediatr.* **75**:1037–1040, 1969.
7 Crouzon, O., Dysostose cranio-faciale héréditaire. *Bull. Soc. Méd. Hôp. Paris* **33**:545–555, 1912.
8 Crouzon, O., Dysostose cranio-faciale héréditaire. *Arch. Méd. Inf.* **18**:529–539, 1915.
9 Crouzon, O., Une nouvelle famille atteinte de dysostose cranio-faciale héréditaire. *Arch. Méd. Inf.* **18**:540–543, 1915.
10 Dodge, H. W., et al., Craniofacial Dysostosis: Crouzon's Disease. *Pediatrics* **23**:98–106, 1959.
11 Flippen, J. H., Jr., Cranio-facial Dysostosis of Crouzon: Report of a Case in Which the Malformation Occurred in Four Generations. *Pediatrics* **5**:90–96, 1950.
12 Fogh-Andersen, P., Dysostosis craniofacialis (Crouzon) som dominant arvelig lidelse. *Nord. Med.* **18**:993–996, 1943.

13 Franceschetti, A., Dysostose crânienne avec calotte cérébriforme (pseudo-Crouzon). *Confinia Neurol.* **13**:161–166, 1953.
14 Hall, B. D., et al., Kleeblattschädel (Cloverleaf) Syndrome: Severe Form of Crouzon's Disease? *J. Pediatr.* **80**:526–527, 1972.
15 Heuyer, G., et al., A propos de la dysostose cranio-faciale (ou maladie de Crouzon). *Actual. Odontostomatol. (Paris)* **16**:413–428, 1951.
16 Jones, K. E., and Cohen, M. M., Jr., The Crouzon Syndrome. *J. Med. Genet.* **10**:398, 1973.
17 Juberg, R. C., and Chambers, S. R., An Autosomal Recessive Form of Craniofacial Dysostosis (The Crouzon Syndrome). *J. Med. Genet.* **10**:89–93, 1973.
18 Kelln, E. E., et al., Oral Manifestations of Crouzon's Disease. *Oral Surg.* **13**:1245–1248, 1960.
19 Koziak, P. H., Craniostenosis: Report on 22 cases. *Am. J. Ophthalmol.* **37**:380–390, 1954.
20 Krause, A. C., and Buchanan, D. N., Dysostosis Craniofacialis (Crouzon). *Am. J. Ophthalmol.* **22**, Ser. 3:140–144, 1939.
21 Lake, M. S., and Kuppinger, J. C., Craniofacial Dysostosis (Crouzon's Disease): Report of Three Cases. *Arch. Ophthalmol.* **44**:37–46, 1950.
22 Nager, F. R., and Reynier, J. de, Das Gehörorgan bei den angeborenen Kopfmissbildungen. *Pract. Otorhinolaryngol. (Basel)* **10** (Suppl. 2):1–128, 1948.
23 Pinkerton, O. D., and Pinkerton, F. J., Hereditary Craniofacial Dysplasia. *Am. J. Ophthalmol.* **35**:500–506, 1952.

24 Schiller, J. G., Craniofacial Dysostosis of Crouzon: A Case Report and Pedigree with Emphasis on Heredity. *Pediatrics* **23:**107–112, 1959.

25 Terrahi, K., Das Gehörorgan bei den kraniofazialen Missbildungensyndromen nach Crouzon und Apert. *Z. Laryng. Rhinol.* **50:**794–802, 1971.

26 Vichi, F., I caratteri clinici della sindrome disostosica craniofacciale di Crouzon. *Minerva Stomatol.* **8:**211–220, 1959.

27 Vogt, A., Dyskephalie (Dysostosis craniofacialis, Maladie de Crouzon, 1912) und eine neuartige Kombination dieser Krankheit mit Syndaktylie der 4 Extremitäten (Dyskephalodaktylie). *Klin. Monatsbl. Augenheilkd.* **90:**441–454, 1933.

28 Vulliamy, D. G., and Normandale, P. A., Craniofacial Dysostosis in a Dorset Family. *Arch. Dis. Child.* **41:**375–382, 1966.

29 Wiegand, R., Dysostosis craniofacialis (Morbus Crouzon, 1912) mit beidseitiger (häutiger) Gehörgangsatresie. *Arch. Ohr. Nas. Kehlk. Heilk.* **166:**128–139, 1954.

40

Craniosynostosis Syndromes—Unusual Variants

In addition to the more well-known craniosynostosis conditions, such as the *Apert syndrome, Pfeiffer syndrome, Saethre-Chotzen syndrome, Carpenter syndrome, Crouzon syndrome,* and the *Kleeblattschädel anomalad,* several unusual craniosynostosis syndromes are known to occur. These have been thoroughly reviewed by Cohen (5).

CRANIOSYNOSTOSIS, VARIABLE SYNDACTYLY, AND OBESITY (SUMMITT SYNDROME)

In 1969, Summitt (18) reported a syndrome consisting of craniosynostosis and variable syndactyly. Obesity of the trunk and moderate gynecomastia were evident. Intelligence was normal. Two affected sibs and parental consanguinity suggest autosomal recessive inheritance (Fig. 40-1).

Acrocephaly and occipital irregularity were observed. Scaphocephaly was noted in one case. Epicanthal folds and strabismus were also described. The palate was narrow and highly arched, and delayed dental eruption was reported.

Anomalies of the hands and feet varied from severe syndactyly to mild syndactyly and clinodactyly. In one case, bilateral complete 2 to 5 syndactyly of the hands, brachymesophalangy of digits 2 through 5, fusion of the third and fourth distal phalanges, medial deviation of the second and third digits, and lateral deviation of the fourth and fifth digits were observed. In these

respects, the hand abnormalities were similar to those found in the Apert syndrome. The thumbs, however, were normal. Syndactyly of all five

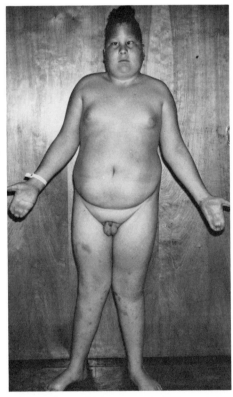

Figure 40-1. *Summitt syndrome.* Note acrocephaly, strabismus, obesity, syndactyly of hands, and genu valgum. (*From R. L. Summitt,* Birth Defects 5(3):35, 1969.)

toes was noted, varying from partial to complete, with normal toenails. Two phalanges were present in each toe. The proximal phalanges of the great toes were triangular, with deviation of the distal phalanges. In the other case, partial 2-3-4 syndactyly of the hands and brachymesophalangy and clinodactyly of digits 2 and 5 were noted, together with partial 2-3 syndactyly of the toes. Genu valgum and coxa valga were also observed.

CRANIOSYNOSTOSIS AND RADIAL APLASIA (BALLER-GEROLD SYNDROME)

Baller (3) and Gerold (9) reported a syndrome consisting of craniosynostosis and radial aplasia. Consanguinity was noted in Baller's case, and affected sibs were reported by Gerold. Thus, autosomal recessive transmission seems likely.

Craniosynostosis involving the coronal suture was evident, the skull being turribrachycephalic. Steep forehead, high nasal bridge, and long philtrum were noted. Epicanthic folds and dysplastic ears were also described. Intelligence was normal (Fig. 40-2).

Absent or hypoplastic radius, short curved ulna, radially deviated hands, missing carpal bones, fused carpal bones, hypoplastic or absent thumb, and hypoplastic or absent first metacarpal were noted. A vertebral anomaly was mentioned by Gerold.

Another case was reported by Greitzer et al. (11). The patient had fusion of the metopic suture, ocular hypotelorism, high nasal bridge, dysplastic ears, absent radii, three digits on each hand, polymicrogyria, and subaortic valvular hypertrophy.

The condition should be distinguished from

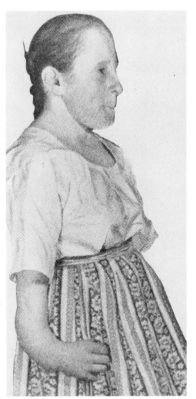
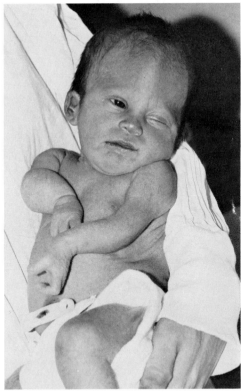

A   *B*

Figure 40-2. *Craniosynostosis and radial aplasia* (Baller-Gerold syndrome). (*A from F. Baller. Z. Menschl. Vererb, Konstit-Lehre* **29:**782, 1950.) (*B*). Example personally seen. Note metopic ridging, short forearms (absent radii), and three fingers on each hand.

the radial aplasia-thrombocytopenia syndrome, the Holt-Oram syndrome, and the Fanconi syndrome.

CRANIOSYNOSTOSIS AND FIBULAR APLASIA (LOWRY SYNDROME)

Lowry (15) described two male sibs with craniosynostosis and bilateral fibular aplasia. Consanguinity was also noted, suggesting autosomal recessive transmission.

In one patient, both coronal and sagittal sutures were synostosed. In the other child, only the coronal suture was involved. The eyes were prominent in both sibs, and strabismus was noted in one case. A partial cleft of the hard palate was observed in one sib, a highly arched palate in the other (Fig. 40-3A).

The fingers were normal, and bilateral simian creases were noted in both sibs. Bilaterally absent fibulas, talipes equinovarus, and normal toes were reported in both children (Fig. 40-3B).

Other findings included cryptorchism in both sibs, short sternum, pilonidal dimple, and normal intelligence in one sib, and large posterior fontanel, Wormian bones, low-set ears with pointed helices, short webbed neck, and mild chordee of the penis in the other sib.

CRANIOSYNOSTOSIS, MIDFACE HYPOPLASIA, HYPERTRICHOSIS, AND ANOMALIES OF THE EYES, TEETH, HEART, AND EXTERNAL GENITALIA (GORLIN-CHAUDHRY-MOSS SYNDROME)

In 1960, Gorlin et al. (10) described a syndrome in two female sibs consisting of craniosynostosis,

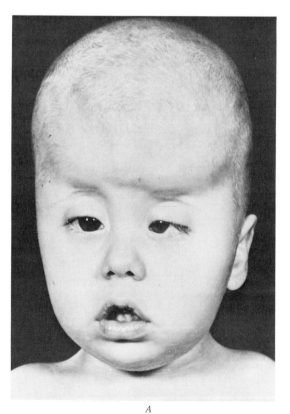
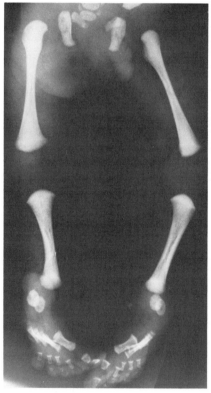

A *B*

Figure 40-3. *Craniosynostosis and fibular aplasia (Lowry syndrome). (A). Note tower skull, ptosis of eyelids, and strabismus. (B). Fibular aplasia and talipes equinovarus. (From R. B. Lowry, J. Med. Genet. 9:227, 1972.)*

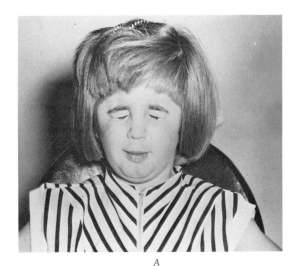

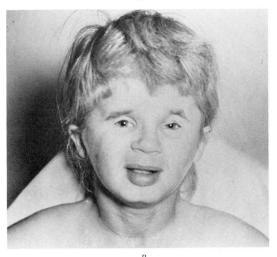

A

B

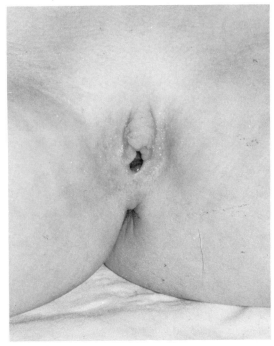

C

Figure 40-4. *Craniosynostosis, midface hypoplasia, hypertrichosis, cardiac and genital anomalies* (*Gorlin-Chaudhry-Moss syndrome*). (*A, B*). Note hypertrichosis, severe midface hypoplasia, and eyelid ptosis. (*C*). Hypoplasia of labia majora. (*From R. J. Gorlin et al.,* J. Pediatr. **56:**778, 1960.)

midface hypoplasia, hypertrichosis, and anomalies of the eyes, teeth, heart, and external genitalia. There was no parental consanguinity. The disorder possibly has autosomal recessive transmission (Fig. 40-4*A–C*).

Both sibs were short but of stocky build. Both held their heads in mild anteflexion when walking. Pronounced midface hypoplasia and depressed supraorbital ridges were observed in both, but were more pronounced in the older sib. Hypertrichosis of the scalp, arms, legs, and back was noted. The scalp hair line was lower than normal. Antimongoloid obliquity, inability fully

to open or close the eyes, upper-eyelid colobomas, microphthalmia, and hyperopia were reported. The younger sib had unilateral persistence of the iridopupillary membrane. Bilateral conductive hearing loss was noted in both sibs.

Oral anomalies consisted of class III malocclusion, highly arched narrow palate, hypodontia, microdontia, and abnormally shaped teeth.

Other findings included patent ductus arteriosus, pronounced hypoplasia of the labia majora, and umbilical hernia.

Roentgenographic examination of the skull revealed premature synostosis of the coronal suture, brachycephaly, hypoplastic maxillary and nasal bones, ocular hypertelorism, lordosis of the petrous ridges, clival hypoplasia, and elevation of the lesser sphenoidal wings.

CRANIOSYNOSTOSIS, ARTHROGRYPOSIS, AND CLEFT PALATE (CHRISTIAN-ANDREWS-CONNEALLY-MULLER SYNDROME)

In 1971, Christian et al. (5) reported an autosomal recessive disorder consisting of craniosynostosis, arthrogryposis, and cleft palate.

Findings included craniosynostosis with microcephaly, prominent occiput, ocular hypertelorism, antimongoloid obliquity, ophthalmoplegia, abnormal ear placement, and cleft palate or bifid uvula.

Also observed were adducted thumbs, camptodactyly of other digits in some cases, limited extension at the elbows and knees in one case, talipes equinovarus, and pectus excavatum (Fig. 40-5A–E). Dysphagia, laryngomalacia, and muscle fibrillation were also noted. Neuropathologic studies of one affected infant revealed dysmyelination with excessive glial proliferation in the white matter.

Many features of this syndrome are secondary to abnormal development of the central nervous system. Hypertelorism and cleft palate, however, are pleiotropic effects.

CRANIOSYNOSTOSIS, BRACHYSYNDACTYLY OF HANDS, AND ABSENT TOES (HERRMANN-OPITZ SYNDROME)

In 1969, Herrmann and Opitz (12) and Herrmann et al. (13) reported a sporadic malformation syn-

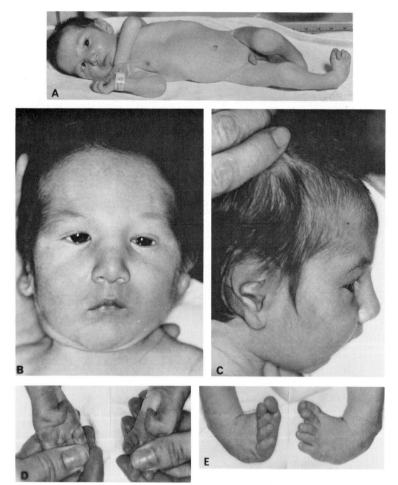

Figure 40-5. *Craniosynostosis, arthrogryposis, and cleft palate* (*Christian syndrome*). (*A–E*). Pectus excavatum, facial asymmetry with telecanthus and antimongoloid obliquity of palpebral fissure, hirsutism, micrognathia, posteriorly rotated ears, adducted thumbs, and talipes equinovarus. (*From J. C. Christian et al.,* Clin. Genet. **2**:95, 1971.)

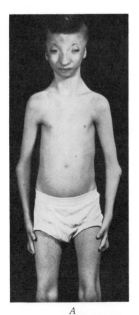

A

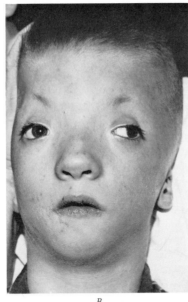

B

Figure 40-6. *Craniosynostosis, brachydactyly of hands, and absent toes (Herrmann-Opitz syndrome). (A–E).* Craniofacial anomalies, ocular hypertelorism, subluxation of radial heads, soft-tissue syndactyly of fingers, absence of toes other than halluces. *(From J. Herrmann et al.,* Birth Defects **5**(3):39, 1969, *and J. Opitz, Madison, Wis.)*

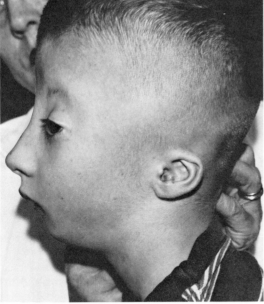

C

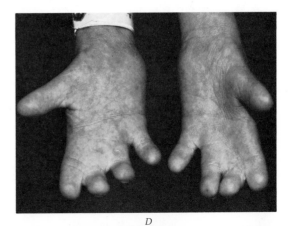

D

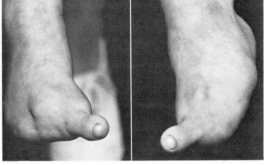

E

drome consisting of craniosynostosis, brachysyndactyly of the hands, and absent toes. A chromosome study was normal. The height and weight were consistently below the 3d percentile, and mental retardation was noted.

The head was turribrachycephalic with hypoplastic supraorbital ridges and bitemporal flattening. Ocular hypertelorism, prominent eyes, exotropia, posteriorly rotated ears with incompletely formed helices, micrognathia, and highly arched palate were also noted. Roentgenographic examination of the skull revealed a large defect in the posterior parietal area, ossification defects of the frontal bone, and small mastoid sinuses.

Extension and rotation at the elbow joints were limited. Symmetric cutaneous syndactyly of the second to fourth fingers was observed, extending to the distal interphalangeal joints. Cutaneous syndactyly of lesser degree was noted between the fourth and fifth fingers. Simian creases and distally placed axial triradii were reported. Roentgenographic examination revealed no osseous syndactyly or symphalangism. A defect of the proximal phalangeal epiphysis of both thumbs was noted.

A single digit was present on each foot. Roentgenographic examination revealed two phalanges in each digit and four metatarsals in each foot, one larger than the other three in association with the single digit (Fig. 40-6A–E).

We have observed a similar case in which unsuccessful abortion had been attempted with methotrexate.

CRANIOSYNOSTOSIS, SEVERE SYMMETRICALLY MALFORMED EXTREMITIES, AND CLEFT LIP-PALATE (HERRMANN-PALLISTER-OPITZ SYNDROME)

Herrmann et al. (13) described an 11-year-old boy with craniosynostosis, severe symmetrically malformed extremities, and cleft lip-palate. A chromosome study revealed no abnormality.

The skull was microbrachycephalic. Synostosis involved mainly the coronal suture, the sagittal and lambdoidal sutures remaining partly open. The metopic suture was patent. Ocular hypertelorism, occipital capillary hemangioma, protruding dysplastic ears, deviation of the nasal septum, and cleft lip-palate were observed. Severe mental retardation was noted.

Radial aplasia and shortened ulna were observed bilaterally. The hands were situated in valgus position. Both fused and missing carpal bones were noted. Three metacarpals and three fingers were present on each hand, the fourth and fifth metacarpals and fingers being absent. Two epiphyses were present in each metacarpal. The third finger was split, with two separate fingernails (Fig. 40-7A, B).

Congenital hip dislocation, dysplasia of the femoral heads and necks, ankylosis of the knees, and absent fibulas were reported. The feet were held in varus position, and the third and fourth toes on each foot were hypoplastic.

Other findings included narrow shoulders and thorax, slight depression of the lower part of the sternum, and cryptorchism.

ACROCEPHALOPOLYSYNDACTYLY, SHORT LIMBS, CONGENITAL HEART DISEASE, EAR ANOMALIES, AND SKIN DEFECTS (SAKATI-NYHAN-TISDALE SYNDROME)

Sakati et al. (17) described a sporadic malformation syndrome consisting of acrocephalopolysyndactyly, short limbs, congenital heart disease, ear anomalies, and skin defects. A chromosome study revealed no abnormality.

A large calvaria with disproportionately small face was noted. The orbits were shallow, and the eyes prominent. All cranial sutures were synostosed. The ears were dysplastic and low-set. A unilateral ear tag was noted. Patches of alopecia with atrophic skin were present above the ears. Linear scarlike lesions were observed in the submental area. The palate was narrow and highly arched. Maxillary hypoplasia and crowding of the upper teeth were reported. The neck was short, and the hairline was low.

Short arms, cubitus valgus, and short broad hands were evident. Fusion of the proximal interphalangeal joints of the fourth fingers, radial deviation of the distal phalanx of the fifth fingers, and proximally placed thumbs were observed. A sixth digit had been surgically removed from the right hand.

Extreme shortening of the legs and adducted feet were observed, together with polysyndactyly there being seven toes on the right foot and six

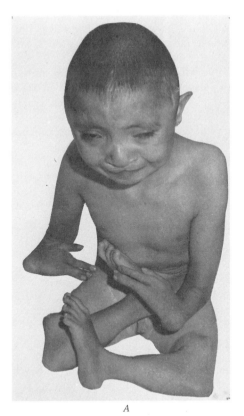 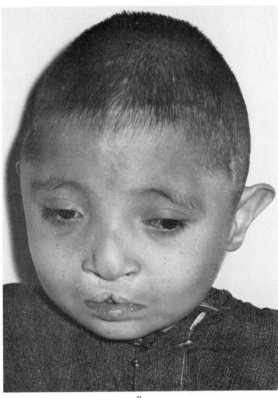

A   B

Figure 40-7. *Craniosynostosis, severe symmetrically malformed extremities, and cleft lip-palate (Herrmann-Pallister-Opitz syndrome).* (A–B). Note symmetric limb malformations, microbrachycephaly, ocular hypertelorism, repaired cleft lip. (*From J. Herrmann et al.,* Rocky Mt. Med. J. **66**:45, 1969.)

toes on the left foot. Roentgenographic examination revealed bilateral coxa valga, lateral bowing of both femurs, hypoplastic tibias, deformity and displacement of the fibulas, and abnormal malposed tarsals and metatarsals. There were six metatarsals in each foot (Fig. 40-8).

Other findings included congenital heart disease, widely spaced nipples, cryptorchism, small phallus, and inguinal hernia. Intelligence was normal.

CRANIOSYNOSTOSIS AND RADIOULNAR SYNOSTOSIS (BERANT SYNDROME)

Berant and Berant (4) described an autosomal dominant condition in which craniosynostosis occurred together with radioulnar synostosis.

Involvement of the sagittal suture and concomitant dolichocephaly were observed.

CRANIOSYNOSTOSIS, DWARFISM, RETINITIS PIGMENTOSA AND OTHER ANOMALIES (ARMENDARES SYNDROME)

Armendares et al. (2) reported a presumably autosomal recessive or X-linked recessive condition characterized by postnatal onset growth deficiency, microcephaly, cranial asymmetry, craniosynostosis, small face, scant eyebrows, short nose, micrognathia, highly arched palate, ptosis of eyelids, epicanthal folds, retinitis pigmentosa, malformed auricles, short fifth fingers, and simian creases.

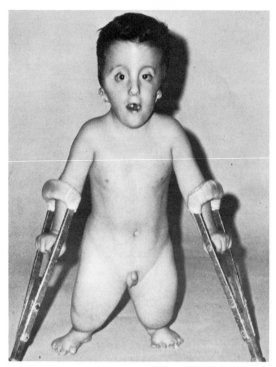

Figure 40-8. *Acrocephalopolysyndactyly, short limbs, congenital heart disease, ear anomalies, and skin defects (Sakati-Nyhan-Tisdale syndrome).* Unusual facies, bizarre low-set pinnas, shortened limbs, and polysyndactyly of feet. *(From N. Sakati et al.,* J. Pediatr. **79:**104, 1971.)

CRANIOSYNOSTOSIS AND FOOT ANOMALIES (WEISS SYNDROME)

Weiss (20) reported an autosomal dominant syndrome consisting of craniosynostosis and medially deviated great toes with alterations in tarsal morphogenesis. Some patients exhibited mild syndactyly. Wide variability of craniofacial involvement ranged from severe oxycephaly to no obvious alteration. Individual members of this pedigree could easily be mistaken as examples of Pfeiffer syndrome or Crouzon syndrome.

CRANIOSYNOSTOSIS, BRACHY-DACTYLY, AND FAILURE OF TOOTH ERUPTION (FAIRBANKS SYNDROME)

Fairbanks (8) described a short male (124 cm) adult patient with stubby hands and fingers. His head was turribrachycephalic with a supraorbital

transverse depression. The eyes were exophthalmic. His legs were short. There was limited extension at the knees and elbows and lumbar lordosis.

Roentgenographic studies at 10 years showed digital impressions in the calvaria, enlarged sella, short phalanges with cone-shaped epiphyses and cystic alterations in the lower metaphyses of the femurs. The digital impressions and cystic changes disappeared with age. The phalanges and metacarpals became short and wide. The teeth never erupted. A patient having virtually identical changes was seen by T. Keats (personal communication, 1975).

CRANIOSYNOSTOSIS AND 7p— KARYOTYPE

Only four instances of craniosynostosis with 7p— or 7r karyotype are known to date. Phenotypic expression has been variable and may be related to the extent of deletion. The disorder needs to be further delineated. Findings have included craniosynostosis, high forehead, flat occiput, microcephaly, mental deficiency, growth retardation, upslanting or downslanting palpebral fissures, ptosis of the eyelids, ocular hypotelorism, proptosis, microcornea, depressed nasal bridge, anteverted nostrils, low-set ears, submucous cleft palate, bifid uvula, widely spaced nipples, sacral dimple, genital anomalies, long slender fingers and toes, square hands with shortened third fingers, and talipes equinovarus (21, 22, J. Hall, personal communication, 1975).

CRANIOSYNOSTOSIS, ECTODERMAL DYSPLASIA, AND SHORT STATURE

Andersen and Pindborg (1) described a girl with cranial dysostosis, blindness, short stature, impacted teeth, hair defects, dry skin, saddle nose, and everted lips.

CRANIOSYNOSTOSIS, SKELETAL ANOMALIES, AND LIMB DEFECTS

Waardenburg (19) reported a patient with craniosynostosis, hydrophthalmos, cleft palate, malposed clavicles, contractures at the elbows and knees, multiple defects of the hands and feet, genital abnormalities, and congenital heart disease.

CRANIOSYNOSTOSIS AND KNEE DISLOCATION

We have observed a sporadic instance of a distinctive syndrome consisting of craniosynostosis with marked scaphocephaly, mental deficiency, cardiovascular defect, camptodactyly of the fingers, deviation of the fingers to the ulnar side, short first metacarpals with proximally placed thumbs, complete anterior dislocation of the tibia and fibula, and clubfeet.

CRANIOSYNOSTOSIS, EAR TAGS, AND SKELETAL ANOMALIES

We have also observed a sporadic occurrence of an unusual syndrome characterized by cranio-synostosis with scaphocephaly, mental deficiency, downslanting palpebral fissures, beaked nose, small low-set and posteriorly rotated ears, large ear tags, micrognathia, long neck, sloping shoulders, narrow thorax, pectus carinatum, winging of the scapulas, and cubitus valgus.

OTHER SYNDROMES WITH CRANIOSYNOSTOSIS

Other disorders in which craniosynostosis is either an occasional or secondary abnormality have been presented elsewhere (7, 14, 16). Many of these conditions have been reviewed by Duggan et al. (7).

REFERENCES

1 Andersen, T. H., and Pindborg, J. J., Et tilfaelde af total "pseudo-anodonti" i forbindelse med kraniedeformitet, dvaergvaekst og ektodermal dysplasi. *Odont. T.* **55:**472–483, 1947.

2 Armendares, S., et al., A Newly Recognized Inherited Syndrome of Dwarfism, Craniosynostosis, Retinitis Pigmentosa, and Multiple Congenital Malformations. *J. Pediatr.* **85:**872–873, 1974.

3 Baller, F., Radiusaplasie und Inzucht. *Z. Menschl. Vererb. Konstit. Lehre* **29:**782–790, 1950.

4 Berant, W., and Berant, N., Radioulnar Synostosis and Craniosynostosis Syndromes. *Birth Defects* **11**(2):137–189, 1973.

5 Christian, J. C., et al., The Adducted Thumbs Syndrome: An Autosomal Recessive Disease with Arthrogryposis Dysmyelination, Craniostenosis, and Cleft Palate. *Clin. Genet.* **2:**95–103, 1971.

6 Cohen, M. M., Jr., An Etiologic and Nosologic Overview of Craniosynostosis Syndromes. *Birth Defects* **11**(2):137–189, 1975.

7 Duggan, C. A., et al., Secondary Craniosynotosis. *Am. J. Roentgenol.* **109:**277–293, 1970.

8 Fairbanks, T., Acrocephaly with Abnormalities of the Extremities. *An Atlas of General Affections of the Skeleton,* 1951, E. and S. Livingstone, Ltd., Edinburgh and London (Case 84).

9 Gerold, M., Frakturheilung bei einen seltenen Fall kongenitaler Anomalie der oberen Gliedmassen. *Zentralbl. Chir.* **84:**831–834, 1959.

10 Gorlin, R. J., et al., Craniofacial Dysostosis, Patent Ductus Arteriosus, Hypertrichosis, Hypoplasia of Labia Majora, Dental and Eye Anomalies – A New Syndrome? *J. Pediatr.* **56:**778–785, 1960.

11 Greitzer, L., et al., Craniosynostosis – Radial Aplasia Syndrome. *J. Pediatr.* **84:**723–724, 1974.

12 Herrmann, J., and Opitz, J. M., An Unusual Form of Acrocephalosyndactyly. *Birth Defects* **5**(3):39–42, 1969.

13 Herrmann, J., et al., Craniosynostosis and Craniosynostosis Syndromes. *Rocky Mt. Med. J.* **66:**45–56, 1969.

14 Hootnick, D., and Holmes, L. B., Familial Polysyndactyly and Craniofacial Anomalies. *Clin. Genet.* **3:**128–134, 1972.

15 Lowry, R. B., Congenital Absence of the Fibula and Craniosynostosis in Sibs. *J. Med. Genet.* **9:**227–229, 1972.

16 Opitz, J. M., and Kaveggia, E. G., The FG Syndrome. An X-Linked Recessive Syndrome of Multiple Congenital Anomalies and Mental Retardation. *Z. Kinderheilkd.,* in press.

17 Sakati, N., et al., A New Syndrome with Acrocephalopolysyndactyly, Cardiac Disease, and Distinctive Defects of the Ear, Skin, and Lower Limbs. *J. Pediatr.* **79:**104–109, 1971.

18 Summitt, R. L., Recessive Acrocephalosyndactyly with Normal Intelligence. *Birth Defects* **5**(3):35–38, 1969.

19 Waardenburg, P. J., Eine merkwürdige Kombination von angeborenen Missbildugen: Doppelseitiger Hydrophthalmus Nerbunden mit Akrokephalosyndaktylie, Herzfehler, Pseudomermaphroditismus und anderen Abweichungen. *Klin. Mbl. Augenheilk.* **92:**29, 1934.

20 Weiss, L., cited in Smith, D. W., Syndromes II, Birth Defects, *Proc. 4th Int. Conf.,* Vienna, Austria, September 2–8, 1973, Excerpta Medica, Amsterdam, 1974, pp. 309–310.

21 Wilson, M. G., et al., Giant Satellites or Translocation? *Cytogen. Cell Genet.* **12:**209–214, 1973.

22 Zachai, E. H., and Breg, W. R., Ring Chromosome 7 with Variable Phenotypic Expression (Abstract). *Ped. Res.* **6:**358, 1972.

41

Craniotubular Bone Dysplasias
and Hyperostoses

There has been much confusion attendant to genetic disorders of bone characterized by modeling errors of tubular and cranial bones. Gorlin et al. (1) divided the craniotubular dysplasias into Pyle disease, craniometaphyseal dysplasia, craniodiaphyseal dysplasia, frontometaphyseal dysplasia, Schwarz-Lélek syndrome, dysosteosclerosis, and oculodentoosseous dysplasia. The craniotubular hyperostoses consist of van Buchem disease, sclerosteosis, congenital hyperphosphatasia, and Camurati-Engelmann disease.

Within the compass of this text, only a few of these conditions can be considered, and these only in abbreviated form. Frontometaphyseal dysplasia is considered elsewhere in this text, since it may represent a metabolic (storage) disease. Others, such as Pyle disease, dysosteosclerosis, and Camurati-Engelmann disease, will not be discussed here since they have no orofacial manifestations.

CRANIOMETAPHYSEAL DYSPLASIA

This disorder, often erroneously reported as Pyle disease, is characterized by a bizarre facies. Usually within the first year of life, the root of the nose begins to broaden and often hypertelorism becomes evident.

Increasing bony sclerosis narrows the nasal lumen, leading to obstruction, with resultant open mouth (Fig. 41-1A, B). Alterations in the temporal bone and pyramid frequently produce disturbances of sound conduction or perception. Deafness usually becomes evident before puberty. Rarely, defective vision or facial paralysis is noted.

Roentgenographically, the calvaria exhibits frontal and occipital hyperostosis or sclerosis. Most marked is frontonasal hyperostosis (Fig. 41-1C). The long bones have a "club-shaped" metaphyseal flare that is far milder than that seen in Pyle disease and may be minimal during the first years of life. Diaphyseal sclerosis is noted in the young but disappears with age. The short tubular bones exhibit the same changes as those noted in long bones (Fig. 41-1D, E).

Craniometaphyseal dysplasia may have both autosomal dominant (2–12) and recessive (13–21) transmission. In the recessive form of craniometaphyseal dysplasia, the clinical alterations are more severe than those noted in the dominant form (Fig. 41-2A–C). Nasal obstruction is usually complete, resulting in permanently open mouth. The skull is larger and thicker, and a history of cranial nerve alteration is far more common than in the dominant type. In sporadic cases, the authors cannot distinguish the dominant from the recessive form on a clinical basis.

CRANIODIAPHYSEAL DYSPLASIA

Gorlin et al. (1) employed the term "craniodiaphyseal dysplasia" to designate a severe bone

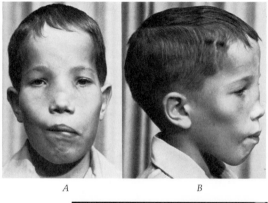

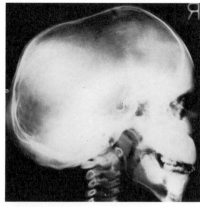

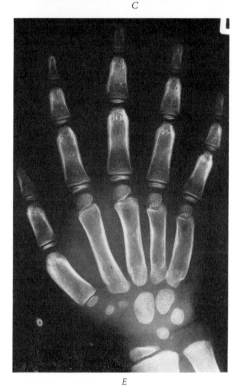

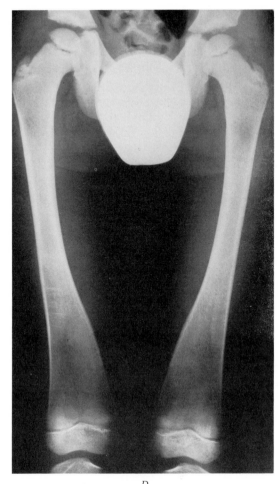

Figure 41-1. *Craniometaphyseal dysplasia—dominant form.* (*A, B*). Eleven-year-old boy with progressive mixed deafness. Note widened nasal bridge, left facial palsy. Mother and sister were similarly affected. (*C*). Skull of six-year-old male showing frontooccipital hyperostosis, sclerosis of skull base and facial bones, underpneumatization of sinuses and mastoids, and dolichocephaly with postcoronal depression of parietal bones. (*D*). Femurs of same child showing club-shaped metaphyseal flare, minimal diaphyseal sclerosis. (*E*). Hands of same child exhibiting under-modeling of short tubular bones, with distal cortical sclerosis of phalanges.

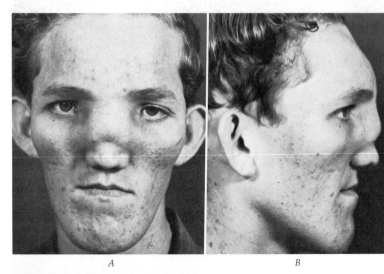

Figure 41-2. *Craniometaphyseal dysplasia — recessive form.* (*A, B*). Seventeen-year-old boy exhibiting bony overgrowth of frontal, nasal, and maxillary bones, ocular hypertelorism, and mild mandibular prognathism. Sister was more severely affected. (*C*). Marked bony overgrowth, especially of maxillary, nasal, and frontal areas. (*From D. R. Millard et al.* Am. J. Surg. **113:**615, 1967.)

A   *B*

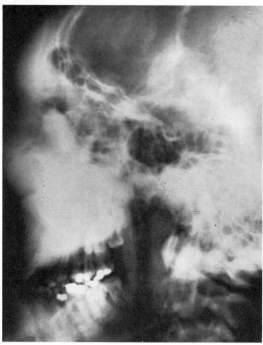

C

disorder characterized by massive generalized hyperostosis and sclerosis, especially involving the skull and facial bones (Fig. 41-3*A, B*).

Facial and cranial thickening, distortion, and enlargement are severe (22–25). Mental retardation has been present in most cases. Nasal obstruction appears within the first few years of life followed by marked bony thickening. Seizures, failure of vision, and deafness have been noted, as well as retardation of growth and absence of sexual maturity.

Roentgenographically, the skull and facial bones as well as the mandible are severely sclerotic and hyperostotic. There are moderate thickening and marked sclerosis of ribs and clavicles. The long tubular bones do not exhibit metaphyseal flare but have the shape of a policeman's nightstick and show diaphyseal endostosis (Fig. 41-3*C, D*).

Autosomal recessive inheritance appears to be most likely.

SCHWARZ-LÉLEK SYNDROME

The patients described by Schwarz (27) and Lélek (26) appear to have a distinct syndrome comprising severe genu varum and marked frontal bossing (Fig. 41-4*A*).

Roentgenographically, the changes in the humerus, hands, clavicles, and ribs were similar to those in Pyle disease. However, there was massive internal bowing of the femur, with radiolucent splaying of the metaphyseal area (Fig. 41-4*B*). Hyperostosis and mild sclerosis of the skull, especially in the frontal and occipital areas, as well as in the maxilla and mandible, were marked. The paranasal sinuses were obliterated. Serum alkaline phosphatase level was elevated. Both cases were isolated examples.

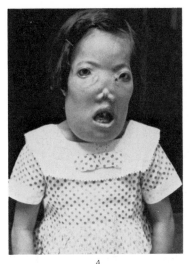

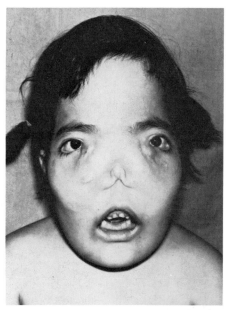

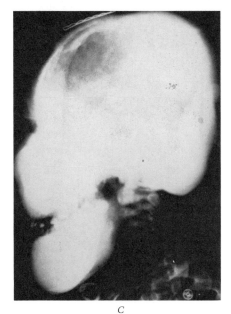

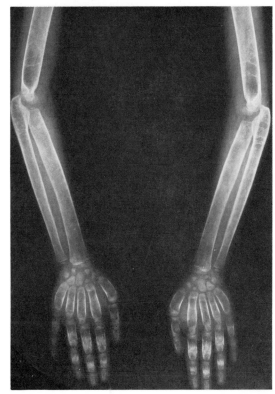

Figure 41-3. *Craniodiaphyseal dysplasia.* (*A*). Fourteen-year-old girl with severe distortion of face and skull. Head circumference was 57 cm. (*B*). Similar facial changes in another patient (from R. I. Macpherson. *J. Can. Assoc. Radiol.* **25**:22, 1974). (*C*). Marked thickening and sclerosis of all craniofacial bones. (*D*). Osteoporosis, "policeman's nightstick" appearance, lack of normal modeling. (*From E. Stransky et al.,* Ann. Paediatr. **199**:393, 1962.)

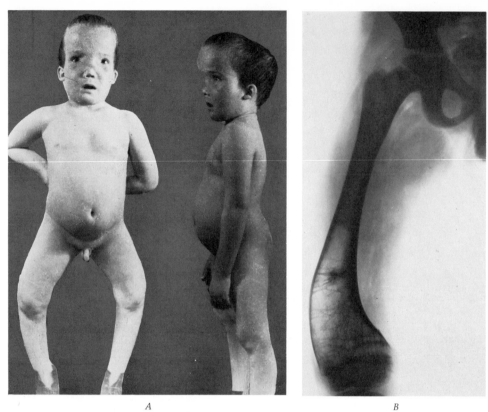

A   *B*

Figure 41.4. *Schwarz-Lélek syndrome.* (*A*). Nine-year-old male, 122 cm tall. Note large skull, frontal bossing, severe genu varum. (*B*). Femur is symmetrically broadened and bent inward in distal portion. Proximal femur is sclerotic, distal femur thinned, genu varum. (*From I. Lélek*, Fortschr. Röntgenstr. **94:**702, 1965.)

VAN BUCHEM DISEASE

Van Buchem disease, or "generalized cortical hyperostosis," is characterized by mandibular enlargement and diaphyseal thickening. The disorder exhibits autosomal recessive inheritance (28–31).

Facial changes develop slowly but usually become apparent before the second decade. The most characteristic alteration is broadening and prominence of the mandible, but the teeth are usually in normal occlusion. Occasionally there is mild exophthalmos.

Patients experience headache, unilateral or rarely bilateral facial paralysis, optic atrophy, and progressive sensorineural hearing loss. Thickening of the calvaria and increased density of the skull base are constant features. The body of the mandible is greatly enlarged in all measurements; the angle is obtuse. The long tubular bones exhibit diaphyseal thickening and are rough-textured. The cortical hyperostosis is predominantly endosteal in character, and in severe cases, the medullary cavity is occluded. The transverse diameter of the diaphysis is normal or increased (Fig. 41-5*A*–*C*).

Alkaline phosphatase values are increased from 50 to 250 percent above normal.

SCLEROSTEOSIS

Hansen (33) described a disorder characterized by generalized osteosclerosis with hyperostosis of the calvaria, mandible, clavicles, and pelvis different from that observed in Van Buchem dis-

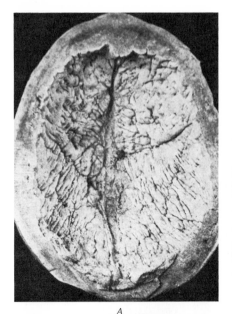

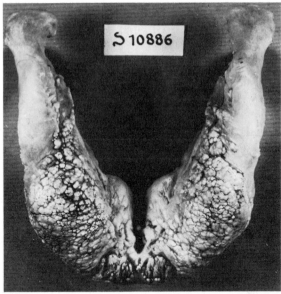

A

B

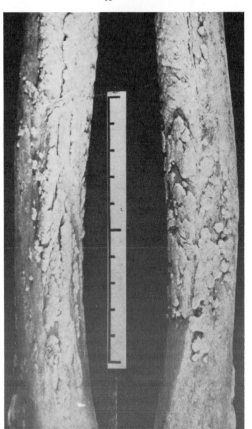

C

Figure 41-5. *Van Buchem disease.* (*A*). Marked thickening of calvaria. (*From F. S. P. van Buchem*, Acta Radiol. (Stockh.) **44**:109, 1955.) (*B*). Undersurface of mandible, showing marked broadening and osteophytic formation. (*From F. S. P van Buchem and H. N. Hadders*, Schweiz. Med. Wochenschr. **87**:231, 1957.) (*C*). Sclerosis and thickening of long bones with osteophytic formation. (*Courtesy of F. S. P. van Buchem, Haarlem, The Netherlands.*)

ease. It has been combined with syndactyly and other abnormalities of the digits in a number of cases (32–40).

Sclerosteosis is inherited as an autosomal recessive trait.

The typical facies, evident in infancy, is characterized by a steep high forehead, hypertelorism, broad flat nasal root, and a prognathic, broadened, squared mandible. Head circumference is enlarged (Fig. 41-6*A–C*). In many cases, sensorineural deafness appears early in infancy. Facial nerve paralysis appears later but is almost as frequent in occurrence. Characteristically, it is unilateral for many years. Optic atrophy, reduced visual fields, convergent strabismus, nystagmus, exophthalmos, chronic headache, and decreased sensory function of the trigeminal nerve have been described.

Body height and proportions are normal. Commonly there is asymmetric cutaneous syn-

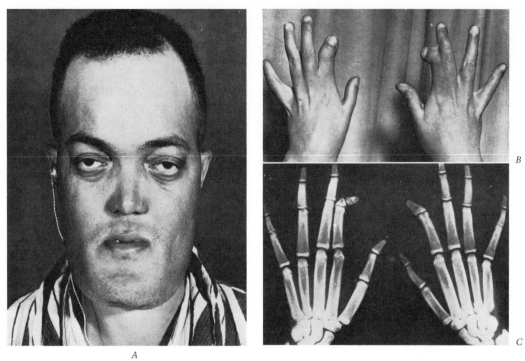

Figure 41-6. *Sclerosteosis.* (*A*). Square appearance of mandible, due in part to flattening of mandibular plane. Patient was deaf and had facial palsy. (*Courtesy of C. J. Witkop, Jr., Minneapolis, Minn.*) (*B*). Soft-tissue syndactyly of second and third fingers bilaterally. Third and fourth fingers partly fused unilaterally. Radial clinodactyly of index fingers. (*C*). Roentgenogram showing absent middle phalanx of one index finger and delta phalanx of other index finger, as well as general lack of modeling of tubular bones. (B and C from *A. S. Truswell*, J. Bone Joint Surg. **40B**:208, 1958.)

dactyly of the index and middle fingers. This often extends only to the proximal interphalangeal joint and there is radial deviation of the distal phalanx of the index fingers. Syndactyly of the toes is more variable.

Roentgenographically, the calvaria is greatly thickened and the tables are obliterated. The skull base is especially thickened. The inner acoustic meatus and optic canals are narrowed. The body of the mandible is greatly thickened and prognathic, and the angle is obtuse. The clavicles and ribs are broadened because of cortical thickening. The scapulas, pelvis, and vertebral bodies are uniformly sclerotic. The tubular bones, in addition to increased density, exhibit a lack of diaphyseal modeling. The index finger may have no middle phalanx or only a small triangular bone (delta phalanx).

CONGENITAL HYPERPHOSPHATASIA

This autosomal recessive disorder is characterized by hyperostosis affecting the skull and tubular bones, with replacement of the cortical bone by trabecular bone. It becomes manifest in early childhood with fever, bone pain, multiple fractures, and premature shedding of the teeth. Patients are dwarfed, with a large head, short neck, pigeon breast, and anteriorly bowed limbs. They exhibit blue scleras and tight skin. Hearing loss and retinal degeneration have been described in several cases (41–48) (Fig. 41-7A).

Roentgenographic changes include marked irregular thickening of the calvaria without sclerosis, coarse trabeculation of the mandible, and considerable expansion of the diaphyses of tubular bones. Generalized loss of bone results in

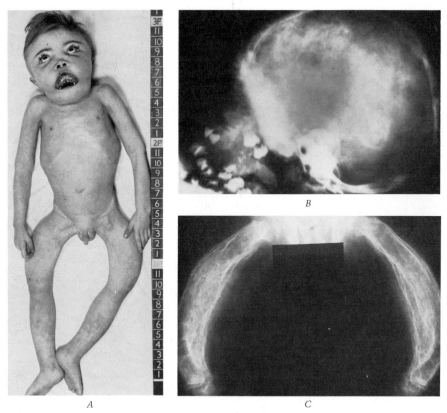

Figure 41-7. *Congenital hyperphosphatasia.* (*A*). Four-year-old child exhibiting enlargement of skull, obstruction of upper air passages, bowing of lower extremities, and extensive enlargement of maxilla. (*B*). Note changes similar to those observed in Paget's disease. (*C*). Marked thickening and bending of femurs with diaphyseal widening due to periosteal new bone formation. (*Courtesy of W. C. Marshall, London, England.*)

flattening of vertebral bodies, protrusion of the femoral heads into the pelvis, and bowing of long bones (Fig. 41-7B, C).

Alkaline phosphatase level is consistently elevated, and high levels of uric acid have been reported.

REFERENCES

GENERAL ASPECTS

1 Gorlin, R. J., et al., Genetic Craniotubular Bone Dysplasias and Hyperostoses. A Critical Analysis. *Birth Defects* **5**(4):79–95, 1969.

CRANIOMETAPHYSEAL DYSPLASIA — DOMINANT FORM

2 Brown, A., and Harper, R., Craniofacial Dysostosis: The Significance of Ocular Hypertelorism. *Q. J. Med.* **15**:171–182, 1946.

3 Guibaud, P., et al., La dysplasie cranio-métaphysaire. *Pédiatrie* **28**:149–161, 1973.

4 Holt, J. F., The Evolution of Cranio-metaphyseal Dysplasia. *Ann. Radiol. (Paris)* **9**:209–224, 1966.

5 Jackson, W. P. U., et al., Metaphyseal Dysplasia, Epiphyseal Dysplasia, Diaphyseal Dysplasia and Related Constitutions. *Arch. Intern. Med.* **94**:871–885, 1954 (cases 1–3).

6 Komins, C., Familial Metaphyseal Dysplasia. *Br. J. Radiol.* **27**:670–675, 1954.

7 Lejeune, E., et al., Une nouvelle observation de dysplasie

cranio-metaphysaire familiale. *J. Radiol. Electrol.* **49:** 493–498, 1968.

8 Mitchell, R. G., and Macleod, W., Leontiasis Ossea Due to Albers-Schönberg's Disease. *Br. J. Radiol.* **25:**442–445, 1952.

9 Paulsen, K., et al., Otorhinologische Gesichtspunkte bei der kraniometaphysären Dysplasie (Pyle-Syndrom). *Z. Laryngol. Rhinol.* **46:**916–927, 1967.

10 Rimoin, D. L., et al., Craniometaphyseal Dysplasia (Pyle's Disease): Autosomal Dominant Inheritance in a Large Kindred. *Birth Defects* 5(4):96–104, 1969.

11 Spranger, J., et al., Die kraniometaphysäre Dysplasie (Pyle). *Z. Kinderheilkd.* **93:**64–79, 1965.

12 Walker, N., Pyle's Disease or Cranio-metaphyseal Dysplasia. *Ann. Radiol. (Paris)* **9:**197–207, 1966.

CRANIOMETAPHYSEAL DYSPLASIA — RECESSIVE FORM

13 Graf, K., Die Bedeutung des Pyle-Syndroms (Leontiasis ossea) für die Oto-Rhino-Laryngologie. *Z. Laryngol. Rhinol.* **44:**438–445, 1965.

14 Jackson, W. P. U., et al., Metaphyseal Dysplasia, Epiphyseal Dysplasia, Diaphyseal Dysplasia and Related Constitutions. *Arch. Intern. Med.* **94:**871–885, 1954.

15 Lehmann, E. C. H., Familial Osteodystrophy of the Skull and Face. *J. Bone Joint Surg.* **39B:**313–315, 1957.

16 Lièvre, J. A., and Fischgold, H., Léontiasis ossea chez l'enfant (ostéopétrose partielle probable). *Presse Méd.* **64:**763–765, 1956.

17 Millard, D. R., et al., Craniofacial Surgery in Craniometaphyseal Dysplasia. *Am. J. Surg.* **113:**615–621, 1967.

18 Neuhauser, E. B. D., Growth, Differentiation and Disease. *Am. J. Roentgenol.* **69:**723–737, 1953.

19 Ross, M. W., and Altman, D. H., Familial Metaphyseal Dysplasia: Review of the Clinical and Radiological Features of Pyle's Disease. *Clin. Pediatr. (Bologna)* **6:**143–149, 1967.

20 Sommer, F., Eine besondere Form einer generalisierten Hyperostose mit Leontiasis ossea faciei et cranii. *Radiol. Clin. (Basel)* **23:**65–75, 1954.

21 Thoma, K. H., and Goldman, H. M., *Oral Pathology.* 5th ed., Mosby, St. Louis, 1960, pp. 627–634.

CRANIODIAPHYSEAL DYSPLASIA

22 Halliday, J., A Rare Case of Bone Dysplasia. *Br. J. Surg.* **37:**52–63, 1949–1950.

23 Joseph, R., et al., Dysplasie cranio-diaphysaire progressive: Ses relations avec la dysplasie diaphysaire progressive de Camurati-Engelmann. *Ann. Radiol. (Paris)* **1:**477–490, 1927.

24 Macpherson, R. I., Craniodiaphyseal Dysplasia, a Disease or Group of Diseases? *J. Can. Assoc. Radiol.* **25:**22–33, 1974 (Case 1).

25 Stransky, E., et al., On Paget's Disease with Leontiasis Ossea and Hypothyreosis Starting in Early Childhood. *Ann. Paediatr.* **199:**393–408, 1962.

SCHWARZ-LÉLEK SYNDROME

26 Lélek, I., Camurati-Engelmann'sche Erkrankung. *Fortschr. Röntgenstr.* **94:**702–712, 1961.

27 Schwarz, E., Craniometaphyseal Dysplasia. *Am. J. Roentgenol.* **94:**461–466, 1960.

VAN BUCHEM DISEASE

28 Fosmoe, R. J., et al., Van Buchem's Disease (Hyperostosis Corticalis Generalisata Familiaris). *Radiology* **90:**771–774, 1968.

29 Garland, L. H., Generalized Leontasis Ossea. *Am. J. Roentgenol.* **55:**37–43, 1946.

30 Van Buchem, F. S. P., et al., Hyperostosis Corticalis Generalisata Familiaris. *Acta Radiol.* **33:**109–119, 1955.

31 Van Buchem, F. S. P., et al., Hyperostosis Corticalis Generalisata: Report of Seven Cases. *Am. J. Med.* **33:**387–397, 1962.

SCLEROSTEOSIS

32 Falconer, A. W., and Ryrie, B. J., Report on a Familial Type of Generalized Osteosclerosis. *Presse Méd.* **195:**12–14, 1937.

33 Hansen, H. G., Sklerosteose, in H. Opitz and F. Schmid (eds.), *Handbuch der Kinderheilkunde,* Vol. 6. Berlin, Gottingen, Heidelberg, New York, 1967, Springer-Verlag, pp. 351–355.

34 Higinbotham, N. L., and Alexander, S. F., Osteopetrosis: Four Cases in One Family. *Am. J. Surg.* **53:**444–454, 1941.

35 Hirsch, I. S., Generalized Osteitis Fibrosa. *Radiology* **13:**44–84, 1929.

36 Kelley, C. H., and Lawlah, J. W., Albers-Schönberg Disease: A Familial Survey. *Radiology* **47:**507–513, 1946.

37 Klintworth, G. K., Neurologic Manifestations of Osteopetrosis (Albers-Schönberg's Disease). *Neurology* **13:**512–519, 1963.

38 Pietruschka, G., Weitere Mitteilungen über die Marmorknochenkrankheit. (Albers-Schönbergsche Krankheit) nebst Bemerkungen zur Differential-Diagnose. *Klin. Monatsbl. Augenheilk.* **132:**509–525, 1958.

38a Sugiura, Y., and Yasuhara, T., Sclerosteosis. *J. Bone Joint Surg.* **57A:**273–276, 1975.

39 Truswell, A. S., Osteopetrosis with Syndactyly: A Morphologic Variant of Albers-Schönberg's Disease. *J. Bone Joint Surg.* **40B:**208–218, 1958.

40 Witkop, C. J., Genetic Disease of the Oral Cavity, in R. W. Tiecke (ed.), *Oral Pathology.* McGraw-Hill, New York, 1965 [same kindred as in Kelley and Lawlah (36)].

CONGENITAL HYPERPHOSPHATASIA

41 Bakwin, H., and Eiger, M. S., Fragile Bones and Macrocranium. *J. Pediatr.* **49:**558–564, 1956.

42 Bakwin, H., et al., Familial Osteoectasia with Macrocranium. *Am. J. Roentgenol.* **91:**609–617, 1964.

43 Caffey, J., *Pediatric X-ray Diagnosis.* 4th ed., Year Book, Chicago, 1961, pp. 1042–1044.

44 Choremis, C., et al., Osteitis Deformans (Paget's Disease) in an 11-year-old Boy. *Helv. Paediatr. Acta* **13:**185–188, 1958.

45 Eyring, E. J., and Eisenberg, E., Congenital Hyperphosphatasia. *J. Bone Joint Surg.* **50A:**1099–1117, 1968.

46 Fanconi, G., et al., Osteochalasia desmalis familaris. *Helv. Paediatr. Acta* **19:**279–295, 1964.

47 Sorrel, E., and LeGrand, L., Dystrophie osseuse généralisée. *Bull. Soc. Pédiat. Paris* **36:**89–92, 1938.

48 Swoboda, W., Hyperostosis corticalis deformans juvenilis: Ungewöhnliche generalisierte Osteopathie bei zwei Geschwistern. *Helv. Paediatr. Acta* **13:**292–312, 1958.

42

Cryptophthalmos Syndrome

First described by Zehender (11) in 1872, the cryptophthalmos syndrome consists of (a) extension of the skin of the forehead to cover one or both eyes completely, (b) total or partial soft-tissue syndactyly of fingers and/or toes, (c) coloboma of the alae nasi, (d) unusual hairline, and (e) various urogenital abnormalities.

About 50 cases have been reported under a variety of names. The syndrome is inherited in an autosomal recessive pattern. Parental consanguinity has been present in at least 18 percent of patients. Especially good reviews are those of Ide and Wollschlaeger (5), Sugar (8), Otradovec and Janovsky (6), François (2), and Schönenberg (7).

SYSTEMIC MANIFESTATIONS

Facies and eyes. The face is not uncommonly asymmetric. The eyebrows may be completely or partially missing (12). The globes can be seen and felt beneath the skin covering which extends from the forehead over the eyes. In about 65 percent of the cases, cryptophthalmos is bilateral (Fig. 42-1A, B). Exposure to strong light may induce reflex wrinkling of the skin because of contraction of the orbicularis muscles. In case of unilateral cryptophthalmos, the opposite eye may exhibit upper lid coloboma, microphthalmia, epibulbar dermoid, or supernumerary eyebrows (8, 9). The conjunctival sac is partially or completely obliterated, and there is no sign of lashes, meibomian glands, or lacrimal glands. The cornea has been shown to be differentiated from the sclera. The lens may be absent, hypoplastic, or calcified and displaced. Orbicularis and levator palpebrae muscles are normal, however (12). Histopathologic alterations are especially well reviewed by François (2).

The hairline is bizarre in at least 25 percent of patients, extending over the entire temple area and tapering to a point in the skin of the forehead overlying the eyes.

Ear. The pinnas are small in at least 30 percent of the cases, and they may be low-set. Not uncommonly, the skin of the upper part of the helix is continuous with that of the scalp. The external auditory meatuses are narrowed (3, 5, 6, 10). There is usually conduction loss, and malformed ossicles have been noted (5).

Nose. Nasal abnormalities are seen in about half the patients. In most cases, there are malformed conchas and colobomas of the alae nasi, with a groove extending to the nasal tip (1, 3, 4, 8, 10, 11). The coloboma may be unilateral or bilateral.

Genitalia. Malformations of the genitals have included small penis, cryptorchism, chordee, hypospadias, and hypertrophy of the clitoris with vaginal atresia and incomplete labial development, i.e., female pseudohermaphroditism (3, 6, 10).

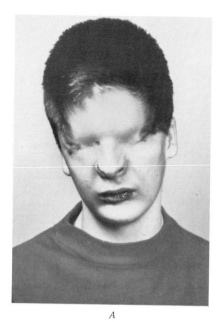

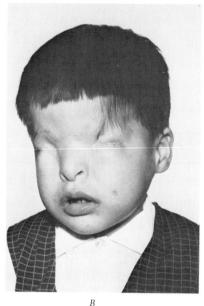

Figure 42-1. *Cryptophthalmos. (A). Skin extends from forehead covering eyes. Note tongue-shaped hair extensions. (From C. H. Ide and P. B. Wollschlaeger, Columbia, Mo.) (B). Similar alterations in Greenland boy. (From M. Warburg, Birth Defects* **7**(3):136, 1971.)

A *B*

Central Nervous System. Malformed parietal and temporal bones have been noted in about 20 percent of cases. Some patients have exhibited calcification of the falx cerebri. Ide and Wollschlaeger (5) found the foramen magnum to be heart-shaped with incomplete closure of the exoccipital portion of the occipital bone. Meningoencephalocele has been described in about 10 percent of cases (11, 12). A small percentage of patients have been found to be mentally retarded (5).

Extremities. Marked soft-tissue syndactyly has been present in about 40 percent of cases. It may include both fingers and toes (1, 5, 8, 9, 11, 12).

Miscellaneous anomalies. Anal atresia, umbilical hernia, and renal anomalies have been evident in 10 percent of patients (2, 3, 7, 10, 11).

Oral manifestations. Cleft lip and/or cleft palate and ankyloglossia have been noted in about 10 percent of the cases (1, 4, 5, 12). Laryngeal atresia or hypoplasia has also been present in about 10 percent (1, 10).

DIFFERENTIAL DIAGNOSIS

This disorder is so striking that other conditions would not be considered.

LABORATORY AIDS

None is known.

REFERENCES

1 Azevedo, E. S., et. al., Cryptophthalmos in Two Families from Bahia, Brazil. *J. Med. Genet.* **10**:389–392, 1973.

1a Dinno, N. D., et. al., The Cryptophthalmos-Syndactyly Syndrome. *Clin. Pediat.* **13**:219–224, 1974.

2 François, J., Syndrome malformatif avec cryptophtalmie. *Acta Genet. Med. (Roma)* **18**:18–50, 1969.

3 Gupta, S. P., and Saxena, R. C., Cryptophthalmos. *Br. J. Ophthalmol.* **46**:629–632, 1962.

4 Guttmann, A., Einseitiger Kryptophthalmos. *Zentralbl. Prakt. Augenheilkd.* **33**:264, 1909.

5 Ide, C. H., and Wollschlaeger, P. B., Multiple Congenital Abnormalities Associated with Cryptophthalmia. *Arch.*

Ophthalmol. **81**:640–644, 1969.

6 Otradovec, J., and Janovsky, M., Cryptophthalmos. *Čs. Oftal.* **18**:128–138, 1962.

7 Schönenberg, H., Kryptophthalmus-Syndrom. *Klin. Pediätr.* **185**:165–172, 1973.

8 Sugar, H. S., The Cryptophthalmos-Syndactyly Syndrome. *Am. J. Ophthalmol.* **66**:897–899, 1968.

9 Waring, G. O., and Shields, J. A., Partial Unilateral Cryptophthalmos with Syndactyly. Brachydactyly, and Renal Anomalies. *Am. J. Ophthalmol.* **79**:437–440, 1975.

10 Viallefont, H., et al., Un cas de cryptophtalmie. *Bull. Soc. Ophtal. Fr.* **65**:329–332, 1965.

11 Zehender, W., Eine Missgeburt mit hautüberwachsenen Augen oder Kryptophthalmus. *Klin. Monatsbl. Augenheilkd.* **10**:225–234, 1872.

12 Zinn, S., Kryptophthalmia. *Am. J. Ophthalmol.* **40**:219–223, 1955.

43

Cutis Laxa Syndromes

(Generalized Elastolysis)

Cutis laxa syndromes are characterized by (a) skin which hangs in loose folds, (b) emphysema, (c) hernia, and often (d) diverticulas of various organs. The first recorded cases are those of Variot and Cailliau (42) and Vaglio (41). Goltz and coworkers (15, 16) clearly separated this condition from other disorders.

Cutis laxa should not be confused with the Ehlers-Danlos syndromes. In cutis laxa, the skin although hyperextensible is also lax. There is an acquired postinflammatory type of cutis laxa. However, our discussion is limited to the congenital forms.

To date there are three known genetic forms of cutis laxa. A severe autosomal recessive form, in which affected sibs (9, 16, 26, 35, 36, 40, 45) and parental consanguinity (9, 26, 35, 40) have been reported, is known to occur. Less commonly observed is a relatively benign autosomal dominant form (3, 5, 19, 22, 35, 39). Several sporadic instances of mild involvement probably represent this form of the disorder (23, 24, 27, 31, 37, 41). Byers et al. (8) reported an X-linked form of cutis laxa in which there is deficiency of Lysyl oxidase, the collagen and elastin cross-linking enzyme. Lysyl oxidase activity in the mother of an affected male was intermediate between the control and the affected levels.

SYSTEMIC MANIFESTATIONS

Somatic as well as mental retardation (26, 28, 34) has been described. Most other aspects of the syndrome can be explained on the basis of generalized elastolysis.

Facies. The drooping and ectropion of the eyelids, together with the sagging facial skin (jowls) and accentuation of the nasolabial and other facial folds, produce a "bloodhound" or aged appearance (Figs. 43-1, 43-2). The nose is often hooked, the nostrils are everted, and the philtrum is long in the dominant type (Fig. 43-2). An affected pubertal child will often look older than his unaffected parents!

Skin. The skin of the entire body appears too large for the individual, often hanging in folds. It is not hyperplastic and there is no fragility or difficulty in healing.

Cardiorespiratory. Emphysema has been one of the more common features (2, 9, 16, 18, 27, 33, 36, 38), resulting from the generalized elastolysis. This causes right ventricular enlargement, bundle branch block, cor pulmonale, and often death at an early age (15, 16). Pulmonary stenosis (19, 21, 26) and extremely tortuous blood vessels (19, 44) have been described in the recessive type.

Musculoskeletal alterations. A few children have exhibited late closure of the anterior fontanel (14, 40, 45). In some, somatic growth has been retarded (21, 26, 40, 45) and muscles have been hypotonic (34, 45). Hip dislocation (40, 45), joint hyperextensibility (35, 45), and inguinal (3,

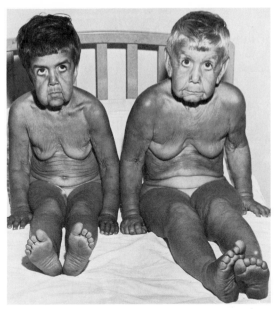

Figure 43-1. *Cutis laxa.* Affected sibs with autosomal recessive type of cutis laxa look much older than their chronologic ages of five and six years. (*From F. A. Balboni, Garden City, N.Y.*)

9, 26, 35, 36, 38, 39), diaphragmatic (11, 16, 33), and umbilical (16, 36) hernias have been described.

Gastrointestinal tract. Diverticulas of the gastrointestinal tract [esophagus (16), stomach (16), and intestine (11, 36)] and prolapse of the gastric

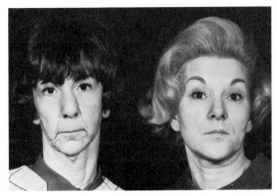

Figure 43-2. Autosomal dominant type of cutis laxa in fifteen-year-old girl who looks older than her middle-aged mother. (*From P. E. Beighton, Br. J. Plast. Surg.* **23**:285, 1970.)

(16, 36) and rectal (16, 26) mucosa have been noted.

Genitourinary system. Bladder diverticulas have been described by several authors (15, 16, 33, 36).

Eye. Other than ectropion (16, 18, 33) of the lids, which results from the generalized elastolysis, a wide variety of uncommon changes has been observed, including hypertelorism (40, 45), iris hypoplasia (34, 45), blue scleras, and microcornea (45).

Oral manifestations. Several authors have recorded micrognathia and delayed or bizarre tooth eruption (34, 40, 45). The voice is usually deep and resonant in quality, resulting from laxity of vocal cords (5, 16, 24, 37). Our limited experience suggests thickening of the oral and pharyngeal mucosa (16).

DIFFERENTIAL DIAGNOSIS

So-called "acquired cutis laxa" may follow cutaneous inflammation. A number of cases have been described and especially well reviewed by Marshall (23), Reed et al. (29), and Verhagen and Woerdeman (42a). It should be noted that in the case of Jablonska (20), the patient subsequently developed pulmonary emphysema. Bettman's patient (6) did not develop cutis laxa until forty-nine years of age. In addition to grotesque cutaneous changes, he exhibited multiple hernias and intestinal and oral diverticulas.

Braun-Falco et al. (7) were dealing with a case of prune-belly. We cannot classify the case of deBarsay et al. (4). Tracheobronchiomegaly (Mounier-Kuhn syndrome) is characterized by dilatation and diverticulas of the trachea and bronchi (1, 45) with blephalochalasis and redundancy of oral mucosa (Ascher syndrome?).

An unusual disorder, *gerodermia osteodysplastica,* inherited as an X-linked trait, is characterized by generalized hyperlaxity, atrophy, and aging of the skin, hyperlaxity of joints, growth retardation, predisposition to skeletal fractures, and platyspondyly.

Debré et al. (12), Fittke (14), and Kaye and Fisher (20a) described cutis laxa with wide-open fontanels and various other skeletal alterations. This probably represents a separate syndrome.

Also to be excluded are the "wrinkly skin syndrome," a recessively inherited disorder characterized by congenital wrinkling of the skin of the chest, abdomen, and dorsa of the hands and feet (14a).

Cutis laxa has also been found in association with a dominantly inherited syndrome of corneal lattice dystrophy, cranial nerve palsy, and nephropathy. Blepharochalasis may be marked (26a).

LABORATORY AIDS

With orcein or other elastic fiber stain, absence or marked diminution of elastic fibers has been observed histologically (16–18).

Several investigators have found low serum copper levels (16, 18).

In the X-linked form of cutis laxa, lysyl oxidase deficiency can be demonstrated in dermal fibroblasts; intermediate activity can be demonstrated in carrier mothers (8).

REFERENCES

1 Aaby, G. V., and Blake, H. A., Tracheobronchiomegaly. *Ann. Thorac. Surg.* **2**:64–70, 1966.

2 Bakker, B. J., Cutis laxa universalis und Lungenemphysem. *Hautarzt* **10**:271–272, 1959.

3 Balboni, F. A., Cutis Laxa and Multiple Vascular Anomalies. Including Coarctation of the Aorta. *Bull, St. Francis Hosp. (Roslyn)* **19**:26–34, 1963.

4 de Barsy, A. M., et al., Dwarfism, Oligophrenia and Degeneration of the Elastic Tissue in Skin and Cornea: A New Syndrome? *Helv. Paediatr. Acta* **23**:305–313, 1968.

5 Beighton, P., et al., The Dominant and Recessive Forms of Cutis Laxa. *J. Med. Genet.* **9**:216–221, 1972.

6 Bettman, A. G., Excessively Relaxed Skin and the Pituitary Gland. *Plast. Reconstr. Surg.* **15**:489–501, 1955.

7 Braun-Falco, O., et al., Angeborene Dermatochalasis als Leitsymptom eines Symptomkomplexes. *Arch. Klin. Exp. Dermatol.* **220**:166–182, 1964.

8 Byers, P. H., et al., An X-linked Form of Cutis Laxa Due to Deficiency of Lysyl Oxidase; the Collagen and Elastin Crosslinking Enzyme. *Birth Defects*, in press.

9 Cashman, M. E., Cutis Laxa. *Proc. R. Soc. Med.* **50**:719–720, 1957.

10 Chatfield, H. W., Cutis Laxa. *Br. J. Dermatol.* **81**:387–388, 1969.

11 Christiaens, L., et al., Emphyseme congénital et cutis laxa. *Presse Méd.* **62**:1799–1801, 1954.

12 Debré, R., et al., "Cutis laxa" avec dystrophies osseuses. *Bull. Soc. Méd. Hôp. Paris* **53**:1038–1039, 1937.

13 Dingman, R. O., et al., Cutis Laxa Congenita – Generalized Elastosis. *Plast. Reconstr. Surg.* **44**:431–435, 1969.

14 Fittke, H., Über eine ungewöhnliche Form "multipler Erbabartung" (Chalodermie und Dysostose). *Z. Kinderheilkd.* **63**:510–523, 1942.

14a Gazit, E., et al., The Wrinkly Skin Syndrome: A New Heritable Disorder of Connective Tissue. *Clin. Genet.* **4**:186–192, 1973.

15 Goltz, R. W. and Hult, A. M., Generalized Elastolysis (Cutis Laxa) and Ehlers-Danlos Syndrome (Cutis Hyperelastica). *South. Med. J.* **58**:848–854, 1965.

16 Goltz, R. W., et al., Cutix Laxa, a Manifestation of Generalized Elastolysis. *Arch. Dermatol.* **92**:373–387, 1965.

17 Grahame, R., and Beighton, P., The Physical Properties of Skin in Cutis Laxa. *Br. J. Dermatol.* **84**:326–329, 1971.

18 Hajjar, B. A., and Joyner, E. W., Congenital Cutis Laxa with Advanced Cardiopulmonary Disease. *J. Pediatr.* **73**:116–118, 1968.

19 Hayden, J. G., et al., Cutis Laxa Associated with Pulmonary Artery Stenosis. *J. Pediatr.* **72**:506–509, 1968.

20 Jablonska, S., Inflammatorische Hautveränderungen, die einer erworbenen Cutis laxa vorausgehen. *Hautarzt* **17**:341–346, 1966.

20a Kaye, C. I., and Fisher, D. E., Cutis Laxa and Associated Anomalies. *Birth Defects* **11**(2):130–131, 1975.

21 Koblenzer, P. J., and Lo Presti, P. J., Dermatochalasia (Dermatomegaly) and Congenital Pulmonic Stenosis. *Arch. Dermatol.* **97**:602–603, 1968.

22 Lewis, E., Cutis Laxa. *Proc. R. Soc. Med.* **41**:864–865, 1948.

23 Marshall, J., et al., Post Inflammatory Elastolysis and Cutis Laxa. *S. Afr. Med. J.* **40**:1016–1022, 1966.

24 Maxwell, E., and Esterly, N. B., Cutis Laxa. *Am. J. Dis. Child.* **117**:479–482, 1969.

25 McCarthy, C. F., et al., Loose Skin (Cutis Laxa) Associated with Systemic Abnormalities. *Arch. Intern. Med.* **115**:625–627, 1965.

26 Mendoza, H. R., Cutis laxa. *Rev. Esp. Pediatr.* **24**:735–740, 1968.

26a Meretoja, J., Genetic Aspects of Familial Amyloidosis with Corneal Lattice Dystrophy and Cranial Neuropathy. *Clin. Genet.* **4**:173–185, 1973.

27 Nitishin, A., Cutis Laxa with Bilateral Pulmonary Emphysema. *Arch. Dermatol.* **95**:334–336, 1967.

28 Raspi, M., Di un caso di cutis laxa. *Riv. Clin. Pediatr.* **25**:648–649, 1927.

29 Reed, W. B., et al., Acquired Cutis Laxa. *Arch. Dermatol.* **103**:661–669, 1971.

30 Reidy, J. P., Cutis Hyperelastica (Ehlers-Danlos) and Cutis Laxa. *Br. J. Plast. Surg.* **16**:84–89, 1963.

31 Robinson, H. M., and Ellis, F. A., Cutis Laxa. *Arch. Dermatol.* **77**:656–665, 1958.

32 Rossbach, M. J., Ein merkwürdiger Fall von griesenhafter Veränderung der allgemeinen Körperdecke bei einem achtzehnjährigen Jüngling. *Arch. Klin. Med.* **36**:197–203, 1884.

33 Schreiber, M. M., and Tilley, J. C.: Cutis Laxa (Case 4). *Arch. Dermatol.* **84:**266–272, 1961.

34 Schirren, C., et al., Ektodermale Dysplasie mit Hypohidrosis, Hypotrichosis, und Hypodontie. *Hautarzt* **11:**70–75, 1960.

35 Sestak, Z., Ehlers-Danlos Syndrome and Cutis Laxa: An Account of Families in the Oxford Area. *Ann. Hum. Genet.* **25:**313–321, 1962.

36 Siegmund, L., Über das sogennante Oedema lymphangiectaticum. *Zentralbl. Allg. Pathol.* **70:**243, 1938.

37 Siemens, H. W., and Eindhoven, C. A., Über Chalasis cutis universalis congenita und über secondäre Chalasis cutis bei Cutis elastica. *Arch. Dermatol. Syphilol.* (*Berl.*) **183:**135–141, 1942–1943.

38 Spyropulos, N., Gerodermia generalisata congenita mit Hypoplasie und Hypotonie der Muskulatur. *Kinderärztl. Prax.* **12:**72–76, 1941.

39 Talbot, F. B., Metabolism Study of a Case Simulating Premature Senility. *Monatsschr. Kinderheilkd.* **25:**643–646, 1923.

40 Theopold, W., and Wildhack, R., Dermatochalasis in Rahmen multipler Abartungen. *Monatsschr. Kinderheilkd.* **99:**213–218, 1951.

41 Vaglio, R., Uno caso di cutis laxa. *Pediatria* (*Napoli*) **31:**321–323, 1923.

42 Variot, –, and Cailliau, –, Peau ridée sénile chez un enfant de deux ans. Agénésie des réseux élastique du derme. *Bull. Soc. Méd. Hôp. Paris* **43:**989–994, 1919.

42a Verhagen, A. R., and Woerdeman, M. J., Post-inflammatory Elastolysis and Cutis Laxa. *Br. J. Dermatol.* **92:**183–190, 1975.

43 Wagstaff, L. A., et al., Vascular Abnormalities in Congenital Generalized Elastolysis (Cutis Laxa). *S. Afr. Med. J.* **44:**1125–1127, 1970.

44 Wanderer, A. A., et al., Tracheobronchiomegaly and Acquired Cutis Laxa in a Child. *Pediatrics* **44:**709–715, 1969.

45 Wiedemann, H. R., Über einige progeroide Krankheitsbilder und deren diagnostische Einordnung (Case 2). *Z. Kinderheilkd.* **107:**91–106, 1969.

44

Diastrophic Dwarfism

amy and Morateaux (5) used the term "diastrophic dwarfism" to describe a syndrome consisting of (a) micromelic dwarfism, (b) progressive scoliosis, (c) bilateral talipes equinovarus and various deformities of the digits, (d) hip dysplasia, (e) characteristic external ear deformities, and, frequently, (f) cleft palate. Over 120 cases have been described (17). Early examples are those of Schenk (12) in 1910 and Duken (2) in 1921. The most complete survey is that of Walker et al. (17).

The syndrome has autosomal recessive inheritance. Its occurrence in sibs and parental consanguinity have been observed (10, 15). Fertility seems to be reduced (17).

Prior to the delineation of this syndrome in 1960, cases in infants were generally classified as examples of "achondroplasia with clubbed feet," and in adults, as the Morquio syndrome (2, 4).

In the so-called "diastrophic variant," the patient is taller, general skeletal deformity is less marked, and the clubfoot is not so resistant to treatment (17).

SYSTEMIC MANIFESTATIONS

About 25 percent of these patients die in infancy of aspiration pneumonia or respiratory distress. The somewhat hoarse cry, noted in several infants, may be related to abnormal laryngeal cartilages which may, in turn, be related to poor prognosis (17). Intelligence is normal.

Facies. The face tends to be square, with a narrow nasal bridge, broad midnose, flared nostrils, and circumoral fullness (17). The external auditory canals may be narrowed.

Musculoskeletal alterations. Mesomelic dwarfism is a constant feature. Mean birth length is

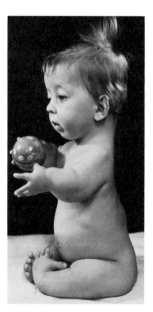

Figure 44-1. *Diastrophic dwarfism.* Infant showing micromelic dwarfism, scoliosis, bilateral talipes equinovarus, deviated thumbs, and halluces. (*From J. Spranger and H. Gerken,* Z. Kinderheilkd. **98**:227, 1967).

250

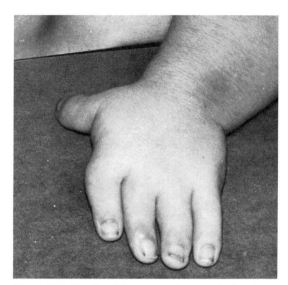

Figure 44-2. Hand and fingers are short, with thumb proximally placed.

about 33 cm. Mean adult height is about 112 cm with males ranging from 86 to 127 cm and females from 104 to 122 cm (17). There is shortening of all limbs (Fig. 44-1). Bilateral talipes equinovarus is severe, becomes worse with age, is resistant to treatment, and tends to recur after therapy. The patients bear their weight on their toes; thus walking is limited.

The thumbs are proximally inserted, hypermobile, and laterally displaced ("hitchhiker's thumb"). The broad hands and shortened fingers often exhibit ulnar deviation, and frequent webbing, contractures, and fixation of the interphalangeal finger joints occur (Fig. 44-2).

Scoliosis is not present at birth but is progressive and often is present within the first few years of life. Kyphosis is occasionally associated, and lordosis is frequent. Flexion contracture and/or subluxation or dislocation, especially of the hips, and to a lesser extent of the knees and shoulders, are common and progressive, further reducing height (17). Inguinal hernia has also been described (16, 17).

Roentgenographic changes include shortening and thickening of nearly all tubular bones. The epiphyses have delayed appearance and are flattened and distorted. With time the metaphyses become widened, irregular, and deformed. The

humerus is less shortened than the radius and ulna. The thumb is proximally placed, and the first metacarpal is small and rounded. Synostosis of the proximal interphalangeal joints is a constant feature. Carpal development is accelerated, but secondary centers for the metacarpals, metatarsals, and phalanges are retarded in appearance. The metacarpals are broader at the distal end than at the proximal end. The first metatarsal is broader and wider than the others (1, 6, 15, 18) (Fig. 44-3).

Dislocation or subluxation of the hips and coxa vara are associated with flattening of the acetabular roof and delayed appearance and poor development of the capital femoral epiphysis. The patella is often subluxated. Progressive kyphosis of the cervical region of the spine, with subluxation of the second and third cervical ver-

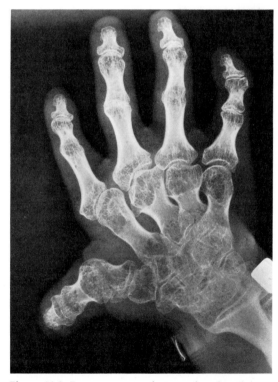

Figure 44-3. Roentgenogram showing short broad metacarpals with widened metaphyses. First metacarpal is especially shortened. Fusion is evident at proximal interphalangeal joint of second to fourth fingers. (*From J. Spranger and H. Gerken,* Z. Kinderheilkd. **98:**227, 1967.)

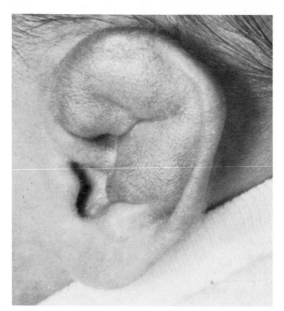

Figure 44-4. Cystic ear during hemorrhagic phase, which resolves, leaving pinnas calcified and distorted in form.

tebras, is frequent and may result in spinal cord compression (6).

Precocious ossification of costal cartilages and calcification of pinnal cartilage occur. Intracranial calcification has also been described (17).

Histopathologic study of bones has shown a generalized degenerative disorder of cartilage, with focal death of cells followed by matrix dis-

solution, cyst formation, fibrovascular scarring, and dystrophic ossification (11).

Facial and oral manifestations. Bilateral, but at times asymmetric, deformity of the pinnas has been noted in over 80 percent of cases (17). It may be evident within the first few days or weeks of life as a cystic swelling from which serosanguineous fluid may be extracted (4, 17) (Fig. 44-4). This resolves within a month, but the architecture of the pinna becomes distorted with calcification of the cartilage.

The mouth is full and broad, with the lower lip slightly larger than the upper.

Cleft palate has been found in over 50 percent of cases that we have recently surveyed. A similar estimate was made by Spranger and Gerken (13). A lower estimate (27 percent) was made by Walker et al. (17). The mandible is usually small.

DIFFERENTIAL DIAGNOSIS

The disorder may be confused with a plethora of chondrodysplastic and other disorders, such as arthrogryposis multiplex congenita, *achondroplasia,* and *cartilage-hair hypoplasia* (6, 17).

Pinnal calcification can rarely be seen in other disorders such as ochronosis, Addison disease, acromegaly, systemic chondromalacia, and familial cold hypersensitivity (17).

LABORATORY AIDS

None is known.

REFERENCES

1 Amuso, S. J., Diastrophic Dwarfism. *J. Bone Joint Surg.* **50A:**113–118, 1968.
2 Duken, J., Zur Frage der mechanischen Entstehung der Chondrodystrophie. *Monatsschr. Kinderheilkd.* **22:**348–355, 1921.
3 Kaplan, M., et al., Etude d'un nouveau cas de nanisme diastrophique. *Arch. Fr. Pédiatr.* **18:**981–1001, 1961.
4 Kratz, R. C., Congenital Perichondritis Associated with Achondroplasia. *Laryngoscope* **66:**93–97, 1956.
5 Lamy, M., and Maroteaux, P., Le nanisme diastrophique. *Presse Méd.* **68:**1977–1980, 1960.
6 Langer, L. O., Diastrophic Dwarfism in Early Infancy. *Am. J. Roentgenol.* **93:**399–404, 1965.
7 Lasserre, J., et al., Deux cas de nanisme diastrophique. *J. Méd. Bordeaux* **142:**1898–1900, 1965.
8 Monnet, P., et al., Le nanisme diastrophique. *Ann. Pédiatr.* **14:**483–489, 1967.
9 Neimann, N., et al., A propos d'un nouveau cas de nan-

isme diastrophique. *Arch. Fr. Pédiatr.* **21:**957–971, 1964.
10 Paul, S. S., et al., Diastropic Dwarfism: A Little Known Disease Entity. *Clin. Pediatr.* **4:**95–101, 1965.
11 Rimoin, D., Histopathology and Ultrastructure of Cartilage in the Chondrodystrophies. *Birth Defects* **10**(9):1–18, 1974.
12 Schenk, A. K., cited by Lamy and Maroteaux (5).
13 Spranger, J., and Gerken, H., Diastrophischer Zwergwuchs. *Z. Kinderheilkd.* **98:**227–234, 1967.
14 Stover, C. N., et al., Diastrophic Dwarfism. *Am. J. Roentgenol.* **89:**914–922, 1963.
15 Taybi, H., Diastrophic Dwarfism. *Radiology* **80:**1–10, 1963.
16 Vazquez, A. M., and Lee, F. A., Diastrophic Dwarfism. *J. Pediatr.* **72:**234–242, 1968.
17 Walker, B. A., et al., Diastrophic Dwarfism. *Medicine* **51:**41–59, 1972.
18 Wilson, D. W., et al., Diastrophic Dwarfism. *Arch. Dis. Child.* **44:**48–59, 1969.

45

Double Lip, Blepharochalasis, and Nontoxic Thyroid Enlargement

(Ascher Syndrome)

Though the combination of double lip and blepharochalasis was described by Laffler (14) in 1909, credit goes to Ascher (1, 2) for bringing to the attention of ophthalmologists in 1920–1922 the syndrome of blepharochalasis, double lip, and thyroid struma. Subsequently, additional cases of the complete syndrome were reported (7, 8, 11–13, 18, 19). Other investigators reported the combination of blepharochalasis and either double lip or thyroid enlargement (3–5, 9, 10, 22, 25). Examination of the published pictures of other patients with double lip reveals evidence of blepharochalasis (3). Some reports of isolated double lip have appeared in the literature (6, 23).

The cause of the syndrome is unknown, although many suggestions have been made, including hormonal dysfunction (7, 11, 13, 19, 24) and vasomotor instability (8, 13, 19).

Autosomal dominant transmission has been suggested (3, 10, 17, 21).

SYSTEMIC MANIFESTATIONS

Facies. The abnormal facies, produced by the combination of sagging eyelids and abnormal lip, is seen during smiling or talking (Figs. 45-1, 45-2, 45-3).

Eyes. The upper lids, rarely the lower, are characterized by relaxation of the supratarsal fold, which allows the tissue between the eyebrow and the edge of the lid to hang slack over the pal-pebral fissure. The lid skin is markedly thin and atrophic. The atrophy and drooping of the lid often follow repeated angioneurotic edema-like episodes. In several cases, swelling of the lids has appeared during the first 8 years of life. In others, its occurrence was noted at about the time of puberty (13, 19). The swelling of the lids and the enlargement of the lips may occur simultaneously (7, 18).

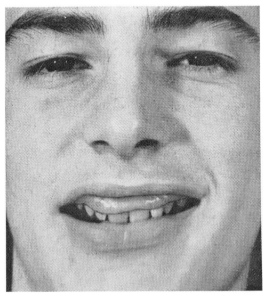

Figure 45-1. *Double lip, blepharochalasis, and nontoxic thyroid enlargement, or Ascher syndrome.* Note transverse crease with "doubling" of upper lip and sagging of lateral portion of upper eyelids. (*From M. C. Oldfield,* Br. J. Surg. **47**:58, 1959.)

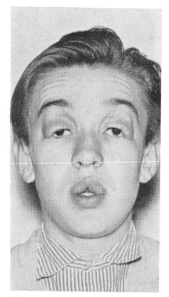

Figure 45-2. Patient with appearance similar to that of patient in Fig. 45-1. (*From K. Stehr, Dtsch. Med. Wochenschr.* **87**:1148, 1962.)

Gross surgical examination of tissue removed from the relaxed skin of the lid has shown prolapsed orbital fat or, more frequently, hyperplastic lacrimal gland tissue. The lids, on microscopic examination, have exhibited an increased number of blood vessels, but no unanimity of opinion exists concerning changes in the elastic fibers (16).

Thyroid. Thyroid gland enlargement is variable and not associated with toxic symptoms. It may appear several years after eyelid involvement (2) but usually appears during the second decade. It may be evident only on scanning with radioactive iodine (18).

Oral manifestations. The lip, almost always the upper, is the site of a horizontally running duplication located between the inner (pars villosa) and outer (pars glabrosa) parts of the lip (16). The fold cannot be seen when the lips are closed, only when the patient is smiling or talking. The enlargement of the lip may exist from childhood (3, 4, 10). Rarely, the lower lip is also enlarged (6, 10).

Microscopic examination of the excessive labial tissue usually reveals loose areolar tissue and hyperplastic mucous glands, numerous blood-filled capillaries, and perivascular infiltration with plasma cells and lymphocytes (3, 4, 6, 9, 12).

DIFFERENTIAL DIAGNOSIS

Double lip may occur as an isolated anomaly.

The *Melkersson-Rosenthal syndrome* (cheilitis glandularis, facial paralysis, and fissured tongue) and vascular neoplasms (hemangioma, lymphangioma) should be considered.

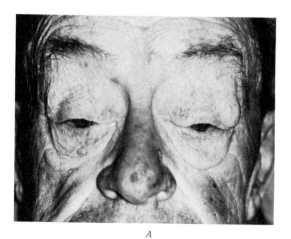
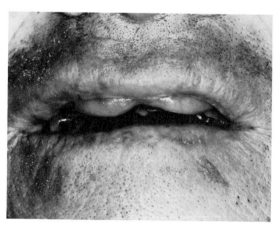

A   *B*

Figure 45-3. (*A, B*). Compare similar alterations in older patient. (*Courtesy of A. F. Morgan, Seattle, Wash.*)

LABORATORY AIDS

None is known.

REFERENCES

1 Ascher, K. W., Blepharochalasis mit Struma und Doppellippe. *Klin. Monatsbl. Augenheilkd.* **65**:86–97, 1920.

2 Ascher, K. W., Das Syndrom Blepharochalasis, Struma und Doppellippe. *Klin. Wochenschr.* **1**:2287–2288, 1922.

3 Barnett, M. L., et al., Double Lip and Double Lip with Blepharochalasis (Ascher's Syndrome). *Oral Surg.* **34**:727–733, 1972.

4 Calnan, J., Congenital Double Lip: Record of a Case with a Note on the Embryology. *Br. J. Plast. Surg.* **5**:197–202, 1952–1953.

5 Delaire, J., et al., Les doubles lèvres. *Actual. Odontostomatol.* (Paris) **87**:365–380, 1969.

6 Dingman, R. O., and Billman, H. R., Double Lip. *J. Oral Surg.* **5**:146–148, 1947.

7 Eigel, W., Blepharochalasis und Doppellippe, ein thyreotoxisches Oedem? *Dtsch. Med. Wochenschr.* **51**:1947–1949, 1925.

8 Eisenstodt, M. D., Blepharochalasis and Double Lip. *Am. J. Ophthalmol.* **32**:128–130, 1949.

9 Findlay, G. H., Idiopathic Enlargements of the Lips: Cheilitis Granulomatosa, Ascher's Syndrome and Double Lip. *Br. J. Dermatol.* **66**:129–138, 1954.

10 Franceschetti, A., Manifestation de blépharochalasis chez le père associé à des doubles lèvres apparaissant également chez sa filette âgée d'un mois. *J. Génét. Hum.* **4**:181–182, 1955.

11 Hartmann, K., Blepharochalasis mit Struma und Doppellippe. *Klin. Monatsbl. Augenheilkd.* **89**:376–380, 1932.

12 Hausamen, J. E., et al., Klinischer Beitrag zum Ascher-Syndrom. *Dtsch. Zahnärztl. Z.* **24**:983–987, 1969.

13 Klemens, F., Blepharochalasis, Struma und Doppellippe. *Klin. Monatsbl. Augenheilkd.* **105**:474–482, 1940.

14 Laffler, W. B., Blepharochalasis: Report of a Case of This Trophoneurosis Involving Also the Upper Lip. *Cleveland Med. J.* **8**:131–135, 1909.

15 Mouly, R., Correction of Hypertrophy of the Upper Lip (Case 1). *Plast. Reconstr. Surg.* **46**:262–264, 1970.

16 Neurstaetter, O., Über den Lippensaum beim Menschen: seinen Bau, seine Entwicklung und seine Bedeutung. *Jena Z. Med. Naturw.* **29**:345–390, 1895.

17 Panneton, P., La blépharo-chalazis. *Arch. Ophtalmol.* (Paris) **53**:729–755, 1936.

18 Papanayatou, P. H., and Hatziotis, J. C., Ascher's Syndrome. *Oral Surg.* **35**:467–471, 1973.

19 Schimpf, A., Das Ascher Syndrom. *Dermatol. Wochenschr.* **132**:1077–1086, 1955.

20 Segal, P., and Jablonska, S., Le syndrome d'Ascher. *Ann. Ocul.* **194**:511–526, 1961.

21 Stehr, K., et al., Pathogenese und Therapie des Ascher Syndroms. *Dtsch. Med. Wochenschr.* **87**:1148–1154, 1962.

22 Stein, R., Blepharochalasis der Unterlides. *Klin. Monatsbl. Augenheilkd.* **84**:846–851, 1930.

23 Swerdloff, G., Double Lip. *Oral Surg.* **13**:627–629, 1960.

24 Tapasztó, I., et al., Some Data on the Pathogenesis of Blepharochalasis (Case 1). *Acta Ophthalmol.* (Kbh.) **41**:167–175, 1963.

25 Wirths, M., Beiderseitige Lidgeschwulst, kombiniert mit Geschwulstbildung der Oberlippe. *Z. Augenheilkd.* **44**:176–178, 1920.

46

Dubowitz Syndrome

In 1965, Dubowitz reported a syndrome consisting of (a) primordial shortness of stature, (b) microcephaly, (c) eczema, (d) mental retardation, (e) high-pitched voice, and (f) characteristic facial appearance. The syndrome was further documented by Grosse et al. (2) and Opitz et al. (4).

Autosomal recessive mode of transmission seems likely, because of multiple sib involvement and parental consanguinity (2, 4). Fewer than a dozen cases have been described to date.

SYSTEMIC MANIFESTATIONS

Facies. Head circumference is disproportionately small for age and height. The forehead is high with flat supraorbital ridges. Facial asymmetry may be noted in some cases. The nasal bridge has been described as relatively high. Dystopia canthorum or true ocular hypertelorism is present, together with blepharophimosis. Ptosis and slight mongoloid or antimongoloid obliquity has been observed. Micrognathia has been present in all cases. The ears may be prominent or low-set in some instances (1, 2, 4) (Fig. 46-1, 46-2).

Skeletal system. Intrauterine growth retardation with primordial shortness of stature has been evident in all cases. Slightly retarded bone age has also been noted. Periosteal hyperostosis of long bones, various rib anomalies, metatarsus varus, pes planus, and pes planovalgus have been

reported. Preaxial polydactyly and clinodactyly of the fifth fingers have been noted occasionally (1, 2).

Integumentary system. An eczematous skin eruption, especially of the face and extremities, has been observed during infancy in a few cases (1, 2). Chronic rhinorrhea and serous otitis

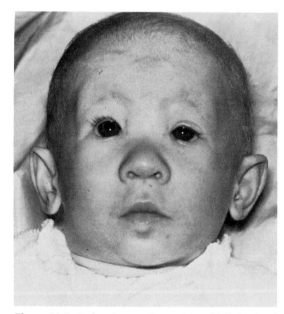

Figure 46-1. *Dubowitz syndrome.* Note high forehead with flat supraorbital ridges, widely spaced eyes, blepharophimosis, and small mandible.

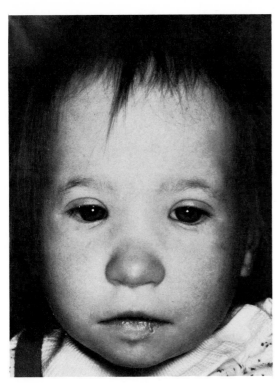

Figure 46-2. Sister of patient shown in Fig. 46-1 having similar facies.

Central nervous system. Mild mental retardation and behavioral problems have been reported. However, several patients have normal intelligence in spite of markedly reduced head circumference! Hyperactivity, short attention span, stubbornness, and shyness have been noted (1, 2).

Other findings. High-pitched voice, diarrhea during infancy, pilonidal dimples, hypospadias, and cryptorchism have been described (1, 2, 4).

Oral manifestations. Submucous cleft palate, highly arched palate, bifid uvula, delayed dental eruption, and severe dental caries have been reported (1, 2, 4).

DIFFERENTIAL DIAGNOSIS

The Dubowitz syndrome may be confused with *Bloom syndrome,* or the *fetal alcohol syndrome,* in which there are intrauterine growth retardation, microcephaly, and sparse hair. However, these patients have sharp upper epicanthal folds and short palpebral fissures not seen in the Dubowitz syndrome (3).

LABORATORY AIDS

Microcytic, normochromic, or mildly hypochromic anemia has been described (4).

media have also been noted in several cases (1, 2, 4). The scalp hair is sparse, and hypoplasia of the eyebrows has been observed (1, 2).

REFERENCES

1 Dubowitz, V., Familial Low Birthweight Dwarfism with an Unusual Facies and a Skin Eruption. *J. Med. Genet.* **2:**12–17, 1965.
2 Grosse, R., et al., The Dubowitz Syndrome. *Z. Kinderheilkd.* **110:**175–187, 1971.
3 Jones K. L., et al., Pattern of Malformation in Offspring of Chronic Alcoholic Mothers. *Lancet* **1:**1267–1271, 1973.
4 Opitz, J., et al., The Dubowitz Syndrome: Further Observations. *Z. Kinderheilkd.* **116:**1–12, 1973.

47

Dyskeratosis Congenita

(Zinsser-Engman-Cole Syndrome)

Zinsser (30) in 1906 reported what appears to be the first case of a syndrome comprising "reticular atrophy of the skin with pigmentation, dystrophy of the nails, and oral leukoplakia." His report went unrecognized, and, in 1926, the same syndrome was reported under almost the same title by Engman, Sr. (9). Cole et al. (7) developed the syndrome, bringing it to the attention of dermatologists. Wilgram and Weinstock (29) pointed out that the oral lesions are characterized by a decreased number of keratinosomes associated with a decreased epithelial cell turnover. Thus, the disorder is not really a dyskeratosis.

The hereditary pattern of the disorder is not clear. Although an overwhelming percentage of the patients are male and there is clearly X-linked inheritance in one report (4), a few fully expressed examples of the condition have been described in females (1, 19, 26). There have been several affected male sibs (2, 4, 9, 11, 17), and in two cases a brother and sister have been affected (1,19). This suggests possible genetic heterogeneity, there being X-linked and autosomal recessive forms of the disorder. The condition described by Moon-Adams and Slatkin (21) is probably not dyskeratosis congenita. About 35 cases have been published (15).

SYSTEMIC MANIFESTATIONS

There are generalized growth retardation and frailty.

Skin and skin appendages. The most prominent skin changes closely resemble those seen in poikiloderma vasculare atrophicans, involving especially the face, neck, and chest and appearing approximately at puberty (5). A prominent reticulated hyperpigmentation of skin, usually described as gunmetal in color, involves the same areas (Fig. 47-1*A*, *B*). Microscopically, there is atrophy of the epidermis and subcutaneous tissues, accompanied by capillary hyperplasia. Melanin pigment is heavily deposited, especially near blood vessels (16). There is characteristically no inflammatory exudate.

Hyperhidrosis of the palms and soles but generalized hypohidrosis elsewhere have been noted in over half the cases, and palmar keratoses have been mentioned (8, 24). Several observers have remarked on the occurrence of cutaneous bullae and/or the tendency of the hands to be subject to trauma (6, 8, 16). Acrocyanosis of the hands and feet appears to be exceedingly common. In most cases the fingernails and toenails become dystrophic at about puberty (Fig. 47-2). Hypotrichosis and/or premature canities have been noted in about 20 percent of the cases (15).

Eyes and ears. Chronic blepharitis and ectropion (6, 8, 9, 12, 22, 24), profuse tearing due to keratinization with obstruction of the lacrimal points (12, 16, 22, 24), and loss of eyelashes have been described (24). Thinning of the eardrum and malformation of the middle ear (20) have also been reported (8).

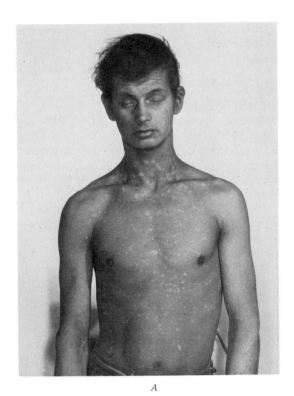
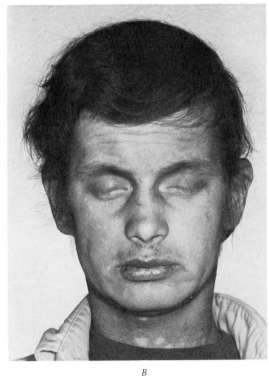

A   *B*

Figure 47-1. *Dyskeratosis congenita.* (*A*). Whitish, irregular atrophic areas, increased pigmentation, and telangiectasia, producing picture that resembles poikiloderma vasculare atrophicans. (*B*). Sparse scalp hair, blepharitis due to absence of lacrimal puncta.

Blood. Several authors have noted the association of aplastic anemia and hypersplenism in their patients (1–4, 6, 12, 15, 18, 27).

Central nervous system. Mental retardation or schizophrenia has been reported in about 30 percent of patients (8, 12, 13).

Other findings. Small testes have been described in about 15 percent of cases. Enlarged thyroid gland has been noted occasionally (15).

Oral manifestations. Crops of vesicles and bullae appear on the oral mucosa, most frequently during the five- to seven-year-old

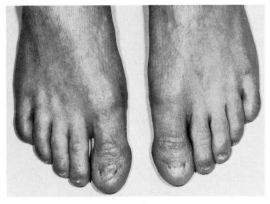

A   *B*

Figure 47-2. (*A, B*). Note shriveled, shrunken appearance of nails.

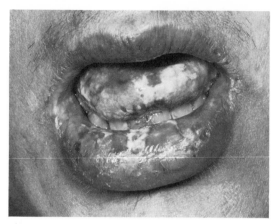

Figure 47-3. Thick white plaques of labial and lingual mucosa.

period or, in some cases, earlier. These flaccid bullae are recurrent and essentially painless. Because of moisture and maceration, they rupture early, leaving ulcerated areas, with epithelial tags along the margin. After several attacks, the mucosa becomes atrophic and the tongue loses its papillae and becomes smooth. Under ultraviolet light, the normal orange fluorescence of the tongue is missing. Eventually, the mucosa becomes thickened, fissured, and white (Fig. 47-3). About 20 percent of patients complain of dysphagia, and esophageal diverticula have been noted with increased frequency. Addison and Rice (1), Cannell (5), Sorrow and Hitch (26), and Milgrom et al. (20) reported large verrucous carcinomatous lesions on the buccal and cervical mucosa of patients with this syndrome. Microscopically, dyskeratotic changes may be seen. Carcinomatous or premalignant changes have been reported in the urethral and anal mucosa (8, 24), and one of the patients reported by Garb (11) developed anal carcinoma. Mucosal atrophy or stenosis has been described in the mouth, esophagus, anus, urethra, and vagina.

The teeth are said to be subject to early decay (24), periodontal disease (8, 28, 30), malforma-tion, and malposition (8, 24). These changes with rare exception have not been well documented and merit further investigation.

DIFFERENTIAL DIAGNOSIS

Differential diagnosis covers the wide spectrum of ectodermal dysplasis, including *xeroderma pigmentosum, pachyonychia congenita,* the Siemen syndrome, Schaefer syndrome, Kummer-Loos syndrome, several palmar-plantar hyper-keratotic syndromes, congenital ichthyosiform erythroderma, *epidermolysis bullosa, incontinentia pigmenti,* keratosis with poikiloderma, etc. See the differential diagnosis by Greither (13).

The Naegeli syndrome, though marked by reticular pigmentation, palmar and plantar hyperkeratoses, ocular malformation, and mottled teeth, in contrast to dyskeratosis congenita, has diminished sweat gland function (17).

Focal dermal hypoplasia consists of a congenital poikiloderma-like condition, syndactyly, missing digits, scoliosis, and hypohidrosis. The nails are thin, and the teeth are small, often missing, and defective.

LABORATORY AIDS

Demonstration of pancytopenia (2, 6, 12, 16, 18, 28), low serum gamma globulins, and thymic dysplasia (23) may aid in the diagnosis.

Steier et al. (27) and many authors have pointed out similarities and differences between dyskeratosis congenita and Fanconi anemia. More prominent in dyskeratosis congenita are cutaneous telangiectatic erythema and atrophy; exocrine, ungual, and dental dysplasias; mucosal leukoplakia, carcinomatosis and stenosis, and esophageal diverticula. Prominent in Fanconi anemia but absent in dyskeratosis congenita are the renal and skeletal anomalies.

REFERENCES

1 Addison, M., and Rice, M. S., The Association of Dyskeratosis Congenita and Fanconi's Anemia. *Med. J. Aust.* **1:**797–799, 1965.

2 Bazex, A., and Dupré, A., Dyskératose congénitale (type Zinsser-Cole-Engman) associée à une myélopathie constitutionelle (purpura thrombopénique et neutropénie). *Ann. Dermatol. Syphiligr.* (*Paris*) **84:**497–513, 1957.

3 Bodalski, J., et al., Fanconi's Anemia and Dyskeratosis

Congenita as a Syndrome. *Dermatologica* **127**:330–342, 1963.

4 Bryan, H. G., and Nixon, R. K., Dyskeratosis Congenita and Familial Pancytopenia. *J.A.M.A.* **192**:203–208, 1965.

5 Cannell, H., Dyskeratosis Congenita. *Br. J. Oral Surg.* **9**:8–20, 1971.

6 Cole, H. N., et al., Dyskeratosis Congenita with Pigmentation, Dystrophia Unguis and Leukokeratosis Oris. *Arch. Dermatol. Syphilol. (Chic.)* **21**:71–95, 1930.

7 Cole, H. N., et al., Dyskeratosis Congenita. *Arch. Dermatol.* **76**:712–719, 1957.

8 Costello, M. J., and Buncke, C. M., Dyskeratosis Congenita. *Arch. Dermatol.* **73**:123–132, 1956 (questionable case).

9 Engman, M. F., Sr., A Unique Case of Reticular Pigmentation of the Skin with Atrophy. *Arch. Dermatol. Syphilol. (Chic.)* **13**:685–687, 1926.

10 Engman, M. F., Jr., Congenital Atrophy of the Skin, with Reticular Pigmentation. *J.A.M.A.* **105**:1252–1256, 1935.

11 Garb, J., Dyskeratosis Congenita with Pigmentation, Dystrophia Unguium and Leukoplakia Oris: A Follow-up Report of Two Brothers. *Arch. Dermatol.* **77**:704–712, 1958.

12 Garb, J., and Rubin, G., Dyskeratosis Congenita with Pigmentation, Dystrophia Unguium and Leukoplakia Oris (Cole and Others). *Arch. Dermatol. Syphilol. (Chic.)* **50**:191–198, 1944.

13 Greither, A., Über eine mit Keratosen und Pigmentstörungen einhergehende erbliche Dysplasie der Haut. *Hautarzt* **9**:364–369, 1958.

14 Grekin, J. N., and Schwartz, O. D., Dyskeratosis Congenita with Pigmentation, Dystrophia Unguium and Leukokeratosis oris. *Arch. Dermatol.* **85**:124–215, 1962.

15 Inoue, S., et al., Dyskeratosis Congenita with Pancytopenia. *Am. J. Dis. Child.* **126**:389–396, 1973.

16 Jansen, L. H., The So-called "Dyskeratosis Congenita." *Dermatologica* **103**:167–177, 1951.

17 Kitamura, K., and Hirako, T., Über zwei japanische Fälle einer eigenartigen retikulären Pigmentierung (Case 2). *Dermatologica* **110**:97–107, 1955.

18 Koszewski, B. J., and Hubbard, T. F., Congenital Anemia in Hereditary Ectodermal Dysplasia. *Arch. Dermatol.* **74**:159–166, 1956.

19 Marshall, J., and van der Meulen, H., Dyskeratosis Congenita - Its Occurrence in the Female. *Br. J. Dermatol.* **77**:162, 1965.

20 Milgrom, H., et al., Dyskeratosis Congenita. *Arch. Dermatol.* **89**:345–349, 1964.

21 Moon-Adams, D., and Slatkin, M. H., Familial Pigmentation with Dystrophy of the Nails. *Arch. Dermatol.* **71**:591–598, 1955.

22 Orfanos, C., and Gartmann, H., Leukoplakien, Pigmentverschiebungen und Nageldystrophie. *Med. Welt* **48**:2589–2594, 1966.

23 Ortega, J. A., et al., Congenital Dyskeratosis. *Am. J. Dis. Child.* **124**:701–705, 1972.

24 Pastinszky, I., et al., Ein Beitrag zur Pathologie der "Dyskeratosis congenita" Cole-Rauschkolb-Toomey. *Dermatol. Wochenschr.* **135**:587–593, 1957.

25 Ramos e Silva, J., Syndrome de Zinsser-Fanconi. *Ann. Dermatol. Syphilol.* **93**:497–502, 1966.

26 Sorrow, J. M., and Hitch, J. M., Dyskeratosis Congenita. *Arch. Dermatol.* **88**:340–347, 1963.

27 Steier, W., et al., Dyskeratosis Congenita: Relationship to Fanconi's Anemia. *Blood* **39**:510–521, 1972.

28 Wald, C., and Diner, H., Dyskeratosis Congenita with Associated Periodontal Disease. *Oral Surg.* **37**:736–744, 1974.

29 Wilgram, G. F., and Weinstock, A., Advances in Genetic Dermatology. *Arch. Dermatol.* **94**:456–479, 1966.

30 Zinsser, F., Atrophica cutis reticularis cum pigmentatione, dystrophia unguium et leukoplakia oris. *Ikonograph Derm. Kioto*, pp. 219–223, 1906.

48

Ehlers-Danlos Syndromes

The syndrome had been described, in part, as early as the seventeenth century in Holland by van Meekeren (27). Ehlers (14), in 1901, reported the association of (a) hyperelastic skin, (b) skin hemorrhages, and (c) loose-jointedness. Danlos (12), in 1908, added (d) cutaneous pseudotumors and fragility, and Weber and Aitken (35), a fifth component, (e) subcutaneous spherules. Actually, the syndrome had been described in toto by Tschernogobow (34) in 1892. At least 400 cases have been reported (19). Several of those affected had jobs as "human pretzels" and "Indian rubber men" at circus sideshows (11). Comprehensive surveys are those of McKusick (27) and Beighton et al. (9).

There are at least seven variants of the syndrome, three of which are characterized by autosomal dominant inheritance. The fifth type is X-linked. The other three have autosomal recessive inheritance (Table 48-1). Beighton et al. (9) estimated their approximate frequency as follows: severe—30 percent; mild—45 percent; benign hypermobile—10 percent; ecchymotic—5 percent; and X-linked—10 percent. The interested reader is also referred to the classification of Barabas (2). In a sixth and uncommon autosomal recessive form, patients exhibit the dermal and joint changes seen in the Ehlers-Danlos syndrome of moderate severity but have a tendency to serious ophthalmologic complications, including scleral perforation, retinal detachment, blue sclerae, and myopia (5, 22, 29).

The basic defect is not known in types I to III, but a defect in elastin has again recently been suggested (21), a view which we do not share. McKusick (27) has argued convincingly that the disorder appears to be one of collagen, possibly one of defective cross-linkage. Type IV is due to a deficiency in type 3 collagen (30a). The cause of the X-linked form (type V) is uncertain at present. In the sixth form, the collagen has been shown to be hydroxylysine-deficient (15a, 31, 32a). A seventh type, marked by floppiness or loose-jointedness, short stature, and moderate stretchability and bruisability and inherited as an autosomal recessive trait, exhibits deficiency of procollagen peptidase (26a).

SYSTEMIC MANIFESTATION

Prematurity, due to early rupture of fetal membranes, is frequently observed in the severe form. Death in youth or early adulthood may occur in the ecchymotic type. Friable tissues and operative difficulties due to abnormal bleeding have been seen in both the severe and ecchymotic forms.

Facies. The facies is not characteristic; scars on the forehead and chin are the most constant among the facial stigmata but are present in only about one-half the cases (4). The ears may project outward and somewhat downward ("lop ears") (15). They are frequently stretchable, but not in the ecchymotic form. Epicanthal folds are

Table 48-1. Characteristics of seven types of the Ehlers-Danlos syndrome

Type of EDS	Skin hyperextensibility	Joint hypermobility	Skin fragility	Bruising	Major complications	Inheritance	Basic defect
Severe (type I)	Marked	Marked	Marked	Moderate	Musculoskeletal deformities common; varicose veins; prematurity due to ruptured membranes	Autosomal dominant	Unknown
Mild (type II)	Moderate	Moderate	Moderate	Moderate		Autosomal dominant	Unknown
Benign hypermobile (type III)	Variable; usually marked	Marked	Minimal	Minimal		Autosomal dominant	Unknown
Ecchymotic (type IV)	Minimal	Limited to digits	Moderate	Marked	Death from arterial rupture, aortic dissection, intestinal perforation; musculoskeletal abnormalities absent	Autosomal recessive	Type 3 collagen deficiency
X-linked (type V)	Marked	Limited to digits	Minimal	Minimal	Musculoskeletal disorders common	X-linked	Lysyl-* oxidase deficiency(?)
Ocular variety (type VI)	Marked	Marked	Minimal	Minimal	Fragility of cornea and sclera; retinal detachment; severe scoliosis	Autosomal recessive	Lysyl hydroxylase deficiency
Arthrochalasis multiplex congenita (type VII)	Moderate	Marked	Moderate	Moderate	Marked short stature and multiple joint dislocations	Autosomal recessive	Procollagen peptidase deficiency

SOURCE: Modified from P. Beighton et al., *Ann. Rheum. Dis.* **28:**228, 1969, and V. A. McKusick and G. R. Martin, *Ann. Intern. Med.* **82:**585, 1975.
* Suggested (12a) but not confirmed.

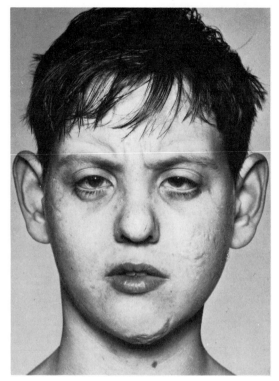

Figure 48-1. *Ehlers-Danlos syndrome.* Numerous "cigarette paper" scars of face, epicanthal folds, flat nasal bridge. (From *G. M. Barabas and A. P. Barabas* Br. Dent. J. **123**:473, 1967.)

frequent (11, 24, 27), causing the nasal bridge to appear wide (Fig. 48-1).

Skin. The skin has a velvety feel and is hyperelastic, especially over the major joints. After being stretched, it returns to its normal position (Fig. 48-2). The hyperextensible skin fold in the X-linked form is thicker than that in the severe variety.

The skin, demonstrated to be thinner than normal (19), is also brittle and fragile, and minimal trauma produces gaping wounds. After healing, pigmented papyraceous scars result (Fig. 48-1). The skin is especially translucent in the ecchymotic form, the subcutaneous venous pattern being quite evident, and elastosis perforans is more frequently found in this form. These can usually be detected over the forehead, chin, knees, shins, or elbows. Bruising in the severe form is variable in degree but is particularly

marked in the ecchymotic type (Fig. 48-5). Goodman et al. (18) have demonstrated secondary skin creases in the palms.

Molluscoid or raisin-like pseudotumors over the heels and major joints are not uncommon, and there is often redundancy of the skin of the hands and feet (11, 24) (Fig. 48-4). Calcified, cystlike structures, 2 to 10 mm in diameter, may be found subcutaneously, especially over bony prominences of the forearms and shins, in about 30 percent of patients (7). Varicose veins are common in both the severe and X-linked forms. Acrocyanosis has been noted with increased frequency.

Musculoskeletal system. Hyperextensibility of joints, a weak hand clasp, and pes planus are usually present (6, 13) in the severe form of the syndrome (Fig. 48-3). Genu recurvatum has been

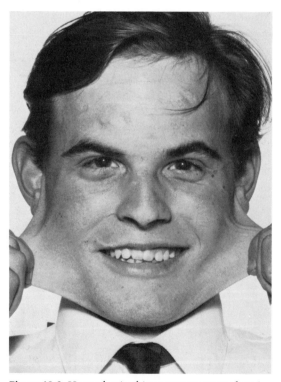

Figure 48-2. Hyperelastic skin returns to normal position after being stretched. (*From P. E. Beighton,* The Ehlers-Danlos Syndrome. Heinemann Med. Books, Ltd, London, 1972.)

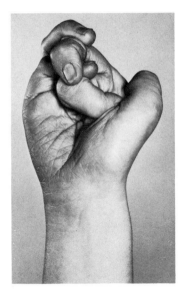

Figure 48-3. Extreme joint hypermobility. (*From G. M. Barabas and A. P. Barabas*, Br. Dent. J. **123**:473, 1967.)

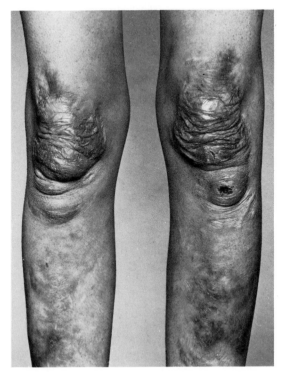

Figure 48-4. Papyraceous scars of knees, with pseudo-tumor below left knee. (*From G. M. Barabas and A. P. Barabas*, Br. Dent. J. **123**:473, 1967.)

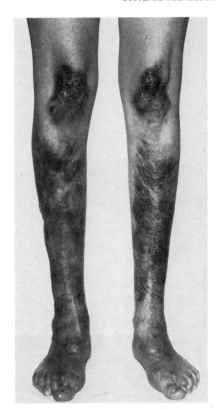

Figure 48-5. Ecchymotic type showing severe bruising following minor trauma over knees and shins. Elbows also commonly involved. Skin and joint hyperextensibility are less marked than in severe type (see Table 48-1). (*From P. E. Beighton*, The Ehlers-Danlos Syndrome. *Heinemann Med. Books, Ltd.*, London, 1972.)

noted in about 25 percent of cases, and there may be recurrent joint dislocations. Talipes has been noted in about 5 percent of patients. The ulnar styloid process may be elongated. Kyphoscoliosis and thoracic asymmetry are found in 15 to 20 percent of cases but are usually not severe (7, 13). Hernia, either inguinal or umbilical, has been found in about 10 to 20 percent of cases (8).

Eyes. Epicanthal folds are seen in about 25 percent of these patients (5). Blue scleras are noted in much less than 10 percent of them, being far less frequent than in patients with osteogenesis imperfecta (11, 13, 24, 25). Myopia and strabismus have been seen with far greater frequency than blue scleras. Also noted in iso-

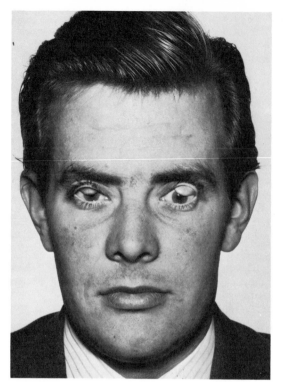

Figure 48-6. Easy eversion of upper lids (Méténier sign). *(From P. E. Beighton, The Ehlers-Danlós Syndrome. Heinemann Med. Books, Ltd.,* London, 1972.)

lated cases have been microcornea, retinal detachment, keratoconus, and angioid streaks (20, 29). The hyperextensibility of the skin allows for easy eversion of the upper lids (Méténier sign) (9) (Fig. 48-6).

Other findings. Various gastrointestinal complications have been observed, including hiatus hernia, intestinal diverticula, diaphragmatic eventration, and rectal prolapse during infancy. Rarely, there is spontaneous perforation of the intestine or massive gastrointestinal hemorrhage, especially in the ecchymotic form (8).

Also in the ecchymotic type, patients may die suddenly of arterial rupture or aortic dissection (8). Multiple arterial lesions and peripheral pulmonary artery stenoses have also been described (16, 23).

Medullary sponge kidney has been noted in several cases (27).

Oral manifestations. The oral mucosa is of normal color but excessively fragile and easily bruised. It does not hold sutures satisfactorily. Healing may be slightly retarded, since the edges of the wound draw apart, but there is no evidence of abnormal healing or excessive scar formation in the mouth (4). The gingiva are said to be more liable to injury, and periodontal disease occurs at an early age (11, 24). These observations have also been made by the authors. In addition, severe bleeding has been noted following tooth extraction (24).

Recurrent subluxation of the temporomandibular joint has been reported (6, 17, 33).

Barabas and Barabas (4) found that premolar and molar teeth had high cusps and deep occlusal fissures. Roentgenographically, the teeth may have stunted and deformed roots and large pulp stones in the coronal part of the pulp chamber. This observation was first made in 1965 by Selliseth (32) and later confirmed by Barabas and Barabas (4) and Pindborg (30) (Fig. 48-7A, B). In 1969, Barabas (3) found hypoplastic areas in the enamel; irregularities of amelodentinal and cementodentinal junctions; and formation of pathologic dentin, occurring more often in the root than in the crown and containing vascular inclusions, dentinal tubules following abnormal courses, and many denticles. The finding of abnormalities in the dentin indicates that collagenous tissue is affected regardless of whether elastic tissue is present, dentin having no significant elastic tissue content. One of us (R. J. G.), however, has not been able to find these changes in any of a series of six patients.

The authors have observed that at least 50 percent of patients with the Ehlers-Danlos syndrome have the ability to touch the nose with the tongue, an ability manifested by about 8 to 10 percent of ostensibly normal persons (Fig. 48-7C).

DIFFERENTIAL DIAGNOSIS

Unfortunately, the term "cutis laxa" has been applied by some authors to Ehlers-Danlos syndrome. In true *cutis laxa,* the skin hangs in loose, inelastic folds, the voice is deep, and often there are emphysema and hernia. No oral anom-

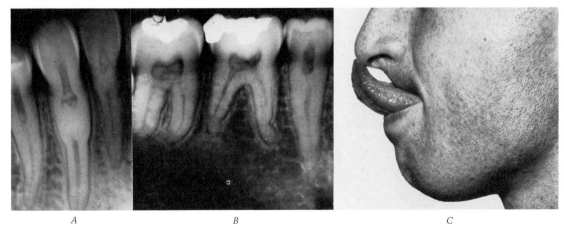

A   B   C

Figure 48-7. (*A, B*). Stunted and deformed roots and large pulp stones in coronal portion of pulp chamber. *From J. J. Pindborg*, Pathology of the Hard Dental Tissues, *Saunders, Philadelphia, 1970.*) (*C*). Ability to touch nose with tongue tip, present in 50 percent of those with Ehlers-Danlos syndrome, occurs in less than 10 percent of normal persons. (*From P. E. Beighton*, The Ehlers-Danlos Syndrome. *Heinemann Med. Books, Ltd., London, 1972.*)

alies have been documented in association with this condition.

Joint hypermobility may occur as an isolated finding or in association with various disorders such as *Marfan syndrome, osteogenesis imperfecta, Down syndrome, Larsen syndrome,* and a host of other syndromes. Incidentally, it may also be associated with familial transverse nasal groove (1).

To be excluded are patients with autosomal dominantly inherited generalized hypermobility (Marfanoid hypermobility syndrome) but with no skin hyperextensibility, splitting, or scarring (11) (Fig. 48-8).

A possible additional ocular form of Ehlers-Danlos syndrome was reviewed by Greenfield et al. (20a). This autosomal recessively inherited disorder is characterized by keratoconus or keratoglobus with fragile cornea, blue scleras, loose ligaments, and, at times, conduction deafness. Beasley and Cohen (4a) noted two sibs from a consanguineous mating who had joint hyperextensibility, dislocated hips, inguinal hernia, lopears, mental retardation, "small eyes," cataracts, and deafness. Skin biopsies were negative for hydroxylysine deficiency and procollagen peptidase deficiency. A sporadic instance of the same disorder was observed by J. Hall (personal communication, 1975).

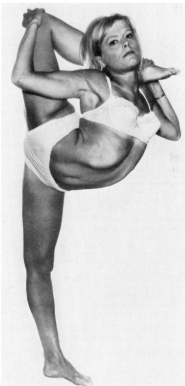

Figure 48-8. Familial generalized articular hypermobility should not be confused with Ehlers-Danlos syndrome. Proposita is an acrobatic dancer. (*From P. H. Beighton et al.*, J. Bone Joint Surg. **52B:**145, 1970.)

LABORATORY AIDS

The basic defect can be demonstrated in several types (12a, 26a, 30a, 31). Joint mobility may be tested by the Ellis-Bundick method (16), and skin elasticity by the "pinchmeter" of Olmstead et al. (28) and by the method of Graham and Beighton (19).

REFERENCES

1 Anderson, P. C., Familial Transverse Nasal Groove. *Arch. Dermatol.* **84:**316–317, 1961.

2 Barabas, A. P., Heterogeneity of the Ehlers-Danlos Syndrome: Description of Three Clinical Types and a Hypothesis to Explain the Basic Defects. *Br. Med. J.* **2:**612–613, 1967.

3 Barabas, G. M., The Ehlers-Danlos Syndrome: Abnormalities of the Enamel, Dentine, Cementum and the Dental Pulp: A Histological Examination of 13 Teeth from 6 Patients. *Br. Dent. J.* **126:**509–515, 1969.

4 Barabas, G. M., and Barabas, A. P., The Ehlers-Danlos Syndrome: A Report of the Oral and Haematological Findings in Nine Cases. *Br. Dent. J.* **123:**473–479, 1967.

4a Beasley, R. P., and Cohen, M. M., Jr., A New Form of the Ehlers-Danlos Syndrome, personal observation, 1975.

5 Beighton, P., Serious Ophthalmological Complications in the Ehlers-Danlos Syndrome. *Br. J. Ophthalmol.* **54:**263–268, 1970.

6 Beighton, P., and Horan, F., Orthopaedic Aspects of the Ehlers-Danlos Syndrome. *J. Bone Joint Surg.* **51B:**444–453, 1969.

7 Beighton, P., and Thomas, M. L., The Radiology of the Ehlers-Danlos Syndrome. *Clin. Radiol.* **20:**354–361, 1969.

8 Beighton, P. H., et al., Gastrointestinal Complications of the Ehlers-Danlos Syndrome. *Gut* **10:**1004–1008, 1969.

9 Beighton, P., et al., Variants of the Ehlers-Danlos Syndrome: Clinical, Biochemical, Haematological, and Chromosomal Features of 100 Patients. *Ann. Rheum. Dis.* **28:**228–245, 1969.

10 Beighton, P. H., et al., Dominant Inheritance in Familial Generalized Articular Hypermobility. *J. Bone Joint Surg.* **52B:**145–147, 1970.

11 Benjamin, B., and Weiner, H., Syndrome of Cutaneous Fragility and Hyperelasticity and Articular Hyperlaxity. *Am. J. Dis. Child.* **65:**247–257, 1943.

12 Danlos, H., Un cas de cutis laxa avec tumeurs par contusion chronique des coudes et des genoux. *Bull. Soc. Fr. Dermatol. Syphiligr.* **19:**70–72, 1908.

12a Di Ferrante, N., et al., Lysyl Oxidase Deficiency in Ehlers-Danlos Syndrome Type V. *Conn. Tissue Res.,* in press.

13 Durham, D. G., Cutis Hyperelastica (Ehlers-Danlos Syndrome) with Blue Scleras, Microcornea and Glaucoma. *Arch. Ophthalmol.* **49:**220–221, 1953.

14 Ehlers, E., Cutis laxa, Neigung zu Hemorrhagien in der Haut, Lockerung mehrerer Artikulationen. *Dermatol. Z.* **8:**173–174, 1901.

15 Ellis, F. E., and Bundick, W. R., Cutaneous Elasticity and Hyperelasticity. *Arch. Dermatol.* **74:**22–32, 1956.

15a Elsas, L. J., et al., Hydroxylysine-deficient Collagen Disease: Effect of Ascorbic Acid. *Am. J. Hum. Genet.* **26:**28, 1974.

16 Frieden, J., et al., Ruptured Aortic Cusp Associated with an Heritable Disorder of Connective Tissue. *Am. J. Med.* **33:**615–618, 1962.

17 Goodman, R. M., and Allison, M. L., Chronic Temporomandibular Joint Subluxation in Ehlers-Danlos Syndrome. *J. Oral Surg.* **27:**659–661, 1969.

18 Goodman, R. M., et al., Evolution of Palmar Skin Creases in the Ehlers-Danlos Syndrome. *Clin. Genet.* **3:**67–72, 1972.

19 Grahame, R., and Beighton, P., Physical Properties of the Skin in the Ehlers-Danlos Syndrome. *Ann. Rheum. Dis.* **28:**246–251, 1969.

20 Green, W. R., et al., Angioid Streaks in Ehlers-Danlos Syndrome. *Arch. Ophthalmol.* **76:**197–204, 1966.

20a Greenfield, G., et al., Blue Sclerae and Keratoconus: Key Features of a Distinct Heritable Disorder of Connective Tissue. *Clin. Genet.* **4:**8–16, 1973.

21 Heilman, K., et al., Das Ehlers-Danlos-Syndrom als morphologischer und chemischer Sicht. *Virchows Arch.* [*Pathol. Anat.*] **354:**268–284, 1971.

22 Hyams, S. W., et al., Blue Sclerae and Keratoglobus. *Br. J. Ophthalmol.* **53:**53–58, 1969.

23 Imahori, S., et al., Ehlers-Danlos Syndrome with Multiple Arterial Lesions. *Am. J. Med.* **47:**967–977, 1969.

24 Johnson, S. A. M., and Falls, H. F., Ehlers-Danlos Syndrome: A Clinical and Genetic Study. *Arch. Dermatol. Syph.* (*Chic.*) **60:**82–104, 1949.

25 Kanof, A., Ehlers-Danlos Syndrome: Report of a Case with Suggestion of a Possible Causal Mechanism. *Am. J. Dis. Child.* **83:**197–202, 1952.

26 Lees, M. H., et al., Ehlers-Danlos Syndrome Associated with Multiple Pulmonary Artery Stenoses and Tortuous Systemic Arteries. *J. Pediatr.* **75:**1031–1036, 1969.

26a Lichtenstein, J. R., et al., Defect in Conversion of Procollagen to Collagen in a Form of Ehlers-Danlos Syndrome. *Science* **182:**298–300, 1973.

27 McKusick, V. A., *Heritable Disorders of Connective Tissue.* 4th ed. Mosby, St. Louis, 1972.

27a McKusick, V. A., and Martin, G. R., Molecular Defects in Collagen. *Ann. Intern. Med.* **82:**585–586, 1975.

28 Olmstead, F., et al., A Device for Objective Clinical Measurement of Cutaneous Elasticity: A "Pinchmeter." *Am. J. Med. Sci.* **222:**73–75, 1951.

29 Pemberton, J. W., et al., Familial Retinal Detachment and the Ehlers-Danlos Syndrome. *Arch. Ophthalmol.* **76:**817–824, 1966.

30 Pindborg, J. J., *Pathology of the Dental Hard Tissues.* Saunders, Philadelphia, 1970.

30a Pope, M., et al., Patients with Ehlers-Danlos Syndrome Type IV Lack Type 3 Collagen, *Proc. Nat. Acad. Sci.* **72:**1314–1316, 1975.

31 Pinnell, S. R., et al., A Heritable Disorder of Connective Tissue: Hydroxylysine Deficiency of Collagen Disease. *N.*

Engl. J. Med. **286:**1013–1021, 1972.

32 Selliseth, N. E., Odontologische Befunde bei einer Patientin mit Ehlers-Danlos Syndrom. *Acta Odontol. Scand.* **23:**91–101, 1965.

32a Sussman, M. D., et al., Hydroxylysine-deficient Skin Collagen in a Patient with a Form of the Ehlers-Danlos Syndrome. *J. Bone Joint Surg.* **56A:**1228–1234, 1974.

33 Thexton, A., A Case of Ehlers-Danlos Syndrome Presenting with Recurrent Dislocation of the Temporomandibular Joint. *Br. J. Oral Surg.* **2:**190–193, 1965.

34 Tschernogobow, A., Cutis Laxa. *Monatsh. Prakt. Dermatol.* **14:**76, 1892.

35 Weber, F. P., and Aitken, J. K., Nature of Subcutaneous Spherules in Some Cases of Ehlers-Danlos Syndrome. *Lancet* **1:**198–199, 1938.

36 Wechsler, H. L., and Fisher, E. R., Ehlers-Danlos Syndrome: Pathologic, Histochemical and Electron Microscopic Observations. *Arch. Pathol.* (*Chic.*) **77:**613–619, 1964.

49

Endocrine-Candidosis Syndrome

Addison Disease, Juvenile Hypoparathyroidism, Keratoconjunctivitis,
and Superficial Candidosis

The association of candidosis with idiopathic hypoparathyroidism (5, 7, 24) and Addison disease (7, 27) has been known for several years, the first reference probably being the report by Thorpe and Handley (28) in 1929. However, it has been only within the past two decades that enough cases have been reported for analysis to yield a recognizable pattern of the "endocrine-candidosis syndrome" (20).

It now appears that several of the earlier cases either were incomplete forms of the syndrome or were followed for too short a period of time. Several authors have described the association of three of the components, and Carter et al. (2) suggested that hypothyroidism may be still another. In some patients with the syndrome, one or more of the following disorders may be present: a celiac-like condition (5), malabsorption, chronic liver disease, achlorhydria, pernicious anemia, malfunction of the thyroid gland (such as Hashimoto disease), and pulmonary infiltrates of undetermined cause (1, 13, 17). However, it should also be emphasized that not all the cardinal elements of the syndrome need be present in the same individual or in a single family.

Defective delayed hypersensitivity to *Candida albicans* has been demonstrated in patients with the syndrome (3, 4, 18, 19). Congenital abnormalities of the thymus may also be associated with mucocutaneous candidosis (13). Defective lymphocyte function has been demonstrated *in vitro* (18, 19). Excellent reviews of this autoimmune syndrome are those of Gass (8), Hermans and Ritts (13), and Kirkpatrick (18).

Several examples of the complete syndrome have occurred in sibs, which suggests that the syndrome is inherited as an autosomal recessive condition (17, 23, 24, 29, 30).

SYSTEMIC MANIFESTATIONS

Not all components of the syndrome appear simultaneously. Review of the cases reported to date clearly marks the syndrome as juvenile.

Candidosis is nearly always the first component to appear, most observers recording its presence during the first 6 years of life. It is followed from 3 months to 13 years later by the other components. The hypoparathyroidism and hypoadrenal corticism become manifest most frequently during the prepubescent period, the former at a mean of about 5 years, the latter at a mean of 8.5 years.

Endocrine system. Hypoparathyroidism is nearly always manifested by tetany. The serum calcium level is reduced and the serum phosphorus level elevated in the absence of significant disease of the genitourinary and gastrointestinal systems. Furthermore, parathyroid hormone injection results in an increase in the level of serum calcium and in elevated urinary phosphorus excretion. Candidosis does not complicate the hypocalcemia seen in chronic tetany owing to inadvertent parathyroidectomy in the course of thyroidectomy (13). At necropsy, absence of the parathyroid glands or their replacement with fat has been noted.

Addison disease makes itself apparent soon after the appearance of hypoparathyroidism. Lassitude, anorexia, progressive weakness, hypotension, and progressive pigmentation of the skin and mucous membrane signal its onset, and laboratory findings confirm the low serum sodium and high potassium levels. Death from adrenal crisis is a common outcome, and necropsy shows adrenocortical atrophy of the "cytotoxic type." Castells et al. (3) have demonstrated poor ACTH reserve in three sibs with this syndrome.

Hypothyroidism has been infrequently diagnosed (2, 30). It has been shown to be primary, since thyroid-stimulating hormone (TSH) does not produce a rise in thyroid ^{131}I uptake or alter the protein-bound iodine (PBI) level.

The relation of the *Candida* infection to the endocrine glands is not known. It has been suggested that the candidosis is a superficial expression of undetermined abnormalities which are already present in the host and which favor the development of the infection as well as the endocrinopathies (13). It is of significance that possibly as many as 15 percent of patients with endocrine candidosis develop thymonas late in life.

Skin and skin appendages. The skin is dry, and the hair of both body and scalp is usually brittle and diminished (Fig. 49-1). The eyebrows and axillary and pubic hair are remarkably sparse. Total alopecia may develop, most notably after therapy with dihydrotachysterol. The fingernails and toenails are frequently thin, ridged, and brittle and are often the site of *Candida* infection (Fig. 49-2). If infected, they become brown, irregular, and thickened, with a crumbled outer edge.

Central and peripheral nervous systems. Increased cerebrospinal fluid pressure, associated with papilledema, intracranial calcification (Fig. 49-3), epileptiform seizures, and mental retardation, have been noted (8). Muscle twitchings and cramps, tetany, abdominal pain, paresthesias, and rigidity are seen. The neurologic findings have been especially well reviewed by Jordan and Kelsall (16).

Other findings. Keratoconjunctivitis, photophobia, cataracts, hoarseness, laryngospasm, and wheezing have been noted (8) (Fig. 49-4). Hetzel and Robson (14) and Craig et al. (7) have commented on the posthepatitic changes found in the liver and the elevated serum gammaglobulin concentration. Pernicious anemia has also been described in several cases (15, 25).

Oral manifestations. The candidosis may be superficial or deep-seated and may involve the lips, tongue, buccal mucosa, palate, and larynx with thick creamy-white plaques (Fig. 49-5A). The mucosa between the plaques is often hy-

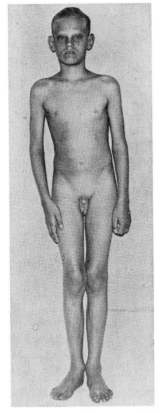

Figure 49-1. *Endocrine-candidosis syndrome.* Note generalized skin pigmentation, especially marked over face, midtrunk, and knees. (*Courtesy of J. A. Whitaker,* J. Clin. Endocrinol. **16:**1374, 1956.)

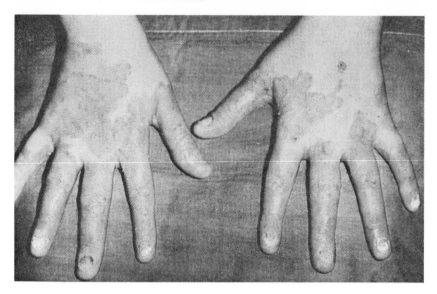

Figure 49-2. Candidosis of hands and fingernails. (*From J. D. B. Gass*, Am. J. Ophthalmol. **54:**660, 1962.)

peremic, and the tongue may be smooth and devoid of papillae. Perleche, or angular stomatitis, may extend over a considerable portion of the perioral skin. Similar involvement of the anal and vaginal mucosa has been described.

With the advent of Addison disease, areas of splotchy melanin pigment are seen in the mouth, especially on the buccal mucosa and palate.

The teeth are chalky, with pitted crowns or transverse grooves of enamel hypoplasia (8, 22, 25) (Fig. 49-5B). The involvement, however, is usually of mild degree (12, 13, 16, 30). Hurwitz (15) observed thickening and increased density of the lamina dura—the opposite of that seen in hyperparathyroidism. Hurwitz (15) further remarked that the tooth roots were incompletely developed and stumpy and that the teeth were

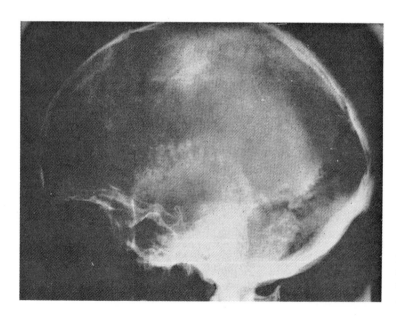

Figure 49-3. Skull roentgenogram exhibiting extensive basal ganglion calcification. (*From J. D. B. Gass,* Am. J. Ophthalmol. **54:**660, 1962.)

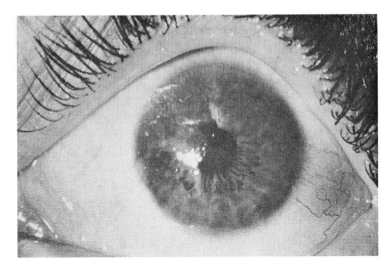

Figure 49-4. Keratoconjunctivitis. Note peripheral corneal vascularization and irregular, slightly raised, confluent nodular opacities in midperiphery of cornea. Lower paracentral cornea is not involved. (*From J. D. B. Gass,* Am. J. Ophthalmol. **54**:660, 1962.)

widely separated. He estimated that the dental age of his nineteen-year-old patient was eight to nine years. Jordan and Kelsall (16) and Mortell (21) suggested late dental eruption. Richman et al. (24) reported the occurrence of squamous cell carcinoma of the oral cavity in their patient.

DIFFERENTIAL DIAGNOSIS

Because of the wide spectrum of this syndrome, differential diagnosis must include the differential diagnosis of each of its components. This runs an exceedingly wide gamut, including *hypohidrotic ectodermal dysplasia, pseudohypoparathyroidism,* and renal tubular acidosis.

Oral and perioral candidosis, possibly as a secondary factor, may also be seen in association with an underlying malignant process (leukemia, lymphoma, and iatrogenically prolonged antibiotic or corticosteroid therapy). It is also seen in *acrodermatitis enteropathica.* Addison disease may occur in association with thyroiditis, diabetes mellitus, and various other disorders. Hypoparathyroidism, primary ovarian failure, and pernicious anemia can occur as part of the Schmidt syndrome (9, 11). Increased suscepti-

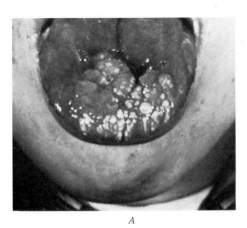

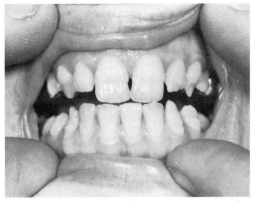

A

B

Figure 49-5. (*A*). Monilial granuloma of tongue. (*B*). Treated hypoparathyroidism in sister of boy seen in *A*. Note hypoplasia of enamel toward the incisal edge of several teeth.

bility to chronic mucocutaneous candidosis has also been observed in association with delayed hypersensitivity in Swiss-type agammaglobulinemia and in the DiGeorge syndrome (6).

LABORATORY AIDS

There are no specific diagnostic aids for the syndrome other than those used in the diagnosis of the individual components. Laboratory examinations to determine the calcium and phosphorus levels, tests for kidney function, and the Ellsworth-Howard test and levels of serum parathyroid hormone are necessary to establish the diagnosis of idiopathic hypoparathyroidism. The Chvostek and Trousseau signs are positive when the calcium level is sufficiently low. Hypoadrenalcorticism is established on the basis of the clinical findings, the low serum sodium and high potassium levels, and the failure of ACTH to alter the serum values of cortisol and the urinary excretion of 17-hydroxycorticosteroids. The hypothyroidism is established upon finding low serum and thyroxine and high serum thyrotropin.

REFERENCES

1 Blizzard, R. M., and Gibbs, J. H., Candidosis: Studies Pertaining to Its Association with Endocrinopathies and Pernicious Anemia. *Pediatrics* **42**:231–237, 1968.

2 Carter, A. C., et al., An Unusual Case of Idiopathic Hypoparathyroidism, Adrenal Insufficiency, Hypothyroidism and Metastatic Calcification. *J. Clin. Endocrinol.* **19**:1633–1641, 1959.

3 Castells, S., et al., Familial Moniliasis, Defective Delayed Hypersensitivity and Adrenocorticotropic Hormone Deficiency. *J. Pediatr.* **79**:72–79, 1971.

4 Chilgren, R. A., et al., Chronic Mucocutaneous Candidosis, Deficiency of Delayed Hypersensitivity and Selective Local Defect. *Lancet* **2**:688–693, 1967.

5 Collins-Williams, C., Idiopathic Hypoparathyroid with Papilledema in a Boy of 6 Years of Age: Report of a Case Associated with Moniliasis and Celiac Syndrome and Brief Review of the Literature. *Pediatrics* **5**:998–1007, 1950.

6 Cooper, M. D., et al., A New Concept of the Cellular Basis of Immunity. *J. Pediatr.* **67**:907–908, 1965.

7 Craig, J. M., et al., Chronic Moniliasis Associated with Addison's Disease. *Am. J. Dis. Child.* **89**:669–684, 1955.

8 Gass, J. D., The Syndrome of Keratoconjunctivitis, Superficial Moniliasis, Idiopathic Hypoparathyroidism and Addison's Disease. *Am. J. Ophthalmol.* **54**:660–674, 1962.

9 Genant, H. K., Addison's Disease and Hypothyroidism (Schmidt's Syndrome). *Metabolism* **16**:189–194, 1967.

10 Gharib, H., and Gastineau, C. F., Coexisting Addison's Disease and Diabetes Mellitus. *Mayo Clin. Proc.* **44**:217–227, 1969.

11 Golonka, J. E., and Goodman, A. D., Coexistence of Primary Ovarian Insufficiency, Primary Adrenocortical Insufficiency and Idiopathic Hypoparathyroidism. *J. Clin. Endocrinol.* **28**:79–82, 1968.

12 Greenberg, M. S., et al., Idiopathic Hypoparathyroidism, Chronic Candidosis and Dental Hypoplasia. *Oral Surg.* **28**:42–53, 1969.

13 Hermans, P. E., and Ritts, R. E., Chronic Mucocutaneous Candidiasis: Its Association with Immunologic and Endocrine Abnormalities. *Minn. Med.* **53**:75–80, 1970.

14 Hetzel, B. S., and Robson, H. N., The Syndrome of Hypoparathyroidism, Addison's Disease and Moniliasis. *Aust. Ann. Med.* **7**:27–33, 1958.

15 Hurwitz, L. J., Spontaneous Hypoparathyroidism with Megaloblastic Anemia. *Lancet* **1**:234–235, 1956.

16 Jordan, A., and Kelsall, A. R., Observations on a Case of Idiopathic Hypoparathyroidism. *Arch. Intern. Med.* **87**:242–258, 1951.

17 Kenny, F. M., and Holliday, M. A., Hypoparathyroidism, Moniliasis, Addison's and Hashimoto's Diseases. *N. Engl. J. Med.* **271**:708–713, 1964.

18 Kirkpatrick, C. H., et al., Chronic Mucocutaneous Moniliasis with Impaired Delayed Hypersensitivity. *Clin. Exp. Immunol.*, **6**:375–385, 1970.

19 Kirkpatrick, C. H., et al., Chronic Mucocutaneous Candidiasis: Model-Building in Cellular Immunity. *Ann. Intern. Med.* **74**:955–978, 1971.

20 Lehner, T., Classification and Clinicopathological Features of Candida Infections in the Mouth, in H. I. Winner and R. Hurley (eds.), *Symposium on Candida Infections*, E. & S. Livingstone, Edinburgh, 1966, p. 119.

21 Mortell, E. J., Idiopathic Hypoparathyroidism with Mental Deterioration: Effect of Treatment on Intellectual Function. *J. Clin. Endocrinol.* **6**:266–274, 1946.

22 Nally, F. F., Idiopathic Juvenile Hypoparathyroidism with Superficial Moniliasis. *Oral Surg.* **30**:356–365, 1970.

23 Perheentupa, J., and Hiekkala, H., Twenty Cases of the Syndrome of Autoimmune Endocrinopathy and Candidiasis, *Acta Paediatr. Scand.* **62**:110–111, 1973.

24 Richman, R. A., et al., Candidiasis and Multiple Endocrinopathies. *Arch. Dermatol.* **111**:625–627, 1975.

25 Sjöberg, K. H., Monihasis—an Internal Disease. *Acta Med. Scand.* **179**:157–166, 1966.

26 Spinner, M. W., et al., Clinical and Genetic Heterogeneity in Idiopathic Addison's Disease and Hypoparathyroidism. *J. Clin. Endocrinol.* **3**:625–634, 1943.

27 Talbot, N. B., et al., The Effect of Testosterone and Allied Compounds on the Mineral, Nitrogen and Carbohydrate Metabolism of a Girl with Addison's Disease. *J. Clin. In-*

vest. **22:**583–593, 1943.

28 Thorpe, E. S., and Handley, H. E., Chronic Tetany and Chronic Mycelial Stomatitis in a Child Aged 4½ years. *Am. J. Dis. Child.* **38:**328–338, 1929.

29 Wells, R. S., Chronic Oral Candidiasis (Autosomal Recessive Inheritance). *Proc. R. Soc. Med.* **63:**10–11, 1970.

30 Whitaker, J., et al., The Syndrome of Familial Juvenile Hypoadrenalcorticism, Hypoparathyroidism and Superficial Moniliasis. *J. Clin. Endocrinol.* **16:**1374–1387, 1956.

31 Wuepper, K. D., and Fudenberg, H. H., Moniliasis, "Autoimmune" Polyendocrinopathy, an Immunologic Family Study. *Clin. Exp. Immunol.* **2:**71–82, 1967.

50

Epidermal Nevus Syndrome

(Linear Sebaceous Nevus Syndrome)

In 1962, Feuerstein and Mims (5) described two patients with (a) linear epidermal nevus, (b) convulsions, (c) mental retardation. An earlier example is that of Berg and Crome (1). Marden and Venters (13) and Monahan et al. (16) noted patients with similar findings. Less certain, because of incomplete information, are the cases of Sherman (18), Gördüren (7), and Lall (10).

All cases reported to date have been sporadic. However, Berg and Crome (1) and Bianchine (2) noted relatives with either seizures or mental retardation. We concur with Solomon et al. (19) that the name "epidermal nevus syndrome" is more appropriate than "linear sebaceous nevus syndrome" since sebaceous elements may be absent.

SYSTEMIC MANIFESTATIONS

Facies. The facies is characterized by an extensive unilateral or (less commonly) bilateral linear epidermal nevus, which often extends from the crown of the scalp to the nose or lip.

Eye and ear. The palpebral fissures may have an antimongoloid slant. Dermoid or lipodermoid of the conjunctiva; eyelid ptosis; choroidal, iris, or upper eyelid colobomas; and nystagmus may be present (1, 4, 5, 9, 13, 15a, 17, 20). One patient had slanted pinnas and deafness (13).

Skin. The most prominent feature of the syndrome is an extensive congenital linear epidermal nevus (Fig. 50-1A–D). This lesion is a form of epithelial dysplasia, a prominent component of which may be sebaceous glands. The latter impart a yellow-brown appearance and a greasy consistency to the verrucous plaque. In most cases, the nevus occurs on the head, with a special predilection for the sutural areas of the scalp and the region around the ears, temple, and forehead (Fig. 50-2A, B).

A unilateral arrangement of pigmented nevi, blue nevi, and mongolian spots has been observed in one patient (20). Macular pigmented lesions were noted on the neck, trunk, and limbs of another individual (13, 16).

Central nervous system. Nearly all patients with epidermal nevus syndrome have mental retardation, frequent focal, myoclonic, or generalized seizures which appear during the first few years of life, and occasionally hemiparesis (9, 10a). No calcifications have been detected in the brain. The ventricles usually are enlarged, with cerebral atrophy. Hydrocephaly has been described (13, 16). A single gliotic focus with giant nerve cells in the temporal lobe has been noted (1).

Some patients have exhibited asymmetry of the skull and premature closure of the spheno-frontal suture (16, 17, 20).

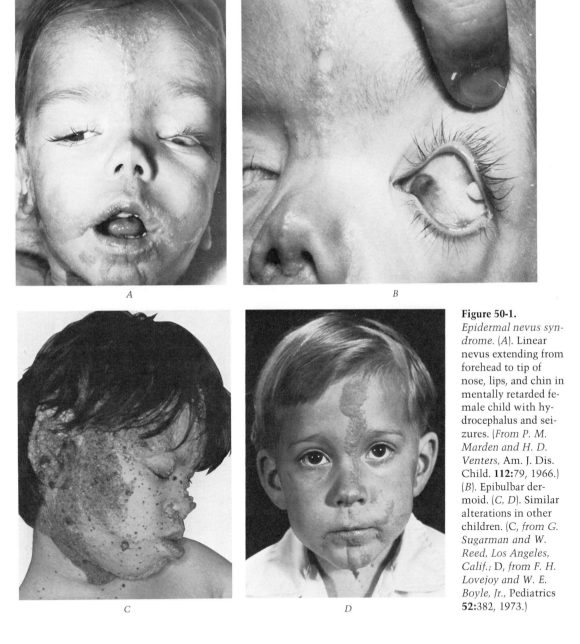

A

B

C

D

Figure 50-1.
Epidermal nevus syndrome. (*A*). Linear nevus extending from forehead to tip of nose, lips, and chin in mentally retarded female child with hydrocephalus and seizures. (*From P. M. Marden and H. D. Venters, Am. J. Dis. Child.* **112**:79, 1966.) (*B*). Epibulbar dermoid. (*C, D*). Similar alterations in other children. (*C, from G. Sugarman and W. Reed, Los Angeles, Calif.; D, from F. H. Lovejoy and W. E. Boyle, Jr., Pediatrics* **52**:382, 1973.)

Other organs. Coarctation and hypoplasia of the aorta and bizarre origin of the subclavian artery were noted (13). A bilateral lytic defect of the eighth, ninth, and tenth ribs and gross malformation of the clavicles have been described (20).

Defects of the humerus were noted by Gorduren (7) and by Moynahan and Wolff (17).

Oral manifestations. The epidermal nevus may, by extension, involve the upper lip and hard pal-

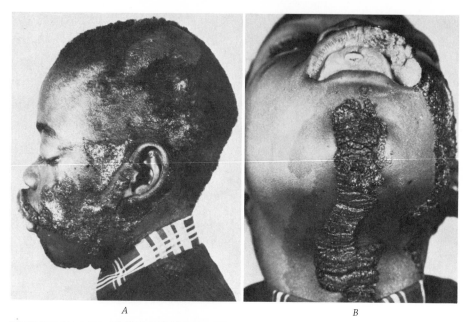

A   *B*

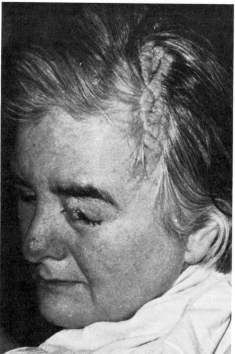

C

Figure 50-2. (*A, B*). Ten-year-old male with epidermal nevus syndrome. Note linear distribution, focal alopecia, hyperpigmented areas. Patient was blind and had epileptiform seizures. (*From J. E. Kelley et al., Oral Surg.* **34**:774, 1972.) (*C*). Same disorder in forty-five-year-old mentally retarded woman. Associated were coloboma of upper eyelid, epibulbar dermoid, hyperostosis of skull, ipsilateral cerebral atrophy. (*From J. Jancar, Bristol, England.*)

ate (1, 3, 13, 16, 22) (Fig. 50-3*A, B*). The patient described by Berg and Crome (1) had cleft palate, and that of Jancar (9) had bifid uvula. The teeth in the involved area are frequently hypoplastic (2, 13, 16) and may resemble teeth having odontodysplasia (Fig. 50-3*C*).

DIFFERENTIAL DIAGNOSIS

In two large series of patients with isolated sebaceous nevus, there were no instances of mental deficiency or convulsions (14, 23). The epidermal nevus may occasionally be associated with congenital skeletal disorders and central nervous system disease. Of 35 such patients reviewed by Solomon and associates (19), 13 exhibited skeletal abnormalities; nine, central nervous system abnormalities; and eight, both.

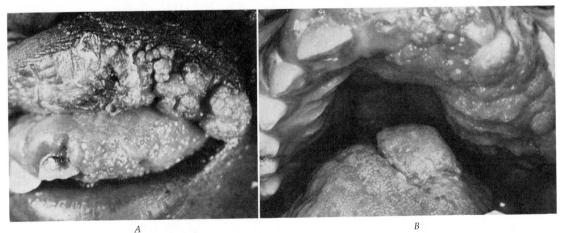

A

B

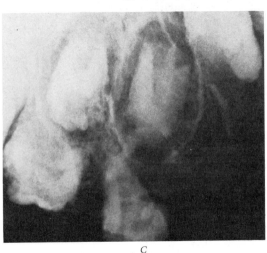

C

Figure 50-3. (*A*). Labial and gingival involvement. (*B*). Unilateral involvement of maxillary alveolar ridge, palate, and tongue. (*C*). Roentgenogram of teeth showing hypoplasia of enamel and dentin reminiscent of odontodysplasia. (*From J. E. Kelley et al.*, Oral Surg. **34:**774, 1972.)

Nevus unius lateris, bilateral linear epidermal nevi, and ichthyosis hystrix may be grouped under the general category of epidermal nevi. Nevus unius lateris was described in association with brain tumor and diencephalic syndrome (15).

LABORATORY AIDS

Biopsy of the epidermal nevus.

REFERENCES

1 Berg, J. M., and Crome, J., A Possible Case of Atypical Tuberous Sclerosis. *J. Ment. Defic. Res.* **4:**24–31, 1960.

2 Bianchine, J., The Nevus Sebaceous (*sic*) of Jadassohn: A Neurocutaneous Syndrome and a Potentially Premalignant Lesion. *Am. J. Dis. Child.* **120:**223–228, 1970.

3 Bitter, K., Über die Erstbeobachtung eines angeborenen Naevus sebaceus im Trigeminusbereich mit Gehirnmissbildungen und Riesenzellgeschwülsten des Ober- und Unterkiefers. *Dtsch. Zahn Mund Kieferheilkd.* **56:**17–24, 1971.

4 Chaurasia, B. D., and Goswami, H. K., Congenitally Malformed Female Infant with Hairy Ears. *Clin. Genet.* **2:**111–114, 1971.

5 Feuerstein, R. C., and Mims, L. C., Linear Nevus Sebaceus with Convulsions and Mental Retardation. *Am. J. Dis. Child.* **104:**675–679, 1962.

6 Gellis, S. S., and Feingold, M., Linear Nevus Sebaceous (*sic*) Syndrome. *Am. J. Dis. Child.* **120:**139–140, 1970.

7 Gördüren, S., Aberrant Lacrimal Gland Associated with Other Congenital Abnormalities. *Br. J. Ophthalmol.* **46:**277–280, 1962.

8 Herbst, B. A., and Cohen, M. E., Linear Nevus Sebaceus. *Arch. Neurol.* (*Chic.*) **24:**317–322, 1971.

8a Holden, K. R., et al. Neurological Involvement in Nevus Unius Lateris and Nevus Linearis Sebaceus. *Neurology* (*Minneap.*) **22:**879–897, 1972.

9 Jancar, J., Naevus Syringocystadenomatosus Papilliferus with Skull and Brain Lesions, Hemiparesis, Epilepsy and Mental Retardation. *Br. J. Dermatol.* **82:**402–406, 1970.

10 Lall, K., Teratoma of Conjunctiva (Associated with Nevus Systematicus and Epilepsia Symptomatica). *Acta Ophthalmol.* (*Kbh.*) **40:**555–558, 1962.

10a Lansky, L. L., et al., Linear Sebaceous Nevus Syndrome. *Am. J. Dis. Child.* **128:**587–590, 1972.

11 Lantis, S., et al., Nevus Sebaceus of Jadassohn: Part of a New Neurocutaneous Syndrome. *Arch. Dermatol.* **98:**117–123, 1968.

12 Lovejoy, F. H., and Boyle, W. E., Linear Nevus Sebaceous (*sic*) Syndrome. *Pediatrics* **52:**382–387, 1973.

13 Marden, P. M., and Venters, H. D., A New Neurocutaneous Syndrome. *Am. J. Dis. Child.* **112:**79–81, 1966.

14 Mehregan, H., and Pinkus, H., Life History of Organoid Nevi. *Arch. Dermatol.* **91:**564–588, 1965.

15 Meyerson, L. B., Nevus Unius Lateralis, Brain Tumor, and Diencephalic Syndrome. *Arch. Dermatol.* **95:**501–504, 1967.

15a Mollica, F., et al., Linear Sebaceous Nevus in a Newborn. *Am. J. Dis. Child.* **128:**868–871, 1974.

16 Monahan, R. H., et al., Multiple Choristomas, Convulsion and Mental Retardation as a New Neurocutaneous Syndrome. *Am. J. Ophthalmol.* **64:**529–532, 1967.

17 Moynahan, E. J., and Wolff, O. H., A New Neurocutaneous Syndrome (Skin, Eye, Brain) Consisting of Linear Nevus, Bilateral Lipodermoids of the Conjunctiva, Cranial Thickening, Cerebral Cortical Atrophy, and Mental Retardation. *Br. J. Dermatol.* **79:**651–652, 1967.

18 Sherman, A. R., Teratoid Tumor of the Conjunctiva with Other Developmental Anomalies with Naevus Verrucosus of Scalp. *Arch. Ophthalmol.* **29:**441–445, 1943.

19 Solomon, L. M., et al., The Epidermal Nevus Syndrome. *Arch. Dermatol.* **97:**273–285, 1968.

20 Sugarman, G. I., and Reed, W. B., Two Unusual Neurocutaneous Disorders with Facial Cutaneous Signs (Case 1). *Arch. Neurol. (Chic.)* **21:**242–247, 1969.

21 Tripp, J. H., A New "Neurocutaneous" Syndrome (Skin, Eye, Brain, and Heart Syndrome. *Proc. R. Soc. Med.* **64:**23–24, 1971.

22 Wauschkuhn, J., and Rohde, B., Systematisierte Talgdrüsen-, Pigment- und epitheliale Naevi mit neurologischer Symptomatik; Feuerstein-Mimssches Neuroektodermales Syndrom. *Hautarzt* **22:**10–13, 1971.

23 Wilson Jones, E., and Heyl, T., Naevus Sebaceus: A Report of 140 Cases with Special Regard to Development of Secondary Malignant Tumours. *Br. J. Dermatol.* **82:**99–117, 1970.

51

Epidermolysis Bullosa

Epidermolysis bullosa includes several hereditary vesicular disorders that involve skin and often oral and other mucosas. The vesicles usually arise at points of trauma. For some types, however, heat may be the precipitating factor, or the blisters may arise spontaneously.

The interested reader is referred to the works of Bergenholtz and Olsson (9), Schnyder and coworkers (37, 38), and Gedde-Dahl (18) for a detailed historical review.

Epidermolysis bullosa is classified into autosomal dominant and recessive forms (see Table 51-1), each of which may be divided into two or more types (15, 29, 30). These will be considered separately.

DOMINANT SIMPLEX FORM

Systemic manifestations. Sites of friction or trauma are most frequently involved. Nails are affected in about 20 percent of cases. Scarring and/or pigmentation do not result after healing. The disorder, which usually appears neonatally or during infancy when the child begins to crawl, principally involves the feet, hands, and neck, rarely the ankles, knees, trunk, and elbows (Fig. 51-1A). After the third year of life, usually only the hands and feet are affected. The nails are normal. Generally, the condition improves markedly at puberty. Heat also seems to be an important precipitating factor in blister production (16). Most authors attempt to separate generalized involvement (Koebner type) from a group in which only the feet are affected (Weber-Cockayne type). This latter form more commonly (70 percent as against 40 percent) appears at less than one year of age.

Oral manifestations. Although 2 percent of patients are stated to have oral bullae (39), there is not sufficient documentation of this claim. Davidson (16) and Tilsley and Beard (42), for example, found no oral involvement. Gedde-Dahl (18) noted lingual and/or palatal lesions in several patients (Fig. 51-1B).

Histologic study reveals cleavage through the basal layer, with nuclei on the blister floor, i.e., above the PAS-positive basement membrane. Adjacent to areas of separation, the basal cells are vacuolated, with displacement of the nucleus to the epidermal end of the cell. These alterations have been confirmed ultrastructurally (31, 32). No histochemical abnormality has been observed (25).

DOMINANT DYSTROPHIC (HYPERTROPHIC) FORM

Systemic manifestations. This form of epidermolysis bullosa (Cockayne-Touraine type) is characterized by flat, pink, scar-producing bullae of the ankles, knees, hands, elbows, and feet, in decreasing order of frequency (16). Milia are common but less numerous than in the recessive dysplastic type. The nails are usually (in 80

Table 51-1. Epidermolysis bullosa

			Site of lesions							
Type	Inheritance	Age of onset	Extremities	Mucous membranes	Nails	Trunk	Teeth	Residual scarring	Physical and mental development	Prognosis
Simple	Dominant	Infancy or childhood	+	0	0	0	0	0	Normal	Often clears at puberty
Dystrophic	Dominant	Birth or early infancy	+	±	+	±	0	+	Normal	May clear at puberty
Dystrophic	Recessive	Birth or early infancy	+	+	+	±	+	+	Retarded	Most patients die in childhood
Lethal	Recessive	Birth	+	+	+	+	−	0	....	Most patients die in early infancy

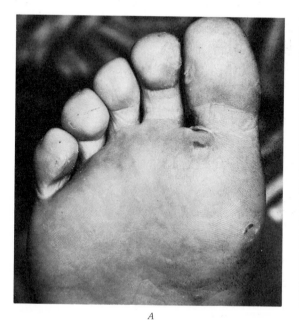
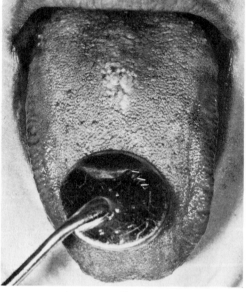

A   B

Figure 51-1. *Epidermolysis bullosa, dominant simplex type.* (*A*). Nonscarring blisters of feet. (*B*). Oral vesicles, seen in about 2 percent of patients.

RECESSIVE DYSTROPHIC TYPE

Systemic manifestations. The extensive studies of Gedde-Dahl (18) suggest that this disorder is a genetic heterogeneity. The reader is referred to his text for a discussion of the many subtypes.

Bullae are usually manifested at or shortly after birth, arising at sites of pressure or trauma or appearing spontaneously. In infants, the most commonly affected areas are the feet, buttocks, scapulas, elbows, fingers, and occiput. In older children, the hands, feet, knees, and elbows are most often involved. When a bulla ruptures or its roof peels off, a raw painful surface is evident. The fluid contained in the bulla is at first sterile but may become secondarily infected and bloody. Upon healing, the bullae often are followed by keloidal scars, causing contraction, and by various degrees of pigmentation or depigmentation. They are frequently associated with miliumlike cysts. The scars may lead to loss of bony structures or to interference with growth and resultant dwarfism. Formation of clawhand and the enclosure of the hand in a glovelike epidermal sac have been noted frequently (12) (Fig. 51-3A). The Nikolsky sign is often present. The nails may be extremely involved, often being dystrophic or absent (18) (Fig. 51-3B, C). Hyperhidrosis of palms and soles is an inconsistent finding but may be marked. Hair may be deficient.

The eyes have been subject to a number of changes: essential shrinkage of the conjunctiva, nonspecific blepharitis, symblepharon, conjunctivitis, and keratitis with corneal opacity and vesicle formation (18).

Hoarseness and, rarely, aphonia and dysphagia may occur as a result of bullae of the larynx or pharynx. Laryngeal stenosis may eventuate from the scarring. Involvement of the esophagus may result in complete obstruction (8).

Changes are essentially limited to the hands, feet, and esophagus. The esophagus (most often the upper half) may become segmentally stenotic in childhood, with consequent dysphagia (8, 45). The metacarpals become slender and overconstricted, and the distal phalanges become pointed and clawlike (12).

Oral manifestations. Although a considerable number of authors have remarked on the teeth

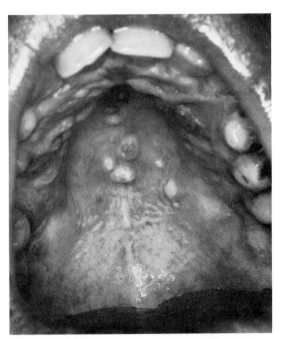

Figure 51-2. *Dominant dystrophic type.* Milia of palate. (*From J. O. Andreasen et al.*, Acta Pathol. Microbiol. Scand. **63**:37, 1965.)

percent of cases) thick and dystrophic. In contrast to what happens in the recessive dystrophic cases, the conjunctiva and cornea are never involved. About 20 percent of patients show changes before the age of one year (37). Improvement seems to occur with age. Hyperhidrosis of the palms and soles may also occur. Bart et al. (6, 7) described localized absence of skin associated with what may be dominant dystrophic epidermolysis bullosa or may, on the other hand, represent a new syndrome, the latter possibility being more likely.

Oral manifestations. The consensus favors the view that teeth are not affected. Touraine's oft-quoted statement (43) that 20 percent of patients manifest oral bullae would appear to be essentially substantiated by other studies (16, 37), but the series have been small. Oral milia were noted by Andreasen and associates (2) (Fig. 51-2). These milia are not retention cysts, but epidermoid cysts which originate from detached islands of epithelium in areas of earlier bulla formation.

having hypoplastic enamel with great susceptibility to dental caries, delayed eruption, and frequent retention, there is little documentation concerning frequency of these manifestations (21, 27, 46). We share with Rodermund (35) the belief that there is no correlation between the degree of cutaneous involvement and the degree of dental involvement. Pockmarked alteration of the enamel was handsomely illustrated by Rodermund (35) (Fig. 51-3G). Excellent histologic studies of unerupted teeth have been published by Delaire and colleagues (17) and by Arwill and coworkers (4). Both groups noted hypoplasia of enamel with absence of prismatic structure. The dentin is probably not significantly affected (4).

Oral mucosal involvement occurs soon after birth, vesicles apparently forming from the negative pressure involved in the sucking reflex (Fig. 51-3D). Although oral bullae are said to occur in at least 16 percent of cases (39), our impression is that the percentage is much higher. The lingual mucosa appears thick, gray, and smooth and may become bound down (47) (Fig. 51-3E, F). The sulci may become obliterated, with much scarring, microstomia, and immobility of the lips (Fig. 51-3F). Even routine dental management may cause the eruption of bullae on the lips and oral mucosa. The slightest abrasion from normal toothbrushing may cause serious sequelae. Other oral changes, the frequencies of which have not been established, are atrophy of the maxilla with resultant relative mandibular prognathism, increased mandibular angle (1, 12), and oral carcinoma (22, 34, 36).

Histopathologic changes in the oral mucosa were well demonstrated by Arwill and associates (3). As shown in skin by Vogel and Schnyder (44) and by Lowe (25), the bullae occur below the PAS-positive basement membrane. Hemidesmosomes and tonofibrils are absent or decreased in numbers. Lowe (25) also noted an increase in elastic and preelastic fibers in the corium. Hitchin (19) described defective cementum.

EPIDERMOLYSIS BULLOSA LETALIS

Systemic manifestations. The criteria for diagnosis of the Herlitz lethal type are (a) neonatal onset, (b) death within the first 3 months of life, and (c) absence of milia, pigmentary changes, and scarring (Fig. 51-4). Several authors (23, 25, 28) view the lethal type as a severe form of the dystrophic recessive disorder. The two disorders may represent different alleles of the same gene (18). Though the ultrastructural studies of Pearson (31) suggest that they are distinct, those of Lapière and colleagues (24) challenge his findings. At the present time, we have only clinical criteria, such as early death and absence of scarring, pigmentation, and/or milia, to separate the two forms. To compound the confusion further, there are a few examples in which scarring occurred after several months (9). Histochemical or biochemical differences have not been found (25).

Usually the vesicles, often hemorrhagic, are noted at the base of the fingernails within the first few hours of life. The nails soon become loose and are shed. This is followed by involvement of the trunk, umbilicus, face, scalp, and extremities. The palms and soles are never affected. There seems to be an absence of reaction to traumatic provocation.

Light-microscope examination demonstrates epidermal-dermal cleavage which follows the rete ridge contour. Inflammatory changes are not originally present (26, 33). Vesicles at the dermoepidermal junction in the stratum germinativum of intact skin have been demonstrated (9, 33).

Electron microscopic study was carried out by Pearson (31), who suggested that in the lethal form separation occurred between the plasma membrane of the basal cell and the basement membrane. In contrast, he found that in patients with the recessive dystrophic type, the initial alterations occurred in the basal cell layer. However, this view was not sustained by the ultrastructural studies of Lapière and colleagues (24), who described changes in the cytoplasm of juxtadermal cells, or by Vogel and Schnyder (44), who noted the same changes described by Pearson in recessive dystrophic cases.

Oral manifestations. Bullae which are remarkably fragile and hemorrhagic are found in nearly all patients, especially at the junction between the hard and soft palates (5). Histologic

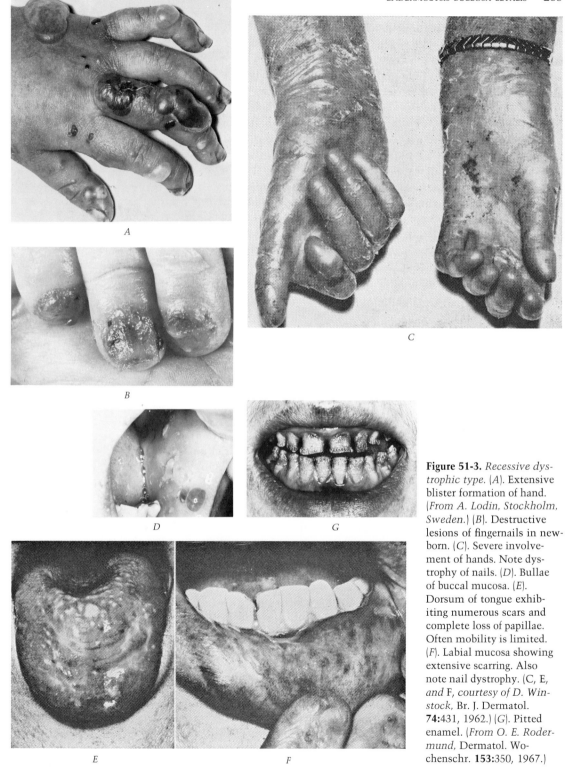

Figure 51-3. *Recessive dystrophic type.* (*A*). Extensive blister formation of hand. (*From A. Lodin, Stockholm, Sweden.*) (*B*). Destructive lesions of fingernails in newborn. (*C*). Severe involvement of hands. Note dystrophy of nails. (*D*). Bullae of buccal mucosa. (*E*). Dorsum of tongue exhibiting numerous scars and complete loss of papillae. Often mobility is limited. (*F*). Labial mucosa showing extensive scarring. Also note nail dystrophy. (C, E, and F, *courtesy of D. Winstock,* Br. J. Dermatol. **74**:431, 1962.) (*G*). Pitted enamel. (*From O. E. Rodermund,* Dermatol. Wochenschr. **153**:350, 1967.)

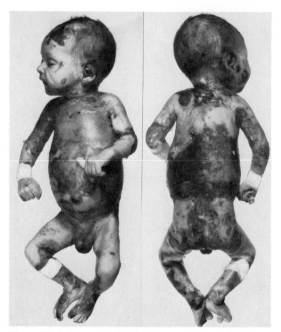

Figure 51-4. *Recessive letalis type.* Extensive skin involvement. *(From E. B. Brain and J. S. Wigglesworth,* Br. Dent. J. **124:**255, 1968.)

study reveals cleavage between the epithelium and connective tissue or within the epithelium between the basal layer and the stratum spinosum. The cells of the basal layer seem quite palisaded as a result of extracellular vacuolization.

Arwill and coworkers (5) investigated skin as well as oral mucosa ultrastructurally in four cases of the letalis form. They found that, in contrast to findings in the normal infant, the gingiva and skin exhibited fewer hemidesmosomes and tonofilaments. The initial changes consisted of edema of the subepithelial connective tissue; degeneration of mitochondria; an electron-opaque perinuclear zone which, upon dissolution, frees remnants of tonofibrils and mitochondria; and widened intercellular spaces between epithelial basal cells. Although the desmosomes remained intact, minute vesicles were found between the basement membrane and the basal cell membrane in the intermediate zone. The lamellated pattern of the hemidesmosomes disappeared, with replacement by a granular substance.

Arwill and colleagues (4) appear to have been the first to have done microscopic and microradiographic studies on the teeth of patients with the lethal form of the disease. The enamel, lamellar in appearance, varied in thickness from 50 to 400 μ, the outer and inner zones being more markedly mineralized than the intermediate zone. Outside and at varied distances from the surface were free globular structures exhibiting variable mineralization. The cervical enamel was more highly mineralized than the incisal edge. In the permanent teeth there was folding at the dentinoenamel junction, which was normal in the deciduous teeth.

Decalcified sections showed intense proliferation of the dental lamina and the inner and outer enamel epithelium. The latter also manifested metaplasia to stratified squamous epithelium. Numerous vacuoles containing epithelium were observed. The enamel stroma was hyalinized, lamellar, and, at times, globular. Vascular proliferation was marked about the tooth germs, and hemorrhage was noted in the dental sac and stellate reticulum.

Brain and Wigglesworth (11) also investigated the deciduous dentition of an infant with the lethal form of epidermolysis bullosa, and noted that the enamel was greatly reduced in quantity, being only 40 μ thick. There was no organized prism structure, and some parts appeared laminated. Globules resembling enamel were distributed between the hypoplastic layer of enamel and the outer enamel epithelium. The reduced enamel epithelium was extensively disorganized. Vesicle-like structures were present adjacent to tooth crowns.

DIFFERENTIAL DIAGNOSIS

Recognition of the disease is seldom difficult, even without assessing the entire clinical, genetic, and histologic character of the disease. In infants and children, the syndrome may be confused with conditions such as bullous impetigo (so-called "pemphigus neonatorum"), Ritter disease, porphyria congenita, congenital syphilis, or juvenile bullous dermatitis herpetiformis. In older patients, differential diagnosis includes pemphigus, drug eruptions, dermatitis herpetiformis, and bullous *erythema multiforme.*

It has been noted that in epidermolysis bullosa, pulling up of a strip of cellophane adhesive tape will cause the top layers of the skin to adhere to the tape. This phenomenon is not seen in Ritter disease or in generalized impetigo. The lesions of porphyria are generally confined to chronically sun-exposed areas, and only exposed skin is fragile; epidermolysis bullosa shows no localization of skin fragility.

LABORATORY AIDS

Microscopically, bullae are subepithelial in the recessive dystrophic and lethal forms; thus, in the simple type, they are most often observed within the epidermis beneath the stratum corneum. Capillary dilatation and the development of new vessels together with nonspecific inflammatory reaction are present, and the organization of this granulation tissue is thought to account for the final scarring. Absence of elastic tissue in the dystrophic form is probably not primary but is the result of destruction by the inflammatory process. Studies of normal elastic tissue indicate that it plays no part in the coherence between epidermis and dermis. The milia-like lesions found in the dystrophic form consist of small intradermally located epidermal cysts. Sweat glands and hair follicles are reduced in number.

Electron microscopic studies have indicated the possibility of distinguishing the lethal form, the recessive dystrophic form, and porphyria cutanea tarda.

REFERENCES

1 Alpert, M., Roentgen Manifestations of Epidermolysis Bullosa. *Am. J. Roentgenol.* **78**:66–72, 1957.

2 Andreasen, J. O., et al., Milia Formation in Oral Lesions in Epidermolysis Bullosa. *Acta Pathol. Microbiol. Scand.* **63**:37–41, 1965.

3 Arwill, T., et al., Epidermolysis Bullosa Hereditaria. IV. Histologic Changes of the Oral Mucosa in the Polydysplastic, Dystrophica, and the Letalis Forms. *Odontol. Rev.* **16**:101–111, 1965.

4 Arwill, T., et al., Epidermolysis Bullosa Hereditaria. III. Histologic Study of Changes in Teeth in the Polydysplastic, Dystrophic, and Lethal Forms. *Oral Surg.* **19**:723–744, 1965.

5 Arwill, T., et al., Epidermolysis Bullosa Hereditaria. V. The Ultrastructure of Oral Mucosa and Skin in Four Cases of the Letalis Form. *Acta Pathol. Microbiol. Scand.* **74**:311–324, 1968.

6 Bart, B., Epidermolysis Bullosa and Congenital Localized Absence of Skin. *Arch. Dermatol.* **101**:78–81, 1970.

7 Bart, B. J., et al., Localized Absence of Skin and Associated Abnormalities Resembling Epidermolysis Bullosa. *Arch. Dermatol.* **93**:296–304, 1966.

8 Becker, M. H., and Swinyard, C. A., Epidermolysis Bullosa Dystrophica in Children; Radiologic Manifestations. *Radiology* **90**:124–128, 1968.

9 Bergenholtz, A., and Olsson, O., Epidermolysis Bullosa Hereditaria. I. Epidermolysis Bullosa Hereditaria Letalis; A Survey of the Literature and Report of 11 Cases, *Acta Derm. Venereol.* (*Stockh.*) **48**:220–241, 1968.

10 Bergenholtz, A., et al., Die Epidermolysis bullosa hereditaria dystrophica mit Oesophagusveränderungen. *Arch. Klin. Exp. Dermatol.* **217**:518–533, 1963.

11 Brain, E. B., and Wigglesworth, J. S., Developing Teeth in Epidermolysis Bullosa Hereditaria Letalis; A Histologic Study. *Br. Dent. J.* **124**:255–260, 1968.

12 Brinn, L. B., and Khilnam, M. T., Epidermolysis Bullosa with Characteristic Hand Deformities. *Radiology* **89**:272–274, 1967.

13 Bülow, K., and Nörholm-Pedersen, A., Epidermolysis bullosa hereditaria. *Ugeskr. Laeger* **115**:479–487, 1953.

14 Crikelair, G. F., et al., Skin Homografts in Epidermolysis Bullosa Dystrophica. *Plast. Reconstr. Surg.* **46**:89–92, 1970.

15 Cross, H. E., et al., Inheritance in Epidermolysis Bullosa Hereditaria. *J. Med. Genet.* **5**:189–196, 1968.

16 Davidson, B. C. C., Epidermolysis Bullosa. *J. Med. Genet.* **2**:233–242, 1965.

17 Delaire, J., et al., Manifestation buccodentaires des epidermolyses bulleuses. *Rev. Stomatol.* (*Paris*) **61**:189–200, 1960.

18 Gedde-Dahl, T., Jr., *Epidermolysis Bullosa: A Clinical, Genetic, and Epidemiologic Study.* Johns Hopkins, Baltimore, 1971.

19 Hitchin, A. D., The Defects of Cementum in Epidermolysis Bullosa Dystrophica. *Br. Dent. J.* **135**:437–441, 1973.

20 Keller, L., Silver Nitrate Therapy in Epidermolysis Bullosa Hereditaria of the Newborn. *J. Pediatr.* **72**:854–856, 1968.

21 Kinast, H., and Schuh, E., Die Epidermolysis Bullosa und ihre orale Erscheinungsform. *Oest. Z. Stomatol.* **70**:166–175, 1973.

22 Klausner, E., Zungenkrebs als Folgestand bei einem Falle von Epidermolysis bullosa (dystrophische Form). *Arch. Dermatol. Syphilol.* (*Berl.*) **116**:71–78, 1913.

23 Klunker, W., Zur nosologischen Stellung der Epidermolysis bullosa hereditaria letalis Herlitz (mit Kasuistik). *Arch. Klin. Exp. Dermatol.* **216**:74–100, 1963.

24 Lapière, S., et al., Elektronenmikroskopische Untersuchungen über die Ultrastruktur der Epidermolysis bullosa letalis bei einem Saügling mit familiärer Belastung. *Hautarzt* **15**:30–33, 1964.

25 Lowe, L. B., Hereditary Epidermolysis Bullosa. *Arch. Dermatol.* **95:**587–595, 1967.

26 Maddison, T. G., and Barter, R. A., Epidermolysis Bullosa Hereditaria Letalis. *Arch. Dis. Child.* **36:**337–339, 1961.

27 Matras, H., Ein Beitrag zur Epidermolysis bullosa dystrophica mit Zahn- und Mundschleimhautveränderungen. *Oest. Z. Stomatol.* **60:**138–145, 1963.

28 Muggler, F., Häufung von Epidermolysis bullosa hereditaria dystrophica recessiva in einer grossen Aargauer Sippe. *Helv. Paediatr. Acta* **18:**323–338, 1963.

29 Noojin, R. D., et al., Genetic Study of Hereditary Type of Epidermolysis Bullosa Simplex. *Arch. Dermatol.* **65:**477–483, 1963.

30 Passarge, E., Epidermolysis Bullosa Hereditaria Simplex. *J. Pediatr.* **67:**819–825, 1963.

31 Pearson, R. W., Epidermolysis Bullosa Hereditaria Letalis. *Arch. Dermatol.* **109:**349–355, 1974.

32 Ritzenfeld, P., Zur Histogenese und Differentialdiagnose hereditären Epidermolysen. *Arch. Klin. Exp. Dermatol.* **224:**128–137, 1966.

33 Roberts, M. H., et al., Epidermolysis Bullosa Letalis; Report of Three Cases with Particular Reference to the Histopathology of the Skin. *Pediatrics* **25:**283–290, 1960.

34 Röckl, H., Carcinom bei Epidermolysis bullosa dystrophica. *Hautarzt* **7:**463–464, 1956.

35 Rodermund, O. E., Zahnveränderungen bei Epidermolysis bullosa. *Dermatol. Wochenschr.* **153:**350–357, 1967.

36 Schiller, F., Zungencarcinom bei Epidermolysis bullosa dystrophica, *Arch. Klin. Exp. Dermatol.* **209:**643–651, 1960.

37 Schnyder, U. W., and Eichhoff, D., Zur Klinik und Genetik der dominant dystrophische Epidermolysis bullosa hereditaria. *Arch. Klin. Exp. Dermatol.* **218:**62–90, 1964.

38 Schnyder, Y. W., et al., Zur Klassifizierung, Histogenetik, Gerinnungsphysiologie und Therapie der hereditären Epidermolysen. *Arch. Klin. Exp. Dermatol.* **220:**38–59, 1964.

39 Schuermann, H., *Krankheiten der Mundschleimhaut und der Lippen,* 2d ed., Urban & Schwarzenberg, Berlin, 1958.

40 Severin, G. L., and Farber, E. M., The Management of Epidermolysis Bullosa in Children; Effective Topical Steroid Treatment. *Arch. Dermatol.* **95:**302–307, 1967.

41 Silver, H. K., Epidermolysis Bullosa Hereditaria Letalis. *Arch. Dis. Child.* **32:**216–219, 1957.

42 Tilsley, D. A., and Beard, T. C., Epidermolysis Bullosa Simplex in Tasmania. *Lancet* **2:**905–907, 1963.

43 Touraine, M. A., Classification des epidermolyses bulleuses. *Ann. Dermatol. Syphiligr.* (*Paris*) **2:**309–312, 1942.

44 Vogel, A., and Schnyder, U. W., Feinstrukturelle Untersuchungen an rezessivdystrophischer Epidermolysis bullosa hereditaria. *Dermatologica* **135:**149–172, 1967.

45 Wey, W., and Schnyder, U. W., Über Ösophagustenosen bei Epidermolysis bullosa hereditaria und ihre Busehandlung. *Dermatologica* **128:**173–183, 1964.

46 Winstock, D., Oral Aspects of Epidermolysis Bullosa. *Br. J. Dermatol.* **74:**431–438, 1962.

52

Erythema Multiforme

(Stevens-Johnson Syndrome)

Because of the great variation in clinical manifestations, the terminology of erythema multiforme has been, and still is, very confusing. In 1860, Hebra (11) coined the term "erythema multiforme exudativum" in an attempt to describe a new entity characterized by cutaneous lesions and constitutional symptoms, but he made no mention of mucosal involvement. In 1876, Fuchs (9) described the mucosal lesions; subsequently, the condition was known as the Fuchs syndrome. Fiessinger and Rendu (7), in 1917, observing a number of similar cases occurring in soldiers on the French front, suggested the name "ectodermosis erosiva pluriorificialis" (8). In 1922, Stevens and Johnson (25) described what they thought was a new entity and designated it "eruptive fever associated with stomatitis and ophthalmia." Since this report, many authors, particularly those in the English-speaking world, have applied the term "Stevens-Johnson syndrome" when referring to cases of the more severe type of erythema multiforme. In the German-speaking countries, the term "Baader's dermatostomatitis" has been widely accepted for the same condition (1).

Thomas (28) suggested that "erythema multiforme exudativum minor" and "erythema multiforme exudativum major" be applied to the mild and severe cases, respectively. Other authors use the term "minor" for patients who primarily present cutaneous and oromucosal lesions, and the term "major" for those presenting not only cutaneous and oromucosal lesions but also fever and ocular and genital involvement (14). Most authors, however, consider the above-mentioned conditions to be the same basic disease with a great variety of clinical manifestations.

One reason for the confusion is the obscure etiology (10). Many precipitating factors are known, of which herpes simplex infection is an important one (17, 20). The majority of cases, however, are idiopathic. Apart from viral etiology, other infectious agents and an allergic mechanism, particularly associated with drugs, may play etiologic roles (27). Recent observations have emphasized the significance of *Mycoplasma pneumoniae* (17). The role of drugs as etiologic factors in erythema multiforme has been studied in 138 cases by Bianchine et al. (2). Various antibiotics, especially sulfa drugs, were most frequently associated with the syndrome.

A recurrence rate of 25 percent has been reported (26). No definite rules concerning time of recurrence can be given. The degree of severity may vary in the same patient during different attacks (28). Each attack may be characterized by a different form of skin lesion. The episodes may flare in certain parts of the year, usually in spring and fall, perhaps because of the seasonal variation in humidity which has been demonstrated to occur (Table 52-1).

SYSTEMIC MANIFESTATIONS

In the following description of erythema multiforme, we shall not make any attempt to sepa-

Table 52-1. Frequency of oral manifestations and seasonal proclivity from larger surveys of erythema multiforme

Investigator	Country	Year	No. of cases	Frequency of oral manifestations %	Seasonal proclivity
Jersild	Denmark	1945	25	100	Feb.–Mar.
Stanyon and Warner	Canada	1945	17	100	Spring and fall
Soll	United States	1947	20	100	Jan.–July
Löffler	Switzerland	1947	30	80	(No information)
Ustvedt	Norway	1949	219	39	April–June and Dec.–Jan.
Costello and Vandow	United States	1948	111	40	May–July
Hauge	Norway	1952	28	96	(No information)
Lynch	United States	1955	171	. . .	Mar.–June

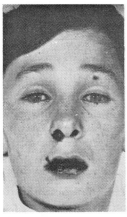

Figure 52-1. *Erythema multiforme.* Note conjunctival, nasal, and oral mucosal involvement in early stage. (*Courtesy of A. Proppe, Kiel, Germany.*)

rate the major type and minor type, since no sharp line exists between them.

The disease, primarily seen in young adults and found more frequently in males, has an acute onset and runs a self-limited course from one to several weeks. Frequently, there is a preceding upper respiratory infection combined with headache, malaise, nausea, and/or arthralgia. Often during the early stage of the illness there is fever.

Skin. A few days after the prodromal stage, the cutaneous lesions develop. They may appear anywhere on the body but have a predilection for the dorsa of the hands and feet. The cutaneous lesions vary in size and form from maculopapular to vesiculobullous eruptions, often symmetrically distributed. Some are even nodular. The basic pattern is an annular lesion. Secondary and tertiary rings in red or bluish colors may result in a "target" appearance of concentric rings, often described as having "iris" form (Fig. 52-2).

Eyes. The eye lesions may assume a wide variety of types; there is no condition of the eyes

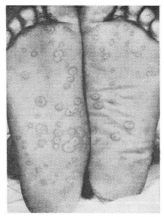

Figure 52-2. Soles of feet exhibiting typical iris-like lesions.

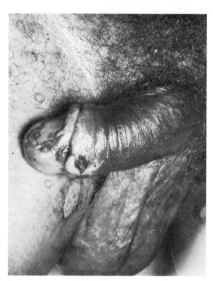

Figure 52-3. Balanitis, a sign often overlooked. (*Courtesy of A. Proppe, Kiel, Germany.*)

that is pathognomonic of the disease. Two main forms of conjunctival involvement are described—a fibromembranous type and a papulovesicular type, the former occurring more frequently (Fig. 52-4).

Other mucous membranes. Other mucous membranes may be involved, those of the penis and vulva being most frequently affected. Balanitis, nonspecific urethritis, and vulvovaginitis have also been described (14, 24) (Fig. 53-3).

The disease may spread through the respiratory tract, resulting in bronchitis which in some cases is complicated by bronchopneumonia. In a number of cases, extensive involvement of internal organs has been accompanied by ulceration of the gastrointestinal tract with colitis, proctitis, nephritis, and cystitis (18, 23). Some cases have been fatal.

Oral manifestations. The frequency of oral manifestations may vary from about 40 to 100 percent (Table 52-1). Oral lesions usually appear after the skin eruption. However, some cases have been described in which this sequence was reversed; the authors also have observed this reverse sequence. Furthermore, it has been reported that some patients never develop skin lesions (6, 13, 15).

Oral lesions may be found on the lips, buccal and gingival mucosa, tongue, and hard and soft palates (Fig. 52-5C). Because of the humid environment and movements of the mucosal tissues during mastication, the oral lesions are not so well defined as the cutaneous. The development of oral lesions can be divided into five distinct stages: macular, bullous, sloughing, pseudomembranous, and healing (30). The initial stage in the development of the oral lesion is a small erythematous plaque or macule, which is soon followed by a vesicle or bulla, present but for a brief time and, therefore, infrequently observed. The ruptured vesicles or bullae become confluent, forming shallow erosions covered by slough, giving rise to the pseudomembranous stage. The oral lesions become extremely painful as the vesicles rupture and the ulcerated areas become secondarily infected. Swallowing may be difficult if lesions are present in the oropharynx (22). It is characteristic for extensive crust formation to occur on the lips (Figs. 52-1, 52-5A, B). The appearance of this crusting can be helpful in making the diagnosis. Marked halitosis may be present. When the gingiva is affected by the disease, a peculiar mixture of catarrhal and necrotic gingivitis may result. The lesions usually complete their course within 2 weeks.

The oral changes may be complicated by sialorrhea, dysphagia, and enlarged cervical lymph nodes. Because of severe pain on swallowing and the formation of crusts with attendant bleeding and fissuring, the patient may often be in great discomfort.

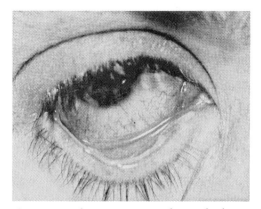

Figure 52-4. Edema, injection, and vesicular formation in conjunctiva.

292

PATHOLOGY

Histopathologic findings are varied, and disagreement exists concerning the etiology of the blisters on both the skin and oral mucosa. In the skin, the changes seen are primarily due to edema. Spongiosis and intracellular edema are frequently observed in the epithelium, giving rise to subepidermal bullae. The blister formation may also be explained on the basis of disintegration of the basement membrane (29). The bullae are filled with polymorphonuclear neutrophilic leukocytes. The connective tissue, especially that of the papillae, is edematous and exhibits a marked dilatation of its vessels with perivascular cell infiltration. In the oral mucosa, the vesicles may develop as subepithelial lesions caused by the accumulation of fluid beneath the epithelium, or as intraepithelial lesions resulting from extensive hydropic degeneration of the epithelial cells of the stratum spinosum. Electron microscopic studies show both intercellular and intracellular edema (4).

DIFFERENTIAL DIAGNOSIS

Erythema multiforme may present diagnostic problems because of the varied clinical picture. Among the more important diseases which may resemble erythema multiforme are benign mucous membrane pemphigoid, epizootic stomatitis, the *Behçet syndrome,* and the *Reiter syndrome.* In benign mucous membrane pemphigoid, the skin lesions are scarce and do not exhibit the iris sign. Furthermore, the patients are not constitutionally ill. In epizootic stomatitis, conjunctivitis and balanitis may be present but the changes about the nails and the demonstration of a virus in the lesions lead to the proper diagnosis. The Behçet syndrome is considered by some authors to represent a variant of erythema multiforme; however, several features of the Behçet syndrome are distinctive. The lesions are chronic and smaller, resembling aphthous lesions, and eye complications are more severe. The Reiter syndrome has also been considered part of erythema multiforme. However, the oral manifestations are not widespread

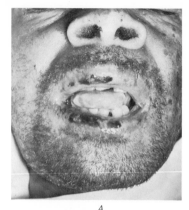

A

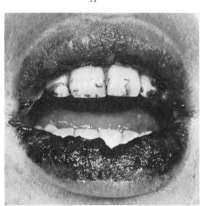

B

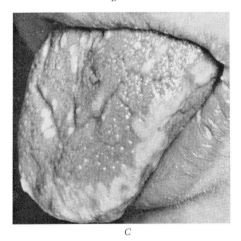

C

Figure 52-5. (*A*). Multiple bullous formation and erosions on the lips. The anterior margin of the tongue may be almost denuded. (*B*). Extensive crusting and erosion of lips. (*C*). Multiple coalesced vesicles on anterior and lateral margins of tongue, small lesions on dorsum. (*C, courtesy of A. Lodin, Stockholm, Sweden.*)

in the Reiter syndrome and keratosis blennorrhagica-like lesions are typically present.

There are striking similarities (12) between erythema multiforme and the Lyell syndrome (toxic epidermal necrolysis), and it has been suggested that the latter is the most severe form of erythema multiforme, but this view is inconsistent with the mild and localized examples of the Lyell syndrome (17).

In patients having only oral lesions, two more conditions should be considered, viz., necrotic ulcerative gingivitis and herpetic stomatitis. In necrotic ulcerative gingivitis, the lesions are predominantly limited to the interdental papillae and marginal gingiva and have a punched-out appearance, in contrast to the more diffuse lesions of erythema multiforme. With regard to herpetic stomatitis, the differential diagnosis can be made because of the missing skin eruption (the Kaposi type of varicelliform eruption is exempted) and the well-defined herpes simplex virus which can be cultivated from the lesions, as well as characteristic Pap smears.

DIAGNOSTIC AIDS

If possible, biopsy of a small lesion should be performed, since valuable information may be obtained from a specimen taken near the location of the blister formation. Complement-fixing antibodies to *Mycoplasma pneumoniae* may be demonstrated in titers of 1/256 or higher in some cases (5, 16).

REFERENCES

1 Baader, E., Dermatostomatitis. *Arch. Dermatol. Syph. (Berl.)* **149**:261–268, 1925.

2 Bianchine, J. R., et al., Drugs as Etiologic Factors in the Stevens-Johnson Syndrome. *Am. J. Med.* **44**:390–405, 1968.

3 Brandtzaeg, P., Erythema Multiforme Exudativum: A Review of the Literature with Special Reference to Oral Manifestations. *Odontol. Tidskr.* **72**:363–390, 1964.

4 von Bülow, F. A., et al., An Electronmicroscopic Study of Oral Mucosal Lesions in Erythema Multiforme Exudativum. *Acta Pathol. Microbiol. Scand.* **66**:145–153, 1966.

5 Cannell, H., et al., Stevens-Johnson Syndrome Associated with *Mycoplasma Pneumoniae* Infection. *Br. J. Dermatol.* **81**:196–199, 1969.

6 Cooke, B. E. D., The Diagnosis of Bullous Lesions Affecting the Oral Mucosa. *Br. Dent. J.* **109**:83–96 and 131–138, 1960.

7 Fiessinger, N., and Rendu, R., Sur un syndrome caractérisé par l'inflammation simultanée de toutes les muqueuses externes coexistant avec une éruption vésiculeuse des quatre membres, non douloureuse et non recidivante. *Paris Méd.* **25**:54–58, 1917.

8 Fiessinger, N., et al., Ectodermose érosive pluri-orificielle. *Bull. Soc. Méd. Hôp. Paris* Ser. 3, **47**:446–449, 1923.

9 Fuchs, E., Herpes iris conjunctivae. *Klin. Augenheilkd.* **14**:333–351, 1876.

10 Gädeke, R., Erythema exudativum multiforme major. *Hippokrates* **41**:323–336, 1970.

11 Hebra, F., Acute Exantheme und Hautkrankheiten, in R. Virchow (ed.), *Handbuch der speziellen Pathologie und Therapie*, vol. 3. Ferdinand Enke, Stuttgart, 1860.

12 Held, A., Stevens-Johnson-Syndrome, Lyell-Syndrom oder "polymorphe Ektodermosen"? *Med. Klin.* **63**:167–173, 1968.

13 Kennett, S., Erythema Multiforme Affecting the Oral Cavity. *Oral Surg.* **25**:366–373, 1968.

14 Kwapis, B. W., Erythema Multiforme Exudativum. *Oral Surg.* **10**:363–369, 1957.

15 Lighterman, I., Erythema Multiforme Limited to the Oral Cavity. *Oral Surg.* **11**:1237–1243, 1958.

16 Ludlam, G. B., Association of Stevens-Johnson Syndrome with Antibody for *Mycoplasma Pneumoniae. Lancet* **1**:958–959, 1964.

17 Lyell, A., Erythema Multiforme and Toxic Epidermal Necrolysis, in T. B. Fitzpatrick et al. (eds.), *Dermatology in General Medicine.* McGraw-Hill, New York, 1971, pp. 598–608.

18 Müller, W. A., and Hartenstein, H., Die Beteiligung innerer Organe beim Erythema exudativum multiforme maius. *Dtsch. Med. Wochenschr.* **85**:879–882, 1960.

19 Rendu, R., Sur un syndrome caractérisé par l'inflammation simultanée de toutes les muqueuses externes (conjunctivale, nasale, linguale, buccopharyngée, ovale et balano-préputiale) coexistant avec une éruption varicelliforme puis purpurique des quatre membres. *Rev. Gén. Clin. Thérap.* **30**:351–358, 1916.

20 Schmidt, H., Isolation of Herpes Simplex Virus from Blisters of a Patient with Stevens-Johnson Syndrome. *Acta Derm. Venereol. (Stockh.)* **41**:53–55, 1961.

21 Shklar, G., Oral Lesions of Erythema Multiforme. *Arch. Dermatol.* **92**:495–500, 1965.

22 Shklar, G., and McCarthy, P. L., Oral Manifestations of Erythema Multiforme in Children. *Oral Surg.* **21**:713–723, 1966.

23 Short, I. A., Stevens-Johnson Syndrome: A Report of Five Cases and a Discussion on Aetiology and Treatment. *Lancet* **1**:290–294, 1957.

24 Soll, S. N., Eruptive Fever with Involvement of the Respiratory Tract, Conjunctivitis, Stomatitis and Balanitis: An Acute Clinical Entity, Probably of Infectious Origin: Report of Twenty Cases and Review of the Literature. *Arch.*

Intern. Med. **79:**475–500, 1947.

25 Stevens, A. M., and Johnson, C. F., A New Eruptive Fever Associated with Stomatitis and Ophthalmia. *Am. J. Dis. Child.* **24:**526–533, 1922.

26 Stillman, M. T., Stevens-Johnson Syndrome. *Minn. Med.* **51:**273–280, 1968.

27 Ström, J., Febrile Mucocutaneous Syndromes (Ectodermosis Erosiva Pluriorificialis, Stevens-Johnson's Syndrome, etc.) In Adenovirus Infections. *Acta Derm. Venereol. (Stockh.)* **47:**281–286, 1967.

28 Thomas, B. A., The So-called Stevens-Johnson Syndrome. *Br. Med. J.* **1:**1393–1397, 1950.

29 Van der Meiren, L., Zur Klinik und Histologie des Erythema exudativum multiforme. *Hautarzt* **11:**246–249, 1960.

30 Wooten, J. W., et al., Development of Oral Lesions in Erythema Multiforme Exudativum. *Oral Surg.* **24:**808–816, 1967.

53

Fabry Syndrome

(Angiokeratoma Corporis Diffusum Universale)

The clinical syndrome was described independently in 1898 by Anderson (1) in England and by Fabry (14) in Germany. The characteristic cutaneous lesions led Fabry subsequently to term this disease *angiokeratoma corporis diffusum universale.* The disorder is characterized by the systemic accumulation of the glycosphingolipid trihexosyl ceramide, particularly in the cardiovascular-renal system (5, 30). The primary metabolic defect is the deficient activity of the specific α-galactosidase (11, 21), ceramide trihexosidase (2), which normally catabolizes the accumulated glycosphingolipid.

Opitz et al. (25) documented the X-linked transmission with complete penetrance and variable clinical expressivity of this disease in hemizygous males. Although most heterozygous females are asymptomatic, some have been reported as expressing all manifestations of the disease (30). Studies (19, 25) have demonstrated that the loci for Xg^a and Fabry syndrome are linked. Over 200 cases have been described. Recent comprehensive reviews are available (20, 30).

SYSTEMIC MANIFESTATIONS

Facies. There is no pathognomonic facies; however, frontal bossing and prominent lower jaw and lips have been reported in several male patients (15, 35). Many patients appear young for their chronologic age (35).

Skin. The cutaneous, vascular lesions (angiokeratoma corporis diffusum) are telangiectases; they do not blanch with pressure, and usually appear as clusters of individual macular to papular punctate, dark-red angiectases in the superficial layers of the skin. There may be moderate keratosis over these lesions. They usually appear during childhood and progressively increase in size and number with age. Characteristically, they are most dense over the iliosacral area, scrotum, posterior thorax, thighs, buttocks, and umbilicus (30) (Figs. 53-1, 53-2*A, B*). Some of the larger lesions are slightly raised. The face, with the exception of the submental area, may be involved.

Variants without the characteristic skin lesions have been recently observed (4, 30). Hypohidrosis is a common symptom, and atrophic or sparse sweat and sebaceous glands have been reported (31). Males shave infrequently, and their body hair may be slight.

Eyes. Ocular manifestations include aneurysmal dilatation and tortuosity of conjunctival and retinal vessels with corneal opacities in males. The opacities are characterized by diffuse haziness or whorled streaks in the corneal epithelium, resembling changes seen in chloroquine intoxication, and must be observed by slit lamp microscopy (33, 35). They occur in all hemizygous males and in many heterozygous females. The corneal dystrophy and vascular tortuosity result from deposition of glycosphingolipid in the corneal epithelium (17, 34) and

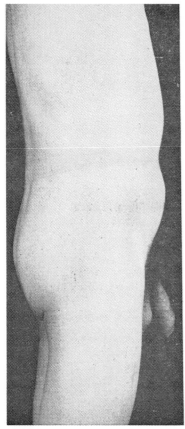

Figure 53-1. *Fabry disease.* Note distribution of skin lesions in twenty-seven-year-old man. (*From A. Rahmen,* Trans. Assoc. Am. Physicians **75:**371, 1961.)

vascular endothelium (17, 18, 34). These lesions do not impair vision.

Cardiovascular-renal system. With increasing age, the major symptoms result from involvement of the cardiovascular-renal system. Early in the course of the disease, casts, red cells, and lipid inclusions with characteristic birefringent "Maltese crosses" appear in the urinary sediment. Proteinuria, isosthenuria, and gradual deterioration of renal function and development of azotemia occur in the second to fourth decades of life (5, 30). Cardiovascular findings in late maturity may include hypertension, left ventricular hypertrophy, myocardial ischemia or infarction, and cerebral vascular disease. Death most often results from uremia or vascular dis-

ease of the heart or brain during the fourth decade (30).

Microscopic examination of various tissues demonstrates the accumulation of the glycosphingolipid, predominantly in endothelial, perithelial, and smooth-muscle cells of blood vessels, epithelial cells of the cornea and of glomeruli and tubules of the kidney, in muscle fibers of the heart, in ganglion cells of the autonomic nervous system, and in peripheral Schwann cells. Foamy, lipid-laden macrophages are seen in the bone marrow and lymph nodes (15).

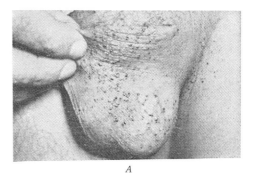

A

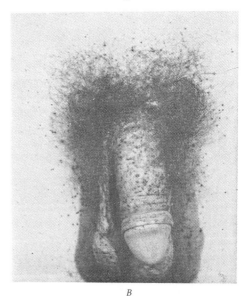

B

Figure 53-2. (*A, B*). Small, somewhat raised, vascular lesions on scrotum and penis of patients. (A, *from A. Rahmen,* Trans. Assoc. Am. Physicians **75:**371, 1961.)

Other clinical features. Onset of the disease in hemizygous males usually occurs during childhood or adolescence and is characterized by periodic, excruciating acroparesthesias which may become more frequent and severe with age. These painful episodes may last several days and are associated with low-grade fever and elevation of the erythrocyte sedimentation rate; these symptoms have infrequently led to the misdiagnosis of rheumatic fever. During the second and third decades of life, these recurrent episodes become progressively more painful and may occur weekly, usually lasting 12 to 24 hours, but occasionally persisting for 1 to 2 weeks. Affected individuals may be incapacitated for prolonged periods of time. Loss of small peripheral sensory neurons has been reported (24a).

Nausea, vomiting, diarrhea, and abdominal or flank pain are common gastrointestinal symptoms (27). Other less frequent features include massive lymphedema of the legs (Fig. 53-3), hypohidrosis, and dyspnea. Musculoskeletal system findings have included a permanent deformity of the distal interphalangeal joints of the fingers (35) and avascular necrosis of the head of the femur and talus (16, 26). Mild normochromic, normocytic anemia, presumably due to decreased red cell survival, has been observed. Many hemizygotes appear to have growth retardation or delayed puberty.

Oral manifestations. The majority of patients have symmetric, pinpoint, macular, purplish

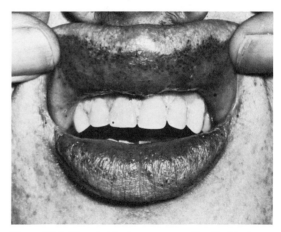

Figure 53-4. Pinpoint lesions on upper lip. Oral lesions are generally limited to the lips and do not involve the tongue. (*From A. I. Rae et al.,* J. Clin. Pathol. **20:**21, 1967.)

spots on the lips, especially on the lower lip near the skin-mucosal junction, on either side of the midline (5, 15, 26, 29, 35) (Fig. 53-4). The lesions are smaller than those on the skin. The buccal mucosa appears to be involved to a lesser degree (15, 30, 35). Only rarely are other oral tissues—gingiva (29), soft palate, and uvula (22, 35)—involved. The tongue is not affected. The nasal mucosa has been affected, with resultant epistaxis (35). Glycosphingolipid accumulation has been demonstrated in dental pulp from hemizygous males (13).

DIFFERENTIAL DIAGNOSIS

The condition can be diagnosed in hemizygotes by a history of acroparesthesias, the presence of characteristic skin lesions and corneal opacities, and increased erythrocyte sedimentation rate; heterozygotes may be asymptomatic or may manifest attentuated symptoms, particularly corneal lesions.

The skin lesions are so characteristic in distribution that the need for differential diagnosis is extremely limited. The lesions of *hereditary hemorrhagic telangiectasia* are larger, do not involve the lower trunk and thighs, and are less numerous and more irregular. The Fordyce type of angiokeratoma is usually limited to the

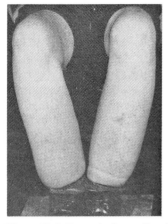

Figure 53-3. Extensively swollen lower legs.

scrotum, and the Mibelli type forms warty lesions on the extremities or ears (30, 35).

LABORATORY AIDS

Birefringent lipid inclusions can be observed histologically in biopsied tissues, bone marrow macrophages, or urinary sediment. All cases should be confirmed biochemically by the demonstration of increased levels of trihexosyl ceramide in urinary sediment (8, 9), plasma (32), or cultured fibroblasts (24), or deficient activity of the specific enzyme, ceramide trihexosidase (2, 23), or nonspecific α-galactosidase in plasma (11), leukocytes (11, 21), biopsied tissue (11), or cultured fibroblasts (3, 6, 12, 27). Prenatal detection can be accomplished by the demonstration of deficient α-galactosidase in cultured cells (3, 7, 12) obtained by amniocentesis. Fibroblasts from skin biopsy show characteristic crystalline cytoplasmic inclusions (23).

REFERENCES

1 Anderson, W., A Case of "Angiokeratoma." *Br. J. Dermatol.* **10**:113–117, 1898.

2 Brady, R. O., et al., Enzymatic Defect in Fabry's Disease: Ceramide Trihexosidase Deficiency. *N. Engl. J. Med.* **275**:1163–1167, 1967.

3. Brady, R. O., et al., Fabry's Disease: Antenatal Diagnosis. *Science* **172**:172–175, 1971.

4 Clarke, J. T. R., et al., Ceramide Trihexosidosis (Fabry's Disease) without Skin Lesions. *N. Engl. J. Med.* **284**:233–235, 1971.

5 Colley, L., et al., The Renal Lesion in Angiokeratoma Corporis Diffusum. *Br. Med. J.* **1**:1266–1268, 1958.

6 Dawson, G., et al., Enzyme Replacement in Fabry's Disease: Treatment of Cultured Skin Fibroblasts with a Purified α-Galactosidase from Ficin, in R. J. Desnick, R. W. Bernlohr, and W. Krivit (eds), *Enzyme Therapy in Genetic Diseases. Birth Defects* **9**(2):97–101, 1973.

7 Desnick, R. J., and Sweeley, C. C., Prenatal Diagnosis of Fabry's Disease, in A. Dorfman (ed.), *Antenatal Diagnosis*, 1972, U. of Chicago Press, Chicago, pp. 185–192.

8 Desnick, R. J., et al., A Method for the Quantitative Determination of the Neutral Glycosphingolipids in Urine Sediment. *J. Lipid Res.* **11**:31–37, 1970.

9 Desnick, R. J., et al., Diagnosis of Glycosphingolipidoses by Urinary Sediment Analysis. *N. Engl. J. Med.* **284**:739–744, 1971.

10 Desnick, R. J., et al., Treatment of Fabry's Disease: Correction of the Enzymatic Deficiency by Renal Transplantation. *J. Lab. Clin. Med.* **78**:989–990, 1971.

11 Desnick, R. J., et al., Fabry's Disease: Enzymatic Diagnosis of Hemizygotes and Heterozygotes: alpha-Galactosidase Activities in Plasma, Serum Urine, and Leukocytes, *J. Lab. Clin. Med.* **81**:157–171, 1973.

12 Desnick, R. J., et al., Fabry's Disease: Biochemical and Ultrastructural Studies of an Affected Fetus, in preparation.

13 Desnick, S. J., et al., Fabry's Disease (Ceramide Trihexosidase Deficiency): Diagnostic Confirmation by Analysis of Dental Pulp. *Arch. Oral Biol.* **17**:1473–1479, 1972.

14 Fabry, J., Ein Beitrag zur Kenntnis der Purpura haemorrhagica nodularis (Purpura papulosa hemorrhagica Hebrae). *Arch. Dermatol. Syphilol.* (*Berl.*) **43**:187–200, 1898.

15 Fessas, P., et al., Angiokeratoma Corporis Diffusum Universale (Fabry). *Arch. Intern. Med.* **95**:469–481, 1955.

16 Fone, D. J., and King, W. E., Angiokeratoma Corporis Diffusum (Fabry's Syndrome). *Aust. Ann. Med.* **13**:339–348, 1964.

17 Font, R. L., and Fine, B. S., Ocular Pathology in Fabry's Disease: Histochemical and Electron Microscopic Observations. *Am. J. Ophthalmol.* **73**:419–430, 1972.

18 Frost, P., et al., Fabry's Disease—Glycolipid Lipidosis: Histochemical and Electron Microscopic Studies of Two Cases. *Am. J. Med.* **40**:618–627, 1966.

19 Johnston, A. W., et al., Linkage Relationships of the Angiokeratoma (Fabry) Locus. *Ann. Hum. Genet.* **32**:369–374, 1969.

20 Kahlke, W., Angiokeratoma Corporis Diffusum (Fabry's Disease), in G. Schettler (ed.), *Lipids and Lipidoses.* Springer, Berlin, 1967, pp. 332–351.

21 Kint, J. A., Fabry's Disease: α-Galactosidase Deficiency. *Science* **167**:1268–1269, 1970.

22 Kuang-Yuan, Y., Angiokeratoma Corporis Diffusum Universalis (Fabry): Report of a Case with Lipoiduria. *Chinese Med. J.* **74**:478–488, 1956.

23 McLean, J., and Stewart, G., Fabry's Disease: Specific Inclusions Found on Electron Microscopy of Fibroblast Cultures. *J. Med. Genet.* **11**:133–135, 1974.

24 Matalon, R., et al., Glycolipid and Mucopolysaccharide Abnormality in Fibroblasts of Fabry's Disease. *Science* **164**:1522–1523, 1969.

24a Ohnishi, A., and Dyck, P. J., Loss of Small Peripheral Sensory Neurons in Fabry Disease. *Arch. Neurol.* **31**:120–127, 1974.

25 Opitz, J. M., et al., The Genetics of Angiokeratoma Corporis Diffusum (Fabry's Disease), and Its Linkage with Xg(a) Locus. *Am. J. Hum. Genet.* **17**:325–342, 1965.

26 Pittelkow, R. B., et al., Angiokeratoma Corporis Diffusum. *Arch. Dermatol.* **72**:556–561, 1955; **75**:59–64, 1957.

27 Rowe, J. W., et al., Intestinal Manifestations of Fabry's Disease, *Ann. Intern. Med.* **81**:628–631, 1974.

28 Schibanoff, J. M., et al., Tissue Distribution of Glycosphingolipids in a Case of Fabry's Disease. *J. Lipid Res.* **10**:515–520, 1969.

29 Steiner, L., and Voerner, H., Angiomatosis Miliaris: "Eine idiopathische Gefässerkrankung." *Dtsch. Arch. Klin. Med.* **96**:105–116, 1909.

30 Sweeley, C. C., et al., Fabry's Disease, in J. B. Stanbury, J.

B. Wyngaarden, and D. S. Fredrickson (eds.), *The Metabolic Basis of Inherited Disease.* McGraw-Hill, New York, 1972, pp. 663–687.

31 Uono, M., Fabry's Disease—from the Standpoint of Neuronal Lipidosis. *Jap. J. Clin. Med.* **25:**1587–1594, 1967.

32 Vance, D. E., et al., Concentrations of Glycosyl Ceramides in Plasma and Red Cells in Fabry's Disease. *J. Lipid Res.* **10:**188–192, 1969.

33 Wallace, H. J., Anderson-Fabry Disease. *Br. J. Dermatol.* **88:**1–24, 1973.

34 Weingeist, T. A., and Blodi, F. C., Fabry's Disease: Ocular Findings in a Female Carrier: A Light and Electron Microscopic Study. *Arch. Ophthalmol.* **85:**169–175, 1971.

35 Wise, D., et al., Angiokeratoma Corporis Diffusum: A Clinical Study of Eight Affected Families. *Q. J. Med.* **31:**177–206, 1962.

54

Familial Dysautonomia

(Riley-Day Syndrome)

A syndrome consisting of (*a*) absence of overflow tears, (*b*) vasomotor instability, (*c*) hypoactive deep-tendon reflexes, (*d*) relative indifference to pain, (*e*) feeding difficulties, and (*f*) absence of lingual fungiform papillae was first described by Riley et al. (27) in 1949. Subsequently, Riley and coworkers (26, 28) presented thorough reviews of its clinical picture.

Genetic studies have shown autosomal recessive inheritance. Virtually all patients have Ashkenazic Jewish ancestry, the great majority stemming from eastern Europe (Galicia, Ukraine, Romania) (6). According to McKusick et al. (21), about one American Jew in 10,000 to 20,000 has familial dysautonomia. The frequency is similar among Israeli Jews of Ashkenazic extraction. Parental consanguinity has been noted in at least 5 percent of cases.

Carriers do not have any clinical signs of the disorder, but their urinary vanillylmandelic acid (VMA) concentration is lower than in healthy adults (22). Over 200 patients have been described with this syndrome (6).

Smith and associates (31–33) proposed that this disorder is due to a derangement in catecholamine metabolism, suggesting that there is a deficiency of release at the peripheral sensory level. Goodall et al. (14) opined a defect at the cell membrane level. Andersson et al. (2) indicated that the disorder resulted from an imbalance between the adrenergic and cholinergic systems due to a defect in dopamine β-hydroxylase activity.

SYSTEMIC MANIFESTATIONS

About 25 percent have breech presentation in contrast to 3–8 percent of normal infants (2a). Stature is small even at birth, and psychic development is delayed. About 25 percent die of pulmonary infection by the age of ten years. Recurrent bronchopneumonia is common, probably because food is frequently aspirated.

Facies. A frightened fixed expression with a slit-like mouth and a peculiar "working" of the tongue is typical (20, 28) (Figs. 54-1, 54-3). The face is thin, frequently asymmetric, with a pale to grayish color except during excitement. External strabismus is common.

Nervous system. Difficulties in swallowing and regurgitation appear soon after birth (15), and the infant fails to produce overflow tears with the usual stimuli (19). Other virtually constant signs are absent to hyporeactive deep-tendon reflexes, motor retardation and/or motor incoordination, breath-holding spells, postural hypotension, paroxysmal hypertension, emotional lability, and relative indifference to pain (28). On the other hand, many of these children do not like their feet or scalp to be touched (dysesthesia). The indifference to pain may result in Charcot joints as the child grows older. The patient is relatively insensitive to hypercapnia and hypoxia (8). Skin blotching, abnormal sweating, erratic temperature control, and episodic vom-

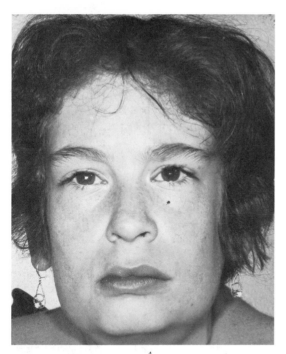

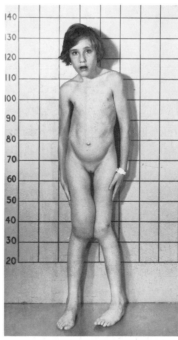

A   *B*

Figure 54-1. *Familial dysautonomia.* Fixed expression, asymmetric thorax, scoliosis, genu valgum due to Charcot joint-like changes (B, *courtesy of V. A. McKusick, Baltimore, Md.*)

iting are frequently seen (19). Many of these patients (about 80 percent) exhibit growth retardation and severe progressive scoliosis (about 55 percent) which appears around the eighth or ninth year of life (22, 28). Intelligence is usually normal. Speech is often monotonous and slurred, with an unusual nasal quality (6). Defective nerve conduction (4) and a reduction in the number of unmyelinated nerve fibers, no myelinated nerve fibers greater than 12 μ in diameter, and abnormally short internodal length of small myelinated nerves have been demonstrated (1).

Skin. A macular erythema, varying in color from pink to bright orange and located principally on the trunk and limbs, especially during periods of emotional excitement, is common. Acrocyanosis and excessive sweating are constant features (22). Severe burns have resulted from indifference to pain in some patients. There may be spotty alopecia and seborrheic dermatitis (12).

Eyes. Constant features are decreased tearing, absent corneal reflex, and absent pupillary constriction in response to subconjunctival instillation of methacholine (28, 31). Neuroparalytic keratitis, mild keratitis sicca, or corneal ulceration has been noted in at least 30 percent of cases. The eye changes can be so severe that blindness may result (11). Myopia and retinal vascular tortuosity are also frequently observed (6, 18).

Oral manifestations. Quite characteristically the mouth is transversely elongated into a horizontal slit (Fig. 54-3). Smith and Dancis (34, 35) reported absence of fungiform papillae on the tongue (Fig. 54-2A, B). Henkin and Kopin (16) and Moses et al. (22) reported that circumvallate papillae were also absent or greatly diminished in number. Sensitivity to sweet and bitter taste is reduced in these patients and provides the first anatomic evidence of a peripheral sensory defect in the disease. Some parents may have decreased numbers of fungiform papillae (23, 28).

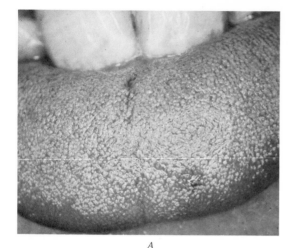

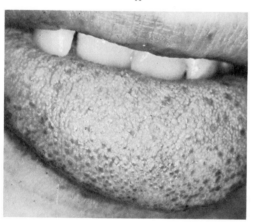

Figure 54-2. (*A*). Tongue in familial dysautonomia. Note absence of fungiform papillae. (*B*). Normal tongue for comparison. Observe presence of fungiform papillae. (*Courtesy of A. A. Smith, New York.*)

Excessive drooling and diminished gag reflex or swallowing disturbance occur in about 80 percent of patients (22).

Dental caries is infrequent, perhaps because of the reduced taste sensibility and consequent lowered desire for sweets (25). However, periodontal disease, malocclusion, and dental arch crowding are common (6).

DIFFERENTIAL DIAGNOSIS

No disorder exactly mimics familial dysautonomia, but many progressive sensory neurop-

athies have similar features (6, 17) (Table 54-1). Absence of fungiform and circumvallate papillae is an important specific clinical finding. Fungiform papillae may also be absent in the *Behçet syndrome.*

Schmidt and associates (30) reported two sisters of consanguineous parents of Sephardic Jewish origin with clinical findings similar to those of the Riley-Day syndrome, such as ophthalmic lesions, absence of tears, vasomotor disturbances, ataxia, and mental retardation. However, they had neither the metabolic defect nor the absence of fungiform papillae. Of interest was the finding of irregular pupillary margins in both girls.

Wolfe and Henkin (39) have suggested that the term "familial dysautonomia, type II" be applied to congenital sensory neuropathy with anhidrosis (5, 24), a disorder characterized by sensory deficit (diminished knee jerks, deficient taste discrimination, failure of axon flare after histamine injection) but differing from familial dysautonomia in that it exhibits normal tear secretion and failure to produce miosis or alter taste thresholds after methacholine administration (36). We agree with Dancis and Smith (9) that use of the term "familial dysautonomia, type II" should not be encouraged.

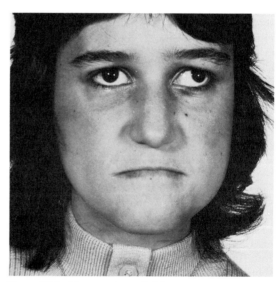

Figure 54-3. Characteristic slitlike mouth. (*Courtesy of A. A. Reitman, Garden City, N.Y.*)

Table 54-1. Comparison of familial dysautonomia with other conditions in which pain sensation is impaired

Characteristic	Familial dysautonomia	Congenital indifference to pain (7)	Asymbolia for pain (29)	Radicular sensory neuropathy (10)	Sensory neuropathy with anhidrosis (5, 24)	Congenital sensory neuropathy (3)
Inheritance	Autosomal recessive	Autosomal recessive	None	Autosomal dominant(?)	Autosomal recessive	Autosomal recessive(?)
Features present at birth	Yes	Yes	Probably not	No	Yes	Yes
Sensory loss other than pain:						
Temperature	Abnormal	Normal	Normal	Abnormal	Abnormal	Abnormal
Touch	Abnormal	Normal	Normal	Abnormal	Abnormal	Abnormal
Physiologic reactions to pain	Reduced	Normal	Normal	Reduced	Reduced	Reduced
Axon reflex	Absent	Normal	Normal	Absent	Absent	Absent
Distribution of sensory loss	Variable	Universal	Universal	Predominantly distal limbs	Incomplete	Incomplete
Intelligence	Dull to normal	Dull to normal	Normal	Normal	Defective	Dull to normal
Demonstrable pathologic changes	None consistent	None	Parietal lobe	Abnormal nerve roots	Possibly changes in Lissauer's tract	Absence of dermal nerve networks

LABORATORY AIDS

These patients show little to no pain or axon flare on intracutaneous injection of 0.01 ml of 1:10,000 histamine sulfate (31), or scratch test (6), and a strong reaction to norepinephrine and related drugs. Some children fail to respond to a pinprick. There is immediate pupillary constriction with 2.5 percent methacholine eyedrops. This test is good but not pathognomonic. Taste acuity for salty and sweet foods, absent in familial dysautonomia, becomes normal with parenterally administered methacholine (16).

An increased homovanillic acid (HVA/VMA) ratio has been reported in the urine of affected patients (13, 21, 28). Heterozygotes had normal ratios (13). Andersson et al. (2) noted high HVA levels in the spinal fluid. Moses et al. (22), however, found normal HVA values, and Brunt and McKusick (6) have failed to confirm an altered HVA/VMA ratio. Skin or mucous membrane biopsy is of no value (14).

Weinshilboum and Axelrod (37) noted absent plasma dopamine-β-hydroxylase activity in about 25 percent of children with this disorder. Mothers of these children had decreased activity of the enzymes.

REFERENCES

1 Aguayo, A. J., et al., Peripheral Nerve Abnormalities in the Riley-Day Syndrome. *Arch. Neurol.* **24:**106–116, 1971.

2 Andersson, H., et al., Homovanillic Acid and 5-Hydroxyindoleacetic Acid in Cerebrospinal Fluid of a Child with Familial Dysautonomia. *Acta Paediatr. Scand.* **62:**46–47, 1973.

2a Axelrod, F. B., et al., Breech Presentation of Infants with Familial Dysautonomia. *J. Pediatr.* **84:**107–109, 1975.

3 Bourlond, A., and Winkelmann, R. K., A Study of Cutaneous Innervation in Congenital Anesthesia. *Arch. Neurol.* **14:**223–227, 1966.

4 Brown, J. C., Nerve Conduction in Familial Dysautonomia (Riley-Day Syndrome). *J.A.M.A.* **201:**200–203, 1967.

5 Brown, J. W., and Podosin, R., A Syndrome of the Neural Crest. *Arch. Neurol.* **15:**294–301, 1966.

6 Brunt, P. W., and McKusick, V. A., Familial Dysautonomia: A Report of Genetic and Clinical Studies with a Review of the Literature. *Medicine* **49:**343–374, 1970.

7 Critchley, M., Congenital Indifference to Pain. *Ann. Intern. Med.* **45:**737–747, 1956.

8 Dancis, J., and Smith, A. A., Familial Dysautonomia. *N. Engl. J. Med.* **274:**207–209, 1966.

9 Dancis, J., and Smith, A. A., Familial Dysautonomia. *J. Pediatr.* **77:**174–175, 1970.

10 Denny-Brown, D., Hereditary Sensory Radicular Neuropathy. *J. Neurol. Neurosurg. Psychiatr.* **14:**237–252, 1951.

11 Edwards, T. S., Familial Dysautonomia, a Rare Cause of Corneal Ulcers. *J. Pediatr. Ophthalmol.* **1:**51–56, 1964.

12 Fellner, M. J., Manifestations of Familial Autonomic Dysautonomia. *Arch. Dermatol.* **89:**190–195, 884–887, 1964.

13 Gitlow, S. E., et al., Excretion of Catecholamine Metabolites by Children with Familial Dysautonomia. *Pediatrics* **46:**513–522, 1970.

14 Goodall, J., et al., Early Diagnosis of Familial Dysautonomia. *Arch. Dis. Child.* **43:**455–458, 1968.

15 Gyepes, M. T., and Linde, L. M., Familial Dysautonomia: The Mechanism of Aspiration. *Radiology* **91:**471–475, 1968.

16 Henkin, R., and Kopin, I., Abnormalities of Taste and Smell Thresholds in Familial Dysautonomia: Improvement with Methacholine. *Life Sci.* **3:**1319–1325, 1964.

17 Johnson, R. J., and Spalding, J. M., Progressive Sensory Neuropathy in Children. *J. Neurol. Neurosurg. Psychiatr.* **27:**125–130, 1964.

18 Keith, C. G., Riley-Day Syndrome. *Br. J. Ophthalmol.* **49:**667–672, 1965.

19 Mahloudi, M., et al., Clinical Neurological Aspects of Familial Dysautonomia. *J. Neurol. Sci.* **11:**383–395, 1970.

20 McKendrick, T., Familial Dysautonomia. *Arch. Dis. Child.* **33:**465–468, 1958.

21 McKusick, V. A., et al., The Riley-Day Syndrome: Observations on Genetics and Survivorship. *Israel J. Med. Sci.* **3:**372–379, 1967.

21a Mensher, J. H., Familial Dysautonomia. Report of a Case in a Non-Jewish Child. *J. Pediatr. Ophthalmol.* **12:**40–48, 1975.

22 Moses, S. W., et al., A Clinical, Genetic and Biochemical Study of Familial Dysautonomia in Israel. *Israel J. Med. Sci.* **3:**358–369, 1967.

23 Pearson, J., et al., The Tongue and Taste in Familial Dysautonomia. *Pediatrics* **45:**739–745, 1970.

24 Pinsky, L., and DiGeorge, A. M., Congenital Familial Sensory Neuropathy with Anhidrosis. *J. Pediatr.* **68:**1–13, 1966.

25 Reitman, A. A., et al., Clinical Evaluation of the Dental Aspects of Familial Dysautonomia. *J. Am. Dent. Assoc.* **71:**1436–1446, 1965.

26 Riley, C. M., Familial Dysautonomia. *Adv. Pediatr.* **9:**157–190, 1957.

27 Riley, C. M., et al., Central Autonomic Dysfunction with Defective Lacrimation. *Pediatrics* **3:**468–481, 1949.

28 Riley, C. M., and Moore, R. H., Familial Dysautonomia Differentiated from Related Disorders. *Pediatrics* **37:**435–446, 1966.

29 Schilder, P., and Stengel, E., Asymbolia for Pain. *Arch. Neurol. Psychiatr.* **25:**598–600, 1931.

30 Schmidt, R., et al., A Clinical Entity Simulating Familial Dysautonomia in a North African Jewish Family. *J. Pediatr.* **76:**283–288, 1970.

31 Smith, A. A., and Dancis, J., Physiologic Studies in Familial Dysautonomia. *J. Pediatr.* **63:**838–840, 1963.

32 Smith, A. A., and Dancis, J., Catecholamine Release in

Familial Dysautonomia. *N. Engl. J. Med.* **277:**61–64, 1967.

33 Smith, A. A., et al., Abnormal Catecholamine Metabolism in Familial Dysautonomia. *N. Engl. J. Med.* **268:**705–707, 1963.

34 Smith, A., et al., Absence of Taste-bud Papillae in Familial Dysautonomia. *Science* **147:**1040–1041, 1965.

35 Smith, A. A., et al., Tongue in Familial Dysautonomia. *Am. J. Dis. Child.* **110:**152–154, 1965.

36 Smith, A. A., et al., Responses to Infused Methacholine in Familial Dysautonomia. *Pediatrics* **36:**225–230, 1965.

37 Weinshilboum, R. M., and Axelrod, J., Reduced Dopamine-β-Hydroxylase Activity in Familial Dysautonomia. *N. Engl. J. Med.* **285:**938–942, 1971.

38 Westlake, R. J., et al., Cathecholamine Metabolite Excretion by Patients with Familial Dysautonomia and Their Mothers. *Clin. Res.* **13:**336, 1965.

39 Wolfe, S. M., and Henkin, R. I., Absence of Taste in Type II Familial Dysautonomia: Unresponsiveness to Methacholine Despite the Presence of Taste Buds. *J. Pediatr.* **77:**103–108, 1970.

55

Fetal Face Syndrome

(Robinow Syndrome)

Described initially by Robinow et al. (7) in 1969, the syndrome consists of (a) characteristic facies, (b) forearm brachymelia, and (c) hypoplastic genitalia. Since then, there have been several examples reported (1–6, 8–12).

The syndrome has been observed to follow autosomal dominant transmission (7). However, two affected sibs with normal parents (12) and three affected sibs with normal but consanguineous parents (J. Opitz, personal communication, 1975) suggest genetic heterogeneity, with an autosomal recessive type.

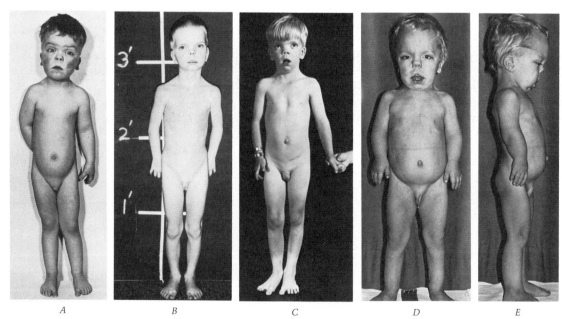

| A | B | C | D | E |

Figure 55-1. *Fetal face syndrome.* (*A*). Flattened facies, micropenis. (*From R. A. Pfeiffer*, Pädiatr. Pädol. **6:**262, 1971.) (*B*). Short stature, mesomelia, and micropenis. (*From M. Robinson, Yellow Springs, Ohio.*) (*C*). Compare with boy seen in Fig. 55-1*A*. (*Courtesy of H. N. Needleman, Boston, Mass.*) (*D, E*). Note marked similarity in phenotype among patients. (*From R. E. Seel et al.*, Monatschr. Kinderheilkd. **122:**663, 1974.)

SYSTEMIC MANIFESTATIONS

Facies. The facies resembles that of a fetus at 8 weeks, i.e., there are a disproportionately large neurocranium, bulging forehead, ocular hypertelorism, S-shaped lower eyelids, short upturned nose with anteverted nostrils, and triangular mouth with downturned angles (Figs. 55-1*A–E*, 55-2).

Skeletal alterations. Growth is at the lower level of normal at birth and during the neonatal period, but falls below the 3d percentile by the third year of life.

Forearm brachymelia is a common feature, the ratios of the upper to lower arm length and height to span being excessive (Fig. 55-1*A–E*).

Hemivertebras, fused vertebras, scoliosis, and anomalies of the radius, ulna, and metacarpals and bifid terminal thumb phalanx (5, 6) have been noted (Fig. 55-3*A–C*). Most patients have exhibited some degree of clinodactyly and brachydactyly of the fifth fingers.

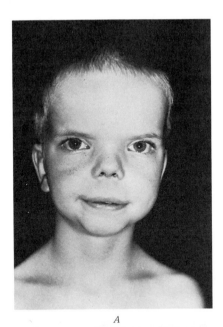

A

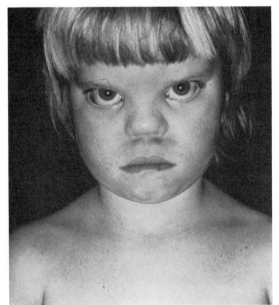

B

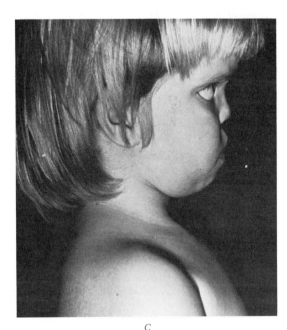

C

Figure 55-2. (*A*). Close-up of face showing fetal proportions. (*B, C*). Sister of boy seen in A. Note S-shaped lower eyelids, ocular hypertelorism, and midface hypoplasia. (*A–C from M. Robinow, Yellow Springs, Ohio.*)

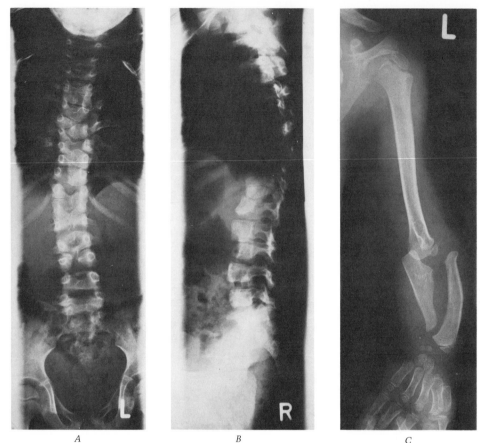

A   *B*   *C*

Figure 55-3. (*A–C*). Radiographs showing keel-shaped vertebras, hemivertebras, and fused vertebras. Note short, plump, and bent radius and ulna but normal humerus. (*From R. E. Seel et al.*, Monatschr. Kinderheilkd. **122**:663, 1974.)

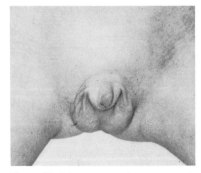

Figure 55-4. Micropenis. (*From M. Robinow, Yellow Springs, Ohio.*)

Genitals. The micropenis may not be apparent at birth. With time, it becomes less hypoplastic (Fig. 55-4). Cryptorchism and absent penis have been observed (11). The clitoris and labia minora are hypoplastic in affected females.

Oral manifestations. The maxillary arch is trapezoidal, and the teeth are crowded. Cleft lip, cleft palate, and minor clefting of the lower lip and tongue have been noted (1, 4, 10, 12).

Gingival enlargement and macroglossia have been reported in several cases (1, 2, 5, 6, 8, 10, 12).

DIFFERENTIAL DIAGNOSIS

The combination is so striking and characteristic that no other condition with the possible exception of *Aarskog syndrome* and *acrodysostosis* need be considered.

LABORATORY AIDS

Roentgenographic studies of the vertebral column and upper extremities should be carried out.

REFERENCES

1 Cohen, M. M., Jr., et al., The Fetal Face Syndrome. *J. Med. Genet.*, in press.
2 Feingold, M., and Bull, M., Case Report 4. *Syndrome Identification* 1(1):14–16, 1973.
3 Harms, S., and Kracht, H., Seltene Fehlbildung des Genitale bei einem Jungen mit multiplen Anomalien im Bereich des Skelett- and Muskelsystems. *Z. Kinderchir.* **12:**128–134, 1973. [Same case as that of Seel et al. (9).]
4 Hornblass, A., and Dolan, R., Oculofacial Anomalies and Corneal Ulceration. *Ann. Ophthalmol.* **6:**575–579, 1974.
5 Kelly, T. E., et al., The Robinow Syndrome. *Am. J. Dis. Child.* **129:**383–386, 1975.
6 Pfeiffer, R. A., Ein Komplex multipler Missbildungen bei zwei nicht verwandten Kindern. *Pädiatr. Pädol.* **6:**262–267, 1971.
7 Robinow, M., et al., A Newly Recognized Dwarfing Syndrome. *Am. J. Dis. Child.* **117:**645–651, 1969.
8 Schinzel, A., et al., Fetal Face Syndrome with Acral Dysostosis. *Helv. Paediat. Acta* **29:**55–60, 1974.
9 Seel, R. E., et al., Das Fetalgesicht-Minderwuchs-Syndrom nach Robinow. *Monatschr. Kinderheilk.* **122:**663–664, 1974.
10 Seemanova, E., et al., Fetal Face Syndrome with Mental Retardation. *Humangenetik* **23:**79–81, 1974.
11 Vera-Roman, J. M., Robinow Dwarfism Accompanied by Penile Agenesis and Hemivertebrae. *Am. J. Dis. Child.* **126:**206–208, 1973.
12 Wadlington, W. B., et al., Mesomelic Dwarfism with Hemivertebrae and Small Genitalia (the Robinow Syndrome). *Am. J. Dis. Child.* **126:**202–205, 1973.

56

Focal Dermal Hypoplasia Syndrome

(Goltz Syndrome)

Goltz (8) in 1962 and Gorlin et al. (10) in 1963 defined a syndrome consisting of (*a*) atrophy and linear hyperpigmentation of the skin; (*b*) localized deposits of superficial fat; (*c*) multiple papillomas of mucous membranes or periorificial skin; (*d*) abnormalities of the extremities; and (*e*) anomalies of the nails. The earliest reported case may be that of Jessner (15) in 1928. The most complete reviews to date are those of Goltz et al. (9), Ginsburg et al. (7), and Walbaum et al. (27).

All cases described thus far, except two (7, 9), have been isolated examples. It is possible that this condition is inherited as an X-linked dominant trait, lethal in the male (6, 8, 20) and producing markedly reduced fertility in the female. However, affected males have been described (6, 9, 25a, 27). Karyotypes have shown no evidence of gross chromosomal abnormalities (9, 10, 14).

SYSTEMIC MANIFESTATIONS

Skin and skin appendages. Asymmetric skin lesions are usually present at birth, manifesting as scarlike abnormalities, streaky hyperpigmentation, atrophy, and telangiectasia (6, 9). Occasionally "blisters" are present at birth, evolving into scarlike lesions (6, 9). The iliac crest area, groin, and posterior aspect of the thigh frequently show fatty collections, varying in color from tan to yellow or pinkish-yellow

(Fig. 56-2*A*, *B*). A few patients have exhibited papillomatosis of the skin (15, 18, 22) (Fig. 56-1).

Hypotrichosis (3, 6, 9, 10, 16, 19, 21, 28, 29) and dystrophic nails (1, 7–10, 14, 15, 19–21, 23–29) are very common (Fig. 56-3). Photosensi-

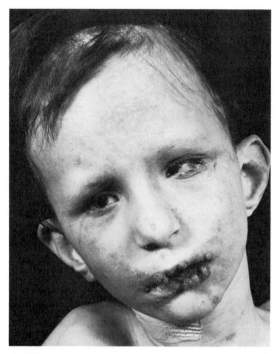

Figure 56-1. *Focal dermal hypoplasia.* Note multiple frambesiform lesions on lips, coloboma of iris, strabismus, thin hair.

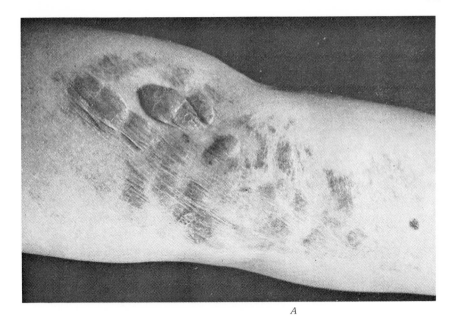

A

B

Figure 56-2. (*A*). Multiple saccular growths presenting in antecubitae area. (*B*). Photomicrograph of focal dermal defect showing subcutaneous fat covered only by epithelium.

tivity (18, 21) has also been described. The epidermal ridges of the fingertips may be hypoplastic (29).

Musculoskeletal system. Bilateral syndactyly, especially between the third and fourth fingers, has been the most common finding (2, 7–10). Polydactyly (7, 8, 10, 27), oligodactyly and adac-

tyly (6, 9, 14, 16, 20, 21, 28), and syndactyly (1, 3, 6–10, 14, 16, 18–21, 28) are also common. The extremities, or parts thereof, may be shortened (1, 6, 7, 9, 10, 16, 18, 22, 25). Brachydactyly can result from shortened phalanges, metacarpals, or metatarsals (4, 10, 14, 23, 28). Clinodactyly (1, 16, 25) and rib anomalies (6, 20, 25) have been reported. Midclavicular aplasia or hypoplasia

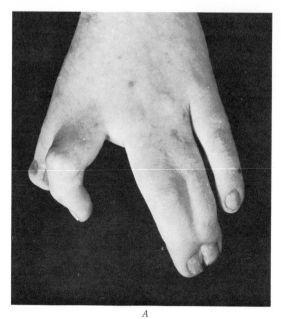
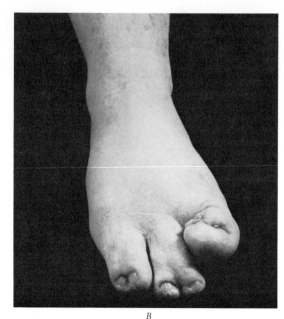

A *B*

Figure 56-3. (*A, B*). Syndactyly of digits, bizarre nail formation.

occurs, apparently limited to the right side (6, 7, 14, 26, 27).

Scoliosis is frequent (6, 10, 25, 25a, 28), as are spina bifida occulta (10, 25) and "failure of segmentation" (10). A constant finding is osteopathia striata (13a, 17, 22, 26a) (Fig. 56-4). Selzer et al. (24) noted multiple giant cell tumor-like lesions in bone in their patient.

Eyes and ears. Chorioretinal coloboma (2, 9, 16, 20) and iris coloboma (9, 16, 26, 28) are the most frequent ocular findings. Other eye anomalies include strabismus (7, 9), nystagmus (6–9, 16), obstructed tear ducts (2, 6), microphthalmia (6, 9, 10, 16, 25), and unilateral anophthalmia (5, 11, 16, 17).

Reported anomalies of the ears include poorly modeled pinnas (1, 6, 7, 25, 29), hypoplastic ear cartilages (4, 6), and deafness (7, 10, 23, 25a) (Fig. 56-1).

Central nervous system. Microcephaly is not uncommon (8, 9, 23). In addition to physical retardation, mental retardation is frequent (6–9, 23, 25a).

Other findings. Hypoplasia of the genital system

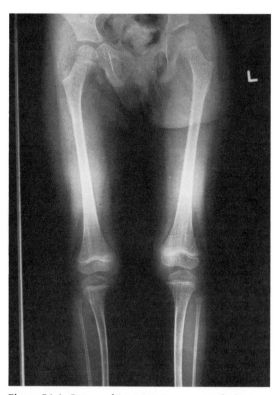

Figure 56-4. Osteopathia striata is constant finding.

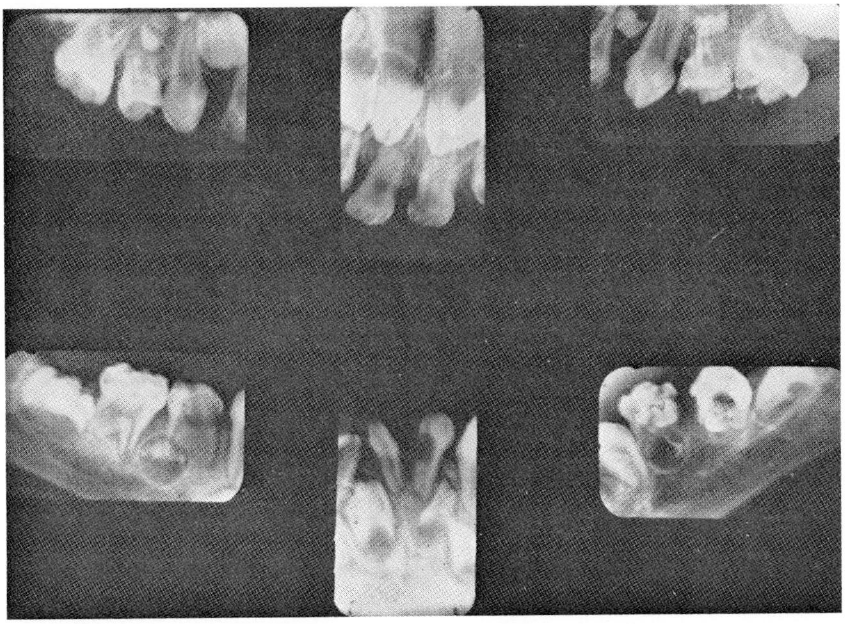

Figure 56-5. Roentgenogram exhibiting severe hypoplasia of teeth.

(1, 6, 18, 25, 28) and small breasts (19, 28) have been reported.

Oral manifestations. The most frequent dental finding is hypodontia or oligodontia (4, 6, 16, 25, 29). Other features include microdontia (6, 9, 14, 16, 18), retarded eruption (19), and enamel fragility (2–4, 13) (Fig. 56-5).

Aborescent papillomas of the oral mucosa and/or lips (1–6, 9, 10, 14, 20–23), perianal region (1, 4, 10, 15, 21, 25), and genital mucosa (4, 21, 28) also occur. Bilateral cleft lip and palate have also been observed (6, 26).

DIFFERENTIAL DIAGNOSIS

Nevus lipomatosus superficialis (Hoffman-Zurhelle) is characterized by neutral fat-bearing cells adjacent to blood vessels in the middle and upper layers of the skin (13). In differential diagnosis, *incontinentia pigmenti* and *Rothmund-Thomson syndrome* should be excluded.

Congenital pseudoarthrosis apparently nearly always is a right-sided anomaly (in the one left-sided example, there was dextrocardia) and in some cases is inherited as an autosomal dominant trait. Rarely is it bilateral (6a, 20a).

LABORATORY AIDS

Skin biopsy of a fatty lesion demonstrates normal adipose cells in the corium. Less specific changes are found in the scarlike areas (7, 12). Roentgenographic studies show osteopathia striata and numerous skeletal changes described above.

REFERENCES

1 Barta, L., and Lengyel, J., Über ein Syndrom mit naeviformen Hautatrophien (systematisierte naeviforme Atrophodermie). *Ann. Paediatr. (Basel)* **207**:258–268, 1966.

1a Becker, S. W., and Lindsay, D. G., A Case for Diagnosis. *Arch. Dermatol.* **77**:620–621, 1958.

2 Beurey, J., et al., Hypoplasie dermique en aires et dysplasie méso-ectodermique. *Bull. Soc. Fr. Dermatol. Syphiligr.* **74**:7–9, 1967.

3 Braun-Falco, O., and Marghescu, S., Über eine systematisierte naeviforme Atrophodermie. *Arch. Klin. Exp. Der-*

matol. **221**:549–565, 1965.

4 Daly, J. G., Focal Dermal Hypoplasia. *Cutis* **4**:1354–1359, 1968.

5 Fazekas, A., et al., Goltzsches Syndrom–Osteo-, Okulo-, Dermale Dysplasie. *Z. Haut Geschlechtskr.* **48**:307–316, 1973.

6 Ferrara, A., Goltz's Syndrome. *Am. J. Dis. Child.* **123**:263, 1972.

6a Gibson, D. A., and Carroll, N., Congenital Pseudoarthrosis of the Clavicle. *J. Bone Joint Surg.* **52B**:629–643, 1970.

7 Ginsburg, L. D., et al., Focal Dermal Hypoplasia Syndrome. *Am. J. Roentgenol.* **110**:561–571, 1970.

8 Goltz, R. W., Focal Dermal Hypoplasia. *Arch. Dermatol.* **86**:708–717, 1962.

9 Goltz, R. W., et al., Focal Dermal Hypoplasia Syndrome. *Arch. Dermatol.* **101**:1–11, 1970.

10 Gorlin, R. J., et al., Focal Dermal Hypoplasia Syndrome. *Acta Derm. Venereol. (Stockh.)* **43**:421–440, 1963.

11 Gottlieb, S. K., et al., Focal Dermal Hypoplasia. *Arch. Dermatol.* **108**:551–553, 1973.

11a Hailey, H., et al. Poikiloderma congenitale. *Arch. Dermatol.* **44**:345–348, 1941.

12 Holden, J. D., and Akers, W. A., Goltz's Syndrome: Facial Dermal Hypoplasia: Combined Mesoectodermal Dysplasia. *Am. J. Dis. Child.* **114**:292–300, 1967.

13 Howell, J. B., Nevus Angiolipomatosus vs. Focal Dermal Hypoplasia. *Arch. Dermatol.* **92**:238–248, 1965.

13a Howell, J. B., and Reynolds, J., Osteopathia Striata. *Trans. St. John's Hosp. Dermatol. Soc.* **60**:178–182, 1974.

14 Ishibashi, A., and Kurihara, Y., Goltz's Syndrome: Focal Dermal Hypoplasia Syndrome. *Dermatologica* **144**:156–167, 1972.

15 Jessner, M., Naeviforme, poikilodermie-artige Hautveränderungen mit Missbildungen (Schwimmhautbildung an den Fingern, Papillome am Anus). *Zbl. Haut Geschlechtskr.* **27**:46, 1928.

16 Lanzieri, M., Su di una rara associazione di sindrome malformativa craniofacciale e di assenza congenita del perone. *Ann. Ottalmol. Clin. Ocul.* **87**:667–678, 1961.

17 Larregue, M., et al., L'osteopathie striée, symptome radiologique de l'hypoplasie dermique en aires. *Ann. Radiol. (Paris)* **15**:287–295, 1972.

18 Liebermann, S. L., Atrophodermia linearis maculosa et papillomatosis congenitalis. *Acta Derm. Venereol. (Stockh.)* **16**:476–484, 1935.

19 Mandel, E. H., Poikiloderma Congenitale (Rothmund-Thomson Syndrome). *Arch. Dermatol.* **91**:678–679, 1965.

20 Martin-Scott, I., Congenital Focal Dermal Hypoplasia. *Br. J. Dermatol.* **77**:60–62, 1965.

20a Owen, R., Congenital Pseudoarthrosis of the Clavicle. *J. Bone Joint Surg.* **52B**:644–652, 1970.

21 Orbaneja, J. G., and De Castro Torres, A., Un nuevo caso de hipoplasia dermica focal. *Acta Dermo-sifilol.* **58**:93–100, 1969.

22 Rochiccioli, P., et al., Hypoplasie dermique en aire, osteopathie striée et nanisme. *Pédiatrie* **30**:271–280, 1975.

23 Ruiz-Maldonado, R., et al., Focal Dermal Hypoplasia. *Clin. Genet.* **6**:36–45, 1974.

24 Selzer, G., et al., Goltz Syndrome with Multiple Giant-Cell Tumor-like Lesions in Bones. *Ann. Intern. Med.* **80**:714–717, 1974.

25 Stollmann, K., Bisher noch nicht beschriebene Befunde bei Incontinentia pigmenti. *Dermatol. Wochenschr.* **153**:489–496, 1967.

25a Toro-Sola, M. A., et al., Focal Dermal Hypoplasia Syndrome in a Male. *Clin. Genet.* **7**:325–327, 1975.

26 Valerius, N. H., A Case of Focal Dermal Hypoplasia Syndrome (Goltz) with Bilateral Cheilo-Gnatho-Palatoschisis. *Acta Paediat. Scand.* **63**:287–288, 1974.

26a Verger, P., et al., Hypoplasie dermique en aires et ostéopathie striée. *Ann. Pédiat.* **16**:349–354, 1975.

27 Walbaum, R., et al., Syndrome de Goltz chez un garçon. *Pédiatrie* **25**:911–920, 1970.

28 Warburg, M., Focal Dermato-phalangeal Dysplasia. *Acta Ophthalmol. (Kbh.)* **46**:137, 1968.

29 Zergollern, L., et al., Focal Dermal Hypoplasia. *Dermatologia* **148**:240–246, 1974.

57

Frontometaphyseal Dysplasia

Gorlin and Cohen (3) in 1969 separated frontometaphyseal dysplasia from a number of other craniotubular dysplasias. The condition consists of (a) pronounced bony supraorbital ridge, (b) deafness, and (c) other skeletal alterations. Similar cases were described by Lischi (8), Holt et al. (6), Walker (10), Danks et al. (2), and others (7, 9, 11).

Inheritance may be autosomal dominant, since the disorder was found in a mother and son (11). However, possibly genetic heterogeneity exists since it was reported in two mentally

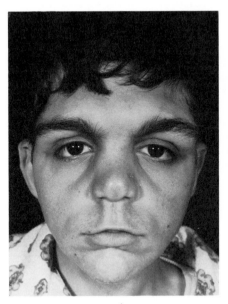 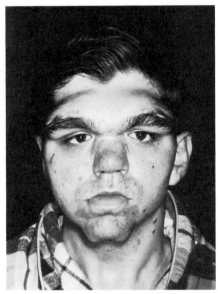

A   B

Figure 57-1. *Frontometaphyseal dysplasia.* (*A*). Facies is marked by pronounced supraorbital ridge, wide nasal bridge, small chin. (*From D. Danks et al.,* Am. J. Dis. Child. **123:**254, 1972.) (*B*). Note similar but more marked changes in older patient. (*From R. J. Gorlin and M. M. Cohen, Jr.,* Am. J. Dis. Child. **118:**287, 1969.)

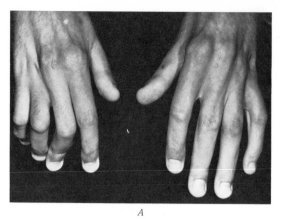
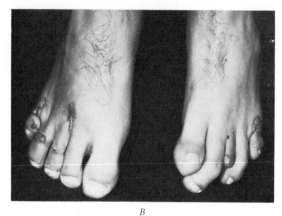

A   *B*

Figure 57-2. (*A*). Wasting of muscles of hands, flexion deformities of fingers, progressive ulnar deviation of wrists. (*B*). Hammertoes and keloid formation. (*A and B from R. J. Gorlin and M. M. Cohen, Jr., Am. J. Dis. Child.* **118:**287, 1969.)

retarded half-brothers whose mother was normal (7).

SYSTEMIC MANIFESTATIONS

Facies. The marked supraorbital ridge, wide nasal bridge, and small pointed chin give the patient a striking appearance. Enlargement of the supraorbital ridge becomes evident before puberty (2) (Fig. 57-1*A*, *B*).

Musculoskeletal alterations. There is wasting of muscles of the arms and legs, especially the hypothenar and interosseous muscles of the hands. Dorsiflexion of the wrist and extension of the elbows are reduced, with pronation and supination being extremely limited. Flexion deformities of the fingers and ulnar deviation of the wrist are progressive. Finger mobility is essentially limited to the metacarpophalangeal joints. Hammertoes have been also noted (Fig. 57-2*A*, *B*).

Roentgenographic examination demonstrates a thick torus-like frontal ridge, absence of frontal sinuses, "Hershey kiss" or "top of the mosque" defects of supraorbital rims, arched superior border of maxillary sinuses, and antegonial notching along the lower border of the body of the mandible with marked hypoplasia of the

angle and condyloid process (1, 3, 6) (Fig. 57-3*A*). The foramen magnum is greatly enlarged, and numerous cervical vertebral anomalies have been noted, e.g., the odontoid process is located too far anteriorly, the atlas has no posterior arch. There are fusion of the 2d and 3d cervical vertebras, and subluxation of the 3d and 4th vertebras. The long bones manifest increased density in the diaphyseal region, with lack of modeling in the metaphyseal area producing an Erlenmeyer flask deformity (Fig. 57-3*B*). Marked flaring of the iliac bones and coxa valga are noted, as well as fused and eroded carpal bones, wide elongated middle phalanges, and increased interpediculate distances in the lumbar region of the spine (2, 3, 9, 11) (Fig. 57-3*C*). The ribs and vertebras are irregularly contoured (6) or scoliotic (10).

Ear. Progressive mixed deafness has been reported (1, 3, 9–11).

Other findings. One patient (3) had a small penis and cryptorchism. Bundle branch block has been described (2).

Oral manifestations. Missing permanent teeth and retained deciduous teeth were noted (1–3, 8, 9, 11), as well as a bifid uvula (2) (Fig. 57-4).

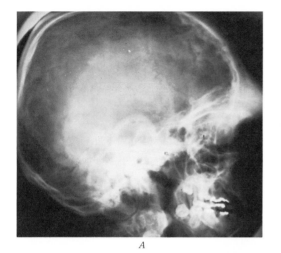

A

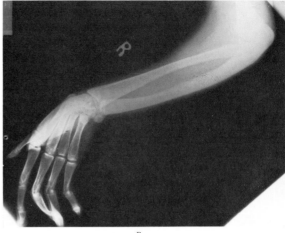

B

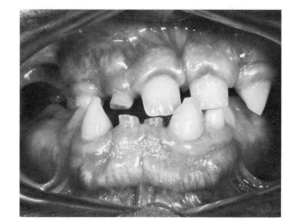

C

Figure 57-3. (*A*). Supraorbital torus, hypoplastic mandible with irregular lower border. (*B*). Relative absence of metaphyseal modeling. (*C*). Marked flaring of the iliac bones and coxa valga. (A, B, *and* C *from R. J. Gorlin and M. M. Cohen, Jr.,* Am. J. Dis. Child. **118:**287, 1969.)

LABORATORY AIDS

Danks et al. (2) found metachromasia in cultured fibroblasts.

DIFFERENTIAL DIAGNOSIS

Other craniotubular dysplasias, such as *craniometaphyseal dysplasia* and *craniodiaphyseal dysplasia*, should be excluded: These disorders are discussed at length by Gorlin et al. (3, 4).

A thick torus-like frontal ridge has been noted in the end stage of Jansen metaphyseal chondrodysplasia (5), a bone disorder otherwise quite different.

Figure 57-4. Missing permanent teeth, retained deciduous teeth, teeth with conical crown form in eighteen-year-old patient.

REFERENCES

1 Arenberg, I. K., et al., Otolaryngologic Manifestations of Frontometaphyseal Dysplasia. The Gorlin-Holt Syndrome. *Arch. Otolaryngol.* **99:**52–58, 1974.

2 Danks, D. M., et al., Fronto-Metaphyseal Dysplasia. *Am. J. Dis. Child.* **123:**254–258, 1972.

3 Gorlin, R. J., and Cohen, M. M., Jr., Frontometaphyseal Dysplasia: A New Syndrome. *Am. J. Dis. Child.* **118:**487–494, 1969.

4 Gorlin, R. J., et al., Genetic Craniotubular Bone Dysplasias and Hyperostoses: A Critical Analysis. *Birth Defects* **5**(4):79–95, 1969.

5 de Haas, W. H., et al., Metaphyseal Dysostosis. *J. Bone Joint Surg.* **51B:**290–299, 1969.

6 Holt, J. F., et al., Frontometaphyseal Dysplasia. *Radiol. Clin. N. Am.* **10:**225–243, 1972.

7 Jerris, G. A., and Jenkins, E. C., Frontometaphyseal Dysplasia. *Syndrome Identification* **3**(1):18–19, 1975.

8 Lischi, G., Le torus supraorbitalis: Variation crânienne rare. *J. Radiol. Électrol.* **48:**463–466, 1967.

9 Sauvegrain, J., et al., Dysplasie fronto-métaphysaire. *Ann. Radiol.* **18:**155–162, 1975.

10 Walker, B. A., A Craniodiaphyseal Dysplasia or Craniometaphyseal Dysplasia, ? Type. *Birth Defects* **5**(4):298–300, 1969.

11 Weiss, L., et al., Frontometaphyseal Dysplasia—Evidence for Dominant Inheritance. *Birth Defects* **11**(5):55–56, 1975.

58

Frontonasal Dysplasia

(*Median Cleft Face Syndrome*)

This condition, probably first described by Hoppe (12) in 1859, consists of (a) ocular hypertelorism, (b) broad nasal root, (c) lack of formation of the nasal tip, (d) widow's peak scalp-hair anomaly, and (e) anterior cranium bifidum occultum. Associated defects may include (f) median clefting of the nose or of both nose and upper lip and, rarely, palate, and (g) unilateral or bilateral notching or clefting of the nasal alae. The most complete reviews are those of Sedano et al. (22), who called the condition "frontonasal dysplasia," and of DeMyer (7), who used the term "median cleft face syndrome."

The primary set of anomalies may be explained as a single syndromic malformation. Embryologically, if the nasal capsule fails to develop properly, the primitive brain vesicle fills the space normally occupied by the capsule, thus producing anterior cranium bifidum occultum, a morphokinetic arrest in the positioning of the eyes, and lack of formation of the nasal tip. The widow's peak scalp-hair anomaly results from ocular hypertelorism, since the two periocular fields of hair-growth suppression are also further apart than usual. Thus, the fields fail to overlap sufficiently high on the forehead, resulting in a widow's peak (23).

We consider frontonasal dysplasia not to be a well-defined syndrome, but a nonspecific developmental field complex in which the defect occurs with notching of the nasal alae, and a host of low-frequency anomalies (*vide infra*), resulting in broader patterns of abnormalities.

Almost all cases are sporadic (7, 22). However, familial instances have been noted. Cohen et al. (5) cited a personal communication which suggested autosomal dominant transmission, and he noted two other possible instances in the literature. Pendl and Zimprich (18) noted two possibly affected half-sibs. In all these instances, no more than one severely affected individual was present in each family. Warkany et al. (25) reported two severely affected half-sisters. Although dominant inheritance (with most cases representing fresh mutations together with reduced genetic fitness) and polygenic inheritance are both conceivable, the authors believe that the condition most likely has a multiplicity of causes. For example, the same set of facial features may be observed with large anterior encephalocele, frontal lipoma, and frontal teratoma. Furthermore, the host of extracephalic low-frequency anomalies found with frontonasal dysplasia suggests that a variety of multiple congenital anomaly syndromes may be present within the frontonasal dysplasia category. To date, however, no true multiple congenital anomaly syndromes have been isolated or identified.

The number of instances of twinning is greater in families with frontonasal dysplasia than in the general population (22). We have no explanation for this phenomenon. Although some clinicians have maintained that frontonasal dysplasia represents an incomplete form of twinning, we cannot accept this view. Twinning of the head results from anterior duplication of the notochord. Doubling of the hypophysis constitutes the mildest form of anterior duplication. In diprosopia, a more extensive duplication, there may be doubling of the hypophysis, mouth, and nose. Doubling may lead to formation of two lateral eyes and a median eye. There is no evidence of duplication of any structure in frontonasal dysplasia to our knowledge.

SYSTEMIC MANIFESTATIONS

Facies. The clinical appearance of the face has been classified on a somewhat different basis by DeMyer (7) and Sedano et al. (22). Facial malformation can be graded from mild to severe (Figs. 58-1 to 58-8).

Eyes. Ocular hypertelorism is a constant finding. Secondary telecanthus, or narrowing of the palpebral fissures, may be observed in severe cases. Epibulbar dermoids have been observed in several cases (5, 8, 9, 11, 16). Rarely documented

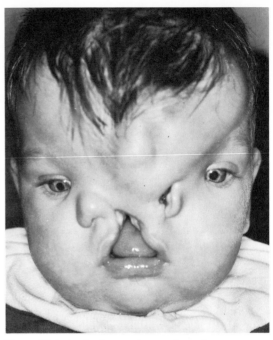

Figure 58-2. Ocular hypertelorism, frontal encephalomeningocele, separated nostrils. (*From W. DeMyer,* Neurology (Minneap.) **17:**961, 1967.)

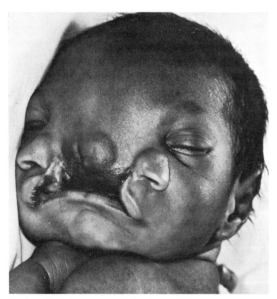

Figure 58-1. *Frontonasal dysplasia.* Most extreme example showing marked ocular hypertelorism, separated nasal halves, rectangular oronasal opening, absence of premaxilla. (*From W. DeMyer,* Neurology (Minneap.) **17:**961, 1967.)

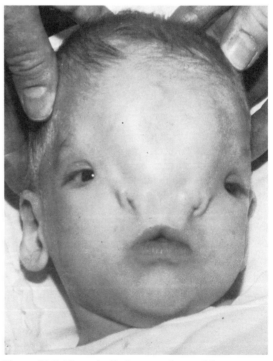

Figure 58-3. Note similarity to embryonal face.

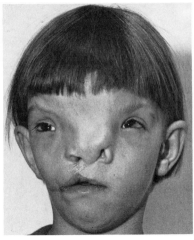 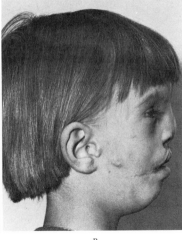

A   *B*

Figure 58-4. (*A, B*). Facies similar to that in Fig. 58-3 but with coloboma of upper left eyelid and epibulbar dermoid, repaired cleft lip, repaired macrostomia, remnants of ear tags (oculoauriculovertebral syndrome). (*From A. Fleischer-Peters*, Dtsch. Zahnärztl. Z. **24**:545, 1969.)

are congenital cataracts (22), upper eyelid colobomas (9, 16, 23), microphthalmia, and anophthalmia (22).

Nose. In severe cases, the nose may be flattened, with widely spaced nostrils and broad nasal root. In other cases, clefting of the nose may be observed. Notching or clefting of the nasal alae is present in some cases. When notching occurs bilaterally, the nose appears square (Fig. 58-6). Nose tags have also been noted (20).

Ears. Preauricular tags (3, 9, 11, 19, 23) have been observed. Low-set ears, absent tragus, and conductive deafness (22) have also been reported.

Central nervous system. Mental deficiency is present in some cases (4, 8, 26, 27). Of clinical importance, especially at birth, is DeMyer's observation (7) that when extracephalic anomalies occur or when hypertelorism is severe, the probability of mental deficiency is increased. Conversely, when extracephalic anomalies are absent

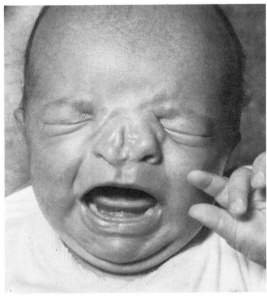

Figure 58-5. Ocular hypertelorism, bifid nose. (*From W. DeMyer*, Neurology (Minneap.) **17**:961, 1967.)

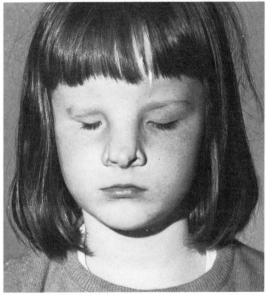

Figure 58-6. Colobomas of nostrils, wide nasal bridge, unilateral anophthalmia, microphthalmia on left.

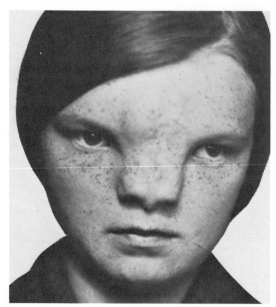

Figure 58-7. Ocular hypertelorism, broad nose. (*Courtesy of F. Burian, Prague, Czechoslovakia.*)

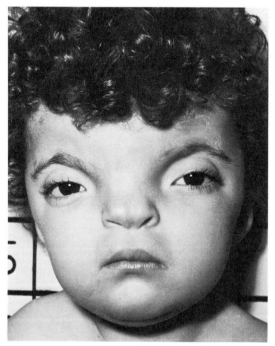

Figure 58-8. Least severely affected example. (*Courtesy of S. Cocuzza and E. Zoratto, Torino, Italy.*)

and hypertelorism is mild, the probability of mental deficiency is low.

Anterior cranium bifidum is seen roentgenographically. The frontal sinuses have been noted to be hypoplastic in a number of instances (13, 24). Large anterior encephalocele and, rarely, lipoma or teratoma may be associated with the condition (22).

Coronal craniosynostosis and brachycephaly have been noted in several patients (17, 22, 26, personal observation). Also reported have been absence of the corpus callosum (7, 25), hydrocephalus (22), and early occlusive anterior and middle cerebral artery disease (personal observation).

Other findings. Occasionally polydactyly (4, 22), syndactyly (4), clinodactyly (7, 26, 27), brachydactyly (personal observation), umbilical hernia (2, 4), cryptorchism (7, 22, personal observation), and other anomalies (7, 22) have been reported.

Oral manifestations. Median cleft of the upper lip is present in some cases. Rarely, cleft palate is observed (16, 22).

DIFFERENTIAL DIAGNOSIS

The syndrome known as "ocular hypertelorism of Greig" can no longer be regarded as a distinct entity. Rather, ocular hypertelorism should be regarded as a nonspecific malformation that may occur in a variety of different syndromes. Peterson et al. (19) have tabulated a large number of disorders in which ocular hypertelorism or dystopia canthorum is a feature.

Bifid nose may occur without ocular hypertelorism, and a number of familial instances are known (10, 25).

Since epibulbar dermoids, and sometimes upper eyelid colobomas and preauricular tags, may occur in association with frontonasal dysplasia, differentiation from *oculoauriculovertebral dysplasia* (*Goldenhar syndrome*) should be kept in mind.

LABORATORY AIDS

None is known.

REFERENCES

1 Borges, A. F., and Alexander, J. E., Plastic Surgical Improvement of Rare Congenital Deformities. *Va. Med. Mon.* **91:**448–457, 1964.

2 Bougon, –, and Derocque, –, Fissure médiane de la face. *Rev. Orthop. (Paris)* **9:**219–224, 1908.

3 Burian, F., Median Clefts of the Nose. *Acta Chir. Plast. (Praha)* **2:**180–189, 1960.

4 Cocozza, G., and Ferola, R., Considerazioni sulla sindrome ipertelorica di Greig nei suoi rapporti con altre craniosinostosis patologiche. *Pediatria (Napoli)* **66:**592–613, 1958.

5 Cohen, M. M., Jr., et al., Frontonasal Dysplasia (Median Cleft Face Syndrome): Comments on Etiology and Pathogenesis. *Birth Defects* **7**(7):117–119, 1971.

6 Converse, J. M., et al., The Use of Tomography in the Diagnosis of Unusual and Occult Clefts of the Palate. *Cleft Palate J.* **5:**311–316, 1968.

7 DeMyer, W., The Median Cleft Face Syndrome: Differential Diagnosis of Cranium Bifidum Occultum, Hypertelorism, and Median Cleft Nose, Lip and Palate. *Neurology (Minneap.)* **17:**961–971, 1967.

8 Edwards, W. C., et al., Median Cleft Face Syndrome. *Am. J. Ophthalmol.* **72:**202–205, 1971.

9 Fleischer-Peters, A., Goldenhar Syndrom und Kiefermissbildungen. *Dtsch. Zahnärztl. Z.* **24:**545–551, 1969.

10 Francesconi, G., and Fortunato, G., Median Dysraphia of the Face. *Plast. Reconstr. Surg.* **43:**481–491, 1969.

11 Gupta, J. S., et al., Oculo-auricular-cranial Dysplasia. *Br. J. Ophthalmol.* **52:**346–347, 1968.

12 Hoppe, I., Eine angeborene Spaltung der Nase. *Preuss. Med.-Ztg., Berl.* **2:**164–165, 1859.

13 Kazanjian, V., and Holmes, E., Treatment of Median Cleft Lip Associated with Bifid Nose and Hypertelorism. *Plast. Reconstr. Surg.* **24:**582–587, 1959.

14 Kitlowski, E. A., Congenital Anomaly of the Face: Inclusion Cyst Arising from Mucous Membrane of Pharynx with Deformity of Nose and Cleft Lip and Palate. *Plast. Reconstr. Surg.* **23:**64–68, 1959.

15 Kurlander, G. F., et al., Roentgenology of the Median Cleft Face Syndrome. *Radiology* **88:**473–478, 1967.

16 Lyford, J. H., and Roy, F. H., Arhinencephaly Unilateralis, Uveal Coloboma and Lens Reduplication. *Am. J. Ophthalmol.* **77:**315–318, 1974.

17 McCowatt, M. T., Hereditary Hypertelorism without Mental Deficiency. *Arch. Dis. Child.* **4:**381–384, 1929.

18 Pendl, G., and Zimprich, H., Ein Beitrag zum Syndrom des Hypertelorismus Greig. *Helv. Paediatr. Acta* **26:**319–325, 1971.

19 Peterson, M. O., et al., Comments on Frontonasal Dysplasia, Ocular Hypertelorism and Dystopia Canthorum. *Birth Defects* **7**(7):120–124, 1971.

20 Rohasco, S. A., and Massa, J. L., Frontonasal Syndrome. *Br. J. Plast. Surg.* **21:**244–249, 1968.

21 Sauvegrain, J., and Nahum, H., Hypertelorisme essentiel. *J. Radiol. Électrol.* **43:**528–531, 1962.

22 Sedano, H. O., et al., Frontonasal Dysplasia. *J. Pediatr.* **76:**906–913, 1970.

23 Smith, D. W., and Cohen, M. M., Jr., Widow's Peak, Scalp-hair Anomaly and Its Relation to Ocular Hypertelorism. *Lancet* **2:**1127–1128, 1973.

24 Viezens, A., and Willenberg, W., Zwei seltene Gesichtsmissbildungen im Hals- Nasen- Ohrenbereich: Doppelnase und Dysostosis mandibulofacialis. *Dtsch. Med. J.* **7:**457–461, 1956.

25 Warkany, J., et al., Median Facial Cleft Syndrome in Half-sisters. Dilemmas in Genetic Counseling. *Teratology* **8:**273–286, 1973.

26 Webster, J., and Deming, E., The Surgical Treatment of the Bifid Nose. *Plast. Reconstr. Surg.* **6:**1–37, 1950.

27 Zunin, C., Hipertelorismo di Greig e suoi rapporti con le sindromi di disostosicraniche e facciali. *Minerva Pediatr.* **7:**71–79, 1955.

59

Gardner Syndrome

(Osteomatosis-Intestinal Polyposis Syndrome)

ardner and coworkers (15, 30), in 1953–1954, recognized a syndrome of (a) multiple osteomas, especially of the facial bones, (b) epidermoid cysts of the skin, (c) multiple polyposis of the large intestine, and (d) desmoids or fibromas of the skin. Earlier case reports of the syndrome have been documented (2, 10, 11, 23).

Others subsequently reported mesenteric desmoids, lipomas (5, 21, 34), leiomyomas (5, 16), and odontomas (10).

The syndrome has autosomal dominant inheritance with at least 80 percent penetrance and markedly variable expressivity (29). The incidence has been estimated at 1 per 14,000 people (29).

SYSTEMIC MANIFESTATIONS

Facies. The facies may be altered if osteomas of sufficient size are present in the mandible, maxilla, or frontal bones (31) (Fig. 59-1).

Skin and skin appendages. Epidermoid inclusion cysts of the skin occur in about 50 percent of the cases, but may be present in nearly all those affected in some families (40). They may appear anywhere on the scalp, face, trunk, or extremities (Fig. 59-2). The age at which the cysts first appear seems to be variable, although on the average they become manifest about the age of thirteen years, prior to the appearance of the

intestinal polyposis (16, 21a). New cysts appear periodically (16, 40).

Fibrous tumors of the skin (fibromas and desmoids) commonly occur in association with polyposis of the colon (22, 33, 35). The desmoid tumors frequently arise in the abdominal scar after resection for colonic surgery (Fig. 59-3).

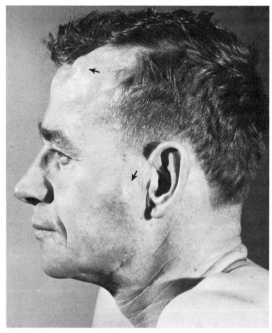

Figure 59-1. *Gardner syndrome.* Arrows point to osteomas of frontal bone and mandibular condylar area.

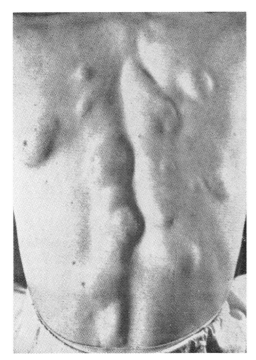

Figure 59-2. Multiple epidermoid inclusion cysts over dorsal region. (*From M. C. Oldfield*, Br. J. Surg. **41**:534, 1954.)

They may, however, arise on the skin in the absence of any prior surgery. Lipoma or lipofibroma of the skin may also be found (4, 5, 21, 34).

Gastrointestinal system and allied structures. Multiple intestinal polyposis of the colon and rectum, with a marked tendency to rapid

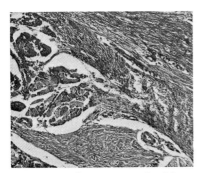

Figure 59-3. Photomicrograph of desmoid tumor in rectus muscle, showing muscle remnants.

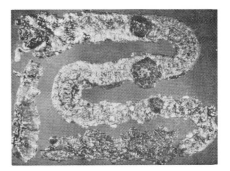

Figure 59-4. Multiple polyps of colon undergoing malignant transformation to adenocarcinoma.

malignant degeneration, is characteristic (4) (Fig. 59-4). Small-intestine involvement has been reported by only a few investigators (4, 8, 16, 17, 25) but there is marked malignant propensity at this site. The polyps may occur before puberty (4). By 20 years, about 50 percent have demon-

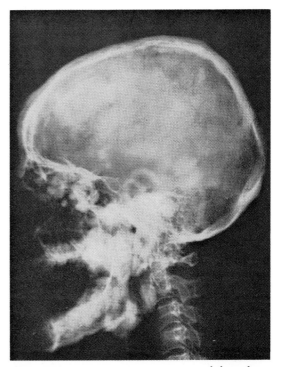

Figure 59-5. Numerous osteomas scattered throughout jaws and skull.

strated polyps, and at time of surgery about half the patients exhibit malignant degeneration of one or more polyps. Lymphoid hyperplasia of the terminal ileum has been reported (4, 8, 32a, 35, 38).

Desmoid tumors may be found scattered throughout the mesentery (33). They may be single or multiple and may be found in 10 to 30 percent (19, 22, 40). Gorlin and Chaudhry (16) reported one patient with 40 such fibromatous growths. Postoperative adhesions are especially severe, frequently resulting in obstruction (16, 33). Leiomyomas, both retroperitoneal and within the stomach and ileum, have also been observed (5, 17).

Other findings. Papillary adenocarcinoma of the thyroid has been described in sibs with the Gardner syndrome (2, 34).

Oral manifestations. Multiple osteomas may be scattered throughout the calvaria and facial skeleton (Fig. 59-5). In most cases, the osteomas appear around puberty and precede the appearance of intestinal polyposis (3). In the more completely reported bone surveys, the frontal bone, maxilla, mandibular angle, and the lower border of the mandible below the teeth were most frequently involved (16, 31). The osteomas may project into the paranasal sinuses. Microscopically, the bone is mature, consisting of well-developed Haversian systems.

Long bones, most often radius, ulna, and metacarpals, may be the site of small osteomas, but involvement, in contrast to that of the facial skeleton, is minimal and bony thickening is

usually subperiosteal and rather diffuse. In a few cases, however, the osteomas have been small and well defined (3, 19, 35). Early involvement may simulate osteomyelitis (3, 31).

Compound odontomas, unerupted teeth, and/or hypercementosis have been described in about 50 percent of cases (3, 4, 8, 9, 10, 14, 19) (Fig. 59-6).

DIFFERENTIAL DIAGNOSIS

Multiple polyps of the intestines have been described in a number of disorders:

Familial adenomatous polyposis of the colon. Inherited as an autosomal dominant trait, this is probably the most common of all polypoid disorders. The polyps appear between the ages of ten to forty years and usually develop adenocarcinomatous changes. Marked lymphoid hyperplasia of the terminal ileum may be noted (24, 32a, 42).

Juvenile polyposis of the colon. Juvenile polyps of the colon may be inherited as an autosomal dominant trait (13a, 39). The polyps are hamartomatous and not precancerous.

Generalized juvenile gastrointestinal polyposis. Sachatello et al. (32) described the autosomal dominant inheritance of juvenile polyps of the stomach, small intestine, colon, or rectum. They are associated with melena and intussusception. The juvenile polyps consist of an epithelial component surrounded by a mesen-

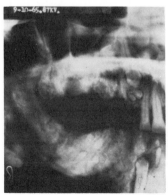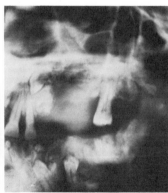

Figure 59-6. Panorex of jaws showing osteomas and supernumerary teeth. (*From C. J. Witkop, Jr., Minneapolis, Minn.*)

chymal-appearing connective tissue. The epithelial element is arranged in tubules associated with an overproduction or retention of mucus.

Turcot syndrome. The association of glioblastoma multiforme and/or medulloblastoma with colonic polyposis has been described as autosomal recessive (1, 6, 24, 27, 37, 40). It may be a spurious entity.

Peutz-Jeghers syndrome. This autosomal dominant syndrome, characterized by generalized gastrointestinal hamartomatous polyps and macular pigmentation of the face, lips, and oral mucosa, is described in detail in Chap. 117. The typical polyp contains muscularis mucosa, and the epithelial element is related to the smooth muscle in the same manner as in normal mucous membrane.

Cronkheit-Canada syndrome. Generalized gastrointestinal polyposis in middle-aged to elderly individuals may be associated with edema, malabsorption, diarrhea, protein-losing enteropathy, generalized alopecia, and nail dystrophy. Brownish skin pigmentation may be diffuse over the face, neck, and hands, including palmar creases (18, 20, 28). The disorder is not hereditary. Most patients are females. Pigmentation of the oral mucosa has also been noted (18). The tongue may be devoid of papillae. Most patients have presented anemia, hypoalbuminemia, and depression of the levels of serum calcium, magnesium, and potassium, with resultant death in a cachectic state (28).

Other multiple intestinal syndromes. Zanca (43) noted multiple cartilaginous exostoses of several bones and colonic polyposis, a possible chance association. Fraumeni (12) described a multiple polyposis family with various sarcomas. There are several inherited examples of associated polyposis of stomach and colon (24). Solitary polyps of the colon and rectum have also been noted to be inherited as an autosomal dominant trait (24). Yonemoto et al. (42) described familial polyposis of the entire gastrointestinal tract. Polyposis of the large intestine may be seen in the *multiple hamartoma syndrome.*

The presence of multiple epidermoid inclusion cysts, desmoid, or bony growths, especially of the facial skeleton, should lead to a complete search for the intestinal component. Recording of these incidental findings should be just as mandatory as roentgenographic search for additional intestinal polyps if a single rectal polyp is detected. The discovery of multiple polyps, or of any other component, also places the onus of responsibility upon the investigator to search other relatives thoroughly for stigmata. Since a negative report does not mean that polyps or other components will not appear in future years, periodic reexamination of all persons with a parent or sib who had one or more signs is necessary.

Endosteomas or occult hyperostoses of the mandible have been described in patients with familial polyposis coli without other stigmata of Gardner syndrome (37a).

LABORATORY AIDS

Roentgenographic survey, especially of the facial skeleton, and barium studies of the large and small intestine are mandatory.

Trygstad et al. (36) described resistance to parathormone in adult patients with the Gardner syndrome. This, however, has not been confirmed.

REFERENCES

1 Baughman, F. A., Jr., et al., The Glioma-polyposis Syndrome. *N. Engl. J. Med.* **281**:1345–1346, 1969.

2 Camiel, M. R., et al., Thyroid Carcinoma with Gardner's Syndrome in Siblings. *N. Engl. J. Med.* **278**:1056–1058, 1968.

3 Chang, C. H., et al., Bone Abnormalities in Gardner's Syndrome. *Am. J. Roentgenol.* **102**:645–652, 1968.

4 Coli, R. D., et al., Gardner's Syndrome. *Am. J. Dig. Dis.* **15**:551–568, 1970.

5 Collins, D. C., Frequent Association of Other Body

Tumors with Familial Polyposis. *Am. J. Gastroenterol.* **31:**376–381, 1959.

6 Crail, H. W., Multiple Primary Malignancies Arising in the Rectum, Brain and Thyroid. *U.S. Naval Med. Bull.* **49:**123–128, 1949.

7 Devic, A., and Bussy, M. M., Un cas de polypose adenomateuse generalisée a tout l'intestin. *Arch. Mal. Appar. Dig.* **6:**278–289, 1912.

8 Duncan, B. R., et al., The Gardner Syndrome: Need for Early Diagnosis. *J. Pediatr.* **72:**497–505, 1968.

9 Fader, M., et al., Gardner's Syndrome (Intestinal Polyposis, Osteomas, Sebaceous Cysts) and a New Dental Discovery. *Oral Surg.* **15:**153–172, 1962.

10 Fitzgerald, G. M., Multiple Composite Odontomas Coincidental with Other Tumorous Conditions. *J. Am. Dent. Assoc.* **30:**1408–1417, 1943.

11 Frangenheim, P., Familiäre Hyperostosen der Kiefer. *Bruns Beitr. Klin. Chir.* **90:**139–151, 1914.

12 Fraumeni, J. F., Sarcomas and Multiple Polyposis in a Kindred: A Genetic Variety of Hereditary Polyposis? *Arch. Intern. Med.* **121:**57–61, 1968.

13 Fuhrmann, W., et al., Gardner's Syndrome without Polyposis. *Humangenetik* **5:**59–64, 1967.

13a Gathwright, J. B., Jr., and Cofer, T. W., Jr., Familial Incidence of Juvenile Polyposis Coli. *Surg. Gynecol. Obstet.* **138:**185–188, 1974.

14 Gardner, E. J., Follow-up Study of a Family Group Exhibiting Dominant Inheritance for a Syndrome Including Intestinal Polyposis, Osteomas, Fibromas and Epidermal Cysts. *Am. J. Hum. Genet.* **14:**376–390, 1962.

15 Gardner, E. J., and Richard, R. C., Multiple Cutaneous and Subcutaneous Lesions Occurring Simultaneously with Hereditary Polyposis and Osteomatosis. *Am. J. Hum. Genet.* **5:**139–147, 1953.

16 Gorlin, R. J., and Chaudhry, A. P., Multiple Osteomatosis, Fibromas, Lipomas, and Fibrosarcomas of the Skin and Mesentery, Epidermoid Inclusion Cysts of the Skin, Leiomyomas and Multiple Intestinal Polyposis. *N. Engl. J. Med.* **263:**1151–1158, 1960.

17 Gumpel, R. C., and Carballo, J. D., New Concept of Familial Adenomatosis. *Ann. Intern. Med.* **45:**1045–1058, 1956.

18 Johnston, M. M., et al., Gastrointestinal Polyposis Associated with Alopecia, Pigmentation and Atrophy of the Fingernails and Toenails. *Ann. Intern. Med.* **56:**935–940, 1962.

19 Jones, E. L., et al., Gardner's Syndrome. *Arch. Surg.* **92:**287–300, 1966.

20 Koehler, P. R., et al., Diffuse Gastrointestinal Polyposis with Ectodermal Changes. *Radiology* **103:**589–594, 1972.

21 Laberge, M. Y., et al., Soft Tissue Tumors Associated with Familial Polyposis: Report of Case. *Mayo Clin. Proc.* **32:**749–752, 1957.

21a Leppard, B., and Bussey, H. J. R., Epidermoid Cysts, Polyposis Coli, and Gardner's Syndrome. *Br. J. Surg.* **62:**387–393, 1975.

22 McAdam, W. A. F., and Goligher, J. C., The Occurrence of Desmoids in Patients with Familial Polyposis Coli. *Br. J. Surg.* **57:**618–631, 1970.

23 McKittrick, L. S., et al., Case 21061. *N. Engl. J. Med.* **212:**263–267, 1935.

24 McKusick, V. A., Genetic Factors in Intestinal Polyposis. *J.A.M.A.* **182:**271–277, 1962.

25 Melmed, R. N., and Boucher, I. A. D., Duodenal Involvement in Gardner's Syndrome. *Gut* **13:**524–527, 1972.

26 Murphey, E. S., et al., Familial Polyposis of Colon and Gastric Carcinoma. *J.A.M.A.* **179:**1026–1028, 1962.

27 Nuyts, J. P., et al., Le syndrome gliome-polypose. *Arch. Fr. Pédiat.* **30:**210, 1973.

28 Orimo, H., et al., Gastrointestinal Polyposis with Proteinlosing Enteropathy, Abnormal Skin Pigmentation and Loss of Hair and Nails (Cronkheit-Canada syndrome). *Am. J. Med.* **47:**445–449, 1969.

29 Pierce, E. R., et al., Gardner's Syndrome: Formal Genetics and Statistical Analysis of a Large Canadian Kindred. *Clin. Genet.* **1:**65–80, 1970.

30 Plenk, H. P., and Gardner, E. J., Osteomatosis (Leontiasis Ossea): Hereditary Disease of Membranous Bone Formation Associated in One Family with Polyposis of Colon. *Radiology* **62:**830–840, 1954.

31 Rayne, J., Gardner's Syndrome. *Br. J. Oral Surg.* **6:**11–17, 1968.

32 Sachatello, C. R., et al., Generalized Juvenile Gastrointestinal Polyposis. *Gastroenterology* **58:**699–708, 1970.

32a Schull, L. N., and Fitts, C. T., Lymphoid Polyposis Associated with Familial Polyposis and Gardner's Syndrome. *Ann. Surg.* **180:**319–322, 1974.

33 Simpson, R. D., et al., Mesenteric Fibromatosis in Familial Polyposis: A Variant of Gardner's Syndrome. *Cancer* **17:**526–534, 1964.

34 Smith, W. G., and Kern, B. B., The Nature of the Mutation in Familial Multiple Polyposis. Papillary Carcinoma of the Thyroid, Brain Tumors and Familial Multiple Polyposis. *Dis. Colon Rectum* **16:**264–271, 1973.

35 Thomas, K. E., et al., Natural History of Gardner's Syndrome. *Am. J. Surg.* **115:**218–226, 1968.

36 Trygstad, C. W., et al., Resistance to Parathyroid Extract of Gardner's Syndrome. *J. Clin. Endocrinol.* **28:**1153–1159, 1968.

37 Turcot, J., et al., Malignant Tumors of Central Nervous System Associated with Familial Polyposis of the Colon. *Dis. Colon Rectum* **2:**465–468, 1959.

37a Utsunomiya, J., and Nakamura, T., The Occult Osteomatous Changes in the Mandible in Patients with Familial Polyposis Coli. *Br. J. Surg.* **62:**45–51, 1975.

38 Vanhoutte, J. J., Polypoid Lymphoid Hyperplasia of the Terminal Ileum in Patients with Familial Polyposis Coli and with Gardner's Syndrome. *Am. J. Roentgenol.* **110:**340–342, 1970.

39 Veale, A. M. O., et al., Juvenile Polyposis Coli. *J. Med. Genet.* **3:**5–16, 1966.

40 Weary, P. E., et al., Gardner's Syndrome. *Arch. Dermatol.* **90:**20–30, 1964.

41 Yaffee, H. S., Gastric Polyposis and Soft Tissue Tumors (a Variant of Gardner's Syndrome). *Arch. Dermatol.* **89:**806–808, 1964.

42 Yonemoto, R. H., et al., Familial Polyposis of the Entire Gastrointestinal Tract. *Arch. Surg.* **99:**427–434, 1969.

43 Zanca, P., Multiple Hereditary Cartilaginous Exostoses with Polyposis of the Colon. *U.S. Armed Forces Med. J.* **7:**116–120, 1956.

60

Gingival Fibromatosis and Its Syndromes

Gingival fibromatosis may exist as an iso-lated finding or as part of a syndrome. As an isolated finding, it may be inherited as an autosomal dominant trait (1–12).

GINGIVAL FIBROMATOSIS, HYPERTRICHOSIS, EPILEPSY, AND MENTAL RETARDATION

This is the most common syndrome of gingival fibromatosis. Epilepsy and mental retardation are not present, however, in all cases. The binary combination of gingival enlargement and hyper-trichosis (5–7, 9, 10, 12, 16–18) would appear to be far less common than is isolated gingival fibromatosis. The syndrome appears to be in-herited as an autosomal dominant trait (16, 17). The hypertrichosis is usually generalized, in-volving the eyebrows, extremities, and sacral and genital areas (Fig. 60-1A–C).

Associated mental retardation and/or epilepsy have been noted by a few authors (1, 2, 5, 8, 11, 13, 15, 18), and it is possible that this combina-tion represents a genetic heterogeneity, some ex-amples possibly being inherited as an autosomal recessive trait (4). Other possibly aleatory skel-etal alterations, such as narrow second cervical vertebra, long odontoid process, and abnormal first ribs, were described by Anderson (1). The gingival enlargement usually occurs at less than five years of age (13).

We are uncertain how to classify the unusual case reported by Vontobel (14). Features in-cluded acromegaloid features, marked hyper-trichosis, hyperconvex nails, and gingival fibro-matosis.

GINGIVAL FIBROMATOSIS WITH MULTIPLE HYALINE FIBROMAS (MURRAY-PURETIĆ-DRESCHER SYNDROME)

Multiple hyaline fibrous tumors of the scalp, back, fingers, thighs, and legs were described by Murray (6) in 1873. The same patients were rede-scribed by Whitfield and Robinson (11). Other examples were identified by Puretić et al. (7, 8), Drescher (1), Ishikawa and Hori (3), Enjoji et al. (2), Kitano et al. (5), and Schmidt et al. (9).

The condition is inherited as an autosomal recessive trait. Affected sibs of consanguineous parents were described in several reports.

The hyaline, fibrous, painless tumors appear within the first few years of life and slowly en-large to the size of a small orange. Some regress slowly over a period of several years, while others calcify, ulcerate, and gradually disappear, leaving barely visible scars (Fig. 60-2A, B).

Histologically, the tumors vary, some having abundant connective tissue cells, others being rich in pseudocartilaginous hyaline matrix, which is homogeneous, acidophilic, and PAS-positive (4, 8, 12). Between the cells there are argyrophilic fibers (Fig. 60-2C). The collagen

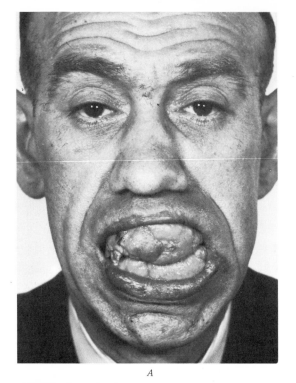

A

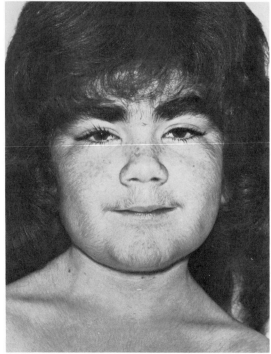

B

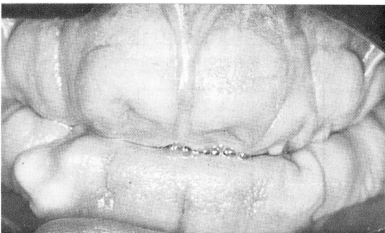

C

Figure 60-1. *Gingival fibromatosis-hypertrichosis.* (*A*). Extensive gingival fibromatosis. Patient cannot close lips over hyperplastic gingival masses. (*From A. McIndoe and B. O. Smith,* Br. J. Plast. Surg. **11**:62, 1959). (*B*). Note marked facial hypertrichosis. (*From G. B. Winter and M. J. Simpkiss,* Arch. Dis. Child. **49**:394, 1974.) (*C*). Massive gingival overgrowth in seven-year-old boy, covering all but the incisal edges of some teeth. Excessive overgrowth of hair on face and limbs. (*From M. Rushton,* Dent. Pract. Dent. Rec. **7**:136, 1957.)

fibers are thicker than normal. Ultrastructural studies were carried out by Woyke et al. (12) and by Kitano et al. (5), who also cultured tumor cells which stored a metachromatic substance. Ishikawa and Mori (4) found an increased amount of chondroitin-6-sulfate in the skin. The patient reported by Suschke and Kunze (10) was noted to have elevated amounts of hyaluronic acid and dermatan sulfate in the urine, suggesting that this is a mucopolysaccharidosis.

Painful progressive flexion contractures of the knees, elbows, hips, and shoulders appear within the first year of life (3, 5, 7, 8). Osteolysis of the terminal phalanges and small cystic lesions of long bones have been noted, as well as generalized osteoporosis and thoracolumbar scoliosis (8). Height and weight are reduced, and skeletal and sexual maturation is delayed.

There appears to be a marked tendency to suppurative infections of the skin and mucous membranes. The skin undergoes poikilodermatous and sclerodermatous changes.

GINGIVAL FIBROMATOSIS AND CORNEAL DYSTROPHY (RUTHERFURD SYNDROME)

Relatively mild gingival enlargement was described in three generations as an autosomal dominant trait by Rutherfurd (2). This family was followed up and reported on again by Houston and Shotts (1) in 1966. Associated anomalies were mental retardation, aggressive behavior, curtain-like corneal opacities involving the superior part of the cornea, and failure of eruption of the teeth, which exhibit root resorption (1). Dentigerous cyst development occurred around the unerupted first permanent molars.

GINGIVAL FIBROMATOSIS, EAR, NOSE, BONE, AND NAIL DEFECTS, AND HEPATOSPLENOMEGALY (LABAND SYNDROME)

In addition to the (a) gingival fibromatosis which is manifested at birth or within the first few months of life (6), there are (b) striking hypoplastic changes in the terminal phalanges of the fingers and toes.

The syndrome appears to be inherited as an autosomal dominant trait (1, 4).

Facies. The nose and pinnas are large and poorly structured, because of the soft consistency of the cartilage (1, 3, 4, 6). This change is striking, but has been seen in patients with gingival fibromatosis only (2) (Fig. 60-3A).

Skin. Mild hirsutism in the form of synophrys, hairy arms and legs, or increased sacral hair has been noted (3, 6).

Skeletal alterations. The thumb nails are hypoplastic or absent (Fig. 60-3B). The second to the fifth fingers usually exhibit missing nails and terminal phalanges. In most cases, all toes lack terminal phalanges, the first and second toes often having only one phalanx (1, 3, 4, 6). Pes cavus was noted in about half the kindred described by Laband (4). Joint hypermobility, especially involving the metacarpophalangeal, shoulder, and knee joints (1, 4), is common. Spina bifida occulta of the fifth lumbar vertebra was described in a few cases (3, 6). The third thoracic vertebra has been divided sagittally into two segments, with the fourth thoracic vertebra flattened (3).

Hepatosplenomegaly. Hepatomegaly (1) and splenomegaly (4) have been noted. Laband (4) suggested that splenomegaly might become more marked with age. On the other hand, enlargement of the liver and spleen has been specifically denied (6).

Other findings. Mental retardation (6) has been described in one case.

Oral. Gingival fibromatosis is a constant feature (Fig. 60-3C).

GINGIVAL FIBROMATOSIS, MICROPHTHALMIA, MENTAL RETARDATION, ATHETOSIS, AND HYPOPIGMENTATION (CROSS SYNDROME)

Cross et al. (1) described three sibs, the product of a consanguineous union, who exhibited microphthalmia, cloudy cornea, and hypopigmented skin (Fig. 60-4). By the third month, there were signs of spasticity and mental retardation. Reduced tyrosinase-active melanosomes demonstrated by Witkop (2, 3). He noted gingival fibromatosis in two of three sibs. Autosomal recessive inheritance is likely.

DIFFERENTIAL DIAGNOSIS

The presence of a complete syndrome usually gives the clinician little diagnostic difficulty.

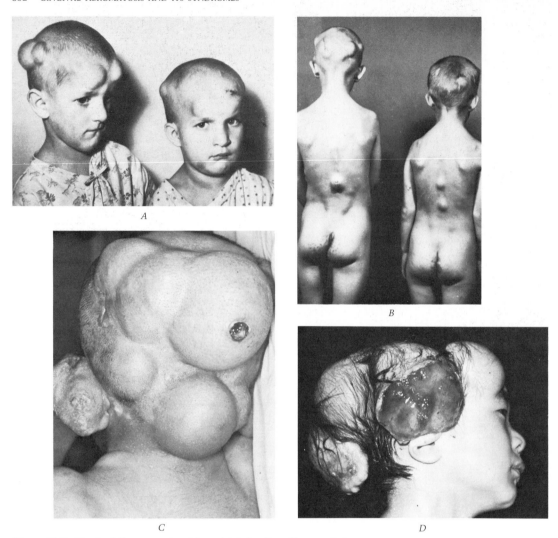

Figure 60-2. *Gingival fibromatosis with multiple hyaline fibromas (Murray-Puretić-Drescher syndrome)*. *(A)*. Tumors of the head in five-year-old male and four-year-old female sibs. Tumors first appeared when children were two years of age. *(B)*. Note tumors of the head, along spine, and in elbow region. Some have been removed. *(C)*. Skin tumors of head of thirteen-year-old boy. *(D)*. Tumors of head of seven-year-old boy.

Although the gingiva are enlarged in a number of other conditions (inflammation, Dilantin hyperplasia, pregnancy, leukemia, etc.), they are not enlarged to the degree seen in these syndromes and they are usually softer and considerably more vascular. Coverage of the teeth by the gingiva may suggest anodontia.

Hirsutism may result from a plethora of causes. These have been thoroughly discussed by Muller (7) and Felgenhauer (4). Acquired hypertrichosis may occasionally be a sign of malignancy (6, 9).

Extreme hypertrichosis with true anodontia was described by a number of authors (1, 5, 8, 10,

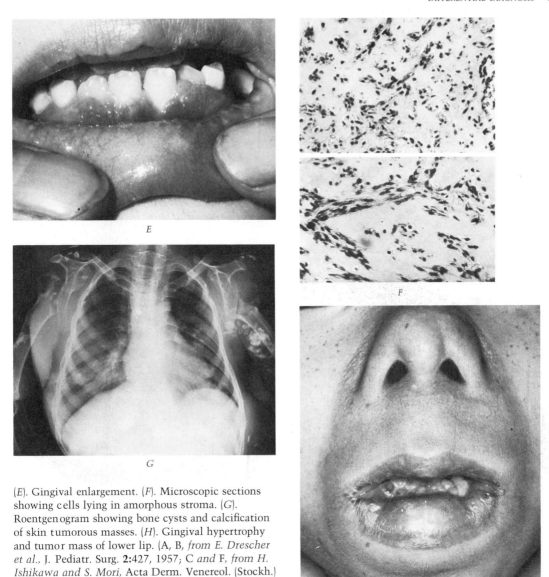

(E). Gingival enlargement. (F). Microscopic sections showing cells lying in amorphous stroma. (G). Roentgenogram showing bone cysts and calcification of skin tumorous masses. (H). Gingival hypertrophy and tumor mass of lower lip. (A, B, *from E. Drescher et al.,* J. Pediatr. Surg. **2:**427, 1957; C *and* F, *from H. Ishikawa and S. Mori,* Acta Derm. Venereol. (Stockh.) **53:**185, 1973; D *and* E, *from Y. Kitano et al.* Arch. Dermatol. **106:**877, 1972.)

11). The hair has been so profuse that some individuals have been exhibited as "dog-face" men and women (2–4). With rare exceptions (Juliana Pastrana), these persons have not exhibited gingival enlargement.

One of the authors (M. M. C.) has observed an isolated patient with marked gingival fibromatosis, hypertrichosis, prominent frontal bone, and alterations in the ribs and metacarpals and axillary pterygia.

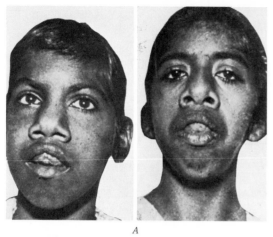

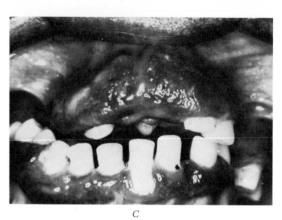

A

C

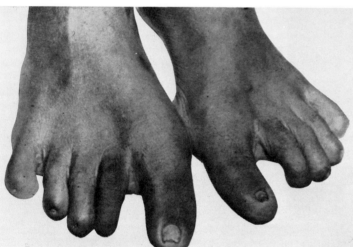

B

Figure 60-3. *Gingival fibromatosis, ear, nose, bone, and nail defects and hepatosplenomegaly (Laband syndrome).* (*A*). Nose and pinnas large and poorly formed because of soft cartilage. Note marked gingival enlargement. (*B*). Hypoplastic nails and terminal phalanges of toes. (*C*). Hyperplastic gingiva. Gingivectomy has been performed on lower arch. (A, B, *from P. F. Laband,* Oral Surg. **17:**339, 1964; C, *courtesy of C. J. Witkop, Jr., Minneapolis, Minn.*)

LABORATORY AIDS

Other than jaw roentgenograms to ascertain the presence of teeth, no diagnostic aids are needed. Endocrine studies performed on these patients have not shown abnormal values.

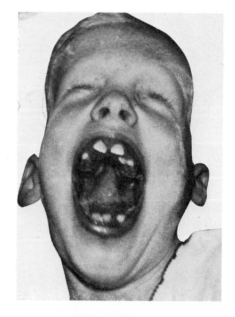

Figure 60-4. *Gingival fibromatosis, microphthalmia, mental retardation, athetosis and hypopigmentation (Cross syndrome).* Note microphthalmia, hypopigmented skin, enlarged gingiva. (*From H. E. Cross et al.,* J. Pediatr. **70:**398, 1967.)

REFERENCES

GINGIVAL FIBROMATOSIS, GENERAL ASPECTS

1 Biegel, H., Über abnorme Haarentwicklung beim Menschen. *Virchows Arch. Pathol. Anat.* **44**:418–427, 1868.
2 Danforth, C. H., Studies on Hair with Special Reference to Hypertrichosis. *Arch. Dermatol. Syph.* (*Chic.*) **12**:380–401, 528–537, 1925.
3 Fauvelle, −, Un cas de pilosisme chez un jeune laotienne. *Bull. Soc. Anthropol.* **9**:439–488, 1886.
4 Felgenhauer, W. R., Hypertrichosis lanuginosa universalis. *J. Génét. Hum.* **17**:1–44, 1969.
5 Gross, S. D., Case of Hypertrophy of the Gums. *Louisville Rev.* **1**:232–237, 1856.
6 Hensley, G. T., and Glynn, K. P., Hypertrichosis Lanuginosa as a Sign of Internal Malignancy. *Cancer* **24**:1051–1056, 1969.
7 Muller, S. A., Hirsutism. *Am. J. Med.* **46**:803–817, 1969.
8 Parreidt, J., Über die Bezahnung bei Menschen mit abnormer Behaarung. *Dtsch. Monatsschr. Zahnheilkd.* **4**:41–54, 1886.
9 Van der Lugt, L., and Dudok de Wit, C., Hypertrichosis lanuginosa acquisita. *Dermatologica* **146**:46–54, 1973.
10 Virchow, R., Die russischen Haarmenschen. *Berl. Klin. Wochenschr.* **10**:337–339, 1873.
11 White, J. W., Periscope. *Dent. Cosmos* **16**:43–46, 1874.
12 Witkop, C. J., Jr., Heterogeneity in Gingival Fibromatosis. *Birth Defects* **7**(7):210–221, 1971.

GINGIVAL FIBROMATOSIS, HYPERTRICHOSIS, EPILEPSY, AND MENTAL RETARDATION

1 Anderson, J., et al., Gingival Fibromatosis. *Br. Med. J.* **3**:218–219, 1969.
2 Araiche, M., and Brode, H., A Case of Fibromatosis Gingivae. *Oral Surg.* **12**:1307–1310, 1959.
3 Balestra, M., and Gnudi, A., Contributo alla conoscenza de un raro caso di iperplasia osteo-fibro-mucosa a carattere famigliare. *Ann. Stomatol.* (*Roma*) **11**:609–635, 1962.
4 Jorgensen, R. J., and Cocker, M. E., Variation in the Inheritance and Expression of Gingival Fibromatosis. *J. Periodontol.* **45**:472–477, 1974.
5 Kerageorgis, B. P., Elephantiasis des gingives. *Rev. Chir.* (*Paris*) **87**:308–320, 1949.
6 McIndoe, A., and Smith, B. O., Congenital Familial Fibromatosis of the Gums with the Teeth as a Probably Etiological Factor. *Br. J. Plast. Surg.* **11**:62–71, 1958.
6a Miles, A. E. W., Julia Pastrana, The Bearded Lady. *Proc. R. Soc. Med.* **67**:160–164, 1974.
7 Perkoff, D., Primary Generalized Hypertrophy of the Gums. *Lancet* **1**:1294–1297, 1929.
8 Ramon, Y., et al., Gingival Fibromatosis Combined with Cherubism. *Oral Surg.* **24**:435–448, 1967.
9 Ray, A. K., Hypertrichosis Terminalis with Simian Characteristics. *J. Med. Genet.* **3**:156, 1966.
10 Rushton, M. A., Hereditary or Idiopathic Hyperplasia of the Gums. *Dent. Pract. Dent. Rec.* **7**:136–146, 1957.
11 Snyder, C. H., Syndrome of Gingival Hyperplasia, Hirsutism and Convulsions. *J. Pediatr.* **67**:499–502, 1965.
12 Thoma, K. H., and Goldman, H., *Oral Pathology*, 5th ed., Mosby, St. Louis, 1960, pp. 1365–1366.

13 Villa, V. G., and Zarate, A. L., Extensive Fibromatosis of the Gingivae in the Maxilla and in the Mandible in a 6-year-old Boy. *Oral Surg.* **6**:1228–1229, 1953.
14 Vontobel, F., Idiopathic Gingival Hyperplasia and Hypertrichosis Associated with Acromegaloid Features. *Helv. Pediatr. Acta* **28**:401–411, 1973.
15 Waterman, T., Diseases of the Jaws. *Boston Med. Surg. J.* **81**:165–168, 1869.
16 Willert, E., Ein seltener Fall einer echten Fibromatosis gingivae. *Oest. Z. Stomatol.* **51**:663–666, 1954.
17 Winstock, D., Hereditary Gingivofibromatosis. *Br. J. Oral Surg.* **2**:59–64, 1964 (same cases as in Ref. 6).
18 Winter, G. B., and Simpkiss, M. J., Hypertrichosis with Hereditary Gingival Hyperplasia. *Arch. Dis. Child.* **49**:394–399, 1974.

GINGIVAL FIBROMATOSIS WITH MULTIPLE HYALINE FIBROMAS (MURRAY-PURETIĆ-DRESCHER SYNDROME)

1 Drescher, E., et al., Juvenile Fibromatosis in Siblings. *J. Pediatr. Surg.* **2**:427–430, 1967.
2 Enjoji, M., et al., Juvenile Fibromatosis of the Scalp in Siblings. *Acta Med. Univ. Kagoshima* (*Suppl.*) **10**:145–151, 1968.
3 Ishikawa, H., and Hori, Y., Systematisierte Hyalinose im Zusammenhang mit Epidermolysis bullosa polydystrophica und Hyalinosis cutis et mucosae. *Arch. Klin. Exp. Dermatol.* **218**:30–51, 1964.
4 Ishikawa, H., and Mori, S., Systemic Hyalinosis or Fibromatosis Multiplex Juvenilis as a Congenital Syndrome. *Acta Derm. Venereol.* (*Stockh.*) **53**:185–191, 1973.
5 Kitano, Y., et al., Two Cases of Juvenile Hyaline Fibromatosis: Some Histological, Electron Microscopic, and Tissue Culture Observations. *Arch. Dermatol.* **106**:877–883, 1972.
6 Murray, J., On Three Peculiar Cases of Molluscum Fibrosum in One Family. *Med.-Chir. Trans. London* **56**:235–238, 1873.
7 Puretić, S., et al., An Unusual Form of Mesenchymal Dysplasia. *Br. J. Dermatol.* **74**:8–19, 1962.
8 Puretić, S., and Puretić, S., Clinical and Histopathological Observations on Systemic Familial Mesenchymatosis. *Proc. 13th Int. Congr. Pediatr. Vienna*, 1971, **5**:373–381, 1971.
9 Schmidt, B. J., et al., Hemangiomatose sclerosante atypique. *Arch. Fr. Pédiatr.* **26**:213–219, 1969.
10 Suschke, J., and Kunze, D., Ein neuer Mucopolysaccharidose-Typ. *Dtsch. Med. Wochenschr.* **96**:1941–1943, 1971.
11 Whitfield, A., and Robinson, A. H., A Further Report on the Remarkable Series of Cases of Molluscum Fibrosum in Children Communicated to the Society by Dr. John Murray in 1873. *Med.-Chir. Trans. London* **86**:293–301, 1903.
12 Woyke, S., et al., Ultrastructure of a Fibromatosis Hyalinica Multiplex Juvenilis. *Cancer* **26**:1157–1168, 1970.

GINGIVAL FIBROMATOSIS AND CORNEAL DYSTROPHY (RUTHERFURD SYNDROME)

1   Houston, I. B., and Shotts, N., Rutherfurd's Syndrome: A Familial Oculodental Disorder. *Acta Paediatr. Scand.* **55:**233–238, 1966.

2   Rutherfurd, M. E., Three Generations of Inherited Dental Defect. *Br. Med. J.* **2:**9–11, 1931.

GINGIVAL FIBROMATOSIS, EAR, NOSE, BONE, AND NAIL DEFECTS, AND HEPATO-SPLENOMEGALY (LABAND SYNDROME)

1   Alavandar, G., Elephantiasis Gingivae: Report of an Affected Family with Associated Hepatomegaly, Soft Tissue and Skeletal Abnormalities. *J. All-India Dent. Assoc.* **37:**349–353, 1965.

2   Henefer, E. P., and Kay, L. A., Congenital Idiopathic Gingival Fibromatosis in the Deciduous Dentition. *Oral Surg.* **24:**65–70, 1967.

3   Jacoby, N. M., et al., Partial Anonychia (Recessive) with Hypertrophy of the Gums and Multiple Abnormalities of the Osseous System. *Guy's Hosp. Rep.* **90:**34–40, 1940.

4   Laband, P. F., et al., Hereditary Gingival Fibromatosis: Report of an Affected Family with Associated Splenomegaly and Skeletal and Soft Tissue Abnormalities. *Oral Surg.* **17:**339–351, 1964.

5   Lawn, A., Über die Elephantiasis der Gingiva und ihre operative Behandlung. *Wien. Med. Wochenschr.* **79:**607–610, 1929.

6   Zimmermann, –, Über Anomalien des Ektoderms (Cases 1 and 2). *Vjschr. Zahnheilkd.* **44:**419–434, 1928.

GINGIVAL FIBROMATOSIS, MICROPHTHALMIA, MENTAL RETARDATION, ATHETOSIS, AND HYPERPIGMENTATION (CROSS SYNDROME)

1   Cross, H. E., et al., A New Oculocerebral Syndrome with Hypopigmentation. *J. Pediatr.* **70:**398–406, 1967.

2   Witkop, C. J., Jr., Heterogeneity in Gingival Fibromatosis. *Birth Defects* **7**(7):210–221, 1971.

3   Witkop, C. J., Jr., Personal communication, 1975.

61

Heerfordt Syndrome

(*Uveoparotitic Paralysis*)

Though this disorder had been reported earlier by several investigators (6, 9), credit is usually given to Heerfordt (15), a Danish ophthalmologist who, in 1909, described a syndrome of (a) uveitis, (b) parotid enlargement, (c) fever, and (d) facial palsy. Between 1935 and 1937, a number of investigators identified the syndrome as a form of sarcoidosis (26, 36).

In general, Heerfordt syndrome occurs in only about 5 to 8 percent of cases of sarcoidosis. The syndrome is far more common in the Southeastern part of the United States (5) and far more frequent (18:1) in Negroes (12, 21).

The reader is referred to several excellent reviews (1, 8, 10, 11, 16, 18, 21, 22, 29).

SYSTEMIC MANIFESTATIONS

Prodromal symptoms may arise a few days to several months prior to the appearance of the syndrome. These may include weakness, cough, polyuria, dry mouth, gastrointestinal distress, joint pain, and mild fever. Fever is present in only about 25 percent of patients and usually appears only during the prodromal period. It seldom exceeds 38.5°C.

The syndrome principally affects persons in their second and third decades. Garland and Thompson (11) and Savin (29) found that 65 percent of patients were under thirty years of age.

Eyes. Uveitis (iridocyclitis type) is the most common eye finding, frequently preceding enlargement of the parotid salivary glands. It is the first sign in somewhat fewer than 25 percent of the cases (3, 13, 21). It may appear suddenly or gradually with minimal pain; although both eyes become involved, they usually do not do so at the same time. Frequent relapses occur, even after 2 years (31), often resulting in total blindness. Permanent pupillary changes (fixity, irregularity, inequality) as well as posterior synechiae are common (in about 40 percent of cases) (29). Iris nodules are seen in about one-third of the patients, and vitreous opacities in about half (29). Lacrimal gland enlargement occurs in less than 5 percent of cases (13a, 21).

Nervous system. Levin (18) indicated that the nervous system becomes involved in over half the patients. Recent studies would indicate that fewer than 5 percent of patients with sarcoidosis have neurologic manifestations (17, 37). The most common neurologic finding is facial paralysis (30 to 50 percent), principally involving the lower branches (10, 28, 29); it is bilateral in over one-third of the cases (11, 29) (Figs. 61-1, 61-2).

The facial palsy usually follows enlargement of the parotid gland by a few days, though it may take as long as a year (18, 38). On occasion, it has preceded the parotid swelling, or it may appear long after all signs of the swelling are gone

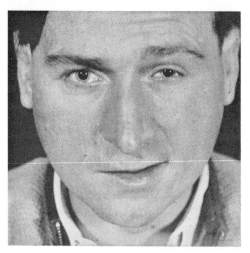

Figure 61-1. *Heerfordt syndrome.* Patient has iridocyclitis and optic neuritis, bilateral parotitis, paralysis of right facial nerve, enlarged lymph nodes, etc. (*From R. Zeilhofer and E. Schmid,* Ärtzl. Wochenschr. **12:**285, 1957.)

(27). The paralysis usually resolves within 2 months, although some patients have never improved (38). Taste may also be impaired (6, 15, 23).

Other cranial nerves may be involved as well. Paralysis of the soft palate (15, 23, 27, 34) and vocal cords (15, 34) has been noted. Nerve deafness of the central type (11, 23, 33), ptosis of the eyelids (4, 18, 27), and alteration of the sen-

sory portion of the trigeminal nerve (17, 39) have been reported.

In addition, common findings are loss of deep reflexes and polyneuritis (4, 7, 11, 22, 23, 27, 33, 34). Dysphagia has been reported by several authors (4, 15, 27), but it is likely that this is predicated upon the attendant xerostomia. Polyuria is also seen, but it may be related to the excessive consumption of water because of the feeling of dry mouth (1, 11, 18, 22). Hypercalcemia is an important cause of polyuria and renal failure in sarcoidosis.

Skin. An erythema nodosum–like rash appears in about 25 percent of patients (7, 22, 27, 33, 39).

Oral manifestations. The parotid glands (rarely, the submandibular, sublingual, or lacrimal glands) enlarge bilaterally, but not necessarily symmetrically in about 80 percent of the cases. There may be unilateral enlargement (4, 11, 13, 38). This is usually the first sign of the syndrome (11). The glands are firm, nodular, and painless, but somewhat sensitive to pressure. They never suppurate. Resolution takes place within 8 to 12 weeks, but may occur 2 weeks or as long as 3 years after onset of the symptom (13). The salivary flow is greatly decreased, and xerostomia may be severe (13, 38).

Mucous membrane involvement is not common in uveoparotitic paralysis. Mild cer-

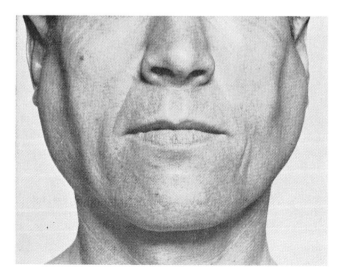

Figure 61-2. Patient has bilateral painless swelling of parotid and lacrimal glands. (*From G. C. Manning,* Br. J. Clin. Pract. **16:**541, 1962.)

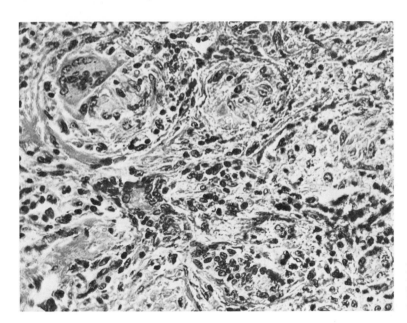

Figure 61-3. Parenchyma of parotid salivary gland is replaced by numerous noncaseating granulomas with giant cells.

vical lymphadenopathy is occasionally noted (11).

Microscopically, one observes that the acini are atrophic and displaced by numerous miliary, partly confluent, epithelioid, noncaseating tubercles. Giant cells, with or without inclusions, are not uncommon. There may be a moderate degree of proliferation of salivary duct epithelium (14, 20) (Fig. 61-3). Similar lesions have been found in the eye. Palatal paralysis, due to involvement of the vagus nerve, is a rather uncommon but striking finding (4, 23, 27, 34).

In lymph nodes, in addition to the granulomas, a paramyloid subcapsular deposit is not uncommon.

DIFFERENTIAL DIAGNOSIS

The diagnosis of generalized sarcoidosis is usually based on a combination of roentgenographic, clinical, immunologic, and laboratory data. By means of any one method alone, diagnosis is difficult, if not impossible. In spite of widespread organ involvement, symptoms are mild.

Death may, however, occur from pulmonary fibrosis, myocardial infiltration, or renal failure.

In Heerfordt syndrome, one must consider the *Sjögren syndrome* and the differential diagnosis of each of the components (uveitis, parotid enlargement, facial palsy) that constitute the Heerfordt syndrome.

DIAGNOSTIC AIDS

Microscopic examination of the involved salivary gland reveals noncaseating granulomas.

The Nickerson-Kveim test is positive in about 85 percent of cases with active sarcoidosis. If good antigen is employed, only about 5 percent false-positive results are obtained (24, 32, 35). The antigen is a saline suspension of sarcoid tissue, usually lymph node, injected intradermally. Biopsy of the resultant nodule in 3 to 4 weeks reveals sarcoid tissue. A hemagglutinin reaction has also been employed (25).

Secretion volume and salivary amylase and kallikrein content have been shown to be greatly reduced (2).

REFERENCES

1 Arbuse, D., and Madonick, M., Uveoparotid Fever (Heerfordt's Syndrome). Neurologic Manifestations. *Am. J. Med. Sci.* **196**:222–232, 1938.

2 Bhoola, K. D., et al., Changes in Salivary Enzymes in Patients with Sarcoidosis. *N. Engl. J. Med.* **281**:877–879, 1969.

3 Crick, R., et al., The Eyes in Sarcoidosis. *Br. J. Ophthalmol.* **45**:461–481, 1961.

4 Critcheley, M., and Philips, P., A Case of Uveo-parotitic Paralysis. *Lancet* **2**:906–907, 1924.

5 Cummings, M. M., et al., Epidemiologic and Clinical Observations in Sarcoidosis. *Ann. Intern. Med.* **50**:879–890, 1959.

6 Daireaux, P., Paralysie faciale et iritis d'origine ourlienne. Des neurites ourliennes. *Bull. Méd. (Paris)* **13**:227–228, 1899.

7 Feiling, A., and Viner, G., Iridocyclitis, Parotitis, Polyneuritis. A New Syndrome. *J. Neurol. Psychiatr.* **2**:353–358, 1922.

8 Ferguson, R. H., and Paris, J., Sarcoidosis. Study of Twenty-nine Cases with a Review of Splenic, Hepatic, Mucous-membrane, Retinal and Joint Manifestations. *Arch. Intern. Med.* **101**:1065–1084, 1958.

9 Fleischer, B., Über epithelioidzellige Granulomatose. *Albrecht von Graefes Arch. Klin. Ophthalmol.* **143**:435–455, 1941.

10 Folger, H. P., Uveoparotitis (Heerfordt). Report of a Case. *Arch. Ophthalmol.* **15**:1098–1116, 1936.

11 Garland, H. G., and Thompson, J. G., Uveo-parotid Tuberculosis (Febris Uveo-parotidea of Heerfordt). *Q. J. Med.* **26**:157–177, 1933.

12 Gentry, J. G., et al., Studies on the Epidemiology of Sarcoidosis in the U.S. *J. Clin. Invest.* **34**:1839–1856, 1955.

13 Greenberg, G., et al., Enlargement of Parotid Gland due to Sarcoidosis. *Br. Med. J.* **2**:861–862, 1964.

13a Gupta, R., et al., Dacro-sialo-adenitis in Sarcoidosis. *Can. J. Ophthalmol.* **9**:381–383, 1974.

14 Hamner, J. E., III, and Scofield, H. H., Cervical Lymphadenopathy and Parotid Swelling in Sarcoidosis: A Study of 31 Cases. *J. Am. Dent. Assoc.* **74**:1224–1230, 1967.

15 Heerfordt, C. F., Über eine "Febris uveo-parotidea subchronica," an der Glandula parotis und der Uvea des Auges lokalisiert und häufig mit Paresen cerebrospinaler Nerven kompliziert. *Albrecht von Graefes Arch. Klin. Ophthalmol.* **70**:254–273, 1909.

16 Israel, H. L., and Sones, M., Sarcoidosis: Clinical Observations on One Hundred and Sixty Cases. *Arch. Intern. Med.* **102**:766–776, 1958.

17 Lambert, V., and Richards, S. H., Facial Palsy in Heerfordt's Syndrome. *J. Laryngol.* **78**:684–693, 1964.

18 Levin, P. M., Neurological Aspects of Uveoparotid Fever. *J. Nerv. Ment. Dis.* **81**:176–191, 1935.

19 Löfgren, S., Diagnosis and Incidence of Sarcoidosis. *Br. J. Tuberc.* **51**:8–13, 1957.

20 Manning, G. C., Mukulicz's Syndrome Due to Sarcoidosis. *Br. J. Clin. Pract.* **16**:541–543, 1962.

21 Maycock, R. L., et al., Manifestations of Sarcoidosis. *Am. J. Med.* **35**:67–89, 1963.

22 Merrill, H. G., and Oaks, L. W., Uveoparotitis (Heerfordt) with Case Report. *Am. J. Ophthalmol.* **14**:15–22, 1931.

23 Mohn, A., Ein Fall von Febris Uveo-parotidea (Heerfordt). *Acta Ophthalmol. (Kbh.)* **11**:397–403, 1933.

24 Nelson, C. T., and Schwimmer, B., The Specificity of the Kveim Reaction. *J. Invest. Dermatol.* **28**:56–61, 1957.

25 Nielsen, R. H., Ocular Sarcoidosis. *Arch. Ophthalmol.* **61**:657–663, 1959.

26 Pautrier, L. M.: Syndrome de Heerfordt et maladie de Besnier-Boeck-Schaumann. *Bull. Soc. Méd. Hôp. Paris* **54**:1608–1620, 1937.

27 Ramsey, A. M., Case of Cyclitis with Swelling of the Parotids and Paralysis of Cranial Nerves. *Trans. Ophthalmol. Soc. U.K.* **41**:194–209, 1921.

28 Roos, B., Cerebral Manifestations of Lymphogranulomatosis Benigna (Schaumann) and Uveoparotid Fever (Heerfordt). *Acta Med. Scand.* **104**:123–130, 1940.

29 Savin, L. H., An Analysis of the Signs and Symptoms of 66 Published Cases of the Uveoparotid Syndrome with Details of an Additional Case. *Trans. Ophthalmol. Soc. U.K.* **54**:549–566, 1934.

30 Schönholzer, G., Morbus Besnier-Boeck-Schaumann und Armeedurchleuchtung. *Schweiz. Med. Wochenschr.* **77**:585–588, 1947.

31 Schou, S., Demonstration eines Patienten mit Febris uveoparotidea subchronica. *Klin. Monatsbl. Augenheilkd.* **1**:281–282, 1914.

32 Siltzbach, L. E., and Ehrlich, J. C., The Nickerson-Kveim Reaction in Sarcoidosis. *Am. J. Med.* **16**:790–803, 1954.

33 Souter, W. C., A Case of Uveo-parotid Fever with Autopsy Findings. *Trans. Ophthalmol. Soc. U.K.* **49**:113–128, 1929.

34 Tait, C. B. V., Uveo-parotitis. *Lancet* **2**:748–749, 1934.

35 Talbot, F. J., et al., Broncho-pulmonary Sarcoidosis: Some Unusual Manifestations and the Serious Complications Thereof. *Am. J. Med.* **26**:341–355, 1959.

36 Tillgren, J., Diabetes Insipidus as a Symptom of Schaumann's Disease. *Br. J. Dermatol.* **47**:223–229, 1935.

37 Wiederholt, W. C., and Siekert, R. G., Neurologic Manifestations of Sarcoidosis. *Neurology* **15**:1147–1154, 1965.

38 Wilson, H. L., Facial Paralysis in the Uveoparotid Fever of Boeck's Sarcoid. *Ann. Otol. Rhinol. Laryngol.* **66**:164–172, 1957.

39 Zeilhofer, R., and Schmid, E., Klinische Beobachtungen bei einer seltener Sonderform des Morbus Boeck (Heerfordt Syndrom). *Ärztl. Wochenschr.* **12**:285–290, 1957.

62

Hemifacial Atrophy

(Romberg Syndrome)

Although the disorder was mentioned as early as 1825 by Parry (18), credit for its delineation is usually given to Romberg (20), who described classic cases in 1846. The name "progressive facial hemiatrophy" was applied to the condition by Eulenberg in 1871. We prefer hemifacial atrophy. The condition consists of (*a*) slowly progressive atrophy of the soft tissues of essentially half the face, accompanied most often by (*b*) contralateral Jacksonian epilepsy, (*c*) trigeminal neuralgia, and (*d*) changes in the eyes and hair. Occasionally (in about 7 percent of cases), there may be (*e*) associated atrophy of half the body (1). Comprehensive surveys have been carried out by several authors (1, 8, 16, 27, 28).

Nearly all cases have been sporadic, but a few familial instances have been noted (11, 13, 28).

Theories of origin have been numerous (1, 27). A number of affected persons have had a history of prior trauma (7). Most emphasis has been placed on alterations in the peripheral trophic sympathetic system (28). Moss and Crikelair (15) produced a condition in rats by unilateral cervical sympathectomy that resembled the condition in man.

SYSTEMIC MANIFESTATIONS

Facies and skin. In the advanced case, the facies is quite distinct (Fig. 62-1A–C). The ear may become misshapen and smaller than normal or, because of lack of supporting tissues, may pro-

ject from the head (12). An alteration in the basal skull angle (kyphosis) has been described (7). A complete cephalometric study was carried out by Berkman (3).

The first facial change, usually appearing during the first decade (Fig. 62-1), involves the paramedian area of the face and slowly spreads, so that atrophy of the underlying muscle, bone, and cartilage soon becomes apparent. From the initial site, usually in the area covered by the temporal or buccinator muscles, the process extends to involve the brow, angle of the mouth, neck, or even half the body (1, 27) (Fig. 62-2). There is a marked predilection for involvement of the left side of the face (23). The overlying skin often becomes darkly pigmented (12). As a rule, the condition slowly progresses for several years and then becomes stationary for the remainder of life. The average progress of the disease lasts about 3 years (7).

There has been long-standing debate on the relationship between progressive hemifacial atrophy and scleroderma, several authors stoutly defending the position that the coup-de-sabre form of scleroderma is only a special type of progressive hemifacial atrophy (1, 26, 28). Others state that the two conditions may occur simultaneously (17). It should be pointed out that in some cases the skin is spared while only the fat and subcutaneous tissues disappear. Occasionally, vitiligo accompanies the disorder (24).

Changes in the hair may precede those in the skin (1, 28, 29). The scalp on the affected side

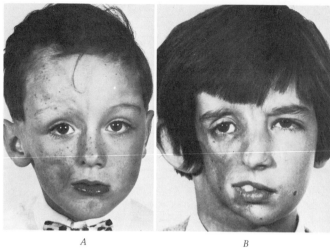

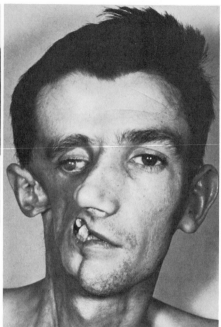

A   *B*

Figure 62-1. *Hemifacial atrophy.* (*A, B,* and *C*). Increased severity of disorder in patients illustrated from left to right. (A, B, *from D. Glass,* Br. J. Oral Surg. **1:**194, 1963–1964; C, *courtesy of P. Cernea, Paris, France.*)

C

may exhibit circumscribed but complete alopecia limited to the paramedian area, eyelashes, and median portion of the eyebrow (28). Poliosis, or blanching of the hair, has also been noted (27).

Central nervous system. The most common neurologic finding is epilepsy or epileptiform phenomena, most often of the sensory Jacksonian type, which often appear late (1, 9, 19, 26, 28, 30). On the other hand, trigeminal neuralgia and/or facial paresthesia appear early and may precede the rest of the changes. Migraine has also been a common finding (9, 28, 30).

Eyes. The eye is often involved. Loss of periorbital fat produces enophthalmos (27). Loss of underlying bone may cause the outer canthus to be displaced downward. Muscular paralysis has been noted by several authors (10, 11), as well as lagophthalmos and ptosis (1, 10, 29). The Horner syndrome, heterochromia iridis, and dilated and fixed pupil have also have described. Inflammatory processes involving the eyes, such as neuroparalytic keratitis, iritis, iridocyclitis, choroiditis, cataract, and pupillary edema (11, 28), are

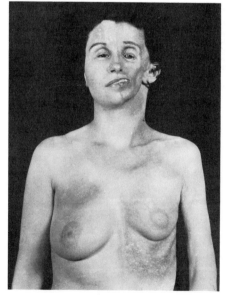

Figure 62-2. Involvement of half of body. (*From A. J. Barksy et al.,* Principles and Practice of Plastic Surgery, 2d ed., *McGraw-Hill, New York, 1964.*)

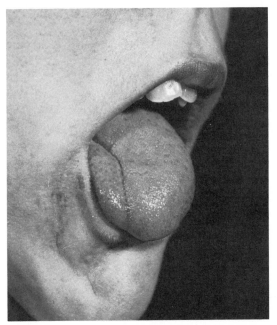

Figure 62-3. Atrophy of right side of tongue.

Oral manifestations. Atrophy of half of the upper lip and tongue (10, 26, 30) are usual. The maxillary teeth on the involved side are exposed (Fig. 62-3). Spontaneous fracture of the involved mandible has also been noted (4).

Roentgenographic study of the jaws has revealed that the body and ramus of the mandible were shorter on the involved side and that there was a delay in development of the angle (12), with resultant malocclusion. The teeth on the involved side may be retarded in eruption or may have atrophic roots (12, 21, 24, 27).

DIFFERENTIAL DIAGNOSIS

Differential diagnosis includes congenital facial hypoplasia. Its natal appearance and diminution in the size of teeth on the involved side (2, 5, 22), aid in differentiation. Scleroderma (25), fat necrosis, and *oculoauriculovertebral syndrome* should also be considered.

common. All changes cited above may occasionally affect the eye on the noninvolved side (11).

LABORATORY AIDS

None is known.

REFERENCES

1 Archambault, L., and Fromm, N. K., Progressive Facial Hemiatrophy. *Arch. Neurol. Psychiatr.* **27**:529–584, 1932.

2 Bates, J. F., Unilateral Facial Hypoplasia. *Br. Dent. J.* **104**:453–454, 1958.

3 Berkman, M. D., *Craniofacial Changes in Progressive Hemifacial Atrophy.* Thesis, Columbia University, 1972.

4 Bromley, P., and Forbes, A., A Case of Progressive Hemiatrophy Presenting with Spontaneous Fractures of the Lower Jaw. *Br. Med. J.* **1**:1476–1478, 1960.

5 Burke, P. H., Unilateral Facial Hypoplasia Affecting Tooth Size. *Br. Dent. J.* **103**:41–44, 1957.

6 Calmettes, L., et al., L'hemiatrophie faciale (maladie de Romberg) et ses manifestations oculaires. *Rev. Otoneuroophthalmol.* **31**:215–241, 1959.

7 Crikelair, G. F., et al., Facial Hemiatrophy. *Plast. Reconstructr. Surg.* **29**:5–13, 1962.

8 Dechaume, M., et al., L'hemiatrophie faciale progressive. *Rev. Stomatol.* (Paris) **55**:12–44, 1954.

9 Dieler, T., A Case Exhibiting Symptoms of Facial Hemiatrophy and Jacksonian Sensory Epilepsy. *J. Nerv. Ment. Dis.* **20**:284–289, 1895.

10 Finesilver, B., and Rosow, H., Total Hemiatrophy. *J.A.M.A.* **110**:366–368, 1938.

11 Franceschetti, A., and Koenig, H., L'importance du facteur heredodegeneratif dans l'hemiatrophie faciale progressive (Romberg). Etude des complications oculaires dans ce syndrome. *J. Génét. Hum.* **1**:27–64, 1952.

12 Glass, D., Hemifacial Atrophy. *Br. J. Oral Surg.* **1**:194–199, 1963–1964.

13 Klingman, T., Facial Hemiatrophy. *J.A.M.A.* **49**:1888–1891, 1907.

14 Meline, F., Hemiatrophie faciale progressive. *Ann. Chir. Plast.* **7**:49–60, 1962.

15 Moss, M. L., and Crikelair, G. F., Progressive Facial Hemiatrophy Following Cervical Sympathectomy in the Rat. *Arch. Oral Biol.* **1**:254–258, 1960.

16 Mussinelli, G., et al., L'emiatrophia facciale progressiva. Malattia de Parry-Romberg. *Rev. Otoneuroophthal.* **39**:3–52, 283–303, 477–526, 583–638, 1964; **40**:105–197, 1965.

17 Osborne, E. D., Morphea Associated with Hemiatrophy of the Face. *Arch. Dermatol. Syph.* (Chic.) **6**:27–34, 1922.

18 Parry, C. H., *Collections from Unpublished Papers,* vol. 1, Underwood, London, 1825, p. 478.

19 Pollock, L. J., Progressive Facial Hemiatrophy. *Arch. Neurol. Psychiatr.* **33:**888–889, 1935.

19a Rees, T. D., et al., Silicone Fluid Injections for Facial Atrophy. A Ten-Year Study. *Plast. Reconstr. Surg.* **52:**118–127, 1973.

20 Romberg, M. H., Trophoneurosen. *Klinische Ergebnisse,* A. Forstner, Berlin, 1846, pp. 75–81.

21 Rushton, M. A., An Early Case of Facial Hemiatrophy. *Oral Surg.* **4:**1457–1460, 1951.

22 Rushton, M. A., Asymmetry of Tooth Size in Congenital Hypoplasia of One Side of the Body. *Br. Dent. J.* **95:**309–311, 1953.

23 Schnall, B. S., and Smith, D. W., Nonrandom Laterality of Malformations in Paired Structures. *J. Pediatr.* **85:**509–511, 1974.

24 Schneider, G., Ein Beitrag zur Hemihypertrophia und Hemiatrophia faciei. *Dtsch. Zahn Mund Kieferheilkd.* **12:**43–66, 1949.

25 Singh, G., and Bajpai, H. S., Progressive Facial Hemiatrophy. *Dermatologica* **138:**288–291, 1969.

26 Tauber, E. B., and Goldman, L., Hemiatrophia faciei progressiva. *Arch. Dermatol. Syph.* **39:**696–704, 1939.

27 Walsh, F. B., Facial Hemiatrophy. *Am. J. Ophthalmol.* **22:**1–10, 1939.

28 Wartenberg, R., Progressive Facial Hemiatrophy. *Arch. Neurol. Psychiatr.* **54:**75–96, 1945.

29 Wolfe, M. O., and Weber, M. L., Progressive Facial Hemiatrophy. *J. Nerv. Ment. Dis.* **91:**595–607, 1940.

30 Wolff, H. G., Progressive Facial Hemiatrophy. *Arch. Otolaryngol.* **7:**580–582, 1928.

63

Hemihypertrophy

Hemihypertrophy, described in 1822 by Meckel (17) and in 1839 by Wagner (26), gained widespread recognition after the studies of Gesell (10) and Lenstrup (15) during the 1920s. Comprehensive reviews were undertaken by Wakefield and Hines (27), Ward and Lerner (28), and Ringrose et al. (22).

A tendency toward dizygous twinning has been observed in some cases (8). Chromosomal anomalies, including diploid-triploid mosaicism (14), trisomy 18 mosaicism, partial G and B monosomy with B/G translocation, and abnormally large chromosome 3 have been reported (8).

Many other theories have been advanced to explain hemihypertrophy, including anatomic and functional vascular or lymphatic abnormalities, lesions of the central nervous system leading to altered neurotrophic action, endocrine abnormalities, asymmetric cell division and deviation of the twinning process, fusion of two eggs following fertilization leading to unequal regulative ability in the two halves, and mitochondrial damage to an overripened egg leading to overregeneration. These theories have been especially well reviewed by Noé and Berman (19).

The range and variability of clinical abnormalities, together with the large number of sporadic cases, means certain etiologic heterogeneity. None of the proposed theories, some of which are quite fanciful, explains adequately all cases of hemihypertrophy, even by excluding those conditions discussed under Differential

Diagnosis. Hemihypertrophy is not a disorder *sui generis,* but a nonspecific sign which may be observed in a variety of different disorders. Almost all cases appear to be sporadic. Familial instances (1, 2, 7, 16, 18, 23), frequently incompletely documented, may represent other disorders, particularly neurofibromatosis.

In hemihypertrophy, the enlarged area may vary from a single digit, a single limb, or unilateral facial enlargement to involvement of half of the body (10). Hemihypertrophy may be segmental, unilateral, or crossed. In some cases, the defect is limited to a single system, e.g., muscular, vascular, skeletal, or nervous system, but it may frequently involve multiple systems (28). Asymmetry is usually evident at birth and may become accentuated with age, especially at puberty. Occasionally, asymmetry has been stated not to be present at birth, but to develop later (3). However, such observations are valid only when measurements are taken at birth. In total hemihypertrophy, the right side is more often involved (10, 15) and males are more frequently affected (10, 27).

SYSTEMIC MANIFESTATIONS

Facies. In some patients, only the face is involved (Fig. 63-1). In others, unilateral facial enlargement is accompanied by hypertrophy of half the body (11) (Fig. 63-2).

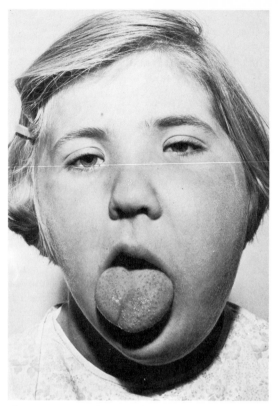

Figure 63-1. *Hemihypertrophy.* Unilateral hypertrophy of face and tongue.

Integumentary system. Thickened skin in the affected area, excessive secretion of sebaceous and sweat glands, vascular and pigmentary defects, hirsutism, hypertrichosis on the affected side, abnormal nail growth, and polythelia have been reported (5, 10, 12, 13, 22). A medusa-like complex of the lower part of the abdomen or groin has also been observed (5).

Skeletal system. The bones have been found to be unilaterally enlarged, and increased bone age on the affected side has been reported. Other abnormalities of the skeletal system may include macrodactyly, syndactyly, polydactyly, compensatory scoliosis, and a variety of other skeletal defects (10, 22, 27, 28).

Central nervous system. Central nervous system defects may include unilateral enlargement of a cerebral hemisphere, mental retarda-

tion (about 15 to 20 percent), and epilepsy (10, 22, 27). Other abnormalities of the central nervous system which may occur have been tabulated by Ringrose et al. (22).

Other findings. Various tumors (see below), umbilical hernia, congenital heart defects, hypospadias, cryptorchism, and a large variety of low-frequency anomalies have been discussed by Ringrose et al. (22) and by Parker and Skalko (20). Medullary sponge kidney has been noted in several cases (6). Ipsilateral nephromegaly has been reported (15a).

Associated neoplasia. Adrenal cortical carcinoma, nephroblastoma, and hepatoblastoma have been occasionally associated with this disorder (7). Since these tumors have embryonal origin, study of their relationship to the teratogenic aspects of hemihypertrophy may lead to more specific information on oncogenic mechanisms. There is no relationship between the laterality of hemihypertrophy and any of the solid tumors reported. When the oncogenic stimulus does not lateralize to the enlarged side, it is possible that such cases may represent "occult"

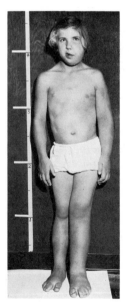

Figure 63-2. Note asymmetry of body, with complete left-sided hypertrophy. Note also syndactyly of toes.

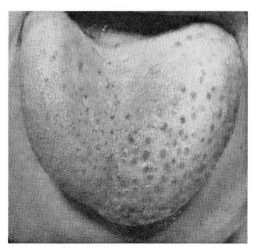

Figure 63-3. Marked hemihypertrophy of tongue with enlargement of fungiform papillae. Note sharp demarcation at midline.

crossed hemihypertrophy, affecting the internal organs of the contralateral side.

Sexual precocity may accompany adrenal cortical tumors. Adrenogenital syndrome, virilization, and adrenal calcification have been noted in some cases of hemihypertrophy. Adrenal adenoma, adrenal neuroblastoma, and undifferentiated sarcoma of the lung have also been reported (7, 8, 11, 20).

Oral manifestations. Cases in which the oral changes have been especially well documented have been ones in which hemihypertrophy was largely restricted to the head. Macroglossia may

be unilateral or diffuse. When one side of the tongue is affected, the fungiform papillae may be hypertrophic (Fig.63-3). The lips, palate, maxilla, and mandible may also be enlarged on the affected side. Polypoid excrescences resembling lipomas may be observed in some cases on the lower lips and buccal mucosa (11).

The permanent dentition is more strikingly affected than the deciduous dentition, with increased mesiodistal and buccolingual diameters on the affected side (Fig. 63-4). In the permanent dentition, the incisors and second and third molars are usually spared. In the deciduous dentition, the changes are frequently restricted to the second molars. On the affected side, premature exfoliation of deciduous teeth with early eruption of permanent teeth has been observed. Abnormal roots have also been reported (11, 24).

DIFFERENTIAL DIAGNOSIS

Hemihypertrophy may occur as an isolated finding or in association with various embryonal tumors and a host of other anomalies. Asymmetry may also occur with arteriovenous aneurysm, congenital lymphedema, *neurofibromatosis, Russell-Silver syndrome, McCune-Albright syndrome, Beckwith-Wiedemann syndrome, Klippel-Trénaunay-Weber syndrome,* multiple exostoses, *Langer-Giedion syndrome,* Ollier syndrome, *Maffucci syndrome,* and facial tumors of childhood (9). Hemihypertrophy

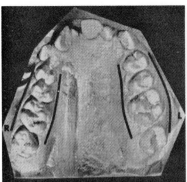
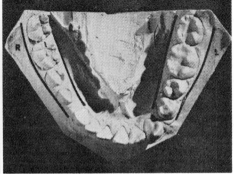

Figure 63-4. Casts of jaws. Note differences in width of bone and size of teeth on affected and normal sides. (*From R. Gorlin and L. Meskin,* J. Pediatr. **61**:870, 1962.)

should be distinguished from hemiatrophy, which may be secondary to early intrauterine central nervous system defect and may also occur in the *Romberg syndrome*, the *Sturge-Weber anomalad*, or with unilateral ichthyosiform erythroderma (4).

A dominant form of hemifacial hyperplasia associated with strabismus and amblyopia has been described (2).

LABORATORY AIDS

Cytogenetic studies may rarely reveal chromosomal anomalies.

REFERENCES

1 Arnold, E. B., Case of Hemiacromegaly. *Int. J. Orthod.* **22**:1228–1233, 1933.

2 Bencze, J., et al., Dominant Inheritance of Hemifacial Hyperplasia Associated with Strabismus. *Oral Surg.* **35**:489–501, 1973.

3 Boxer, L. A., and Smith, D. L., Wilms' Tumor Prior to Onset of Hemihypertrophy. *Am. J. Dis. Child.* **120**:564–565, 1970.

4 Cullen, S. I., et al., Congenital Unilateral Ichthyosiform Erythroderma. *Arch. Dermatol.* **99**:724–729, 1969.

5 Curtis, F., Kongenitaler partieller Riesenwuchs mit endokrinen Störungen. *Dtsch. Arch. Klin. Med.* **147**:310–319, 1925.

6 Eisenberg, R. L., and Pfister, R. C., Medullary Sponge Kidney Associated with Congenital Hemihypertrophy (Asymmetry). *Am. J. Roentgenol.* **116**:773–777, 1972.

7 Fraumeni, J. F., and Miller, R. W., Adrenocortical Neoplasms with Hemihypertrophy, Brain Tumors, and Other Disorders. *J. Pediatr.* **70**:129–138, 1967.

8 Fraumeni, J. F., et al., Wilms' Tumor and Congenital Hemihypertrophy: Report of Five New Cases and Review of Literature. *Pediatrics* **40**:886–899, 1967.

9 Furnas, D. W., et al., Congenital Hemihypertrophy of the Face: Impersonator of Childhood Facial Tumors. *J. Pediatr. Surg.* **5**:344–348, 1970.

10 Gesell, A., Hemihypertrophy and Twinning: Further Study of the Nature of Hemihypertrophy with Report of a New Case. *Am. J. Med. Sci.* **173**:542–555, 1927.

11 Gorlin, R. J., and Meskin, L. H., Congenital Hemihypertrophy. *J. Pediatr.* **61**:870–879, 1962.

12 Haicken, B. N., Congenital Hemihypertrophy. *Am. J. Dis. Child.* **120**:372–373, 1970.

13 Hurwitz, S., and Klaus, S. N., Congenital Hemihypertrophy with Hypertrichosis. *Arch. Dermatol.* **103**:98–100, 1971.

14 Johnston, A. W., and Penrose, L. S., Congenital Asymmetry. *J. Med. Genet.* **3**:77–85, 1966.

15 Lenstrup, E., Eight Cases of Hemihypertrophy. *Acta Paediatr.* **6**:205–213, 1926.

15a Kirks, D. R., and Shackeford, G. D., Idiopathic Hemihypertrophy with Associated Ipsilateral Benign Nephromegaly. *Radiology* **115**:145–148, 1975.

16 Levy, M., et al., Hemihypertrophy and Medullary Sponge Kidney. *Can. Med. Assoc. J.* **96**:1322–1326, 1967.

17 Meckel, J. F., *Über die seitliche Asymmetrie im tierischen Körper, anatomische physiologische Beobachtungen und Untersuchungen.* Renger, Halle, 1822, p. 147.

18 Morris, J. V., and MacGillivray, R. C., Mental Deficiency and Hemihypertrophy. *Am. J. Ment. Defic.* **59**:644–651, 1955.

19 Noé, O., and Berman, H. H., The Etiology of Congenital Hemihypertrophy and One Case Report. *Arch. Pediatr.* **79**:278–288, 1962.

20 Parker, D. A., and Skalko, R. G., Congenital Asymmetry: Report of 10 Cases with Associated Developmental Abnormalities. *Pediatrics* **44**:584–589, 1969.

21 Reed, E. A., Congenital Total Hemihypertrophy. *Arch. Neurol Psychiatr.* **14**:824–827, 1925.

22 Ringrose, R. E., et al., Hemihypertrophy. *Pediatrics* **36**:434–448, 1965.

23 Rudolph, C. E., and Norvold, R. W., Congenital Partial Hemihypertrophy Involving Marked Malocclusion. *J. Dent. Res.* **23**:133–139, 1944.

24 Rushton, M. A., A Dental Abnormality of Size and Race. *Proc. R. Soc. Med.* **41**:490–496, 1948.

25 Schnall, B. S., and Smith, D. W., Nonrandom Laterality of Malformations in Paired Structures. *J. Pediatr.* **85**:509–511, 1974.

26 Wagner, R., see H. L. Kottmeier, Über Hemihypertrophia und Hemiatrophia corporis totalis nebst spontane Extremitätengangräne bei Saüglingen im Anschluss zu einem ungewöhnlichen Fall. *Acta Paediatr.* **20**:543, 1938.

27 Wakefield, E. G., and Hines, E. A., Jr., Congenital Hemihypertrophy: A Report of Eight Cases. *Am. J. Med. Sci.* **185**:493–500, 1933.

28 Ward, J., and Lerner, H. H., A Review of the Subject of Congenital Hemihypertrophy and a Complete Case Report. *J. Pediatr.* **31**:403–414, 1947.

64

Hereditary Benign Intraepithelial Dyskeratosis

(Witkop-von Sallmann Syndrome)

The syndrome of hereditary benign intraepithelial dyskeratosis was described in a North Carolina triracial isolate (Caucasian-Negro-Indian) in 1960 by Witkop et al. (4) and by von Sallmann and Paton (2). The chief components are (*a*) plaques of the bulbar conjunctiva and (*b*) oral mucosal thickenings clinically similar to white folded hypertrophy (white sponge nevus of Cannon).

The syndrome is inherited as an autosomal dominant trait with a high degree of penetrance (4). Attempts to link this trait with several blood groups have met with negative results (1).

SYSTEMIC MANIFESTATIONS

Eyes. About the limbus, both nasally and temporally, there are foamy gelatinous plaques, more superficial than pterygia, on a hyperemic bulbar conjuctiva (Fig. 64-1). The eye lesion is usually noted within the first year of life (2).

The dyskeratotic process may involve the cornea, producing blindness from shedding and resultant vascularization of this structure. Photophobia, especially in children, is common.

Oral manifestations. The oral mucosal thickenings are asymptomatic. They appear as soft white folds and plaques, resembling the lesion described by Cannon in 1935 as white sponge nevus (7, 8). Though the thickenings appear at birth, they are mild, increasing in severity to

about fifteen years of age. There does not appear to be a tendency for the plaques to undergo malignant degeneration (Fig. 64-2).

DIFFERENTIAL DIAGNOSIS

The white sponge nevus and the oral lesions of *pachyonychia congenita* bear a distinct clinical resemblance to those of hereditary benign intraepithelial dyskeratosis.

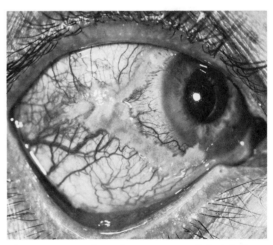

Figure 64-1. *Hereditary benign intraepithelial dyskeratosis.* Superficial gelatinous plaques on hyperemic bulbar conjunctiva involving limbus and cornea.

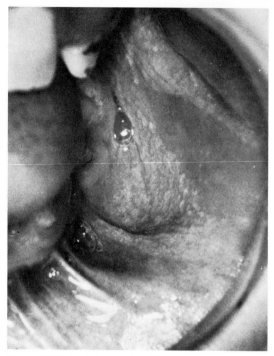

Figure 64-2. Leukokeratosis of buccal mucosa.

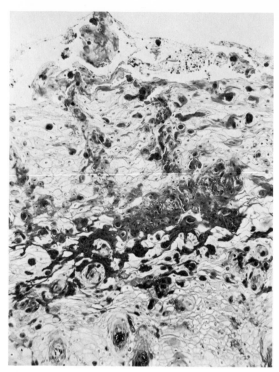

Figure 64-3. Section of buccal mucosa demonstrating dyskeratotic eosinophilic cells in acanthotic epithelium (Giemsa stain).

LABORATORY AIDS

Tissue sections of buccal mucosal or conjunctival scrapings treated with Giemsa stain are characteristic (Fig. 64-3).

Acanthosis, vacuolization of the stratum spinosum, and intraepithelial dyskeratosis characterized by waxy eosinophilic cells called "tobacco cells" and a "cell-within-a-cell" pattern are noted. These latter changes are especially evident in Papanicolaou stained smears (2) (Fig. 64-4).

Witkop and Gorlin (5) found similarities in oral smears from hereditary benign intraepithelial dyskeratosis and keratosis follicularis (Darier-White disease). The grains of the latter resemble the so-called "tobacco cells" of the former, and the corps ronds of the latter resemble the "cell-within-a-cell" body seen in the syndrome under discussion. However, the cell-within-a-cell is far more common in oral

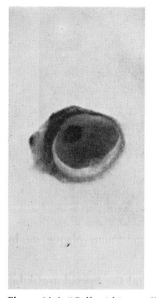

Figure 64-4. "Cell-within-a-cell" phenomenon, Papanicolaou smear. (Figs. 64-1 to 4, *courtesy of C. J. Witkop, Jr., Minneapolis, Minn.*)

smears of hereditary benign intraepithelial dyskeratosis, and, in addition, one rarely sees the small blue parabasilar cells so often seen in keratosis follicularis. Witkop (3) pointed out that

patients receiving methotrexate and 5-fluorouracil also exhibit the "cell-within-a-cell" phenomenon in exfoliated buccal cells.

REFERENCES

1 Pollitzer, W. S., et al., Hereditary Benign Intraepithelial Dyskeratosis—a Linkage Study. *Am. J. Hum. Genet.* **17:**104–108, 1965.

2 Sallmann, L., von, and Paton, D., Hereditary Benign Intraepithelial Dyskeratosis: I. Ocular Manifestations. *Arch. Ophthalmol.* **63:**421–429, 1960.

3 Witkop, C. J., Jr., Epithelial Intracellular Bodies Associated with Hereditary Dyskeratoses and Cancer Therapy in *Proc. First Internat.* Cong. Exfoliative Cytology (Ed., G. L. Wied). Vienna, Austria, 1961. Published by J. B. Lippincott, Philadelphia, 1962.

4 Witkop, C. J., et al., Hereditary Benign Intraepithelial Dyskeratosis: II. Oral Manifestations and Hereditary Transmission. *Arch. Pathol.* **70:**696–711, 1960.

5 Witkop, C. J., and Gorlin, R. J., Four Hereditary Mucosal Syndromes. *Arch. Dermatol.* **84:**762–771, 1961.

6 Yanoff, M., Hereditary Benign Intraepithelial Dyskeratosis. *Arch. Ophthalmol.* **79:**291–293, 1968.

7 Zegarelli, E. V., and Kutscher, A. H., Familial White Folded Hypertrophy of the Mucous Membranes. *Oral Surg.* **10:**262–270, 1957.

8 Zegarelli, E. V., et al., Familial White Folded Hypertrophy of the Mucous Membranes. *Arch. Dermatol.* **80:**97–103, 1959.

65

Hereditary Hemorrhagic Telangiectasia

(Osler-Rendu-Weber Syndrome)

The syndrome characterized by familial occurrence of multiple capillary and venous dilatations of skin and mucous membranes with repeated hemorrhage was mentioned in 1864 by Sutton (40) and in 1865 by Babington (3). Rendu (33), in 1896, reported a man suffering from recurrent epistaxis and numerous dilated vessels on the face and oral mucosa. Osler (28), in 1901, gave a full account of the syndrome, and Weber (46), in 1907, pointed out that the condition becomes worse with age. The descriptive term "hereditary hemorrhagic telangiectasia" was suggested by Hanes (17), in 1909, and is now widely used, although various eponyms are still employed.

Hereditary hemorrhagic telangiectasia is not extremely rare. In 1950, Garland and Anning (14), in an extensive review of the literature, found 264 affected families, with approximately 1,500 persons involved. Its frequency in Germany has been estimated at about 1 or 2 per 100,000 population (43). The syndrome is very rare among blacks (11). Garland and Anning (14) found it relatively more common among Jews.

The mode of transmission of the syndrome is autosomal dominant (8, 14, 43). We cannot accept as valid the so-called lethal homozygotic state (38).

SYSTEMIC MANIFESTATIONS

The telangiectasia observed in the syndrome may vary in appearance. Thus, Osler (29), in 1907, distinguished three types: (*a*) pinpoint, (*b*) spider-like, and (*c*) nodular. The lesions are bright red, violaceous or purple. When a glass slab is pressed upon them, they blanch. Often the patients are pale, and they may have a history of fatigue and weakness caused by bleeding from the telangiectases, with resultant anemia. The hemorrhage, often nontraumatic, is the most severe complication and becomes more frequent with advancing age. It has been postulated that the hemorrhages are aggravated by anemia, thus producing a vicious cycle.

Skin. Telangiectases are observed on the facial skin, especially on the cheeks, ears, and nasal orifices, in about 60 percent of cases (39) (Fig. 65-1). They may also occur on the fingers, toes, and nail beds in about 30 percent. They usually appear in the second to third decades of life and increase in number and size with age. The lesions may be purpuric. In elderly persons, spider-like configurations may be seen.

Nasal mucosa. Telangiectasis of the nasal mucosa is common and in 80 to 90 percent of cases results in recurrent epistaxis, which tends to become more severe with time. As a rule, epistaxis precedes the appearance of telangiectasia on the skin, often appearing in childhood. Bleeding from the nose may be oozing, sometimes persisting continuously for several days, or profuse hemorrhage may be initiated by sneezing or coughing. Hemorrhagic death has resulted in 2 to 4 percent of patients (25, 39).

Oral manifestations. The lips and tongue (frequently the dorsum and tip) are sites of telangiectasia in about 60 percent of the cases (34) (Fig. 65-2). The palate, gingiva, buccal mucosa, and mucocutaneous junctions may be similarly affected in about 20 percent. Recognition of oral lesions has often led to the correct diagnosis. Bleeding from the mouth is second in frequency to epistaxis (25), having been noted in about 20 percent of cases (8). Hemorrhage from the gingiva and buccal mucosa occurs less frequently than from the lips and tongue. A dramatic report of bleeding from telangiectasia of the tongue has been given by Bird et al. (8). That oral hemorrhage may be serious is evident from the report of Philips (30), who mentioned a fatal outcome after gingival bleeding. Gingival hemorrhages may become manifest at a rather late age. Labial lesions are more common (about 85 percent) in those with gastrointestinal bleeding. Dental prophylaxis has caused bleeding from lip telangiectases (30). Even toothbrushing should be carried out with great care in patients with gingival telangiectasia.

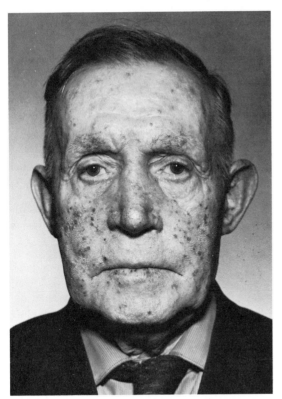

Figure 65-1. *Hereditary hemorrhagic telangiectasia.* Note numerous telangiectases on face and lips.

Other mucous membranes. The gastric mucosa is often involved (16, 27a), resulting in melena and hematemesis which increase with age in about 20 percent of the cases (8, 39). Other areas of the gastrointestinal tract (pharynx, esophagus, jejunum, sigmoid colon) or the conjunctiva (12, 16, 24) may be the seat of telangiectasia. When located in the bladder, vagina, or uterus, the telangiectases may lead to genitourinary bleeding (18, 31).

Other findings. Almost any organ may be affected by angiodysplasias: liver, brain, spinal cord, and lungs (16, 25, 27a, 31, 42). Attention has been called to the rather high incidence of pulmonary and intrahepatic arteriovenous fistulas (7, 16, 19). Duodenal ulcer has been noted in about 5 percent of the patients but in almost 20 percent of those with gastrointestinal bleeding (16).

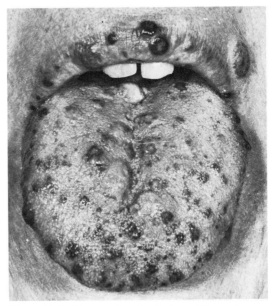

Figure 65-2. Close-up showing lesions of lips and tongue.

PATHOLOGY

Histologically, the telangiectases are found just beneath the epidermis. Their walls are extremely thin, consisting of a single layer of endothelial cells on a continuous basement membrane. The telangiectases are not associated with new formation of vessels but consist solely in the dilatation of these vessels. A detailed analysis of the course of the dilated vessels has been given by Nödl (27). Jahnke (21) and Hashimoto and Pritzker (18) studied these vessels ultrastructurally, suggesting that they were primarily weak, rather than thin, because of defective overlapping of terminal villi of extended cytoplasm of endothelial cells, with resultant gaps.

DIFFERENTIAL DIAGNOSIS

Scrotal angiokeratomas are present in 10 to 20 percent of normal males over fifty years of age (5, 32).

Sublingual phlebectases (caviar spots) are present in about 15 percent of healthy males under 40 years (32) and in 50 percent of males and 20 percent of females between fifty and sixty years of age. Caviar spots increase with age, so that 60 percent of males and 75 percent of females between seventy and seventy-nine years of age have them (5).

Spider nevi have been noted in over 45 percent of healthy schoolchildren (1) and in about 15 percent of normal adults (5).

Cherry angiomas (de Morgan spots) are seen in 90 percent of patients over 40 years of age (37).

Phlebectasia of the lips or oral mucosa was noted by Bean (5) in about 50 percent of normal individuals over forty years of age.

There is a plethora of types of angiomatosis that may affect oral structures. The interested reader should carefully peruse the works of Bean (5, 6).

Labial involvement is common in *Fabry syndrome*, and oral angiomas occasionally occur in the *Maffucci syndrome*. Oral and cutaneous telangiectases indistinguishable from those in hereditary hemorrhagic telangiectasia are seen in the *CRST syndrome*.

Multiple phlebectasia of the oral cavity, jejunum, and scrotum is a nongenetic, age-dependent association first described by Rappaport and Shiffman (32). Most patients have been males over forty years of age. The scrotal lesions (Fordyce angiokeratomas) are round, raised, red to black, well-defined lesions less than 4 mm in diameter. Phlebectatic lesions are present in the wall of the jejunum, less often of the ileum or cecum. A number of patients have also had gastric or duodenal ulcer (26, 32, 37). Phlebectatic lesions have been observed beneath the tongue or on the lower lip, buccal mucosa, or palate. Gius et al. (15) found that 25 percent of patients with peptic ulcers exhibit phlebectatic lesions of the lower lip.

Bean (5, 6) defined the *blue rubber bleb nevus syndrome* as multiple, vascular, nipple or bladderlike lesions of the skin and mucous membranes which may be accompanied by gastrointestinal bleeding and hepatic and pulmonary angiomas. In several families the disorder has been inherited as an autosomal dominant trait. Oral angiomas have been noted in several cases (13, 34, 35).

Multilocular hemangiomatosis, separable from the above by the tendency of these lesions to disappear before the second year of life, may also involve the mouth (10, 20, 44).

Katz and Askin (22) described oral lesions in a patient with multiple hemangiomas with thrombopenia, a variant of the Kasabach-Merritt syndrome. Also present were intraosseous angiomas and hepatosplenomegaly. LaDow et al. (23) noted a maxillary angioma in a patient with von Hippel syndrome, and Tasanen (41) described oral, retinal, and encephalic angiomatosis in a patient with thrombocytopenia. Arteriovenous aneurysms of the mandible and retina with hematemesis and epistaxis were described by Bower et al. (9).

LABORATORY AIDS

The blood should be examined to exclude blood dyscrasias. The hemoglobin and erythrocyte count may be lowered because of hemorrhage. When telangiectases are suspected in the gastrointestinal tract, gastroscopy and sigmoidoscopy may be done.

REFERENCES

1 Alderson, M. R., Spider Naevi: Their Incidence in Healthy School-children. *Arch. Dis. Child.* **38**:286–288, 1963.

2 Babej, K., Multilokuläre Hämangiomatose. *Monatsschr. Kinderheilkd.* **116**:107–110, 1968.

3 Babington, B. G., Hereditary Epistaxis. *Lancet* **2**:362–363, 1865.

4 Bartholomew, L. G., et al., Cutaneous Manifestations of Gastrointestinal Disease. *Postgrad. Med.* **36**:247–259, 1964.

5 Bean, W. B., *Vascular Spiders and Related Lesions of the Skin.* Charles C Thomas, Springfield, Ill., 1958.

6 Bean, W. B., *Rare Diseases and Lesions.* Charles C Thomas, Springfield, Ill., 1967.

7 Berquist, N., et al., Arteriovenous Pulmonary Aneurysms in Osler's Disease (Telangiectasia Hereditaria Haemorrhagica): Report of Four Cases in the Same Family. *Acta Med. Scand.* **171**:301–309, 1962.

8 Bird, R. M., et al., A Family Reunion: A Study of Hereditary Hemorrhagic Telangiectasia. *N. Engl. J. Med.* **257**:105–109, 1957.

9 Bower, L. E., et al., Arteriovenous Angioma of Mandible and Retina with Pronounced Hematemesis and Epistaxis. *Am. J. Dis. Child.* **64**:1023–1029, 1942.

10 Burman, D., et al., Miliary Haemangiomata in the Newborn. *Arch. Dis. Child.* **42**:193–197, 1967.

11 Durocher, R. T., et al., Oral Manifestations of Hereditary Hemorrhagic Telangiectasia. *Oral Surg.* **14**:550–555, 1961.

12 Ecker, J. A., et al., Gastrointestinal Bleeding in Hereditary Hemorrhagic Telangiectasia. *Am. J. Gastroenterol.* **33**:411–421, 1960.

13 Fretzin, D. F., and Potter, B., Blue Rubber Bleb Nevus. *Arch. Intern. Med.* **116**:924–949, 1965.

14 Garland, H. G., and Anning, S. T., Hereditary Hemorrhagic Telangiectasia: A Genetic and Bibliographical Study. *Br. J. Dermatol.* **62**:289–310, 1950.

15 Gius, J. A., et al., Vascular Formations of the Lip and Peptic Ulcer. *J.A.M.A.* **183**:725–729, 1963.

16 Halperin, M., et al., Angiodysplasias of the Abdominal Viscera Associated with Hereditary Hemorrhagic Telangiectasia. *Am. J. Roentgenol.* **102**:783–789, 1968.

17 Hanes, F. M., Multiple Hereditary Telangiectases Causing Hemorrhage (Hereditary Hemorrhagic Telangiectasia). *Bull. Johns Hopkins Hosp.* **20**:63–73, 1909.

18 Hashimoto, K., and Pritzker, M. S., Hereditary Hemorrhagic Telangiectasia. *Oral Surg.* **34**:751–768, 1972.

19 Hodgson, C. H., et al., Hereditary Hemorrhagic Telangiectasia and Pulmonary Arteriovenous Fistulas. *N. Engl. J. Med.* **261**:625–636, 1959.

20 Holden, K. L., and Alexander, F., Diffuse Neonatal Hemangiomatosis. *Pediatrics* **46**:411–421, 1970.

21 Jahnke, V., Ultrastructure of Hereditary Telangiectasia. *Arch. Otolaryngol.* **91**:262–265, 1970.

22 Katz, H. P., and Askin, J., Multiple Hemangiomata with Thrombopenia. *Am. J. Dis. Child.* **115**:351–357, 1968.

23 LaDow, C. S., et al., Central Hemangioma of the Maxilla with von Hippel's Disease. *J. Oral Surg.* **22**:252–259, 1964.

24 Landau, J., et al., Hereditary Hemorrhagic Telangiectasia with Retinal and Conjunctival Lesions. *Lancet* **2**:230–231, 1956.

25 Larson, D. L., et al., Hereditary Hemorrhagic Telangiec-

tasia: Rendu-Osler-Weber's Disease. *Wisconsin Med. J.* **61**:229–236, 1962.

26 Miller, D. A., and Akers, W. A., Multiple Phlebectasia of the Jejunum, Oral Cavity and Scrotum. *Arch. Intern. Med.* **121**:180–182, 1968.

27 Nödl, F., Zur Histopathogenese der Telangiectasia hereditaria hämorrhagica Rendu-Osler. *Arch. Klin. Exp. Dermatol.* **204**:213–235, 1957.

27a Novak, D., Telangiectasia hereditaria haemorrhagica (Morbus Rendu-Osler-Weber). Angiographischer Nachweis der Lungen-, Leber- und Magen-Manifestation. *Fortschr. Roentgenstr.* **120**:491–494, 1974.

28 Osler, W., On a Family Form of Recurring Epistaxis, Associated with Multiple Telangiectases of the Skin and Mucous Membranes. *Bull. Johns Hopkins Hosp.* **12**:333–337, 1901.

29 Osler, W., On Multiple Hereditary Telangiectases with Recurring Haemorrhages. *Q. J. Med.* **1**:53–58, 1907.

30 Philips, S., Multiple Telangiectases. *Proc. R. Soc. Med.* **1** (Clin. Sec.):64, 1908.

31 Quickel, K. E., and Whalen, R. J., Subarachnoid Hemorrhage in a Telangiectasis. *Neurology* **17**:716–719, 1967.

32 Rappaport, I., and Shiffman, M. A., Multiple Phlebectasia Involving Jejunum, Oral Cavity and Scrotum. *J.A.M.A.* 437–440, 1963.

33 Rendu, M., Epistaxis répétées chez un sujet porteur de petits angiomes cutanés et muqueux. *Bull. Soc. Méd.* (Paris) **13**:731–733, 1896.

34 Rice, J. S., and Fischer, D. S., Blue Rubber Bleb Nevus Syndrome. *Arch. Dermatol.* **86**:503–511, 1962.

35 Richter, G., "Blue Rubber-Bleb Nevus Syndrom" als Anämieursache. *Z. Haut Geschlechtskr.* **39**:256–261, 1965.

36 Saunders, W. H., Hereditary Hemorrhagic Telangiectasia. *Arch. Otolaryngol.* **76**:245–260, 1962.

37 Shiffman, M. A., and Rappaport, I., Multiple Phlebectasia. *Arch. Surg.* **94**:771–775, 1967.

38 Snyder, L. H., and Doan, C. A., Studies in Human Inheritance: Is Homozygous Form of Multiple Telangiectasia Lethal? *J. Lab. Clin. Med.* **29**:1211–1216, 1944.

39 Stecker, R. H., and Lake, C. F., Hereditary Hemorrhagic Telangiectasia. *Arch. Otolaryngol.* **82**:522–526, 1965.

40 Sutton, H. G., Epistaxis as an Indication of Impaired Nutrition and of Degeneration of the Vascular System. *Med. Mirror* **1**:769–781, 1864.

41 Tasanen, A., Bonnet-Dechaume-Blanc Syndrome Accompanied by Mandibular Angiomatosis and Thrombocytopenia. *Br. J. Oral Surg.* **4**:213–217, 1967.

42 Trell, E., et al., Familial Pulmonary Hypertension and Multiple Abnormalities of Large Systemic Arteries in Osler's Disease. *Am. J. Med.* **53**:50–63, 1972.

43 Tünte, W., Klinik und Genetik der Oslerschen Krankheit. *Z. Menschl. Vererb. Konstit. Lehre* **37**:221–250, 1964.

44 Vogel, C., Beitrag zur angeborenen multilokulären Hämangiomatose. *Hautarzt* **17**:504–507, 1961.

45 Wallis, L. A., et al., Diffuse Skeletal Hemangiomatosis: Report of Two Cases and Review of the Literature. *Am. J. Med.* **37**:545–563, 1964.

46 Weber, F. P., Multiple Hereditary Developmental Angiomata (Telangiectases) of the Skin and Mucous Membranes Associated with Recurring Hemorrhages. *Lancet* **2**:160–162, 1907.

66

Holoprosencephaly and Facial Dysmorphic Syndromes

Holoprosencephaly is frequently, but not always, associated with facial dysmorphia; together, these anomalies may be said to constitute a single developmental field. Because the abnormalities within this field represent a spectrum and because they may be associated with various patterned groups of extracephalic anomalies, they should not, as a rule, be considered a disorder *sui generis,* but an anomalad which may occur in a variety of disorders. However, there is no a priori reason why anomalies within this developmental field cannot occur without other associated abnormalities, and a few such cases are known (10).

Etiologic heterogeneity is a sine qua non of holoprosencephaly with facial dysmorphia (26a). Several distinct chromosomal syndromes which may be associated with holoprosencephaly and facial dysmorphia include trisomy 13 syndrome, 18p– syndrome, and 13q– syndrome (3, 8, 10, 22, 32, 35, 44). Various other abnormal karyotypes have been reported in association with holoprosencephaly and facial dysmorphia including trisomy 18, triploidy, and a variety of unusual karyotypes (7, 26a, 38, 45). Normal karyotypes have also been reported (9, 10–12, 14, 26, 30).

Most cases of holoprosencephaly with severe facial dysmorphia are sporadic. However, cases have occurred in sibs and in twins (9, 13, 15, 16a, 17, 21a, 26, 27, 29, 38a). In some cases, sibs and twins were of similar facial type; in other cases, sibs and twins were of different facial type. Holoprosencephalic infants and several sibs with clefts have been reported (9, 10, 15). It has been suggested that some cases of holoprosencephaly with facial dysmorphia may follow an autosomal recessive mode of transmission (18). Several reports of affected sibs and consanguinity noted in three instances (10) tend to support this notion. Cohen (10a) suggested that several pedigrees were compatible with autosomal dominant transmission, incomplete penetrance and remarkably variable expressivity (10a, 10b, 23, 31a). Minimal involvement may include mild ocular hypotelorism, anosmia or hyposmia, asymmetric nose, or single permanent maxillary incisor (31a).

Holoprosencephaly and facial dysmorphia may be observed in some cases of the Meckel syndrome. Arhincephaly with anosmia may be part of the Kallmann syndrome, an etiologic heterogeneity. Various teratogenic agents have been used to produce the condition experimentally in animals (28). Possible environmental causes in human beings have also been considered (29a).

In an extensive analysis of 30 families in which holoprosencephaly occurred (38a), Roach et al. estimated the incidence of lobar and alobar types to be 1/16,000 live births. This should be considered a minimal estimate since ascertainment was probably not complete. Furthermore, cases associated with chromosomal anomalies were excluded from consideration. The empiric recurrence risk was calculated to be 6 percent. Nonchromosomal cases also seemed to cluster in families of poverty-level socioeconomic status. Other factors such as mental deficiency, mental illness, endocrine disorders, and an increased twinning rate were noted in families of probands with holoprosencephaly. There was a 3:1 female-to-male sex ratio in alobar holoprosencephaly, whereas the sex ratio was approximately 1:1 for the lobar type. Patients with a severe degree of holoprosencephaly rarely survive infancy (12, 38a). Several papers deal with pathogenesis (1, 10, 43).

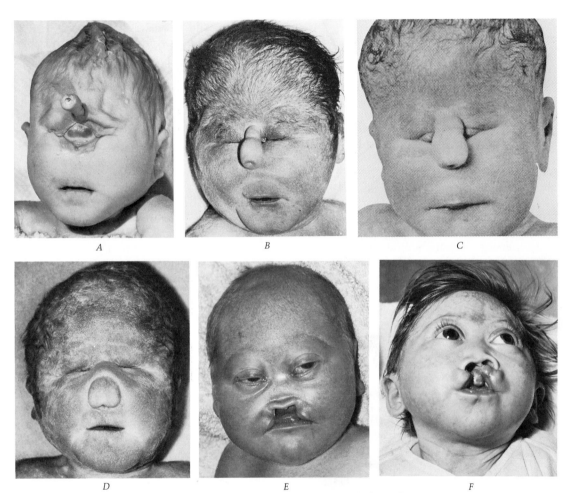

A   *B*   *C*

D   *E*   *F*

Figure 66-1. (*A*). *Cyclopia.* Note central eye where root of nose is normally located. Proboscis with single opening is located above eye. (*B*). *Cyclopia-ethmocephaly.* Intermediate form having separate palpebral fissures but single bony orbit; infant had trisomy 13. (*From K. Taysi and K. Tinaztepe, Am. J. Dis. Child.* **124:**170, 1972.) (*C*). *Ethmocephaly.* Separate eye sockets, probosets located above eye. (*From W. B. Davis, Surg. Gynecol. Obstet.* **61:**209, 1935.) (*D*). *Cebocephaly.* Microphthalmia, ocular hypotelorism, single-nostril nose. (*From P. E. Conen, Can. Med. Assoc. J.* **87:**709, 1962.) (*E*). *Premaxillary agenesis.* Ocular hypotelorism, mongoloid obliquity of palpebral fissures, absence of nasal bones and cartilages, and agenesis of philtrum area. (*F*). *Partial premaxillary agenesis.* Note ocular hypotelorism, hypoplasia of nasal cartilages and philtrum area. (*From W. DeMyer et al., Pediatrics* **34:**2563, 1964.)

SYSTEMIC MANIFESTATIONS

Facies. Different facial anomalies may be associated with holoprosencephaly. In *cyclopia,* the most extreme variant, a single median eye globe with varying degrees of doubling of the intrinsic ocular structures is associated with arhinia and usually with proboscis formation. Absent proboscis, hypognathia, and even anophthalmia may occur in some instances (Fig. 66-1*A*). In *ethmocephaly,* two separate hypoteloric eyes are associated with arhinia and usually with proboscis formation (41) (Fig. 66-1*B, C*). In *cebocephaly,* ocular hypotelorism is associated with a single-nostril nose (Fig. 66-1*D*). In *premaxillary agenesis,* ocular hypotelorism is associated with a flat nose and a median pseudocleft of the upper lip (Fig. 66-1*E*). Less severe forms of holoprosencephaly may occur together with less severe facial dysmorphia (10) (Fig. 66-1*F*). In cases of semilobar or lobar holoprosencephaly, the severe facial dysmorphia of cyclopia, ethmocephaly, cebocephaly, or premaxillary agenesis, is usually not present. Hypotelorism is sometimes associated with semilobar holoprosencephaly, and arhinencephaly may occur without severe facial dysmorphia (6a, 12). Table 66-1 presents a classification of holoprosencephalic facies. It should be noted that transitional forms of these facies are known to occur. Combination with anencephaly has also been noted (42).

Central nervous system. In holoprosencephaly, impaired midline cleavage of the embryonic forebrain is the basic feature. The term "holoprosencephaly" was coined by DeMyer (14) to replace the term "arhinencephaly" because the former more accurately reflects these brain anomalies. Thus, the embryonic forebrain fails to cleave sagittally into cerebral hemispheres, transversally into telencephalon and diencephalon, and horizontally into olfactory and optic bulbs (Fig. 66-2*A, B*).

DeMyer (12) distinguished between alobar, semilobar, and lobar holoprosencephaly. A monoventricular forebrain lacking interhemispheric division is present in alobar holoprosencephaly. Rudimentary cerebral lobes are present in semilobar holoprosencephaly, and in some cases, a posterior interhemispheric fissure. Well-formed lobes and a distinct interhemispheric

Table 66-1. Holoprosencephalic facies*

Facial type†	Main facial features‡	Brain
Cyclopia	Median monophthalmia, synophthalmia, or anophthalmia. Proboscis may be single, double, or absent. Hypognathia in some cases	Alobar holoprosencephaly
Ethmocephaly	Ocular hypotelorism. Proboscis may be single, double, or absent	Alobar holoprosencephaly
Cebocephaly	Ocular hypotelorism and single-nostril nose	Usually alobar holoprosencephaly
Premaxillary agenesis	Ocular hypotelorism, flat nose, and median cleft lip	Usually alobar holoprosencephaly
Less severe facial dysmorphia	Variable features, including ocular hypotelorism or hypertelorism, flat nose, unilateral or bilateral cleft lip, iris coloboma, or other anomalies. Minimal facial dysmorphia in some cases	Semilobar or lobar holoprosencephaly

* Modified after DeMyer et al. (13).

† Transitional facial forms are known to occur.

‡ Only the main distinguishing features are listed here. Features such as microcephaly, various eye anomalies, ear anomalies, and other defects also occur.

SOURCE: From M. M. Cohen, Jr., et al. (10).

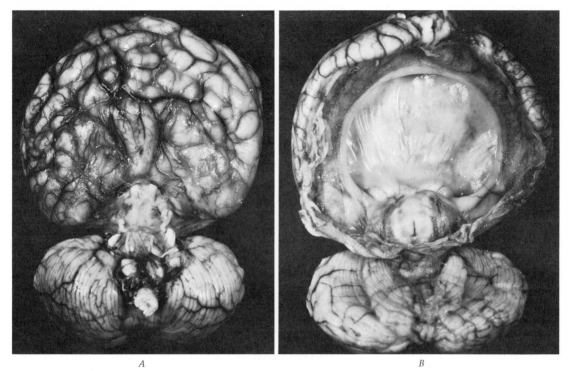

A   *B*

Figure 66-2. *Holoprosencephalic brain, alobar type.* (*A*). Dorsal view showing pancake-like structure without corpus callosum or septum pellucidum. Diencephalon and telencephalon are uncleft. (*B*). Ventral view showing absent olfactory bulbs and tracts and no interhemispheric fissure. (*From W. DeMyer and P. T. White,* Arch. Neurol. **11**:507, 1964.)

fissure which may be interrupted anteriorly are found in lobar holoprosencephaly. The central nervous system anomalies have been extensively described by Yakovlev (43), DeMyer (11–14), and Opitz (35).

Skeletal system. In holoprosencephaly with severe facial dysmorphia, the ethmoid, middle portion of the sphenoid, vomer, premaxilla and turbinate, nasal, and lacrimal bones are absent. Polydactyly, syndactyly, agenesis or hypoplasia of the thumb, talipes equinovarus, and spina bifida have been associated with various cases of holoprosencephaly (10, 39). Infants with extracephalic anomalies probably represent examples of chromosomal aneuploidy.

Other findings. A wide spectrum of other anomalies has been reported (16, 19, 34, 35, 39, 40), including a host of different cardiovascular and genitourinary abnormalities, aplastic or hypoplastic endocrine glands, hirsutism, dermatoglyphic abnormalities, lung anomalies, diaphragmatic anomalies, situs inversus viscerum, diastasis recti, umbilical hernia, Meckel diverticulum, intestinal malrotation anomalies, stenotic colon, anal atresia, liver malformations, and dystopic gallbladder. This list is by no means exhaustive. Many of these infants probably had chromosomal aneuploidy.

Oral manifestations. In holoprosencephaly with severe facial dysmorphia, the philtrum and maxillary frenulum are absent. In cyclopia and ethmocephaly, a concave groove is frequently present above the upper lip. Median pseudoclefting is seen in premaxillary agenesis. Unilateral or bilateral cleft lip, and cleft palate or bifid uvula may be observed in some cases of holoprosencephaly (10, 14). In cyclopia, the maxillary incisor teeth are absent and at times a single, conical tooth may be erupted at birth in the midline of the maxillary ridge (6, 24). Sedano and Gorlin (39) suggested that the conical tooth may arise from central fusion of the two anlagen of the lateral incisors. Rarely, aglossia, bifid tongue, and hypoplasia of the parotid glands and muscles of mastication may be observed in cyclopia. Microstomia or astomia and hypoplasia or absence of the mandible may occur in cyclopia hypognathus (39). A single permanent maxillary central incisor was noted in a minimally affected mother of a holoprosencephalic infant with median pseudocleft (31a).

DIFFERENTIAL DIAGNOSIS

Diagnosis of alobar holoprosencephaly usually presents little challenge because of the attendant facial dysmorphia. Semilobar holoprosencephaly and lobar holoprosencephaly are associated with less severe facial dysmorphia, and in some cases, the facial changes may be minimal. Otocephaly should be distinguished from cyclopia hypognathus. Occasionally, asymmetric monophthalmia has been confused with cyclopia. In this condition, one normal eye is present in its normal position, the other eye has failed to form, and a proboscis may be located in its place (39). Holoprosencephaly has not been reported in association with asymmetric monophthalmia.

Furthermore, other conditions with failure of olfactory placode development or with dystopic olfactory placodes leading to proboscis formation may occur independently of holoprosencephaly. Arhinencephaly has been observed in association with eunuchoidism. Although trigonocephaly sometimes occurs with holoprosencephaly, it may also occur without cerebral malformations (10).

LABORATORY AIDS

A number of procedures may be used to confirm the diagnosis of alobar holoprosencephaly. Absence of crista galli and absence or hypoplasia of the nasal septum, revealed by skull roentgenograms or planigrams, are consistent with holoprosencephaly. Transillumination of the skull may be useful. Electroencephalograms are invariably abnormal, showing multiple independent spikes, paroxysmal hypersynchrony, and, often, flattening over the areas of transillumination. Pneumoencephalography should be reserved for cases in which semilobar or lobar holoprosencephaly is suspected (4, 15).

Since hypothalamic-pituitary dysfunction has been reported in siblings of patients with holoprosencephaly (38b), neuroendocrine studies may be advisable in seemingly normal sibs of affected infants.

REFERENCES

1 Adelmann, H. B., The Problem of Cyclopia. Q. Rev. Biol. **11**:161–182, 284–304, 1936.

2 Araki, D. T., and Waxman, S. H., Trisomy D in a Cyclops. J. Pediatr. **74**:620–622, 1969.

3 Batts, J. A., et al., A Case of Cyclopia. Am. J. Obstet. Gynecol. **112**:657–661, 1972.

4 Bligh, A. S., and Lawrence, K. M., The Radiological Appearances in Arhinencephaly. Clin. Radiol. **18**:383–393, 1967.

5 Bock, E., Beschreibung eines atypischen Cyclops. Klin. Monatsbl. Augenheilkd. **27**:508–522, 1889.

6 Breckwoldt, H., Über die Zahnverhältnisse bei Zyklopie und Gesichtsspalte. Beitr. Pathol. Anat. **98**:115–135, 1936.

6a Carrier, H., et al., A propos d'un cas d'arhinencephalie. Ann. Pédiat. **21**:96–100, 1974.

7 Cohen, M. M., Chromosomal Mosaicism Associated with a Case of Cyclopia. J. Pediatr. **69**:793–798, 1966.

8 Cohen, M. M., et al., A Ring Chromosome (No. 18) in a Cyclops Clin. Genet. **3**:249–252, 1972.

9 Cohen, M. M., Jr., and Gorlin, R. J., Genetic Considerations in a Sibship of Cyclopia and Clefts. Birth Defects **5**(2):113–118, 1969.

10 Cohen, M. M., Jr., et al., Holoprosencephaly and Facial Dysmorphia: Nosology, Etiology and Pathogenesis. Birth Defects **7**(7):125–135, 1971.

10a Cohen, M. M. Jr., Holoprosencephaly Revisited. Am. J. Dis. Child. **127**:597, 1974.

10b Dallaire, L., et al., Familial Holoprosencephaly. Birth Defects **7**(7):136–147, 1971.

11 DeMyer, W., A 46 Chromosome Cebocephaly with Remarks on the Relation of 13–15 Trisomy to Holoprosencephaly (Arhinencephaly). Ann. Paediatr. (Basel) **203**:169–177, 1964.

12 DeMyer, W. E., and Zeman, W., Alobar Holoprosencephaly

(Arhinencephaly) with Median Cleft Lip and Palate: Clinical, Electroencephalographic and Nosologic Considerations. *Confin. Neurol.* **23**:1–36, 1963.

13 DeMyer, W. E., et al., Familial Alobar Holoprosencephaly (Arhinencephaly) with Median Cleft Lip and Palate. *Neurology* **13**:913–918, 1963.

14 DeMyer, W. E., et al., The Face Predicts the Brain: Diagnostic Significance of Median Facial Anomalies for Holoprosencephaly (Arhinencephaly). *Pediatrics* **34**:256–263, 1964.

15 Deveze, J., and Jezequel, C., Les cyclopes: Étude clinique et anatomique d'une cyclopie familiale. *Arch. Fr. Pédiatr.* **28**:321–337, 1971. (Also reviews literature.)

16 Diebold, J., et al., Trisomie 13–15: Étude anatomo-pathologique d'une forme rare avec ethmocéphale. *Arch. Anat. Pathol.* **15**:277–287, 1967.

16a Dominok, G., and Kirchmair, H., Familiäre Häufung von Fehlbildungen der Arbinencephaliegrieppe. *Z. Kinderheilkd.* **85**:19–30, 1961.

17 Ellis, R., On a Rare Form of Twin Monstrosity. *Trans. Obstet. Soc. London* **7**:160–164, 1865.

18 François, J., *Heredity in Ophthalmology.* C. V. Mosby, St. Louis, 1961, pp. 173–176.

19 Frutiger, P., Zur Frage der Arhinencephalie. *Acta Anat. (Basel)* **73**:410–430, 1969.

20 Gardner, D. G., and Lim, H., The Oral Manifestations of Cyclopia. *Oral Surg.* **32**:910–917, 1971.

21 Gerken, H., and Wiedemann, H. R., Cyclopie. *Z. Menschl. Vererb. Konstit. Lehre* **37**:602–610, 1964.

21a Godeano, D., et al., Familial Holoprosencephaly with Median Cleft Lip. *J. Génét. Hum.* **21**:223–228, 1973.

22 Gorlin, R. J., et al., Short Arm Deletion of Chromosome 18 in Cebocephaly. *Am. J. Dis. Child.* **115**:473–476, 1968.

23 Grebe, H., Zur Ätiologie der Arhinencephalie. *Erbarzt* **12**:138–145, 1944.

24 Grimmer, T., Histologische Untersuchungen zweier Fälle von Zyklopie. *Dtsch. Zahn Mund Kieferheilkd.* **2**:349–358, 1935.

25 Hill, E., Cyclopia, Its Bearing upon Certain Problems of Teratogenesis, and of Normal Embryology with a Description of a Cyclocephalic Monster. *Arch. Ophthalmol.* **49**:597–620, 1920; **50**:52–80, 1921.

26 Hintz, R. L., et al., Familial Holoprosencephaly with Endocrine Dysgenesis. *J. Pediatr.* **72**:81–87, 1968.

26a Holmes, L. B., et al., Genetic Heterogeneity of Cebocephaly. *J. Med. Genet.* **11**:35–40, 1974.

27 James, E., and Van Leeuwen, G., Familial Cebocephaly. *Clin. Pediatr.* **9**:491–493, 1970.

28 Keeler, R. F., and Binns, W., Teratogenic Compounds of *Veratrum californicum. Teratology* **1**:5–10, 1968.

29 Khan, M., et al., Familial Holoprosencephaly. *Dev. Med. Child. Neurol.* **12**:71–76, 1970.

29a Khudr, G., and Olding, L., Cyclopia. *Am. J. Dis. Child.* **125**:120–122, 1973.

30 Kotte, W., and Kunze, P., Alobäre Holoprosencephalie (Arhinencephalie) mit medianer Lippenkieferspalte und normalem Karyotyp. *Zentralbl. Allg. Pathol.* **114**:173–184, 1971.

31 Kuhlenbeck, H., The Human Diencephalon. *Confin. Neurol. (Suppl.)* **14**:1–230, 1954.

31a Lowry, R. B., Holoprosencephaly. *Am. J. Dis. Child.* **128**:887, 1974.

32 McDermott, A., et al., Arrhinencephaly Associated with a Deficiency Involving Chromosome 18. *J. Med. Genet.* **5**:60–67, 1968.

33 Mettler, F., Congenital Malformation of the Brain. *J. Neuropathol. Exp. Neurol.* **6**:98, 1947.

34 Ognew, B. W., Die Zyklopie im Zusammenhang mit Anomalien anderer Organe. *Anat. Anz.* **70**:241–246, 1930.

35 Opitz, J. M., et al., Report of a Patient with a Presumed Dq− Syndrome. *Birth Defects* **5**(5):93–99, 1969.

36 Ostertag, B., *Handbuch der speziellen pathologischen Anatomie und Histologie.* Springer, Berlin, 1956.

37 Patel, H., et al., Holoprosencephaly with Median Cleft Lip. *Am. J. Dis. Child.* **124**:217–225, 1972.

38 Pfitzer, P., and Müntefering, H., Cyclopism as a Hereditary Malformation. *Nature* **217**:1071–1072, 1968.

38a Roach, E., et al., Holoprosencephaly: Birth Data, Genetic and Demographic Analyses of 30 Families. *Birth Defects* **11**(2):294–313, 1975.

38b Romshe, C. A., and Sotos, J. F., Hypothalamic-Pituitary Dysfunction in Siblings of Patients with Holoprosencephaly. *J. Pediatr.* **83**:1088–1090, 1973.

39 Sedano, H. O., and Gorlin, R. J., The Oral Manifestations of Cyclopia. *Oral Surg.* **16**:823–838, 1963.

40 Toews, H. A., and Jones, H. W., Jr., Cyclopia in Association with D Trisomy and Gonadal Agenesis. *Am. J. Obstet. Gynecol.* **102**:53–56, 1968.

41 White, G. M., and Foster, T. A., A Case of Cyclops. *Can. Med. Assoc. J.* **72**:213–214, 1955.

42 Wolter, J. R., et al., Synophthalmus and Anencephaly. *J. Pediatr. Ophthalmol.* **5**:217–223, 1968.

43 Yakovlev, P., Pathoarchitectonic Studies of Cerebral Malformations. *J. Neuropathol. Exp. Neurol.* **18**:22–55, 1959.

44 Yanoff, M., et al., Ocular and Cerebral Abnormalities in Chromosome 18 Deletion Defect. *Am. J. Ophthalmol.* **70**:391–402, 1970.

45 Zergollern, L., et al., A Liveborn Infant with Triploidy (69, XXX). *Z. Kinderheilkd.* **112**:293–300, 1972.

67

Homocystinuria

(Cystathionine Synthase Deficiency)

Homocystinuria, known also as cysta-thionine synthase deficiency, is a disorder characterized by (a) ectopia lentis, (b) thromboembolic episodes involving medium-sized arteries and veins, (c) malar flushing and livedo reticularis, and (d) osteoporosis together with frequent (e) dolichostenomelia, (f) pectus carinatum, and (g) mental retardation. In 1962, cystathionine synthase deficiency was clearly separated from the Marfan syndrome by Carson and Neill (8) and by Gerritson et al. (18). Further important studies were carried out by Mudd et al. (29, 30), Finkelstein et al. (12), Brenton et al. (4, 5), and Brenton and Cusworth (3).

The disorder follows an autosomal recessive mode of transmission. Deficiency of cysta-thionine synthase (residual activity of 2 to 3 percent) has been demonstrated in liver, brain, skin fibroblasts, and phytohemagglutinin-stimulated lymphocytes of homozygotes (13a, 21, 29, 30), and reduced activity has been observed in heterozygous carriers (3a, 12, 13a). Prenatal diagnosis has also been demonstrated. Normal amniotic cells must be used for a control (13a).

Affected individuals have sometimes been reported as having the Marfan syndrome (19, 22, 23). It has been suggested that Marfan's original patient had cystathionine synthase deficiency (2). However, congenital contractural arachno-dactyly is a more likely diagnosis.

Although the disorder has been known as "homocystinuria," the term "cystathionine synthase deficiency" is more appropriate, since homocystinuria is only one of several biochemical consequences of the disorder. Levels of plasma methionine and homolanthionine are elevated. Furthermore, homocystinuria may be found in other disorders, such as a defect in coenzyme B_{12} synthesis, N-5,10-methylenetet-rahydrofolate reductase, or in intestinal resorption of vitamin B_{12} (13).

Accumulation of homocystine proximal to the enzymatic block seems to be implicated in the development of arteriosclerotic lesions (24), abnormal platelet adhesiveness (25), and activation of the Hageman factor (34). Furthermore, the connective tissue changes observed in the skeleton, vascular system, and eye may possibly be related to reduced collagen cross-linking caused by homocysteine interference (20, 26). It is also possible that increased excretion of sulfur-containing compounds may lead to deficiency of sulfate donor, resulting in faulty metabolism of glycosaminoglycans (26).

Deficiency of cystathionine distal to the enzymatic block may bear some relationship to the mental retardation frequently reported in this disorder, since the normal brain is known to contain a considerable amount of this enzyme (4, 11, 16). Ectopia lentis may possibly be a consequence of deficient cystine and cysteine, since the normal lens contains high concentrations of cystine and glutathione, a cysteine-containing tripeptide (26, 32).

Perry et al. (31) suggested that the disorder

might arise not from the absence of cysta-thionine synthase, but from an altered form of the enzyme which has greater activity for the presence of homoserine than for serine, its normal substrate. It is also conceivable that cysta-thionine synthase deficiency might result from impaired production of either an essential enzyme or an essential enzyme activator (6). Recently, evidence has been presented favoring two types of cystathionine synthase deficiency—pyridoxine-responsive and pyridoxine-unresponsive (5a, 38). This has evoked further comment by Frimpter (14). The basic defect and pathogenesis of the disorder deserve further study.

SYSTEMIC MANIFESTATIONS

Skeletal system. A Marfanoid appearance has been described in only about 35 percent of patients (28) (Fig. 67-1). Joint laxity, genu valgum, pes planus, pes cavus, kyphoscoliosis, pectus carinatum, dolichostenomelia, and arachnodactyly have been reported (1, 28, 36) with about the same frequency. Restricted joint mobility of the fingers and contractures also have been observed. Generalized osteoporosis is present in at least one-third of affected adults. Probably more have codfish vertebras and some collapse of vertebral bodies occurs in older patients (36). An increased frequency of fracture has been noted (28). Poor growth has been reported in severely affected individuals (26, 34a, 35). Calcific streaks or spicules may be present in the radius or ulna of children (5a).

Skin. Malar flushing is a feature in about 50 percent of patients (Fig. 67-2). On exertion, flushing becomes intense. Facial skin in older patients is coarse, with large pores. Elsewhere, the skin may be red and blotchy or display livedo reticularis. Sparse, fine, blond or red hair has been observed in some cases (9, 26).

Eyes. Ectopia lentis is present in about 90 percent of cases, and in several instances, displacement of the lens was shown to be progressive. Displacement in over 50 percent of cases is nasal, inferonasal, or inferior (Fig. 67-3). The lens

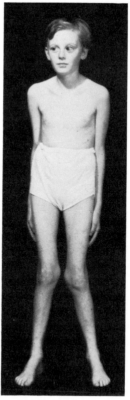

Figure 67-1. *Homocystinuria.* Marfanoid habitus and genu valgum.

was initially in the vitreous body in almost 20 percent of patients, and in the anterior chamber in about 10 percent. Iridodonesis, zonular cataracts, cystic degeneration of the retina with detachment, myopia, optic atrophy, and glaucoma have been reported (10, 17, 23, 33).

Cardiovascular system. Thrombosis of medium-sized arteries, especially the coronary and renal arteries and the main aortic branches supplying the limbs and brain, constitutes the main cardiovascular disorder seen in about 40 to 50 percent of adult patients (16). Venous thrombosis has also been reported. Sequelae have been discussed by McKusick (26). Platelet cytoplasm is vacuolated, suggesting that the coagulation disorder is thrombocytogenic (19).

Central nervous system. Mental retardation is a frequent finding, although there is normal in-

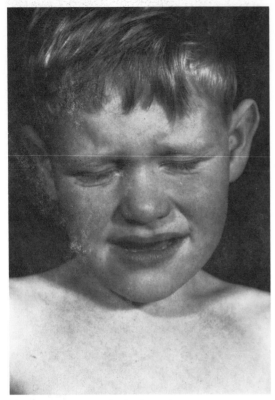

Figure 67-2. Note malar flushing. (*From N. A. J. Carson and G. Gaull, New York.*)

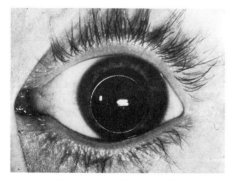

Figure 67-3. Inferior dislocation of lens associated with acute glaucoma. (*From M. C. Carey, Am. J. Med.* **45**:7, 1968.)

telligence in about 30 percent of cases. Some patients have been noted to be excessively nervous, and a diagnosis of schizophrenia has been occasionally made (26). Seizures have been observed in 15 to 50 percent of patients (9). Spasticity, hyperreflexia (17), electroencephalographic abnormalities, and neurologic signs attributable to intracranial arterial and/or venous thrombosis (26) have also been reported. Neuroblastoma has been noted in one case (27).

Other findings. Bilateral inguinal hernias and omphalocele have been reported (17, 26).

Oral manifestations. The palate may be narrow and highly arched. The teeth have been reported to be crowded and irregularly aligned (26). Mandibular prognathism has also been noted, but its frequency has not been assessed (1).

PATHOLOGY

Arterial lesions are distinctive, with partial luminal obstruction, thinning of the media, and dilatation. The elastic lamellas of the aortic media may be abnormal in some cases. Fibroelastic endocardial thickening of the left atrium has been found in autopsied cases. Focal necrosis, gliosis, and spongy degeneration of the brain with micropolygyria and hypoplasia of the corpus callosum have also been reported. Degenerative changes of the zonular fibers of the lens have been described. Fatty degeneration of the liver has been noted in autopsied cases (9, 26, 35).

DIFFERENTIAL DIAGNOSIS

Cystathionine synthase deficiency should be distinguished from *Marfan syndrome* and other disorders with Marfanoid habitus, such as congenital contractural arachnodactyly, Marfanoid hypermobility syndrome, *Klinefelter syndrome,* XYY syndrome, sickle cell anemia, *multiple basal cell carcinoma syndrome,* and *multiple mucosal neuroma syndrome.* In homocystinuria with methylmalonic aciduria, the clinical course is fulminant, with death in early infancy (13).

LABORATORY AIDS

The cyanide-nitroprusside test is positive for both cystinuria and homocystinuria. Cystine and homocystine can be distinguished by high-voltage electrophoresis or by specific assay with a Stein-Moore column chromatographic automatic amino acid analyzer (26). Platelet cytoplasm is vacuolated (19).

REFERENCES

1 Beals, R. K., Homocystinuria: A Report of Two Cases and Review of the Literature. *J. Bone Joint Surg.* **51A:**1564–1572, 1969.

2 Bianchine, J. W., The Marfan Syndrome Revisited. *J. Pediatr.* **79:**717–718, 1971.

3 Brenton, D. P., and Cusworth, D. C., Homocystinuria: Metabolism of ^{35}S Methionine. *Clin. Sci.* **31:**197–206, 1966.

3a Bittles, A. H., and Carson, N., Tissue Culture Techniques as a Aid to Prenatal Diagnosis and Genetic Counselling in Homocystinuria. *J. Med. Genet.* **10:**120–123, 1973.

4 Brenton, D. P., et al., Homocystinuria: Biochemical Studies of Tissues Including a Comparison with Cystathioninuria. *Pediatrics* **35:**50–56, 1965.

5 Brenton, D. P., et al., Homocystinuria, Clinical and Dietary Studies. *Q. J. Med.* **35:**325–346, 1966.

5a Brill, P. W., et al., Homocystinuria due to Cystathionine Synthase Deficiency: Clinical Roentgenologic Correlations. *Am. J. Roentgenol.* **121:**45–54, 1974.

6 Butterworth, C. E., et al., Studies on the Absorption and Metabolism of Folic Acid. II. Homocystinuria. *Ala. J. Med. Sci.* **8:**30–43, 1971.

7 Carey, M. C., et al., Homocystinuria. *Am. J. Med.* **45:**7–25, 1968.

8 Carson, N. A. J., and Neill, D. W., Metabolic Abnormalities Detected in a Survey of Mentally Backward Individuals in Northern Ireland. *Arch. Dis. Child.* **37:**505–513, 1962.

9 Carson, N. A. J., et al., Homocystinuria. *J. Pediatr.* **66:**565–583, 1965.

10 Cross, H. E., and Jensen, A. D., Ocular Manifestations in the Marfan Syndrome and Homocystinuria. *Am. J. Ophthalmol.* **75:**405–419, 1973.

11 Cusworth, D. C., and Dent, C. E., Homocystinuria. *Br. Med. Bull.* **25:**42–47, 1969.

12 Finkelstein, J. D., et al., Homocystinuria Due to Cystathionine Synthetase Deficiency: The Model of Inheritance. *Science* **146:**785–787, 1964.

13 Finkelstein, J. D., et al., Homocystinuria. *Clin. Proc. Child. Hosp. (Washington, D.C.)* **25:**291–307, 1969.

13a Fleisher, L. D., et al., Homocystinuria: Investigations of Cystathionine Synthase in Cultured Fetal Cells and the Prenatal Determination of Genetic Status. *J. Pediatr.* **85:**677–680, 1974.

14 Frimpter, G. W., Homocystinuria: Vitamin B_6 Dependent or Not? *Ann. Intern. Med.* **71:**209–211, 1969.

15 Gaull, G., Homocystinuria. *Adv. Teratol.* **2:**101–126, 1967.

16 Gerritsen, T., and Waisman, H. A., Homocystinuria: Absence of Cystathionine in the Brain. *Science* **145:**588, 1964.

17 Gerritsen, T., and Waisman, H. A., Homocystinuria, an Error in the Metabolism of Methionine. *Pediatrics* **33:**413–420, 1964.

18 Gerritsen, T., et al., The Identification of Homocystine in the Urine. *Biochem. Biophys. Res. Commun.* **9:**493–496, 1962.

19 Gröbe, H., and von Bassewitz, D. B., Thromboembolische Komplikationen und Thrombocytenanomalien bei Homocystinurie. *Z. Kinderheilkd.* **112:**309–320, 1972.

20 Harris, E. D., Jr., and Sjoerdsma, A., Collagen Profile in Various Clinical Conditions. *Lancet* **2:**707–711, 1966.

21 Laster, L., et al., Homocystinuria Due to Cystathionine Synthase Deficiency. *Ann. Intern. Med.* **63:**1117–1142, 1965.

22 Loughridge, L. W., Renal Abnormalities in the Marfan Syndrome. *Q. J. Med.* **28:**531–544, 1959.

23 Lynas, M. A., Marfan's Syndrome in Northern Ireland: An Account of Thirteen Families. *Ann. Hum. Genet.* **22:**289–301, 1958.

24 McCully, K. S., and Ragsdale, B. D., Production of Arteriosclerosis by Homocystinuria. *Am. J. Pathol.* **61:**1–8, 1970.

25 McDonald, L., et al., Homocystinuria, Thrombosis and the Blood-platelets. *Lancet* **1:**745–746, 1964.

26 McKusick, V. A., *Heritable Disorders of Connective Tissue*, 4th ed., Mosby, 1972, pp. 224–276.

27 Mönch, E., et al., Neuroblastoma Typ Pepper mit Homocystinurie. *Helv. Paediat. Acta* **25:**530–541, 1970.

28 Morreels, S. H., et al., The Roentgenographic Features of Homocystinuria. *Radiology* **90:**1150–1158, 1968.

29 Mudd, S. H., et al., Homocystinuria: An Enzymatic Defect. *Science* **143:**1443–1445, 1964.

30 Mudd, S. H., et al., Homocystinuria Due to Cystathionine Synthase Deficiency: The Effect of Pyridoxine. *J. Clin. Invest.* **49:**1762–1773, 1970.

31 Perry, T. L., et al., Homolanthionine Excretion of Homocystinuria. *Science* **152:**1750–1752, 1966.

32 Pirie, A., and van Heyningen, R., *Biochemistry of the Eye.* Charles C Thomas, Springfield, Ill., 1956, pp. 12–31, 60–63.

33 Presley, G. D., et al., Homocystinuria at the North Carolina State School for the Blind. *Am. J. Ophthalmol.* **66:**884–889, 1968.

34 Ratnoff, O. D., Activation of Hageman Factor by L-Homocystine. *Science* **162:**1007–1009, 1968.

34a Schedewie, H., et al., Skeletal Findings in Homocystinuria. *Pediatr. Radiol.* **1:**12–23, 1973.

35 Schimke, R. N., et al., Homocystinuria. *J.A.M.A.* **193:**711–719, 1965.

36 Smith, S. W., Roentgen Findings in Homocystinuria. *Am. J. Roentgenol.* **100:**147–154, 1967.

37 White, H. H., et al., Homocystinuria. *Arch. Neurol.* **13:**455–470, 1965.

38 Yoshida, T. K., et al., Homocystinuria of Vitamin B-6 Dependent Type. *Tohoku J. Exp. Med.* **96:**235–242, 1968.

68

Hyalinosis Cutis et Mucosae

(Urbach-Wiethe Syndrome, Lipoid Proteinosis)

The syndrome, consisting of (a) yellowish nodular infiltration of skin and mucous membranes, and (b) hoarseness, was first described by Siebenmann (19) in 1908. Other cases were described in the 1920s, but credit is usually given to Urbach and Wiethe (23, 24, 26), who defined the condition and applied the terms "lipoidosis cutis et mucosae" and "lipoid proteinosis" (11). The history of the syndrome has been reviewed by Laymon and Hill (11), and Gordon (4). About 200 cases have been described to date (2, 3, 4, 6, 11).

The syndrome is transmitted as an autosomal recessive trait. It has appeared in sibs (3, 6, 8, 17, 21, 24), and in about 20 percent of the cases there has been parental consanguinity (1, 2, 12). Many patients have been of German extraction.

SYSTEMIC MANIFESTATIONS

Skin and skin appendages. Discrete or confluent yellowish-ivory or waxy nodules, from pinhead to matchhead in size, usually occur on the face, neck, axillas, and hands early in life. Some patients develop pustular or bullous lesions of the face and upper extremities; on healing, these lesions leave mauve, pitted, atrophic patches (4) (Fig. 68-1).

On the margin of the eyelids, beadlike excrescences appear in about 50 percent of patients followed by loss of cilia (11, 16) (Fig. 68-2A). Brownish-yellow, wartlike hyperkeratotic le-sions appear on the knees, elbows, and proxi-mal interarticular surfaces of the fingers (4) (Fig. 68-2B).

Diffuse, nonscarring alopecia, often in the occipital area, or thinning of the scalp hair and beard, at times transient, has been noted by several authors (2, 20, 21). Eyelashes are often lost.

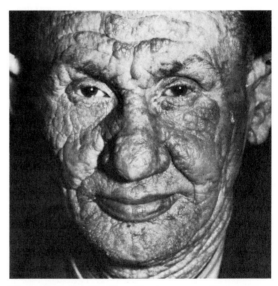

Figure 68-1. *Hyalinosis cutis et mucosae.* Note numerous raised yellowish nodules. (*Courtesy of K. H. Holtz,* Arch. Klin. Exp. Dermatol. **214**:289, 1962.)

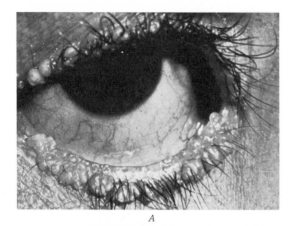

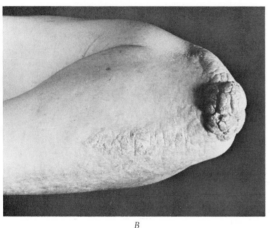

A

B

Figure 68-2. (*A*). Beadlike excrescences along eyelid margins. (*From A. R. Rosenthal and J. R. Duke,* Am. J. Ophthalmol. **64:**1120, 1967.) (*B*). Verrucous lesion of elbow. (*From R. C. Juberg et al.,* J. Med. Genet. **12:**116, 1975.)

Central nervous system. Intracranial calcification, found in at least 70 percent of cases, has been located above the pituitary fossa in the hippocampus, falx cerebri, or temporal lobes (2, 4, 5, 8, 11, 13, 17, 25), and may be more often seen in individuals over the age of ten years (4). It has also been associated with psychomotor and grand mal epilepsy or rage attacks (2, 11–13) (Fig. 68-3). Specifically it has been found in the caudate nucleus, globus pallidus, and amygdaloid nucleus (13).

Larynx and other mucosal involvement. The voice may be hoarse from birth or within the

first few years of life. The inability to cry at birth in the majority of cases testifies to early laryngeal involvement. Laryngoscopic examination reveals yellowish-white plaques on the epiglottis, aryepiglottic folds, and interarytenoid region (4, 7a, 14). The cords are thickened and nodular, and closure is insufficient. Dyspnea may be severe, and laryngectomy may be necessary (1).

Other mucosal surfaces, such as the vulva, esophagus, stomach, and rectum are rarely affected (2, 4, 7, 24).

Oral manifestations. The mouth is the most extensively involved area. Nearly all oral tissues become infiltrated with yellowish-white, elevated, pea-size plaques, which appear most frequently before puberty and gradually increase in severity. The lower lip, usually more severely affected, assumes a cobblestone appearance (Fig. 68-4*A*). Radiating fissures may appear at the angles of the mouth (11).

The tongue becomes firm or woody, thick, large, and bound to the floor of the mouth, with marked infiltration of the frenum and sublingual and fimbriated plicae, which become inelastic

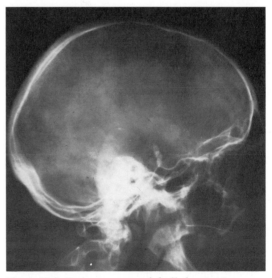

Figure 68-3. Roentgenogram of skull showing intracranial calcification in the region of the dorsum sellae. Calcification can also occur in the temporal lobes of the brain, with resultant epilepsy. (*Courtesy of K. H. Holtz,* Arch. Klin. Exp. Dermatol. **214:**289, 1962.)

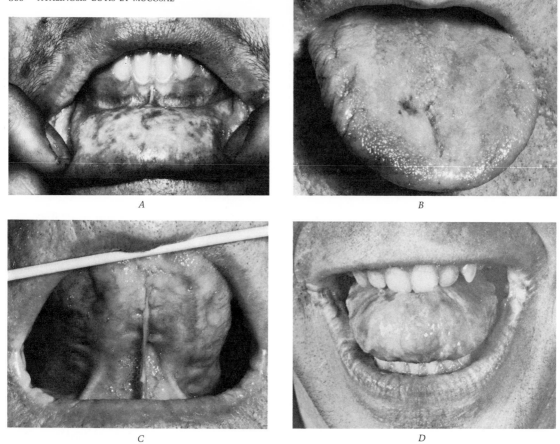

Figure 68-4. (*A*). Extensive infiltration of lower lip. (*From J. A. Keipert*, Aust. Paediatr. J. **6**:135, 1970.) (*B, C*). Tongue is thickened and indurated with plaques on dorsum, sides, and undersurface. (*From R. F. Dickey and S. Davis*, Ann. Otol. Rhinol. Laryngol. **73**:287, 1964.) (*D*). Advance infiltration of tongue in adult. (*From R. C. Juberg et al.*, J. Med. Genet. **12**:110, 1975.)

cords. The dorsum loses its papillae. Ulcers may develop (1, 27) (Fig. 68-4*B, C, D*).

With infiltration of the buccal mucosa, the opening of the parotid duct may become stenosed, with ensuing retrograde parotitis (1, 5, 11, 12, 20). Extension of the infiltration to the tonsils and pharynx may result in dysphagia. The uvula is involved and usually retracted (Fig. 68-5).

Teeth may fail to develop or may be hypoplastic, especially the upper lateral incisors, canines, and upper or lower second premolar teeth (4, 6–9, 11); or the enamel may be severely hypoplastic (16, 23).

DIFFERENTIAL DIAGNOSIS

Conditions to be considered include systematized amyloidosis, colloid milium, adenoma sebaceum, and *pseudoxanthoma elasticum*.

LABORATORY AIDS

A diabetic tendency has been stated to be part of the syndrome (20, 23), but there is insufficient evidence to support this contention (7). A slight elevation in phospholipid level has been reported in some patients (5). Several investigators have

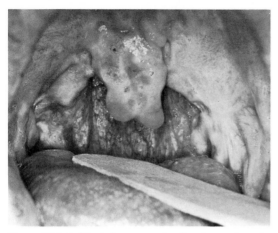

Figure 68-5. Infiltrated mucosa of soft palate and uvula. (*From W. Mootz, Homburg, Saar, Germany.*)

noted an increase in alpha 2- and gamma-globulin levels and a diminution in the concentration of albumins (4, 5, 8), but these changes have been denied by others (11).

Microscopically, there is hyalinosis of the upper layers of the corium or dermis, beginning about the small arterioles or sweat glands and by extension to infiltrate the entire subepithelial area (Fig. 68-6*A*, *B*). Visceral involvement has also been demonstrated (2). Histochemical study (5) has revealed the presence of carbohydrate but few or no lipids. The hyaline material stains intensely with the PAS procedure (22), thus appearing to be a glycoprotein either free or loosely bound to collagen (3, 7, 18). Ultrastructural studies have been carried out on the hyaline material (6, 10, 15). Hashimoto et al. (6) and Newton et al. (13) have suggested that it represents an altered collagen.

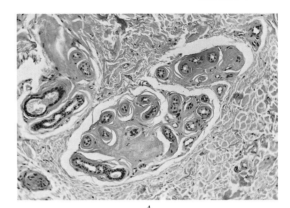

A

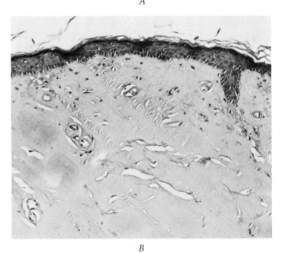

B

Figure 68-6. (*A*). Deposition of hyaline material around sweat glands in lower dermis. (*From R. Shore,* Arch. Dermatol. **110**:591, 1974.) (*B*). Amorphous deposits lying directly beneath epithelium. (*From A. R. Rosenthal and J. R. Dukes,* Am. J. Ophthalmol. **64**:1120, 1967.)

REFERENCES

1 Burnett, J. W., and Marcy, S. M., Lipoid Proteinosis. *Am. J. Dis. Child.* **105**:81–84, 1963.

2 Caplan, R. M., Visceral Involvement in Lipoid Proteinosis. *Arch. Dermatol.* **95**:149–155, 1967.

3 Fleischmayer, R., et al., Hyalinosis Cutis et Mucosae: A Histochemical Staining and Analytical Biochemical Study. *J. Invest. Dermatol.* **52**:495–503, 1969.

4 Gordon, H., et al., Lipoid Proteinosis. *Birth Defects* **7**(8):164–177, 1972.

5 Grosfeld, J. C. M., et al., Hyalinosis Cutis et Mucosae (Lipoid Proteinosis Urbach-Wiethe). *Dermatologica* **130**:239–266, 1965.

6 Hashimoto, K., et al., Hyalinosis Cutis et Mucosae: An Electronmicroscopic Study. *Acta Derm. Venereol* (Stockh.) **52**:179–195, 1972.

7 Hofer, P., Urbach-Wiethe Disease. *Acta Derm. Venereol.* (Stockh.) **53**:(Suppl. 71):1–52, 1973.

7a Hofer, P. A., and Öhman, J., Laryngeal Lesions in Urbach-Wiethe Disease. *Acta Pathol. Microbiol. Scand.* **82A**:547–558, 1974.

8 Holtz, K. H., Über Gehirn-und Augenveränderungen bei Hyalinosis cutis et mucosae mit Autopsiebefund. *Arch. Klin. Exp. Dermatol.* **214**:289–306, 1962.

9 Jensen, A., Lipoidosis Cutis et Mucosae (Lipoid Pro-

teinosis) in 2 Brothers. *Acta Derm. Venereol. (Stockh.)* **42:**164–166, 1962.

9a Juberg, R. C., et al., A Case of Hyalinosis Cutis et Mucosae with Common Ancestors in Four Remote Generations. *J. Med. Genet.* **12:**110–112, 1975.

10 König, W. F., Elektronenmikroskopische Untersuchungen bei Hyalinosis cutis et mucosae. *Z. Laryngol. Rhinol.* **45:**672–675, 1966.

11 Laymon, C. W., and Hill, E. M., An Appraisal of Hyalinosis Cutis et Mucosae. *Arch. Dermatol.* **75:**55–65, 1957.

12 Macleod, W., Hyalinosis Cutis et Mucosae. *Ann. Radiol.* **9:**305–310, 1966.

13 Newton, F. H., et al., Neurologic Involvement in Urbach-Wiethe's Disease. *Neurology (Minneap.)* **21:**1205–1213, 1971.

14 Richards, S. H., and Bull, P. D., Lipoid Proteinosis. *J. Laryngol. Otol.* **87:**187–190, 1973.

15 Rodermund, O. E., and Klingmüller, G., Elektronenmikroskopische Befunde des Hyalins bei Hyalinosis cutis et mucosae. *Arch. Klin. Exp. Dermatol.* **236:**238–249, 1970.

16 Rosenthal, A. R., and Duke, J. R., Lipoid Proteinosis: Case Report of Direct Lineal Transmission. *Am. J. Ophthalmol.* **64:**1120–1125, 1967.

17 Scott, F. P., and Findlay, G. H., Hyalinosis Cutis et Mucosae (Lipoid Proteinosis). *S. Afr. Med. J.* **34:**189–195, 1960.

18 Shore, R. N., et al., Lipoid Proteinosis. *Arch. Dermatol.* **110:**591–594, 1974.

19 Siebenmann, F., Über Mitbeteiligung der Schleimhaut bei allgemeiner Hyperkeratose der Haut. *Arch. Laryngol.* **20:**101–109, 1908.

20 Tompkins, J., and Weinstein, I. M., Lipoid Proteinosis: Two Case Reports Including Liver Biopsies, Special Blood Lipid Analysis and Treatment with a Lipotropic Agent. *Ann. Intern. Med.* **41:**163–171, 1954.

21 Tripp, R. N., Lipoidosis Cutis et Mucosae. *N.Y. State J. Med.* **36:**619–626, 1936.

22 Ungar, H., and Katzenellenbogen, I., Hyalinosis of Skin and Mucous Membrane (Urbach-Wiethe's Lipoid Proteinosis). *Arch. Pathol.* **63:**65–74, 1957.

23 Urbach, E., Über eine familiäre lokale Lipoidose der Haut und der Schleimhaute auf Grundlage einer diabetischen Stoffwechselstörung. *Arch. Dermatol. Syph. (Berl.)* **159:**451–466, 1929.

24 Urbach, E., and Wiethe, C., Lipoidosis Cutis et Mucosae. *Virchows Arch. [Pathol. Anat.]* **273:**285–319, 1929.

25 Weidner, W. A., et al., Roentgenographic Findings in Lipoid Proteinosis. *Am. J. Roentgenol.* **110:**457–461, 1970.

26 Wiethe, C., Kongenitale diffuse Hyalinablagerungen in den oberen Luftwegen familiärer auftretend. *Z. Hals. Nas. Ohrenheilkd.*, **10:**359–362, 1924.

27 Wile, W. J., and Snow, J. S., Lipoid Proteinosis. *Arch. Dermatol. Syph. (Chic.)* **43:**134–144, 1941.

28 Wood, M. G., et al., Histochemical Study of a Case of Lipoid Proteinosis. *J. Invest. Dermatol.* **26:**263–274, 1956.

69

Hyperkeratosis Palmoplantaris and Attached Gingival Hyperkeratosis

Raphael et al. (5) reported the combination of hyperkeratosis palmophantaris and attached gingival hyperkeratosis in a kindred involving several generations. In 1974, while visiting Athens, Greece, one of us (R. J. G.) had the opportunity to see another family with the same disorder and, in 1975, examined a large affected kindred in Minneapolis (3). Other examples were reported by Fred et al. (1) and James and Beggs (4).

Autosomal dominant inheritance is indicated by transmission of the disorder through several generations. There was male-to-male transmission in all kindreds.

SYSTEMIC MANIFESTATIONS

Skin and skin appendages. Focal hyperkeratosis of the soles was more marked over the weight-bearing areas: the heels, toe pads, and metatarsal heads (Fig. 69-1). Hyperkeratosis of the palms also seemed trauma-related (Fig. 69-2). Hyperhidrosis was noted in the hyperkeratotic areas. The hyperkeratotic areas appeared around puberty in most patients. Involvement of the distal portion of the finger and toe nails with keratin deposits first involved the toes at four to five years of age followed by fingernail changes at eight to nine years of age.

Oral manifestations. Sharply marginated hyperkeratosis involved the labial and lingual at-tached gingiva (Fig. 69-3). The hyperkeratotic area appeared in early childhood and increased in severity with age.

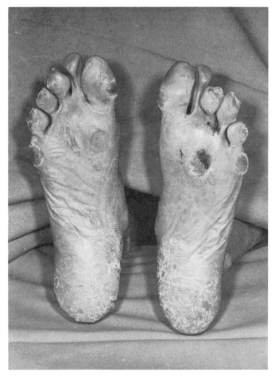

Figure 69-1. *Hyperkeratosis palmoplantaris and attached gingival hyperkeratosis.* Numerous focal hyperkeratoses of soles, especially over pressure points.

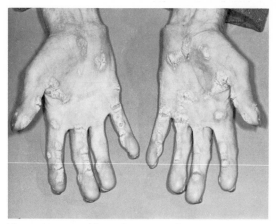

Figure 69-2. Focal hyperkeratoses of palms.

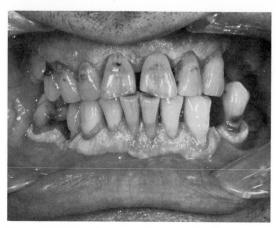

Figure 69-3. Hyperkeratosis limited to fixed gingiva.

DIFFERENTIAL DIAGNOSIS

As indicated in Chap. 70, there is a plethora of disorders which may be associated with hyperkeratosis palmoplantaris (2). Generalized oral hyperkeratosis has been noted in patients with autosomal dominant tylosis and esophageal carcinoma (6).

LABORATORY AIDS

Biopsy is of no value in establishing the diagnosis.

REFERENCES

1 Fred, H. L., et al., Keratosis palmaris et plantaris. *Arch. Intern. Med.* **113:**866–871, 1974.
2 Gibbs, R. C., and Costello, M. J., *The Palms and Soles in Medicine.* Charles C Thomas, Springfield, Ill., 1967.
3 Gorlin, R. J., Hyperkeratosis Palmoplantaris and Attached Gingival Hyperkeratosis. *Birth Defects* (in press).
4 James, P., and Beggs, D., Tylosis: A Case Report. *Br. J. Oral Surg.* **11:**143–145, 1973.

5 Raphael, A. L., et al., Hyperkeratosis of Gingival and Plantar Surfaces. *Periodontics* **6:**118–120, 1968.
6 Tyldesley, W. R., Oral Leukoplakia Associated with Tylosis and Esophageal Carcinoma. *J. Oral Pathol.* **3:**62–70, 1974.

70

Hyperkeratosis Palmoplantaris
and Periodontoclasia in Childhood

(Papillon-Lefèvre Syndrome)

Papillon and Lefèvre (19), in 1924, described a syndrome consisting of (a) hyperkeratosis of palms and soles, and (b) destruction of the supporting tissues of both primary and secondary dentitions. They conceived of the disorder as a variant of mal de Meleda.

The syndrome is inherited as an autosomal recessive trait (9). In several cases there has been evidence of parental consanguinity (1, 2, 7, 16, 19).

SYSTEMIC MANIFESTATIONS

Skin. At approximately the same time that periodontal involvement first occurs, i.e., sometime between the second and fourth years of life, or on rare occasions even earlier (1, 4, 5), the palms and soles become red and scaly. The hyperkeratotic involvement of the palms is usually quite well demarcated, extending to the edges and over the thenar eminences. The soles are usually more severely involved, the process frequently spilling over the edges, where it may be most marked, extending to the Achilles tendon (Fig. 70-1A–C). Occasionally, the external malleoli, tibial tuberosities, and dorsal finger and toe joints may exhibit a scaly redness. The degree of hyperkeratosis is not severe, but the normal skin markings become accentuated and the skin assumes a parchment-like quality. The degree of involvement seems to fluctuate. Some authors have indicated that this fluctua-

tion is seasonal (1, 4). It should be pointed out, however, that some degree of palmoplantar hyperkeratosis remains throughout life. Greither (11) noted improvement after exfoliation of teeth. Nails are rarely, if ever, involved.

Other findings. Calcium deposits in the attachment of the tentorium and choroid (4–6, 10, 16, 20, 21) have been reported, but it is uncertain whether this finding is significant.

Oral manifestations. The development and eruption of the deciduous teeth proceed normally, but almost simultaneously with the appearance of palmar and plantar hyperkeratosis, the gingiva swell and become boggy, and marked halitosis develops. Destruction of the periodontium follows almost immediately the eruption of the last primary molar tooth. The teeth are involved in roughly the same order in which they erupt. Deep periodontal pocket formation precedes the exfoliation of teeth. By the age of four years, nearly all primary teeth have been lost. After exfoliation, the inflammation subsides and the gingiva resumes its normal appearance. The mouth then appears normal until the secondary (permanent) dentition erupts, when the process is repeated in essentially the same manner. Only the third molars do not exfoliate. Bony destruction is usually severe, and the alveolar process is often completely destroyed. Even during the stage of active periodontal breakdown, the rest

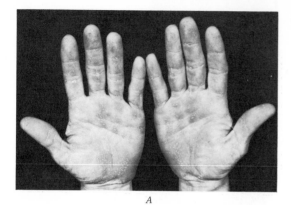

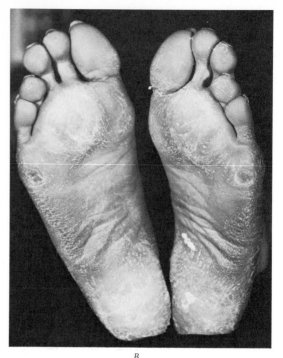

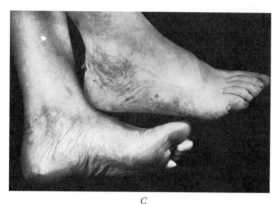

A

C

B

Figure 70-1. *Hyperkeratosis palmoplantaris and perio-dontoclasia in childhood* (Papillon-Lefèvre syndrome). (*A–C*). Sharply demarcated hyperkeratosis of hands and feet. (*C, from R. K. Hall,* Aust. Dent. J. **8:**185, 1963.)

of the oral tissue appears perfectly normal (Fig. 70-2*A, B*).

DIFFERENTIAL DIAGNOSIS

Premature loss of deciduous and/or permanent teeth occurs with trauma and in *acrodynia,* histiocytosis X, hypophosphatasia, leukemia, the neutropenias, acatalasia, *Chediak-Higashi syndrome,* and idiopathic periodontosis (8, 18).

Premature tooth loss may be observed in hypophosphatasia, a condition transmitted as an autosomal recessive trait which, because of a deficiency in alkaline phosphatase, produces a rickets-like condition. In addition to genu valgum, bowing of the femurs and tibias, enlarged wrists, and other signs, the teeth are prematurely shed, often hypoplastic, and deficient in cementum. There is an increased amount of phosphoethanolamine in the urine (3, 15).

Acatalasia is transmitted as an autosomal recessive trait and has rarely been observed outside Japan. It is characterized by progressive gangrenous lesions involving the gingiva and alveolar bone, resulting in exfoliation of teeth (24).

Hyperkeratosis palmaris has been seen in association with a dentinogenesis imperfecta-like condition (27) and a host of other disorders (8, 9). It may also occur in the syndrome of *hyperkeratosis palmoplantaris and attached gingival hyperkeratosis.*

Haim and Munk (12) and Smith and Rosenzweig (22) reported several members in three related families with an unusual syndrome consisting of congenital palmoplantar keratosis, progressive periodontal disease, arachnodactyly, and a peculiar deformity of the fingers, consisting of tapered pointed phalangeal ends and a claw-like volar curve. In all these patients, the skin manifestations were severe, with involvement

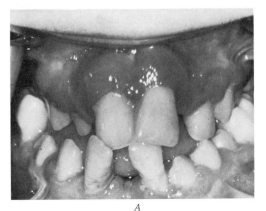 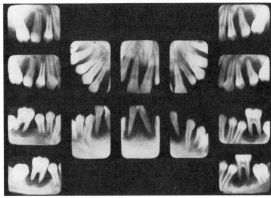

A	B

Figure 70-2. (*A*). Severe periodontal disease in seven-year-old child. (*B*). Roentgenogram showing extensive periodontal destruction. (*From J. S. Giansanti et al.*, Oral Surg., *in press.*)

of other sites as well. The periodontium was less severely affected than in the Papillon-Lefèvre syndrome.

LABORATORY AIDS

None is known.

REFERENCES

1 Bach, J. N., and Levan, N. E., Papillon-Lefèvre Syndrome. *Arch. Dermatol.* **97:**154–158, 1968.
2 Barriere, H., and Delaire, –, Keratodermie, type Papillon-Lefèvre. *Bull. Soc. Fr. Dermatol. Syphiligr.* **65:**114–115, 1958.
3 Beumer, J., et al., Childhood Hypophosphatasia and the Premature Loss of Teeth. *Oral Surg.* **35:**631–640, 1973.
4 Brownstein, M. H., and Skolnik, P., Papillon-Lefèvre Syndrome. *Arch. Dermatol.* **106:**533–534, 1972.
5 Corson, E. F., Keratosis Palmaris et Plantaris with Dental Alteration. *Arch. Dermatol. Syph.* **40:**639, 1939.
6 Dekker, G., and Jansen, L. H., Periodontosis in a Child with Hyperkeratosis Palmo-plantares *J. Periodontol.* **29:**266–271, 1958.
7 Galanter, D., and Bradford, S., Hyperkeratosis Palmo-plantaris and Periodontosis. *J. Periodontol.* **40:**40–47, 1969.
8 Giansanti, J. S., et al., Palmar-plantar Hyperkeratosis and Concomitant Periodontal Destruction (Papillon-Lefèvre Syndrome). *Oral Surg.* **36:**40–48, 1973.
9 Gorlin, R. J., and Chaudhry, A. P., The Oral Manifestations of Cyclic Neutropenia. *Arch. Dermatol.* **82:**344–348, 1960.
10 Gorlin, R. J., et al., The Syndrome of Palmar-plantar Hyperkeratosis and Premature Periodontal Destruction of the Teeth. *J. Pediatr.* **65:**895–908, 1964.
11 Greither, A., Keratosis palmo-plantaris mit Periodontopathie (Papillon-Lefèvre). *Dermatologica* **119:**248–263, 1959.
12 Haim, S., and Munk, J., Keratosis Palmo-plantaris Congenita, with Periodontosis, Arachnodactyly and Peculiar Deformity of the Terminal Phalanges. *Br. J. Dermatol.* **77:**42–54, 1965.
13 Hall, R. K., Papillon-Lefèvre Syndrome. *Australian Dent. J.* **8:**185–188, 1963.
14 Herforth, A., et al., Juvenile Parodontopathien und Hauterkrankungen. *Dtsch. Zahnärztl. Z.* **28:**242–246, 1973.
15 Illingsworth, R. S., and Gardiner, J. H., Premature Loss of Deciduous Teeth. *Arch. Dis. Child.* **30:**449–452, 1955.
16 Jansen, L. H., and Dekker, G., Hyperkeratosis Palmo-plantaris with Periodontosis (Papillon-Lefèvre). *Dermatologica* **113:**207–219, 1956.
17 Lalis, R. R., et al., A Case of Papillon-Lefevre Syndrome. *Periodontics* **3:**292–295, 1965.
18 Manson, J. D., and Lehner, T., Clinical Features of Juvenile Periodontitis (Periodontosis). *J. Periodontol.* **45:**636–640, 1974.
19 Papillon, –, and Lefèvre, P., Deux cas de kératodermie palmaire et plantaire symétrique familiale (maladie de Meleda) chez le frère et la soeur. Coexistence dans les deux cas d'altérations dentaires graves. *Bull. Soc. Fr. Dermatol. Syphiligr.* **31:**82–84, 1924.
20 Piquet, B., et al., Kératodermie palmaire et plantaire (Papillon-Lefèvre syndrome). *Rev. Stomatol. (Paris)* **70:**446–459, 1969.
21 Rosenthal, S. L., Periodontosis in a Child Resulting in Exfoliation of the Teeth. *J. Periodontol.* **22:**101–104, 1951.
22 Smith, P., and Rosenzweig, K. A., Seven Cases of Papillon-

Lefevre Syndrome. *Periodontics* **5**:42–46, 1967.

23 Stevanovic, D. V., Keratoderma with Periodontopathy. *Dermatologica* **123**:119–128, 1961.

24 Takahara, S., Acotalasemia and Hypocatalasemia in the Orient. *Seminars Hematol.* **8**:397–416, 1971.

25 Woods, E. C., and Wallace, W. R. J., A Case of Alveolar Atrophy of Unknown Origin in a Child. *Oral Surg.* **27**:676, 1941.

26 Zellner, R., Die Klinik und Morphologie der Capdepontischen Erkrankung. *Dtsch. Zahnärztl. Z.* **15**:479–486, 1960.

27 Ziprkowski, L., et al., Hyperkeratosis Palmo-plantaris with Periodontosis (Papillon-Lèfevre). *Arch. Dermatol.* **88**:207–209, 1967.

71

Hypertelorism-Hypospadias Syndrome

(*Opitz Syndrome*)

In 1965 Opitz et al. (3) reported a syndrome consisting of (*a*) hypertelorism, (*b*) hypospadias, and (*c*) other anomalies. Subsequently, Opitz et al. (4) described their findings in detail. Christian et al. (1) reported a family with possibly the same syndrome.

Autosomal dominant inheritance, incomplete penetrance, variable expressivity, and predominant male sex limitation seem likely. The most severe manifestations of the syndrome are observed in affected males. Hypertelorism may be the only expression in affected females, and some female transmitters of the gene show no manifestations of the disorder. One instance of male-to-male transmission was reported by Opitz et al. (4).

It is possible that some sporadic and some familial cases of hypertelorism or hypospadias with or without some of the less common findings may represent examples of this syndrome (4). However, it may be difficult or impossible to establish diagnosis with certainty in such cases. Further studies are necessary to delineate the complete spectrum of anomalies that may be associated with the hypertelorism-hypospadias syndrome.

SYSTEMIC MANIFESTATIONS

Eyes. Hypertelorism is the most commonly observed manifestation. Slight mongoloid or antimongoloid obliquity, epicanthic folds, and strabismus have been observed occasionally (1, 3, 4) (Fig. 71-1).

Ears. Posteriorly rotated ears have been reported in a few instances (2, 4).

Cranium. Cranial asymmetry was noted in several cases by Christian et al. (1). Brachycephaly, prominent forehead, prominent metopic suture,

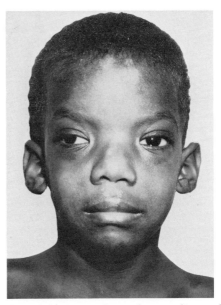

Figure 71-1. *Hypertelorism-hypospadias syndrome.* Wide-spaced eyes. (*From J. M. Opitz et al.,* Birth Defects 5(2):82, 1969.)

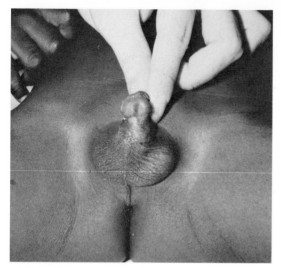

Figure 71-2. Hypospadias. *(From J. M. Opitz et al.* Birth Defects **5**(2):82, 1969.)

widow's peak, and low-set anterior and posterior scalp line have been observed occasionally (1, 4). Nevus flammeus has also been noted (1).

Central nervous system. Mild to moderate mental deficiency was reported by Opitz et al. (4) and by Michaelis and Mortimer (2).

Genitourinary system. Hypospadias is the most commonly observed anomaly in affected males (Fig. 71-2). Cryptorchism, ureteral stenosis, urethrocolic fistula, and inguinal hernia have also been noted (1, 4, 5).

Other findings. Coarctation of the aorta, atrial septal defect, imperforate anus, diastasis recti, multiple lipomas, and slight hyperextensibility of joints have been observed in some instances (1, 4, 5). Distally placed axial triradii, increased number of arches, and bridged simian creases have been reported occasionally (3).

Oral manifestations. Cleft lip-palate, micrognathia, fused and supernumerary teeth, and malocclusion have been noted in some cases (1, 2, 4, 5).

DIFFERENTIAL DIAGNOSIS

Hypertelorism and hypospadias may be observed in the *hypospadias-dysphagia syndrome.* However, neuromuscular defect of the esophagus and swallowing mechanism together with the overall pattern of anomalies observed in the hypospadias-dysphagia syndrome clearly distinguish it from the hypertelorism-hypospadias syndrome. Hypertelorism and hypospadias may each be observed as isolated anomalies or in association with various other malformation syndromes.

LABORATORY AIDS

None is known.

REFERENCES

1 Christian, J. C., et al., Familial Telecanthus with Associated Congenital Anomalies. *Birth Defects* **5**(2):82–85, 1969.
2 Michaelis, E., and Mortimer, W., Association of Hypertelorism and Hypospadias in the BBB Syndrome. *Helv. Paediatr. Acta* **27**:575–581, 1972.
3 Opitz, J. M., et al., Hypertelorism and Hypospadias: A Newly Recognized Hereditary Malformation Syndrome. (Abstr.) *J. Pediatr.* **67**:968, 1965.
4 Opitz, J. M., et al., The BBB Syndrome: Familial Telecanthus with Associated Congenital Anomalies. *Birth Defects* **5**(2):86–94, 1969.
5 Sanchez Cascos, A., Genetics of Atrial Septal Defect. *Arch. Dis. Child.* **47**:581–588, 1972.

72

Hypohidrotic Ectodermal Dysplasia

(Anhidrotic Ectodermal Dysplasia)

This syndrome, ordinarily considered to be a triad of (a) hypodontia, (b) hypotrichosis, and (c) hypohidrosis, is usually associated with other components resulting from defective development of structures of ectodermal origin (3).

Charles Darwin (10) cited Wedderburn as having found this complex among a closely inbred Indian group as early as 1838, and it may have been recorded as early as 1792 by Danz, according to Perabo (40). Christ (5), in 1913, further defined it as a "congenital ectodermal defect," and Weech (55), in 1929, impressed by the depression of sweat gland function, coined the term "anhidrotic ectodermal dysplasia." Felsher (12), in 1944, pointed out that the skin is rarely, if ever, completely anhidrotic, and suggested the adjective "hypohidrotic," which appears to be a far better choice. The reader is referred to the study of Perabo (40) for an excellent analysis of sign and symptom frequency.

Analysis of over 300 cases reveals that the syndrome is usually transmitted as an X-linked trait, the gene being carried by the female and manifested in the male (35, 52). However, at least 35 females have exhibited the complete syndrome, and it is probable that most of these cases are examples of the autosomal recessive form of the condition (20, 28, 39).

In the X-linked form, the carrier mothers exhibit minimal expression of the gene in the form of hypodontia and/or conical crowned teeth and spottily reduced sweating. This is consistent with the Lyon hypothesis for variability of expression (27, 29).

Several unorthodox patterns of inheritance have been reported. These cases have been reviewed by Gorlin et al. (20) and by Franceschetti (14). Dominant hidrotic forms of ectodermal dysplasia are discussed under Differential Diagnosis.

SYSTEMIC MANIFESTATIONS

Facies. Though the physiognomy is quite characteristic and affected individuals from different families look enough alike to be sibs, the condition may not be apparent until the second year of life. The skull resembles an inverted triangle. The combination of frontal bossing, usually marked, and a depressed nasal bridge—somewhat resembling the saddle nose of congenital syphilis—gives the observer the impression that the face is small. The lips are protuberant, and the ears may be inserted obliquely into the head, causing them to stand out (40, 43) (Fig. 72-1A–C).

Skin and skin appendages. The most remarkable characteristic of this disorder is hypohidrosis. Because the physical features are not so apparent in the first year, the child may present with a "fever of unknown origin." The inability to sweat, predicated upon marked aplasia of eccrine sweat glands, results in intolerance to heat, with severe incapacitation and hyperpyrexia after only mild exertion or even following meals.

The skin is soft and thin. Dryness is often severe, because of the absence of sebaceous glands (26), and flexural eczema of atopic type is common, especially during the early years of

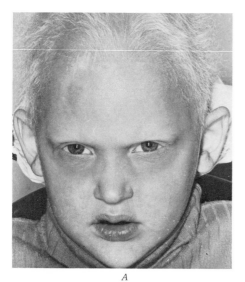

A

life. Fine, linear wrinkles and increased pigmentation are often noted about the eyes and mouth. The palms and soles are frequently the sites of small hyperkeratoses. The body is usually devoid of lanugo hair, and after puberty, although the beard is usually normal, the axillary and pubic hair is frequently scant. The scalp hair is often blond, fine, stiff, and short. The eyelashes and, especially, the eyebrows are often missing (43).

The nails are usually normal or somewhat spoon-shaped (55), but the mammary glands have been noted by several observers to be aplastic or hypoplastic (38, 52). Dermatoglyphic alterations have been described (41, 53).

Eyes. Lacrimal gland function has been diminished in a few cases (21, 31). Congenital glaucoma has been occasionally noted (25, 47).

Other findings. Beahrs (2) pointed out the increased susceptibility of these individuals to allergic disorders, especially asthma and eczema, as noted above.

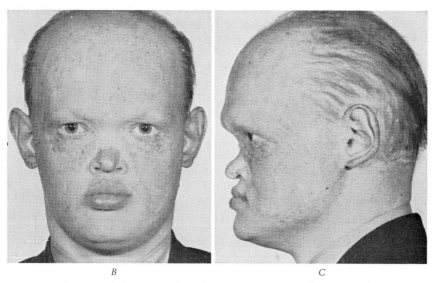

B   *C*

Figure 72-1. (*A*). *Hypohidrotic ectodermal dysplasia.* Female with autosomal recessive type. Note sparse hair and fine linear wrinkling around eyes. (*From R. J. Gorlin et al.,* Z. Kinderheilkd. **108**:1, 1970.) (*B*, *C*). X-linked recessive inherited form. Facies is characterized by frontal bossing, depressed nasal bridge, outstanding ears, thin hair, and pouting lips.

Oral manifestations. The most striking oral alteration is hypodontia or, in many cases, anodontia, reflecting complete suppression of dental ectoderm. The few teeth that may be present are often retarded in eruption. Because of the hypodontia and the resultant loss of vertical dimension, the lips are protuberant. The vermilion border is indistinct and pseudorhagades may be present (40, 52).

The alveolar process does not develop in the absence of teeth and, hence, is missing (11, 37, 45, 48, 51). However, cephalometric studies by Sarnat et al. (48) have indicated that apart from defective alveolar growth, jaw and facial development are essentially normal. Cephalometric study has also been carried out by Lipshutz (30).

The incisors, canines, and premolars, when present, often have conical crowns (Fig. 72-2*A*, *B*). The shape of the crown is determined by the inner enamel or ameloblastic layer of the tooth germ. Why this particular form eventuates is not known, but it apparently represents incomplete expression of anodontia.

It has been stated by a few investigators that the oral mucosa appears "dry." Histopathologic studies of Fleischmann (13), Everett et al. (11), Sackett et al. (45), and Capitanio et al. (4) have shown aplasia of the labial and buccal mucous glands and those of the lower part of the respiratory tract. Pharyngeal and laryngeal mucosa may be atrophic, resulting in dysphonia. Several authors have described atrophy of the nasal mu-

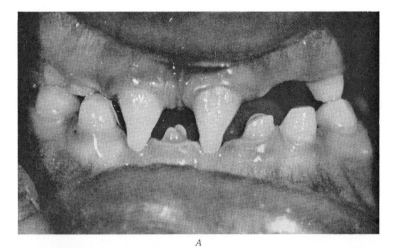

A

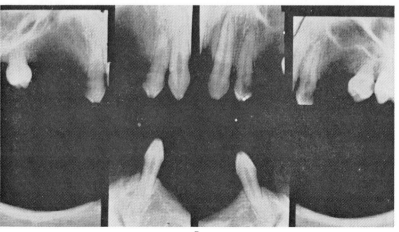

B

Figure 72-2. (*A*). Hypodontia and conical crown tooth form in fourteen-year-old female. No other stigmata present; possible carrier of trait. (*B*). Dental roentgenograms of patient seen in Fig. 72-1*B, C*. Note hypodontia and conical form of tooth crowns.

cosa associated with severe crusting and marked ozena, characterized by a fetid green secretion (13, 40). Scintilligraphic and biochemical studies (33) have suggested an inflammatory process in the parotid glands.

DIFFERENTIAL DIAGNOSIS

Although the physiognomy is distinctive, several facets of the syndrome resemble those of other disorders. The term "ectodermal dysplasia" has been employed in the generic sense to describe disorders that are clearly unrelated to hypohidrotic ectodermal dysplasia (7, 16, 46).

The nasal deformity and linear perioral scarring may suggest congenital syphilis. The conical teeth are virtually identical with those seen in idiopathic oligodontia, *chondroectodermal dysplasia, Rieger syndrome,* and *incontinentia pigmenti.* Witkop (59), Hinrichsen (24), and Redpath and Winter (42) described autosomal dominantly inherited hypodontia and nail dysplasia (*tooth-nail syndrome*). An apparently unique disorder, described by Andersen and Pindborg (1), consists of hypohidrotic ectodermal dysplasia, pituitary deficiency, and a craniofacial dysostosis.

Oligodontia occurs in combination with taurodontism and somewhat sparse scalp hair as an autosomal recessive trait (49, 50). We have also seen an example of this syndrome. Oligodontia or anodontia has been seen in association with facial clefts and nail dysplasia (54). Related syndromes are discussed in Chaps. 24, 29, and 144. Total absence of permanent teeth is inherited as an autosomal recessive trait (4a, 8, 19a, 53a). Lack of eruption of permanent teeth may be seen in *cleidocranial dysplasia* and as an autosomal dominant trait (48a).

An autosomal dominant form of hidrotic ectodermal dysplasia exists in a family of French extraction which migrated to Canada, Scotland, and northern United States (3, 6, 14, 35, 56–58). Most patients, in contrast to those exhibiting the hypohidrotic form, have (a) normal sweat and sebaceous gland function, (b) total alopecia, (c) severe nail dystrophy, (d) pigmentation of skin, especially over the joints, and (e) normal teeth. Other findings have included stra-

bismus, mental deficiency, clubbing of fingers, tufting of distal phalanges, and palmar and plantar hyperkeratoses.

Another form of dominantly inherited hidrotic ectodermal dysplasia has been described in which the tooth crowns were conical. In association were sensorineural deafness, polydactyly, syndactyly, and nail dystrophy (32, 44). The patients described by Mannkopf and Hanney (36) as having ectodermal dysplasia were of several types. Their case 7 had *focal dermal hypoplasia.* Patients possibly similarly involved are those described by Šalamon and Miličević (46) and by Friedrich and Seitz (16).

Anhidrosis together with neurolabyrinthitis which develops in middle life has been described as an autosomal trait (23). Isolated amastia may be inherited as a dominant trait (19).

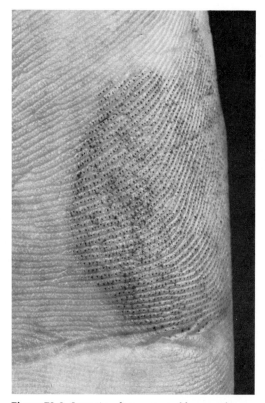

Figure 72-3. Sweating demonstrated by use of *o*-phthalaldialdehyde. (*From J. Verbov,* Br. J. Dermatol. **83:**341, 1970.)

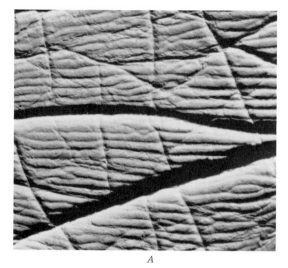

A

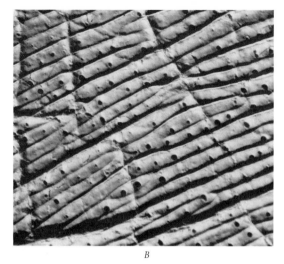

B

Figure 72-4. Sweating using silicone rubber technique. (*A*). Affected male. (*B*). Female heterozygote. (*C*). Normal individual. (*From J. Verbov*, Br. J. Dermatol. **83:**341, 1970.)

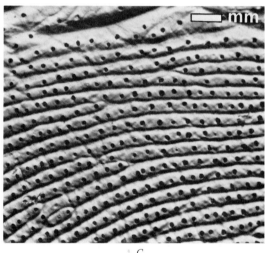

C

DIAGNOSTIC AIDS

The dental roentgenogram is of invaluable service in ascertaining the presence of hypo- or anodontia and in ruling out pseudoanodontia.

Decreased secretion of sweat may be demonstrated by the starch-iodine method (Minor test) (11, 12), by the use of agar plates containing silver nitrate and potassium chromate devised by Schwachman and Gahm (see 18), by the altered electrical resistance of the skin (29), or by use of *o*-phthalaldialdehyde in xylene (53) (Fig. 72-3).

Frias and Smith (15) advocated counting sweat pores per linear centimeter, the normal number decreasing from about 40 in infancy to 20 in old age. They suggested that carrier mothers had fewer sweat pores, a finding concurred in by Verbov (53), but denied by Crump and Danks (9). The latter authors found no sweat pores in males with the X-linked form but a decreased number in males and females with the autosomal recessive type.

Sweat pore counting may be carried out by direct observation or by use of silicone rubber or cellulose pellicles (9, 15, 53) (Fig. 72-4*A*–*C*).

REFERENCES

1 Andersen, T. H., and Pindborg, J. J., Et tilfaelde af total "pseudo-anodonti" i forbindelse med kraniedeformitet, dvaergvaekst, og ektodermal dysplasi. *Odontol. Tidskr.* **55:**484–493, 1947.

2 Beahrs, J. O., Anhidrotic Ectodermal Dysplasia: Predisposition to Bronchial Disease. *Ann. Intern. Med.* **74:**92–96, 1971.

3 Blattner, R. J., Hereditary Ectodermal Dysplasia. *J. Pediatr.*

73:444–447, 1968.

4 Capitanio, M. A., et al., Congenital Anhidrotic Ectodermal Dysplasia. *Am. J. Roentgenol.* **103**:168–172, 1968.

4a Coutley, H. L., Abnormalities of Human Dentition. *Br. Dent. J.* **49**:669, 1928.

5 Christ, J., Über die Korrelationen der kongenitalen Defekte des Ektoderms untereinander, mit besonderer Berücksichtigung ihrer Beziehungen zum Auge. *Zentralbl. Haut Geschlechtskr.* **40**:1–21, 1932.

6 Clouston, H. R., The Major Forms of Hereditary Ectodermal Dysplasia. *Can. Med. Assoc. J.* **40**:1–7, 1939.

7 Cole, H. M., et al., Congenital Cataracts in Sisters with Congenital Ectodermal Dysplasia. *J.A.M.A.* **129**:723–728, 1945.

8 Cramer, M., Case Report of Complete Anodontia of the Permanent Teeth. *Am. J. Orthodont.* **33**:760–764, 1947.

9 Crump, J. A., and Danks, D. M., Hypohidrotic Ectodermal Dysplasia. *J. Pediatr.* **78**:466–473, 1971.

10 Darwin, C., *The Variations of Plants and Animals under Domestication*, vol. 2. Appleton, New York, 1893, p. 319.

11 Everett, F. G., et al., Anhidrotic Ectodermal Dysplasia with Anodontia: A Study of Two Families. *J. Am. Dent. Assoc.* **44**:173–186, 1952.

12 Felsher, Z., Hereditary Ectodermal Dysplasia. Report of a Case with Experimental Study. *Arch. Dermatol. Syph.* (*Chic.*) **49**:410–414, 1944.

13 Fleischmann, O., Angeborener Schweissdrüsenmangel und Ozäna. *Z. Laryngol. Rhinol.* **20**:503–537, 1931.

14 Franceschetti, A., Les dysplasies ectodermiques et les syndromes héréditaires apparentés. *Dermatologica* **106**:129–156, 1953.

15 Frias, J. L., and Smith, D. W., Diminished Sweat Pores in Hypohidrotic Ectodermal Dysplasia: A New Method of Assessment. *J. Pediatr.* **72**:606–610, 1968.

16 Friedrich, H. C., and Seitz, R., Über eine Form der ektodermalen Dysplasie unter dem Bilde der Pili torti mit Augenbeteiligung und Störungen der Schweisssekretion. *Dermatol. Wochenschr.* **131**:277–283, 1955.

17 Glasstone, S., Development of Tooth Germs in Vitro. *J. Anat.* **70**:260–266, 1935–1936.

18 Glicklich, L. B., and Rosenthal, I. M., Anhidrotic Ectodermal Dysplasia: Use of Silver Nitrate Plate to Detect Anhidrosis. *J. Pediatr.* **54**:19–26, 1959.

19 Goldenring, H., and Creling, E. S., Mother and Daughter with Bilateral Congenital Amastia. *Yale J. Biol. Med.* **33**:466, 1961.

19a Goose, D. H., Anodontia. *Br. Dent. J.* **137**:477, 1974.

20 Gorlin, R. J., et al., Hypohidrotic Ectodermal Dysplasia in Females: A Critical Analysis and Argument for Genetic Heterogeneity. *Z. Kinderheilkd.* **108**:1–11, 1970.

21 Grant, R., and Falls, H. F., Anodontia: Report of a Case Associated with Ectodermal Dysplasia of the Anhidrotic Type. *Am. J. Orthodont.* **30**:661–672, 1944.

22 Hartwell, S. W. J., et al., Congenital Anhidrotic Ectodermal Dysplasia. *Clin. Pediatr.* **4**:383–386, 1965.

23 Helweg-Larsen, H. J., and Ludvigsen, K., Congenital Familial Anhidrosis and Neurolabyrinthitis. *Acta Derm. Venereol.* (*Stockh.*) **26**:489–505, 1946.

24 Hinrichsen, C. F. L., Ectodermal Dysplasia. *Aust. Dent. J.* **8**:101–105, 1963.

25 Jerndal, T., Ectodermal Dysplasia with Infantile Congenital Glaucoma. *J. Pediatr. Ophthalmol.* **7**:29–32, 1970.

26 Katz, S. I., and Penneys, N. S., Sebaceous Gland Papules in Anhidrotic Ectodermal Dysplasia. *Arch. Dermatol.* **103**:507–509, 1971.

27 Kerr, C. B., et al., Genetic Effect in Carriers of Anhidrotic Ectodermal Dysplasia. *J. Med. Genet.* **3**:169–176, 1966.

28 Kratzsch, R., Ektodermale Dysplasie von anhidrotischen Typ bei zwei Schwestern. *Klin. Pädiatr.* **184**:328–332, 1972.

29 Levit, S. G., The Problem of Dominance in Man. *J. Genet.* **33**:411–434, 1936.

30 Lipshutz, H., Anhidrotic Ectodermal Dysplasia. *J. Albert Einstein Med. Cent.* **11**:33–37, 1963.

31 Lowenburg, H., and Grimes, E. L., Ectodermal Dysplasia of the Anhidrotic Type. *Am. J. Dis. Child.* **63**:357–365, 1942.

32 Lowry, R. B., et al., Hereditary Ectodermal Dysplasia. *Clin. Pediatr.* **5**:395–402, 1966.

33 Machtens, E., et al., Klinische Aspekte der ektodermalen Dysplasie. *Z. Kinderheilkd.* **112**:265–280, 1972.

34 Mahloudji, J., and Livingston, K. E., Familial and Congenital Simple Anhidrosis. *Am. J. Dis. Child.* **113**:477–479, 1967.

35 Mallmann-Mühlberger, E., and Helwig, H., Familiäre ektodermale Dysplasie von hidrotischen Typ. *Ann. Paediatr.* (*Basel*) **202**:358–370, 1964.

36 Mannkopf, H., and Hanney, F., Zum Erscheinungsbild der kongenitalen ektodermalen Dysplasien. *Albrecht v. Graefes Arch. Ophthalmol.* **159**:643–661, 1957.

37 Metson, B. F., and Williams, B. K., Hereditary Ectodermal Dysplasia of the Anhidrotic Type. *J. Pediatr.* **40**:303–309, 1952.

38 Osbourn, R. A., Congenital Ectodermal Dysplasia with Amastia. *J.A.M.A.* **148**:644–645, 1952.

39 Passarge, E. C., et al., Anhidrotic Ectodermal Dysplasia as Autosomal Recessive Trait in an Inbred Kindred. *Humangenetik* **3**:181–185, 1966.

40 Perabo, F., et al., Ektodermale Dysplasie von anhidrotischen Typus. *Helv. Paediatr. Acta* **11**:604–639, 1956.

41 Priest, J., Dermatoglyphics in Ectodermal Dysplasia. *Lancet* **2**:1093, 1967.

42 Redpath, T. H., and Winter, G. B., Autosomal Dominant Ectodermal Dysplasia with Significant Dental Defects. *Br. Dent. J.* **126**:123–128, 1969.

43 Reed, W. B., et al., Clinical Spectrum of Anhidrotic Ectodermal Dysplasia. *Arch. Dermatol.* **102**:134–143, 1970.

44 Robinson, G. C., et al., Familial Ectodermal Dysplasia with Sensory Neural Deafness and Other Anomalies. *Pediatrics* **30**:797–802, 1962.

45 Sackett, L. M., et al., Congenital Ectodermal Dysplasia of the Anhidrotic Type. *Oral Surg.* **9**:659–665, 1956.

46 Šalamon, T., and Miličevič, M., Über eine besondere Form der ektodermalen Dysplasie mit Hypohidrosis, Hypotrichosis, Hornhautveränderungen, Nagel- und anderen Anomalien. *Arch. Klin. Exp. Dermatol.* **220**:564–575, 1964.

47 Samuelson, G., Hypohidrotic Ectodermal Dysplasia. *Acta Paediatr. Scand.* **59**:94–99, 1970.

48 Sarnat, B. G., et al., Fourteen Year Report of Facial Growth in Case of Complete Anodontia with Ectodermal Dysplasia. *Am. J. Dis. Child.* **86**:162–169, 1953.

48a Shokeir, M. H. K., Complete Failure of Eruption of All Permanent Teeth: An Autosomal Dominant Disorder. *Clin. Genet.* **5**:322–326, 1974.

49 Stenvik, A., et al., Taurodontism and Concomitant Hypo-

dontia in Siblings. *Oral Surg.* **33:**841–845, 1972.

50 Stoy, P. J., Taurodontism Associated with Other Dental Abnormalities. *Dent. Pract. Dent. Rec.* **10:**202–205, 1960.

51 Thoma, K. H., and Allen, F. W., Anodontia in Ectodermal Dysplasia. *Am. J. Orthodont.* **26:**503–507, 1940.

52 Upshaw, B. Y., and Montgomery, H., Hereditary Anhidrotic Ectodermal Dysplasia: A Clinical and Pathologic Study. *Arch. Dermatol. Syph. (Chic.)* **60:**1170–1183, 1949.

53 Verbov, J., Hypohidrotic (or Anhidrotic) Ectodermal Dysplasia: An Appraisal of Diagnostic Methods. *Br. J. Dermatol.* **83:**341–348, 1970.

53a Warr, V. C., A Case of Complete Absence of Permanent Dentition. *Br. Dent. J.* **64:**327–328, 1938.

54 Watson, R. M., and Hardwick, C. E., Hypodontia As-sociated with Cleft Palate. *Br. Dent. J.* **130:**77–80, 1971.

55 Weech, A. A., Hereditary Ectodermal Dysplasia. *Am. J. Dis. Child.* **37:**766–790, 1929.

56. White, A. G., Hereditary Ectodermal Dysplasia with Megaloblastic Anemia. *Br. J. Clin. Pract.* **18:**541–545, 1964.

57 Wilkey, W. D., and Stevenson, G. H., A Family with Inherited Ectodermal Dystrophy. *Can. Med. Assoc. J.* **53:**226–230, 1945.

58 Williams, M., and Fraser, F. C., Hidrotic Ectodermal Dysplasia in Clouston's Family Revisited. *Can. Med. Assoc. J.* **96:**36–38, 1967.

59 Witkop, C. J., in R. W. Tiecke (ed.), *Oral Pathology,* McGraw-Hill, New York, 1959, p. 786.

73

Hypospadias-Dysphagia Syndrome

(G Syndrome)

The disorder initially described and named the "G syndrome" by Opitz et al. (7) appears to be uncommon, only a few examples having been noted (1–3, 5, 7). The designation stems from the surname of the first affected family. The term "hypospadias-dysphagia syndrome" has also been used but should not imply that all affected patients necessarily have these two manifestations.

It appears that the disorder has autosomal dominant inheritance (5, 8).

SYSTEMIC MANIFESTATIONS

Severely affected infants have usually been born after uneventful pregnancy of normal duration. In surviving children, growth and intelligence are normal.

Facies. The facial appearance at birth is characteristic. The infant may have prominence of the occipital and parietal eminences, apparent hypertelorism, relatively narrow slitlike palpebral fissures usually having a slight antimongoloid slant, and epicanthal folds (2, 6) (Fig. 73-1). An accessory fold may follow the lid part way to the outer canthus. Some patients have exhibited relative entropion of the lower lid. The nasal bridge is flattened, the nostrils are often anteverted (Fig. 73-1), the philtrum is rather flat and inapparent, and there is usually mild, rarely severe, micrognathia. The pinnas may show some de-

gree of posterior rotation and occasionally abnormal modeling, primarily affecting the helix (2).

Genitourinary manifestations. The male genital and anal anomalies are so unusual that they alone may suggest the correct diagnosis. The degree of hypospadias varies from a mild coronal to a scrotal type with an associated ventral urethral groove. In mild cases, the scrotum appears normal; in severe examples, the scrotum is cleft and chordee may be so severe as to draw the tip of the glans to the anterior edge of the anus (Fig. 73-2). In all cases, the testes are descended and appear to be of normal size. One patient had imperforate anus with rectourethral fistula (7). Bilateral ureteral reflex has also been seen. Affected females have normal genitalia.

Respiratory system. Respiration usually begins spontaneously at birth, and the infant generally has a normal Apgar score. In some infants, stridorous respiration and a hoarse cry may be noted even before the first feeding. In severe cases, the infant sucks eagerly but seems to have difficulty in swallowing, since he chokes, coughs, and becomes cyanotic. This may be followed by respiratory distress, increase in stridor, apparent aspiration pneumonia, patchy atelectasis and emphysema, and, in chronic cases, bronchiectasis. Cinefluoroscopic studies have shown apparent neuromuscular dysfunction of the swallowing mechanism, with up to half of each

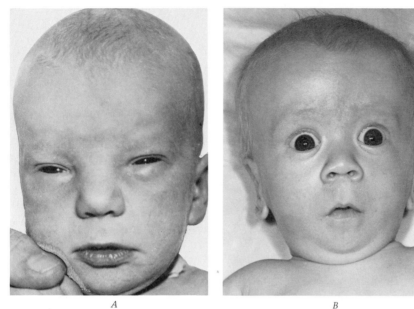

Figure 73-1. *Hypospadias-dysphagia (G syndrome)*. (*A*). Ocular hypertelorism, narrow palpebral fissures, anteverted nostrils. (*From J. Opitz et al.*, Birth Defects **5**(2):95, 1969.) (*B*). Patient of one of the authors (R. J. G.)

mouthful entering the tracheobronchial tree with gastroesophageal reflex (2) (Fig. 73-3). Achalasia may also be present. In one family, this was associated with complex malforma- tions: short trachea with high carina and supra- clavicular tracheal bifurcation, severe hypo- plasia of one lung, epiglottis, vocal cords, and larynx, with absence of the dorsal portions of

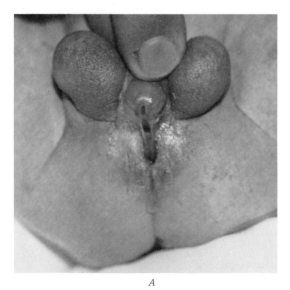

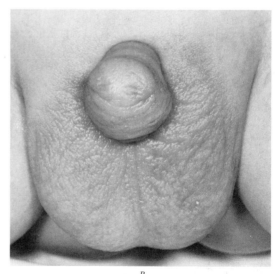

Figure 73-2. (*A*). Cleft scrotum with anterior displacement, severe chordee deformity of hypoplastic phallus. (*From J. Opitz et al.*, Birth Defects **5**(2):95, 1969.) (*B*). Hypospadias, chordee.

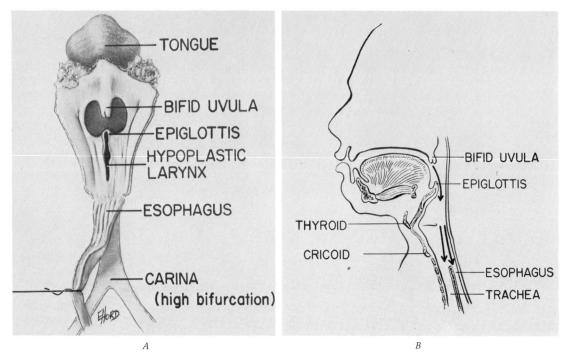

Figure 73-3. (*A, B*). Artist's conception of defects of soft palate, larynx, and hypopharynx. Note absence of posterior wall of larynx and presence of single, large laryngopharyngeal cavity. Arrows show that solid substances are as likely to enter trachea as to enter esophagus. (*From E. F. Gilbert et al.*, Z. Kinderheilkd. **111**:290, 1972.)

the larynx and first tracheal rings and a single cavity extending from the epiglottis and hypopharynx superiorly to the trachea and inferiorly to the esophagus.

Miscellaneous findings. Anomalous venous return to the heart has been noted, as well as unlobed lungs, midline position of the heart, bifid renal pelvis with double ureter, Meckel diverticulum, patency of the foramen ovale and ductus arteriosus (4), absence of the gallbladder, and duodenal stricture (5). Mild mental retardation was noted in one family (8).

Oral manifestations. The uvula may be broad or bifid, and ankyloglossia or shortened lingual frenum has been observed in some cases. The mandible is often small. Cleft lip-palate has been described (8).

DIFFERENTIAL DIAGNOSIS

The syndrome is quite distinctive, and differentiation from other syndromes is easily made. *Hypertelorism-hypospadias syndrome* should be excluded.

LABORATORY AIDS

Cinefluoroscopic study of swallowing should be carried out.

REFERENCES

1   Beas, F., Pediatric Laboratory, School of Medicine, University of Chile, Santiago, personal communication, 1971.

2   Coburn, T. P., G Syndrome. *Am. J. Dis. Child.* **120**:466, 1970.

3   Frias, J. L., and Rosenbloom, A. L., Two New Familial Cases of the G Syndrome. *Birth Defects* **11**(2):54–57, 1975.

4   Gilbert, E. F., et al., The Pathologic Anatomy of the G Syndrome. *Z. Kinderheilkd.* **111**:290–298, 1972.

5   Kasner, J., et al., The G Syndrome — Further Observations. *Z. Kinderheilkd.* **118**:81–86, 1974.

6   Little, J. R., and Opitz, J. M., The G Syndrome. *Am. J. Dis. Child.* **121**:505–507, 1971.

7   Opitz, J. M., et al., The G Syndrome of Multiple Congenital Anomalies. *Birth Defects* **5**(2):95–101, 1969.

8   Van Biervliet, J. P., and van Hemmel, J. O., Familial Occurrence of the G Syndrome. *Clin. Genet.* **7**:238–244, 1975.

74

Inability To Fully Open the Mouth and Pseudocamptodactyly

The syndrome of (a) limited oral opening and (b) curvature of the fingers at all interphalangeal joints on dorsiflexion of the wrists (pseudocamptodactyly) was described independently in 1969 by Hecht and Beals (2) and by Wilson et al. (9). The family originated in the Netherlands (1, 5, 7, 8). The disorder is inherited as an autosomal dominant trait (1–3, 7, 9).

SYSTEMIC MANIFESTATIONS

The patients are normally proportioned, but stature is reduced below the 3d percentile, the adult male rarely exceeding 160 cm.

Facies. De Jong (1) described blepharochalasis in older individuals, and a quilted appearance of the cheeks (Fig. 74-1).

Musculoskeletal alterations. In addition to mildly reduced stature and limited oral opening discussed below, the distinguishing features of the syndrome are limited to abnormalities of the extremities which result from shortness of various skeletal muscles or tendons.

The hands may be clenched at birth but loosen during infancy and childhood (8). Upon dorsiflexion of the wrist, due to shortening of the flexor tendon-muscle unit, curvature of all fingers at each interphalangeal joint is noted. Upon volar flexion, all fingers are completely ex-

tended (Fig. 74-2A, B). There is no associated muscular weakness, but there is mild limitation of dorsiflexion and supination at the wrist.

Short leg muscles result in a variety of mild foot deformities: talipes equinovarus or calcaneovalgus, metatarsus varus, etc. Shortened hamstring muscles produce pelvic tilt with straight leg raising. Pes planus, hammer toes, and torticollis have also been noted (3, 9).

Oral manifestations. The maximum aperture between the incisal edges of the upper and lower incisors is 1.0 to 1.8 cm. This inhibits mastica-

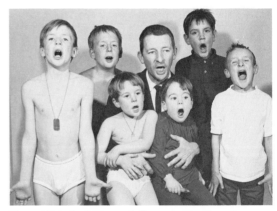

Figure 74-1. *Inability to fully open mouth and pseudocamptodactyly.* Kindred of affected father and several affected and normal children showing attempt to open mouth fully. (*From F. Hect and R. K. Beals,* Birth Defects **5**(3):96, 1969.)

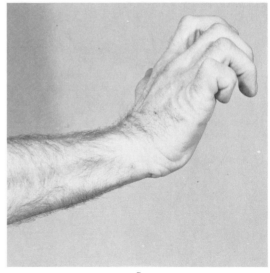
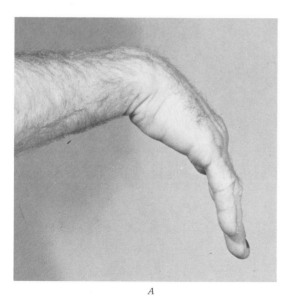

A   *B*

Figure 74-2. (*A*). On volar flexion, all fingers can be completely extended. (*B*). On dorsiflexion of wrist, there is flexion of fingers at interphalangeal joints. (*From F. Hecht and R. K. Beals,* Birth Defects **5**(3):96, 1969.)

tion, an affected individual requiring about twice as much time to consume a meal. The temporomandibular joints have been shown to be normal (3). The coronoid processes are enlarged and are responsible for the inability to open the

mouth widely (7). A hardened nodular cord has been noted in the region of the nasolabial furrow.

DIFFERENTIAL DIAGNOSIS

Inability to open the mouth must be differentiated from microstomia seen in a variety of disorders (*craniocarpotarsal dysplasia, Schwartz-Jampel syndrome,* etc.). Abnormalities, either congenital or acquired, of the temporomandibular joint may result in reduced jaw-opening. Patients with the *temporomandibular joint dysfunction syndrome* cannot open their mouths widely, but this disorder can easily be separated from the syndrome under discussion.

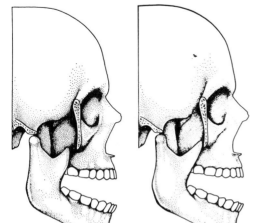

Figure 74-3. *Left,* normal relationship. *Right,* enlarged coronoid process which prevents normal opening of jaws. (*From R. F. Van Hoof, Leiden, The Netherlands.*)

LABORATORY AIDS

Average opening between edges of incisor teeth is 49 mm (range 30 to 70 mm) in normal adults. From eight to twelve years of age, the normal vertical distance is about 40 mm (range 25 to 55 mm) (2, 4, 5). This has also been our experience, but not that of Sheppard and Sheppard (6).

REFERENCES

1   De Jong, J. G. Y., A Family Showing Strongly Reduced Ability to Open the Mouth and Limitation of Some Movements of the Extremities. *Humangenetik* **12:**210–217, 1971. (Same family as that described by ter Haar.)

2   Hecht, F., and Beals, R. K., Inability to Open the Mouth Fully: An Autosomal Dominant Phenotype with Facultative Campylodactyly and Short Stature. *Birth Defects* **5**(3):96–98, 1969.

3   Horowitz, S. L., et al., Limited Intermaxillary Opening - an Inherited Trait. *Oral Surg.* **36:**490–492, 1973.

4   Lignell, L., and Ransjö, K., Maximal gapförmaga. *Sverig. Tandläk. Förb. Tidn.* **59:**859–862, 1967.

5   Mabry, C. C., et al., Trismus-Pseudocamptodactyly Syndrome. *J. Pediatr.* **85:**503–508. 1974

6   Sheppard, I. M., and Sheppard, S. M., Maximal Incisal Opening - Diagnostic Index? *J. Dent. Med.* **20:**13–15, 1965.

7   Ter Haar, B. G., and Van Hoof, R. F., The Trismus-Pseudocampylodactyly Syndrome. *J. Med. Genet.* **11:**41–49, 1974.

8   Van Hoof, R. F., *Enlargement of the Coronoid Process with Special Reference to the Trismus-Pseudocampylodactyly Syndrome.* Stafleu and Tholen, Leiden, 1973.

9   Wilson, R. V., et al., Autosomal Dominant Inheritance of Shortening of the Flexor Profundus Muscle-Tendon Unit with Limitation of Jaw Excursion. *Birth Defects* **5**(3):99–102, 1969.

75

Incontinentia Pigmenti

(Bloch-Sulzberger Syndrome)

Though this disorder was possibly first noticed by Garrod (8) in 1906, credit is usually given to Bardach (2), Bloch (3), Sulzberger (25), and Siemens (24) for clearly defining it in the 1920s. The chief components include (*a*) vesicular, verrucous, and pigmented macular lesions of the skin, and (*b*) anomalies of the eye, central nervous system, skeletal system, and teeth. About 350 cases have been reported to date.

The name "incontinentia pigmenti" was applied to the syndrome by Bloch (3) and has been used almost uniformly. However, several authors have indicated their dissatisfaction with the term (26).

A familial occurrence has been found in about 15 percent of cases. Pfeiffer (19), Lenz (15), and Lucas (16), in very comprehensive reviews, concluded that the syndrome is X-linked dominant, essentially lethal in the male, only about 5 percent of cases being of that sex (20, 21). An increased number of chromosomal breaks has been noted (4, 11, 13).

Pfeiffer (19) found that over half the patients had involvement of systems other than that of the integument.

SYSTEMIC MANIFESTATIONS

Skin. In most patients, two or three days after birth, linear or grouped vesicles containing a honey-colored serum appear on the extremities.

By the end of the first month, the vesicles may disappear, recur, or be replaced by irregularly distributed violaceous papules and inflammatory lesions. In another few weeks, on the dorsal surface of the digits and over the knuckles and joints, hyperkeratotic, warty lesions appear and last for a few months. The inflamed areas eventually heal and may become atrophic, somewhat resembling scleroderma.

Often present at birth (though they may appear much later) are pigmented macules, brownish-gray and arranged in a reticulated pattern or in streaks, whorls, or patches over the trunk and extremities. The sites and degree of pigmentation are not related to the bullous or verrucous formation. Fading of the pigmentation may begin at about the age of two years, though some residuum is often present for life (Fig. 75-1).

Alopecia of the atrophic, scarring (pseudopelade) type is seen near the apex of the crown in the vast majority of affected persons (5) (Fig. 75-2). Rarely, the fingernails are dystrophic (5, 9) and the breasts asymmetric (9).

During the vesicular stage, microscopic examination reveals tense intraepithelial (or occasionally subepithelial) vesicles containing eosinophilic polymorphonuclear leukocytes. The verrucous lesion is nonspecific, manifesting only hyperkeratosis, acanthosis, and a banal subepithelial infiltrate. The later skin changes are nonspecific. There are hydropic changes in individual basal cells and a decrease in the number

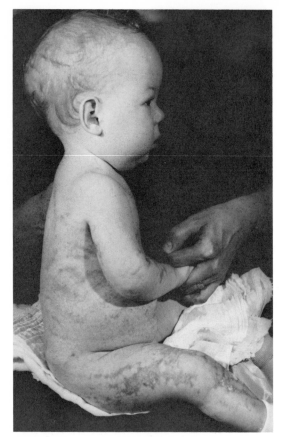

Figure 75-1. *Incontinentia pigmenti.* Ten-month-old female manifesting bullae, verrucae, and whorled and linear distribution of pigment. Also note area of crusting and scarification on thigh.

of pigment granules. The hyperpigmentation is due to numerous melanin-bearing phagocytes located in the upper and middle cutis. Guerrier and Wong (11a, 27) described the evolution of ultrastructural cutaneous changes.

Eyes. Ophthalmologic changes are present in about 25 to 35 percent of patients (7, 14, 16a, 19, 22). The most common alterations include strabismus, cataract, optic atrophy, retinal detachment, and changes similar to those seen in retrolental fibroplasia. Less often, there are blue scleras, metastatic ophthalmitis, myopia, nystagmus, papillitis, microphthalmia, and exudative chorioretinitis.

Central nervous system. There is central nervous system involvement in 35 to 40 percent of affected persons (19). This involvement includes mental retardation, microcephaly, hydrocephalus, spastic and lax paralysis, paresis of eye muscles, and convulsive episodes (5, 6, 14, 17).

Skeletal system. Bony defects are present in about 20 percent of patients, but are not severe (5). They may take the form of hemivertebras, extra ribs, syndactyly, hemiatrophy, and shortening of an arm or leg (5, 20).

Oral manifestations. Oral changes are limited to the teeth and have been noted in 90 percent of cases (12). Delayed tooth eruption, pegged or conical crowned teeth, missing teeth, and malformed teeth have been noted (5, 6, 9, 13, 21, 24, 26) (Fig. 75-3A, B). The dental abnormalities affect both the primary and permanent dentitions, more frequently the latter. The conical crown form is present not only in the incisors but often in the canines and premolars as well. Oligodontia creates spaces or diastemas between the teeth. The reader is referred to the extensive analysis of Hagemann (12) for details on the frequency of various tooth anomalies.

DIFFERENTIAL DIAGNOSIS

Skin changes present in early infancy must be distinguished from those of congenital syphilis,

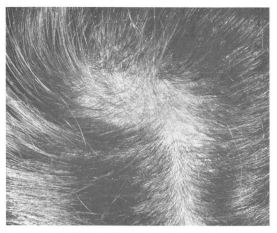

Figure 75-2. Alopecia of pseudopelade type located at crown of head.

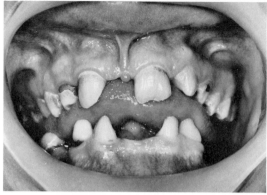

A

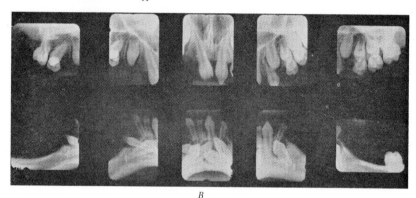

B

Figure 75-3. (*A*). Missing teeth and teeth with conical crown form. (*B*). Dental roentgenograms of patient demonstrating missing teeth, impacted teeth, and conical crown form of several teeth. (*From R. J. Gorlin and J. Anderson,* J. Pediatr. **57:**78, 1960.)

epidermolysis bullosa, bullous impetigo, contact dermatitis, dermatitis herpetiformis, verrucous nevus, and the Naegeli syndrome.

The dental changes are somewhat similar to those seen in congenital syphilis but far more like those of other ectodermal dysplasias, such as *chondroectodermal dysplasia (Ellis-van Creveld syndrome)* and *hypohidrotic ectodermal dysplasia.* In congenital syphilis, the primary dentition is rarely involved (except possibly a deciduous molar), because of the inability of the spirochetes to pass the placental barrier until at least the eighteenth week of pregnancy. The incisors in congenital syphilis are never conical; the incisal edge is simply narrower than the cervical portion of the crown. In hypohidrotic ectodermal dysplasia, the suppresion of dentition

is usually far more marked than in incontinentia pigmenti. In chondroectodermal dysplasia, there are other oral anomalies which are not present in incontinentia pigmenti, such as fusion of the lip and gingiva and notching of the mandibular alveolar process. The teeth in the Naegeli syndrome are not pointed (7, 10).

LABORATORY AIDS

Blood eosinophilia during the vesicular stage or even later may be marked, in some cases reaching over 55 percent (1, 5, 6, 18). Evidence of chromosome instability has been demonstrated (4, 11, 13).

REFERENCES

1 Asboe-Hansen, G., Bullous Keratogenous and Pigmentary Dermatitis with Blood Eosinophilia in Newborn Girls. *Arch. Dermatol. Syph.* (*Chic.*) **67:**152–157, 1953.

2 Bardach, M., Systematisierte Naevusbildungen bei einem eineiigen Zwillingspaar. *Z. Kinderheilkd.* **39:**542–550, 1925.

3 Bloch, B., Eigentümliche, bisher nicht beschriebene Pigmentaffektion (Incontinentia pigmenti). *Schweiz. Med. Wochenschr.* **7:**404–405, 1926.

4 Cantu, J. M., et al., Chromosomal Instability in Incontinentia Pigmenti. *Ann. Génét.* **16:**117–119, 1973.

5 Carney, R. G., and Carney, R. G., Jr., Incontinentia Pigmenti. *Arch. Dermatol.* **102:**157–162, 1970.

6 Findlay, G. H., On the Pathogenesis of Incontinentia Pigmenti: With Observations on an Associated Eye Disturbance Resembling Retrolental Fibroplasia. *Br. J. Dermatol.* **64:**141–146, 1952.

7 Franceschetti, A., and Jadassohn, W., Á propos de l'incontinentia pigmenti, délimitation de deux syndromes différents figurant sous le même terme. *Dermatologica* **108:**1–28, 1954.

8 Garrod, A. E., Peculiar Pigmentations of the Skin of an Infant. *Trans. Clin. Soc. Lond.* **39:**216, 1906.

9 Gorlin, R. J., and Anderson, J. A., The Characteristic Dentition of Incontinentia Pigmenti (Bloch-Sulzberger Syndrome): A Diagnostic Aid. *J. Pediatr.* **57:**78–85, 1960.

10 Greither, A., and Haensch, R., Anhidrotische retikuläre Pigmentdermatose mit blasig erythematösem Anfangsstadium. *Schweiz. Med. Wochenschr.* **100:**228–233, 1970.

11 Grouchy, J., et al., Cassures chromosomiques dans l'incontinentia pigmenti. *Ann. Génét.* **15:**61–66, 1972.

11a Guerrier, C. J. W., and Wong, C. K., Ultrastructural Evolution of the Skin in Incontinentia Pigmentia. *Dermatologica* **149:**10–22, 1974.

12 Hagemann, E., Zahnbefund bei der Incontinentia pigmenti. *Dtsch. Zahnärztl. Z.* **18:**1198–1208, 1262–1268, 1963.

13 Iancu, T., et al., Incontinentia Pigmenti. *Clin. Genet.* **7:**103–110, 1975.

14 Jones, S. T., Retrolental Membrane Associated with Bloch-Sulzberger Syndrome (Incontinentia Pigmenti). *Am. J. Ophthalmol.* **62:**330–334, 1966.

15 Lenz, W., Zur Genetik der Incontinentia pigmenti. *Ann. Paediatr.* (*Basel*) **196:**149–165, 1961.

16 Lucas, D., Beitrag zur Genetik der Incontinentia Pigmenti. *Klin. Pädiat.* **186:**142–147, 1974.

16a Menshaha-Manhart, O., et al., Retinal Pigment Epithelium in Incontinentia Pigmenti. *Am. J. Ophthalmol.* **79:**571–577, 1975.

17 Oldfelt, V., Incontinentia Pigmenti. *J. Pediatr.* **54:**446–458, 1959.

18 Pallisgaard, G., Incontinentia Pigmenti in a Newborn Boy. *Acta Derm. Venereol.* (*Stockh.*) **49:**197–201, 1969.

19 Pfeiffer, R. A., Zur Frage der Vererbung der Incontinentia Pigmenti (Bloch-Siemens). *Z. Menschl. Vererb. Konstit. Lehre* **35:**469–493, 1960.

20 Reed, W. B., et al., Incontinentia Pigmenti. *Dermatologica* **134:**243–250, 1967.

21 Russell, D. L., and Finn, S. B., Incontinentia Pigmenti (Bloch-Sulzberger Syndrome): A Case Report with Emphasis on Dental Manifestations. *J. Dent. Child.* **34:**494–500, 1967.

22 Scott, J., et al., Ocular Changes in the Bloch-Sulzberger Syndrome (Incontinentia Pigmenti). *Br. J. Ophthalmol.* **39:**276–282, 1955.

23 Shotts, N., and Emery, A. E. H., Bloch-Sulzberger Syndrome. *J. Med. Genet.* **3:**148–152, 1966.

24 Siemens, H. W., Die Melanosis corii degenerativa, eine neue Pigmentdermatose. *Arch. Dermatol. Syph.* (*Berl.*) **157:**382–391, 1929.

25 Sulzberger, M. B., Über eine bisher nicht beschriebene congenitale Pigmentanomalie (Incontinentia pigmenti). *Arch. Dermatol. Syph.* (*Berl.*) **154:**19–32, 1928.

26 Undeutsch, U., et al., Die Incontinentia pigmenti als Leitsymptom eines Komplexes multipler Abartung. *Z. Kinderheilkd.* **74:**484–506, 1954.

27 Wong, C. K., et al., An Electron Microscopical Study of Bloch-Sulzberger Syndrome (Incontinentia Pigmenti). *Acta Derm. Venereol.* (*Stockh.*) **51:**161–168, 1971.

76

Infantile Cortical Hyperostosis

(Caffey-Silverman Syndrome)

Though this syndrome was originally described by Roske (18) in 1930, it was not until 1945–1946 that the clinical and roentgenographic studies of Caffey and Silverman (7) and of Smyth et al. (21) brought attention to it. The disorder affects infants under six months of age. Its most constant features are (*a*) bilateral swelling over the mandible or other bones, (*b*) roentgenographic evidence of new bone formation in this area, (*c*) hyperirritability, and (*d*) mild fever. At least 200 cases have been reported to date. A report on 33 cases has been published by Holman (13).

It is possible that the syndrome is caused by a congenital anomaly of the vessels supplying the periosteum of the involved bones, the hypoxia effecting a focal necrosis of the overlying soft tissue and resulting in new subperiosteal bone formation (19, 20).

The disorder has autosomal dominant inheritance (1, 3a, 13, 14, 15, 20, 24). Tampas et al. (22) demonstrated the condition in 11 children in one family. Its occurrence is probably more frequent than suspected, for involvement may be mild and resolution may be rapid. Cayler and Peterson (8) estimated that the syndrome is seen in 3 of every 1,000 registered patients under six months of age. A low mortality rate has been described.

Although the onset in the vast majority of infants is from two to four months of age (average, nine weeks), it has been observed roentgenographically as early as 5 weeks prenatally and as late as 20 months after birth (1, 2, 7, 14, 15).

SYSTEMIC MANIFESTATIONS

Facies. Because of the swelling, the facies is so striking that the condition may be diagnosed with considerable assurance even prior to confirmatory x-ray evidence. The swelling is symmetric and located over the body and ramus of the mandible (Fig. 76-1). Pallor is often observed as well.

Soft tissues. The condition is initiated by tender, soft-tissue swelling over the face, around the orbits, thorax, or extremities; this swelling often undergoes remission and exacerbation (16). It is firm, brawny, and often so painful as to cause pseudoparalysis of an extremity. It is not accompanied by redness or increased heat.

Fever and irritability. Pain, fever of mild degree, and hyperirritability are seen in at least two-thirds of the patients (4, 20). These signs commonly precede the appearance of the swelling and bone involvement. One or all may, however, be absent. Anemia, leukocytosis, and elevation of the sedimentation rate occur in more than half the patients (13).

Skeletal system. The most frequently affected bone is the mandible, at least three of every four patients manifesting mandibular involvement (Fig. 76-2). Less commonly involved are the clavicle, tibia, ulna, femur, rib, humerus, maxilla, and fibula (4, 12, 13, 20). Usually several bones are affected at the same time (Fig. 76-3).

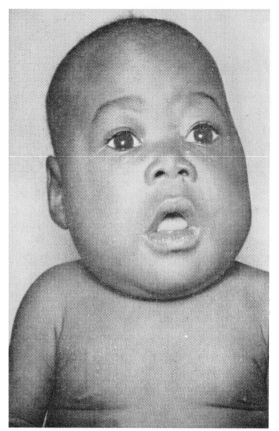

Figure 76-1. *Infantile cortical hyperostosis.* Note bilateral swellings over ramus of mandible.

The new periosteal bone formation, appearing most often during the ninth week, undergoes resolution slowly. Though complete clinical resolution takes place within 3 to 30 months (average, 9 months), roentgenographic evidence may persist for many years (5, 17). Bone bridges between the radius and ulna and between ribs have been described (5). Forward bowing of the tibia is common (15, 24). Pleural effusion has been reported in cases in which there has been rib involvement (7). Late recurrences of the disorder, although uncommon, have occurred (2a).

Oral manifestations. The oral findings have been discussed, in part, above. Involvement of the mandible was formerly thought to be necessary for diagnosis of the condition, but analysis

of large series of cases has revealed that this is not so (20). Nevertheless, swelling of the jaws is the most common presenting sign. In a follow-up survey of 11 cases, Burbank et al. (4) demonstrated that in six cases the mandible was the only bone involved. Follow-up showed that the fever had no effect on the enamel or on the eruption sequence. However, eight of the 11 patients had roentgenographic evidence of residual bony asymmetry of the mandible at the angle and ramus, and some of them had severe malocclusion.

PATHOLOGY

Several microscopic studies have been performed (3), the most comprehensive being that of Eversole et al. (10). In the early stages, foci of polymorphonuclear neutrophilic leukocytes are seen within the periosteum. The periosteum is swollen and mucoid in appearance, losing its well-defined limits and blending into the muscle, fascia, and tendons. At this stage, there is some resemblance to osteosarcoma and erroneous diagnosis and treatment may result. The small arteries of the periosteum and overlying soft tissue show intimal proliferation. In the

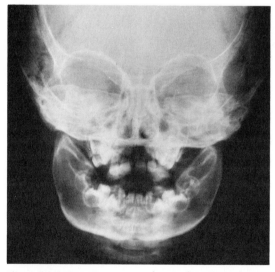

Figure 76-2. Roentgenogram of jaws showing symmetric mandibular enlargement 6 months after onset of infantile cortical hyperostosis. (*From P. M. Burbank et al., Oral Surg.* **11**:1126, 1958.)

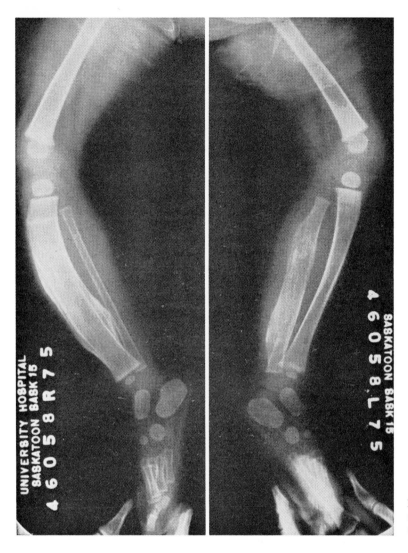

Figure 76-3. Roentgenogram showing thickening of periosteum and new bone formation.

later stages, poorly vascularized and incompletely structured new bone is laid down. Neither hemorrhage nor inflammation is seen at this stage (13).

DIFFERENTIAL DIAGNOSIS

To be considered are epidemic parotitis (mumps), vaccinial and pyogenic osteomyelitis, parotid tumor, rickets, congenital syphilis, subperiosteal hematoma, scurvy, and vitamin A intoxication (9, 14).

LABORATORY AIDS

Roentgenographic study not only of the mandible but of the chest and long bones confirms the clinical impression. Serum alkaline phosphatase level is elevated in cases with marked bone deposition (13). Frequently (in over 80 percent of patients), there is elevation of the sedimentation rate. Anemia and leukocytosis are common. Elevated IgM level and thrombocytopenia have also been noted (23).

REFERENCES

1 Barba, W. P., and Freriks, D. J., The Familial Occurrence of Infantile Cortical Hyperostosis in Utero. *J. Pediatr.* **42:**141–150, 1953.

2 Bennett, H. S., and Nelson, T. R., Prenatal Cortical Hyperostosis. *Br. J. Radiol.* **26:**47–49, 1953.

2a Blank, E., Recurrent Caffey's Cortical Hyperostosis and Persistent Deformity. *Pediatrics* **55:**856–860, 1975.

3 Brooksaler, F., and Miller, J. E., Infantile Cortical Hyperostosis. *J. Pediatr.* **48:**739–753, 1956.

3a Ball, M. J., and Feingold, M., Autosomal Dominant Inheritance of Caffey's Disease. *Birth Defects* **10**(9):139–146, 1974.

4 Burbank, P. M., et al., The Dental Aspects of Infantile Cortical Hyperostosis. *Oral Surg.* **11:**1126–1137, 1958.

5 Caffey, J., On Some Late Skeletal Changes in Chronic Infantile Cortical Hyperostosis. *Radiology* **59:**651–657, 1952.

6 Caffey, J., Infantile Cortical Hyperostosis: Review of Clinical and Roentgenographic Features. *Proc. R. Soc. Med.* **50:**347–354, 1957.

7 Caffey, J., and Silverman, W. A., Infantile Cortical Hyperostosis. *Am. J. Roentgenol.* **54:**1–16, 1945.

8 Cayler, G. C., and Peterson, C. A., Infantile Cortical Hyperostosis: Report of 17 Cases. *Am. J. Dis. Child.* **91:**119–125, 1956.

9 Cochran, W., Infantile Cortical Hyperostosis: A Review with Illustrative Case Report. *Acta Paediatr. Scand.* **51:**442–453, 1962.

10 Eversole, S. L., Jr., et al., Hitherto Undescribed Characteristics of the Pathology of Infantile Cortical Hyperostosis (Caffey's Disease). *Bull. Johns Hopkins Hosp.* **101:**80–100, 1957.

11 Faul, R., Familiäre Auftreten der infantilen kortikalen Hyperostose. *Arch. Kinderheilkd.* **164:**271–276, 1961.

12 Galyean, J., and Robertson, W. O., Caffey's Syndrome: Some Unusual Ocular Manifestations. *Pediatrics* **45:**122–125, 1970.

13 Holman, G. H., Infantile Cortical Hyperostosis: A Review. *Q. Rev. Pediatr.* **17:**24–31, 1962.

14 Käser, H., Das Krankheitsbild der infantilen corticalen Hyperostose. *Helv. Paediatr. Acta* **17:**153–184, 1962.

15 Kühl, J., et al., Ein Beitrag zur Krankheitsbild der infantilen kortikalen Hyperostose. *Arch. Kinderheilkd.* **179:**209–229, 1969.

16 Minton, L. R., and Elliott, J., Ocular Manifestations of Infantile Cortical Hyperostosis. *Am. J. Ophthalmol.* **64:**902–907, 1967.

17 Pajewski, M., and Vure, E., Late Manifestations of Infantile Cortical Hyperostosis (Caffey's Disease). *Br. J. Radiol.* **40:**90–95, 1967.

18 Röske, G., Eine eigenartige Knochenerkrankung im Säuglingsalter. *Monatsschr. Kinderheilkd.* **47:**385–400, 1930.

19 Sidbury, J. B., Infantile Cortical Hyperostosis. *Postgrad. Med.* **22:**211–215, 1957.

20 Sidbury, J. B., Jr., and Sidbury, J. B., Infantile Cortical Hyperostosis: Inquiry into the Etiology and Pathogenesis. *N. Engl. J. Med.* **250:**304–314, 1954.

21 Smyth, F. S., et al., Periosteal Reaction, Fever and Irritability in Young Infants: A New Syndrome? *Am. J. Dis. Child.* **71:**333–350, 1946.

22 Tampas, J. P., et al., Infantile Cortical Hyperostosis. *J.A.M.A.* **175:**491–493, 1961.

23 Temperley, I. J., et al., Raised Immunoglobulin Levels and Thrombocytopenia in Infantile Cortical Hyperostosis. *Arch. Dis. Child.* **47:**982–983, 1972.

24 Van Zeben, W., Infantile Cortical Hyperostoses. *Acta Paediatr. Scand.* **35:**10–20, 1948.

77

Kartagener Syndrome

(Sinusitis, Bronchiectasis, and Situs Inversus Viscerum)

The relationship between situs inversus viscerum and bronchiectasis was pointed out by Siewert (14) in 1904. Kartagener (7, 8), in a series of papers from 1933 through 1935, added chronic rhinosinusitis, i.e., nasal polyposis, chronic hyperplastic rhinitis, and ethmoidomaxillary sinusitis. Numerous investigators have also noted absence or hypoplasia of the frontal sinuses. More than 400 cases have been recorded (3, 5).

The syndrome exhibits autosomal recessive inheritance (9, 10). Knox et al. (11) presented linkage data with the Rh system, but existence of such a connection was denied by Cook et al. (4).

SYSTEMIC MANIFESTATIONS

Respiratory tract. Sinusitis is a frequent but inconstant finding (5) (Fig. 77-1). Similarly, nasal polyps have been reported with situs inversus in the absence of bronchiectasis (16). Agenesis or diminution of the frontal sinuses is common (12) but also is rather frequently seen in bronchiectasis and sinusitis without situs inversus (5), indicating a relationship between the sinuses and the rest of the respiratory tract but not with visceral inversion.

In early infancy, nasal discharge, frequent colds, and chronic bronchitis are observed, as well as recurrent bouts of pneumonia. Nasal catarrh and anosmia soon intervene and are followed in most cases by chronic cough productive of foul-smelling phlegm. In some persons, bronchiectasis seems to precede involvement of the upper part of the respiratory tract. Occasionally, there are accompanying asthma, hemoptysis, and pulmonary osteoarthropathy.

Among cases of situs inversus viscerum (see below), bronchiectasis is present in from 15 to 25 percent. This is far higher than the incidence

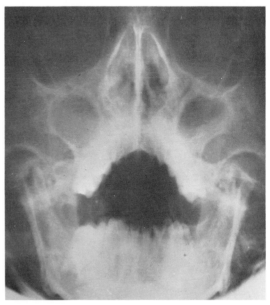

Figure 77-1. *Kartagener syndrome.* Bilateral maxillary sinusitis, more pronounced on right side.

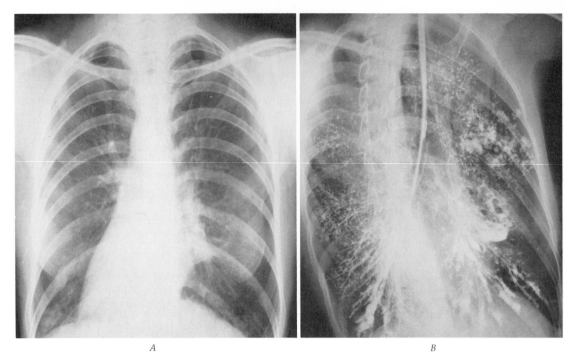

A   *B*

Figure 77-2. (*A*). Dextrocardia. Atelectasis of left middle lobe and right basal infiltration. (*B*). Bronchography showing bronchiectasis of left middle and both lower lobes. (*From A. Glay,* J. Can. Assoc. Radiol. **12:**22, 1961.)

among the general population (0.25 to 0.50 percent) (8).

The bronchiectasis is generally tubular or varicose, rather than cystic. There is still disagreement as to whether the bronchiectasis is of the acquired or congenital type (10) (Fig. 77-2*B*).

Situs Inversus Viscerum. As an isolated phenomenon, situs inversus viscerum occurs once in about 8,000 to 10,000 births (3, 12, 16). There is no unanimity of opinion concerning this most bizarre relationship between visceral inversion and bronchiectasis, but Fornatto et al. (5) believe that some factor predisposes the neonate with situs inversus to defective postnatal lung growth and atelectasis.

Dextrocardia, without further evidence of visceral inversion, has been frequently detected (Fig. 77-2*A*).

Other findings. Rheumatoid arthritis has been reported on at least two occasions (5). Other cases have been reported with anomalous subclavian artery, malformation of retinal vessels,

cardiac and renal anomalies, turricephaly, and absence of the xiphoid process (5). Various associated eye anomalies have been reviewed by Collier (3) and by Segal et al. (13).

DIFFERENTIAL DIAGNOSIS

Thick tenacious sinus and bronchial secretions, nasal polyposis, chronic sinusitis, and bronchiectasis also occur in cystic fibrosis. The histologic appearance of the respiratory epithelium, the bronchial plugging, and the absence of other stigmata (situs inversus viscerum) clearly distinguish cystic fibrosis from Kartagener syndrome (6).

LABORATORY AIDS

Holmes et al. (6) described transient immunoglobulin deficiencies during childhood, i.e., low serum IgA levels, in this syndrome, a finding not supported by Miller and Divertie (11a).

REFERENCES

1 Bergstrom, W. H., et al., Situs Inversus, Bronchiectasis and Sinusitis: Report of Family with Two Cases of Kartagener's Triad and Two Additional Cases of Bronchiectasis among Six Siblings. *Pediatrics* **6**:573–580, 1950.

2 Chang, K. H. R., Kartagener's Triad. *J. Thorac. Cardiovasc. Surg.* **43**:127–134, 1962.

3 Collier, M., Constatations ophthalmologiques dans le syndrome de Kartagener. *Bull. Soc. Fr. Ophthalmol.* **74**: 429–447, 1961.

4 Cook, C. D., et al., Blood Grouping in Three Families with Kartagener's Syndrome. *Am. J. Hum. Genet.* **14**:290–294, 1962.

5 Fornatto, E. J., et al., The Triad of Kartagener: Relation of Upper to Lower Respiratory Pathology. *Laryngoscope* **66**:1202–1220, 1956.

5a Heuckenkamp, P. U., et al., Das Kartagener-Syndrom. *Dtsch. Med. Wochenschr.* **97**:1458–1461, 1972.

6 Holmes, L. B., et al., A Reappraisal of Kartagener's Syndrome. *Am. J. Med. Sci.* **255**:13–28, 1968.

7 Kartagener, M., Zur Pathogenese der Bronchiektasien. Bronchiectasien bei Situs viscerum inversus. *Beitr. Klin. Tuberk.* **83**:489–501, 1933.

8 Kartagener, M., and Horlacher, A., Zur Pathogenese der Bronchiektasien. Situs viscerum inversus und Polyposis nasi in einem Falle familiärer Bronchiektasien. *Beitr. Klin. Tuberk.* **87**:331–333, 1935.

9 Kartagener, M., and Mully, K., Familiäres Vorkommen von Bronchiektasien. *Z. Tuberk.* **13**:221–255, 1956.

10 Kartagener, M., and Stucki, P., Bronchiectasis with Situs Inversus. *Arch. Pediatr.* **79**:193–201, 1962.

11 Knox, G., et al., A Family with Kartagener's Syndrome: Linkage Data. *Ann. Hum. Genet.* **24**:137–140, 1960.

11a Miller, R. D., and Divertie, M. B., Kartagener's Syndrome. *Chest* **62**:130–135, 1972.

12 Overholt, E. L., and Bauman, D. F., Variants of Kartagener's Syndrome in the Same Family. *Ann. Intern. Med.* **48**:574–579, 1958.

12a Pony, J. C., et al., Syndrome de Kartagener et malformations cardiovasculaires. *Ouest. Med.* **25**:2125–2134, 1972.

13 Segal, P., et al., Kartagener's Syndrome with Familial Eye Changes. *Am. J. Ophthalmol.* **55**:1043–1049, 1963.

14 Siewert, A. K., Über einen Fall von Bronchiectasie bei einem Patienten mit Situs inversus viscerum. *Berl. Klin. Wochenschr.* **41**:139–141, 1904.

15 Taiana, J. A., et al., Kartagener's Syndrome. *Int. Surg.* **47**:565–569, 1967.

16 Torgersen, J., Transposition of Viscera, Bronchiectasis and Nasal Polyps: Genetical Analysis and Contribution to the Problem of Constitution. *Acta Radiol. (Stockh.)* **28**: 17–24, 1947.

17 Torgersen, J., The Triad of Kartagener. *Schweiz. Med. Wochenschr.* **82**:770–777, 1952.

78

Kleeblattschädel

(Cloverleaf Skull)

Classically, the Kleeblattschädel anomalad consists of a trilobular skull with craniosynostosis. However, variability in the degree of clinical severity occurs, and different sutures may be involved in different patients. Hydrocephaly is an associated defect. Hypoplastic orbits, nasal bones, and maxilla may also be observed.

Holtermüller and Wiedemann (11) first identified the condition, noting other similar cases (9, 13, 18). At least 45 examples have been recorded to date. Most patients have been of German extraction (1, 15, 19, 20), but this probably represents reporting bias. Nearly all cases have been sporadic, and normal karyotypes have been found (1, 6, 7, 8, 19, 20). An early demise has been noted in most instances. The patient reported by Feingold et al. (Case 1) (8) was fourteen years old.

Kleeblattschädel anomalad is not a disorder *sui generis*, but may be a sign occurring in a variety of disorders. The cloverleaf skull may occur (*a*) as an isolated anomalad or in association with (*b*) bony ankylosis of the limbs, (*c*) thanatophoric dwarfism, (*d*) Crouzon syndrome, (*e*) Carpenter syndrome, (*f*) Pfeiffer syndrome, and (*g*) Apert syndrome. The disorder may also occur (*h*) as an iatrogenic anomaly.

SYSTEMIC MANIFESTATIONS

Partington et al. (15) noted that the Kleeblattschädel anomalad may occur with bony anky-losis of the limbs, especially at the elbows and knees, and further, that the anomalad was also an integral part of some cases of thanatophoric dwarfism (11a, 15, 16, 19). Feingold et al. (8a) reported the anomalad in association with Apert syndrome.

Hall et al. (10), citing the pedigree of the Crouzon syndrome reported by Shiller (17), noted in one case a trilobular skull with roentgenographic calvarial honeycombing, synostosis of all cranial sutures, and facial features of the Crouzon syndrome. They noted that the cranial distortion produced in this patient was far more severe than that usually encountered in the Crouzon syndrome. They further suggested that this patient might well have been interpreted as an example of the Kleeblattschädel anomalad had the case arisen as a fresh mutation rather than in a family affected with Crouzon syndrome. Other affected individuals in this family had mild to moderate cranial involvement with the classic Crouzon appearance (11a).

Cohen (4) reported a case of the Kleeblattschädel anomalad in association with the Carpenter syndrome. Both Cohen (5), Eaton (7), and Hodach et al. (10a) observed the cloverleaf skull in patients with the Pfeiffer syndrome. It may be of interest that all such cases have been isolated examples. It was previously noted that the anomaly may occur with bony ankylosis of limbs (12, 15). Cases with ankylosis or limited extension of the elbows should be evaluated especially carefully, because some of them may represent severe examples of either the Crouzon or the Pfeiffer syndrome. Park and Powers (14) and Hall et al. (10) noted cases of Crouzon syndrome associated with limitation of elbow extension. Asnes and Morehead (2) and Cohen (5) have described cases of Pfeiffer syndrome associated with bony ankylosis of the elbows.

An iatrogenic Kleeblattschädel-like anomaly may rarely be observed in patients subjected to bilateral subtemporal decompression procedures (5).

Skull. Although classically the Kleeblattschädel anomalad presents a trilobular configuration, variability from relatively mild to severe involvement has been observed (Figs. 78-1 to 78-3). Classical trilobular skull has been reported by Holtermüller and Wiedemann (11) and by Comings (6). Severe involvement but with less well-defined trilobular shape has been observed by Wollin et al. (Case 1) (20) and by Cohen (4). Asymmetry may be documented in some cases, with more pronounced involvement on one side of the head. Relatively mild involvement may also occur. Changes in skull configuration have been noted with age. One patient reported by Feingold et al. (Case 1) (8) had a trilobular skull

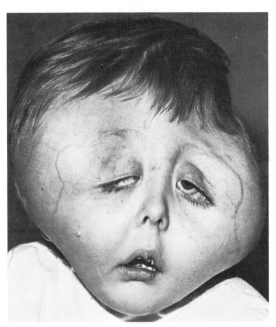

Figure 78-2. Asymmetric deformity of skull. Note severe antimongoloid obliquity of palpebral fissures. (*From D. G. Wollin et al., J. Can. Assoc. Radiol.* **19**:148, 1968.)

at birth, but by the time the patient was fourteen years of age, the skull could no longer be described as trilobular.

When the Kleeblattschädel anomalad is severe, the ears are displaced downward, facing the shoulders. Maxillary hypoplasia and relative mandibular prognathism are frequently encountered. The nasal bridge is depressed and, in some cases, the nose may be beaklike. Severe proptosis, ocular hypertelorism, and antimongoloid obliquity have been reported. The eyelids may fail to close, leading to corneal ulceration and clouding. Venous distention of the scleras, eyelids, periorbital areas, and scalp has been noted (1, 6, 7, 8, 11, 18).

Roentgenographically, the skull classically has a trilobular contour, with marked convolutional impressions and a thin distorted vault, giving a honeycombed appearance (Fig. 78-4). Synostosis of the coronal, lambdoidal, and metopic sutures may be observed, with bulging of the cerebrum through an open sagittal suture, and, in some cases through open squamosal sutures (1, 6, 11, 19). The squamosal and sagittal

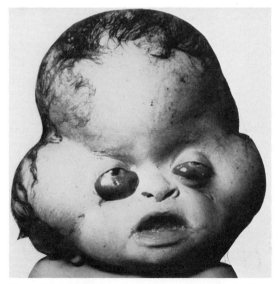

Figure 78-1. *Kleeblattschädel anomalad.* Classical trefoiling of skull. Note subluxation of eyeballs. (*Courtesy of R. T. Guzman, Mexico City, Mexico.*)

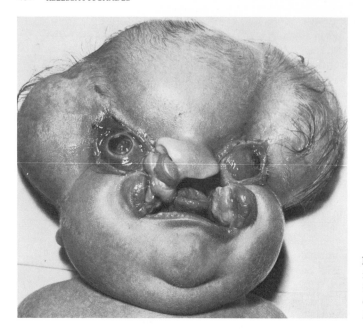

Figure 78-3. Kleeblattschädel anomalad in infant with bilateral oblique facial clefts. Child also had intrauterine amputation of digits. (*From A. Schuch and H. J. Pesch, Z. Kinderheilkd.* **109:**187, 1971.)

sutures may be closed in some cases (8). Cerebral eventration through a widely patent anterior fontanel was observed in one case reported by Feingold et al. (8). Synostosis and shortening of the cranial base have been reported (11). The posterior cranial fossa is small. Maxillary, sphenoid, and ethmoid bones may be underdeveloped and malformed, with shallow orbits. In the case of Comings (6), the orbits and zygomatic arches were absent. Ultrastructural studies have been described (3).

Central nervous system. Hydrocephaly (1, 6, 11), electroencephalographic abnormalities (1, 11), psychomotor and mental retardation (1, 18), small cerebellum (10), cerebellar herniation, and polymicrogyria (10a) have been reported. In some cases, shortening of the cranial base with concomitant distortion of the hindbrain may be responsible for cerebrospinal fluid obstruction at the level of the fourth ventricle, leading to hydrocephaly (1, 11). Obstruction of the cerebral aqueduct was demonstrated in one case (8).

Other findings. Iris coloboma (1, 8), blindness (18), obstructed nasolacrimal duct (8), absent external auditory canals, patent ductus arteriosus, atrial septal defect, bicuspid aortic valve, common mesentery, absent lesser omen-

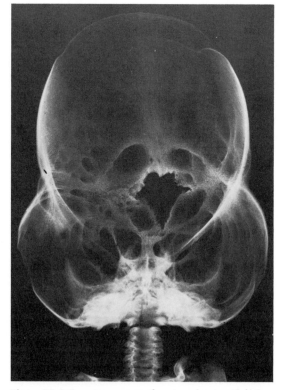

Figure 78-4. Roentgenogram showing classic trilobular skull deformity. (*From M. W. Partington et al.,* Arch. Dis. Child. **46:**656, 1971.)

tum, hypoplastic gallbladder, single umbilical artery, omphalocele, and unilateral hypomelia have been reported (5, 10a).

Oral manifestations. These have included macrostomia, macroglossia (6), highly arched palate, cleft lip-palate, cleft uvula, oblique facial cleft (5, 15a), malocclusion (18), and natal teeth (1, 6, 7).

DIFFERENTIAL DIAGNOSIS

This anomalad is so characteristic that discussion of differential diagnosis is limited to patterns of defects which may occur with Kleeblattschädel.

LABORATORY AIDS

None is known.

REFERENCES

1 Angle, C. R., et al., Cloverleaf Skull: Kleeblattschädel-Deformity Syndrome. *Am. J. Dis. Child.* **114**:198–202, 1967.

2 Asnes, R. S., and Morehead, C. D., Pfeiffer Syndrome. *Birth Defects* **5**(3):198–203, 1969.

3 Bonucci, E., and Nardi, F., The Cloverleaf Skull Syndrome: Histological, Histochemical and Ultrastructural Findings. *Virchows Arch. Pathol. Anat.* **357A**:199–212, 1972.

4 Cohen, M. M., Jr., The Kleeblattschädel Phenomenon—Sign or Syndrome? *Am. J. Dis. Child.* **124**:944, 1972.

5 Cohen, M. M., Jr., An Etiologic and Nosologic Overview of Craniosynostosis Syndromes. *Birth Defects*, **11**(2):137–189, 1975.

6 Comings, D. E., The Kleeblattschädel Syndrome—a Grotesque Form of Hydrocephalus. *J. Pediatr.* **67**:126–129, 1965.

7 Eaton, A., et al., The Kleeblatschädel Anomaly. *Birth Defects*, **11**(2):238–246, 1975.

8 Feingold, M., et al., Kleeblattschädel Syndrome. *Am. J. Dis. Child.* **118**:589–594, 1969.

8a Feingold, M., et al., The Demise of a Syndrome. *Syndrome Identification* **1**(2):21–23, 1973.

9 Gruber, G. B., Über einen akrocephalen Reliefschädel. Ein Beitrag zur Frage der partiellen Chondrodystrophie. *Beitr. Pathol. Anat.* **97**:9–22, 1936.

10 Hall, B. D., et al., Kleeblattschädel (Cloverleaf) Syndrome: Severe Form of Crouzon's Disease? *J. Pediatr.* **80**:526–527, 1972.

10a Hodach, R. J., et al., The Pfeiffer Syndrome, Associated with Kleeblattschädel and Multiple Visceral Anomalies. *Z. Kinderheilkd.* **119**:87–103, 1975.

11 Holtermüller, K., and Wiedemann, H. R., Kleeblatt-schädel-Syndrom. *Med. Monatsschr.* **14**:439–446, 1960.

11a Iannaccone, G., and Gerlini, G., The So-called "Cloverleaf Skull" Syndrome. *Pediatr. Radiol.* **2**:175–184, 1974.

12 Liebaldt, G., "Kleeblatt" Schädel-Syndrom, als Beitrag zur formalen Genese der Entwicklungsstörung des Schädeldaches. *Ergeb. Allg. Pathol.* **45**:23–38, 1964.

13 Meyer, R., Hydrocephalus chondrodystrophicus mit Bemerkungen über den "Perioststreifen" bei Chondrodystrophia. *Virchows Arch. Pathol. Anat.* **235**:766, 1925.

14 Park, E. A., and Powers, G. F., Acrocephaly and Scaphocephaly with Symmetrically Distributed Malformations of the Extremities. *Am. J. Dis. Child.* **20**:235–315, 1920.

14a Pena, S. D. J., Kleeblattschädel Anomaly—Which One? *Syndrome Identification* **2**(1):27, 1974.

15 Partington, M. W., et al., Cloverleaf Skull and Thanatophoric Dwarfism: Report of Four Cases, Two in the Same Sibship. *Arch. Dis. Child.* **46**:656–664, 1971.

15a Schuch, A., and Pesch, H. J., Beitrag zum Kleeblattschädel-Syndrom. *Z. Kinderheilkd.* **109**:187–198, 1971.

16 Shah, K., et al., Thanatophoric Dwarfism. *J. Med. Genet.* **10**:243–252, 1973.

17 Shiller, J. G., Craniofacial Dysostosis of Crouzon: A Case Report and Pedigree with Emphasis on Heredity. *Pediatrics* **23**:107–112, 1959.

18 Welter, H., Zur Frage des Hydrocephalus chondrodystrophicus congenitus. *Beitr. Pathol. Anat.* **97**:1–8, 1936.

19 Wiedemann, H. R., and Ostertag, B., Kleeblattschädel und allgemeine Mikromelie. *Klin. Pädiat.* **186**:261–263, 1974.

20 Wollin, D. G., et al., Cloverleaf Skull. *J. Can. Assoc. Radiol.* **19**:148–154, 1968.

79

Klippel-Feil Anomalad

The association of (*a*) massive fusion of cervical vertebras, (*b*) shortness of the neck, with painless limitation of head movement, and (*c*) low posterior hairline due to cervical abbreviation was described as early as the sixteenth century. Fusion of the second and third cervical vertebras was noted in an Egyptian mummy of about 500 B.C. (14, 27). However, the first adequate clinical and anatomic description of the condition was written by Klippel and Feil (20) in 1912. A particularly severe form is called iniencephaly (6, 12). Feil (10) elaborated on patients who had fusions at one or two interspaces. Some had hemivertebras and occipitoatlantal fusion as well. These entities, unrelated to cases of massive fusion, are discussed briefly under Differential Diagnosis. These other forms of fusion have been considered as examples of the Klippel-Feil anomalad, but we reserve that term to refer only to massive cervical vertebral fusion.

Almost all cases are sporadic. There have been a few examples of familial occurrence (11, 16). Although autosomal recessive inheritance has been suggested (16), we are reluctant to accept this hypothesis. In our analysis of more than 100 case reports of massive cervical vetebral fusion, over 65 percent were women. This sex predilection has been noted by others (8, 12, 28). The frequency of the disorder has been estimated to be approximately 1 per 30,000 to 1 per 40,000 individuals (13, 21).

Many authors have suggested that the condition arises from faulty segmentation of the meso-

dermal somites sometime between the third and seventh weeks in utero (35). There is no evidence of gross chromosomal anomaly (28).

SYSTEMIC MANIFESTATIONS

Facies. The head seems to sit directly on the thorax, without an interposing neck. The flaring trapezius muscles extend from the mastoid areas to the shoulders, producing a pterygium-like effect. Occasionally there is facial asymmetry, with one eye situated lower than the other (26). Posteriorly, the hairline extends to the shoulders (Fig. 79-1*A–D*).

Musculoskeletal system. Characteristically, several, occasionally all, cervical vertebras are fused into a solid mass. Occasionally some upper thoracic vertebras may be involved. Scoliosis, cervical ribs, and/or the Sprengel deformity have been noted in about 30 percent of cases (13, 14, 20, 35). Other common findings include spina bifida occulta, fusion of atlas with occipital bone, cleft vertebras, and hemivertebras (13, 34).

Nervous system. A large number of associated neurologic disturbances have been recorded: spasticity or hyperreflexia, bimanual synkinesis or mirror movements (1, 2, 8, 15), syringomyelia or syringobulbia (26, 35), hemiplegia, paraplegia, triplegia, quadriplegia, and others. The neurologic findings have been thoroughly reviewed by Mosberg (26).

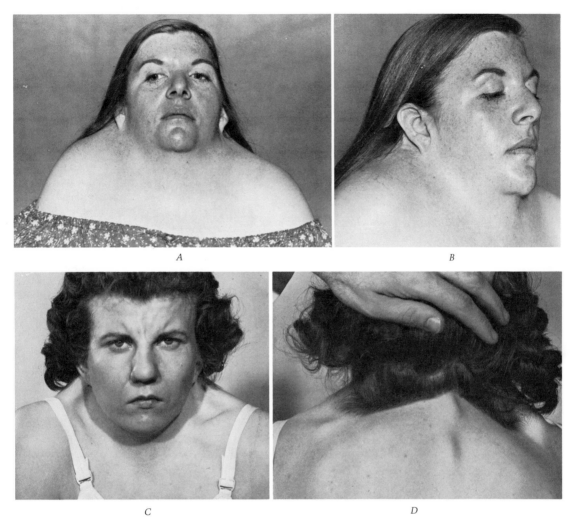

Figure 79-1. *A–D. Klippel-Feil anomalad.* Because of fusion of cervical vertebras, the head appears to rest directly on the thorax, without an intervening neck. The pterygium-like structures are actually the trapezius muscles. Note pulled-down, slanted auricles in *B* and low-set posterior hairline in *D*.

Eyes and ears. The most common eye finding has been convergent strabismus (2). Less frequently found are horizontal nystagmus and chorioretinal atrophy.

About 30 percent of patients have exhibited deafness due to abnormality of development of the inner ear (8, 23, 25, 34), but these may have been cases of the Wildervanck syndrome (vide infra).

Other findings. Congenital heart disease, usually ventricular septal defect, is occasionally noted (1a, 25, 28, 37). Unilateral renal agenesis is a common finding (24).

Oral manifestations. Cleft palate or bifid uvula is present in from 5 to 20 percent of the cases (1, 8, 27–29, 36). A more accurate estimate cannot be made because of the tendency of earlier authors to include several types of cervical fusion under the Klippel-Feil designation.

DIFFERENTIAL DIAGNOSIS

The flaring trapezius muscles give the patient an appearance which may simulate that in *Turner syndrome* or *Noonan syndrome*. The position of the head on the thorax may resemble that seen in tuberculosis of the cervical spine and the *Morquio syndrome*.

A variant, under the name of *cervicooculoacoustic (Wildervanck) syndrome* (Klippel-Feil anomalad, deafness, abducens paralysis, and retraction of the bulb), has been described (9). Most of these patients have been females.

Gunderson et al. (16) convincingly separated autosomal dominantly inherited fusion of the second and third cervical vertebras and variable cervical fusion from the massive cervical fusion usually considered to be the Klippel-Feil anomalad. Less convincing was the posited autosomal recessive inheritance of fusions of the fifth and sixth cervical vertebras. These types of fusion are not exceedingly rare, incidence having been estimated at about 7 per 1,000 individuals (3). *Spondylothoracic dysplasia* is probably a genetic heterogeneity consisting of dominant and recessive forms. The entire vertebral column is involved in fusions, hemivertebras, scoliosis, etc. (5, 19, 32, 38).

A syndrome has been described which included the Klippel-Feil anomalad, conductive deafness due to malformed ossicles, and absent vagina and uterus (1, 31). The Klippel-Feil anomalad has also been reported in association with unilateral renal agenesis, vaginal agenesis, and bicornuate uterus (24).

Mirror movements as an isolated finding may be inherited as an autosomal dominant trait (33).

LABORATORY AIDS

None is known.

REFERENCES

1 Baird, P. A., and Lowry, R. B., Absent Vagina and the Klippel-Feil Anomaly. *Am. J. Obstet. Gynecol.* **118:** 290–291, 1974.

1a Baird, P. A., et al., Klippel-Feil Syndrome: A Study of Mirror Movements Detected by Electromyography. *Am. J. Dis. Child.* 113:546–551, 1967.

2 Bauman, G. I., Absence of the Cervical Spine: Klippel-Feil Syndrome. *J.A.M.A.* **98:**129–132, 1932.

3 Brown, M. W., et al., The Incidence of Acquired and Congenital Fusions in the Cervical Spine. *Am. J. Roentgenol.* **92:**1255–1259, 1964.

4 Canetti, V. A., Sindrome de Klippel-Feil. *Acta Neurol. Lat. Am.* 3:318–353, 1957.

5 Cantu, J. M., et al., Evidence for Autosomal Recessive Inheritance of Costovertebral Dysplasia. *Clin. Genet.* **2:**149–154, 1971.

6 Chawla, S., and Bery, K., Iniencephalus: Prenatal Diagnosis. *Br. J. Radiol.* **42:**29–33, 1969.

7 Cohney, B. C., The Association of Cleft Palate with the Klippel-Feil Syndrome. *Plast. Reconstr. Surg.* **31:**179, 1963.

8 Erskine, C. A., An Analysis of the Klippel-Feil Syndrome. *Arch. Pathol.* **41:**269–281, 1946.

9 Everberg, G., et al., Wildervanck's Syndrome: Klippel-Feil Syndrome Associated with Deafness and Retraction of the Eyeball. *Br. J. Radiol.* **36:**562–567, 1963.

10 Feil, A., *L'absence et la diminution des vertèbres cervicales.* Thesis, Libraire Littéraire et Médicale, Paris, 1919.

11 Gienapp, R., von., Zur Erbbiologie der Klippel-Feilschen Krankheit. *Nervenarzt* 21:74–81, 1950.

12 Gilmour, J. R., The Essential Identity of the Klippel-Feil Syndrome and Iniencephaly. *J. Pathol. Bacteriol.* **53:**117–131, 1941.

13 Gjørup, P. A., and Gjørup, L., Klippel-Feil Syndrome. *Dan. Med. Bull.* **11:**50–53, 1964.

14 Gray, J. W., et al., Congenital Fusion of the Cervical Vertebrae. *Surg. Gynecol. Obstet.* **118:**373–385, 1964.

15 Gunderson, C. H., and Solitare, G. B., Mirror Movements in Patients with the Klippel-Feil Syndrome. *Arch. Neurol.* **18:**675–679, 1968.

16 Gunderson, C. J., et al., The Klippel-Feil Syndrome: Genetic and Clinical Reevaluation of Cervical Fusion. *Medicine* **46:**491–512, 1967.

17 Hadley, L. A., Roentgenographic Studies of the Cervical Spine. *Am. J. Roentgenol.* **52:**173–195, 1944.

18 Heiner, H., Über die Kombination von medianer Gaumenspalte und Klippel-Feil Syndrom. *Dtsch. Stomatol.* **10:** 92–98, 1960.

19 Jarcho, S., and Levin, P. M., Hereditary Malformation of the Vertebral Bodies. *Bull. Johns Hopkins Hosp.* **62:**216–226, 1938.

20 Klippel, M., and Feil, A., Un cêas d'absence des vertèbres cervicales. *Nouv. Iconogr. Salpet.* **25:**223–250, 1912.

21 Luftman, I. I., and Weintraub, S., Klippel-Feil Syndrome in a Full-term Newborn Infant. *N.Y. State J. Med.* **51:**2035–2038, 1951.

22 Martin, B. C., and Trabue, J. C., Klippel-Feil Syndrome with Associated Deformities: A Report of Three Cases. *Plast. Reconstr. Surg.* **9:**59, 1952.

23 McLay, K., and Maran, A. G. D., Deafness and the Klippel-Feil Syndrome. *J. Laryngol.* **83:**175–184, 1969.

24 Moore, W. B., et al., Genitourinary Anomalies Associated with Klippel-Feil Syndrome. *J. Bone Joint Surg.* **57A:**355–357, 1975.

25 Morrison, S. G., et al., Congenital Brevicollis (Klippel-Feil Syndrome) and Cardiovascular Anomalies. *Am. J. Dis. Child.* **115:**614–620, 1968.

26 Mosberg, W. H., The Klippel-Feil Syndrome: Etiology and Treatment of Neurologic Signs. *J. Nerv. Ment. Dis.* **117:**479–491, 1953.

27 Nobel, T. P., and Frawley, J. M., Klippel-Feil Syndrome: Numerical Reduction of Cervical Vertebrae. *Ann. Surg.* **82:**728–734, 1925.

28 Nora, J. J., et al., Klippel-Feil Syndrome with Congenital Heart Disease. *Am. J. Dis. Child.* **102:**858–864, 1961.

29 Nylen, B., and Wahlin, A., Post-operative Complications in Pharyngeal Flap Surgery. *Cleft Palate J.* **3:**347–356, 1966.

30 Palant, D. I., and Carter, B. L., Klippel-Feil Syndrome and Deafness. *Am. J. Dis. Child.* **123:**218–221, 1972.

31 Park, I. J., and Jones, H. W., Jr., A New Syndrome in Two Unrelated Females: Klippel-Feil Deformity, Conductive Deafness and Absent Vagina. *Birth Defects* **7**(6):311–317, 1971.

32 Pochaczevsky, R., et al., Spondylothoracic Dysplasia. *Radiology* **98:**53–58, 1971.

33 Regli, F., et al., Hereditary Mirror Movements. *Arch. Neurol.* **16:**620–623, 1967.

34 Schwarze, K., Zur Frage des Klippel-Feilschen Fehlers der Wirbelsäule. *Arch. Orthop. Unfallchir.* **41:**47–63, 1941.

35 Shoul, M. J., and Ritvo, M., Clinical and Roentgenological Manifestations of Klippel-Feil Syndrome (Congenital Fusion of the Cervical Vertebrae Brevicollis): Report of 8 Additional Cases and Review of the Literature. *Am. J. Roentgenol.* **68:**369–385, 1952.

36 Sommerfeld, R. M., and Schweiger, J. W., Cleft Palate with Klippel-Feil Syndrome. *Oral Surg.* **27:**737–739, 1969.

37 Tveter, K. J., and Kluge, T., Cor Triloculare Biatrium Associated with Klippel-Feil Syndrome. *Acta Paediatr. Scand.* **54:**489–496, 1965.

38 Weber, V., et al., Pathogenetische und genetische Fragen beim Klippel-Feil Syndrom-vergleichende Betrachtungen bei zwei Vettern. *Fortschr. Roentgenstrahl.* **119:**209–215, 1973.

80

Klippel-Trénaunay-Weber Syndrome

(Angioosteohypertrophy)

The syndrome described by Klippel and Trénaunay in 1900 (20) and by Parkes Weber in 1907 (30) has evolved into the most complex of all vascular syndromes. Their original descriptions included unilateral leg hypertrophy with cutaneous and subcutaneous hemangiomas, varicosities, phlebectasia, and, occasionally, arteriovenous fistula. Subsequent reports have expanded these findings to include almost every conceivable body area. Many additional abnormalities have also been recognized, including lymphangiomatous anomalies, macrodactyly, syndactyly, polydactyly, oligodactyly, and abdominal hemangiomas.

Pathologic evaluation of the vascular lesions has shown no consistent pattern (18, 23). Venous abnormalities, such as phlebectasia of superficial and deep venous systems, predominate, but arterial defects are not unusual. Because of the variability of the vascular anomalies this syndrome remains a clinical diagnosis, not a pathologic one.

Most patients are of normal mentality, the exceptions occurring when the vascular abnormalities involve the craniofacial area (12, 16, 23). The majority of these patients present features of the Sturge-Weber anomalad as part of the Klippel-Trénaunay-Weber syndrome (4, 31, 39). There is ample evidence to consider the two disorders as differing only in location of involvement (10, 12).

Koch (21) in 1956 cited from the literature a number of familial cases of the Klippel-Trénaunay-Weber syndrome. Close scrutiny of these cases reveals inadequate documentation of relative degree of involvement; liberal inclusion of relatives of the propositus with minor findings, such as isolated varicosities or posterior neck birthmarks; and other disorders, particularly neurofibromatosis. Among the approximately 135 reported cases (14), only Lindenauer's (24) example of brother-sister involvement is convincing; thus, it appears that almost all other cases show sporadic occurrence.

Although the recurrence risk is seemingly minimal, sporadicity and the wide variety of anomalies observed bespeaks etiologic heterogeneity (2a).

SYSTEMIC MANIFESTATIONS

Facies. Craniofacial involvement, when present, is quite similar to that seen in the Sturge-Weber anomalad, both in degree of variability and distribution of occurrence (10, 27). Hemangiomatous involvement of the craniofacial area places the patient at increased risk for neurologic complications, including mental retardation, as noted above. Macrocephaly has been observed in some instances (38a).

Extremities. Unilateral leg hypertrophy is the most frequent finding (24, 25) (Fig. 80-1). However, the hypertrophy can symmetrically or

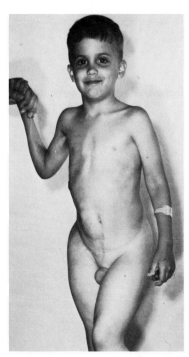

Figure 80-1. *Klippel-Trénaunay-Weber syndrome.*
Asymmetry of legs. Patient had angiomatous lesions
on right lateral aspect of trunk.

asymmetrically involve any or all limbs. The
hypertrophy is usually noted at birth, but may
occur at any age and progressively increase in
degree (21). Circumference and/or length of extremities are usually increased, but rarely, only
the proximal or distal limb segment may be
disproportionately large (24). Infrequently, atrophy of a limb may occur or a hypertrophied limb
may become atrophic over many years (3, 38).
Ultimate height is rarely excessive or stunted
except in severe cases.

In most instances, a visible vascular abnormality is present in the hypertrophied area; however, this is not always the case (13). Hemangiomatous lesions of almost every variety have
been noted, but varicosities, phlebectasia, nevus
flammeus (port-wine mark), and vascular masses
predominate (1, 24, 25). These lesions may minimally involve the extremity, but they can cause
severe distortion. The larger vascular masses
can sometimes cause a generalized bleeding
diathesis of the Kasabach-Merritt variety (17).
The occurrence of arteriovenous fistulas is not

uncommon (25). Lymphectasia in association
with the vascular abnormalities can result in
marked limb swelling with recurrent cellulitis.

Macrodactyly may involve one or many
digits, some assuming gigantic proportions (6,
23, 28a, 29) (Figs. 80-2, 3*A*, *B*). In those instances
in which the digits are not enlarged, they are
often of unequal length. There also may be clinodactyly at the most involved joints and/or relative brachydactyly. Cutaneous syndactyly is
frequent, but rarely involves more than two
digits on any one limb. Polydactyly and oligodactyly are relatively uncommon, usually being
found in patients with more severe and grotesque limb abnormalities (6, 22, 23).

Roentgenographic studies of the hypertrophied extremities usually show enlargement of
subcutaneous tissue, muscle, and bone; however, only one of these tissues may be hypertrophied (3, 33). Phlebectasis, phleboliths,
arteriovenous fistulas, hyperostosis, bony sclerosis, and bone atrophy can readily be demonstrated when present (1, 16, 24, 25, 38).
Roentgenologic manifestations of the craniofacial area are similar to those in Sturge-Weber
anomalad.

Skin. Typically, the various vascular lesions are
distributed over the lower limb (24), with fre-

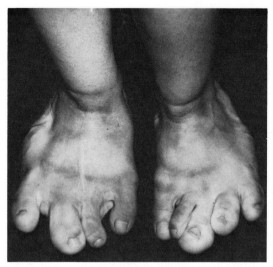

Figure 80-2. Gigantiform toes of patient in Fig. 80-1.
One toe has been surgically removed from the right
foot.

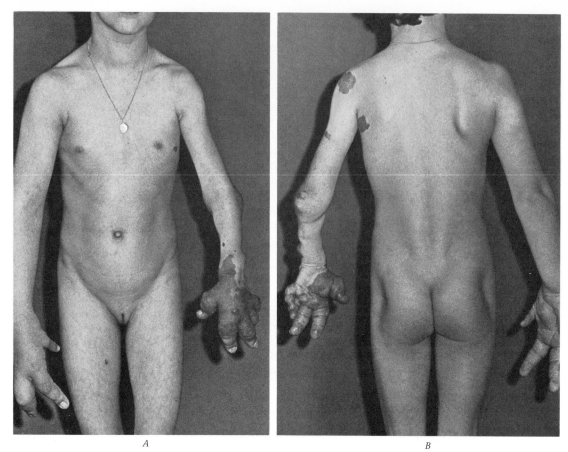

Figure 80-3. *A, B.* Monstrous enlargement of hands, disparity in size of arms, fixation of left elbow joint. (*From E. Nöh and R. Steckenmesser, Z. Orthopäd.* **112:**243, 1974.)

quent extension to the buttocks and less often with involvement of the lower part of the back, flank, lateral area of the chest, and axillary area (21). The upper extremities are sometimes involved, as are the abdomen, chest, neck, and face (5, 10). Telangiectatic spots have been reported (1). Hyperpigmented streaks and spots have been noted particularly in the area of the vascular lesion (18). Rarely, pigmentation of areas has been preceded by a vesicular rash (31). Some patients have had skin ulcers at birth or at a later age (19, 23).

Viscera. Involvement of the viscera is not rare. The major manifestations are hemangiomatous lesions of the gastrointestinal tract (22, 36),

urinary system (15), visceral organs (18), mesentery, and pleura (22). The types of vascular lesions are as varied as those found on the extremities.

Generalized nonspecific visceromegaly has been noted (7), particularly involving the kidney (10, 16). However, it is important to note that no patient with Klippel-Trénaunay-Weber syndrome has had associated Wilms tumor, although one patient with nephroblastomatosis has been described (25a). Abdominal lymphectasia and protein-losing enteropathy secondary to lymphectasia have been reported (8).

Miscellaneous findings. Enlargement of the genitalia with ambiguity secondary to direct he-

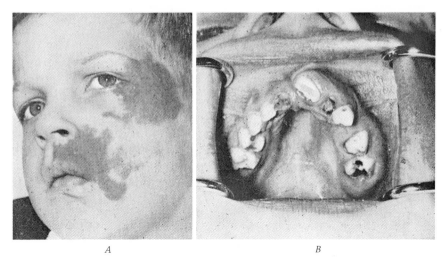

Figure 80-4. (*A*). Flat hemangioma of left maxillary–zygomatic region. (*B*). Enlargement of left upper jaw accompanied by premature eruption of upper left central incisor. (A, B, *courtesy of R. Stellmach*, Fortschr. Kiefer Gesichtschir. **4**:54, 1958.)

mangiomatous involvement has been observed (15). Lipodystrophy involving the upper extremities has occurred in a few severe examples (6, 22). Scoliosis secondary to unequal leg length has been noted (33).

Eye abnormalities have included glaucoma, cataracts, scleral pigmentation, and heterochromia irides (1, 10, 29).

Oral manifestations. The frequency of oral manifestations is unknown. Miescher (26) described oral changes in 33 of 44 cases involving the facial region. The nevus flammeus was located most frequently in the area supplied by the second branch of the trigeminal nerve. The soft and hard palates are most frequently involved (Fig. 80-4*A*, *B*). (These points also apply to the Sturge-Weber anomalad.) Angiomatosis of the tongue and pharynx has also been noted, but in these cases the hemangioma was located in the cervical region. Bony hypertrophy when present may produce asymmetry and malocclusion. In addition, the gingival tissue may also be enlarged. In general, the darker the cutaneous nevus flammeus, the more severe the oral involvement. Stellmach (38) noted accelerated growth and premature eruption of teeth on the involved side, which he believed resulted in malocclusion.

DIFFERENTIAL DIAGNOSIS

Neurofibromatosis must be excluded, since limb hypertrophy and skin hemangiomas may be associated with the disorder (2). A relative lack of multiple discrete café-au-lait spots occurs in Klippel-Trénaunay-Weber syndrome. *Beckwith-Wiedemann syndrome* may have associated hemihypertrophy and skin hemangiomas. However, its usual findings of omphalocele and macroglossia separate it adequately. Cutis marmorata telangiectatica congenita when associated with discrete vascular skin lesions and aberrations of limb size may be difficult to differentiate from the Klippel-Trénaunay-Weber syndrome and may be closely related (9, 40). The *Maffucci syndrome*, with its frequent limb hypertrophy and vascular skin lesions, may cause confusion, but the usual late onset of the vascular lesions and the presence of enchondromatosis clearly separate the two disorders.

Hemihypertrophy can be associated with vascular abnormalities of the skin. Some cases reported under this designation have been examples of the Klippel-Trénaunay-Weber syndrome (32). Large isolated hemangiomas of a limb can cause hypertrophy. Single limb hypertrophy or isolated macrodactyly without hemangiomatous involvement should not be considered as constituting the Klippel-Trénaunay-Weber syndrome. However, such limbs and digits should be watched closely for development of vascular or pigmented skin lesions.

Lipomatosis resembling the Klippel-Trénaunay-Weber syndrome has been reported (2a, 11).

LABORATORY AIDS

None is known.

REFERENCES

1 Arrighi, F., Hamartose ecto-mesodérmique: un cas d'angiomatose diffuse avec fusion de maladie de Sturge-Weber-Krabbe et de maladie de Parkes Weber. *Bull. Soc. Fr. Dermatol. Syphiligr.* **67**:562–563, 1960.

2 Arrighi, F., Hamartose ecto-mesodérmique: un cas de fusion de maladie de Recklinghausen (avec éléphantiasis nevromateux de Virchow) et de maladie de Klippel-Trénaunay-Parkes Weber. *Bull. Soc. Fr. Dermatol. Syphiligr.* **67**:564, 1960.

2a Banhayan, G. A., Lipomatosis, Angiomatosis and Macroencephalia: A Previously Undescribed Congenital Syndrome. *Arch. Pathol.* **92**:1– , 1971.

3 Bereston, E. S., and Roberts, D., Congenital Hypertrophy of Extremities. *South. Med. J.* **58**:302–307, 1965.

4 Bonse, G., Röntgenbefunde bei einer Phakomatose (Sturge-Weber kombiniert mit Klippel-Trénaunay). *Fortschr. Roentgenstr.* **74**:727–729, 1951.

5 Brooksaler, F., The Angioosteohypertrophy Syndrome (Klippel-Trénaunay-Weber Syndrome). *Am. J. Dis. Child.* **112**:161–164, 1966.

6 Buchanec, J., and Galanda, V., Polymalformačny-Klippelov-Trenaunayov-Weberov syndróms progresivnou lipodistrofiou u 6-ročného chlapca. *Čs. Pediatr.* **24**:228–232, 1969.

7 Cagiati, L., Klinischer und pathologischer Beitrag zum Studium der halbseitigen Hypertrophie. *Dtsch. Z. Nervenheilkd.* **32**:282–293, 1907.

8 Caplan, D. B., et al., Angioosteohypertrophy Syndrome with Protein-losing Enteropathy. *J. Pediatr.* **74**:119–123, 1969.

9 Fahrig, H., Zur Cutis marmorata teleangiectatica congenita (Phlebectasia congenita) und ihren Beziehungen zu fakultativ mit Naevi teleangiectatici kombinierten Missbildungen. *Z. Kinderheilkd.* **102**:179–192, 1968.

10 Furukawa, T., et al., Sturge-Weber and Klippel-Trénaunay Syndrome with Nevus of Ota and Ito. *Arch. Dermatol.* **102**:640–645, 1970.

11 Geley, L., et al., Isolierte Gliedmassen-monohypertrophie mit Lipomatosis derselben Körperhälfte-ein neues Syndrom? *Z. Kinderchir.* **12**:101–110, 1973.

12 Gottron, H. A., and Schnyder, U. W., Vererbung von Hautkrankheiten, in *Handbuch der Haut- und Geschlechtskrankheiten*, vol. 7. Springer Verlag, Berlin, 1966, p. 715.

13 Gougerot, H., and Filliol, P., Naevus variquex ostéo-hypertrophique de Klippel ou hémiangiectasie hypertrophique de Parkes Weber. *Arch. Dermatol. Syph.* (*Paris*) **1**:404–411, 1929.

14 Hall, B. D., Bladder Hemangiomas in Klippel-Trénaunay-Weber Syndrome. *N. Engl. J. Med.* **285**:1032–1033, 1971.

15 Hall, B. D., Unpublished data, 1972.

16 Hall, R., A Case of Melorheostosis with Cutaneous Haemangioma and Lymphatic Vesicles. *J. Bone Joint Surg.* **43B**:335–337, 1961.

17 Inceman, S., and Tangün, Y., Chronic Defibrination Syndrome Due to a Giant Hemangioma Associated with Microangiopathic Hemolytic Anemia. *Am. J. Med.* **46**:997–1002, 1969.

18 Inui, M., et al., An Autopsy Case of Klippel-Trénaunay-Weber's Disease. *Acta Pathol. Jap.* **19**:251–263, 1969.

19 Ippen, H., Systematisierte Angiektasie mit Gliedmassenatrophie (Ein Beitrag zum "Klippel-Trénaunay-Syndrom"). *Hautarzt* **8**:317–320, 1959.

20 Klippel, M., and Trénaunay, P., Du naevus variqueux ostéo-hypertrophique. *Arch. Gén. Méd.* **185**:641–672, 1900.

21 Koch, G., Zur Klinik, Symptomatologie, Pathogenese und Erbpathologie des Klippel-Trénaunay-Weber'schen Syndroms. *Acta Genet. Med.* (*Roma*) **5**:326–370, 1956.

22 Kuffer, F. R., et al., Klippel-Trénaunay Syndrome, Visceral Angiomatosis and Thrombocytopenia. *J. Pediatr. Surg.* **3**:65–72, 1968.

23 Lamar, L. M., et al., Klippel-Trénaunay-Weber Syndrome. *Arch. Dermatol.* **91**:58–59, 1965.

24 Lindenauer, S. M., The Klippel-Trénaunay Syndrome: Varicosity, Hypertrophy and Hemangioma with no Arteriovenous Fistula. *Ann. Surg.* **162**:303–314, 1965.

25 Lindenauer, S. M., Congenital Arteriovenous Fistula and the Klippel-Trénaunay Syndrome. *Ann. Surg.* **174**:246–263, 1971.

25a Mankad, V. N., et al., Bilateral Nephroblastomatosis and Klippel-Trénaunay Syndrome. *Cancer* **33**:1462–1467, 1974.

26 Miescher, G., Über plane Angiome (Naevi hyperaemici). *Dermatologica* **106**:176–183, 1958.

27 Nellhaus, G., et al., Sturge-Weber Disease with Bilateral Intracranial Calcifications at Birth and Unusual Pathologic Findings. *Acta Neurol. Scand.* **43**:314–347, 1967.

28 Nöh, E., and Steckenmesser, R., Der angeborene Riesenwuchs, klinische und arteriographische Befunde an Hand und Arm beim Klippel-Trénaunay Syndrom. *Z. Orthopäd.* **112**:243–252, 1974.

29 Noriega-Sanchez, A., et al., Oculocutaneous Melanosis Associated with the Sturge-Weber Syndrome. *Neurology* (*Minneap.*) **22**:256–268, 1972.

30 Parkes Weber, F., Angioma Formation in Connection with Hypertrophy of Limbs and Hemi-hypertrophy. *Br. J. Dermatol.* **19**:231–235, 1907.

31 Rademacher, R., Über einen Fall einer Kombination von Sturge-Weber und Klippel-Trénaunay Syndrom mit kon-

stitutioneller Neurodermitis. *Dermatol. Wochenschr.* **143:**381–386, 1961.

32 Ringrose, R. E., et al., Hemihypertrophy. *Pediatrics* **36:** 434–448, 1965.

33 Rose, L. M., Hypertrophy of the Lower Limbs with Cutaneous Naevus and Varicose Veins. *Arch. Dis. Child.* **25:**162–169, 1950.

34 Sabanas, A. O., and Chatterton, C. C., Crossed Congenital Hemihypertrophy. *J. Bone Joint Surg.* **37A:**871–874, 1955.

35 Schönenberg, H., and Redemann, M., Klippel-Trénaunay-Weber Syndrom. *Klin. Padiatr.* **184:**449–460, 1972.

36 Sheperd, J. A., Angiomatous Conditions of the Gastro-intestinal Tract. *Br. J. Surg.* **40:**409–421, 1953.

37 Silva, M., da, and Neves, H., Über einen Fall von Klippel-Trénaunay-schem Symptomenkomplex, der erfolgreich mit Röntgenstrahlen behandelt wurde. *Fortschr. Roentgenstr.* **90:**475–482, 1959.

38 Stellmach, R., Zwei Beobachtungen von partiellem Riesenwuchs kindlicher Kiefer beim sogenannten planen Hämangiomdes Geischtshaut. *Fortschr. Kiefer Gesichtschir.* **4:**54–57, 1958.

38a Stephan, M. J., et al., Macrocephaly in Association with Unusual Cutaneous Angiomatosis. *J. Pediatr.* (in press).

39 Teller, H., and Lindner, B., Uber Mischformen der phakomatösen Syndrome von Sturge-Weber und Klippel-Trénaunay. *Z. Haut Geschlechtskr.* **13:**113–120, 1952.

40 Way, B. H., et al., Cutis marmorata telangiectatica congenita. *J. Cutaneous Path.* **1:**10–25, 1974.

81

de Lange Syndrome

(Brachmann-de Lange Syndrome, Cornelia de Lange Syndrome)

The syndrome of (*a*) primordial growth deficiency, (*b*) severe mental retardation, (*c*) anomalies of the extremities, and (*d*) characteristic facies was independently described by Brachmann (3) in 1916 and by de Lange (8) in 1933. Excellent reviews are those of Ptacek et al. (14) and Berg et al. (2). At least 250 examples have been reported (1a).

Most cases have been sporadic. The frequency of affected sibs among reported cases is between 2 and 5 percent (1, 1a, 10, 13). There has been no increased rate of parental consanguinity. In a few cases, aleatory chromosomal abnormalities have been noted (5, 13). The disorder was reported in identical twins (12), and we have seen female identical twins with the syndrome.

SYSTEMIC MANIFESTATIONS

Birth weight is usually less than 2,500 g, and both height and weight remain below the 3d percentile for age. There are often recurrent respiratory infections and gastrointestinal upsets (2). Sucking and swallowing ability are diminished. In most cases, the intelligence quotient has been below 50. Seizures have been observed in about 20 percent of the cases. Speech maturation is especially defective. Most patients die before the age of six years.

Facies. Patients resemble one another to a remarkable degree. The skull is microbrachy-cephalic. The eyebrows are confluent (synophrys), the eyelashes long and curly, and the hairline is low. The nose is small with a flat bridge. The nostrils are anteverted, and there is a long philtrum. A bluish hue is often noted about the eyes, nose, and mouth. The temporal and scalp veins may be conspicuous. The typical facies may not be evident during the first year of life (13) (Fig. 81-1*A*, *B*).

Musculoskeletal alterations. In about 35 percent of the cases there is initial hypertonia. The limbs may exhibit characteristic anomalies, but these are usually more variable than facial alterations. Generally, the hands and feet are small. The fingers are often short and tapering, with clinodactylous fifth digits which have only a single flexion crease. The thumbs are proximally placed in about 80 percent of patients (2). About 15 to 20 percent of the patients exhibit oligodactyly or absence or deformity of the bones of the upper limbs. Flexion contractures of the elbow are present in at least 80 percent of cases. Soft-tissue syndactyly of the second and third toes is an almost constant feature (Fig. 81-2*A*, *B*)

Roentgenographic examination shows the skull to be small, with the dorsum sella enlarged. Bone age is delayed, and not uncommonly there is discrepancy in the sequence of development of various centers of ossification (1a). The humerus, radius, and ulna are shortened. There are hypoplasia and dorsal disloca-

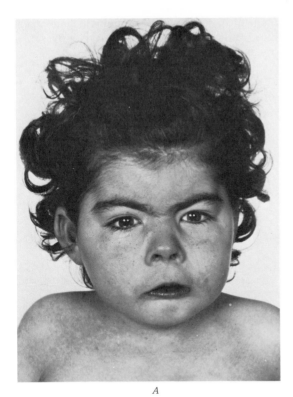
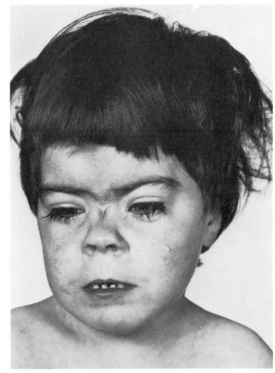

A   *B*

Figure 81-1. *de Lange syndrome.* (*A, B*). Note microcephaly, low hairline, synophrys, small nose with anteverted nostrils, thin lips. (*From B. Schlesinger et al.,* Arch. Dis. Child. **38:**349, 1970.)

tion of the radial head; often the neck of the humerus is elongated (7). In some cases, the forearm bones are absent. The first metacarpal and middle phalanx of the fifth finger are often hypoplastic. The acetabular angle is low, especially when the child is less than one year of age (8). The sternum is short with a reduced number of ossification centers, and the ribs are rather thin.

Skin. Hirsutism is often generalized, but is especially marked by low hairline, synophrys, long and curly eyelashes, and hair whorls over the shoulders, lower back, and extremities (Fig. 81-3*A, B*). The veins on the forehead may be dilated, and there may be circumoral cyanosis. The nipples and umbilicus are frequently hypoplastic.

Dermatoglyphic findings include hypoplastic ridge patterns, simian creases, and increased "atd" palmar angle. There is also an increase in radial loops on the third and fourth fingertips (20) and a palmar interdigital triradius (2). Cutis marmorata is present in at least 50 percent of patients.

Genitourinary. The kidneys are often hypoplastic, dysplastic, or cystic (6). The testes are undescended in over 70 percent of males, and in some there is hypospadias. Female patients commonly have a bicornuate or septate uterus and long narrow ovaries (21).

Other findings. Malrotation of the intestine and various congenital heart defects have been described (6, 15). A variety of miscellaneous findings has been provided by Berg et al. (2).

Oral manifestations. Characteristically there are micrognathia and prominent mental spur. The lips are thin, with the corners of the mouth downturned (so-called "carp mouth"). The philtrum is long, and often there is circumoral cyanosis. Delayed tooth eruption has been reported, and several authors have remarked on the smallness of the teeth, although no measurements have been published to date (5, 11). Our recent analysis of 100 published cases indicates that the palate has been cleft in about 20 percent (1a, 2, 5, 6, 11, 13, 14, 21).

The cry is usually low-pitched and growling. Oral self-mutilation has been described (18).

Russell (16) described a 10-to-30-μ broad acellular zone with gracile fibers around blood vessels in the gingiva. On the basis of his-tochemical study with toluidine blue and alcian blue, this was interpreted as perivascular myxomatous degeneration.

DIFFERENTIAL DIAGNOSIS

The overall pattern is generally diagnostic. Synophrys may be seen in normal individuals and in a number of syndromal conditions such as *Waardenburg syndrome, Down syndrome, gingival fibromatosis–hypertrichosis syndrome*, etc.

Congenital dislocation of the radial head can

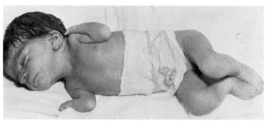

A

Figure 81-2. (*A*). Oligodactyly of upper limbs. (*From G. Lässker, Leipzig, East Germany.*) (*B*). Micromelia with proximally placed thumbs, small fifth fingers with single flexion crease, finger contractures, right simian crease, lack of palmar creases on left. (*From B. Schlesinger et al.*, Arch. Dis. Child. **38**:349, 1970.)

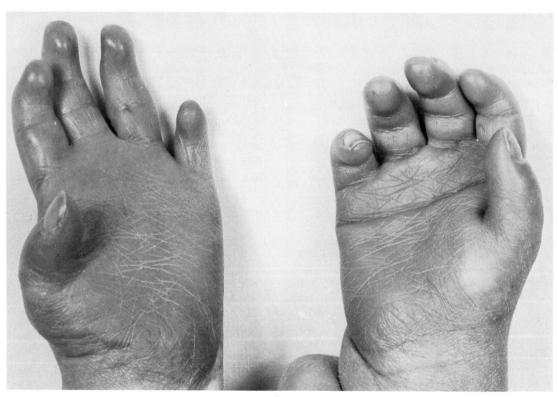

B

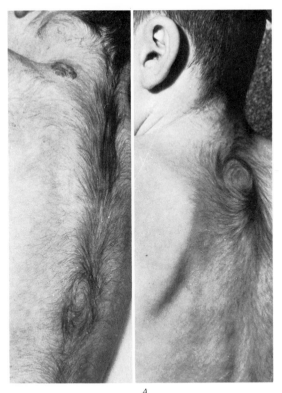 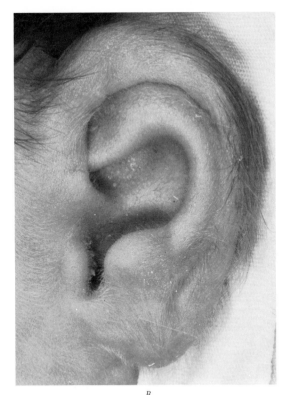

A   B

Figure 81-3. (*A*). Hirsutism of back, with whorling. (*From O. Noé*, Clin. Pediatr. **3:**541, 1964.) (*B*). Hirsutism of pinna.

occur in a large number of disorders: nail-patella syndrome, diaphyseal aclasia, *Ehlers-Danlos syndrome, otopalatodigital syndrome, Klinefelter syndrome*, Nievergelt syndrome, arthrogryposis multiplex congenita, *Apert syndrome*, etc.

LABORATORY AIDS

Elevated serum α-ketoglutarate and glutamate levels have been described (4).

REFERENCES

1 Beck, B., Familial Occurrence of Cornelia de Lange's Syndrome. *Acta Paediatr. Scand.* **63:**225–231, 1974.

1a Beratis, N. G., et al., Familial de Lange Syndrome: Report of Three Cases in a Sibship. *Clin. Genet.* **2:**170–176, 1971.

2 Berg, J. M., et al., *The De Lange Syndrome*. Pergamon, New York, 1970.

3 Brachmann, E., Ein Fall von symmetrischer Monodaktylie durch Ulnadefekt. *Jb. Kinderheilkd.* **84:**224–235, 1916.

4 Daniel, W. L., and Higgins, J. V., Biochemical and Genetic Investigation of the de Lange Syndrome. *Am. J. Dis. Child.* **121:**401–405, 1971.

5 Falek, A., et al., Familial de Lange Syndrome with Chromosome Abnormalities. *Pediatrics* **37:**92–101, 1966.

6 France, N. E., et al., Pathological Features in the de Lange Syndrome. *Acta Paediatr. Scand.* **58:**470–480, 1969.

7 Kurlander, G. J., and DeMyer, W., Roentgenology of the Brachmann-de Lange Syndrome. *Radiology* **88:**101–110, 1967.

8 Lange, C., de, Sur un typ nouveau de dégéneration (typus Amstelodamensis). *Arch. Méd. Enf.* **36:**713–718, 1933.

9 Lee, F., and Kenny, F., Skeletal Changes in the Cornelia de Lange Syndrome. *Am. J. Roentgenol.* **100:**27–39, 1967.

10 Lieber, E., et al., Brachmann-de Lange Syndrome. *Am. J. Dis. Child.* **125:**717–718, 1973.

11 McArthur, R. G., and Edwards, I. H., De Lange Syndrome: Report of 20 Cases. *Can. Med. Assoc. J.* **96:**1185–1198,

1967.

12 Motl, M. L., and Opitz, J. M., Phenotypic and Genetic Studies of the Brachmann-De Lange Syndrome. *Hum. Hered.* **21:**1–16, 1971.

13 Pashayan, H., Variability of the de Lange Syndrome: Report of 3 Cases and Genetic Analysis of 54 Families. *J. Pediatr.* **75:**853–858, 1969.

14 Ptacek, L. J., et al., The Cornelia de Lange Syndrome. *J. Pediatr.* **63:**1000–1020, 1963.

15 Rao, P. S., Congenital Heart Disease in the de Lange Syndrome. *J. Pediatr.* **79:**674–677, 1971.

16 Russell, B. G., The Cornelia de Lange Syndrome. Typus degenerativus Amstelodamensis: Histologic Studies of the Marginal Gingiva. *Scand. J. Dent. Res.* **78:**369–373, 1970.

17 Schlesinger, B., et al., Typus degenerativus Amstelodamensis. *Arch. Dis. Child* **38:**349–357, 1970.

18 Shear, C. S., et al., Self Mutilative Behavior as a Feature of the de Lange Syndrome. *J. Pediatr.* **78:**506–507, 1971.

19 Shuster, D. S., and Johnson, S., Cutaneous Manifestations of the Cornelia de Lange Syndrome. *Arch. Dermatol.* **93:**702–707, 1966.

20 Smith, G. F., A Study of the Dermatoglyphics in the de Lange Syndrome. *J. Ment. Defic. Res.* **10:**241–247, 1966.

21 Vischer, D., Typus degenerativus Amstelodamensis (Cornelia de Lange-Syndrom). *Helv. Paediatr. Acta* **20:**415–445, 1965.

82

Lenz Microphthalmia Syndrome

In 1955, Lenz (4) described a syndrome consisting of (a) microphthalmia, (b) skeletal anomalies of the hands and clavicles, (c) renal anomalies, (d) genital anomalies, and (e) defects of the dentition. The patient reported by Herrmann and Opitz (2) had the same disorder; another probable example is that of Manzitti and Alezzandrini (5). Four cases in a family described by Hoefnagel et al. (3) may also represent the same syndrome.

X-linked recessive transmission seems likely. However, no affected male has reproduced; therefore autosomal dominant inheritance with predominant male sex limitation cannot be excluded. Minor malformations have been noted in female heterozygous carriers in some instances (24). Female carriers have also been noted to have an increased abortion rate, suggesting that many cases may only appear to be sporadic (2, 6).

SYSTEMIC MANIFESTATIONS

Facies. Unilateral or bilateral eye defects ranging from microphthalmia to clinical anophthalmia have been observed (1–4, 6). Mongoloid slanting of the palpebral fissures may be present (2). Microcornea (2), strabismus (4), nystagmus (1, 2), epicanthal folds (3), and other eye defects have been noted. The ears have been observed to be asymmetric, dysplastic, hypoplastic, and protuberant in some cases (1–3, 6) (Fig. 82-1). Micrognathia has also been noted (2).

Central nervous system. Mental retardation has been reported, as well as microcephaly (1–3, 6).

Musculoskeletal system. Camptodactyly of the fifth fingers (2, 4), clinodactyly of the second fingers (2), duplication of the thumb (4), cu-

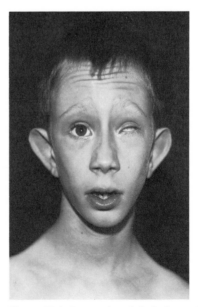

Figure 82-1. *Lenz microphthalmia syndrome.* Eye defects range from microphthalmia to clinical anophthalmia and may be unilateral or bilateral. Note outstanding ears. (*From J. Herrmann and J. M. Opitz, Birth Defects* **5**(2):138, 1969.)

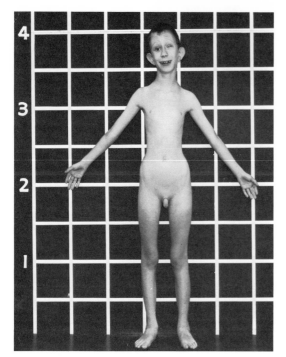

Figure 82-2. Patients are short with cylindric thorax and internally rotated knees. (*From J. Herrmann and J. M. Opitz,* Birth Defects **5**(2):138, 1969.)

taneous syndactyly of the third and fourth toes, wide gap between first and second toes, pseudo-clubbing of the toes, flat foot, calcaneovalgus deformity (2, 6), and varus deformity (3) have been observed.

Short stature (1, 2), cylindrical thorax with sloping shoulders and clavicular defects (2, 4, 6), low scapulas, notching of the vertebral bodies, mild cubitus valgus, limited extension in both hip joints, and mild gena valga with internally rotated knees and prominent fibulas (2) have been reported (Figs. 82-2, 82-3).

Genitourinary system. Unilateral renal agenesis (4), bilateral renal agenesis (3), renal dysgenesis, hydroureters (2), cryptorchism (2, 4, 6), and hypospadias (2) have been described.

Other findings. Congenital heart defect (4), atresia of the ileum (3), umbilical hernia, unusual dermatoglyphics (2), and defective speech (2, 3) have been noted.

Oral manifestations. Highly arched palate, crooked anterior teeth (2, 4), and agenesis of the permanent maxillary lateral incisors (2) have been reported, all probably being aleatory findings.

DIFFERENTIAL DIAGNOSIS

Isolated bilateral anophthalmia is inherited as an autosomal recessive trait. Microphthalmia may be inherited as an autosomal dominant, autosomal recessive, or X-linked recessive trait. Microphthalmia may also occur as an integral part of several different disorders (5).

LABORATORY AIDS

Intravenous pyelograms are indicated in affected individuals.

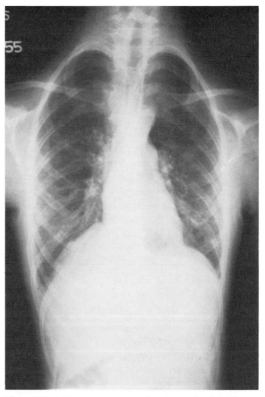

Figure 82-3. Roentgenogram showing cylindric thorax, sloping shoulders, and clavicular defects. (*From J. Herrmann and J. M. Opitz,* Birth Defects **5**(2):138, 1969.)

REFERENCES

1   Goldberg, M. F., and McKusick, V. A., X-linked Colobo-
matous Microphthalmos and Other Congenital Anomalies.
Am. J. Ophthalmol. **71:**1128–1138, 1971.

2   Herrmann, J., and Opitz, J. M., The Lenz Microphthalmia
Syndrome. *Birth Defects* **5**(2):138–143, 1969.

3   Hoefnagel, D., et al., Heredofamilial Bilateral Anophthalmia. *Arch Ophthalmol.* **69:**760–764, 1963.

4   Lenz, W., Recessiv-geschlechtsgebundene Mikrophthalmie

mit multiplen Missbildungen. *Z. Kinderheilkd.* **77:**384–
390, 1955.

5   McKusick, V. A., *Mendelian Inheritance in Man,* 3d ed.
Johns Hopkins Press, Baltimore, 1971.

6   Manzitti, E., and Alezzandrini, A., Syndrome dyscéphalique de François (Case 2). *Ann. Ocul.* **196:**456–465,
1963.

83

Leopard Syndrome

(Multiple Lentigines Syndrome)

The word *leopard* is an acronym which serves as a mnemonic device for remembering the essential features of this disorder. The syndrome as originally described consisted of (*a*) multiple *l*entigines, (*b*) *e*lectrocardiographic conduction abnormalities, (*c*) *o*cular hypertelorism, (*d*) *p*ulmonic stenosis, (*e*) *a*bnormal genitalia, (*f*) *r*etardation of growth, and (*g*) sensorineural *d*eafness. In 1969, Gorlin et al. (6) reviewed the syndrome, noting previously reported cases (3, 11–13, 15, 17, 28–30). One of these families was later reported in greater detail (4). Subsequently, numerous other cases were published (10, 14, 16, 18, 22–25, 27). Several incompletely documented cases are known (1, 2, 5, 8, 9, 19, 21, 26, 31). Extensive reviews have been published by Gorlin et al. (7) and by Polani and Moynahan (20). Pathogenesis has been discussed by the latter authors.

The syndrome clearly follows an autosomal dominant mode of transmission with high penetrance and marked variation in expression. X-linked inheritance has been ruled out by male-to-male transmission (6).

SYSTEMIC MANIFESTATIONS

Facies. The face is usually triangular, with biparietal bossing, hypertelorism, ptosis of the eyelids, epicanthal folds, and low-set ears. Patients frequently exhibit mild pterygium colli (7, 20) (Fig. 83-1).

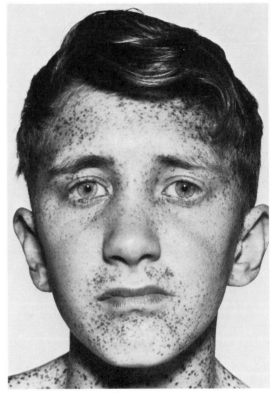

Figure 83-1. *Leopard syndrome.* Ocular hypertelorism, numerous lentigines. *(From P. E. Polani and E. J. Moynahan, Q. J. Med. **41**:205, 1972.)*

Skin. Although multiple lentigines are striking when present, most patients appear not to develop these lesions. When they do occur, they may be present at birth or appear shortly thereafter, increasing in number with age. Lesions may appear anywhere on the skin, being most concentrated on the neck and upper part of the trunk and less dense on the face, scalp, palms, soles, and genitalia. Mucosal surfaces are never involved. A few large "café-noir" spots are often scattered over the trunk (6, 7) (Figs. 83-2, 82-3).

Lentigines differ from common ephelides in appearing earlier, having no relationship to sun exposure, and showing, on microscopic examination, more prominent rete ridges with a larger number of melanocytes per unit area of skin.

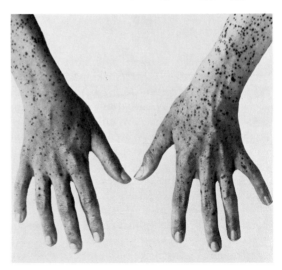

Figure 83-3. Numerous lentigines of hands. (*From P. E. Polani and E. J. Moynahan*, J. Med. **41**:205, 1972.)

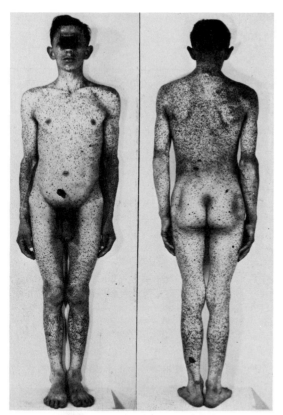

Figure 83-2. (*A, B*). Twenty-seven-year-old with thousands of lentigines widely scattered over body. Lentigines first appeared at four years of age. Also note larger "café-noir" spots. (*From J. J. Herzberg*, Z. Kinderchir. **2**:187, 1965.)

Cardiovascular system. Cardiac defects have been well reviewed by several authors (6, 7, 20, 23, 24). A superiorly oriented mean QRS axis in the frontal plane, generally located between −60 and −120° (S_1, S_2, S_3 pattern), tends to characterize the syndrome, regardless of the type of cardiac malformation. This electrocardiographic finding is not demonstrable in every patient, but is sometimes present even in patients with no structural abnormality of the heart. Complete heart block and complete bundle branch block have been reported.

Valvular pulmonic stenosis, usually of mild degree, is the most common cardiac defect. Typical valvular type and "pulmonary valvular dysplasia" have been reported (10, 16). "Aortic valvular dysplasia" is less commonly seen. Hypertrophic cardiomyopathy, primarily involving the interventricular septum and resulting in both subaortic and subpulmonic stenosis, has been reported (12). Other anomalies have included atrial septal defect, infundibular or supravalvular pulmonic stenosis, muscular subaortic stenosis and atrial myxoma (10, 14, 20a).

Genitorurinary system. Hypospadias is present in half of affected males (6, 7, 17, 28–30). Unilateral or bilateral cryptorchism is frequent. Absence or hypoplasia of an ovary has been reported (6, 17, 20). Late menarche has been common (28, 29).

Skeletal system. Growth retardation is frequently observed, 85 percent of patients being below the 25th percentile for both height and weight (7). Pectus carinatum or excavatum, dorsal kyphosis, and hyperflexible metacarpophalangeal joints have been observed in some patients. Winging of the scapulas is commonly found. Scoliosis is present in about 10 percent of patients (14a). Spina bifida occulta, absent ribs, cubitus valgus, limitation of motion at the elbows, and outer table deficiency of the temporal bone have been noted occasionally (7, 20).

Central nervous system. Sensorineural deafness, usually of profound degree, has been observed in 15 percent of patients (3, 4, 6, 11, 13, 14, 14a). Mild mental retardation (7, 20) and electroencephalographic abnormalities (20) have been noted.

DIFFERENTIAL DIAGNOSIS

The leopard syndrome shows a number of features which overlap with the *Noonan syn-drome*—such as hypertelorism, ptosis of the eyelids, short stature, pulmonic stenosis, cryptorchism, delayed development of secondary sexual characteristics, and skeletal anomalies of the chest. Pulmonic stenosis, abnormal QRS axis, short stature, delayed puberty, and deafness may be observered in the rubella syndrome. Hypertelorism, ptosis of the eyelids, short stature, and cryptorchism are present in the *Aarskog syndrome.*

We suspect that the patient reported by Swanson et al. (25) had a form of Kallmann syndrome.

LABORATORY AIDS

Electrocardiogram and cardiac catheterization may be helpful. Biopsy may be used to confirm lentigo.

REFERENCES

1 Almkvist, −, Zwei Fälle mit reichlicher Ausbreitung von Lentigoflecken, "Lentiginose profuse." *Zentralbl. Haut Geschlechtskr.* **22**:320, 1927.

2 Audry, M., Sur un cas de lentigo infantile profus. *Ann. Dermatol. Syphiligr.* (*Paris*) **4**:343, 1903.

3 Capute, A. J., Congenital Deafness with Multiple Lentigines in Mother and Daughter. *Birth Defects* **5**(2): 226–237, 1969.

4 Capute, A. J., et al., Congenital Deafness and Multiple Lentigines. *Arch. Dermatol.* **100**:207–213, 1969.

5 Fabry, J., Über einen seltener Fall von Naevus spilus. *Arch. Dermatol. Syph.* (*Berl.*) **59**:217–228, 1902.

6 Gorlin, R. J., et al., Multiple Lentigines Syndrome, Complex Comprising Multiple Lentigines, Electrocardiographic Conduction Abnormalities, Ocular Hypertelorism, Pulmonary Stenosis, Abnormalities of Genitalia, Retardation of Growth, Sensorineural Deafness and Autosomal Dominant Hereditary Pattern. *Am. J. Dis. Child.* **117**:652–662, 1969.

7 Gorlin, R. J., et al., The Leopard (Multiple Lentigines) Syndrome Revisited. *Birth Defects* **7**(4):110–115, 1971.

8 Herzberg, J. J., Naevi, Tierfellnaevi, neurocutane Melanosen *Z. Kinderchir.* **2**:187–201, 1965.

9 Jordan, −, Lentigo profuse Darier. *Dermatol. Wochenschr.* **73**:883, 1921.

10 Koretsky, E. D., et al., Congenital Pulmonary Stenosis Due to Valvular Dysplasia. *Circulation* **40**:43–53, 1969.

11 Koroxenidis, G. T., et al., Congenital Heart Disease, Deaf-mutism, and Associated Somatic Malformations Occurring in Several Members of One Family. *Am. J. Med.* **40**:149–155, 1966.

12 Kraunz, R. F., and Blackmon, J. R., Cardiocutaneous Syndrome Continued. *N. Engl. J. Med.* **279**:325, 1968.

13 Lewis, S. M., et al., Familial Pulmonary Stenosis and Deaf-mutism: Clinical and Genetic Considerations. *Am. Heart J.* **55**:458–462, 1958.

14 Lynch, P. J., Leopard Syndrome. *Arch. Dermatol.* **101**:119, 1970.

14a MacEwen, G. D., and Zaharko, W., Multiple Lentigines Syndrome. *Clin. Orthoped.* **97**:34–37, 1973.

15 Matthews, N. L., Lentigo and Electrographic Changes. *N.*

Engl. J. Med. **278**:780–781, 1968.

16 Moller, J. H., et al., A new Form of Pulmonary Stenosis. *Pediatr. Res.* **2**: 288–289, 1968.

17 Moynahan, E. J., Multiple Symmetrical Moles, with Psychic and Somatic Infantilism and Genital Hypoplasia. *Proc. R. Soc. Med.* **55**:959–960, 1962.

18 Moynahan, E. J., and Polani, P., Progressive Profuse Lentiginosis, Progressive Cardiomyopathy, Small Stature with Delayed Puberty, Mental Retardation or Psychic Infantilism and Other Developmental Anomalies: A New Familial Syndrome, in *XIIIth International Dermatologists Congress, Munich.* Springer Verlag, Berlin, 1967, pp. 1543.

19 Pipkin, A. E., and Pipkin, S. W., A Pedigree of Generalized Lentigo. *J. Hered.* **41**:79–82, 1950.

20 Polani, P. E., and Moynahan, E. J., Progressive Cardiomyopathic Lentiginosis. *Q. J. Med.* **41**:205–225, 1972.

20a Rees, J. R., Lentiginosis and Left Atrial Myxoma. *Br. Heart J.* **35**:874–876, 1973.

21 Rosen, I., Lentigines. *Arch. Dermatol. Syph.* (*Chic.*). **45**:979–980, 1942.

22 Selmanowitz, V. J., and Ostenreich, N., Lentiginosis Profusa in Daughter and Mother: Multiple Granular Cell Myoblastomas in the Former. *Arch. Dermatol.* **101**:615, 1970.

23 Smith, R. F., et al., Generalized Lentigo, Electrocardiographic Abnormalities, Conduction Disorders and Arrhythmias in Three Cases. *Am. J. Cardiol.* **25**:501–506, 1970.

24 Somerville, J., and Bonham-Carter, R. E., The Heart in Lentiginosis. *Br. Heart J.* **34**:58–66, 1972.

25 Swanson, S. L., et al., Multiple Lentigines Syndrome: New Findings of Hypogonadotrophism, Hyposmia, and Unilateral Renal Agenesis. *J. Pediatr.* **78**:1037–1039, 1971.

26 Touraine, A., La melanoblastose neurocutanée. *Bull. Soc. Fr. Dermatol. Syphiligr.* **51**:421–431, 1941.

27 Vickers, H. R., and Macmillan, D., Profuse Lentiginosis, Minor Cardiac Abnormality and Small Stature. *Proc. R. Soc. Med.* **62**:1011–1012, 1969.

28 Walther, R. J., et al., Electrocardiographic Abnormalities in a Family with Generalized Lentigo. *N. Engl. J. Med.* **275**:1220–1225, 1966.

29 Walther, R. J., et al., Electrocardiographic Abnormalities in a Family with Generalized Lentigo. Read before the American College of Cardiology, Washington, D.C., Feb. 17, 1967.

30 Watson, G. H., Pulmonary Stenosis, Café-au-lait Spots, and Dull Intelligence. *Arch. Dis. Child.* **42**:303–307, 1967.

31 Zeisler, E. P., and Becker, S. W., Generalized Lentigo. *Arch. Dermatol. Syph.* (*Chic.*) **33**:109–125, 1936.

84

Leprechaunism

(*Donohue Syndrome*)

Described originally by Donohue (4) in 1948, the syndrome consists of (*a*) failure to thrive, (*b*) unusual facies. (*c*) sexual precocity, (*d*) retarded bone age, and (*e*) altered carbohydrate metabolism with hypoglycemia. The term "leprechaunism" was introduced by Donohue and Uchida (5) in 1954.

The disorder has autosomal recessive inheritance. Parental consanguinity has been noted in several cases (3, 5, 7, 12).

SYSTEMIC MANIFESTATIONS

The gestation period tends to be short. Nearly all patients have been marasmic, and the majority have died at ages less than two years.

Facies. The face is gaunt, with large ears and lips. Facial hirsutism may be marked (5, 7, 8, 12–14) (Fig. 84-1).

Musculoskeletal changes. Muscle mass is severely wasted. Bone age is usually retarded. The hands and feet appear disproportionately large (1, 3, 5, 6, 12) (Fig. 84-1).

Skin. Acanthosis nigricans has been observed in several cases (1, 6, 8). Hirsutism may be marked.

Endocrine. In most examples, the breasts and clitoris or penis have been enlarged and there have been alterations in the ovaries or testes.

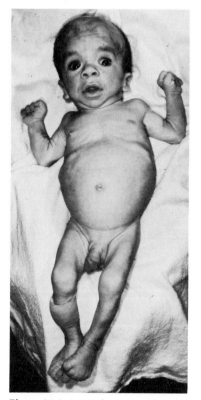

Figure 84-1. *Leprechaunism.* Note hirsutism, large hands, feet, and penis.

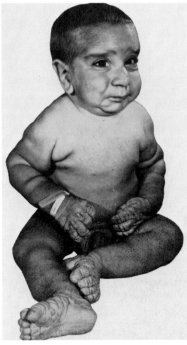
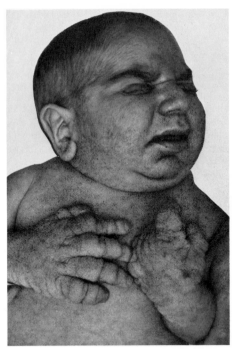

A   *B*

Figure 84-2. (*A*). *Leprechaunoid syndrome.* Large hands and feet in three-year-old male, with redundancy and wrinkling of overlying skin. (*B*). Same child at seven years of age. Note facial hirsutism. Child has had bony changes. (*From J. H. Patterson*, Birth Defects **5**(4):117, 1969.)

Rogers (11) described basophilic hyperplasia of the pituitary gland. Pancreatic islet cell hyperplasia with low fasting blood sugar level has been described (5, 6, 12, 14).

DIFFERENTIAL DIAGNOSIS

It is possible that the condition has been over-diagnosed, since many marasmic infants may develop similar facies. We have been impressed by the clinical resemblance between lepre-chaunism and *lipoatrophic diabetes.* Perhaps there is a similarity in pathogenesis. A lepre-chaunoid disorder was described by Patterson (9, 10). This patient had a cutis laxa-like redundancy of skin of the hands and feet and an underlying skeletal dysplasia (Fig. 84-2*A*, *B*).

LABORATORY AIDS

None is known.

REFERENCES

1 Canlorbe, P., et al., Le leprechaunism. Nouvelle observation et review de la littérature. *Ann. Pédiatr.* **15**:282–291, 1968.
2 Dallaire, L., Leprechaunism. *Birth Defects* **5**(4): 121, 1969.

3 Der Kaloustian, V. M., et al., Leprechaunism. *Am. J. Dis. Child.* **122**:442–445, 1971.
4 Donohue, W. L., Dysendocrinism. *J. Pediatr.* **32**:739–748, 1948.

5 Donohue, W. L., and Uchida, I., Leprechaunism, A Euphemism for a Rare Familial Disorder. *J. Pediatr.* **45**:505–518, 1954.

6 Evans, P. R., Leprechaunism, *Arch. Dis. Child.* **30:** 479–483, 1955.

7 Kálló, A., et al., Leprechaunism. *J. Pediatr.* **66**:372–379, 1965.

8 Kuhlkamp, F., and Helwig, H., Das Krankheitsbild des kongenitalen Dysendokrinismus oder Leprechaunismus. *Z. Kinderheilkd.* **109**:50–63, 1970.

9 Patterson, J. H., Presentation of a Patient with Leprechaunism. *Birth Defects* **5**(4):117–121, 1969.

10 Patterson, J. H., and Watkins, W. L., Leprechaunism in Male Infant. *J. Pediatr.* **60**:730–739, 1962.

11 Rogers, D. R., Leprechaunism (Donohue's Syndrome): A Possible Case with Emphasis on Changes in the Adenohypophysis. *Am. J. Clin. Pathol.* **45**:614–619, 1966.

12 Salmon, M. A., and Webb, J. N., Dystrophic Changes Associated with Leprechaunism in a Male Infant. *Arch. Dis. Child.* **38**:530–535, 1963.

13 Summitt, R. L., and Favara, B., Leprechaunism (Donohue's Syndrome). *J. Pediatr.* **74**:601–610, 1969.

14 Tsujino, G., and Yoshinaga, T., A Case of Leprechaunism as an Analysis of Some Clinical Manifestations of this Syndrome. *Z. Kinderheilkd.* **18**:347–360, 1975.

85

Lesch-Nyhan Syndrome

(HGPRTase Deficiency)

The cardinal clinical features of Lesch-Nyhan syndrome are (a) mental retardation, (b) spastic cerebral palsy, (c) choreoathetosis, and (d) bizarre, self-mutilating, aggressive behavior. Although the disorder had been noted earlier (2, 17), it was not until 1964 that Lesch and Nyhan (12) first described the complete syndrome in two brothers.

Hoefnagel et al. (9) indicated that the syndrome was inherited as an X-linked trait. About 150 patients have been reported (14, 15).

Sass and associates (20) described autopsy findings which indicated that the central nervous system manifestations might be due to uric acid toxicity as well as to uremic poisoning. The defect resides in the absence of hypoxanthine-guanine phosphoribosyltransferase (HGPRTase), an enzyme involved in purine metabolism (19, 21). The condition may be diagnosed in utero as well as in the carrier state (4, 7). "Partial" deficiency has also been described in adult males, the condition being characterized by gouty arthritis, renal complications which may have begun in infancy, and, less often, epilepsy, spasticity, and incoordination (5, 8, 11).

SYSTEMIC MANIFESTATIONS

The patient is normal at birth but by two months of age is noted to be irritable. The signs and symptoms begin to appear during the second year of life. Renal uric acid calculi may develop, leading to infection, eventual uremia, and death before puberty.

Facies. Self-mutilation results in massive destruction of the lower lip and, to a lesser degree, of the upper lip. At first glance, it may appear that the patient has a severely cleft lip (Figs. 85-1 and 85-2).

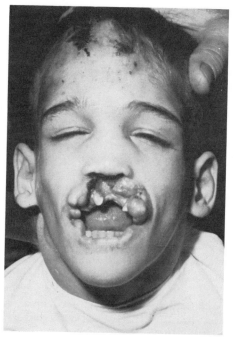

Figure 85-1. *Lesch-Nyhan syndrome.* Self-mutilation of lips. *(Courtesy of D. Hoefnagel, Hanover, N.H.)*

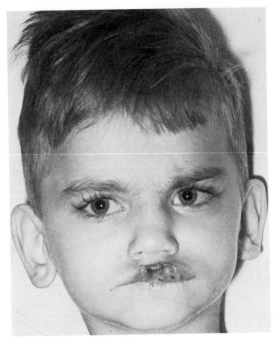

Figure 85-2. This boy and his brother have Lesch-Nyhan syndrome. Brother is more severely affected neurologically. (*Courtesy of B. ter Haar, Nijmegen, The Netherlands.*)

Skin. The patient uses his teeth, tongue, and fingers to mutilate himself (15). The fingers, especially the index fingers, are badly chewed, sometimes to the bone. The ears and nose are occasionally mutilated. There is no loss of pain sensation, and sometimes patients have indicated desire to be restrained (16). Removal of the anterior teeth may be necessary to prevent mutilation (19). Gouty tophi have been noted in the ears (15, 19). The patient of Sass et al. (20) had numerous subcutaneous nodules of uric acid in the lower limbs.

Central nervous system. Despite the severe nature of the central nervous system signs, gross and microscopic findings in the brain are surprisingly discrete, the most consistent change being microcephaly and impaired postnatal development (3). Particularly impressive are the lack of discernible lesions in the basal ganglia and the integrity of the myelin. Rosenbloom et al. (19)

pointed out that high levels of HGPRTase are normally present in basal ganglia. Absence in the Lesch-Nyhan syndrome probably is the basis for the central nervous system signs.

Oral manifestations. Mutilation of the lips has been observed in the majority of cases. Interestingly, the tongue is spared.

DIFFERENTIAL DIAGNOSIS

The Lesch-Nyhan syndrome is clinically quite striking, and in the presence of self-mutilation, one should have little difficulty in recognizing the disorder. In hospitals for the mentally retarded, many patients mutilate themselves but not to the same extent seen in this syndrome. Patients with this condition also have choreoathetosis and the other central nervous system manifestations.

Self-mutilation of the lips has been observed occasionally in the *de Lange syndrome*. In *congenital indifference to pain*, mutation of the lips, tongue, and limbs occurs without mental retardation.

Rosenberg et al. (18) described a syndrome of hyperuricemia, renal insufficiency, ataxia, and deafness. In some affected individuals who did not have renal insufficiency, there were elevated urate levels. The enzymatic defect noted in Lesch-Nyhan syndrome was not present.

Meigel and Braun-Falco (13) described a pseudo-Lesch-Nyhan syndrome.

LABORATORY AIDS

Enzymatic study of skin fibroblasts and cells from amniotic fluid may be used to identify both the hemizygote and the heterozygote, thus providing the basis for therapeutic abortion (1, 4, 7).

Serum uric acid levels, normally 2.5 to 6.0 mg per 100 ml, are raised to 8.5 to 15.0 mg per 100 ml in affected patients. A megaloblastic anemia which disappears with oral adenine administration has been noted by several authors (22). Heterozygotes can easily be detected by electrophoresis of a single hair root lysate (6).

REFERENCES

1 Boyle, J. A., et al., Lesch-Nyhan Syndrome: Preventive Control by Prenatal Diagnosis. *Science* **169**:688–689, 1970.

2 Catel, W., and Schmidt, J., Über familiäre gichtische Diathese in Verbindung mit zerebralen und renalen Symptomen bei einem Kleinkind. *Dtsch. Med. Wochenschr.* **84**:2145–2148, 1959.

3 Crussi, F. G., et al., The Pathological Condition of the Lesch-Nyhan Syndrome. *Am. J. Dis. Child.* **118**:501–506, 1969.

4 DeMars, R., et al., Lesch-Nyhan Mutation: Prenatal Detection with Amniotic Fluid Cells. *Science* **164**:1303–1305, 1969.

5 Emmerson, B. T., and Thompson, L., The Spectrum of Hypoxanthine Guanine Phosphoribosyltransferase Deficiency. *Q. J. Med.* **166**:423–440, 1973.

6 Francke, U., et al., Detection of Heterozygous Carriers of the Lesch-Nyhan Syndrome by Electrophoresis of Hair Root Lysates. *J. Pediatr.* **82**:472–478, 1973.

7 Fujimoto, W. Y., et al., Biochemical Diagnosis of an X-linked Disease in Utero. *Lancet* **2**:511–512, 1968.

8 Greene, M. L., Clinical Features of Patients with the "Partial" Deficiency of the X-linked Uricaciduria Enzyme. *Arch. Intern. Med.* **130**:193–198, 1972.

9 Hoefnagel, D., et al., Hereditary Choreoathetosis, Self-mutilation and Hyperuricemia in Young Males. *N. Engl. J. Med.* **273**:130–135, 1965.

10 Horger, E. O., and Hutchinson, D. L., Diagnostic Use of Amniotic Fluid. *J. Pediatr.* **75**:503–508, 1969.

11 Kelley, W. N., Biochemistry of the X-linked Uricaciduria Enzyme Defect and Its Genetic Variants. *Arch. Intern. Med.* **130**:199–206, 1972.

12 Lesch, M., and Nyhan, W. L., A Familial Disorder of Uric Acid Metabolism and Central Nervous System Function. *Am. J. Med.* **36**:561–570, 1964.

13 Meigel, W., and Braun-Falco, O., Automutilation der Unterlippe, verbunden mit Athetose und Oligophrenie ohne Purinstoffwechelstörung (pseudo-Lesch-Nyhan Syndrom). *Hautarzt* **24**:158–160, 1973.

14 Michener, W. M., Hyperuricemia and Mental Retardation with Athetosis and Self-mutilation. *Am. J. Dis. Child.* **113**:195–206, 1967.

15 Nyhan, W. L., Clinical Features of the Lesch-Nyhan Syndrome. *Arch. Intern. Med.* **130**:186–192, 1972.

16 Reed, W. B., and Fish, C. H., Hyperuricemia with Self-mutilation and Choreoathetosis. *Arch. Dermatol.* **94**: 194–195, 1966.

17 Riley, I. D., Gout and Cerebral Palsy in a Three-year-old Boy. *Am. J. Dis. Child.* **35**:293–295, 1960.

18 Rosenberg, A. L., et al., Hyperuricemia and Neurological Deficits. *N. Engl. J. Med.* **282**:992–996, 1970.

19 Rosenbloom, F. M., et al., Inherited Disorders of Purine Metabolism. *J.A.M.A.* **202**:175–177, 1967.

20 Sass, J. K., et al., Juvenile Gout with Brain Involvement. *Arch. Neurol.* **13**:639–655, 1965.

21 Seegmiller, J. E., et al., Enzyme Defect Associated with a Sex-linked Human Neurological Disorder and Excessive Purine Synthesis. *Science* **155**:1682–1684, 1967.

22 Van der Zee, S. P. M., et al., The Influence of Adenine on the Clinical Features and Purine Metabolism in the Lesch-Nyhan Syndrome. *Acta Paediatr. Scand.* **59**:259–264, 1970.

86

Lipoatrophic Diabetes

(Berardinelli Syndrome, Seip Syndrome,
Generalized Lipodystrophy)

The syndrome of (a) generalized disappearance of body fat, (b) insulin-resistant diabetes, and (c) hepatomegaly occurs in two basic forms: congenital and acquired. Berardinelli (1) in 1954 and Seip (21) in 1959 independently reported cases of the congenital form. Ziegler (28) in 1928 first described the acquired form of generalized lipodystrophy. For a historic review, see Seip (22).

The acquired type is not heritable; the congenital type is inherited as an autosomal recessive trait. Affected sibs and parental consanguinity have been noted in about 25 percent of the congenital cases (1, 2, 17, 22). The sublethal nature of the gene is suggested by the frequent history of miscarriage or death of affected children within the neonatal period. There is a 2:1 female predilection in the acquired type. Mabry et al. (15) postulated a pituitary-hopothalamic dysfunction and utilizing a dopaminergic blocking agent, pimozide, they have reversed the disorder (6).

SYSTEMIC MANIFESTATIONS

A generalized loss of all subcutaneous fat causes the muscles to appear enlarged and the veins to stand out prominently. This is usually evident at birth in the congenital type (21, 22). In the acquired type, fat loss is usually evident before fifteen years of age. Females have a definitely male body build, although the lipodystrophy does not affect breast development in those who have reached puberty. Skeletal growth is often accelerated during the first 10 years of life, during which time patients achieve 90 percent of their growth. However, growth soon tapers off, and they have average or even short stature after puberty. The phenotype is further altered by the enlarged joints of the hands and feet.

Facies. The facies is quite distinctive. Loss of subcutaneous adipose tissue, especially the buccal fat pad, causes the cheeks to have a gaunt appearance (Fig. 86-1 *A*, *B*). This, combined with the large ears, ocular hypertelorism, and hirsutism, give the patient a distinctive appearance.

Viscera. In the congenital type, hepatomegaly may be pronounced in infancy; liver biopsies, taken later in life, have shown fatty infiltration with moderate early fibrosis and increased glycogen deposits. The fatty infiltration is secondary to hypertriglyceridemia and to lack of functional fat storage deposits. Several patients with the acquired form have died of bleeding esophageal varices secondary to cirrhosis of the liver. There is absence of mesenteric and perinephric fat (23, 24). Hypertension and systolic murmur appear to be characteristic of the acquired disease. Patients with the congenital form usually are not hypertensive, but may have cardiac murmurs and cardiomegaly (13, 21, 22). In most patients, the kidneys have been enlarged without apparent histologic cause (17). A few

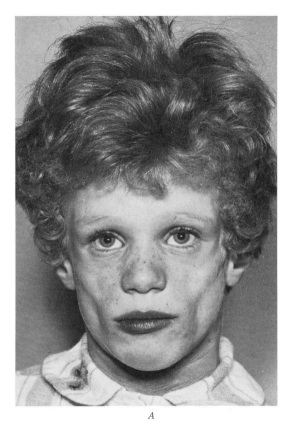
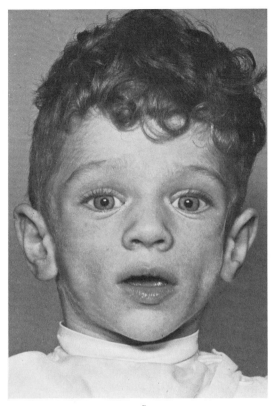

A   *B*

Figure 86-1. *Lipoatrophic diabetes.* (*A, B*). Absence of subcutaneous fat, especially buccal fat pad, produces gaunt appearance.

have had hydronephrosis and hydroureter (17, 18, 25).

Nervous system. Mental retardation of variable degree has been noted in about 50 percent of patients with the congenital form (2, 17, 18, 21, 22, 24).

Musculoskeletal alterations. Muscular prominence, due in part to lack of subcutaneous fat, may be absolute, since some patients exhibit increased urinary creatinine levels (Fig. 86-2*A, B*). Increased skeletal maturation is a common feature during the first 4 years of life, and several patients have exhibited increased bone density (9, 22, 27). An increase in subcutaneous fat may occasionally be noted after puberty.

Genital organs. Enlarged penis or clitoris and cystic ovaries are common features of the con-

genital form (1, 3, 10, 22, 24). Adult females with the acquired form usually develop amenorrhea; oligomenorrhea is common in the congenital type.

Skin. Hirsutism of the face, neck, arms, and legs may be present at birth and increases with age. With the onset of the lipodystrophy, the scalp hair may become excessively curly and thick, the hair growing nearly to the eyebrows. Eruptive xanthomas may be present in the acquired form following hyperlipemia (22).

Acanthosis nigricans is a prominent feature in nearly all patients. It is especially common in the axillas and on the wrists and ankles. It tends to decrease with increasing age and may disappear after puberty (2, 17) (Fig. 86-3).

Oral manifestations. Enlarged tonsils and adenoids are common in the congenital type (2, 22).

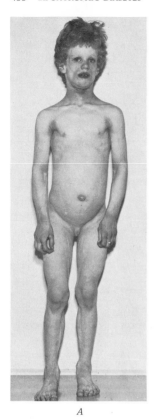
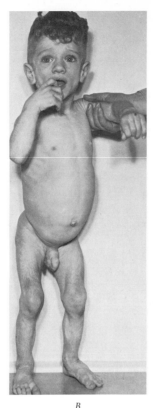

A   *B*

Figure 86-2. (*A, B*). Marked muscular prominence, due in part to lack of subcutaneous fat. Also note evidence of axillary acanthosis nigricans in female. Hirsutism may be marked in some patients. (*From M. Seip*, Acta Paediatr. Scand. **48:**555, 1959.)

DIFFERENTIAL DIAGNOSIS

In partial lipodystrophy there is symmetric absence of facial fat, with retention of distal adipose deposits. Rarely, fat disappears from arms, chest, abdomen, and hips. The characteristic adiposity of the pelvis and legs is seen only in postpubertal women (6, 16). Onset is usually noted between five and fifteen years of age, and the wasting takes place within a period of about 18 months to 6 years. The ratio of females to males is 4 : 1 (2, 16). Renal problems have been noted in over 60 percent of patients (24).

Many features of congenital lipodystrophy have been noted in *leprechaunism:* liver enlargement, lipodystrophy, enlarged clitoris or penis, neurologic damage, hirsutism, and disturbances of glucose metabolism. It is conceivable that leprechaunism represents a lethal form of lipoatrophic diabetes.

The diencephalic syndrome caused by a tumor in the region of the anterior hypothalamus is manifested by profound emaciation with accelerating early growth, increased motor activity, and euphoria (11, 26). The affected infants are normal at birth but become symptomatic with age. Progressive emaciation leads to a loss of subcutaneous fat but without the muscularity of lipodystrophic patients. The hands and feet are often large. Hepatomegaly, genital enlargement, and hyperlipemia have not been reported.

Dunnigan et al. (6) described a dominant form of lipoatrophic diabetes in several females in two families. Onset was at puberty. The lipodystrophy involved the trunk and limbs but the facies was Cushingoid. Acanthosis nigricans, tubero-eruptive xanthomata, insulin-resistant diabetes and type V hyperlipidemia were present in most of the patients.

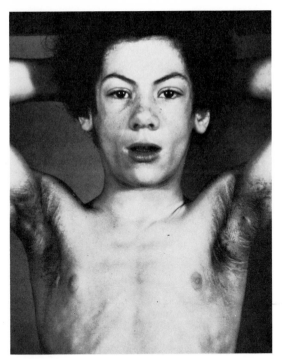

Figure 86-3. Acanthosis nigricans. (*Courtesy of W. Reed, Burbank, Calif.*)

LABORATORY AIDS

Lipoatrophic diabetes is clearly distinct from diabetes mellitus. The diabetes, which is insulin-resistant, appears after the onset of the lipodystrophy, usually between six to twenty years of age (20, 23, 24). Ketosis, however, is rarely present. Infants do not have glycosuria except when challenged with large amounts of glucose.

Hyperlipemia, especially of the triglyceride fraction, is a constant feature. It usually precedes the onset of hyperglycemia. The serum of these patients is intermittently turbid or milky, with increased triglycerides, and contains very low-density lipoprotein. In addition, there is slow turnover of ^{14}C-labeled triglycerides and cholesterol and slow clearance of ingested triglycerides with failure of adipocytes to incorporate triglyceride fatty acids from the blood.

A substance with lipid-mobilizing activity has been isolated from the urine of these patients. Presumably it promotes rapid hydrolysis of triglycerides, inhibiting their accumulation in adipose tissue (14). In turn, the excessive fatty acid mobilization probably leads to insulin resistance and interferes with peripheral glucose utilization.

REFERENCES

1 Berardinelli, W., An Undiagnosed Endocrino-metabolic Syndrome. *J. Clin. Endocrinol.* **14:**193–204, 1954.
2 Brubaker, M. M., et al., Acanthosis Nigricans and Congenital Total Lipodystrophy. *Arch. Dermatol.* **91:**320–325, 1965.
3 Brunzell, J. D., et al., Congenital Generalized Lipodystrophy Accompanied by Cystic Angiomatosis. *Ann. Intern. Med.* **69:**501–516, 1968.
4 Corbin, A., et al., Diencephalic Involvement in Generalized Lipodystrophy: Rationale and Treatment with the Neuroleptic Agent, Pimozide. *Acta Endocrinol. (Kbh.)* **77:**209–220, 1974.
  Curtis, A. C., and Richards, H. J., Acanthosis Nigricans: A Review with Special Emphasis on Associated Endocrinopathies. *Cutis* **3:**147–160, 1967.
6 Dunnigan M. G., et al., Familial Lipoatrophic Diabetes with Dominant Transmission. *Q. J. Med.* **43:**33–48, 1974.
7 Fairnay, A., et al., Total Lipodystrophy. *Arch. Dis. Child.* **44:**368–372, 1969.
8 Gamstory, I., et al., Diencephalic Syndromes of Infancy. *J. Pediatr.* **70:**383–390, 1967.
9 Gold, R. H., and Steinbach, H. L., Lipoatrophic Diabetes Mellitus (Generalized Lipodystrophy): Roentgen Findings in Two Brothers with Congenital Disease. *Am. J. Roentgenol.* **101:**884–896, 1967.
10 Hall, B. E., Congenital Muscular Hypertrophy. *Am. J. Dis. Child.* **52:**773–783, 1936.
11 Hamilton, W., Diencephalic Syndromes of Infancy and Childhood. *Dev. Med. Child. Neurol.* **9:**497–499, 1967.
12 Hamwi, G. J., et al., Lipoatrophic Diabetes. *Diabetes* **15:**262–268, 1966.
13 Lawrence, R. D., Lipodystrophy and Hepatomegaly with Diabetes, Lipaemia and Other Metabolic Disturbances. *Lancet* **1:**724–731, 1946.
14 Louis, L. H., Lipoatrophic Diabetes: An Improved Procedure for the Isolation and Purification of a Diabetogenic Polypeptide from Urine. *Metabolism* **18:**545–555, 1969.
15 Mabry, C. C., et al., Pituitary-hypothalamic Dysfunction in Generalized Lipodystrophy. *J. Pediatr.* **82:**625–633, 1973.
15a Najjar, S. S., et al., Congenital Generalized Lipodystrophy. *Acta Paediatr. Scand.* **64:**273–279, 1975.
16 Poley, J. R., and Stickler, G. B., Progressive Lipodystrophy. *Am. J. Dis. Child.* **106:**356–363, 1963.
17 Reed, W. B., et al., Congenital Lipodystrophic Diabetes with Acanthosis Nigricans: The Seip-Lawrence Syndrome. *Arch. Dermatol.* **91:**326–334, 1965.

18 Reed, W. B., et al., Acanthosis Nigricans in Association with Various Genodermatoses. *Acta Derm. Venereol. (Stockh.)* **48:**465–473, 1968.

19 Ruvalcaba, R. H. A., et al., Lipoatrophic Diabetes. *Am. J. Dis. Child.* **109:**279–294, 1965.

20 Schwartz, R., et al., Generalized Lipoatrophy, Hepatic Cirrhosis, Disturbed Carbohydrate Metabolism, and Accelerated Growth (Lipoatrophic Diabetes). *Am. J. Med.* **28:**973–985, 1960.

21 Seip, M., Lipodystrophy and Gigantism with Associated Endocrine Manifestations. *Acta Pediatr. Scand.* **48:**555–574, 1959.

22 Seip, M., Generalized Lipodystrophy. *Ergeb. Inn. Med. Kinderheilkd.* **31:**59–95, 1971.

23 Senior, B., Lipodystrophic Muscular Hypertrophy. *Arch. Dis. Child.* **36:**426–431, 1961.

24 Senior, B., and Gellis, S. S., The Syndromes of Total Lipodystrophy and of Partial Lipodystrophy. *Pediatrics* **33:**593–612, 1964.

25 Taylor, W. B., and Honeycutt, W. M., Progressive Lipodystrophy and Lipoatrophic Diabetes. *Arch. Dermatol.* **84:**31–36, 1961.

26 Torrey, E. F., and Uyeda, C. I., The Diencephalic Syndrome of Infancy. *Am. J. Dis. Child.* **110:**689–696, 1965.

27 Wesenberg, R. L., et al., The Roentgenographic Findings in Total Lipodystrophy. *Am. J. Roentgenol.* **103:**154–164, 1968.

28 Ziegler, L. H., Lipodystrophies: Report of Seven Cases. *Brain* **51:**147–167, 1928.

87

McCune-Albright Syndrome

(Polyostotic Fibrous Dysplasia, Cutaneous Pigmentation, and Endocrine Disorders)

The syndrome described by McCune (17) in 1936 and by Albright et al. (2) in 1937 was discovered as early as 1922 by Weil (26). The classic triad consists of (*a*) polyostotic fibrous dysplasia, (*b*) abnormal pigmentation of the skin, and (*c*) endocrine dysfunction with somatic and sexual precocity, especially in females. All cases described to date have been isolated examples.

The components of the syndrome are present with variable frequency. Pritchard (19), in a survey of 181 cases of polyostotic fibrous dysplasia, found skin pigmentation in 43 percent. Thirty-seven of 82 females and only five of 83 males exhibited precocious puberty. It has been suggested that the endocrine manifestations of the syndrome result from a hypothalamic abnormality causing overproduction of a variety of releasing hormones (14, 25).

SYSTEMIC MANIFESTATIONS

Facies. The face may be quite normal but is often distorted or grossly asymmetric because of involvement of one or more facial bones (Fig. 87-1).

Bones. Although any bone may be involved, the long bones are most frequently affected, especially the upper end of the femur. A bowing resembling a hockey stick may be produced, resulting in leg-length discrepancy. Seventy percent of patients are seen originally because of

limp, leg pain, or fracture (15). Other bones affected, in descending order of frequency, are the tibia, fibula, pelvis, humerus, radius, and ulna. Bilateral involvement occurs in about half the cases (8, 11) (Fig. 87-2). Occasionally, a single

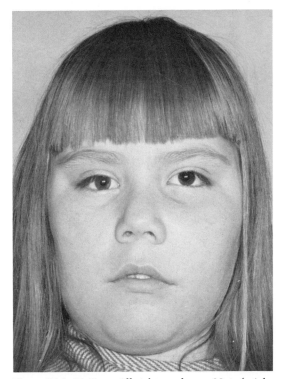

Figure 87-1. *McCune-Albright syndrome.* Note facial asymmetry, fullness of left cheek.

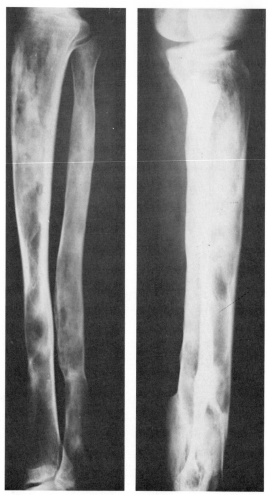

Figure 87-2. Roentgenogram exhibiting thickening and pseudocystic involvement of tibia and fibula.

bone is involved (monostotic). Incipient bowing of the legs may be seen as early as the first year of life and nearly always appears before the end of the first decade (17, 18). The process may be asymptomatic or accompanied by pain and fracture. Fractures may be multiple and recurrent. At least 85 percent of patients have one fracture, and over 40 percent have three or more (15). Occasionally, bones on only one side of the body may be involved (19).

The bone is replaced by a yellowish to redbrown fibrous tissue, its composition varying greatly in different parts of the body. It may be rich or poor in cells. The stroma may vary from a finely fibrillar one with a loose whorled arrangement to one which is densely collagenous. Some areas are edematous, with numerous small cystic spaces. Foci of hemorrhage and multinucleated giant cells may be observed. The trabeculae are irregular in form, and occasionally a few fragments of cartilage are present (Fig. 87-3).

Facial asymmetry occurs in about 25 percent of cases, and may be accompanied by protrusion of the eye, with associated visual disturbances (11, 29). The bony lesions of the skull and facial skeleton, in contrast to the cystic lesions of long bones, are hyperostotic (Fig. 87-4). The skull base becomes thickened and dense, bulging upward into the cranial cavity. The calvaria may also become thickened, with marked occipital and frontal bulging. The bossing may be asymmetric, with unilateral (and occasionally bilateral) obliteration of the sinuses and nasal passages. The overgrowth of bone around the foramens may result in deafness and/or blindness.

Pigmentation. The pigmentation is of the café-au-lait type (Fig. 87-5A, B). Well-defined, generally unilateral, irregular macular spots are scattered over the forehead, nuchal area, and buttocks. Only rarely is the face pigmented. There appears to be a correlation between the amount of pigmentation and the degree of bone involvement (7). It has been stated that ipsilateral pigmentation is more frequent on the side of unilateral bone involvement, although this has been denied (16). The pigment appears from the fourth month to the second year of life, in a few patients it has become evident a few weeks postnatally (5). Only rarely is mucous membrane affected (9, 12, 22, 23).

Endocrine system. The most common feature is precocious puberty in females. The menarche is reached between one and five years of age in 50 percent of females, and between six and ten years in another 33 percent (8). Rarely, vaginal bleeding occurs within the first few months (1–3, 13) or even the first few days of life (5, 13). It is usually irregular, lasts from 2 to 4 days, and may, on occasion, be profuse. There is no evidence that ovulation takes place early, but ample proof that patients of both sexes are subsequently fertile (13).

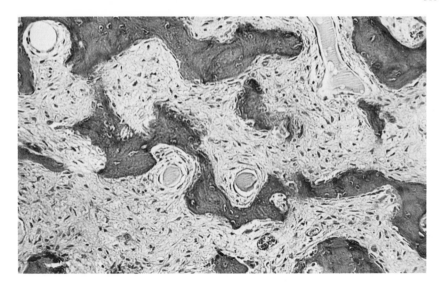

Figure 87-3. C-shaped trabeculae composed of metaplastic woven or fiber bone in fibrous connective stroma.

Breast development and pubic and axillary hair appear after the menarche, usually from the fifth to tenth year, but may be manifested as early as birth (1, 17, 18). Hypertrophy of the external genitalia has also been noted (2, 3). Precocious puberty may occur in males, but far less frequently. It may be accompanied by gynecomastia (11, 19) and spermatogenesis (13).

Skeletal maturation is often rapid, with premature closure of the epiphyses, producing accelerated growth in childhood, but short stature in adulthood.

Hyperthyroidism has been present in about 20 percent of patients, occurring at an early age (3, 18–21) and rarely the Cushing syndrome (14) is found.

Oral manifestations. The jaws may be enlarged, expanded, and distorted. Roentgenographic examination may show a dense mass, especially in the maxilla, extending into and obliterating the sinuses and expanding the buccal plate in the tuberosity areas, or there may be a radiolucent area, more common in the mandible, similar to that seen in long bones. Often there is loss of trabeculae and a "ground-glass" appearance on roentgenographic examination.

Oral pigmentation on the lips and oral mucosa has been noted (9, 12, 20, 22, 23), but either its occurrence is infrequent or its recording is usually neglected (Fig. 87-6*A*, *B*).

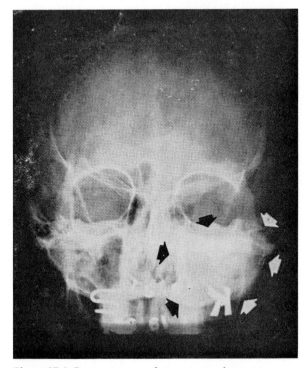

Figure 87-4. Roentgenogram demonstrating hyperostotic involvement of maxillary sinus by fibrous dysplasia.

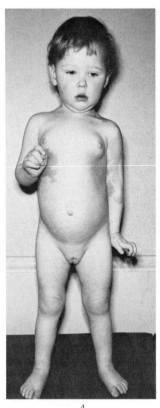 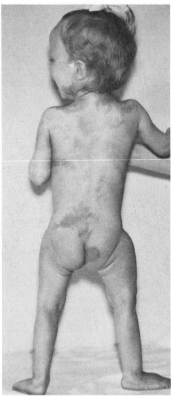

A

B

Figure 87-5. (*A*). Pigmentation and preco-cious puberty. (*From S. Agarwala and J. B. Heycock,* Br. J. Clin. Pract. **22**:339, 1969.) (*B*). Irregular cutaneous pigmenta-tion and hockey-stick deformity. (*From H. Pande, Oslo, Norway.*)

DIFFERENTIAL DIAGNOSIS

The bone lesions should be differentiated from those of hyperparathyroidism, histiocytosis X, multiple myeloma, Paget disease of bone, *neurofibromatosis,* and giant-cell tumor. It is

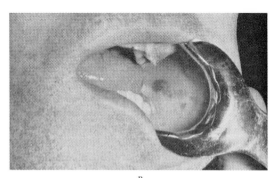

A

B

Figure 87-6. (*A*). Intraoral view of palate of girl shown in Fig. 87-1. (*B*). Buccal and palatal melanotic mucosal pigmentation in patient with Albright syndrome. (*From R. J. Gorlin and A. P. Chaudhry,* Oral Surg. **10**:857, 1957.)

unfortunate that some authors have referred to cherubism as "familial fibrous dysplasia of the jaws," a designation it does not merit.

Skin pigmentation is also seen in neurofibromatosis, but the pigmentation of polyostotic fibrous dysplasia differs from the neurofibromatosis "coast of California" contour in its marked degree of irregular outline ("coast of Maine"). However, exceptions have been noted. Giant pigment granules, characteristically seen in malpighian cells or melanocytes in neurofibromatosis, are very rare in the McCune-Albright syndrome [7]. Precocious puberty occurs in the adrenogenital syndrome, with ovarian granulosa cell tumor, and occasionally in *Peutz-Jeghers syndrome.*

LABORATORY AIDS

Although serum calcium levels have been found to be normal in about 80 percent of the patients, slight elevation (11 to 13.8 per 100 ml) has been recorded in some [8, 19]. The phosphorus level is diminished below 3.5 mg per 100 ml in about 40 percent of affected children [8]. Serum alkaline phosphatase levels are elevated in about 50 percent [19]. Alexander [4] and Verghese [24] described elevated steroid excretion. Husband and Snodgrass [16] noted increased urinary luteinizing hormone and estrogen levels.

REFERENCES

1 Agarwala, S., and Heycock, J. B., A Case of Albright's Syndrome. *Br. J. Clin. Pract.* **23:**339–340, 1969.

2 Albright, F., et al., Syndrome Characterized by Osteitis Fibrosa Disseminata, Areas of Pigmentation and Endocrine Dysfunction with Precocious Puberty in Females. *N. Engl. J. Med.* **216:**727–736, 1937.

3 Albright, F., et al., Syndrome Characterized by Osteitis Fibrosa Disseminata, Areas of Pigmentation and a Gonadal Dysfunction. *Endocrinology* **22:**411–421, 1938.

4 Alexander, F. W., Polyostotic Fibrous Dysplasia with Raised Steroid Excretion. *Arch. Dis. Child.* **46:**91–94, 1971.

5 Arlien-Søborg, U., and Iversen, T., Albright's Syndrome: A Brief Survey and Report of a Case in a Seven-year-old Girl. *Acta Paediatr. Scand.* **45:**558–568, 1956.

6 Benedict, P. H., Sex Precocity and Polyostotic Fibrous Dysplasia. *Am. J. Dis. Child.* **111:**426–429, 1966.

7 Benedict, P. H., et al., Melanotic Macules in Albright's Syndrome and in Neurofibromatosis. *J.A.M.A.* **205:**618–626, 1968.

8 Boenheim, F., and McGavack, T. H., Polyostotische fibröse Dysplasie. *Ergeb. Inn. Med. Kinderheilkd.* **3:**157–184, 1952.

9 Bowerman, J. E., Polyostotic Fibrous Dysplasia with Melanotic Pigmentation. *Br. J. Oral Surg.* **6:**188–191, 1969.

10 Brunt, P., and McKusick, V. A., Fibrous Dysplasia: A Report of Genetic and Clinical Study with a Review of the Literature. *Medicine* **49:**343–374, 1970.

11 Falconer, M. A., et al., Fibrous Dysplasia of Bone with Endocrine Disorders and Cutaneous Pigmentation (Albright's Disease). *Q. J. Med.* **11:**121–154, 1942.

12 Gorlin, R. J., and Chaudhry, A. P., Oral Melanotic Pigmentation in Polyostotic Fibrous Dysplasia: Albright's Syndrome. *Oral Surg.* **10:**857–862, 1957.

13 Hackett, L. J., Jr., and Christopherson, W. M., Polyostotic Fibrous Dysplasia. *J. Pediatr.* **35:**767–771, 1949.

14 Hall, R., and Warrick, C., Hypersecretion of Hypothalamic Releasing Hormones; a Possible Explanation of the Endocrine Manifestations of Polyostotic Fibrous Dysplasia (Albright's Syndrome). *Lancet* **1:**1313–1316, 1972.

15 Harris, W. H., et al., The Natural History of Fibrous Dysplasia: An Orthopedic Pathological and Roentgenographic Study. *J. Bone Joint Surg.* **44A:**207–233, 1962.

16 Husband, P., and Snodgrass, G., McCune-Albright Syndrome with Endocrinological Investigations. *Am. J. Dis. Child.* **119:**164–167, 1970.

17 McCune, D. J., Osteitis Fibrosa Cystica: The Case of a Nine Year Old Girl Who Also Exhibits Precocious Puberty, Multiple Pigmentation of the Skin and Hyperthyroidism. *Am. J. Dis. Child.* **52:**743–747, 1936.

18 McCune, D. J., and Bruch, H., Osteodystrophia Fibrosa. *Am. J. Dis. Child.* **54:**806–848, 1937.

19 Pritchard, J. E., Fibrous Dysplasia of the Bones. *Am. J. Med. Sci.* **222:**313–332, 1951.

20 Robinson, M., Polyostotic Fibrous Dysplasia of Bone. *J. Am. Dent. Assoc.* **42:**47–57, 1951.

21 Samuel, S., et al., Hyperthyroidism in an Infant with McCune-Albright Syndrome: Report of a Case with Myeloid Metaplasia. *J. Pediatr.* **80:**275–278, 1972.

22 Snapper, I., On Lipoid Granulomatosis of the Bones without Symptoms of Schüller-Christian's Disease. *Chinese Med. J.* **56:**303–316, 1939.

23 Thannhauser, S., Jr., and Eltinger, A., cited by K. H. Thoma and H. M. Goldman, in *Oral Pathology,* 5th ed., Mosby, St. Louis, 1960, pp. 580–583.

24 Verghese, A., Albright's Syndrome in the Male with Situs Inversus. *Proc. R. Soc. Med.* **55:**357–358, 1962.

25 Warrick, C. K., Some Aspects of Polyostotic Fibrous Dysplasia: Possible Hypothesis to Account for the Associated Endocrine Changes. *Clin. Radiol.* **24:**125–138, 1973.

26 Weil, –, 9–jähriges Mädchen mit Pubertas praecox und Knochenbrüchigkeit. *Klin. Wochenschr.* **1:**2114–2115, 1922.

88

Macroglobulinemia of Waldenström

In 1944, Waldenström (25) described patients with a pathologic serum globulin fraction of high molecular weight, and in 1948, employed the term "macroglobulinemia," which subsequently has been used mostly in connection with his name (26). In later papers (27–29), Waldenström elaborated on the clinical and hematologic features of the syndrome. Extensive reviews have been made by Kappeler et al. (13) and by Imhof et al. (11).

The macroglobulinemia of Waldenström is an immunoproliferative disorder characterized by the presence of large amounts of monoclonal macroglobulin (IgM) in the serum, apparently produced by abnormally proliferating lymphocytes.

The outcome is usually fatal, although the course may be protracted. Kappeler et al. (13) distinguished two forms of macroglobulinemia: (a) a malignant form leading to early death, and (b) a relatively benign form.

One of the most important ways of judging the ultimate prognosis seems to be the speed of development of the protein alterations. If these remain at the same level for several years, there is a better chance that the condition will remain stationary for a longer period. An increase in globulin values is a serious sign. Patients who have died have always had macroglobulin values of 4 to 7 g per ml (29).

There have been a few examples of the syndrome in parent and child (15).

SYSTEMIC MANIFESTATIONS

The syndrome is more common in patients over the age of fifty years (11, 17), and males are about twice as frequently affected (11, 17, 28).

Initial symptoms are nonspecific, e.g., weakness, general malaise, dyspnea, loss of appetite, and loss of weight. Anemia is present in most cases. A history of vague ill health for several years may be obtained.

Hemorrhagic diathesis. Bleeding has been observed in at least half the patients, especially from the eyes, mouth, and nose, epistaxis often being an early symptom of the syndrome. Bleeding may also be seen from the vagina and gastrointestinal tract and in the skin.

Eyes. Changes in the eyes (21) consist of sludging of the blood flow in conjunctival vessels, marked distension and tortuosity of retinal veins, thrombosis of the central retinal vein (25), multiple retinal hemorrhages and, occasionally, papilledema.

Lymph nodes, spleen, and liver. In about half the cases, the lymph nodes are swollen and the spleen and liver are increased in size. The affected lymph nodes are soft and painless.

Other findings. Neurologic symptoms (aphasia, hemiparesis) have been noted in 13 percent of patients (11). Furthermore, edema, the Raynaud phenomenon, recurrent infections of the upper part of the respiratory tract, and osteoporosis may be observed. Patients with macroglobulinemia appear to have a higher incidence of carcinoma (13, 20).

Oral manifestations. In his first description of the syndrome, Waldenström (25) mentioned the occurrence of gingival bleeding which had caused patients to come to the hospital. In his 1948 paper (26), he dramatically described patients waking in the morning, their mouths filled with blood. Imhof et al. (11) found 21 percent of 107 patients to have gingival bleeding. Persistent hemorrhage following tooth extraction (24, 29), as well as petechiae and ecchymoses of the oral mucosa, have been noted (Fig. 88-1). Gamble and Driscoll (6) and Hjørting-Hansen et al. (9) described peculiar deep and painful ulcerations of the oral mucosa in addition to gingival hemorrhages (Fig. 88-2).

Swelling of the submandibular lymph nodes may also be an initial symptom of macroglobulinemia. Punched-out bone lesions have been seen, and Hörner (10) reported a patient with a destructive lymphocytic tumor of the mandible.

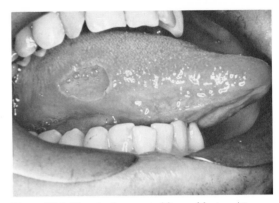

Figure 88-2. Sharply demarcated lingual lesion. (*From J. W. Gamble and E. J. Driscoll*, Oral Surg. **13:**104, 1960.)

PATHOLOGY

The bone marrow is affected in all cases and exhibits a characteristic cell structure. The majority of the cells are small mononuclear cells resembling lymphocytes (29). The lymph nodes, spleen, liver, and other organs may also show infiltration with the same type of cells, including atypical plasma cells (32). Tissue mast cells are also increased in number. Fruhling et al. (5), employing electron microscopy, examined plasmacytic differentiation and found it to be an important morphologic criterion. Grundmann and Amlie (7) suggested that macroglobulinemia is a disease per se in homogeneous deposits of proteins in the bone marrow, liver, and small arteries.

DIFFERENTIAL DIAGNOSIS

Macroglobulinemia, being seen in a number of conditions, led Ritzmann et al. (19) to propose the following classification of macroglobulinemias: (*a*) physiologic macroglobulinemia, (*b*) secondary, or symptomatic, macroglobulinemia (as seen in cirrhosis, lupus erythematosus, and the Sjögren syndrome), and (*c*) primary, idiopathic, or essential macroglobulinemia—or macroglobulinemia of Waldenström.

The syndrome is differentiated from multiple

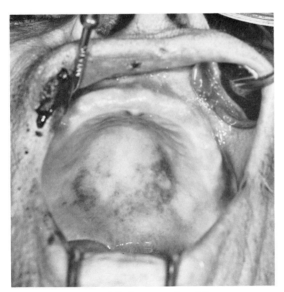

Figure 88-1. *Macroglobulinemia of Waldenström.* Palatal ecchymosis.

myeloma, to which it may be related, by its longer and more benign clinical course, the lack of osteolytic bone lesions, and the infrequent finding of Bence Jones proteinuria (4).

Lymphatic leukemia may present some similarities to macroglobulinemia, and it is still debated whether the two conditions are related.

Mainly because of purpura, hyperviscosity of the serum, and hyperproteinemia, purpura hyperglobulinemia, also described by Waldenström (26), may resemble macroglobulinemia. The differential diagnosis is, however, usually easy (18) because hyperglobulinemia, in contrast to macroglobulinemia, has a mild course and shows a female predominance. The proteinemia is caused by hypergammaglobulinemia, and the mucous membranes never exhibit bleeding. The parotid glands may be enlarged in purpura hyperglobulinemia. Plasmacytoma of the tongue has also been described (22).

LABORATORY AIDS

A large number of laboratory tests is available for diagnosis of macroglobulinemia. For detailed discussion of these methods, the reader is referred to papers by Kappeler et al. (13), Ritzmann et al. (19), and Waldenström (29).

Blood sedimentation rate. In almost all patients with macroglobulinemia, the blood sedimentation rate is extremely high (4). Also conditioned by the presence of macroglobulins is the marked rouleaux formation of red blood cells.

Anemia. The majority of patients—81 percent, according to Imhof et al. (11)—exhibit pronounced anemia. In more than half the patients, the hemoglobin is less than 50 percent of normal. Most frequently found is normochromic anemia. The anemia may be due to loss of blood by hemorrhage or to disturbed erythropoiesis (11).

White blood cells. The number of white blood cells is usually normal or slightly reduced. Sometimes a slight relative lymphocytosis is observed. Quite often pancytopenia is present.

Marrow findings. In many cases the bone marrow findings are abnormal, showing an increase of lymphoid and/or plasma cell elements (4).

Serum proteins. The decisive criterion for the diagnosis of macroglobulinemia is the occurrence of increased levels of macroglobulins in the serum while the total amount of proteins is increased. By means of ultracentrifugation it was demonstrated that the molecular weight of the macroglobulin was about 1,000,000 compared with 150,000 for normal globulin (25). Waldenström (27) stressed that only globulins with a sedimentation constant of 15 S_{20} or over should be regarded as true macroglobulins. In most cases the abnormal protein has been found to migrate electrophoretically as a gamma- or beta-globulin or in the area between normal gamma and beta (4, 23). The macroglobulins are antigenically specific (8). The antiserum that can be produced does not react with proteins in secondary macroglobulinemia (12). A number of cases are reported to be characterized by simultaneous occurrence of cryoglobulin and macroglobulin (15, 23).

The Sia test and viscosity index are also valuable aids.

Urinalysis. Paraproteinuria (often of the Bence Jones type) can be demonstrated in approximately 10 to 20 percent of the cases.

Chromosomal analysis. In 2 to 51 percent of cells from both peripheral lymphoblast culture and bone marrow preparation, a supernumerary marker chromosome has been detected. The marker frequently has been the size of an A, B, or C chromosome, but the position of its centromere has not been constant. Originally called the "W" chromosome (3, 4) and thought to be specific for the Waldenstrom macroglobulinemia, it was later noted to be an inconstant finding. The abnormal chromosome is not present congenitally. It still remains to be demonstrated whether an aneuploid clone of lymphocytes is responsible for the presence of abnormal macroglobulin.

REFERENCES

1 Benirschke, K., et al., Chromosomal Abnormalities in Waldenström's Macroglobulinemia. *Lancet* **2:**594, 1962.

2 Bhoopalam, N., et al., IgM Heavy Chain Fragments in Waldenström's Macroglobulinemia. *Arch. Intern. Med.* **128:**437–440, 1971.

2a Bloch, K. J., and Maki, D. C., Hyperviscosity Syndromes Associated with Immunoglobulin Abnormalities. *Seminars Hematol.* **10:**113–124, 1973.

3 Cervenka, J., and Koulischer, L., *Chromosomes in Human Cancer.* Charles C Thomas, Springfield, Ill., 1973.

4 Cohen, R. J., et al., Waldenström's Macroglobulinemia: A Study of Ten Cases. *Am. J. Med.* **41:**274–284, 1966.

5 Fruhling, L., et al., La maladie de Waldenström. *Ann. Anat. Pathol.* **5:**508–537, 1960.

6 Gamble, J. W., and Driscoll, E. J., Oral Manifestations of Macroglobulinemia of Waldenstrom. *Oral Surg.* **13:**104–110, 1960.

7 Grundmann, E., and Amlie, J. G., Zur pathologischen Anatomie der Makroglobulinämie Waldenström. *Frankfurt Z. Pathol.* **71:**443–452, 1961.

8 Habich, H., Zur Antigenanalyse der Paraproteine bei Makroglobulinämien. *Schweiz. Med. Wochenschr.* **83:**1253–1256, 1953.

9 Hjørting-Hansen, E., et al., Orale manifestationer ved macroglobulinaemia Waldenström. *Ugeskr. Laeger* **124:**133–137, 1962.

10 Hörner, H., Makroglobulinämie Waldenström mit osteolytischen Herden. *Klin. Wochenschr.* **33:**110, 1955.

11 Imhof, J. W., et al., Clinical and Haematological Aspects of Macroglobulinaemia Waldenstrom. *Acta Med. Scand.* **163:**349–366, 1959.

12 Kanzow, U., et al., Serologische Differenzierung von Makroglobulinämien. *Klin. Wochenschr.* **33:**1043–1046, 1955.

13 Kappeler, R., et al., Klinik der Makroglobulinämie Waldenström, in G. Riva (ed.), *Makroglobulinämie Waldenström,* Basel, 1958, pp. 54–152.

14 Lamm, M. E., Macroglobulinemia. *Am. J. Clin. Pathol.* **35:**53–65, 1961.

15 McKusick, V. A., *Mendelian Inheritance in Man,* 4th ed. The Johns Hopkins Press, Baltimore, 1975.

16 Maldonado, J. E., et al., Pathophysiology of the Monoclonal Gammopathies. *Postgrad. Med.* **54:**139–145, 1973.

17 Martin, N. H., Macroglobulinemia. *Q. J. Med.* **29:**179–197, 1960.

18 Quattrin, N., et al., On the Differential Diagnosis and Pathogenesis of the Purpuras With Hypergammaglobulinemia or Macroglobulinemia. *Acta Med. Scand.* **156:**25–38, 1956.

19 Ritzmann, S. E., et al., The Syndrome of Macroglobulinemia. *Arch. Intern. Med.* **105:**939–965, 1960.

20 Schaub, F., Gleichzeitiges Vorkommen von Macroglobulinämie Waldenström und von malignen Tumoren. *Schweiz. Med. Wochenschr.* **52:**1256–1257, 1953.

21 Schwab, P. J., et al., Reversal of Retinopathy in Waldenström's Macroglobulinemia by Plasmapheresis. *Arch. Ophthalmol.* **64:**515–521, 1960.

22 Sheon, R. P., et al., Late Occurrence of Plasmacytoma of the Tongue in "Benign" Hyperglobulinemia Purpura of Waldenström. *Ann. Intern. Med.* **64:**386–390, 1966.

23 Sirridge, M. S., Waldenström's Macroglobulinemia with Cryoglobulinemia. *Arch. Intern. Med.* **53:**380–388, 1960.

24 Voight, A. E., and Frick, P. G., Macroglobulinemia of Waldenström. *Ann. Intern. Med.* **44:**419–425, 1956.

25 Waldenström, J., Incipient Myelomatosis or "Essential" Hyperglobulinemia with Fibrinogenopenia: A New Syndrome? *Acta Med. Scand.* **117:**216–247, 1944.

26 Waldenström, J., Zwei interessante Syndrome mit Hyperglobulinämie, Purpura hyperglobulinamica und Makroglobulinämie. *Schweiz. Med. Wochenschr.* **78:**927–928, 1948.

27 Waldenström, J., Macroglobulinemia. *Triangle* **3:**262–270, 1957–1958.

28 Waldenström, J., Die Makroglobulinämie. *Ergeb. Inn. Med. Kinderheilkd.* **9:**586–621, 1958.

29 Waldenström, J., Macroglobulinemia. *Adv. Metab. Disord.* **2:**115–159, 1965.

30 Wall, R. L., The Use of Serum Protein Electrophoresis in Clinical Medicine. *Arch. Intern. Med.* **102:**618–658, 1958.

31 Wührmann, F., Einige aktuelle klinische Probleme über die Serum-Globuline. *Schweiz. Med. Wochenschr.* **82:**937–940, 1952.

32 Zollinger, H. U., Die pathologische Anatomie der Makroglobulinämie Waldenström, in G. Riva (ed.), *Makroglobulinämie Waldenström,* Basel, 1958, pp. 153–183.

89

Maffucci Syndrome

Enchondromatosis and Hemangiomatosis

The syndrome is characterized by (a) multiple enchondromas with secondary bony deformities, (b) multiple hemangiomas, and (c) phlebolithiasis. The condition was described by Maffucci (12) in 1881 and by Kast and von Recklinghausen (9) in 1889. Fewer than 90 cases have been recorded to date (8). Carleton et al. (5) and Bean (3) have thoroughly reviewed the subject.

Etiology is unknown. All cases reported to date have been sporadic. There is neither racial nor sex predilection (1).

SYSTEMIC MANIFESTATIONS

Skeletal system. Enchondromatosis appears when the child is from one to five years old. The cartilaginous tumors are most numerous in the small bones of the hands and feet but may involve any bone preformed in cartilage (Fig. 89-1A, B). They have been unilateral in approximately 40 percent of the cases (1). The enchondromatosis progresses until puberty, the involved bones frequently becoming grotesque. Chondrosarcomatous changes occur in about 20 percent of the cases (3, 6–8, 11). Multiple fractures have been reported (7).

Hemangiomas. The hemangiomas may be superficial or deeply situated. They appear at approximately the same time as the bone changes, often but not always involving the same areas (3–5). Lesions may be unilateral. Hemangiomas of the hypopharynx, esophagus, ileum, and anal mucosa have been noted (7, 13). It is possible that other viscera may be involved. Phlebectasia has been reported in approximately one-fourth of the cases (1).

Oral manifestations. Oral involvement appears to be limited to occasional hemangiomas (10, 11). They have been most frequently associated with the tongue (Fig. 89-1C), although a number of authors have reported lesions of the cheeks, lips, and soft palate (2, 13–15).

DIFFERENTIAL DIAGNOSIS

The syndrome should not be confused with Ollier disease (multiple enchondromatosis without hemangiomas). Occasionally, difficulty may be encountered in distinguishing the *blue rubber bleb nevus syndrome* from the Maffucci syndrome because the cutaneous vascular lesions of the latter syndrome may, at times, mimic those of the blue rubber bleb nevus syndrome. However, multiple enchondromas are not present. In our opinion, the patient with presumed Maffucci syndrome together with the blue rubber bleb nevus syndrome reported by Sakurane et al. (13) represents simply a case of the Maffucci syndrome.

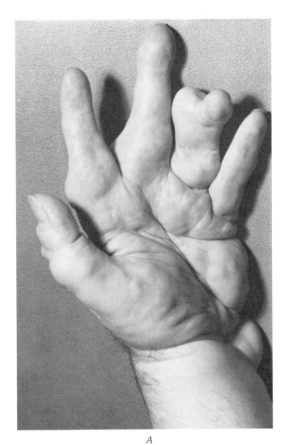

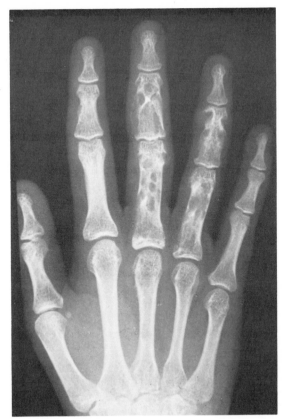

A

B

Figure 89-1. *Maffucci syndrome.* (*A*). Gross distortion of hand due to multiple enchondromas. (*From W. B. Bean*, Arch. Intern. Med. **95**:767, 1955.) (*B*). Enchondromas of several phalanges. (*From W. G. Cauble and H. S. Bowman*, Arch. Surg. **97**:678, 1968.) (*C*). Angiomas of dorsum of tongue. (*From J. G. Kennedy*, Br. Dent. J. **135**:18, 1973.)

LABORATORY AIDS

Hemogram and studies for occult blood in the feces may be indicated in some instances.

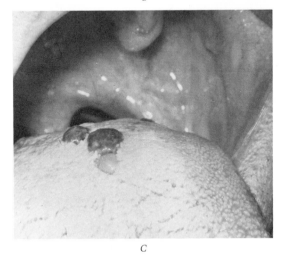

C

REFERENCES

1 Anderson, I. F., Maffucci's Syndrome. *S. Afr. Med. J.* **39**:1066–1070, 1965.

2 Andrén, L., et al., Maffucci's Syndrome. *Acta Chir. Scand.* **126**:397–405, 1963.

3 Bean, W. B., Dyschondroplasia and Hemangiomata (Maffucci's Syndrome). *Arch. Intern. Med.* **177**:299–307, 1965.

4 Berlin, R., Maffucci's Syndrome: Dyschondroplasia with Vascular Hamartomas. *Acta Med. Scand.* **177**:299–307,

1965.

5 Carleton, A., et al., Maffucci's Syndrome: Dyschondroplasia with Haemangiomata. *Q. J. Med.* **11**:203–228, 1942.

6 Elmore, S. M., and Cantrell, W. C., Maffucci's Syndrome. *J. Bone Joint Surg.* **48A**:1607–1613, 1966.

7 Hall, B. D., Intestinal Hemangiomas and Maffucci's Syndrome. *Arch. Dermatol.* **105**:608, 1972.

8 Johnson, J. L., et al., Maffucci's Syndrome (Dyschondroplasia with Hemangiomas). *Am. J. Med.* **28**:864–866, 1960.

9 Kast, –, and von Recklinghausen, –, Ein Fall von Enchondrom mit ungewöhnlicher Multiplication. *Virchows Arch. Pathol. Anat.* **118**:1–18,1889.

10 Kennedy, J. G., Dyschondroplasia and Haemangiomata (Maffucci's Syndrome): Report of a Case with Oral and Intracranial Lesions. *Br. Dent. J.* **135**:18–21, 1973.

11 Lewis, R. J., and Ketcham, A. S., Maffucci's Syndrome: Functional and Neoplastic Significance. *J. Bone Joint Surg.* **55A**:1465–1479, 1973.

12 Maffucci, A., Di un caso di encondroma ed angioma multiplo. *Movimento Med.-chir.* **3**:(2)399–407, 1881.

13 Sakurane, H. F., et al., The Association of Blue Rubber Bleb Nevus and Maffucci's Syndrome. *Arch. Dermatol.* **95**:28–36, 1967.

14 Stang, C., and Rannie, I., Dyschondroplasia and Hemangiomata (Maffucci's Syndrome). *J. Bone Joint Surg.* **32B**:376–383, 1950.

15 Torri, O., Angiome ed encondromi multiple nello individuo. *Clin. Chir. (Milano)* **10**:81–105, 1902.

90

Mandibulofacial Dysostosis

(Treacher Collins Syndrome, Franceschetti-Zwahlen-Klein Syndrome)

Mandibulofacial dysostosis largely involves structures derived from the first branchial arch, groove, and pouch. Although the syndrome was probably first described by Thomson (36) in 1846–1847, credit for its discovery is usually given to Berry (2) or, especially, to Treacher Collins (4) (name often erroneously hyphenated), who described the essential components of the syndrome. Franceschetti and co-workers (7, 8), during the 1940s, published extensive reviews of this syndrome and gave it the name "mandibulofacial dysostosis."

The syndrome is inherited as an autosomal dominant trait with variable expressivity. The gene seems to have a lethal effect, since miscarriage or early postnatal death is common. A number of families have expressed the syndrome in several generations (31, 34, 42). Franceschetti et al. (9), in a review of 63 cases, found 27 with a family history of the syndrome. Possibly 300 or more cases have been published.

The theories of origin of this syndrome are numerous and have been reviewed (7, 19, 21, 33).

SYSTEMIC MANIFESTATIONS

Facies. The facial appearance is characteristic. The downward-sloping palpebral fissures, depressed cheekbones, deformed pinnas, receding chin, and large fishlike mouth present a clinical picture that once seen is unforgettable. Another feature noted in about 25 percent of affected individuals is a tongue-shaped process of hair that extends toward the cheek (Fig. 90-1A–C).

Skull. The calvaria are essentially normal, but roentgenographic studies reveal that the supraorbital ridges are poorly developed, and often there are increased digital markings in the presence of normal suture relationship (23, 34). The body of the malar bones may be totally absent but more often is grossly and symmetrically underdeveloped, with nonfusion of the zygomatic arches. The mastoids are not pneumatized and are frequently sclerotic. The paranasal sinuses are often small and may be completely absent. The lower margin of the orbit has been noted to be defective. An excellent anatomic study has been reported by Lockhart (17).

Eyes. Though vision is usually normal, the palpebral fissures slope laterally downward (antimongoloid obliquity), and, often, there is a coloboma (in about 75 percent of cases) in the outer third of the lower lid (Fig. 90-2). About half the patients have a deficiency of cilia medial to the coloboma. Iridial coloboma may also occur. The lower lacrimal points may be absent (25), as well as the Meibomian glands and intermarginal strip (19, 38). Microphthalmia has also been noted (7, 36). Roentgenographic studies have shown the lower orbital margins to be defective and the orbital cavity to be oval, with the roof inclining downward and outward. The eye anomalies have been especially well reviewed by Franceschetti et al. (9).

Ears. The pinna is often deformed, crumpled forward, or misplaced. In the survey of Stovin et al. (34), 51 of 63 patients had deformed pinna, and over one-third had absence of the external auditory canal or ossicle defect accompanied by conductive deafness (Fig. 90-3). Roentgenographic studies have shown sclerosis of the middle and, very rarely, the inner ear, with poor delineation of their structures. The auditory ossicles and cochlear and vestibular apparatus have been observed to be absent or severely malformed (19, 21, 26). Surgical investigation has corroborated the roentgenographic findings, revealing such abnormalities as fixed malleus, fusion of malformed malleus and incus, monopodal stapes, absence of stapes and oval window, complete absence of middle ear and epitympanic space (21, 33). The space may be filled with connective tissue.

Extra ear tags and blind fistulas may occur anywhere between the tragus and the angle of

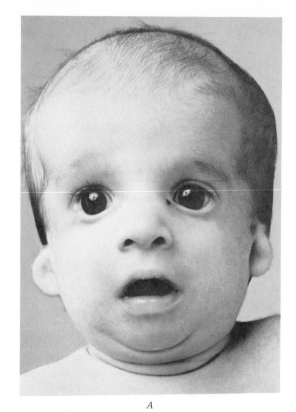

A

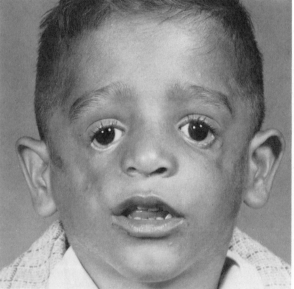

B

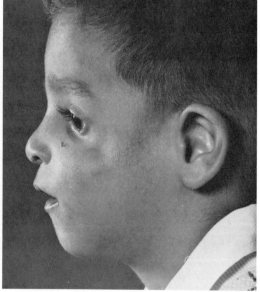

C

Figure 90-1. *Mandibulofacial dysostosis.* (A). Note antimongoloid obliquity of palpebral fissures, coloboma of outer third of lower lids, poor malar and mandibular development, bizarre pinnas. (B, C). Similar feature in older child with less severe alteration of pinnas. (*From B. O. Rogers*, Br. J. Plast. Surg. **17:**109, 1964.)

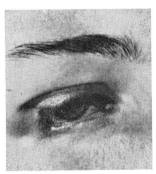

Figure 90-2. Close-up of eye, showing coloboma of lower lid and absence of cilia medial to coloboma.

the mouth. In one case, blind fistulas were found behind the ear lobes (15).

Nose. The nasofrontal angle is usually obliterated, and the bridge of the nose raised. The nose appears large because of the lack of malar development. The nares are often narrow, and the alar cartilages hypoplastic. Choanal atresia has been reported (5, 18, 22, 32, 37).

Mental status. Although Stovin et al. (34) reported that only four of 63 patients were mentally deficient, this estimate seems low. Other investigators have also remarked on mental retardation (13, 15, 40). In some cases, retardation may be secondary to hearing loss.

Other findings. These have been discussed by several authors (5, 14, 20, 23, 35, 37).

Oral manifestations. The mandible is almost always hypoplastic. Roentgenographic studies

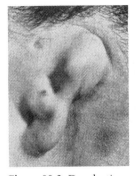

Figure 90-3. Dysplastic ear; note supratragal pit.

have shown that the angle is more obtuse than normal and that the ramus may be deficient. The coronoid and condyloid processes are flat or even aplastic. The undersurface of the body of the mandible is often pronouncedly concave. Grönvall and Olsson (15) reconstructed a model of the mandible. A detailed cephalometric study was carried out by Garner (11).

The palate is cleft in about 30 percent of patients (7, 13, 23, 34, 38). Macrostomia, observed in about 15 percent, may be unilateral or bilateral.

Because of the poor development of the maxilla and the frequency of highly arched or cleft palate, dental malocclusion is frequent. The teeth may be widely separated, hypoplastic, displaced, or associated with open bite (9, 11, 16, 27, 30, 38).

DIFFERENTIAL DIAGNOSIS

The facies is so characteristic that little difficulty in diagnosis should be experienced. However, affected relatives may have minimal signs of the syndrome and must be closely examined. A sporadic case with minimal involvement can present difficulties in diagnosis.

In recent years, it has become evident that "mandibulofacial dysostosis" is etiologically heterogeneous. It is probably best to think of mandibulofacial dysostosis as a nonspecific symptom complex that may occur in several different disorders, the most common being the Treacher Collins syndrome. These other disorders are discussed below.

A distinct entity, acrofacial dysostosis, was first described by Nager and de Reynier (23). It closely resembles Treacher Collins syndrome but has autosomal recessive transmission. The thumbs are hypoplastic or absent, the radius and ulna may be fused or there may be absence or hypoplasia of the radius and/or one or more metacarpals. Lower lid colobomas are rarer, cleft palate more frequent, and the mandible more severely retarded in growth than in mandibulofacial dysostosis. Examples have been described by a number of authors (2a, 3, 10a, 12, 16, 16a, 22–25, 28, 29, 39, 41) (Fig. 90-4*A, B*).

Elsewhere, three patients have been described (1) with many similarities to Nager acrofacial dysostosis. However, all three instances were sporadic, and limb deficiency was predominantly postaxial rather than preaxial as in the Nager syndrome. Further delineation is necessary to determine if this is a separate syndrome and if so what its recurrence risk is.

Parish (26) described what he called the Achard syndrome in which mandibulofacial dysostosis occurs together with features of the Marfan syndrome, particularly arachnodactyly and joint laxity. Since only a single affected patient is known, it is not clear whether this represents a distinct entity or the occurrence of mandibulofacial dysostosis and the Marfan syndrome coincidentally in the same patient.

A number of disorders with some similar features have been described that are difficult to classify. For example, the dominantly inherited maxillofacial dysostosis described by Peters and Hovels (27) consists of bilateral hypoplasia of malar bones, antimongoloid obliquity of lids without colobomas, open bite, and excessive development of the mandible. (These patients appear to have myotonic dystrophy.) The mandibular dysostosis of Nager and de Reynier (23) (bilateral hypoplasia of the ascending ramus, aplasia of the temporomandibular joint, and atresia of external auditory canal without lid anomalies or macrostomia), the otomandibular dysostosis of François and Haustrate (10) (hemifacial microsomia, microphthalmia, coloboma of uveal tract and optic disk), and the oculovertebral syndrome of Weyers and Thier (30) (unilateral anophthalmia or microphthalmia, dysplasia of the maxilla, and rib and vertebral anomalies) may be variants of the *oculoauriculovertebral syndrome.*

Many cases of oculoauriculovertebral syndrome have been erroneously classified as "unilateral mandibulofacial dysostosis."

LABORATORY AIDS

None is known.

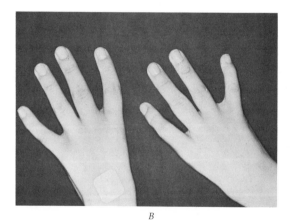

Figure 90-4. (A). *Acrofacial dysostosis of Nager.* Note facies similar to that of mandibulofacial dysostosis. (B). Absence of thumbs. (*From F. A. Walker,* Birth Defects **10**(8):135, 1974.)

REFERENCES

1 Bergsma, D., Case Report 28. *Syndrome Identification* **3**(1):7–13, 1975.

2 Berry, G. A., Note on a Congenital Defect (Coloboma?) of the Lower Lid. *R. Lond. Ophthalmol. Hosp. Rep.* **12**:255–257, 1889.

2a Carter, C. O., personal communication, 1975.

3 Chou, Y. C., Mandibulofacial Dysotosis. *Chin. Med. J.* **80**:373–375, 1960.

4 Collins, E. T., Cases with Symmetrical Congenital Notches in the Outer Part of Each Lid and Defective Development of the Malar Bones. *Trans. Ophthalmol. Soc. U.K.* **20**:190–192, 1900.

5 Fazen, L. E., et al., Mandibulofacial Dysostosis. *Am. J. Dis. Child.* **113**:405–410, 1967.

6 Fernandez, A. O., and Ronis, M. L., The Treacher Collins Syndrome. *Arch. Otolaryngol.* **80**:505–520, 1964.

7 Franceschetti, A., and Klein, D., Mandibulo-facial Dysostosis: New Hereditary Syndrome. *Acta Ophthalmol. (Kbh.)* **27**:143–224, 1949.

8 Franceschetti, A., et al., Dysostose mandibulo-facial unilatérale avec déformations multiples du squelette (Processus paramastoïde, synostose des vertèbres, sacralisation, etc.) et torticolis clonique. *Ophthalmologica* **118**:796–814, 1949.

9 Franceschetti, A., et al., La dysostose mandibulo-faciale dans le cadre des syndrome du premier arc branchial. *Schweiz. Med. Wochenschr.* **89**:478–483, 1959.

10 Francois, J., and Haustrate, L., Anomalies colobomateuses du globe oculaire et syndrome du premier arc. *Ann. Ocul. (Paris)* **187**:340–368, 1954.

10a Herrmann, J., et al., Acrofacial Dysostosis Type Nager. *Birth Defects,* in press.

11 Garner, L. D., Cephalometric Analysis of Berry–Treacher Collins Syndrome. *Oral Surg.* **23**:320–327, 1967.

12 Genée, E., Une forme extensive de dysostose mandibulofaciale. *J. Génêt. Hum.* **17**:42–52, 1969.

13 Gibson, R., Mandibulofacial Dysostosis with Oligophrenia in Siblings. *Am. J. Ment. Defic.* **62**:504–506, 1957–1958.

14 Gottsegen, G., et al., Kammerscheidewanddefekt bei mandibulo-fazialer Dysostose. *Z. Kreislaufforsch.* **45**:499–503, 1956.

15 Grönvall, H., and Olsson, Y., Dysostosis mandibulofacialis. *Acta Ophthalmol. (Kbh.)* **31**:245–252, 1953.

16 Jones, R. G., Mandibulofacial Dysostosis. *Centr. Afr. J. Med.* **14**:193–200, 1968.

16a Klein, D., et al., Sur un forme extensive de dysostose mandibulo-faciale (Franceschetti) accompagnée de malformations des extremites, *Rev. Oto-Neuro-Ophthal.* **42**:422–440, 1970.

17 Lockhart, R. D., Variants Coincident with Congenital Absence of Zygoma (Zygomatic Process of Temporal Bone). *J. Anat.* **63**:233–236, 1928–1929.

18 Lübke, F., von, Über die Beobachtungen einer Dysostosis mandibulofacialis. *Z. Geburtshilfe Gynäkol.* **156**:235–246, 1961.

19 Mann, I., and Kilner, T. P., Deficiency of the Malar Bones with Defect of the Lower Lids. *Br. J. Ophthalmol.* **27**:13–20, 1943.

20 Maran, A. G. D., The Treacher Collins Syndrome. *J. Laryngol.* **78**:135–151, 1964.

20a Mansharamani, R. K., and Badonia, O. P., Mandibulofacial Dysostosis Syndrome. *Indian J. Pediatr.* **33**:344–347, 1966.

21 McKenzie, J., and Craig, J., Mandibulo-facial Dysostosis (Treacher Collins Syndrome). *Arch. Dis. Child.* **30**:391–395, 1955.

22 McNeill, K. A., and Wynter-Wedderburn, L., Choanal Atresia: A Manifestation of the Treacher Collins Syndrome. *J. Laryngol.* **67**:365–369, 1953.

23 Nager, F. R., and de Reynier, J. P., Das Gehörorgan bei den angeborenen Kopfmissbildungen. *Pract. Otorhinolaryngol. (Basel),* suppl. 2, **10**:1–128, 1948.

24 Neidhart, E., *Die Dysostosis mandibulo-facialis in Kombination mit Missbildungen der obern Extremitäten,* Thesis, Zürich, 1968.

25 O'Conner, G. B., and Conway, M. E., Treacher Collins Syndrome (Dysostosis Mandibulo-facialis). *Plast. Reconstr. Surg.* **5**:419–425, 1950.

26 Parish, J. G., Heritable Disorders of Connective Tissue. *Proc. R. Soc. Med.* **53**:515, 1960.

27 Peters, A., and Hövels, O., Die Dysostosis maxillo-facialis, eine erbliche, typische Fehlbildung des l. Visceralbogens. *Z. Menschl. Vererb. Konstit. Lehre* **35**:434–444, 1960.

28 Pfeiffer, R. A., Associated Deformities of the Head and Hands (Case 17). *Birth Defects* **5**(3):18–34, 1969.

29 Piper, H. F., Augenärztliche Befunde bei frühkindlicher Entwicklungsstörung. *Monatsschr. Kinderheilkd.* **105**:170–176, 1957.

30 Rogers, B. O., Berry–Treacher Collins Syndrome: A Review of 200 Cases. *Br. J. Plast. Surg.* **17**:109–137, 1964.

31 Rovin, S., et al., Mandibulofacial Dysostosis: A Familial Study of Five Generations. *J. Pediatr.* **65**:215–221, 1964.

32 Sahawi, E., Beitrag zur Dysostosis mandibulofacialis. *Z. Kinderheilkd.* **94**:195–201, 1965.

33 Snyder, C. C., Bilateral Facial Agenesia (Treacher Collins Syndrome). *Am. J. Surg.* **92**:81–87, 1956.

34 Stovin, J. J., et al., Mandibulofacial Dysostosis. *Radiology* **74**:225–231, 1960.

35 Straith, C. L., and Lewis, J. R., Associated Congenital Defects of the Ears, Eyelids and Malar Bones (Treacher Collins Syndrome). *Plast. Reconstr. Surg.* **4**:204–213, 1949.

36 Thomson, A., Notice of Several Cases of Malformation of the External Ear, Together with Experiments on the State of Hearing in Such Persons. *Monthly J. Med. Sci.* **7**:420, 1846–1847, cited by Klein, D., Dysostose mandibulofaciale. *Prat. Odontol-stomatol. (Geneve),* No. 487–490, pp. 1–8, 1953.

37 Vatré, J., Etude génétique et classification clinique de 154 cas de dysostose mandibulo-faciale (syndrome de Franceschetti) avec description de leurs associations malformatives. *J. Génêt. Hum.* **19**:17–100, 1971. [Same case as Klein (16a).]

38 Walker, D. G., *Malformations of the Face,* E. & S. Livingston, Edinburgh, 1961.

39 Walker, F. A., Apparent Autosomal Recessive Inheritance of the Treacher Collins Syndrome. *Birth Defects* **10**(8):135–139, 1974.

40 Weyers, H., and Thier, C. J., Malformations mandibulo-

faciales et délimitation d'un syndrome oculo-vertébral. *J. Génét. Hum.* **7:**143–173, 1958.

41 Wiedemann, H. R., Missbildungs-Retardierungs-Syndrom mit Fehlen des 5. Strahls an Handenund Füssen, Gaumenspalte, dysplastischen Ohren and Augenlidern und ra-

dioulnärer Synostose, *Klin. Pädiatr.* **185:**181–186, 1973.

42 Wildervanck, L. S., Dysostosis Mandibulo-facialis (Franceschetti-Zwahlen) in Four Generations. *Acta Genet. Med.* (*Roma*) **9:**447–451, 1960.

91

Marfan Syndrome

The main features of the Marfan syndrome include (a) disproportionate skeletal growth with dolichostenomelia and arachnodactyly, (b) ectopia lentis, and (c) fusiform and dissecting aneurysms of the aorta. Although it has been suggested that Marfan's original patient had cystathionine synthase deficiency (homocystinuria) (4), a more convincing argument has been made for congenital contractural arachnodactyly (3).

The disorder is inherited as an autosomal dominant trait with a high degree of penetrance and variable expressivity. Roughly 85 percent of the cases are familial, the rest arising as fresh mutations (20, 22). Advanced paternal age at time of conception is associated with isolated cases (20, 23). The prevalence of the Marfan syndrome is at least 1.5 per 100,000 in the general population, with both sexes being equally affected. It has been suggested that Abraham Lincoln had the disorder (11, 22).

The syndrome is thought to result from a structural defect in protein, particularly the elastic fiber (21, 22). Collagen production is disturbed at the cellular level, and an increase in the ratio of soluble to insoluble collagen has been reported (21).

SYSTEMIC MANIFESTATIONS

Facies. Dolichocephaly usually occurs with prominent supraorbital ridges. Frontal bossing is common, and the eyes often appear sunken, giving the patient a wizened appearance.

Musculoskeletal system. Dolichostenomelia and arachnodactyly are constant features, with the halluces disproportionately elongated. Hallux valgus and hammertoe are frequent.

The lower segment (pubis to sole) is greater than the upper segment (vertex to pubis). The US/LS ratio in the Marfan syndrome averages 0.85, in comparison with the average normal Caucasian value of 0.93 [for normal values of blacks and whites at various ages, see McKusick (22)]. Pectus excavatum and carinatum, late-developing kyphoscoliosis, elongated patellar ligament, spina bifida, and weakness of joint capsules manifested by pes planus and hyperextensibility of joints with habitual dislocation (hips, patella, clavicle) are commonly observed (19, 25, 30). Enlarged vertebras and widened spinal cord have also been noted (14, 19, 25, 39). Hernia (inguinal, femoral) is frequent (31) (Figs. 91-1, 91-2A, B).

Skin. Deficiency of subcutaneous fat and striae distensae have been reported (18, 22). Miescher elastoma, especially on the neck, has been noted with increased frequency.

Eyes. Eye changes seem to be more common in males. Iridodonesis may occur as an early sign of lens dislocation. Ectopia lentis, resulting from weakened or broken suspensory ligaments, is

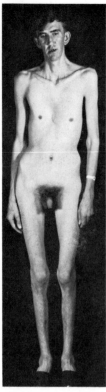

Figure 91-1. *Marfan syndrome.* Patient has tall, thin habitus, arachnodactyly, scoliosis, pectus excavatum, and bilaterally subluxated lenses. (*From N. Tuna and A. P. Thal,* Circulation **24:**1154, 1961.)

present bilaterally in at least 70 percent of patients (2, 7, 20). The dislocated lenses are displaced superiorly, superonasally, or superotemporally in about 70 percent of the cases. Allen and associates (2) described alterations in the chamber angle, ciliary body, and pupil. Ramsey et al. (26) found increased transillumination of the iris diaphragm. Megalocornea, blue scleras, microphakia, spherophakia, and retinal detachment may be observed. Myopia is common (22).

Cardiovascular system. Diffuse, generally progressive dilatation of the ascending aorta with or without dissecting aneurysm may occur and may be a common cause of sudden death in affected individuals even in early adulthood. These changes are preceded by aortic regurgitation and "floppy mitral valve" with mitral regurgitation in at least 65 percent of patients (5, 13, 20, 22, 27, 32, 34). Aneurysms of the thoracic or abdominal aorta or pulmonary artery are less common. An angina-like chest pain is common.

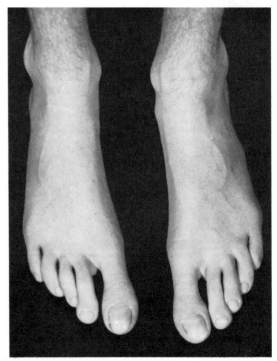

A

B

Figure 91-2. (*A, B*). Arachnodactyly.

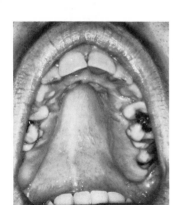

Figure 91-3. High palatal vault.

Aortic coarctation has also been noted with increased frequency (22). Alterations of the renal artery leading to severe hypertension have been reported (14). Microscopically, medial necrosis and intimal thickening of blood vessels have been observed. Occasionally, pulmonary malformations may increase susceptibility to infection in the lower part of the respiratory tract and lead to emphysema (16, 22).

Abnormal bleeding tendency with easy bruising has been observed. Defective giant platelets and an increased number of immature granulocytes have been reported in the peripheral blood (9).

Oral manifestation. Although earlier authors estimated the prevalence of high palatal vault to be between 15 and 40 percent (22), some have observed this condition in all their patients (20) (Fig. 91-3). Cleft palate or bifid uvula has been noted in several instances (20, 22, 37).

The teeth have been noted to be long and narrow (22) and frequently maloccluded (18). Mandibular prognathism is common. Roentgenographically, the maxillary sinuses may be enlarged.

DIFFERENTIAL DIAGNOSIS

A Marfanoid habitus may be observed in *cystathionine synthase deficiency* (*homocystinuria*), congenital contractural arachnodactyly (3, 8), Marfanoid hypermobility syndrome (35), eunuchoidism, *Klinefelter syndrome*, sickle cell anemia, *multiple mucosal neuroma syndrome*, and occasionally in the *multiple nevoid basal cell carcinoma syndrome*. A decreased US/LS ratio is a normal finding in the Nilotic black (22). Ectopia lentis may occur in Weil-Marchesani syndrome (22), *Ehlers-Danlos syndromes, homocystinuria, osteogenesis imperfecta,* and as an isolated autosomal recessive trait (22). In the homocystinuric, the lens tends to dislocate nasally, inferonasally, or inferiorly (7). Aortic dilatation is also seen in Erdheim's cystic medial necrosis and in tertiary syphilis (22). Joint hypermobility is seen in a number of disorders, including *osteogenesis imperfecta,* the *Ehlers-Danlos syndromes, homocystinuria,* the *Stickler syndrome,* and Marfanoid hypermobility syndrome (12, 22).

LABORATORY AIDS

The US/LS ratio (22), metacarpal index (15, 25), relative slenderness index (25), the Walker-Murdoch wrist sign (22), and the Steinberg thumb sign (30) may be helpful. High concentrations of urinary hydroxyproline may occur in some cases, especially during the growth period (17, 22, 28, 29). Increased urinary hydroxyproline levels reflect increased collagen turnover in bone and may be seen in other conditions such as hyperparathyroidism, Paget disease of bone, etc. (29). IgA, IgG, IgM, and alpha-lipoprotein levels were elevated in 9 of 10 patients studied by Suschke et al. (33). Intracytoplasmatic metachromatic inclusions have been observed in fibroblast tissue culture (6) and in fibroblasts cultured from the amniotic fluid of an affected fetus (24).

REFERENCES

1 Adler, R. C., and Nyhan, W. L., An Oculocerebral Syndrome with Aminoaciduria and Keratosis Follicularis.

J. Pediatr. **75:**436–442, 1969.

2 Allen, R. A., et al., Ocular Manifestation of the Marfan

Syndrome. *Trans. Am. Acad. Ophthalmol. Otolaryngol.* **71**:18–38, 1967.

3 Beals, R. K., and Hecht, F., Congenital Contractural Arachnodactyly. *J. Bone Joint Surg.* **53A**:987–993, 1971.

4 Bianchine, J., The Marfan Syndrome Revisited. *J. Pediatr.* **79**:717–719, 1971.

5 Bowden, D. H., et al., Marfan's Syndrome: Accelerated Course in Childhood Associated with Lesions of Mitral Valve and Pulmonary Artery. *Am. Heart J.* **69**:96–99, 1965.

6 Cartwright, E., et al., Metachromatic Fibroblasts in Pseudoxanthoma Elasticum and Marfan's Syndrome. *Lancet* **1**:533–534, 1969.

7 Cross, H. E., and Jensen, A. D., Ocular Manifestations in the Marfan Syndrome and Homocystinuria. *Am. J. Ophthalmol.* **75**:405–420, 1973.

8 Epstein, C. J., et al., Hereditary Dysplasia of Bone with Kyphosis, Contractures and Abnormally Shaped Ears. *J. Pediatr.* **73**:379–386, 1968.

9 Estes, J. W., et al., Marfan's Syndrome. *Arch. Intern. Med.* **116**:889–893, 1965.

10 Ghosh, S., Marfan's Syndrome Associated with Arthrogryposis in a Family. *Indian Pediatr.* **3**:333–335, 1966.

11 Gordon, A. M., Abraham Lincoln – a Medical Appraisal. *J. Kentucky Med. Assoc.* **60**:249–253, 1962.

12 Grahame, R., Joint Hypermobility – Clinical Aspects. *Proc. R. Soc. Med.* **64**:692–694, 1971.

13 Grondin, C. M., et al., Dissecting Aneurysm Complicating Marfan's Syndrome (Arachnodactyly) in a Mother and Son. *Am. Heart J.* **77**:301–306, 1969.

14 Hiragami, H., et al., Marfan's Syndrome Accompanied by Renovascular Hypertension. *Tokuko J. Exp. Med.* **98**:13–20, 1969.

15 Joseph, M. C., and Meadow, S. R., The Metacarpal Index in Infants. *Arch. Dis. Child.* **44**:515–516, 1969.

16 Keech, M. K., et al., Familial Studies of the Marfan Syndrome. *J. Chron. Dis.* **19**:57–83, 1966.

17 Lehmann, O., A Family with Marfan's Syndrome Traced through an Affected Newborn. *Acta Paediatr. Scand.* **49**:540–550, 1960.

18 Loveman, A. B., et al., Marfan's Syndrome: Some Cutaneous Aspects. *Arch. Dermatol.* **87**:428–435, 1963.

19 Lutman, F. C., and Neel, J. V., Inheritance of Arachnodactyly, Ectopia Lentis, and Other Congenital Anomalies (Marfan's Syndrome) in the E Family. *Arch. Ophthalmol. (Chic.)* **41**:276–305, 1949.

20 Lynas, M. A., Marfan's Syndrome in Northern Ireland. *Ann. Hum. Genet.* **22**:289–301, 1958.

21 Macek, M., et al., Study on Fibroblasts in Marfan's Syndrome. *Humangenetik* **3**:87–97, 1966.

22 McKusick, V. A., *Heritable Disorders of Connective Tissue*, 4th ed. Mosby, St. Louis, 1972.

23 Murdoch, J. L., et al., Parental Age Effects on the Occurrence of New Mutations for the Marfan Syndrome. *Ann. Hum. Genet.* **35**:331–336, 1972.

24 Nadler, H. L., Prenatal Detection of Genetic Defects. *J. Pediatr.* **74**:132–143, 1969.

25 Parish, J. G., Skeletal Hand Charts in Inherited Connective Tissue Diseases. *J. Med. Genet.* **4**:227–238, 1967.

26 Ramsey, M. S., et al., The Marfan Syndrome: A Histopathologic Study of Ocular Findings. *Am. J. Ophthalmol.* **76**:102–116, 1973.

27 Rivlin, M. E., Marfan's Syndrome and Pregnancy. *J. Obstet. Gynaecol. Br. Commonw.* **74**:143–144, 1967.

28 Sjoerdsma, A., et al., Increased Excretion of Hydroxyproline in Marfan's Syndrome. *Lancet* **2**:994, 1958.

29 Smith, Q. T., et al., Urinary Hydroxyproline in Various Diseases. *Acta Derm. Venereol. (Stockh.)* **45**:44–49, 1965.

30 Steinberg, I., A Simple Screening Test for the Marfan Syndrome. *Am. J. Roentgenol.* **97**:118–124, 1966.

31 Stinson, H. K., and Cruess, R. L., Marfan's Syndrome with Marked Limb-length Discrepancy. *J. Bone Joint Surg.* **49A**:735–736, 1967.

32 Stone, J. H., Ectopia Lentis, Cardiology and "the Sign of the Trembling Iris." *Am. Heart J.* **72**:466–468, 1966.

33 Suschke, J., et al., Elektrophoretische und immunologische Befunde beim Marfan-Syndrom. *Dtsch. Med. Wochenschr.* **94**:2289–2290, 1969.

34 Traisman, J. S., and Johnson, F. R., Arachnodactyly Associated with Aneurysm of the Aorta. *Am. J. Dis. Child.* **87**:156–166, 1954.

35 Walker, B. A., et al., The Marfanoid Hypermobility Syndrome. *Ann. Intern. Med.* **71**:349–352, 1969.

36 Wilner, H. I., and Finby, N., Skeletal Manifestations in the Marfan Syndrome. *J.A.M.A.* **187**:490–495, 1964.

37 Wilson, R., Marfan's Syndrome: Description of a Family. *Am. J. Med.* **23**:434–444, 1957.

38 Young, D., Familial Dissecting Aneurysm Complicating Marfan's Syndrome. *Am. Heart J.* **78**:577–578, 1969.

39 Zimprich, H., Zur Genetik des Marfan-Syndroms. *Helv. Paediatr. Acta* **19**:483–489, 1964.

Maxillonasal Dysplasia

(Binder Syndrome)

Maxillonasal dysplasia was first recognized as an entity by Binder in 1962 (1). Search of the literature revealed an earlier report of a similar case (4). Less than two dozen examples have been described to date (1–3, 5). However, the condition is probably rather common. We have seen at least a half-dozen cases. The scarcity of reports on the condition is due to absence of markedly striking features.

Consanguinity among parents was noted in a few cases (2, 6), but all cases reported to date have been sporadic. Rival et al. (6) described "familial resemblance" to grandparents, but this was not documented.

SYSTEMIC MANIFESTATIONS

Facies. The face is characterized by a flat vertical nose (Fig. 92-1*A–C*).

Nose. The nasofrontal angle is absent, the nose being hypoplastic with flattened alae and nasal tip. The nostrils are half-moon-shaped when

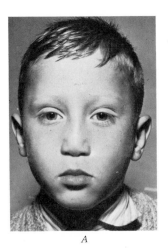 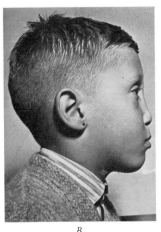 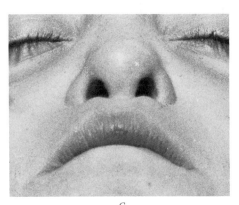

A	*B*	*C*

Figure 92-1. *Maxillonasal dysplasia. (A, B, C).* Flattened nose with depressed subnasal or alar base area and hypoplasia of premaxillary area of upper jaw. Upper lip has convex contour; nostrils are half-moon-shaped. (*From K. H. Binder,* Dtsch. Zahnärztl. Z. **17**:438, 1962.)

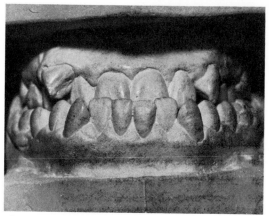

Figure 92-2. Relative mandibular prognathism with reverse overbite. (*From K. Binder,* Dtsch. Zahnärztl. Z. **17:**438, 1962.)

viewed from below. The nasal mucosa has been described as atrophic, but the sense of smell is normal (1).

Roentgenographically, aplasia or hypoplasia of the anterior nasal spine, thinness of the labial plate of alveolar bone over the upper incisors, and an increase in the nasomaxillary angle have been observed. The frontal sinuses are often hypoplastic.

Other findings. No associated anomalies have been described to date. Intelligence is normal.

Oral manifestations. The upper lip has a convex contour with poorly developed philtrum. The premaxillary area is hypoplastic, with flattening of the maxillary base and sagittal shortening of the dental arch. The mandible is of normal width, but the gonial angle is increased and the chin is flattened (2). Because of maxillary shortening, all patients have a relative mandibular prognathism with reverse overbite (class III malocclusion) (Fig. 92-2).

DIFFERENTIAL DIAGNOSIS

Although the facies may appear arrhinencephaloid, no brain abnormalities have been observed in this condition. The sense of smell is completely normal. Absent frontal sinuses and relative mandibular prognathism can be associated with a host of conditions and may also be seen in otherwise normal individuals.

LABORATORY AIDS

None is known.

REFERENCES

1 Binder, K. H., Dysostosis maxillo-nasalis, ein arhinencephaler Missbildungskomplex. *Dtsch. Zahnärztl. Z.* **17:**438–444, 1962.
2 Delaire, J., et al., Le syndrome de Binder (quatre observations). *Rev. Stomatol. (Paris).* **71:**257–269, 1970.
3 Hopkin, G. B., Hypoplasia of the Middle Third of the Face Associated with Congenital Absence of the Anterior Nasal Spine, Depression of the Nasal Bones, and Angle Class III Malocclusion. *Br. J. Plast. Surg.* **16:**146–153, 1963.
4 Noyes, F. B., Case Report. *Angle Orthodont.* **9:**160–165, 1939.
5 Pathenheimer, F., Angeborene Fehlbildungen und Anomalien. 10. Mitteilung: Maxillo-nasales Syndrom. *Med. Monatsschr.* **20:**232–233, 1966.
6 Rival, J. M., et al., Dysostose maxillo-nasale de Binder. A propos de 10 cas. *J. Génét. Hum.* **22:**263–268, 1974.

93

Meckel Syndrome

(Dysencephalia Splanchnocystica, Gruber Syndrome)

Meckel (18), in 1822, was probably the first person to delineate a syndrome which consists of (a) microcephaly, (b) exencephalocele, (c) microphthalmia, (d) congenital heart defects, (e) polydactyly, (f) polycystic kidneys, liver, and pancreas, and (g) clefts of the lip and/or palate. Comprehensive reviews are those of Opitz and Howe (21) and Hsia et al. (13).

The inheritance pattern is autosomal recessive (13, 17). Parental consanguinity (9, 10, 28, 29) and affected sibs (4–6, 9, 13, 14, 17–19, 29) have been noted in several cases.

SYSTEMIC MANIFESTATIONS

The syndrome is lethal, death usually occurring within the first month of life.

Facies. Microcephaly, microphthalmia, and facial clefts characterize the facies (Fig. 93-1). Microphthalmia has been documented in only 15 percent of patients (14, 18).

Central nervous system. Microcephaly (in about 30 percent of cases) with associated holoprosencephaly (9, 16), internal hydrocephalus (25, 29), and occipital encephalocele (in about 80 percent) or meningoencephalocele (6, 9, 16, 23, 26) are frequent features. Anencephaly and/or agenesis or hypoplasia of the cerebellum have been described (9).

Cystic kidneys and cystic liver. Cysts of the kidney (in about 90 percent of patients) and less often cysts of the liver and/or pancreas (in about 20 percent) have been noted (6, 9, 10, 11, 25, 27, 29).

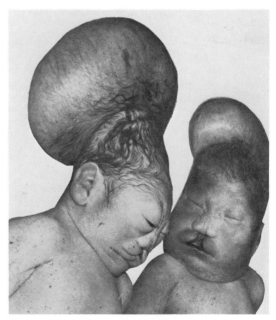

Figure 93-1. *Meckel syndrome.* Microcephaly, occipital exencephalocele, microphthalmia, ocular hypotelorism, premaxillary agenesis in twins. (*From Y. E. Hsia et al.,* Pediatrics **48:**237, 1971.)

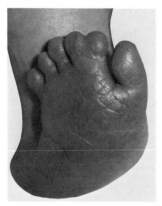

Figure 93-2. Polydactyly, syndactyly, abbreviation of hallux, talipes. (*From J. M. Opitz and J. J. Howe,* Birth Defects **5**(2):167, 1969.)

Skeletal alteration. The most common skeletal alteration is polydactyly. This usually involves all four extremities with hexadactyly, heptadactyly, or an even greater number of postaxial digits (6, 9, 11, 16, 23, 27, 29), and has been observed in 75 percent of patients. Talipes equinovarus has been noted in about 25 percent of cases (19) (Fig. 93-2).

Genital anomalies. Hypoplastic penis and undescended testes (7, 9, 11) and septate vagina and bicornuate uterus (9) have been observed in about 20 percent of cases (Fig. 93-3). The urinary bladder may also be hypoplastic.

Other findings. Malrotation of the intestine, cardiac defects, and a variety of other anomalies have been noted (21).

Oral manifestations. Cleft lip and/or more often cleft palate have been frequent features of the syndrome, being recorded in about 50 percent of the cases (2, 4, 29). Malformation of tongue and larynx has also been noted (9).

DIFFERENTIAL DIAGNOSIS

The disorder may be confused with *trisomy 13* and occasionally with the *Smith-Lemli-Opitz syndrome.* Although not obligatory, the triad of occipital encephalocele, polydactyly, and poly-

cystic kidneys is persuasive in making a diagnosis of Meckel syndrome. In the Meckel syndrome, polydactyly is usually more extreme and may involve all four limbs asymmetrically. Polycystic kidneys and cysts of the liver and pancreas are ordinarily not part of trisomy 13 syndrome. Cystic kidneys may occur alone or in a variety of other syndromes (Zellweger syndrome, Dandy-Walker malformation) or with cystic liver (3).

Majewski et al. (15) described a lethal syndrome of pre- and postaxial polysyndactyly, mesomelic brachymelia (especially short tibia), narrow thorax with short ribs, hypoplastic epiglottis, hypoplasia and incomplete lobulation of lungs, polycystic kidneys, genital anomalies, and, in several cases, cleft lip and/or palate. The skull, vertebras, and pelvis were not remarkably affected. Saldino and Noonan (24) described a lethal syndrome marked by short ribs, postaxial polydactyly, marked shortened flipper-like extremities, and severe metaphyseal dysplasia of tubular bones. Ossification of the calvaria, vertebras, pelvis, and short bones of the hands and

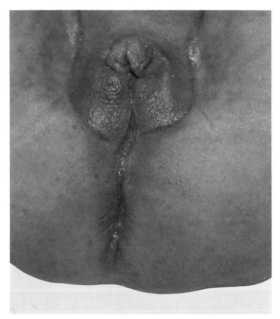

Figure 93-3. Hypoplastic penis, hypospadias. (*From J. M. Opitz and J. H. Howe,* Birth Defects **5**(2):167, 1969.)

feet is defective. Associated anomalies included polycystic kidneys, transposition of great vessels and atretic lesions of the gastrointestinal and genital systems. In contrast, in Meckel syndrome, the thorax is not narrow and the extremities are not short with unossified phalanges. Moreover, exencephalocele, microcephaly, and microphthalmia are not part of either the Majewski or the Saldino-Noonan syndrome.

The so-called Ullrich-Feichtiger syndrome is a spurious entity. All such cases may be resolved into cases of the Meckel syndrome, trisomy 13, or the Smith-Lemli-Opitz syndrome (21).

An apparently incomplete form of Meckel syndrome was described by Fried et al. (9a).

LABORATORY AIDS

Chromosome studies may be helpful in ruling out trisomy 13.

REFERENCES

1 Babes, V., Die Beziehung von Entwicklungsanomalien am Gesicht zu überzahligen Fingern und Zehen. *Verh. Dtsch. Ges. Pathol.* **8**:110–114, 1904.

2 Battaglia, S., and Locatelli, L., Malattia di Gruber e Giordano (dysencephalia splanchnocystica). *Folia Hered. Pathol.* (*Milano*) **5**:259–276, 1956.

3 Blyth, H., and Ockenden, B. G., Polycystic Disease of Kidneys and Liver Presenting in Childhood. *J. Med. Genet.* **8**:257–284, 1971.

4 Bruckner, C., Zweimalige Entbindung derselben Frau von Missgeburten mit vergrösserten Nieren. *Virchows Arch. Pathol. Anat.* **46**:503–506, 1896.

5 Calmann, A., Ein Beitrag zur Casuistik der Missbildungen an Zunge und Kehlkopf. *Virchows Arch. Pathol. Anat.* **134**:337–343, 1893.

6 DeLange, C., Zum Studium der Encephalocele posterior. *Jb. Kinderheilkd.* **126**:253–288, 1930.

7 Ferrier, P., et al., Nonspecific Pseudohermaphroditism. *Helv. Paediatr. Acta* **19**:1–12, 1964.

8 Foerster, A., Zur Casuistik der Hirnkrankheiten. *Würzb. Med. Z.* **3**:193–198, 1862.

9 Fried, K., et al., Polycystic Kidneys Associated with Malformations of Brain, Polydactyly, and Other Birth Defects in Newborn Sibs. *J. Med. Genet.* **8**:285–290, 1971.

9a Fried, K., et al., A Meckel-like Syndrome. *Clin. Genet.* **5**:46–50, 1974.

10 Georgii, A., Zur Frage der Erblichkeit familiär–typischer Fehlbildungskomplexe beim Menschen: Übereinstimmende Kombination von Polydaktylie mit multiplen Abartungen bei Geschwistern (Sektionsbefunde). *Beitr. Pathol. Anat.* **116**:259–272, 1956.

11 Gresham, G. A., Chromosomal Sex Determination in a Male Internal Pseudohermaphrodite. *J. Pathol. Bacteriol.* **70**:546–548, 1955.

12 Gruber, G. B., Beiträge zur Frage "gekoppelter" Missbildung (Akrocephalosyndaktylie und Dysencephalia splanchnocystica). *Beitr. Pathol. Anat.* **93**:459–476, 1934.

13 Hsia, Y. E., et al., Genetics of the Meckel Syndrome (Dysencephalia Splanchnocystica). *Pediatrics* **48**:237–247, 1971.

14 MacRae, D. W., et al., Ocular Manifestations of the Meckel Syndrome. *Arch. Ophthalmol.* **88**:106–113, 1972.

15 Majewski, F., et al., Polysyndaktylie, verkürzte Gliedmassen und Genitalfehlbildungen: Kennzeichen eines selbständigen Syndroms? *Z. Kinderheilkd.* **111**:118–138, 1971.

16 Marshall, R., et al., Features of the 13-15 Trisomy Syndrome with Normal Karyotype. *Lancet* **1**:556, 1964.

17 Mecke, S., and Passarge, E., Encephalocele, Polycystic Kidney and Polydactyly as an Autosomal Recessive Trait Simulating Other Disorders. *Ann. Génét.* **14**:97–103, 1971.

18 Meckel, J. F., Beschreibung zweier durch sehr ähnliche Bildungsabweichung entstellter Geschwister. *Dtsch. Arch. Physiol.* **7**:99–172, 1822.

19 Miller, J. Q., and Selden, R. F., Arhinencephaly, Encephalocele and 13-15 Trisomy Syndrome with Normal Chromosomes. *Neurology* **17**:1087–1091, 1967.

20 Naffah, J., et al., A propos de trois nouveaux cas dans une même fratrie du syndroms de Meckel ou dysencéphalie splanchnocystique de Gruber. *Arch. Fr. Pédiatr.* **29**:1069, 1972.

21 Opitz, J. M., and Howe, J. J., Meckel's Syndrome: Dysencephalia Splanchnocystica, Gruber's Syndrome. *Birth Defects* **5**(2):167–179, 1969.

22 Porak, –, and Couvelaire, –, Foie polycystique cause de dystocie. *Ann. Gynécol. Obstét.* **55**:223–237, 1901.

23 Roscher, F., Über die Häufigkeit, die Art und die pathogene Bedeutung von Missbildungen der Niere und der Harnwege. *Acta Chir. Scand.* **70**:493–540, 1933.

24 Saldino, R. M., and Noonan, C. D., Severe Thoracic Dystrophy with Striking Micromelia, Abnormal Osseous Development Including the Spine and Multiple Visceral Anomalies. *Am. J. Roentgenol.* **114**:257–263, 1972.

25 Simopoulos, A. P., et al., Polycystic Kidneys, Internal Hydrocephalus and Polydactylism in Newborn Siblings. *Pediatrics* **39**:931–934, 1967.

26 Stockard, C. R., Developmental Rate and Structural Expression: An Experimental Study of Twins, "Double Monsters" and Single Deformities and the Interaction among Embryonic Organs during Their Origin and Development (Plate 4). *Am. J. Anat.* **28**:115–277, 1921.

27 Teuscher, M., Über die kongenitale Cystenleber mit Cystennieren und Cystenpankreas. *Beitr. Pathol. Anat.* **75**:459–485, 1926 (reviews earlier literature).

28 Tucker, C. C., et al., Oral-facial-digital Syndrome with Polycystic Kidneys and Liver: Pathological and Cytogenetic Studies. *J. Med. Genet.* **3**:77–158, 1966.

29 Walbaum, R., et al., Polydactylie familiale avec dysplasie neurocrânienne. *Ann. Génét.* **10**:39–41, 1967.

94

Melkersson-Rosenthal Syndrome

Melkersson-Rosenthal syndrome consists of (a) facial paralysis, (b) facial edema, and (c) fissured tongue. It was described in part as early as 1859 by Märt (21). Melkersson (22), in 1928, postulated a relationship between facial paralysis and swelling of the face. Three years later, Rosenthal (29) added lingua plicata to the clinical picture. In 1945, Miescher (23) described several patients with "cheilitis granulomatosa." Most later investigators equated the two conditions (8, 10, 14, 19, 28).

The syndrome has been stated to have no sex predilection (18, 37). However, Schuermann (33) found more women affected, especially when neurologic symptoms and signs are present. Familial occurrence has been described (4, 33, 37) but, in our opinion, single-gene inheritance is unlikely.

Theories of pathogenesis have abounded: allergy (7), angioneurotic phenomena (16), sarcoid and/or tuberculosis (8, 29), virus (5), etc. However, none has met with general acceptance.

SYSTEMIC MANIFESTATIONS

Not all patients have all components of the triad. Mair et al. (21a), studying 23 patients, found the triad in only 9, two signs in 13 patients, and one component in the remaining patient.

Facies. Swelling of the lips, either unilaterally or bilaterally, is the dominant feature of the syndrome (Figs. 94-1, 94-2). The swelling begins suddenly, in most cases prior to facial paralysis (10, 12), but sometimes after or simultaneously with it (16, 17). As a rule, the attack begins during childhood. Kettel (16) and Schuermann (33) reported that some patients observed the swelling after exposure to cold weather. Usually the upper lip is affected, but swelling of the lower lip is also seen, either as an isolated phenomenon or in combination with swelling of the upper lip. The edema may assume a peculiar reddish-brown appearance. It is nontender and

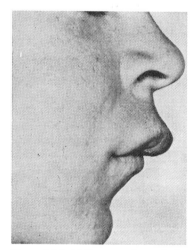

Figure 94-1. *Melkersson-Rosenthal syndrome.* Swelling of upper lip of twenty-year-old man with the syndrome.

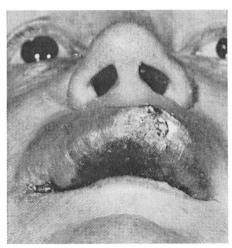

Figure 94-2. Swollen, crusted upper lip of thirty-nine-year-old woman.

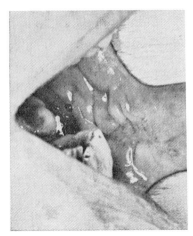

Figure 94-3. Plicated swelling of the buccal mucosa in a patient with Melkersson-Rosenthal syndrome. (*Courtesy of H. Schuermann, Bonn, Germany.*)

nonpitting; occasionally during exacerbation it may be accompanied by slight fever (17). The swollen lip may assume large proportions—at times being three to four times thicker than normal, markedly exposing the vermilion portion. The edema recurs in most patients, often in spring and fall (12), resulting in permanent enlargement of the lips. The lips may be chapped and fissured from the enlargement (26, 34). The eyelids, nose, and chin may also be affected (1).

Facial paralysis. Facial palsy begins suddenly in children or in persons less than twenty years of age (16, 17). It is peripheral and clinically indistinguishable from Bell's palsy. Mair et al. (21a) found the syndrome in about 4.5 percent of patients with idiopathic facial palsy. It may be partial or complete and, in some cases, bilateral. Relapses often occur but most patients ultimately recover (21a). Kettel (16) pointed out that the paralysis may precede attacks of swelling by years. Not always does the paralyzed side correspond to that of the swelling (8). Occasionally, defects in taste along the anterior two-thirds of the tongue are noted (17). Lüscher (20) reported loss of taste and slight visual disturbance one year before the occurrence of facial paralysis.

Other findings. Swelling of the hands, chest, and buttocks occurs, as well as a variety of neurologic symptoms which include acroparesthesia, headache, hyperhidrosis, hypogeusia, hyposialia, blepharospasm, epiphora, and hypacusia (3, 14, 27, 34). Megacolon has also been reported (14, 32), as well as association with Hodgkin disease (24).

Oral manifestations. Simultaneously with the swelling of the skin, the oral mucosa is affected in a similar way in most cases. The swollen buccal mucosa is cushion-like and divided by

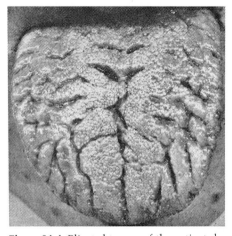

Figure 94-4. Plicated tongue of the patient shown in Fig. 94-1.

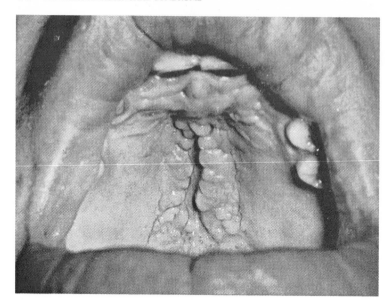

Figure 94-5. Plicated palatal mucosa in another patient with the syndrome. (*Courtesy of A. Lodin, Stockholm, Sweden.*)

furrows of varying depth. The affected mucosa may be slightly red, and atrophy of the tongue papillae may be seen (Fig. 94-3). Swelling of the palate and gingiva has also been reported (34) (Fig. 94-5).

Statements concerning frequency of lingua plicata in the Melkersson-Rosenthal syndrome vary considerably. In a review of 250 recorded cases, Hornstein (14) found folded tongue in one-third of the cases. Plicated tongue is found in about 0.5 to 5 percent of a normal population (Fig. 94-4). The connection between lingua plicata and the other components of the syndrome seems peculiar, and no satisfactory explanation has yet been given. Sometimes the tongue change consists only of a deepened median fissure.

PATHOLOGY

German investigators, particularly, have contributed to the understanding of the pathologic processes underlying the swelling (12, 14, 32, 34). Microscopically, granulomatous changes have been found in most cases. Granulomas of lymphohistiocytic, sarcoidal, or tuberculoid character are located in the lamina propria and are occasionally seen in the muscle (Fig. 94-6). The

granulomas, which may show the presence of inflammation in varying degrees and giant cells of the Langhans type, occur perivascularly and are often surrounded by a connective tissue capsule (8, 12). In the tongue, the granulomatous inflammatory process is sometimes followed by

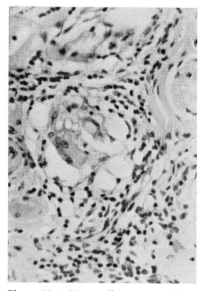

Figure 94-6. Giant cell in a sarcoid-like granuloma in lip of patient seen in Fig. 94-2.

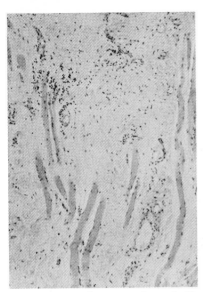

Figure 94-7. Replacement of muscle fibers with edematous fibrous tissue in lip of patient seen in Fig. 94-1.

an increased formation of connective tissue, leading to stiffness (10). Some investigators have stressed the presence of marked edema and round-cell infiltration (16), and Stevens (35) even suggested the term "idiopathic fibroedema" for the syndrome. Figure 94-7 illustrates the replacement of muscle fibers with edematous fibrous tissue. According to Ekbom and Wahlström (6), the swelling, in the chronic stage, is due to dilated lymphatic vessels and sclerotic connective tissue. On the basis of histologic findings, Bazex and Dupré (2) subdivided the Melkersson-Rosenthal syndrome into two groups: the sarcoid type and the lymphedematous type.

DIFFERENTIAL DIAGNOSIS

On glancing at a patient with the Melkersson-Rosenthal syndrome, one has the impression first (apart from congenital malformations associated with macrocheilia–lymphangioma, hemangioma), of an abscess (gumboil, lip furuncle, or insect bite). Simple cheilitis, Quincke edema, and recurrent erysipelas may also simulate the syndrome. Confusion with angioneurotic edema should not occur, because this condition never causes fibrosis, is often associated with urticaria, and is observed largely among patients with an allergic family history (35). If granulomas are found, Boeck sarcoid should be considered. However, cutaneous lesions rarely develop in Melkersson-Rosenthal syndrome. Facial paralysis may occur in the *Heerfordt syndrome.* Uveitis in this latter syndrome, however, separates it from Melkersson-Rosenthal syndrome. Findlay (7) discussed the differential diagnosis between *Ascher syndrome* and cheilitis granulomatosa. Clinically, the two conditions are hard to distinguish. In Ascher syndrome, the upper lip is most often involved and the swelling tends to be more lobulated and discrete. Bazex and Dupré (2) have grouped the two syndromes together because of histologic similarities.

DIAGNOSTIC AIDS

None is known.

REFERENCES

1 Balabanow, K., and Dimitrowa, J., Seltene Lokalisationen und eigentümliche klinische Formen des Melkersson-Rosenthal-Syndroms (Blepharitis granulomatosa et Hemicheilitis granulomatosa). *Dermatol. Wochenschr.* **151:** 101–107, 1965.

2 Bazex, A., and Dupré, A., Les infiltrations lymphoedemateuses, sarcoidiques et adenomateuses chroniques du visage (syndrome de Melkersson-Rosenthal fibroedeme de Stevens, syndrome d'Ascher). *Toulouse Méd.* **58:**89–109, 1957.

3 Broser, F., and Bender, R. M., Über zentral-nervöse Symptome bei Cheilitis granulomatosa Miescher bzw. Mel-

kersson-Rosenthal Syndrom. *Nervenarzt* **29:**21–27, 1958.

4 Carr, R. D., Is the Melkersson-Rosenthal Syndrome Hereditary? *Arch. Dermatol.* **93:**426–427, 1966.

5 Dlabalová, H., and Danda, J., Beitrag zur Ätiologie des Syndroms Melkersson-Rosenthal. *Hautarzt* **19:**256–259, 1968.

6 Ekbom, K. A., and Wahlström, A., Melkersson's Syndrom. *Nord. Med.* **15:**2373–2378, 1942.

7 Findlay, G. H., Idiopathic Enlargements of the Lips: Cheilitis Granulomatosa, Ascher's Syndrome and Double Lip. *Br. J. Dermatol.* **66:**129–138, 1954.

8 Gahlen, W., and Bruckner, B., Beitrag zur Pathogenese des

Melkersson-Rosenthal Syndroms. *Arch. Dermatol. Syph.* (*Berl.*) **192**:468–477, 1951.

9 Gassler, H., and Berthold, H., Ein Beitrag zum Melkersson-Rosenthal Syndrom aus ophthalmologischer Sicht. *Klin. Monatsbl. Augenheilkd.* **193**:44–51, 1961.

10 Hamp, S. E., Melkerssons Syndrom. *Sven. Tandläk. Tidskr.* **59**:65–80, 1966.

11 Hauser, W., Das Melkersson-Rosenthal Syndrom und die Cheilitis granulomatosa. *Dtsch. Zahnärztl. Z.* **8**:986–991, 1953.

12 Hornstein, O., Klinische und histologische Untersuchungen über "Cheilitis granulomatosa" (Miescher) bzw. Melkersson-Rosenthal Syndrom. *Hautarzt* **6**:433–447, 1955.

13 Hornstein, O., Ungewöhnliche Erscheinungsformen des sogenannten Melkersson-Rosenthal Syndroms. *Dtsch. Med. Wochenschr.* **85**:430–433, 1960.

14 Hornstein, O., Über die Pathogenese des sogenannten Melkersson-Rosenthal Syndroms (einschliesslich der "Cheilitis granulomatosa" Miescher). *Arch. Klin. Exp. Dermatol.* **212**:570–605, 1961.

15 Hornstein, O., and Schuermann, H., Das sogenannte Melkersson-Rosenthal Syndrome (einschliesslich "Cheilitis granulomatosa" Miescher). *Ergeb. Inn. Med. Kinderheilkd.* **17**:190–263, 1962.

16 Kettel, K., Melkersson's Syndrome. *Arch. Otolaryngol.* **46**:341–360, 1947.

17 Klaus, S. N., and Brunsting, L. A., Melkersson's Syndrome (Persistent Swelling of the Face, Recurrent Facial Paralysis, and Lingua Plicata). *Mayo Clin. Proc.* **34**:365–370, 1959.

18 Lemoyne, J., et al., Le syndrome de Melkersson-Rosenthal. *Ann. Otolaryngol.* (*Paris*), **77**:640–647, 1960.

19 Luhr, H. G., and Immenkamp, E., Morbus Miescher. Ein Beitrag zur Differential-diagnose der Lippenschwellung. *Dtsch. Zahnärztl. Z.* **24**:949–953, 1969.

20 Lüscher, E., Syndrom von Melkersson-Rosenthal. *Schweiz. Med. Wochenschr.* **79**:1–3, 1949.

21 Märt, E., *Nonnulla de nervi facialis paralysi,* Leipzig, 1859.

21a Mair, I. W. S., et al., Clinical Manifestations of the Melkersson-Rosenthal Syndrome. *Can. J. Otolaryngol.* **3**:123–131, 1974.

22 Melkersson, E., Ett fall av recidiverande facialispares i samband med angioneurotisk ödem. *Hygeia* (*Stockh.*) **90**:737–741, 1928.

23 Miescher, G., Über essentielle granulomatöse Makrocheilie (Cheilitis granulomatosa). *Dermatologica* **91**:57–85, 1945.

24 Mulvihill, J. J., et al., Melkersson-Rosenthal Syndrome, Hodgkin Disease and Corneal Keratopathy. *Ann. Intern. Med.* **132**:116–117, 1973.

25 Nally, F. F., Melkersson-Rosenthal Syndrome. *Oral Surg.* **29**:694–703, 1970.

26 New, G. B., and Kirch, W. A., Permanent Enlargement of the Lips and Face. *J.A.M.A.* **100**:1230–1233, 1933.

27 Rauch, S., Neue Gesichtspunkte zum Melkersson-Rosenthal-Syndrom. *Schweiz. Med. Wochenschr.* **98**:1743–1750, 1968.

28 Rintala, A., et al., Cheilitis granulomatosa. The Melkersson-Rosenthal Syndrome. *Scand. J. Plast. Surg.* **7**:130–136, 1973.

29 Rosenthal, C., Klinischer biologischer Beitrag zur Konstitutionspathologie. Gemeinsames Auftreten von (rezidivierender familiärer) Facialislähmung angioneurotischem Gesichtsödem und Lingua plicata in Arthritismus-Familien. *Z. Gesamte Neurol. Psychiatr.* **131**:475–500, 1931.

30 Saberman, M. N., and Tenta, L. T., The Melkersson-Rosenthal Syndrome. *Arch. Otolaryngol.* **84**:292–296, 1966.

31 Schimpf, A., Ungewöhnliche Schwellungen beim sog. Melkersson-Rosenthal Syndrom. *Dermatol. Wochenschr.* **147**:105–118, 1963.

32 Schröder, H., and Hartmann, G., Melkersson-Rosenthal Syndrom und idiopathischer Megakolon. *Beitr. Klin. Chir.* **205**:208–220, 1962.

33 Schuermann, H., *Krankheiten der Mundschleimhaut und der Lippen,* 2d ed. Urban & Schwarzenberg, Berlin, 1958.

34 Schuppener, H. J., Zum Melkersson-Rosenthal Syndrom. *Dtsch. Gesundheitsw.* **11**:1598–1610, 1956.

35 Stevens, F. A., Streptococci Infection of the "Fibroedema" of Melkersson's Syndrome. *J.A.M.A.* **156**:223–224, 1954.

36 Streeto, J. M., and Watters, F. B., Melkersson's Syndrome: Multiple Recurrence of Bell's Palsy and Episodic Facial Edema. *N. Engl. J. Med.* **271**:308–309, 1964.

95

Melnick-Needles Syndrome

(Osteodysplasty)

Melnick and Needles (5) in 1966 described a syndrome characterized by (a) generalized bone dysplasia and (b) abnormal facies. Similar patients were noted by Coste et al. (1), Stelling and Meunier (6), and Maroteaux et al. (3).

The syndrome is clearly inherited as an autosomal dominant trait.

SYSTEMIC MANIFESTATIONS

Diagnosis is based on roentgenographic findings. Within a single family the unusual facies would suggest the bony alterations.

Early childhood is marked by recurrent respiratory and ear infections.

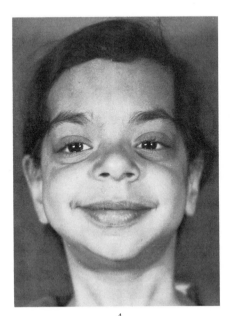
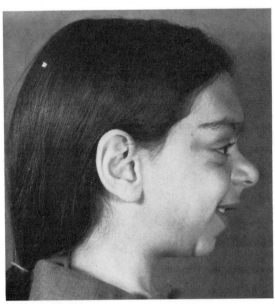

A   *B*

Figure 95-1. *Melnick-Needles syndrome. (A, B).* Note mild prominence of eyes, long neck, small mandible. *(Courtesy of F. H. Stelling and P. Meunier, Greenville, S.C.*

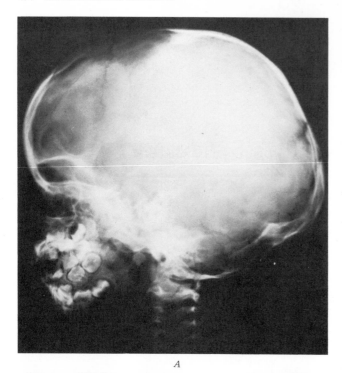

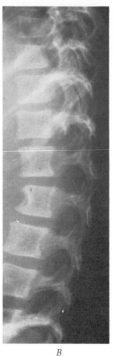

A

B

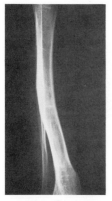

C

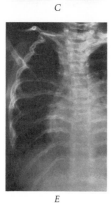

E

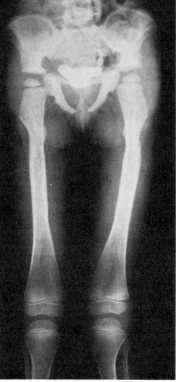

D

Figure 95-2. (*A*). Delayed closure of anterior fontanel; paranasal sinuses underdeveloped. (*B*). Disproportionately tall vertebral bodies having anterior concavity. (*C*). S-shaped bowing of tibia. (*D*). Flared ilia, flat acetabulas, tapered ischial bones, coxa valga, metaphyseal flare. (*E*). Ribbon-like ribs with cortical irregularities. (A, D, *from J. Melnick and C. Needles,* Am. J. Roentgenol. **97:**39, 1966, *and F. H. Stelling and P. Meunier, Greenville, S.C.;* B, C, E, *from B. Leiber, Frankfurt, Germany.*)

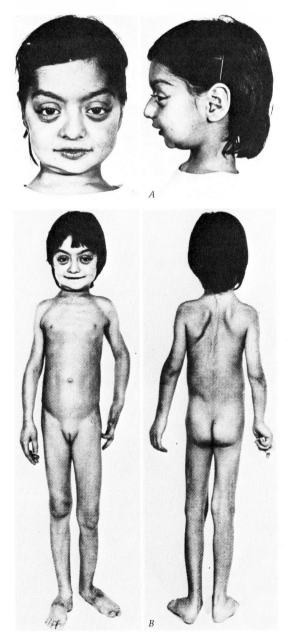

Roentgenographically, delayed closure of the anterior fontanel and sclerosis of the skull base and mastoid processes and, less consistently, the calvaria are found. The paranasal sinuses tend to remain underdeveloped. All vertebral bodies are unusually tall, especially those of the axis, atlas, and occipital condyles. The thoracic vertebras exhibit an anterior concavity with double beaking. The clavicles have cortical irregularity with flaring. Sternal ossification is delayed.

Most striking are the changes in the long bones. Bowing of the radius and tibia produces an S-shaped appearance. The metaphyses at the proximal and distal ends of the humerus, fibula, and tibia are flared. Coxa valga is marked. The iliac bones are flared at the crest and constricted in the supraacetabular area, while the ischial bones are tapered. The ribs are ribbon-like, with cortical irregularity (Fig. 95-2A–E).

Oral manifestations. Micrognathia and marked malocclusion are constant features.

DIFFERENTIAL DIAGNOSIS

The roentgenographic features are so distinctive as to differentiate this syndrome from other disorders in which there is delayed closure of the anterior fontanel.

We see little similarity between the Melnick-Needles syndrome and the so-called autosomal recessive lethal type of "osteodysplasty" reported by Danks et al (2).

LABORATORY FINDINGS

None is known.

REFERENCES

1 Coste, F., et al., Osteodysplasty (Melnick and Needles Syndrome). *Ann. Rheum. Dis.* **27:**360–366, 1968.
2 Danks, D. M., et al., A Precocious Autosomal Recessive Type of Osteodysplasty. *Birth Defects* **10**(12): 124–127, 1974.
3 Maroteaux, P., et al., L'ostéodysplastie (syndrome de Melnick et de Needles). *Presse Méd.* **76:**715–718, 1968.
4 Martin, C., et al., Un cas d'osteodysplastie (syndrome de Melnick et de Needles). *Arch. Fr. Pédiatr.* **28:**446–447, 1971.
5 Melnick, J. C., and Needles, C. F., An Undiagnosed Bone Dysplasia. A 2 Family Study of 4 Generations and 3 Generations. *Am. J. Roentgenol.* **97:**39–48, 1966.
6 Stelling, F. H., and Meunier, P., Melnick-Needles Syndrome. Personal communication, 1971.

Figure 95-3. (A). Note exophthalmos, hypertelorism, outstanding nose, receding chin. (B). Dysplastic habitus, foot dysphases. (*From N. Moelter and A. Walther,* Mschr. Kinderheilkd. **123:**178, 1975.)

Facies. The facies is characterized by micrognathia, full cheeks, prominent eyes, and large ears (Fig. 95-1A, B).

Skeletal alterations. The neck is long, the shoulders narrow, and the upper arms short. Frequently there is abnormal gait and dislocation of the hips is not uncommon.

96

Mucopolysaccharidoses, Mucolipidoses, and Related Disorders

The mucopolysaccharidoses are inherited disorders of mucopolysaccharide metabolism. Defective activity of various genetically controlled pathways of lysosomal degradation leads to intracellular storage of undegraded acid mucopolysaccharides and to a relatively uniform clinical and skeletal phenotype (4, 7, 10). This phenotype is most pronounced in the Hurler and Maroteaux-Lamy syndromes and is less severe in other mucopolysaccharidoses.

The mucopolysaccharidoses have been designated types I through VI (5). However, on the basis of recent knowledge regarding pathogenesis of these disorders, the original classification has been revised (6) and will be used here. With the exception of Hunter syndrome, which is X-linked recessive, all others are autosomal recessive.

Differential diagnostic criteria of the classic mucopolysaccharidoses, some probably genetic variants, and some so-called "mucolipidoses" are summarized in Table 96-1.

In this rapidly changing field, old terms and designations have changed to those in parentheses: chondroitin sulfate B (dermatan sulfate), heparitin sulfate (heparan sulfate), keratosulfate (keratan sulfate), chondroitin sulfate A (chondroitin-4-sulfate), and chondroitin sulfate C (chondroitin-6-sulfate); they will be thus employed in our discussion.

MUCOPOLYSACCHARIDOSIS I-H (HURLER SYNDROME)

Mucopolysaccharidosis I-H (MPS I in McKusick's original classification) was first described in 1919 by Hurler (10) at the suggestion of Pfaundler. It is the classic prototype of the mucopolysaccharidoses, having the following cardinal features: (a) growth failure after infancy, (b) marked mental retardation, (c) characteristic craniofacial dysmorphism and physical habitus, (d) dysostosis multiplex, (e) corneal clouding, (f) histochemical and biochemical evidence of intracellular storage of acid mucopolysaccharides (AMPS), and (g) excessive urinary excretion of AMPS.

In the first months of life there are a few relatively nonspecific findings, such as hernias, macrocephaly, limited hip abduction, and recurrent respiratory infections. The full clinical picture usually develops in the second year of life. Death usually occurs before ten years of age from pneumonia and cardiac failure.

The frequency of mucopolysaccharidosis I-H is approximately 1 : 100,000 births (12). The basic biochemical defect is absence of α-L-iduronidase activity (1, 13). Lack of this activity apparently inhibits intralysosomal degradation of α-L-iduronide-containing mucopolysaccharides. Intracellular accumulation of undegraded or par-

Table 96-1. Differentiation of mucopolysaccharidoses, some mucolipidoses and related disorders

Type	Synonym	Clinical dysmorphism	Skeletal dysplasia	Corneal opacities	Mental retardation	Excessive urinary AMPS	Defective enzyme	Genetic transmission	Type
I-H	Hurler	Severe	Severe	Yes	Yes	DS and HS	α-L-iduronidase	A.R.	I-H
I-S	Scheie	Mild	Mild	Yes	No	DS and HS	α-L-iduronidase	A.R.	I-S
II-A	Hunter A	Late (moderate)	Moderate	No	No	HS and DS	Sulfoiduronate sulfatase	X.R.	II-A
II-B	Hunter B	Early (moderate)	Moderate	No	Yes	DS and HS	Sulfoiduronate sulfatase	X.R.	II-B
III-A	Sanflippo A	Mild	Minimal	No	Yes	HS	HS-N-sulfatase	A.R.	III-A
III-B	Sanflippo B	Mild	Minimal	No	Yes	HS	N-acetyl-α-glucosaminidase	A.R.	III-B
IV	Morquio	Severe	Severe	Yes	No	KS	Chondroitin-6-sulfate N-acetyl-glucosamine-4-sulfate sulfatase	A.R.	IV
† V	....	....	....	...	...	...	....	...	V
VI-A	Maroteaux-Lamy A	Mild to moderate	Moderate	Yes	No	DS	Aryl sulfatase B	A.R.	VI-A
VI-B	Maroteaux-Lamy B	Severe	Severe	Yes	Mild	DS	Aryl sulfatase B	A.R.	VI-B
VII	None	None	None	None	Late	Ch-4-S(?)	β-glucuronidase	A.R.	VII
G_M gangliosidosis I	....	Mild	Severe (type 1) Normal (type 2)	Rare	Yes	No	β-galactosidase A,B,C	A.R.	G_M gangliosidosis
Mucolipidosis I	Lipomucopoly-saccharidosis	Mild	Mild	No	Yes	No	?	A.R.*	Mucolipidosis I
Mucolipidosis II	I-cell disease	Severe	Severe	Rare	Yes	No	Multiple	A.R.*	Mucolipidosis II
Mucolipidosis III	Pseudopolydystrophy	Moderate	Variable	Yes	Yes	No	Multiple	A.R.*	Mucolipidosis III
Fucosidosis	Hurler	Minimal	Mild	No	Yes	No	α-fucosidase	A.R.	Fucosidosis
Mannosidosis	....	Minimal	Mild	Yes	Mild	No	α-mannosidase A & B	A.R.	Mannosidosis

* Probably heterogeneous.
† Type V reclassified as Type I-S.
Note: AMPS, acid mucopolysaccharides; DS, dermatan sulfate; HS, heparan sulfate; KS, keratan sulfate; Ch-4-S, chondroitin-4-sulfate; A.R., autosomal recessive; X.R., X-linked recessive.

tially degraded AMPS interferes with normal function of the affected cells and leads to the characteristic clinical symptoms.

SYSTEMIC MANIFESTATIONS

Facies. Slight coarsening of facial features at three to six months of age is usually the first abnormality noted. The head is large, and the frontal bones bulge. Premature closure of the sagittal and metopic sutures and hyperostosis in this area frequently lead to scaphocephaly. Hirsutism is represented on the face only as synophrys. The nasal bridge is depressed, the tip of the nose is broad, and the nostrils are wide and anteverted. The interpupillary distance is greater than normal. Corneal clouding appears during the third year of life, rarely earlier. The lower eyelids and nasolabial folds are prominent, and the cheeks are full. The earlobes are thick. The lips are enlarged and patulous, and the mouth is usually held open, especially after the age of three years. Chronic nasal discharge is usually marked even between the frequent bouts of upper respiratory infection (Fig. 96-1A, B). Nasal congestion with stertorous breathing through the mouth is severe, being related to hyperplastic adenoid tissue and a deep cranial fossa

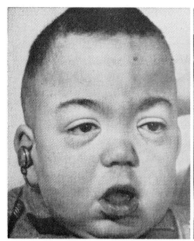
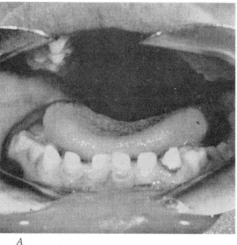

A

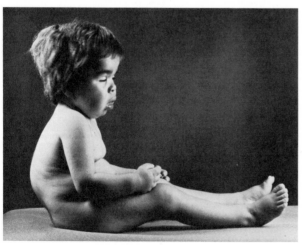

B

Figure 96-1. *Hurler syndrome.* (*A*). Characteristic facies appears during second year of life. Head large with prominent forehead and coarse features. Hypertelorism, heavy lids, flat nasal bridge, snub nose, long philtrum, and open mouth are typical. Progressive deafness is common. (*B*). Two-year-old girl with MPS I-H. Note facies and gibbus.

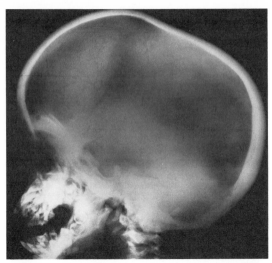

A

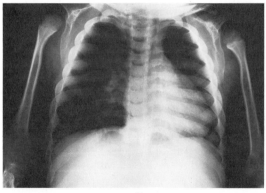

B

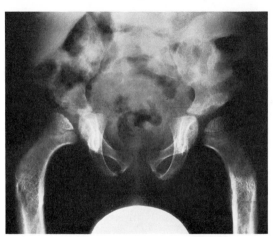

D

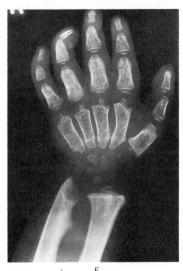

E

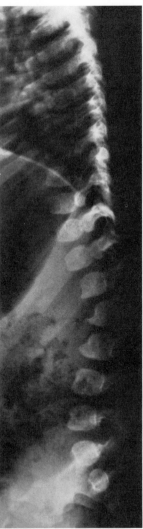

C

Figure 96-2. (*A*). Skull, eight-year-old patient. Macrocephaly, dolichocephaly, thickened calvaria, wide sella. (*B*). Chest of same patient. Wide, oar-shaped ribs, expanded medial portions of clavicle, valgus deformity of humeral neck, submetaphyseal overconstriction of proximal humerus, expansion of distal shaft of humerus. (*C*). Spine of four-year-old patient. Flattening and biconvex end plates of vertebral bodies; hook-shaped configuration of first to third lumbar vertebras. (*D*). Pelvis of eight-year-old patient. Hypoplasia of basilar portion of ilia, flared iliac crest, long femoral neck, coxa valga. (*E*). Hand of six-year-old patient. Expanded shafts of short tubular bones, bullet-shaped phalanges, proximal pointing of second to fifth metacarpals, small carpal bones, tilted distal ends of radius and ulna.

which narrows the airway between the sphenoid bone and the hard palate. Gag and swallowing reflexes become progressively diminished (11).

Musculoskeletal system. Length at birth is not decreased below the norm. The majority of patients with MPS I-H studied between the ages of six and twelve months are at or above the 87th percentile for total body length. Some remain among the tallest babies until 18 months, but growth ceases in all patients before two years of age. By age three years, all MPS I-H patients are below the 3d percentile for stature. The neck is short. Both pectus carinatum and pectus excavatum occur, and usually there is lumbodorsal kyphosis or gibbus. Range of motion is limited in all joints, in the hands resulting in the so-called clawhand deformity (14).

Roentgenographically, in infancy, bone trabeculation is seen to be coarse. In late infancy and early childhood, a pattern of skeletal changes called "dysostosis multiplex" emerges: the skull becomes large and deformed; the sphenoidal plane is depressed; and the sella is J-shaped, possibly from arachnoid cysts (Fig. 96-2A). The sagittal and lambdoidal sutures close prematurely. The cranial base and orbital roofs are especially thick and dense. The orbits are shallow. Communicating hydrocephalus is often present. The ribs are wide in their lateral and ventral portions, with overconstriction at their paravertebral ends. The vertebral bodies are dysplastic, with biconvex end plates and hook-shaped configuration of the lower thoracic and upper lumbar bodies, after twelve to eighteen months of age (Fig. 96-2C). The basilar portions of the ilia are underdeveloped, with flaring of the iliac wings (Fig. 96-2D). The long tubular bones show marked diaphyseal widening and distortion, with small and deformed epiphyses. The shafts of the short tubular bones are underconstricted, with bullet-shaped phalanges and proximal pointing of the second to fifth metacarpals (17) (Fig. 96-2E).

The abdomen protrudes because of hepatic and splenic enlargement, deformity of the chest, shortness of the spine, and laxity of the abdominal wall. These changes are noted during the second year of life. Hepatomegaly may be detected as early as six to twelve months of age.

Inguinal hernia, present at birth or developing within the first 3 months of life, is a constant feature in boys. The hernias tend not to recur following surgery; they are a classic part of the patients' history before diagnosis is established but are not common during the subsequent course of the disorder. Umbilical hernias, usually small at birth in both sexes, gradually reach major proportions. Rarely, intraabdominal complications occur.

Other findings. The skin is pale, coarse, and dry. It is covered by fine, lanugo-like fuzz, particularly on the back and extremities. Mental retardation is conspicuous and progressive. Moderate cardiomegaly, due to deposition of AMPS in the myocardium and valves, is usually present.

Oral manifestations. Oral changes have been reviewed by Gardner (7). The lips are enlarged and patulous, with flattened philtrum, and the upper lip is especially long. The mouth is usually held open, with protruding tongue, from about three years of age. Lip and tongue enlargement becomes marked after the age of five years (11).

The teeth are widely spaced, often exhibiting severe attrition (Fig. 96-3A). The incisors may exhibit some degree of conical crown form but are otherwise normal structurally. Because of macroglossia, there may be anterior open bite. Eruption is probably delayed in at least half the patients (5), especially in areas of bone destruction. The second primary molars or first and second permanent molars are often distoangularly positioned, with the distal surface of the crown being situated more deeply than the mesial. In some cases, there is dilaceration of the distal roots (18). These changes occur more frequently in the mandible.

Extremely common are localized areas of bone destruction which have been designated as "dentigerous cysts." These are often present by three years of age and more often involve the second primary molar and first and second permanent mandibular molars. The margins of the radiolucencies are usually smooth and clearly defined (5, 8, 9) (Fig. 96-3B). In our opinion, they represent pooling of dermatan sulfate in hyperplastic dental follicles, since they also occur in MPS VI but not in MPS III.

The alveolar ridges are nearly always hyper-

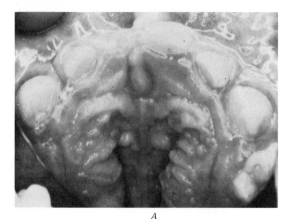

A

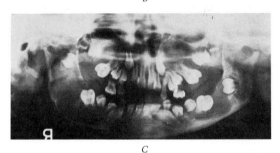

B

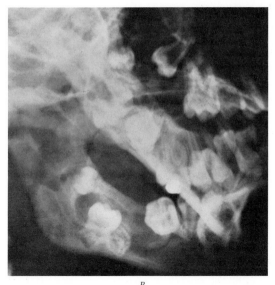

C

Figure 96-3. (*A*). Widened alveolar processes. (*Courtesy of Maj. J. Fay, U.S. Army.*) (*B*). Note distoangular mandibular first molar with dilaceration of distal root, cystic bone destruction around first and second mandibular molars, partially inverted mandibular third molars in ramus, and clearly discernible cleft in mandibular notch. Condyle is hypoplastic. (*From H. M. Worth*, Oral Surg. **22**:21, 1966.) (*C*). More extensive alterations in nine-year-old male with Hurler syndrome. (*From M. A. Germann*, Dtsch. Zahn Mund Kieferheilkd. **59**:59, 1972.)

plastic, resulting in spacing of the teeth. Some patients exhibit hyperplastic gingivitis, because of poor oral hygiene and mouth breathing. Rarely, there is true hyperplastic gingiva with eruption cysts (8). Histochemical study of the gingiva has demonstrated metachromatic cells (7).

The mandible is short and broad, with wide bigonial distance (18). The rami are short and narrow, and the condyle is replaced by a flat inclined surface or cup-shaped excavation. The mandibular notch is irregular or cleft (Fig. 96-3*B*). The temporomandibular joint may exhibit limited motion.

DIFFERENTIAL DIAGNOSIS
The reader is referred to Table 96-1.

LABORATORY AIDS
Histochemical evidence of AMPS storage is found in peripheral leukocytes, bone marrow cells, and in cultured fibroblasts (2, 3). Abnormal amounts of AMPS, most notably dermatan sul-

fate and heparan sulfate, are excreted in the urine. Patients with MPS I-H excrete about twice as much dermatan sulfate as heparan sulfate. Excessive storage of ^{35}S-labeled AMPS is found in cultured fibroblasts. The abnormal intracellular AMPS storage can be corrected by the addition to the culture medium of corrective proteins secreted by normal (non-Hurler) fibroblasts. The corrective proteins have α-L-iduronidase activity and have been isolated from various sources, including human urine (15, 16). Antenatal diagnosis has been described (6).

Several rapid tests have been devised for screening, the most popular of which are the toluidine blue spot test and the gross albumin turbidity test, the latter being far more accurate (4).

MUCOPOLYSACCHARIDOSIS I-S (SCHEIE SYNDROME)

Sibs with mucopolysaccharidosis I-S (MPS V in McKusick's original classification) were described in 1962 by Scheie et al. (3). Patients known in the older European literature as having "late Hurler disease" may have had the same condition (4, 5).

The disease is rarely recognized in childhood. It is characterized by (a) moderately short stature, (b) corneal opacities, (c) clawhands, and (d) biochemical evidence of increased intracellular storage of acid mucopolysaccharides (AMPS) and their excessive urinary excretion.

The disorder is inherited as an autosomal recessive trait. Abnormal intracellular accumulation of AMPS is caused by defective intralysosomal degradation of these substances. The degradation defect is the result of deficient activity of α-L-iduronidase, the same enzyme responsible for the changes in the Hurler syndrome (1). Mucopolysaccharidoses I-H and I-S are probably caused by allelic mutations. The milder clinical changes in MPS I-S (compared to MPS I-H) are best explained by some residual activity of α-L-iduronidase. Later manifestation of the enzyme defect in the former condition is a less likely explanation.

The frequency of the disorder has been estimated at 1 : 500,000 births (2).

SYSTEMIC MANIFESTATIONS

Facies. No major abnormalities are noted in children. In adults, the face is relatively characteristic, but not Hurler-like. It is broad with increased midfacial height and with mandibular prognathism. In most cases, the corners of the mouth are turned downward. Macroglossia may be present. Occasionally, the nose is broad and the nares are wide. Corneal clouding starts in early life, being initially peripheral but by the third or fourth decade severely curtailing vision (Fig. 96-4).

Skeletal system. Patients are moderately short, stocky, and muscular. The neck is short. In some, the trunk is relatively shorter than the extremities. Hands and feet are broad and short,

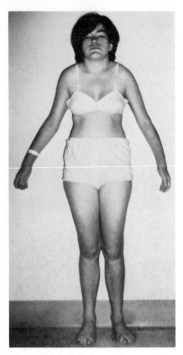

Figure 96-4. *Scheie syndrome.* Fifteen-year-old patient with MPS I-S. Round face, down-turned corners of mouth, relatively coarse facial features. (*Courtesy of R. L. Summitt, Nashville, Tenn.*)

and fingers and toes are fixed in a clawlike position (Fig. 96-5). The range of mobility is limited in all joints. Genu valgum is common.

The most prominent roentgenographic changes are small carpal bones and claw deformity of the fingers. Cystic changes are frequent in the carpals and metacarpals. The carpal tunnel syndrome is common. In addition, there are widened ribs and sometimes mild hypoplasia of the basilar portion of the iliac bones.

Other findings. Intelligence is usually normal. Liver and spleen may be enlarged. Inguinal and/or umbilical hernias are frequently present. Most adult patients show signs of aortic valve involvement.

Oral manifestations. None has been described in this disorder. However, to the best of our knowledge, no special study of the jaws or teeth has been made.

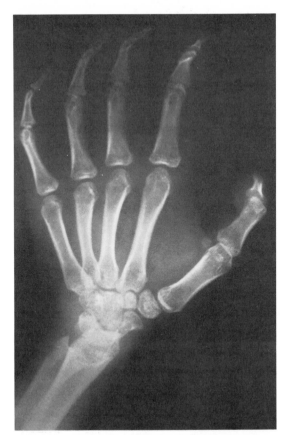

Figure 96-5. Same patient as in Fig. 96-4. Clawing deformities of fingers, small carpal bones with reduced carpal space.

DIFFERENTIAL DIAGNOSIS

See Table 96-1. Mucolipidosis III should be excluded, since the body habitus of patients with this condition is generally identical to that in MPS I-S. However, in ML III the AMPS excretion is normal. There is more severe mental retardation in ML III, and the cornea is clear in the latter disorder. McKusick (2) described patients with the Hurler-Scheie compound, a disorder having an intermediate phenotype.

MUCOPOLYSACCHARIDOSIS II (HUNTER SYNDROME)

The first patients manifesting the X-linked form of MPS were reported by Hunter (5) in 1917. These two brothers were mildly affected at ages

eight and ten years, respectively, with clear corneas and apparently normal intelligence. Although they died at eleven and sixteen years, they probably suffered from the mild type (A) of the disease, which is compatible with survival to adulthood (10). In the severe type (B) one finds rapid psychomotor deterioration and progression of physical deformities after the third year of life, with death usually occurring between four and fourteen years of age (7, 11).

The frequency of Hunter syndrome has been estimated to be higher than that of MPS I-H (8). However, empirical figures are in the range of 0.66 per 100,000 births (8).

Both forms of MPS II are caused by the hemizygous state of a mutant gene located on the X chromosome (3). The mild and severe forms are probably the result of allelic mutations (9). The enzyme defect responsible for the defective intralysosomal degradation of the AMPS has

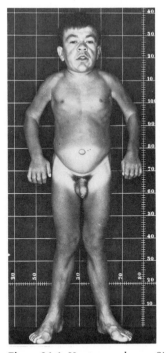

Figure 96-6. *Hunter syndrome.* Sixteen-year-old male with mild (type A) MPS II. Mild coarseness of facies with broad face, depressed nasal bridge, joint contractures, genu valgum. He has mixed hearing loss and normal intelligence. (*From U. N. Wiesmann and S. Rampini,* Helv. Paediatr. Acta **29**:73, 1974.)

been identified as deficiency of sulfoiduronate sulfatase activity (1) in both the mild and severe forms (12). Detection of heterozygotes may be carried out on skin fibroblasts (1a).

SYSTEMIC MANIFESTATIONS

Facies. The head is gross, all measurements being enlarged. The facies tends to develop more slowly and usually is less striking in patients with the mild type than in the severe form (10) (Figs. 96-6, 96-7). The facies of the MPS II patient is different from that of the MPS I patient, even in the fully developed disease. While all Hurler facies are very similar to one another, the facies of any Hunter patient bears a coarse resemblance to the facies of his family members (6).

Skeletal system. The neck is short, the chest is broad, and the abdomen protudes with umbilical hernias. Moderate thoracolumbar kyphosis may be present. The trunk is relatively shorter than the extremities. Joint mobility is restricted, with

clawlike deformities of the fingers. The gait is stiff, with the trunk bent forward. Adults with the mild type (A) reach a height ranging between 120 to 140 cm.

Roentgenographic changes are qualitatively similar to but quantitatively less pronounced than in MPS I-H when compared at identical ages (8).

General body configuration. There is shortness of stature only from about three years of age. Some patients are not dwarfed until five or six years of age. Hunter patients grow faster than normal children during the first 2 to 3 years of life. Average final height of MPS II-B patients is between 105 and 115 cm. At three years of age, few children with the Hunter syndrome are below the 3d percentile, while Hurler patients are (see MPS I-H).

Other findings. Intelligence is only slightly impaired in the mild form. In the the severe type,

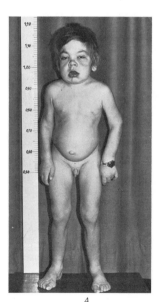
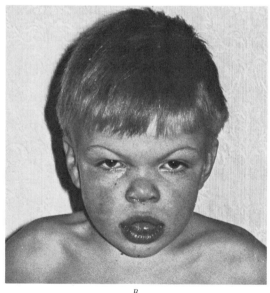

A   *B*

Figure 96-7. (*A*). Thirteen-year-old patient with severe (type B) MPS II. Growth retardation is evident. Abundant and coarse scalp hair, coarse facies, depressed nasal bridge, open mouth provide characteristic phenotype. (*B*). Ten-year-old with severe form of Hunter syndrome. Compare facies with that seen in Fig. 96-7A. (*From E. Passarge et al., Dtsch. Med. Wochenschr.* **99:**144, 1974.)

there is progressive loss of intellectual function after the age of two to three years. It can be seen in retrospect that intellectual function of these patients has never been normal. At three years of age, patients may be brought to a physician because of lack of speech. The patient becomes restless, hyperactive, and destructive (11). Later, muscle tone increases, muscle reflexes become hyperactive, and, within a few years, the patient is bedridden, with flexion contractures and loss of environmental contact. Terminal convulsions are common.

In both forms of the disease, hearing loss is present in about 50 percent of the cases. It is often of the mixed type but may be predominantly conductive or sensorineural. Hepatosplenomegaly, inguinal and/or umbilical hernia, and cardiovascular defects are often found. Skin changes, present in a minority of patients, consist of hard, nontender, irregularly shaped papules varying in size from a few millimeters to a centimeter in diameter located over the posterior upper thorax or arms (10).

Oral manifestations. The teeth are widely spaced. The tongue is enlarged, especially after five years of age. The same bony alterations found in the Hurler syndrome are also found in the severe form of the Hunter syndrome.

DIFFERENTIAL DIAGNOSIS
See Table 96-1.

LABORATORY FINDINGS
Alder-Reilly granulations may be present in peripheral granulocytes and bone marrow cells. Lymphocytes show metachromatic granules within vacuoles following toluidine blue staining. In contrast to patients with MPS I-H, those with MPS II excrete equal amounts of heparan sulfate and dermatan sulfate in the urine. There is abnormal intracellular accumulation of ^{35}S-labeled AMPS in cultured skin fibroblasts (3, 4).

Metachromatic bodies have been demonstrated in fibroblasts, both in affected male hemizygotes and in female heterozygotes. They have been studied ultrastructurally (2).

MUCOPOLYSACCHARIDOSIS III (SANFILIPPO SYNDROME)

The identity of MPS III was established in 1958 by Meyer and Grumbach (10) and later by Meyer and Hoffman (11), Harris (5), and Sanfilippo et al. (14). The condition is characterized by severe mental and sometimes neurologic degeneration, and a relatively mild Hurler-like clinical appearance (2). In our experience, MPS III is the most frequent type of mucopolysaccharidosis but this may be a biased sample.

MPS III is caused by defective degradation and subsequent storage of heparan sulfate. Among the enzymes involved in the degradation of heparan sulfate are a specific heparan sulfate-N-sulfatase and an α-glucosaminidase. Either enzyme has been shown to be involved in the pathogenesis of MPS III: in MPS III-A, there is

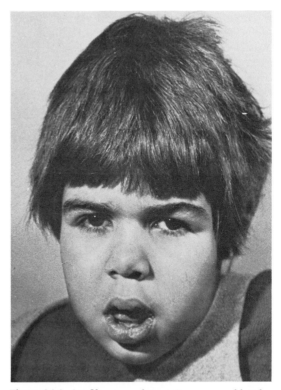

Figure 96-8. *Sanfilippo syndrome.* Seven-year-old girl with MPS III. Note coarse features and thick, abundant scalp hair. (*From E. Passarge et al.,* Dtsch. Med. Wochenschr. **99:**144, 1974.)

deficient activity of heparan sulfate-*N*-sulfatase (8); in MPS III-B, there is deficient activity of *N*-acetyl-α-D-glucosaminidase (4, 12). The two genetically different forms of MPS III cannot be differentiated clinically. They are the result of nonallelic mutations of genes whose defect becomes phenotypically manifest in the homozygous state. Sanfilippo syndrome has been diagnosed in utero (4a).

SYSTEMIC MANIFESTATIONS

Facies. No abnormalities are noted in the young child. Older children may bear some resemblance to patients with the Hurler syndrome, but the facial features never become as strikingly abnormal as in that disorder. About 80 percent of children with MPS III have a dull appearance with a slightly sunken nasal bridge and abundant, coarse scalp hair (13). The latter finding is the most consistent clinical feature even in children without other morphologic alterations. Hairs have been described as triangular in cross section (1). The corneas are clear (Fig. 96-8).

Skeletal system. Height may be slightly reduced or normal. Joint mobility may be mildly restricted in elbows and knees.

Roentgenographically, thickening of the posterior calvaria, sclerotic mastoids, oval-shaped vertebral bodies, and minimal hypoplasia of the supraacetabular portions of the ilia are the most consistent abnormalities (9) (Fig. 96-9). Hands, very abnormal in MPS I-H and MPS II, are normal in MPS III.

Other findings. Behavioral problems, such as restlessness, aggressiveness, diminished attention span, and sleep disturbances, usually become manifest in the second to fifth year of life and are frequently the parents' reason for seeking medical help. Subsequently there is progressive loss of mental and motor skills. Loss of environmental contact is evident prior to a "vegetative" state, with spastic diplegia and death occurring between the ages of ten and twenty years.

Pathologic study of the brain has revealed marked deposition of ceramide polyhexoside and

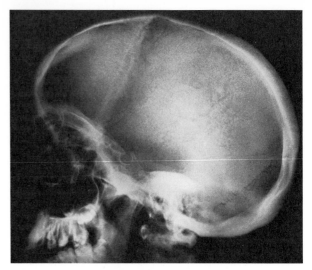

Figure 96-9. Thickening of parietal and occipital portions of cranial vault in eleven-year-old girl with MPS III.

an increase in G_{M_1} ganglioside (2). Hearing loss is frequently suspected but difficult to prove. Hepatomegaly is present in more than 80 percent of patients. Histochemical study of the liver has been carried out (17).

Oral manifestations. There seem to be no remarkable oral manifestations, but tooth abscesses are of major concern during the final stage. The tongue is not large but may protrude late in the disorder.

DIFFERENTIAL DIAGNOSIS
See Table 96-1. The mental deficiency in MPS III is more severe than in MPS II, yet begins later in life than in MPS I-H.

LABORATORY FINDINGS
Clusters of coarse granulations are seen in the cytoplasm of about 35 percent of peripheral lymphocytes and in plasma-cellular and reticulohistiocytic cells of the bone marrow. The granulations are frequently surrounded by areas of diminished stainability. The inclusions stain metachromatically with toluidine blue. Excessive amounts of heparan sulfate are excreted in the urine. There is abnormal intracellular accumulation of ^{35}S-labeled AMPS in cultured fibroblasts.

von Figura et al. (4) described a simplified analysis of the serum of homozygotes and heterozygotes in MPS III-B for decreased levels of *N*-acetyl-α-D-glucosaminidase.

MUCOPOLYSACCHARIDOSIS IV (MORQUIO-BRAILSFORD SYNDROME)

In 1929, Morquio (12) and Brailsford (2) independently reported cases of a disorder characterized by (*a*) marked growth failure, (*b*) progressive spinal deformity, (*c*) short neck, (*d*) pectus carinatum, and (*e*) other skeletal anomalies such as gena valga and pes planus.

The affected child appears normal at birth, but usually by the time he is two years old, growth is stunted.

The disorder is transmitted as an autosomal recessive trait (5, 11, 16). Its frequency has been estimated to be about 1 per 40,000 births (11).

Matalon et al. (9) have discovered a deficiency of chondroitin-6-sulfate *N*-acetyl-glucosamine-4-sulfate sulfatase.

SYSTEMIC MANIFESTATIONS

Facies. The facies is not specific, but the lower half of the face is often outstanding because of shortness and hyperextension of the neck.

Musculoskeletal system. There is reduced height because of shortened neck and trunk and, to a lesser extent, shortened extremities. Adult height rarely exceeds 100 cm (range 80 to 120 cm). The head is essentially normal, but mild scaphocephaly may be present because of premature closure of sutures. The head seems to rest directly on the shoulders. The neck is greatly shortened, with exaggerated cervical curvature and restricted movement. The thorax, after the second year of life, exhibits marked kyphosis or

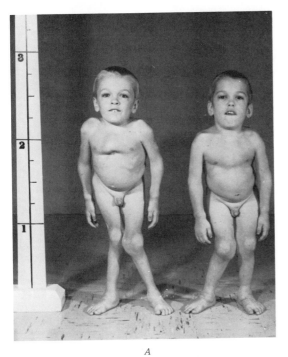
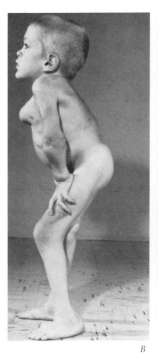
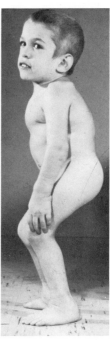

A
B

Figure 96-10. *Morquio syndrome* (MPS IV). (*A, B*). Brothers, aged ten and one-half and nine and one-half, with dwarfism, kyphosis, genu valgum, flexed knees, abnormally short neck, sternal protrusion, and large joints. (*From H. Zellweger et al., J. Pediatr.* **59:**549, 1961.)

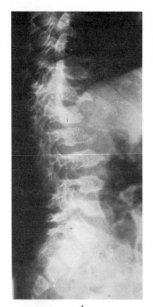

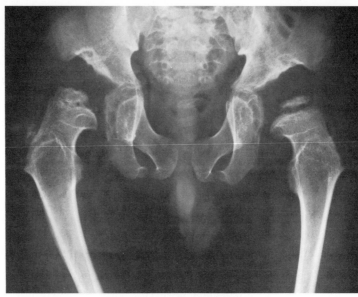

A

B

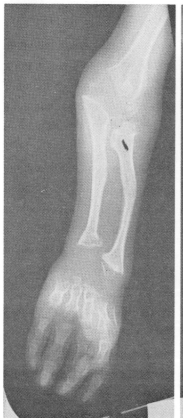

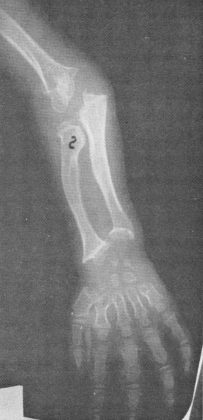

C

Figure 96-11. MPS IV syndrome. (*A*). Platyspondyly of thoracolumbar vertebras. (*B*). Deficiently ossified acetabula, dysplasia of femoral heads, and coxa valga. (*C*). Long bones of upper extremity are more severely involved than those of lower extremity. The humerus, radius, ulna, and metacarpals are short, coarse, curved, and irregularly tubulated, with irregular epiphyseal plates. Also note deficiency of carpal ossification centers. (*From H. Zellweger et al.*, J. Pediatr. **59**:549, 1961.)

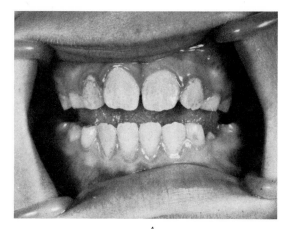

A

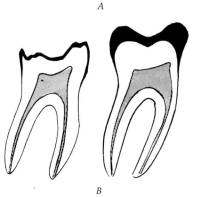

B

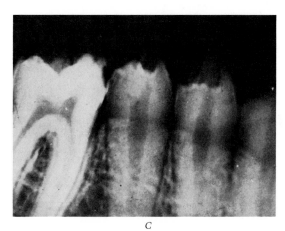

C

Figure 96-12. (*A*). Hypoplasia of enamel in MPS IV. (*B*). Diagram of lower molar showing reduced thickness of enamel layer in affected tooth (left) compared with corresponding tooth in normal sibling. (*From S. M. Garn and V. O. Hurme*, Br. Dent. J. **93**:210, 1952.) (*C*). Dental roentgenogram showing reduced enamel thickness. (*From S. M. Garn and V. O. Hurme*, Br. Dent. J. **93**:210, 1952.)

kyphoscoliosis, with general flattening of vertebras and a characteristic pectus carinatum, the sternum extending almost horizontally from its clavicular junction, then angling downward in midsection. The lumbar region of the spine frequently exhibits a gibbuslike kyphosis or, less often, lordosis in the region of the first lumbar vertebra (Fig. 96-10*A*, *B*). Spinal cord compression may occur in the upper cervical segment as a complication from either atlantoaxial dislocation or subluxation at the thoracolumbar gibbus (1), which may result in death.

Extremities appear disproportionately long. There may be excessive joint mobility, and the wrists are usually enlarged. Genu valgum, thickened knee joints, and pes planus are nearly constant findings (Fig. 96-10*A*, *B*). Stance is semicrouching. Usually there is prominent potbelly.

Roentgenographically, one finds generalized platyspondyly with hypoplasia of the last thoracic and first lumbar vertebras, coxa valga, flared ilia, and progressive femoral head flattening and fragmentation. In the young child, the vertebral bodies are ovoid and the superior acetabula are deficiently ossified. The odontoid process is hypoplastic or absent. The bases of the second to fifth metacarpals are conical, but their shafts are normally constricted (7) (Fig. 96-11*A–C*). The distal ends of the radius and ulna are inclined toward each other. All the bones become markedly osteoporotic.

Other findings. The corneas become slowly but diffusely opacified in the form of a filmy haze. This is rarely obvious to the unaided eye before the tenth year of life (16, 18). Progressive deafness usually begins in adolescence.

Intelligence is nearly always normal. Aortic regurgitation has been reported (11, 14).

Oral manifestations. Both the deciduous and permanent teeth have dull, gray crowns with pitted enamel which is very thin and has a tendency to flake off, causing small diastemas between the teeth. The cusps are small, flattened, and poorly formed, and caries is frequent (4, 8, 15) (Fig. 96-12*A–C*). The mandibular condyles may be flat or concave.

DIFFERENTIAL DIAGNOSIS

Practically all types of short-spine dwarfism

have been confused with Morquio syndrome. In contrast to Morquio syndrome, *achondroplasia* is usually apparent at birth, with skeletal changes entirely different from those in the Morquio syndrome. *Hurler syndrome* has roentgenographic similarities to Morquio syndrome during the first few years of life, but mentality is reduced and the gross physical appearance is strikingly characteristic. Although corneal clouding and deafness were thought to be distinguishing factors, they are also features of Morquio syndrome (18). Multiple epiphyseal dysplasia, a dominantly inherited disorder (3), may also simulate Morquio syndrome, but spinal involvement, if present, is of lesser degree.

Diastrophic dwarfism is characterized by progressive kyphoscoliosis, but normal vertebral body height, micromelia, clubfoot, widening of metaphyses and epiphyses of long bones, some limitation of joint motion, and thickened pinnas easily distinguish the conditions.

Some patients with clinical Morquio syndrome do not excrete keratan sulfate (6, 13).

Children with metatropic dwarfism at first exhibit a long-trunked and later a short-trunked dwarfism. The disorder is characterized by progressive kyphoscoliosis and anisospondyly without hypoplasia of the last thoracic and first lumbar vertebral bodies.

Congenital spondyloepiphyseal dysplasia, inherited as a dominant trait, is a short-trunk dwarfism. There is platyspondyly but no or little involvement of the hands and feet, no corneal clouding, and no keratansulfaturia. Myopia is often severe.

Rickets and hypophosphatasia should also be considered.

Individuals with Dyggve-Melchior-Clausen syndrome somewhat resemble those with Morquio disease in skeletal alterations but do not have corneal clouding, do not excrete keratan sulfate in the urine, and are mentally retarded (17). They do not have enamel deficiency. Pointing of the proximal metacarpals does not occur. Neither is there hypoplasia of the odontoid process nor of the inferior thoracic or lumbar vetebras. The iliac crest has a lacy border. The disorder is inherited as an autosomal recessive trait. Since several patients have had normal intelligence, this disorder may have genetic heterogeneity.

Congenital dysplasia of the odontoid process with atlantoaxial dislocation can be seen in a number of disorders: *Morquio syndrome, Aarskog syndrome,* Dyggve-Melchior-Clausen syndrome, pseudoachondroplasia, *cartilage-hair hypoplasia, congenital spondyloepiphyseal dysplasia,* excess and spondylometaphyseal dysplasia (S. E. Kopits, personal communication, 1972).

LABORATORY AIDS
Marked excretion of keratan sulfate and chondroitin sulfate A in the urine, in childhood, is a constant feature (11). It slowly decreases, reaching normal levels in adults. Increased amounts of chondroitin sulfate C are also excreted. Abnormal granules may be detected in peripheral neutrophilic granulocytes. Ultrastructural studies of epiphyseal plates have been described (10).

MUCOPOLYSACCHARIDOSIS VI (MAROTEAUX-LAMY SYNDROME)

In 1963, Maroteaux and Lamy (3) described a patient with a moderately severe Hurler-like phenotype but normal intelligence and high urinary excretion of dermatan sulfate. The nature of MPS VI was definitely established in 1972 by Barton and Neufeld (1), who discovered a protein which specifically corrects the biochemical defect in Maroteaux-Lamy fibroblasts.

Possibly there exist two forms of mucopolysaccharidosis VI: a mild type (A) and a severe type (B) (1a, 5, 6). Children with type A develop reasonably well until the age of about six years, when small stature and spinal deformities are noted. Hurler-like changes gradually become apparent. The patients usually survive to adulthood. In patients with type B, morphologic changes are noted in early childhood and the disease progresses more rapidly to a state of severe disability with strikingly short stature, marked facial and skeletal abnormalities, severely impaired vision and hearing, and prominent cardiac defects which frequently lead to death in adolescence.

MPS VI is an autosomal recessive condition, the two types possibly being the result of allelic mutations. The clinical and biochemical defects are caused by abnormal intracellular accumula-

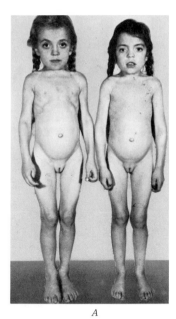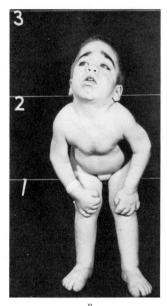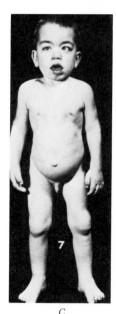

A   *B*   *C*

Figure 96-13. *Maroteaux-Lamy syndrome.* (*A*). Seven- and six-year-old patients with mild form of MPS VI. (*Courtesy of H. R. Wiedemann, Kiel, Germany.*) (*B*). Seven-year-old male with severe form. (*Courtesy of L. Langer, Minneapolis.*) (*C*). Seven-year-old patient with severe form. (*From D. A. Stumpf et al., Am. J. Dis. Child.* **126:**747, 1973.)

tion of AMPS, mostly dermatan sulfate, in mesenchymal cells and, secondarily, in parenchymal cells of internal organs, such as the liver. The basic enzyme defect responsible for the defective degradation of AMPS has been shown to be a deficiency of arylsulfatase B (7).

SYSTEMIC MANIFESTATIONS

Facies. A prominent forehead may be noted at birth. The facies, similar to that in Hurler syndrome, with apparent hypertelorism, depressed nasal bridge, full cheeks and lips, relatively broad jaws, large cranium, and abundant eyebrows and scalp hair, becomes evident about the sixth year of life. Corneal opacities are regularly present (2, 6) (Fig. 96-13*A*, *B*).

Musculoskeletal system. Patients are short. The chest is deformed, with a prominent sternum. Multiple joint contractures and clawhand deformity begin after the first year of life. The roentgenographic changes in severe type B are similar to those of MPS I-H. Ossification of the

superior portion of the femoral capital epiphysis may be markedly defective. In mild type A, there are cranial changes, wide ribs, and pelvic dysplasia but few changes in spine and tubular bones (5) (Fig. 96-14*A*, *B*). Hernias are common.

Other findings. Hepatomegaly is almost invariably present. The spleen is enlarged in about half the cases. Cardiovascular involvement is common, with valvular incompetence and narrowing of the coronary and other arteries.

Hearing defects, both conductive and sensorineural, may be detected audiometrically. Mentation is normal, but impaired vision and hearing, restricted mobility, and secondary psychologic reaction may impede intellectual performance (5, 6).

Oral manifestations. The tongue becomes large as soon as the clinical picture is fully developed. The teeth are frequently widely spaced. Eruption of permanent molar teeth is retarded, and some of them may be deeply buried and angulated in the mandible, surmounted by radiolucent bony

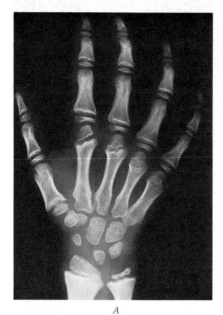

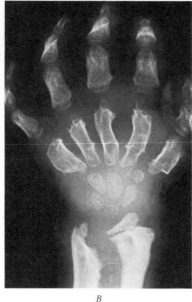

A   *B*

Figure 96-14. (*A*). Mild involvement of short tubular bones in eleven-year-old with MPS VI. (*B*). Severe shortening and distortion of short tubular bones with marked epiphyseal and metaphyseal dysplasia in fourteen-year-old.

defects that represent the accumulation of dermatan sulfate in hyperplastic follicles as in MPS I-H and in MPS II-B.

DIFFERENTIAL DIAGNOSIS
See Table 96-1.

LABORATORY FINDINGS
There is an abundance of coarse, dense inclusions in granulocytes, monocytes, and a large proportion of lymphocytes in peripheral blood smears. Bone marrow preparations exhibit coarse inclusions in reticulohistiocytes, granulocytes, and their precursors. Large quantities of dermatan sulfate are excreted in the urine, but the level decreases with age. Abnormal amounts of ^{35}S-labeled MPS are stored in cultured fibroblasts (1).

MUCOPOLYSACCHARIDOSIS VII (β-GLUCURONIDASE DEFICIENCY)

Beta-glucuronidase deficiency was described by Sly et al. (6) in 1973. A few additional examples have been reported (1, 3). Clinically, the disorder appears to be characterized by (*a*) short stature,

(*b*) hepatosplenomegaly, (*c*) progressive skeletal deformities, and (*d*) progressive mental retardation after the age of two years.

There is virtual absence of β-glucuronidase activity in cultured fibroblasts and in white blood cells (5). Addition of β-glucuronidase to the culture medium corrects the metabolic defect. Intermediate β-glucuronidase activity is found in heterozygotes (6). The absence of β-glucuronidase explains the intracellular accumulation of AMPS-containing glucuronic acid in β linkage.

SYSTEMIC MANIFESTATIONS

Facies. There are moderate Hurler-like changes, with hypertelorism, depressed nasal bridge, prominent alveolar processes, and anteverted nostrils. The corneas appear clear (Fig. 96-15 *A*, *B*).

Skeletal system. Short stature becomes apparent in the second year of life, height falling below the 3d percentile. The head is large, with frontal prominence and premature closure of the sagittal and lambdoidal sutures. Pectus carinatum and thoracolumbar gibbus, already noted in infancy, increase with age (Fig. 96-15A, B). Talipes has also been noted.

Roentgenographically, there are moderately severe changes of dysostosis multiplex with premature closure of cranial sutures, J-shaped sella, oar-shaped ribs, hooklike deformities of the lower thoracic and upper lumbar vertebras, underdevelopment of the basilar portions of the ilia, aseptic necrosis of the femoral heads, shortening of tubular bones, and proximal pointing of metacarpals II through V.

Other findings. Hepatosplenomegaly, inguinal and umbilical hernias, lax skin, and developmental retardation are present after the age of two years. Recurrent pulmonary infections are common.

Oral manifestations. Widened alveolar ridges have been described.

DIFFERENTIAL DIAGNOSIS

Danes and Degnan (2) reported an adult female with β-glucuronidase deficiency who manifested few of the stigmata seen in the infants described above (other than recurrent pulmonary infection and metachromatic granulations in leukocytes).

Whether this genetic heterogeneity reflects allelism is not known.

LABORATORY FINDINGS

Coarse metachromatic inclusions (Alder-Reilly bodies) are present in peripheral granulocytes. Similar inclusions are found in granulocytes and their precursors in bone marrow. There is absence of β-glucuronidase in leukocytes and cultured skin fibroblasts. Cultured fibroblasts accumulate excessive amounts of ^{35}S-labeled MPS. Glaser and Sly (4) described a convenient assay for serum β-glucuronidase.

MISCELLANEOUS MUCOPOLYSACCHARIDOSES

Small amounts of chondroitin 4- and 6-sulfate are normally excreted in the urine. There have been several patients, however, with an excessive output of chondroitin sulfate A and storage of AMPS in leukocytes, bone marrow, and liver (2, 4, 6). Inheritance is autosomal recessive.

There seems to be a common phenotype of essentially normal intelligence, peripheral corneal opacities, short stature, joint contractures,

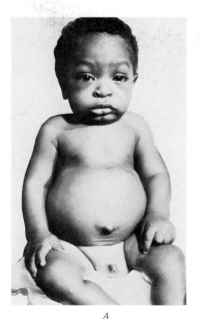
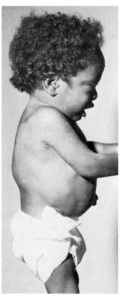

A *B*

Figure 96-15. (*A, B*). *Beta-glucuronidase deficiency.* Coarse facies, potbelly, gibbus. (*From W. S. Sly et al., J. Pediatr.* **82**:249, 1973.)

Table 96-2. Mucolipidoses and related disorders

Name	Storage substance	Enzyme defect
G_{M_1} gangliosidosis, Type 1	G_{M_1} ganglioside and keratan sulfate	β-galactosidases A, B, C
G_{M_1} gangliosidosis, Type 2	G_{M_1} ganglioside and keratan sulfate	β-galactosidases B, C
Fucosidosis	Fucose-containing glycosphingolipid	α-fucosidase
Mucosulfatidosis	Sulfatide and acid mucopolysaccharides	Arylsulfatases A, B, C
Aspartylglucosaminuria	Glycoprotein	Aspartylglucosamine amidohydrolase
Mannosidosis	Glycoprotein	α-mannosidase A, B
Mucolipidosis I	Unknown	Unknown
Mucolipidosis II	Various glycolipids and AMPS	Multiple lysosomal enzymes
Mucolipidosis III	Unknown	Multiple lysosomal enzymes

hepatomegaly, dysostosis multiplex, and survival to adulthood. The facies is normal or somewhat impish.

Excessive chondroitin-4-sulfate and -6-sulfate was reported by Onisawa et al. (1). Their patient, the product of second cousins, had coarse facies, saddle nose, mental retardation, inguinal hernias, joint contractures, dislocated hips, scoliosis, pectus carinatum, and the roentgenographic picture of Morquio syndrome.

Schimke et al. (3) described a child with chondroitin-6-sulfate mucopolysaccharidosis who exhibited growth retardation, lymphopenia, defective cellular immunity, and nephrotic syndrome.

The child described by Suschke and Kunze (5) likely has the Murray-Puretić-Drescher syndrome. Excessive amounts of hyaluronic acid and dermatan sulfate were found in the urine. This is surely an important observation and merits biochemical study of additional patients with this syndrome.

MUCOLIPIDOSES

The term "mucolipidoses" has been proposed for a group of disorders which exhibit clinical and skeletal signs of the mucopolysaccharidoses but differ from them by the normal urinary excretion of uronic acid–containing AMPS (with the exception of mucosulfatidosis) and by the presence of clinical features usually seen in the sphingolipidoses (10). The merit of the term "mucolipidosis" is one of convenience. It is bound to be of temporary usage until the genetic defects of the several entities within the group become known.

This is a heterogeneous group of diseases which includes primary disorders of sphingolipid and mucopolysaccharide metabolism, of glycosphingolipid metabolism, glycoprotein metabolism, and a number of conditions in which the nature of the metabolic defect is not known.

Vacuolated lymphocytes, foam cells in bone marrow and other organs, cherry-red macular spots, and metachromatic myelin degeneration of peripheral nerves may be found in some of the entities.

They are summarized in Table 96-2.

G_{M_1} GANGLIOSIDOSIS, TYPE 1

G_{M_1} gangliosidosis is caused by generalized accumulation of G_{M_1} ganglioside and visceral and mesenchymal storage of a keratan sulfate-like AMPS. The disease was recognized in 1964 by Landing et al. (2).

The condition is manifest at or shortly after

birth. In its full expression, it is characterized by progressive cerebral deterioration, with death usually occurring before the age of two years, and by other clinical and roentgenographic features resembling either I-cell disease or MPS I-H.

G$_{M_1}$ gangliosidosis is the consequence of the homozygous state of the mutant gene which produces a functionally deficient β-galactosidase. Electrophoretic data indicate that all three different β-galactosidase isoenzymes designated as A, B, and C are severely deficient (4). The lack of β-galactosidase activity results in the abnormal intracellular accumulation of its substrates, G$_{M_1}$ ganglioside and keratan sulfate.

SYSTEMIC MANIFESTATIONS

Facies. The facial features are coarse at birth, in contrast to the face in MPS I-H, which is normal for the first 6 months of life. In particular, the nasal bridge is depressed, the philtrum is promi-

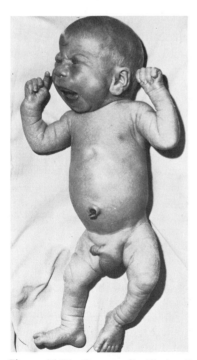

Figure 96-16. G$_{M_1}$ *gangliosidosis.* Coarse facial features, widened alveolar processes, large ears, wrist and ankle deformities were apparent at two weeks of age. (*From C. R. Scott et al.,* J. Pediatr. **71**:357, 1967.)

nent, the cheeks are full, and the eyelids puffy. In mild cases, these facial changes are present only in later infancy. Corneal opacities are rarely found, but cherry-red macular spots are detected in a large number of patients (Fig. 96-16).

Skeletal system. Kyphoscoliosis is an early finding. The hands are short and stubby. There are multiple flexion contractures of the joints.

The roentgenographic changes are those of dysostosis multiplex in an infant. They appear earlier and are more severe than in MPS I-H. The ribs are wide, and the vertebral bodies are short in their anteroposterior diameter, with convex end plates and hook-shaped deformities at the thoracolumbar junction.

The basilar portions of the ilia are hypoplastic. In young infants, there is periosteal cloaking of the shafts of long tubular bones. This is not observed in MPS I-H, but is a well-known early finding in patients with ML II or I-cell disease. In older infants and in young children, the shafts of the long bones are overtubulated, with irregular contours. The short tubular bones appear swollen, with proximal pointing of the second to fourth metacarpals. Bone trabeculation is coarse (1).

Other findings. Hepatosplenomegaly is present in about 80 percent of cases. There is marked psychomotor retardation. After the first year of life, rapid cerebral deterioration occurs, with loss of environmental contact, inability to swallow, tonic-clonic seizures, and blindness.

Oral manifestations. The tongue and alveolar processes are enlarged (2, 6). There is inadequate documentation but some evidence of accumulation of storage material about unerupted first permanent molar teeth (J. Dorst, personal communication, 1972).

DIFFERENTIAL DIAGNOSIS

Cherry-red macular spots can also be found in Tay-Sachs disease, Sandhoff disease, ML I, metachromatic leukodystrophy, infantile Niemann-Pick disease, Goldberg syndrome, and Farber lipogranulomatosis.

Marked dysostosis multiplex-like skeletal anomalies in an infant are more compatible with G_{M_1} *gangliosidosis* or *mucolipidosis II* than with a mucopolysaccharidosis.

Juvenile G_{M_1} gangliosidosis (G_{M_1} gangliosidosis type 2) is thought to be caused by the absent activity of β-galactosidase isoenzymes B and C with preserved activity of only β-galactosidase A (5). The condition is differentiated from G_{M_1} gangliosidosis type 1 by its later manifestation (usually after the age of six months), absence of Hurler-like dysmorphism, absence of skeletal symptoms, and longer survival (usually beyond the age of two years). The differentiation of generalized G_{M_1} gangliosidosis type 1 from other related disorders is summarized in Table 96-1.

LABORATORY FINDINGS

Between 10 and 80 percent of peripheral lymphocytes are vacuolated. Bone marrow preparations show finely vacuolated histiocytic cells. Urinary excretion of AMPS is normal. The activity of acid β-galactosidase is grossly diminished in tissues and body fluids, including leukocytes, cultured fibroblasts, and urine.

MUCOLIPIDOSIS I
(LIPOMUCOPOLYSACCHARIDOSIS)

Mucolipidosis (ML) I, first described in 1968 (5), is characterized by (a) mild Hurler-like clinical changes, (b) moderate mental retardation, (c) normal mucopolysacchariduria, (d) peculiar bone marrow storage cells, and (e) normal activity of various lysosomal enzymes in fibroblasts and elevated activity in liver cells.

Early development is normal. Psychomotor retardation appears toward the end of the first year of life. Later, Hurler-like clinical deformities become manifest.

Probably ML I is heterogeneous. In type A, there is slow progression of the physical and mental changes without signs of neurologic and macular degeneration. In type B, cherry-red macular spots and slowly progressive neurologic degeneration become manifest after the age of about four years, with progressive muscular hypotrophy and hypotonia, and locomotor ataxia.

Mucolipidosis I is an autosomal recessive disorder. Electron microscopy of liver cells reveals polymorphous inclusions limited by unit membranes. The structure of the inclusions is consistent with mucopolysaccharides and lipids (2). Thin layer chromatography of liver glycolipids reveals a small amount of unidentified material migrating with gangliosides (1). One oft-cited case (3) is really mannosidosis.

SYSTEMIC FINDINGS

Facies. The facial features are similar to those in MPS III, with depressed nasal bridge, full cheeks, and lips but without the severe alterations seen in Hurler disease. The facial deformities are slightly more pronounced in type B than in type A. Corneal opacities are not usually found (Fig. 96-17A, B).

Skeletal findings. In children with type A, no major skeletal deformities are evident clinically. In type B, the trunk is short and the musculature hypotrophic. Physical growth is normal until approximately ten years of age but is slow thereafter. Joint mobility is slightly restricted in older children with both types of ML I.

Roentgenographically, mild changes of dysostosis multiplex similar to those in MPS III are noted (5).

Other findings. Hernias and hepatic and/or splenic enlargement are inconsistently present. In younger children the intelligence quotient ranges between 50 and 70 but deteriorates with advancing age. In type B, there are symptoms and signs of progressive peripheral neuropathy and cherry-red macular spots.

Oral manifestations. Teeth have been stated to be spaced (4).

LABORATORY FINDINGS

Peripheral lymphocytes are vacuolated and contain abnormal granules. In the bone marrow, storage cells are found with a peculiar combination of coarse vacuoles and granules. Sural nerve biopsy reveals metachromatic myelin degeneration. In cultured fibroblasts, coarse, regularly refringent inclusions were detected, similar to those in ML II but without the clear perinuclear halo seen in the latter condition. The urinary excretion of AMPS is normal. In fibroblasts and

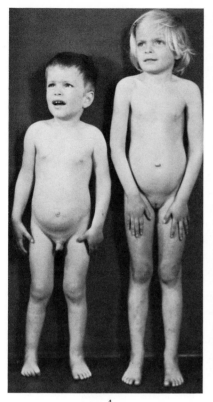
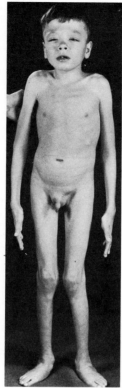

Figure 96-17. *Mucolipidosis I. (A).* Four- and eight-year-old sibs with ML I-A. Round face with coarse features, depressed nasal bridge, relatively large cranium in boy. Girl appears normal. *(B).* Ten-year-old boy with ML I-B. Moderately severe Hurler-like facies, short trunk, muscular hypotrophy. *(Courtesy of H. R. Wiedemann, Kiel, Germany.)*

liver tissue, the activity of numerous lysosomal enzymes, including β-galactosidase, has been found to be normal or increased.

DIFFERENTIAL DIAGNOSIS
See Table 96-1.

MUCOLIPIDOSIS II (I-CELL DISEASE)

Mucolipidosis (ML) II, originally described in 1967 (1a, 5), is characterized by (a) severe psychomotor retardation, (b) marked shortness of stature, (c) facial features reminiscent of MPS I-H, (d) impressive gingival enlargement, (e) slowly progressive course, and (f) death from heart failure usually in early childhood (1). Gilbert et al. (3) have suggested genetic heterogeneity.

Important negative signs and symptoms are absent splenomegaly, equivocal or absent corneal cloudiness, and normal urinary excretion of AMPS (6–8, 10, 12).

Mucolipidosis II is an autosomal recessive condition. It has received the name of (I)nclusion cell disease, because of the numerous granular inclusions in the cytoplasm of all fibroblasts observed under phase contrast microscopy (1a, 5). The inclusions are probably altered lysosomes, according to evidence based on electron microscopic studies on fibroblasts and several visceral organs (2, 4, 12). In cultured fibroblasts, the activity of several lysosomal enzymes is either absent or considerably decreased. The same enzymes have a normal activity in fibroblast cultures derived from the parents of patients (9). Similar multiple enzyme deficiencies have not been found in the brain or in visceral organs. Only β-D-galactosidase has a moderately reduced activity in brain, liver, and kidney (9). No convincing evidence of important storage of either a

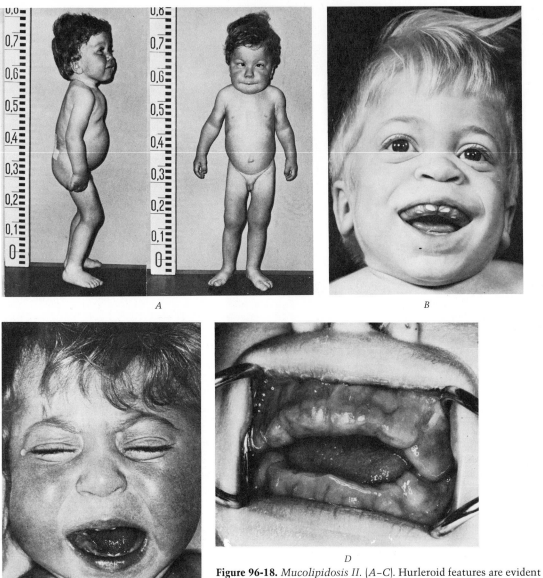

A

B

C

D

Figure 96-18. *Mucolipidosis II. (A–C). Hurleroid features are evident in early infancy. (A, from U. Wiesmann et al., Acta Paediatr. Scand. **63**:9, 1974; B, from C. Scott, Baltimore, Md.; C, from N. S. Gordon, Postgrad. Med. J. **49**:359, 1973.) (D). Marked thickening of gingiva, open anterior bite. (From D. Galili et al., Oral Surg. **37**:533, 1974.)*

specific lipid or mucopolysaccharide has been presented so far.

The medium of cultured I cells and the serum of patients show an increased activity of several acid hydrolases. This phenomenon has been explained by lysosomal leakage (14). Another hypothesis points to an abnormality of intracellular cooperation in I cells due to improperly processed enzyme molecules which would lack sufficient specificity for their uptake from the extracellular compartment into the lysosomes (3a). However, the basic defect of I-cell disease remains unknown.

SYSTEMIC MANIFESTATIONS

At birth there are muscular hypotonia, "orthopedic" symptoms, inguinal hernias in males, and sometimes tight and thickened skin. During the first year, there is a history of recurrent respiratory infections, failure to thrive, and marked lack of psychomotor development. The full clinical picture is reached by one year of age. There is severe shortness of stature. No patient has been taller than 80 cm, and most of them never reach the average height of a one-year-old child. (Note difference with MPS I-H, where excessive growth from six to eighteen months of age has been frequently documented.)

Psychomotor retardation is severe. The patient usually does not accomplish unaided ambulation. The majority of patients never sit upright without support. There are some social responses and early vocalization. This basic level of development is maintained throughout.

Facies. Head circumference remains normal with respect to stature. The facies is reminiscent of that in MPS I-H patients. There are small orbits, puffy eyelids, a slight degree of exophthalmos in most patients, and a pattern of tortuous veins about the orbits and temporal bones [15]. Some patients have exhibited premature lightening of hair color. The supraorbital ridges are inapparent. The cheeks are full and pink, partly because of multiple fine telangiectasias. The lower part of the face is fishlike when viewed in profile, mainly because of enlargement of the gingiva (Fig. 96-18*A, B*).

There is intermittent copious nasal discharge but to a lesser degree than in MPS I-H patients.

In most patients the corneas are clear, but on slit lamp examination all have some degree of corneal opacification.

Musculoskeletal system. There is shortness of the neck and thoracic cage. Umbilical and/or inguinal hernias are common. Considerable restriction of joint mobility, particularly in the shoulders and wrists, is evident. The hands and fingers are stubby and the wrists broadened. Restriction of motion is less impaired in the lower limbs, which appear hypotrophic. Thoracolumbar kyphosis may be present, but is not observed in any patient who can stand upright. The costochondral junctions are knoblike.

Roentgenographically, extensive periosteal cloaking of all long bones is seen in early infancy. This phenomenon is also observed in newborns with G_{M_1} gangliosidosis type 1 and the disorders cannot be differentiated roentgenographically at this stage.

Periosteal bone formation can be observed until four to six months of age. Subsequently, this overgrowth becomes confluent with the underlying cortex and disappears entirely between eight and twelve months of age. From that point "dysostosis multiplex" is observed as in MPS I-H, the bony abnormalities always being more severe in ML II patients at comparable ages. Other differences are minor involvement of calvaria in ML II and minor to moderate degree of diaphyseal widening in long bones, especially of the lower limbs.

Other findings. Hepatomegaly is only minimal to moderate, and splenomegaly apparently does not occur. The parenchyma of the liver is yellow (1, 2).

Oral manifestations. Enlargement of the gingiva and anterior alveolar process is present as early as four months of age. It is slowly progressive. In some patients, it reaches grotesque proportions (1, 2, 6–8, 10) and together with thick tongue (3) prevents proper closure of the mouth (Fig. 96-18*C*). Usually the teeth are deeply buried in the hypertrophied tissue or do not erupt at all. Roentgenographic examination of the teeth reveals that the enamel is quite hypocalcified and that there is accumulation of storage material about the crowns of unerupted first molar teeth.

DIFFERENTIAL DIAGNOSIS
See Table 96-1.

LABORATORY FINDINGS
Peripheral lymphocytes contain large cytoplasmic inclusions (11). The urinary excretion of acid mucopolysaccharides is normal. All cultured fibroblasts contain an abundance of coarse cytoplasmic inclusions with a characteristic inclusion-free perinuclear zone (5).

Several lysosomal acid hydrolases have considerably increased activity (at least twentyfold for some) in the serum of patients (3).

MUCOLIPIDOSIS III

Mucolipidosis (ML) III is characterized by (*a*) mild mental retardation, (*b*) early restriction of joint mobility, (*c*) peculiar bone changes, and (*d*) normal mucopolysacchariduria. Several patients have been reported (1–5). Only sparse histochemical data are available, but the presence of Hurler-like signs and vacuolated bone marrow cells justifies the inclusion of this disease among the mucolipidoses.

The disorder is inherited as an autosomal recessive trait.

SYSTEMIC MANIFESTATIONS

After the second year of life, restricted joint mobility, small stature, short neck, scoliosis, and hip dysplasia are noted. Moderate mental retardation (I.Q. 65 to 85) has been present in half the patients (5).

Facies. Facies has been variable, but in most patients there has been some coarsening of features.

Under slit lamp examinations nearly all patients have manifested corneal clouding which clinically is little more than a slight corneal haze (3) (Fig. 96-19*A*).

Musculoskeletal system. Dwarfism, a decreased upper-to-lower segment ratio, and shortened arm span are present in all patients. The joint stiffness which begins in early life progresses slowly until puberty (3).

Premature closure of cranial sutures is a frequent finding, but the skull is normal in shape. The foramen magnum is small.

The clavicles are short and thick, with the midportions bowed superiorly. Vertebral body alterations are quite variable but generally are mild. There is flaring of the iliac wings, with constriction of the iliac bones and prominent anterior superior iliac spines. The acetabulums are shallow with oblique roofs. Progressive destruction of the capital femoral epiphyses is a striking feature in most patients (Fig. 96-19*B*). The changes in the metacarpals may resemble those seen in the Morquio syndrome. The carpal bones are small and irregular, and they ossify late (Fig. 96-19*C*).

DIFFERENTIAL DIAGNOSIS

See Table 96-1.

LABORATORY FINDINGS

Peripheral leukocytes are normal. Vacuolated plasma cells are often found in the bone marrow. Finely granulated intracytoplasmic material with staining characteristics of AMPS has been found in bone marrow cells. Skin fibroblasts exhibit metachromasia and an increased uronic acid content (3). Ultrastructural studies of fibroblasts have shown vacuoles with membranous lamellas, indicating lipid storage (6). Urinary excretion of AMPS is normal. Thomas et al. (7) demonstrated low levels in fibroblasts but high levels in serum of N-acetyl-β-glucosaminidase, β-galactosidase, α-fucosidase, α-mannosidase, and arylsulfatase A, findings similar to those demonstrated in I-cell disease.

FUCOSIDOSIS

Fucosidosis is a disease caused by the abnormal intracellular accumulation of fucose-containing glycosphingolipids (1). It was first described by Durand et al. in 1966 (2) and more clearly limned in subsequent reports (2, 5, 6). Kousseff et al. (4) described genetic heterogeneity of fucosidosis, there being severe and mild forms.

The severe form becomes manifest during later infancy with symptoms of psychomotor retardation. Progressive neurologic deterioration occurs thereafter, with increasing spasticity, tremor, gradual loss of environmental contact, and death after the fourth year of life. The mild form, which is compatible with life—at least, until adolescence—is marked by psychomotor retardation, long tract, cerebellar, and basal ganglia signs, coarse facies, mild spondyloepiphyseal dysplasia, and *angiokeratoma corporis diffusum* (1).

Fucosidosis is an autosomal recessive disorder. The lack of α-fucosidase results in the abnormal intracellular accumulation of a fucose-containing glycosphingolipid with a molar ratio of fucose/galactose/glucose/N-acetyl-glucosamine/ceramide of $1:2:1:1:1$ (1a).

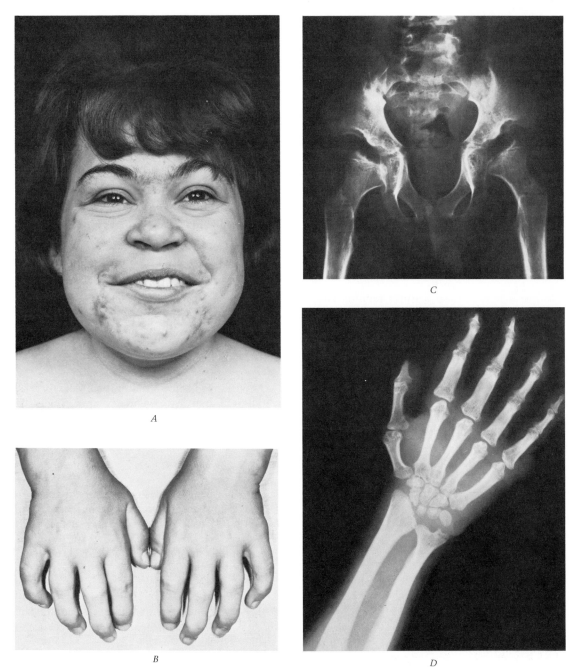

Figure 96-19. *Mucolipidosis III.* (*A*). Patient has had short stature, short neck, restricted joint mobility since early childhood. Facies mildly Hurleroid. (*B*). Fingers cannot be flexed or extended. (*Courtesy of J. Sensenbrenner, Baltimore, Md.*) (*C*). Hypoplastic iliac bodies and femoral heads and necks. (*Courtesy of J. Dorst, Baltimore, Md.*) (*D*). Hand bones coarsely trabeculated. Small proximal carpal bones, irregular distal radius and ulna. (*Courtesy of M. Robinow, Yellow Springs, Ohio.*)

SYSTEMIC MANIFESTATIONS

Facies. The facial features may be coarse, with some resemblance to those of patients with MPS III. The hair, however, is not as coarse. The tongue may be large. The corneas are clear and the fundi unremarkable.

Skeletal system. Clinically, there are no major skeletal alterations. The vertebral bodies are ovoid in lateral projection. There is mild hypoplasia of the supraacetabular portions of the ilia. Bone trabeculation is coarse.

Other findings. The liver is enlarged. Hernias may be present. Recurrent respiratory infections regularly occur.

DIFFERENTIAL DIAGNOSIS

The presence, of clinical features reminiscent of Hurler syndrome in combination with mild skeletal changes of dysostosis multiplex indicates a disturbance in mucopolysaccharide and/or glycoprotein metabolism. It is found in a number of conditions, including MPS III, mucosulfatidosis, *mannosidosis, aspartylglycosaminuria,* and ML I. The differentiation of these disorders frequently requires the use of sophisticated histochemical and biochemical techniques demonstrating the specific storage substances and/or enzyme deficiencies summarized in Table 96-1. Elevated urinary excretion of heparan sulfate is found in MPS III. Excessive urinary AMPS and coarse leukocyte inclusions are present in mucosulfatidosis. Peculiar storage cells are found in bone marrow of patients with ML I. Cherry-red macular spots may be seen in a number of storage diseases [see Mucolipidosis—General References (2)].

LABORATORY FINDINGS

Peripheral lymphocytes are vacuolated. Urinary excretion of AMPS is normal. There is deficient activity of the lysosomal enzyme α-L-fucosidase in all body tissues which have been examined so far, in cultured fibroblasts, white blood cells, serum, and urine (6–8).

MANNOSIDOSIS

Mannosidosis was first characterized in 1967 by Ockerman (4). Autio et al. (1) described several other cases and in personal communication (March 1974) indicated that they had seen adult patients with the disorder. Other authors (2, 3, 5) have reported additional examples.

Inheritance is clearly autosomal recessive.

The children are essentially normal for the first year of life but exhibit a propensity toward recurrent respiratory infections.

SYSTEMIC MANIFESTATIONS

Facies. The coarse facies noted after the first few years of life becomes progressive but not to the degree noted in MPS I nor as early as in ML II. The nasal bridge tends to be low; the forehead and mandible are prominent. The neck is somewhat short (Fig. 96-20).

Central nervous system. There is delayed early motor development, which becomes manifest as clumsy motor function. Speech is delayed. Tendon reflexes are brisk.

Eyes and ears. Wheel-like lens opacities have been noted in several patients (1, 3). Severe high-frequency neural deafness is a common, if not constant, feature (1, 2).

Musculoskeletal system. There is general mild

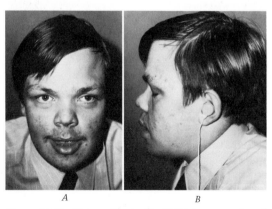

A   *B*

Figure 96-20. *Mannosidosis.* (*A, B*). Note coarsening of facies. Nearly all patients manifest neural deafness. (*From S. Autio, Helsinki, Finland.*)

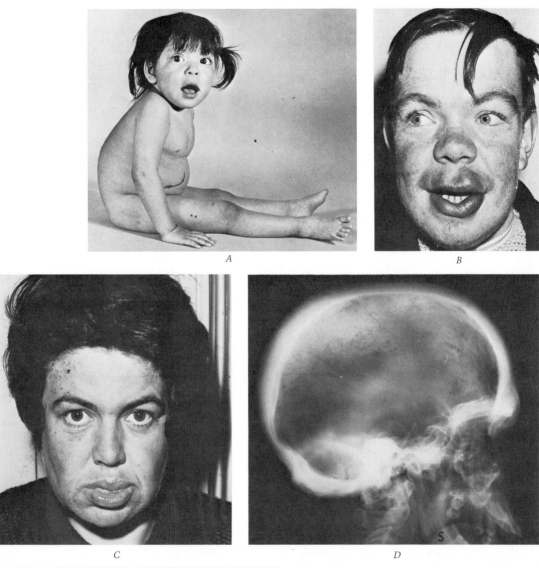

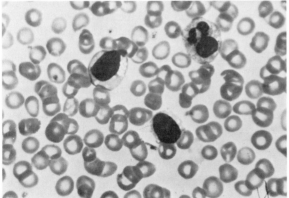

Figure 96-21. *Aspartylglucosaminuria.* (*A*). Five-year-old girl. Note gibbus and hepatomegaly. (*From J. N. Isenberg and H. L. Sharp,* J. Pediatr. **86:**713, 1975.) (*B*). Twenty-four-year-old male with coarse facies, mental retardation, recurrent skin infections, and deafness. (*From R. B. Fountain,* Proc. R. Soc. Med. **67:**878, 1974.) (*C*). Coarsened facies, sagging cheeks. (*From R. J. Pollitt, Sheffield, England.*) (*D*). Radiograph showing thickened calvaria. (*From R. B. Foundation,* Proc. R. Soc. Med. **67:**878, 1974.) (*E*) Vacuolated lymphocytes in peripheral blood smear. (*From J. N. Isenberg and H. L. Sharp,* J. Pediatr. **86:**713, 1975.)

hypotonia. The abdomen is protuberant, but the liver and spleen are not enlarged. Umbilical hernia is apparently common.

The calvaria is thick. The long bones are osteoporotic. The ulna and radius are broad with curved diaphyses and a thin cortex. The upper lumbar vertebras are somewhat trapezoidal in form.

Other findings. Bilateral testicular hydrocele has been described in two of three children (1).

Oral findings. Macroglossia and widely spaced teeth have been noted (4).

LABORATORY AIDS

The peripheral lymphocytes are vacuolated in 20 to 90 percent of the cells counted. Coarse dark granules are present in the neutrophils. The condition is diagnosed by finding reduced α-mannosidase in white blood cells or serum or mannose-rich compounds in the liver and urine (1, 2).

ASPARTYLGLUCOSAMINURIA

Aspartylglucosaminuria was first identified in England by Jenner and Pollitt (6, 8), in Finland by Palo and Mattson (6), and in Minneapolis by Isenberg and Sharp (5). Autio et al. (2, 3) carried out detailed studies on 57 Finnish patients. The four sibs reported by Fountain (4) possibly had this syndrome.

Inheritance is autosomal recessive. Heterozygotes may be identified and prenatal detection is possible (1).

Infancy and childhood are usually characterized by reported bouts of diarrhea and frequent respiratory infections.

Facies. There is a remarkable resemblance among the affected. The skull is frequently asymmetric. The features gradually become coarse during childhood. The nasal bridge is broad and low. The nostrils are anteverted and the lips thickened. Mild ocular hypertelorism and epicanthal folds have been present in but half the cases. The facial skin, especially that of the eyelids and cheeks, has a tendency to sag with age. The face assumes a reddish-brown color. In about one-third of the patients, the voice becomes raspy in adult life. Skin infections, especially of the face, were noted in several patients (Figs. 96-21*A–C*).

Skeletal manifestations. Inguinal and/or, more often, umbilical hernia has been found in over one-third of patients before the age of three months. Muscular hypotonia has been present in about 20 percent of cases. Genu valgum has been noted in at least 75 percent. The long bones have thin cortices. Kyphosis or scoliosis and protuberant abdomen have also been frequently noted. Growth retardation is seen only after fifteen years of age.

The calvaria are characteristically thickened and the frontal sinuses are absent or poorly developed (Fig. 96-21*D*). Osteochondritic alterations in the spine have been common. The ulna is somewhat shortened.

Nervous system. Progressive mental retardation is a constant feature. It usually first becomes evident between one and five years of age. Speech is severely limited. Not uncommonly the voice has a low pitch. Periodic hyperactivity, hyperirritability, and/or aggressive reactions are common.

Mild to moderate hearing loss has been found in about 20 percent of adults with this disorder. Clumsy gait and poor coordination of the hands is noted early in life.

Oral manifestations. The teeth have often been noted to be spread. The gingiva and tongue were stated to be enlarged in about half the cases.

LABORATORY FINDINGS

From 5 to 20 percent of the blood lymphocytes were vacuolated in 75 percent of the patients (Fig. 96-21*E*) and about half exhibited mild neutropenia.

Skin fibroblasts frequently contain metachromatic granules. A decreased prothrombin activity was noted in about half the patients. The definitive diagnosis is made by finding aspartylglycosamine amidohydrolase decreased in the seminal fluid, plasma, leukocyte homogenates, spleen, brain, and liver (5) or aspartylglycosaminuria by chromatographic or electrophoretic methods (3).

REFERENCES

GENERAL

1 Belcher, R. W., Ultrastructure and Cytochemistry of Lymphocytes in the Genetic Mucopolysaccharidoses. *Arch. Pathol.* **93**:1–7, 1972.

2 Danes, B. S., Corneal Clouding in the Genetic Mucopolysaccharidoses: A Cell Culture Study. *Clin. Genet.* **4**:1–7, 1973.

3 Danes, B. S., and Grossman, H., Bone Dysplasia, Including Morquio's Syndrome, Studied in Skin Fibroblast Cultures. *Am. J. Med.* **47**:708–720, 1969.

4 Kenyon, K. R., et al., The Systemic Mucopolysaccharidoses. *Am. J. Ophthalmol.* **73**:811–833, 1972.

5 McKusick, V. A., *Heritable Disorders of Connective Tissue,* 3d ed. Mosby, St. Louis, 1966.

6 McKusick, V. A., *Heritable Disorders of Connective Tissue,* 4th ed. Mosby, St. Louis, 1972.

7 McKusick, V. A., et al., The Genetic Mucopolysaccharidoses. *Medicine (Baltimore)* **44**:445–484, 1965.

8 McKusick, V. A., et al., Allelism, Non-allelism and Genetic Compounds among the Mucopolysacchridoses. *Lancet* **1**:993–995, 1972.

9 Spranger, J., Biochemical Definition of the Mucopolysaccharidoses. *Z. Kinderheilkd.* **108**:17–31, 1970.

10 Spranger, J., The Systemic Mucopolysaccharidoses. *Ergeb. Inn. Med. Kinderheilkd.* **32**:165–265, 1972.

HURLER SYNDROME (MPS I-H)

1 Bach, G., et al., The Defect in the Hurler and Scheie Syndrome: Deficiency of α-L-Iduronidase. *Proc. Natl. Acad. Sci. U.S.A.* **69**:2048–2051, 1972.

2 Bartman, J., and Blanc, W., Fibroblast Cultured in Hurler's and Hunter's Syndromes. *Arch. Pathol.* **89**:279–285, 1970.

3 Belcher, R., Ultrastructure and Cytochemistry of Lymphocytes in the Genetic Mucopolysaccharidoses. *Arch. Pathol.* **93**:1–7, 1972.

4 Carter, C. H., et al., Commonly Used Tests in the Detection of Hurler's Syndrome. *J. Pediatr.* **73**:217–221, 1968.

5 Cawson, R. A., The Oral Changes in Gargoylism. *Proc. R. Soc. Med.* **55**:1066–1070, 1962.

6 Fratantoni, F. C., et al., Intrauterine Diagnosis of the Hurler and Hunter Syndromes. *N. Engl. J. Med.* **280**:686–688, 1969.

7 Gardner, D. G., Metachromatic Cells in the Gingiva in Hurler's Syndrome. *Oral Surg.* **26**:782–789, 1968.

8 Gardner, D. G., The Oral Manifestations of Hurler's Syndrome. *Oral Surg.* **32**:46–57, 1971.

9 Horrigan, W. D., and Baker, D. H., Gargoylism: A Review of the Roentgen Skull Changes with Description of a New Finding. *Am. J. Roentgenol.* **86**:473–477, 1961.

10 Hurler, G., Über einen Typus multipler Abartungen, vorwiegend am Skelettsystem. *Z. Kinderheilkd.* **24**:220–234, 1919.

11 Leroy, J. G., and Crocker, A. C., Clinical Definition of Hurler-Hunter Phenotypes. *Am. J. Dis. Child.* **112**:518–530, 1966.

12 Lowry, R. B., and Renwick, D. H. G., Relative Frequency of the Hurler and Hunter Syndromes. *N. Engl. J. Med.* **284**:221–222, 1971.

13 Matalon, R., and Dorfman, A., Hurler's Syndrome, α-L-Iduronidase Deficiency. *Biochem. Biophys. Res. Commun.* **47**:959–964, 1972.

14 McKusick, V. A., *Heritable Disorders of Connective Tissue,* 4th ed. Mosby, St. Louis, 1972.

15 Neufeld, E. F., and Cantz, M. J., Corrective Factors for Inborn Errors of Mucopolysaccharide Metabolism. *Ann. N.Y. Acad. Sci.* **179**:580–587, 1971.

16 Neufeld, E. F., and Fratantoni, J. C., Inborn Errors of Mucopolysaccharide Metabolism. *Science* **169**:141–145, 1970.

17 Spranger, J., The Systemic Mucopolysaccharidoses. *Ergeb. Inn. Med. Kinderheilkd.* **32**:165–265, 1972.

18 Worth, H. M., Hurler's Syndrome: A Study of Radiologic Appearances in the Jaws. *Oral Surg.* **22**:21–35, 1966.

SCHEIE SYNDROME (MPS I-S)

1 Bach, G., et al., The Defect in the Hurler and Scheive Syndromes: Deficiency of α-L-Iduronidase. *Proc. Natl. Acad. Sci. U.S.A.* **69**:2048–2051, 1972.

2 McKusick, V. A., *Heritable Disorders of Connective Tissue,* 4th ed. Mosby, St. Louis, 1972.

3 Scheie, H. G., et al., A Newly Recognized Forme Fruste of Hurler's Disease (Gargoylism). *Am. J. Ophthalmol.* **53**:733–769, 1962.

4 Schinz, H. R., and Furtwängler, A., Zur Kenntnis einer hereditären Osteo-Arthropathie mit rezessivem Erbgang. *Dtsch. Z. Chir.* **207**:398–416, 1928.

5 Spranger, J., The Systemic Mucopolysaccharidoses. *Ergeb. Inn. Med. Kinderheilkd.* **32**:165–265, 1972.

HUNTER SYNDROME (MPS II)

1 Bach, G., et al., The Defect in the Hunter Syndrome: Deficiency of Sulfoiduronate Sulfatase. *Proc. Natl. Acad. Sci. U.S.A.* **70**:2134–2138, 1973.

1a Booth, C. W., and Nadler, H. L., Demonstration of the Heterozygous State in Hunter's Syndrome. *Pediatrics* **53**:396–399, 1974.

2 Donnelly, P. V., and DiFertante, W., Reliability of the Booth-Nader Technique for the Detection of Hunter Heterozygotes. *Pediatrics* **56**:429–433, 1975.

3 Fratantoni, J. C., et al., The Defect in Hurler's and Hunter's Syndromes: Faulty Degradation of Mucopolysaccharide. *Proc. Natl. Acad. Sci. U.S.A.* **60**:699–706, 1968.

4 Fratantoni, J. C., et al., The Defect in Hurler and Hunter Syndromes. II. Deficiency of Specific Factors Involved in Mucopolysaccharide Degradation. *Proc. Natl. Acad. Sci. U.S.A.* **64**:360–366, 1969.

5 Hunter, C., A Rare Disease in Two Brothers. *Proc. R. Soc. Med.* **10**(pt. 1):104–116, 1917.

6 Leroy, J. G., and Crocker, A. C., Clinical Definition of the Hurler-Hunter Phenotypes. *Am. J. Dis. Child.* **112**: 518–530, 1966.

7 Lichtenstein, J. R., et al., Clinical and Probable Genetic Heterogeneity within Mucopolysaccharidosis II. Report of a Family with a Mild Form. *Johns Hopk. Med. J.* **131**:425–435, 1972.

8 Lowry, R. B., and Renwick, D. H. G., Relative Frequency of the Hurler and Hunter Syndromes. *N. Engl. J. Med.* **284:**221–222, 1971.

9 McKusick, V. A., The Relative Frequency of the Hurler and Hunter Syndromes. *N. Engl. J. Med.* **283:**853–854, 1970.

10 Spranger, J., The Systemic Mucopolysaccharidoses. *Ergeb. Inn. Med. Kinderheilkd.* **32:**165–265, 1972.

11 Thurmon, T. F., et al., Clinical Heterogeneity in Mucopolysaccharidosis II: Evidence for Epistasis. *Birth Defects* **10**(8):125–127, 1974.

12 Wiesmann, U. N., and Rampini, S., Mild Form of the Hunter Syndrome: Identity of the Biochemical Defect with the Severe Type. *Helv. Paediatr. Acta* **29:**73–78, 1974.

SANFILIPPO SYNDROME (MPS III)

1 Crump, I. A., and Danks, D. M., Simple Method for Cutting Transverse Section of Hair: Comments on Shape of Hair in Hurler and Sanfilippo Syndromes. *Arch. Dis. Child.* **46:**383–386, 1971.

2 Danks, D. M., et al., The Sanfilippo Syndrome: Clinical, Biochemical, Radiological, Haematological, and Pathological Features of Nine Cases. *Aust. Paediatr. J.* **8:**174–186, 1972.

3 Dekaban, A. S., and Patton, V. M., Hurler's and Sanfilippo's Variants of Mucopolysaccharidosis. *Arch. Pathol.* **91:**434–443, 1971.

3a Farriaux, J. P., et al., Etude comparative des aspects cliniques, radiologiques, biochimiques et genetiques de la maladie de Sanfilippo de type A et type B. *Helv. Paediatr. Acta* **29:**349–370, 1974.

4 von Figura, K., et al., Sanfilippo B Disease: Serum Assays for Detection of Homozygous and Heterozygous Individuals in Three Families. *J. Pediatr.* **83:**607–611, 1973.

4a Harper, P. S., et al., Sanfilippo A Disease in the Fetus. *J. Med. Genet.* **11:**123–132, 1974.

5 Harris, R. C., Mucopolysaccharide Disorder: A Possible New Genotype of Hurler's Syndrome. *Am. J. Dis. Child.* **102:**741–742, 1961.

6 Haust, M. D., et al., Heparitin Sulfate Mucopolysaccharidosis (Sanfilippo's) Disease: A Case Study with Ultrastructural, Biochemical and Radiological Findings. *Pediatrics* **5:**137–150, 1971.

7 Kresse, H., et al., Biochemical Heterogeneity of the Sanfilippo Syndrome. *Biochem. Biophys. Res. Commun.* **42:**892–898, 1971.

8 Kresse, H., and Neufeld, E. F., The Sanfilippo-A Corrective Factor. *J. Biol. Chem.* **247:**2164–2170, 1972.

9 Langer, L. O., The Radiographic Manifestations of the HS-mucopolysaccharidosis of Sanfilippo. *Ann. Radiol.* **7:**315–325, 1964.

10 Meyer, K., et al., Excretion of Sulfated Mucopolysaccharides in Gargoylism (Hurler's Syndrome). *Proc. Soc. Exp. Biol. Med.* **97:**275–279, 1958.

11 Meyer, K., et al., Sulfated Mucopolysaccharides of Urine and Organs in Gargoylism. *Proc. Soc. Exp. Biol. Med.* **102:**587–590, 1959.

13 Rampini, S., Das Sanfilippo Syndrom. *Helv. Paediatr. Acta* **24:**55–91, 1969.

14 Sanfilippo, S. J., et al., Mental Retardation Associated with Acid Mucopolysacchariduria (Heparitin Sulfate Type). *J. Pediatr.* **63:**837–838, 1963.

15 Spranger, J., et al., Die HS-Mucopolysaccharidose von Sanfilippo (polydystrophe Oligophrenie). Bericht über 10 Patienten. *Z. Kinderheilkd.* **101:**71–84, 1967.

16 Teller, W., et al., Die Heparitinsulfat-Mucopolysaccharidose (Sanfilippo). Klinische, biochemische, genetische und morphologische Untersuchungen. *Klin. Wochenschr.* **45:**497–504, 1967.

17 Wallace, B. J., et al., Mucopolysaccharidosis Type III. *Arch. Pathol.* **82:**462–473, 1966.

MORQUIO-BRAILSFORD SYNDROME (MPS IV)

1 Blaw, M. E., and Langer, L. O., Spinal Cord Compression in Morquio-Brailsford's Disease. *J. Pediatr.* **74:**593–600, 1969.

2 Brailsford, J. F., Chondro-osteo-dystrophy. *Am. J. Surg.* **7:**404–409, 1929.

3 Diamond, L. S., A Family Study of Spondyloepiphyseal Dysplasia. *J. Bone Joint Surg.* **52A:**1587–1594, 1970.

4 Garn, S. M., and Hurme, V. O., Dental Defects in Three Siblings Afflicted with Morquio's Disease. *Br. Dent. J.* **93:**210–212, 1952.

5 Goidanich, I. F., and Lenzi, L., Morquio-Ullrich Disease. *J. Bone Joint Surg.* **46A:**734–746, 1964.

6 Jenkins, P., et al., Morquio-Brailsford Disease. A Report of Four Affected Sisters with Absence of Excessive Keratan Sulfate in the Urine. *Br. J. Radiol.* **46:**668–675, 1973.

7 Langer, L. O., and Carey, L. S., The Roentgenographic Features of the KS Mucopolysaccharidosis of Morquio Disease. *Am. J. Roentgenol.* **97:**1–20, 1966.

8 Levin, L. S., et al., Oral Findings in the Morquio Syndrome (MPS IV). *Oral Surg.* **39:**390–395, 1975.

9 Matalon, R., et al., Morquio's Syndrome: Deficiency of a Chondroitin Sulfate *N*-Acetylhexosamine Sulfate Sulfatase. *Biochem. Biophys. Res. Commun.* **61:**759–765, 1974.

10 Maynard, J. A., et al., Morquio's Disease (Mucopolysaccharidosis Type IV). Ultrastructure of Epiphyseal Plates. *Lab. Invest.* **28:**194–205, 1973.

11 McKusick, V. A., *Heritable Disorders of Connective Tissue*, 4th ed. Mosby, St. Louis, 1972.

12 Morquio, L., Sur une forme de dystrophie osseuse familiale. *Arch. Méd. Enf.* **32:**129–140, 1929.

13 Norman, M. E., Two Brothers with Nonkeratan-Sulfate-Excreting Morquio Syndrome. *Birth Defects* **10**(12):467–469, 1974.

14 Robins, M. M., et al., Morquio's Disease: An Abnormality of Mucopolysaccharide Metabolism. *J. Pediatr.* **62:**881–889, 1963.

15 Sela, M., et al., Oral Manifestations of Morquio's Syndrome. *Oral Surg.* **39:**583–589, 1975.

16 Spranger, J., The Systemic Mucopolysaccharidoses. *Ergeb. Inn. Med. Kinderheilkd.* **32:**166–265, 1972.

17 Spranger, J., et al., The Dyggve-Melchoir-Clausen Syndrome. *Radiology* **114:**415–421, 1975.

18 Von Noorden, G. K., et al., Ocular Findings in the Morquio-Ullrich's Disease. *Arch. Ophthalmol.* **64:**581–591, 1960.

MAROTEAUX-LAMY SYNDROME (MPS VI)

1 Barton, R. W., and Neufeld, E. F., A Distinct Biochemical Deficit in the Maroteaux-Lamy Syndrome (Mucopolysaccharidosis VI). *J. Pediatr.* **80:**114–116, 1972.

1a DiFerrante, N., et al., Mucopolysaccharidosis VI (Maroteaux-Lamy Disease). Clinical and Biochemical Study of a Mild Variant Case. *Johns Hopk. Med. J.* **135:**42–54, 1974.

2 Goldberg, M. F., et al., Hydrocephalus and Papilledema in the Maroteaux-Lamy Syndrome. *Am. J. Ophthalmol.* **69:**969–974, 1970.

3 Maroteaux, M., et al., Une nouvelle dysostose avec élimination urinaire de chondroitin-sulfate B. *Presse Méd.* **71:**1849–1852, 1963.

3a Quigley, H. A., and Kenyon, K. R., Ultrastructural and Histochemical Studies of a Newly Recognized Form of Systemic Mucopolysaccharidosis (Maroteaux-Lamy Syndrome, Mild Type). *Am. J. Ophthalmol.* **77:**809–818, 1974.

4 Rampini, S., and Maroteaux, P., Ein ungewöhnlicher Phanotyp des Hurler Syndroms. *Helv. Paediatr. Acta* **21:**376–386, 1966.

5 Spranger, J., et al., Mucopolysaccharidosis VI (Maroteaux-Lamy Disease). *Helv. Paediatr. Acta* **25:**337–362, 1970.

6 Spranger, J., The Systemic Mucopolysaccharidoses. *Ergeb. Inn. Med. Kinderheilkd.* **32:**165–265, 1972.

7 Stumpf, D. A., et al., Mucopolysaccharidosis Type VI (Maroteaux-Lamy Syndrome). *Am. J. Dis. Child.* **126:** 747–755, 1973.

β-GLUCURONIDASE DEFICIENCY (MPS VII)

1 Beaudet, A. L., et al., Variations in the Phenotypic Expression of β-Glucuronidase Deficiency. *J. Pediatr.* **86:**388–394, 1975.

2 Danes, B. S., and Degnan, M., Different Clinical and Biochemical Phenotypes Associated with β-Glucuronidase Deficiency. *Birth Defects* **10**(12):251–257, 1974.

3 Gehler, J., et al., Mucopolysaccharidosis VII: β-Glucuronidase Deficiency. *Humangenetik* **23:**149–158, 1974.

4 Glaser, J. H., et al., β-Glucuronidase Deficiency Mucopolysaccharidosis: Methods for Enzymatic Diagnosis. *J. Lab. Clin. Med.* **82:**969–977, 1973.

5 Hall, C. W., et al., A β-glucuronidase Deficiency Mucopolysaccharidosis: Studies in Cultured Fibroblasts. *Arch. Biochem. Biophys.* **155:**32–38, 1973.

6 Sly, W. S., et al., Beta-glucuronidase Deficiency: Report of Clinical, Radiologic, and Biochemical Features of a New Mucopolysaccharidosis. *J. Pediatr.* **82:**249–257, 1973.

7 Sly, W. S., et al., β-Glucuronidase Deficiency Mucopolysaccharidosis. *Birth Defects* **10**(12):239–245, 1974.

MISCELLANEOUS MUCOPOLYSACCHARIDOSES

1 Onisawa, J., et al., Chondroitin 4- and 6-sulfaturia in Morquio-Ullrich's Syndrome. *Biochem. Med.* **5:**37–47, 1971.

2 Philippart, M., and Sugarman, G. I., Chondroitin-4-sulfate Mucopolysaccharidosis: A New Variant of Hurler's Syndrome. *Lancet* **2:**854, 1969.

3 Schimke, R. N., et al., Chondroitin-6-sulfate Mucopolysaccharidosis in Conjunction with Lymphopenia, Defective Cellular Immunity and the Nephrotic Syndrome. *Birth Defects* **10**(12):258–266, 1974.

4 Spranger, J. W., et al., Chondroitin-4-sulfate Mucopolysaccharidosis. *Helv. Paediat. Acta* **26:**387–396, 1971.

5 Suschke, J., and Kunze, D., Ein neuer Mucopolysac-

charidose-Typ. *Dtsch. Med. Wochenschr.* **96:**1941–1943, 1971.

6 Thompson, G. R., et al., A Mucopolysaccharidosis with Increased Urinary Excretion of Chondroitin-4-sulfate. *Ann. Intern. Med.* **75:**421–426, 1971.

MUCOLIPIDOSES — GENERAL

1 Autio, S., Aspartylglucosaminuria. *J. Ment. Defic. Res., Monogr. Ser.* I, 1972.

2 Goldberg, M. F., et al., Macular Cherry-red Spot, Corneal Clouding, and β-Galactosidase Deficiency. *Arch. Intern. Med.* **128:**387–397, 1971.

3 Leroy, J. G., et al., I-cell Disease. *J. Pediatr.* **79:**360–365, 1971.

4 Loeb, H., et al., Biochemical and Ultrastructural Studies in a Case of Mucopolysaccharidosis "F" (Fucosidosis). *Helv. Paediatr. Acta* **24:**519–537, 1969.

5 Maroteaux, P., and Lamy, M., La pseudo-polydystrophie de Hurler. *Presse Med.* **74:**2889–2892, 1966.

6 O'Brien, J. S., G$_{M1}$ Gangliosidosis, in J. B. Stanbury et al., *The Metabolic Basis of Inherited Disease,* 3d ed., McGraw-Hill, New York, 1972.

7 Ockerman, P. A., Mannosidosis. *J. Pediatr.* **75:**361–365, 1969.

8 Rampini, S., et al., Die Kombination von metachromatischer Leukodystrophie und Mucopolysaccharidose als selbständiges Krankheitsbild (Mucosulfatidose). *Helv. Paediatr. Acta* **25:**436–461, 1970.

9 Spranger, J., et al., Lipomucopolysaccharidose. *Z. Kinderheilkd.* **103:**285–306, 1968.

10 Spranger, J., and Wiedemann, H. R., The Genetic Mucolipidoses. *Humangenetik* **9:**113–139, 1970.

G$_{M1}$ GANGLIOSIDOSIS

1 Grossman, H., and Danes, B. S., Neurovisceral Storage Disease: Roentgenologic Features and Mode of Inheritance. *Am. J. Roentgenol.* **103:**149–153, 1968.

2 Landing, B. H., et al., Familial Neurovisceral Lipidosis. *Am. J. Dis. Child.* **108:**503–522, 1964.

3 O'Brien, J. S., Generalized Gangliosidosis. *J. Pediatr.* **75:**167–186, 1969.

4 O'Brien, J. S., Five Gangliosidoses. *Lancet* **2:**805, 1969.

5 O'Brien, J., G$_{M1}$ Gangliosidoses, in J. B. Stanbury et al., *The Metabolic Basis of Inherited Disease,* 3d ed. McGraw-Hill, New York, 1972.

6 Scott, C. R., et al., Familial Neurovisceral Lipidosis. *J. Pediatr.* **71:**357–366, 1967.

7 Severi, F., et al., Infantile G$_{M1}$ Gangliosidoses: Histochemical, Ultrastructural and Biochemical Studies. *Helv. Paediatr. Acta* **26:**192–209, 1971.

MUCOLIPIDOSIS I

1 Dawson, G., Personal communication, 1972.

2 Freitag, F., et al., Hepatic Ultrastructure in Mucolipidosis I (Lipomucopolysaccharidosis). *Virchows Arch.* [*Pathol. Anat.*] Abt. B. **7:**189–204, 1971.

3 Loeb, H., et al., Clinical, Biochemical, and Ultrastructural Studies of an Atypical Form of Mucopolysaccharidosis. *Acta Paediatr. Scand.* **58:**220–228, 1969.

4 Pincus, J. H., et al., Delayed Development of Disturbed

Mucopolysaccharide Metabolism in a Hurler Variant. *Arch. Neurol.* **16**:244–253, 1967.

5 Spranger, J., et al., Lipomucopolysaccharidose. *Z. Kinderheilkd.* **103**:285–306, 1968.

6 Spranger, J., and Wiedemann, H. R., Lipomucopolysaccharidosis — a Second Look. *Lancet* **2**:270–271, 1969.

MUCOLIPIDOSIS II

1 Blank, E., and Linder, D., I-cell Disease (ML II): a Lysosomopathy. *Pediatrics* **54**:797–805, 1974.

1a DeMars, R. I., and Leroy, J. G., The Remarkable Cells Cultured from a Human with Hurler's Syndrome. *In Vitro* **2**:107–118, 1967.

2 Galili, D., et al., Massive Gingival Hyperplasia Preceding Dental Eruption in I-Cell Disease. *Oral Surg.* **37**:533–539, 1974.

3 Gilbert, E. F., et al., I-cell Disease, Mucolipidosis II. Pathological, Histochemical, Ultrastructural and Biochemical Observations in Four Cases. *Z. Kinderheilkd.* **114**:259–292, 1973.

3a Hickman, S., and Neufeld, E. F., A Hypothesis for I-cell Disease: Defective Hydrolases That Do Not Enter Lysosomes. *Biochem. Biophys. Res. Commun.* **49**:992–999, 1972.

4 Kenyon, K. R., and Sensenbrenner, J. A., Mucolipidosis II (I-cell Disease): Ultrastructural Observations of Conjunctiva and Skin. *Invest. Ophthalmol.* **10**:555–567, 1971.

5 Leroy, J. G., and DeMars, R. I., Mutant Enzymatic and Cytological Phenotypes in Cultured Human Fibroblasts. *Science* **157**:804–806, 1967.

6 Leroy, J. G., et al., I-cell Disease. *Birth Defects* **5**(4):174–185, 1969.

7 Leroy, J. F., and Spranger, J. W., I-cell Disease Continued. *N. Engl. J. Med.* **283**:598–599, 1970.

8 Leroy, J. G., et al., I-cell Disease: A Clinical Picture. *J. Pediatr.* **73**:360–365, 1971.

9 Leroy, J. G., et al., I-cell Disease: Biochemical Studies. *Pediatr. Res.* **6**:752–757, 1972.

10 de Montis, G., et al., La mucolipidose II (Maladie des cellules à inclusions). *Ann. Pédiat.* **19**:369–379, 1972.

11 Rapola, J., et al., Lymphocytic Inclusions in I-cell Disease. *J. Pediatr.* **85**:88–90, 1974.

12 Tondeur, M., et al., Clinical, Biochemical and Ultrastructural Studies in a Case of Chondrodystrophy Presenting the I-cell Phenotype in Tissue Culture. *J. Pediatr.* **73**:366–378, 1971.

13 Walbaum, R., et al., La mucolipidose de type II (I-cell Disease). *Arch. Fr. Pédiatr.* **30**:577–594, 1973.

14 Wiesmann, U., et al., "I-cell" Disease: Leakage of Lysosomal Enzymes into Extracellular Fluid. *N. Engl. J. Med.* **285**:1090–1091, 1971.

15 Wiesmann, U., et al., Mucolipidosis II (I-cell Disease). A Clinical and Biochemical Study. *Acta Paediatr. Scand.* **63**:9–16, 1974.

MUCOLIPIDOSIS III

1 Maroteaux, P., and Lamy, M., La pseudopolydystrophie de Hurler. *Presse Méd.* **74**:2889–2892, 1966.

2 McKusick, V. A., et al., The Genetic Mucopolysaccharidoses. *Medicine (Baltimore)* **44**:445–484, 1965.

3 Melhem, R., et al., Roentgen Findings in Mucolipidosis III (Pseudo-Hurler Polydystrophy). *Radiology* **166**:153–160, 1973.

4 Steinbach, H. L., The Hurler Syndrome without Abnormal Mucopolysacchariduria. *Radiology* **90**:472–478, 1968.

5 Stern, H., et al., Pseudo-Hurler Polydystrophy (Mucolipidosis 3). A Clinical, Biochemical and Ultrastructural Study. *Israel J. Med. Sci.* **10**:463–475, 1974.

6 Taylor, H. A., Mucolipidosis III (Pseudo-Hurler Polydystrophy): Cytological and Ultrastructural Observations of Cultured Fibroblast Cells. *Clin. Genet.* **4**:388–397, 1973.

7 Thomas, G. H., et al., Mucolipidosis III (Pseudo-Hurler Polydystrophy): Multiple Lysosomal Enzyme Abnormalities in Skin and Cultured Fibroblasts. *Pediatr. Res.* **7**:751–756, 1973.

FUCOSIDOSIS

1 Borrone, C., et al., Fucosidosis: Clinical Biochemical Immunologic and Genetic Studies in Two New Cases. *J. Pediatr.* **84**:727–730, 1974.

1a Dawson, G., and Spranger, J. W., Fucosidosis: A Glycosphingolipidosis. *N. Engl. J. Med.* **285**:122, 1971.

2 Durand, P., A New Mucopolysaccharide Lipid Storage Disease. *Lancet* **2**:1313, 1966.

3 Durand, P., et al., Fucosidosis. *J. Pediatr.* **75**:665–674, 1969.

4 Kousseff, B. G., et al., Genetic Heterogeneity in Fucosidosis. *Lancet* **2**:1387–1388, 1973.

5 Loeb, H., et al., Biochemical and Ultrastructural Studies in a Case of Mucopolysaccharidosis "F". *Helv. Paediatr. Acta* **24**:519–537, 1969.

6 Voelz, C., et al., Fucosidose. *Monatsschr. Kinderheilkd.* **119**:352–355, 1971.

7 Zielke, K., Fucosidosis: Deficiency of α-L-Fucosidase in Cultured Skin Fibroblasts. *J. Exp. Med.* **136**:197–199, 1972.

8 Zielke, K., et al., Fucosidosis: Diagnosis by Serum Assay of α-L-Fucosidase. *J. Lab. Clin. Med.* **79**:164–169, 1972.

MANNOSIDOSIS

1 Autio, S., et al., Mannosidosis: Clinical, Fine-structural and Biochemical Findings in Three Cases. *Acta Paediatr. Scand.* **62**:555–565, 1973.

2 Farriaux, J. P., et al., La mannosidose. *Nour. Presse Med.* **4**:1867–1870, 1975.

3 Loeb, H., et al., Clinical, Biochemical and Ultrastructural Studies of an Atypical Form of Mucopolysaccharidosis. *Acta Paediatr. Scand.* **58**:220–228, 1969.

4 Öckerman, P. A., A Generalized Storage Disorder Resembling Hurler's Syndrome. *Lancet* **2**:239–241, 1967.

5 Tsay, G. C., et al., Excretion of Mannose-rich Complex Carbohydrates by a Patient with Alpha-Mannosidose Deficiency (Mannosidosis). *J. Pediatr.* **84**:865–869, 1974.

ASPARTYLGLUCOSAMINURIA

1 Acula, P., et al., Aspartylglucosaminuria: Deficiency of Aspartylglucosaminidase in Cultured Fibroblasts of Patients and Their Heterozygous Parents. *Clin. Genet.* **4**:297–300, 1973.

2 Autio, S., Aspartylglycosaminuria. Analysis of Thirty-Four Patients. *J. Ment. Defic. Res. Monograph Ser.* **I**:1–93, 1972.

3 Autio, S., et al., Aspartylglucosaminuria (AGU). Further Aspects of its Clinical Picture Mode of Inheritance and Epidemiology based on a Series of 57 Patients. *Ann. Clin. Res.* **5:**149–155, 1973.

4 Fountain, R. B., Familial Bone Abnormalities, Deaf Mutism, Mental Retardation and Skin Granuloma. *Proc. R. Soc. Med.* **67:**878–879, 1974.

5 Isenberg, J. N., and Sharp, H. L., Aspartylglucosaminuria: Psychomotor Retardation Masquerading as a Mucopolysaccharidosis. *J. Pediatr.* **86:**713–718, 1975.

6 Jenner, F. A., and Pollitt, R. J., Large Quantities of 2-acetamido-1-(-L-aspartamido)-1,2-dideoxyglucose in the Urine of Mentally Retarded Siblings. *Biochem. J.* **103:**48, 1967.

7 Palo, J., and Mattson, K., Eleven New Cases of Aspartylglucosaminuria. *J. Ment. Defic. Res.* **14:**168–173, 1970.

8 Pollitt, R. J., et al., Aspartylglycosaminuria: An Inborn Error of Metabolism Associated with Mental Defect. *Lancet* **2:**253–255, 1968.

97

Multiple Hamartoma and Neoplasia Syndrome

(Cowden Syndrome)

This, as yet, probably incompletely defined syndrome was first described by Lloyd and Dennis (6) in 1963. Weary et al. (9) and Gentry et al. (4, 4a) published several examples of the disorder, emphasizing its hamartomatous character and suggesting that it involves principally the skin, gastrointestinal tract, breasts, and thyroid.

The syndrome exhibits autosomal dominant inheritance (4, 6, 9).

SYSTEMIC MANIFESTATIONS

Breasts. Fibroadenomatosis, virginal hypertrophy, and breast carcinoma (4–7, 9) have been described (Fig. 97-1).

Thyroid. Thyroid alteration has included fetal adenoma, follicular adenocarcinoma, and "goiter" (3, 4, 7, 9) (Fig. 97-2).

Other tumors. A wide variety of neoplasms has been noted: ovarian cysts, colonic polyposis and/or diverticulosis, colonic cancer, meningioma of the ear canal, angiomatous lesions of soft and hard tissues, and lipomas, both subcutaneous and retroperitoneal (3–5, 7, 9). The colonic polyps are of different histologic types: ganglioneuromatous, retention, hyperplastic, adenomatous, and, rarely, carcinoma in situ arising in adenomatous polyps. Angiomyomas have been described in the extremities (4, 5).

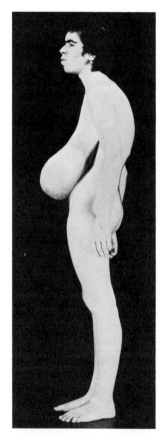

Figure 97-1. *Multiple hamartoma syndrome.* Huge fibroadenomatous breasts, producing secondary kyphosis. *(From L. Ackerman, St. Louis, Mo.)*

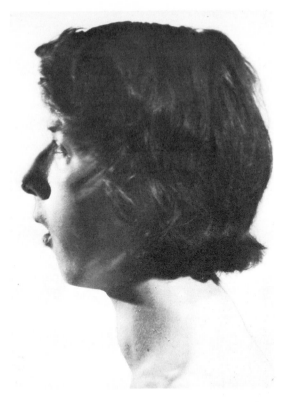

Figure 97-2. Note thyroid enlargement. (*From K. M. Lloyd and M. Dennis,* Ann. Intern. Med. **58:**136, 1963.)

Skin. The pinnas, lateral neck, nasal, periorbital, glabellar and perioral areas and the dorsa of hands and forearms are the most frequently involved sites of lichenoid and papillomatous lesions (4, 9) (Figs. 97-3*A, B*). Histologic examination suggests that they are hamartomas of hair

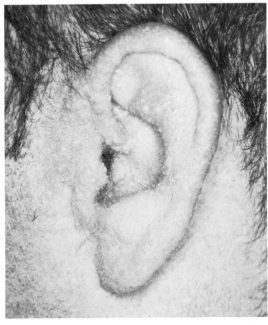

A

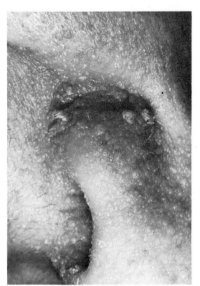

B

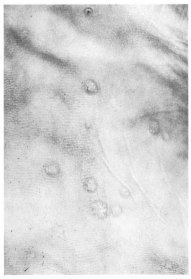

C

Figure 97-3. (*A*). Papillomatous lesions of pinna. (*From P. Weary et al.,* Arch. Dermatol. **106:**682, 1972.) (*B*). Papillomatous lesions near nasal ala. (*From M. Rosenbluth,* Periodontics **1:**81, 1963.) (*C*). Punctate kyperkeratoses of palms. (*From M. Rosenbluth,* Periodontics **1:**81, 1963.)

follicle origin, similar to inverted follicular keratoses (9).

The palms may exhibit waxy punctate keratoderma (4, 7, 8) (Fig. 97-3C).

Other findings. Hydronephrosis has been described (5, 8). However, in one case (5) it was thought to be secondary to a huge retroperitoneal lipoma. Transitional cell carcinoma of the renal pelvis has been reported (7).

Oral manifestations. Papular lesions of the lips and gingiva and, to a lesser extent, the palate as well as papillomatous lesions of the buccal, faucial, and oropharyngeal mucosa have been noted in most patients (1–4, 6, 8) (Fig. 97-4A, B). The tongue is pebbly and fissured.

DIFFERENTIAL DIAGNOSIS

Patients reported by Ackerman (1) and Byars and Jurkiewicz (2) exhibited giant fibroadenomas of the breast, secondary kyphosis, hypertrichosis, and gingival fibromatosis. This may represent another disorder.

The cutaneous lesions in the multiple hamartoma syndrome clinically resemble to some degree those of Darier disease and tuberous sclerosis. The lesions at the angles of the mouth simulate those of *acanthosis nigricans.*

Polyps of the colon are seen in a number of disorders (see Chap. 59).

LABORATORY AIDS

Biopsy of cutaneous lesions should aid in differential diagnosis.

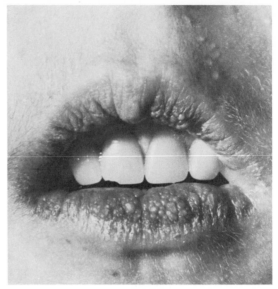

A

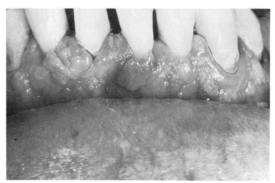

B

Figure 97-4. (*A*). Papillomatous lesion of lips. (*From K. M. Lloyd and M. Dennis,* Ann. Intern. Med. **58:**136, 1963.) (*B*). Papillomatosis of gingiva. (*From M. Rosenbluth,* Periodontics **1:**81, 1963.)

REFERENCES

1 Ackerman, L., Personal communication, 1969.
2 Byars, L. T., and Jurkiewicz, M., Congenital Macrogingivae and Hypertrichosis with Subsequent Giant Fibroadenomas of the Breasts. *Plast. Reconstr. Surg.* **27:** 608–612, 1961.
3 Carlier, G., et al., Sclérose tubéreuse de Bourneville avec papillomatose de la muqueuse buccale. *Rev. Stomatol. (Paris)* **72:**607–614, 1971.
4 Gentry, W. F., et al., Multiple Hamartoma Syndrome (Cowden's Disease). *Arch Dermatol.* **109:**521–530, 1974.
4a Gentry, W. C., et al., Cowden Syndrome. *Birth Defects* **11**(4):137–141, 1975.

5 Lattes, R., New York, N.Y., and Gellmani, S., and Zuflacht, J., Valley Stream, N.Y., Personal communication, 1974.
6 Lloyd, K. M., and Dennis, M., Cowden's Disease: A Possible New Symptom Complex with Multiple System Involvement. *Ann. Intern. Med.* **58:**136–142, 1963.
7 Mulvihill, J. J., Personal communication, 1975.
8 Rosenbluth, M., Multiple Noduli Cutanei: An Unusual Case of Multiple Noduli Cutanei with Gingival Manifestations. *Periodontics* **1:**81–83, 1963.
9 Weary, P., et al., The Multiple Hamartoma Syndrome (Cowden's Disease). *Arch. Dermatol.* **106:**682–690, 1972.

98

Multiple Mucosal Neuromas, Pheochromocytoma, and Medullary Thyroid Carcinoma

(Multiple Endocrine Neoplasia, Type 3)

Initially described in part by Wagenmann (39) and by Froboese (12) in 1922–1923, the syndrome of (a) multiple mucosal neuromas, (b) pheochromocytoma, (c) medullary carcinoma of the thyroid, and (d) asthenic build with muscle wasting of the extremities was enlarged by Williams and Pollock (41), Gorlin et al. (15–17), Schimke et al. (32), Levy et al. (24), and Khairi et al. (20a).

The syndrome has autosomal dominant inheritance. An analysis of 44 cases was carried out by Gorlin and Mirkin (15). Additional cases were analyzed by Khairi et al. (20a). Most aspects of the syndrome can be explained by hyperplasia and/or neoplasia of neural crest derivatives.

SYSTEMIC MANIFESTATIONS

Facies. The distinct facies is characterized by large nodular lips and thickening and often eversion of the upper eyelids (Fig. 98-1).

Mucosal Neuromas

(a) Oral. The mucosal neuromas principally involve the lips and tongue, although buccal, gingival, palatal, pharyngeal, nasal, conjunctival, and other mucosal surfaces may be the site of these lesions (15–17) (Fig. 98-2A, B). Both lips are extensively enlarged and nodular. They have been described as blubbery. The lingual lesions are largely limited to the anterior dorsal surface of the tongue and appear as pink pedunculated nodules. Oral and labial involvement is the first

component of the syndrome to appear, almost invariably before the eighth year of life. In several cases, the neuromas were either congenital or were noticed in early infancy (15–17).

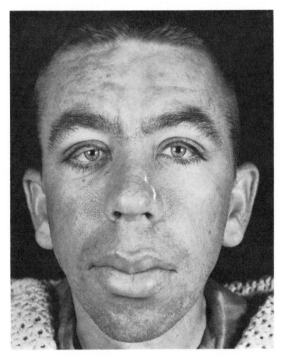

Figure 98-1. *Multiple mucosal neuromas, pheochromocytoma, medullary thyroid carcinoma, asthenic body build with muscle wasting.* Facies is characterized by coarse features, large nodular lips, eversion of upper eyelids. *(From R. N. Schimke et al., N. Engl. J. Med. **279**:1, 1968.)*

513

Microscopically, the mucosal nodules are plexiform neuromas, i.e., unencapsulated masses of convoluted myelinated and unmyelinated nerves (Fig. 98-2*C*) which elaborate calcitonin (38). Histochemical investigation demonstrates absence of both specific and nonspecific cholinesterase activity, in sharp contrast to neurofibroma, which rarely contains axons but is cholinesterase-positive (1).

(*b*) *Eyes.* The eyelid margins are thickened and often everted (6a, 17, 20a, 24). Pedunculated nodules, up to 6 mm in diameter, are present on the palpebral conjunctiva, eyelid margins, or rarely the cornea in about 60 percent of patients.

The cornea is the site of white medullated nerve fibers (1, 3, 5, 6, 6a, 12, 20a, 21, 26, 28, 32, 39, 40) which can easily be seen under slit lamp examination using low power with a broad beam of light. They extend into the pupillary area, where they anastomose (Fig. 98-3*A*).

(*c*) *Other.* Nasal and laryngeal mucosa may also be the site of neuromas (3, 6a, 20a, 28, 30,

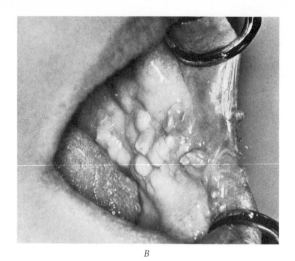

B

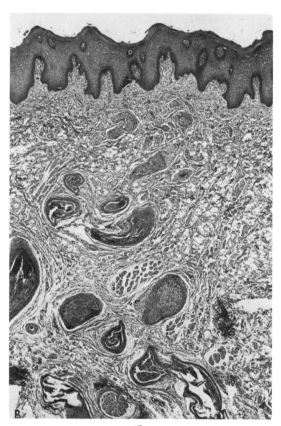

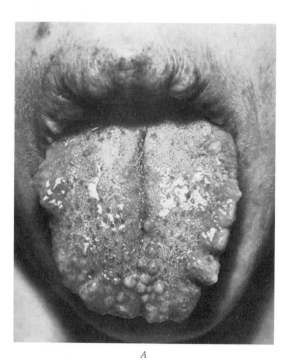

A

C

Figure 98-2. (*A*). Mucosal neuromas of lips and anterior and lateral dorsum of tongue. (*From K. W. Bruce,* Oral Surg. **7:**1150, 1954.) (*B*). Neuromas of buccal mucosa. (*From H. E. Simpson,* Oral Surg. **19:**228, 1965.) (*C*). Congeries of axons of nerves. Histochemically, these are cholinesterase-negative.

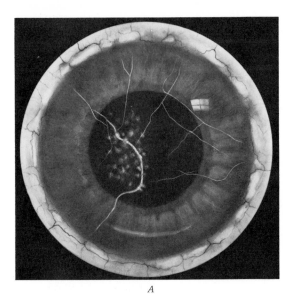

A

Figure 98-3. (*A*). White medullated corneal nerve fibers which anastomose in pupillary area. (*From D. L. Knox*, Birth Defects **7**(3):161, 1971.) (*B*). Hyperplastic neurofibromatous infiltrate with ganglion cells in intestinal wall between muscle layers.

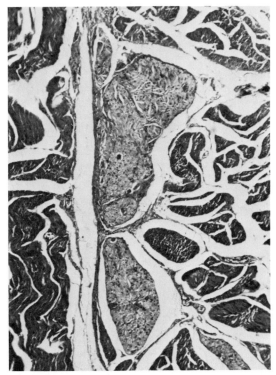

B

36, 40). In addition to hyperplasia of neurenteric ganglion cells throughout the entire gastrointestinal tract wall, similar changes have been observed in the bronchi, bladder, or spinal nerve roots (31, 32) (Fig. 98-3*B*).

Pheochromocytoma. The presence of pheochromocytomas is often heralded by weakness, flushing, pounding headache, nausea, hypertension, dyspnea, palpitation, flatulence, paresthesia, blanching of the extremities, profuse sweating, and intractable diarrhea. Abdominal discomfort or cramping is frequently experienced.

Pheochromocytomas arise from cells derived from the neural crest. They are often multiple and frequently bilateral when associated with medullary carcinoma of the thyroid. Varying in size from a few millimeters to several centimeters in diameter, they are red or dark brown when large and gray when small.

Microscopically, the tumor is seen to consist of bands or nests or polyhedral cells separated by thin connective tissue strands rich in blood vessels. The cytoplasm is abundant, finely granular, and basophilic. The nuclei vary markedly in size (Fig. 98-4*A*). Immersion of the tumor in a dichromate solution causes it to assume a dark brown color. In addition to catecholamines, it may elaborate calcitonin (38).

Pheochromocytoma has been diagnosed in about 50 percent of cases, most often becoming evident during the second and third decades of life. Some may be extra-adrenal (26a).

Medullary carcinoma of the thyroid. Medullary carcinoma of the thyroid is yellowish, consisting of sheets of round to spindle-shaped cells in varying proportions without follicle formation or papillae. The cells are rather uniform and frequently binucleated, with eosinophilic granular cytoplasm and few mitoses. Fibrous masses divide the sheets of neoplastic cells into compartments of different sizes, producing an organoid pattern. Masses of amyloid scattered among the cells or in the stroma may become calcified (Fig. 98-4*B*).

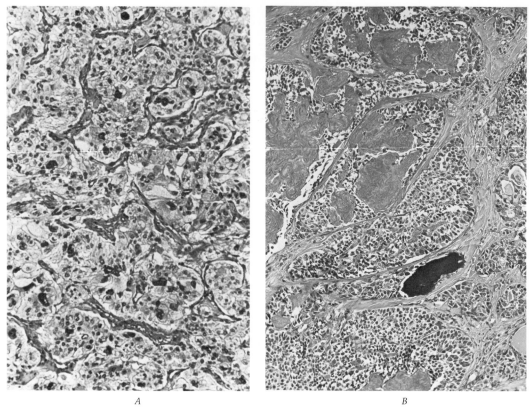

A *B*

Figure 98-4. (*A*). Pheochromocytoma consisting of polyhedral cells separated by thin connective tissue septa, rich in blood vessels. (*B*). Medullary carcinoma of thyroid. Sheets of round to spindle-shaped cells among which there are masses of amyloid. (*From G. H. Friedell,* Cancer **15:**241, 1962.)

Medullary carcinoma of the thyroid comprises about 6 to 10 percent of thyroid cancer. It arises from parafollicular cells which have their origin in the embryonic ultimobranchial body, which in turn is derived at least in part from the neural crest (10, 13, 15, 22). In addition to elaborating calcitonin, medullary thyroid carcinoma may produce serotonin, 5-hydroxyindole acetic acid, histaminase, various prostaglandins, dopa decarboxylase, and an ACTH-like peptide (1a, 15, 38).

The tumor occurs with equal frequency in both sexes and tends to spread through the lymphatic vessels to the cervical lymph nodes and mediastinum. Multiple tumors often arise simultaneously within the same or different lobes of the thyroid gland.

Medullary carcinoma of the thyroid has been diagnosed in over 85 percent of patients with the syndrome. Most of these patients have been between eighteen and twenty-five years of age at the time of initial appearance of the tumor. Rarely has the tumor become clinically manifest before the twelfth year of life.

Gastrointestinal tract. Many patients have some intestinal complaint: persistent diarrhea, megacolon, diverticulosis. Histopathologic study has revealed intestinal ganglioneuromatosis. Rectal carcinoid has also been found (11a).

Musculoskeletal alterations. At least 75 percent of patients have exhibited an asthenic or somewhat Marfanoid build with severe muscular wasting, especially of the extremities, simulating a myopathic state (6a, 8, 9, 15, 19, 20, 24,

27, 28, 37). A host of skeletal alterations has been noted: pes cavum, severe lordosis, aseptic necrosis of the lumbar spine, kyphosis, scoliosis, and increased mobility of joints (Fig. 98-5). These have been reviewed by Gorlin and Mirkin (15). Mandibular prognathism has been noted in several patients (20a).

Other findings. Melanotic skin pigmentation has been reported, possibly reflecting elaboration of an MSH-like peptide (10a, 32).

DIFFERENTIAL DIAGNOSIS

Pheochromocytoma may be observed as an isolated tumor or as an autosomal dominant trait. The tumor is also associated with *neurofibromatosis* in about 5 percent of cases of the latter. It may also be seen with von Hippel-Lindau syndrome and with various brain tumors including cerebellar hemangioblastoma, ependymoma, astrocytoma, meningioma, and spongioblastoma. Medullary carcinoma of the thyroid may occur as an isolated tumor or as an autosomal dominant trait. The binary combination of pheochromocytoma and medullary carcinoma of the thyroid (Sipple syndrome) is known to follow an autosomal dominant mode of transmission. Some cases have been noted to have parathyroid adenomas in addition. In most cases these are secondary to medullary carcinoma of the thyroid—the calcitonin "driving" the parathyroid gland into producing an adenoma. In a few instances, parathyroid adenoma has been noted to precede the medullary carcinoma of the thyroid or to occur without medullary carcinoma of the thyroid at all, suggesting a more primary pleiotropic effect as the cause of the adenoma in these cases. It is possible that in such instances we are dealing with a separate nosologic entity (16, 17, 34).

LABORATORY AIDS

Elevated calcitonin levels may be expected if medullary carcinoma of the thyroid is present (4, 11) even if the tumor is clinically inapparent.

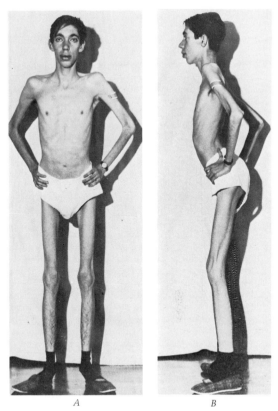

A   *B*

Figure 98-5. (*A, B*). Asthenic body build with muscle wasting and lumbar lordosis. (*From M. Levy et al.,* Arch. Fr. Pédiatr. **27:**561, 1970.)

Both serum and urinary assays are available (4). The pentagastrin stimulation test seems to be an effective technique for producing maximum calcitonin secretion (33a). Intradermal injection of 1 : 1,000 histamine produces a wheal but no flare in patients with medullary carcinoma of the thyroid, a finding which, in our opinion, is not related to its high histaminase content (3, 14) since normal flare response does not return following tumor removal.

Increased vanilmandelic acid production occurs with pheochromocytoma (7). Occasionally, egg-shell calcification signifies a pheochromocytoma (18). Adrenal enlargement is usually noted on perirenal air insufflation studies.

REFERENCES

1 Anderson, T. E., et al., Roentgen Findings in Intestinal Ganglioneuromatosis: Its Association with Medullary Thyroid Carcinoma and Pheochromocytoma. *Radiology* **101**:93–96, 1971.

1a Atkins, F. L., et al. Dopa Decarboxylase in Medullary Carcinoma of the Thyroid. *N. Engl. J. Med.* **289**:545–548, 1973.

2 Bartlett, A., et al., A Neuropolyendocrine Syndrome: Mucosal Neuromas, Pheochromocytoma and Medullary Thyroid Carcinoma. *Oral Surg.* **31**:206–220, 1971.

3 Baum, J. L., Histamine Test in Pheochromocytoma, Medullary Thyroid Carcinoma Syndrome. *N. Engl. J. Med.* **284**:963–964, 1971.

4 Baylin, S. B., et al., Elevated Histaminase Activity in Medullary Carcinoma of the Thyroid Gland. *N. Engl. J. Med.* **283**:1239–1244, 1970.

5 Bazex, A., and Dupré, A., Neuromes myéliniques muqueux à localisation centrofaciale et laryngée-neuromes des lèvres, de la langue, des paupières, des narines, du larynx (entité nouvelle?). *Ann. Dermatol. Syphiligr.* (Paris) **85**:613–641, 1958.

6 Braley, A. E., Medullated Corneal Nerves and Plexiform Neuromas Associated with Pheochromocytoma. *Trans. Am. Ophthalmol. Soc.* **52**:189–197, 1954.

6a Brown, R. S., et al., The Syndrome of Multiple Mucosal Neuromas and Medullary Carcinoma of the Thyroid in Childhood. *J. Pediatr.* **86**:77–83, 1975.

7 Brown, W. G., et al., Vanilmandelic Acid Screening Test for Pheochromocytoma and Neuroblastoma. *Am. J. Clin. Pathol.* **46**:599–602, 1966.

8 Calmettes, L., et al., Manifestations oculo-palpébrales des neuromes myéliniques muqueux. *Arch. Ophthalmol.* **19**:257–269, 1959.

9 Cernea, P., et al., Neuromes myéliniques muqueux de la cavité buccale. *Rev. Stomatol.* (Paris) **68**:103–116, 1967.

10 Chibon, P., Capacité de régulation des excédents dans la crête neurale d'Amphibien. *J. Embryol. Exp. Morphol.* **24**:479–496, 1970.

10a Cunliffe, W. J., et al., A Calcitonin Secreting Medullary Thyroid Carcinoma Associated with Mucosal Neuromas, Marfanoid Features, Myopathy and Pigmentation. *Am. J. Med.* **48**:120–126, 1970.

11 Dubé, W. J., et al., Thyrocalcitonin Activity in Metastatic Medullary Thyroid Carcinoma: Further Evidence for Its Parafollicular Cell Origin. *Arch. Intern. Med.* **123**:423–427, 1969.

11a Dunn, E. L., et al., Medullary Carcinoma of the Thyroid Gland. *Surgery* **73**:848–858, 1973.

12 Froboese, C., Das aus markhaltigen Nervenfascern bestehende, ganglienzellenlose echte Neurom in Rankenform—zugleich ein Beitrag zu den nervösen Geschwülsten der Zunge und des Augenlides. *Virchows Arch. Pathol. Anat.* **240**:312–327, 1923 (same as Wagenmann).

13 Gonzalez-Licea, A., et al., Medullary Carcinoma of the Thyroid, Ultrastructural Evidence of its Origin from the Parafollicular Cell and Its Possible Relation to Carcinoid Tumors. *Am. J. Clin. Pathol.* **49**:512–520, 1968.

14 Gorlin, R. J., Skin Test for Medullary Thyroid Carcinoma. *N. Engl. J. Med.* **284**:983–984, 1971.

15 Gorlin, R. J., and Mirkin, B., Multiple Mucosal Neuromas, Medullary Carcinoma of the Thyroid, Pheochromocytoma and Marfanoid Body Build with Muscle Wasting. *Z. Kinderheilkd.*, **113**:313–325, 1972.

16 Gorlin, R. J., and Vickers, R. A., Multiple Mucosal Neuromas, Pheochromocytoma, Medullary Carcinoma of the Thyroid and Marfanoid Body Build with Muscle Wasting: Reexamination of a Syndrome of Neural Crest Malmigration. *Birth Defects* **7**(6):69–72, 1971.

17 Gorlin, R. J., et al., Multiple Mucosal Neuromas, Pheochromocytoma and Medullary Carcinoma of the Thyroid. A Syndrome. *Cancer* **22**:293–299, 1968.

18 Grainger, R. G., et al., Egg-shell Calcification: A Sign of Pheochromocytoma. *Clin. Radiol.* **18**:282–286, 1967.

19 Grandbois, J., and Tchou, P. K., Mucous Membrane Manifestations of Neurofibromatosis with Malignant Tumors of Endocrine Glands. *Cutis* **5**:1235–1239, 1969.

20 Jacobi, H., and Kleine-Natrop, H. E., Beitrag zum Syndrom der angeborenen fibrillaren Neurome. *Dermatol. Monatschr.* **156**:644–652, 1970.

20a Khairi, M. R., et al., Mucosal Neuroma, Pheochromocytoma and Medullary Thyroid Carcinoma: Multiple Endocrine Neoplasia, Type 3. *Medicine* **54**:89–112, 1975.

20b Kilp, H., and Walzer, P., Ein Neurolemmom der Bindehaut und der Lider mit Veranderungen der Zunge und des Nasenraumes. *Klin. Monatsbl. Augenheilkd.* **162**:251–254, 1973.

21 Koke, M. P., and Braley, A. E., Bilateral Plexiform Neuromata of the Conjunctiva and Medullated Corneal Nerves. *Am. J. Ophthalmol.* **23**:179–182, 1940 (same as Van Epps et al.).

22 Le Dourin, N., and Le Lièvre, C., Démonstration de l'origine neurale des cellules à calcitonine du corps ultimobranchial chez l'embryon de poulet. *C. R. Acad. Sci.* [D] (Paris) **270**:2857–2860, 1970.

23 Levin, D. L., et al., Medullary Carcinoma of the Thyroid Gland: The Complete Syndrome in a Child. *Pediatrics* **52**:192–196, 1973.

24 Levy, M., et al., Neuromatose et épithélioma à stroma amyloïde de la thyroïde chez l'enfant. *Arch. Fr. Pédiatr.* **27**:561–583, 1970.

25 Ljungberg, O., et al., Medullary Thyroid Carcinoma and Pheochromocytoma—a Familial Chromaffinomatosis. *Br. Med. J.* **1**:279–281, 1967.

26 Loos, F., Über doppelseitige Neurofibromatosis der Lider, Konjunctiva und Kornea, der Lippen und der Zunge. *Klin. Monatsbl. Augenheilkd.* **89**:184–189, 1932.

26a Marks, A. D., and Channick, B. J., Extra-adrenal Pheochromocytoma and Medullary Thyroid Carcinoma with Pheochromocytoma. *Arch. Intern. Med.* **134**:1106–1112, 1974.

27 Michalowski, R., Multiple fibrilläre Neurome der Augenlider, Lippen und Zunge mit Genitalhypoplasie und Gelenkanomalien. Beitrag zur Kenntnis der centro-facialen Neuromatosis. *Arch. Klin. Exp. Dermatol.* **231**:20–27, 1967.

28 Mielke, J. E., et al., Diverticulitis of the Colon in a Young Man with Marfan's Syndrome—Associated with Carcinoma of the Thyroid Gland and Neurofibromas of the

Tongue and Lips. *Gastroenterology* **48**:379–382, 1965.

29 Normann, T., and Otnes, B., Intestinal Ganglioneuromatosis: Diarrhea and Medullary Thyroid Carcinoma. *Scand. J. Gastroenterol.* **4**:553–559, 1969.

30 Rappaport, H. M., Neurofibromatosis of the Oral Cavity. *Oral Surg.* **6**:599–604, 1953.

31 Ruppert, R. D., et al., Pheochromocytoma, Neurofibromatosis and Thyroid Carcinoma. *Metabolism* **15**:537–541, 1966.

32 Schimke, R. N., et al., Syndrome of Bilateral Pheochromocytoma, Medullary Thyroid Carcinoma and Multiple Neuromas: A Possible Regulatory Defect in the Differentiation of Chromaffin Tissues. *N. Engl. J. Med.* **279**:1–7, 1968.

33 Schocket, E., and Teloh, H. A., Aganglionic Megacolon, Pheochromocytoma, Megaloureter and Neurofibroma: Co-occurrence of Several Neural Abnormalities. *Am. J. Dis. Child.* **94**:185–191, 1957.

33a Sizemore, G. W., and Go, V. L. W., Stimulation Tests for Diagnosis of Medullary Thyroid Carcinoma. *Mayo Clin. Proc.* **50**:53–56, 1975.

34 Steiner, A. L., et al., Study of a Kindred with Pheochromocytoma, Medullary Thyroid Carcinoma, Hyperparathyroidism and Cushing's Disease. Multiple Endocrine Neoplasms, Type 2. *Medicine* **47**:371–410, 1968.

35 Sturtz, G. S., and Brown, R. B., Medullary Carcinoma of the Thyroid: Bumpy Lip Syndrome. *Clin. Pediatr.* **10**:81–85, 1971.

36 Thies, W., Multiple echte fibrilläre Neurome (Rankenneurome) der Haut und Schleimhaut. *Arch. Klin. Exp. Dermatol.* **218**:561–573, 1964.

37 Van Epps, E. F., et al., Clinical Manifestations of Paroxysmal Hypertension Associated with Pheochromocytoma of Adrenal. *Arch. Intern. Med.* **65**:1123–1129, 1940.

38 Voelkel, E. F., et al., Concentrations of Calcitonin and Catecholamines in Pheochromocytomas, a Mucosal Neuroma and Medullary Thyroid Carcinoma. *J. Clin. Endocrinol. Metab.* **37**:297–307, 1973.

39 Wagenmann, A., Multiple Neurome des Auges und der Zunge. *Ber. Dtsch. Ophthalmol. Ges.* **43**:282–285, 1922.

40 Walker, D. M., Oral Mucosal Neuroma – Medullary Thyroid Carcinoma Syndrome. *Br. J. Dermatol.* **88**:599–604, 1973.

41 Williams, E. D., and Pollock, D. J., Multiple Mucosal Neuromata with Endocrine Tumors – a Syndrome Allied to von Recklinghausen's Disease. *J. Pathol. Bacteriol.* **91**:71–80, 1966.

99

Multiple Nevoid Basal Cell
Carcinoma Syndrome

The syndrome consists principally of (a) multiple nevoid basal cell carcinomas, (b) cysts of the jaws, (c) vertebral and rib anomalies, and (d) intracranial calcification.

It was possibly described first by Jarisch (18) in 1894, but there is evidence that the syndrome existed even in early Egyptian times (29). Early American reports are those of Binkley and Johnson (2), Howell and Caro (17), and Gorlin and Goltz (11). Extremely comprehensive reviews are those of Gorlin and Sedano (12) and Rittersma (28).

The syndrome clearly exhibits autosomal dominant inheritance. Its incidence has not been firmly established, but probably is present in about 0.5 percent of patients with basal cell carcinoma. In over 100 publications, approximately 250 individuals have been described.

SYSTEMIC MANIFESTATIONS

Facies. Frontal and temporoparietal bossing, giving the skull a somewhat pagetoid appearance, and increased cranial circumference are frequent. The eyes may appear widely separated. About 40 percent of patients appear to have true ocular hypertelorism. Several patients have exhibited mild mandibular prognathism (Fig. 99-1*A*, *B*).

Skin. Multiple nevoid basal cell carcinomas usually appear in childhood, more frequently between puberty and the 35th year but occurring as early as the second year of life, and most often involve, in decreasing order of frequency, the face and neck, back and thorax, and abdomen and upper extremities. They appear as papules, varying from flesh-colored to pale brown (Fig. 99-2), 1 mm to 1 cm in diameter.

It should be emphasized that in large kindreds carefully examined for all stigmata, only about half the affected individuals twenty years or older manifest skin tumors (9).

Microscopically, the tumors cannot be differentiated from ordinary basal cell carcinomas. Multiple lesions taken from the skin of a single patient have covered a wide spectrum: superficial, multicentric, pigmented, solid, cystic, adenoid, and lattice-like, resembling the fibroepithelioma of Pinkus (21).

Cysts of the skin vary in size from minute milia common to the face, to those 1 to 2 cm in size, more often found on the extremities. They are found in most patients who are carefully examined. Several authors have described chalazion and comedones.

Palmar-plantar pits have been noted in over 60 percent of cases and have been well illustrated microscopically by Pollitzer (26) and Zackheim et al. (41). They may also occur on the dorsa and sides of the fingers and toes. Transmission and scanning electron microscopic studies have demonstrated normal cornified cells but an increased number of basal cells, a reduction of desmosomal attachments, lumpy tonofilament

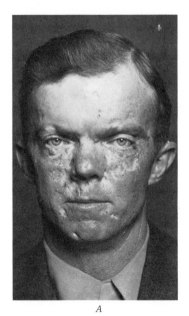
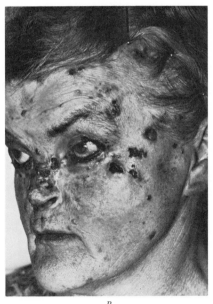

A   *B*

Figure 99-1. (*A*). *Multiple nevoid basal cell carcinoma syndrome.* Facies is characterized by frontal and temporoparietal bossing, apparent ocular hypertelorism, numerous basal cell skin cancers. (*Courtesy of W. D. Maddox, Thesis, University of Minnesota*, 1963.) (*B*). Numerous basal cell carcinomas. (*From U. Berendes, Hautarzt* **22**:261, 1971.)

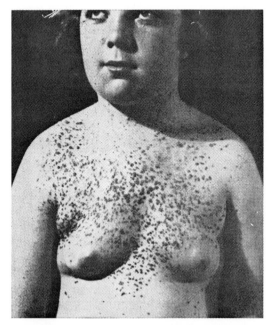

Figure 99-2. Multiple nevoid basal cell carcinomas scattered over chest. (*From J. B. Howell and M. R. Caro,* Arch. Dermatol. **79**:67, 1959.)

fibrils, formation of plasmalemmal microvilli, and a disturbance in the maturation of keratohyaline granules and keratinosomes (39, 41). Basal cell carcinomas have occurred on the palms or soles in a few cases, developing at the base of the pits (16).

Musculoskeletal anomalies. Skeletal anomalies are common, being present in 60 to 75 percent of patients. Among the more common abnormalities are splayed and/or bifurcated rib (in ca. 40 percent of cases). Bifurcation may involve several ribs and may be bilateral (Fig. 99-3). Other costal anomalies include synostosis, partial agenesis, pseudoarthrosis, and cervical rudimentary ribs (22).

Kyphoscoliosis has been observed in at least 50 percent of affected individuals. Cervical and/or upper thoracic vertebral fusion or lack of segmentation have also been noted (22, 23), as well as bridging of the vertebral sulcus of the atlas (28). Spina bifida occulta also commonly (in about 40 percent of patients) involves these same vertebras.

The Sprengel deformity and medial hooking or dysplasia of the scapulas have been noted (12, 20a). Pectus excavatum and carinatum have also been described but possibly are the result of

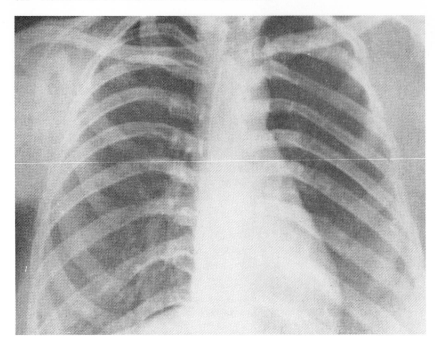

Figure 99-3. Bilateral bifurcation of ribs in thirty-eight-year-old woman. This patient, her mother, and three of her five children had the syndrome.

kyphoscoliosis which, as noted earlier, occurs in at least half of the affected (8).

Shortened metacarpals, especially the fourth, have been seen by several authors (5). It should be noted, however, that about 10 percent of the normal population has a positive metacarpal sign (4). Other low-frequency anomalies have included polydactyly, arachnodactyly, hallux valgus, minor cortical defects of long bones, and bilateral syndactyly of the second and third fingers.

Frontal bossing has already been mentioned. It is usually combined with biparietal bossing, producing a head circumference in adults of approximately 60 cm or more. Broadened nasal root has been noted in at least one-fourth of these patients and may exist without increased distance between inner canthi or without increased distance between the pupils.

Bridging of the sella has been stated to occur in 60 to 80 percent of patients (23, 28), a far higher incidence than in the normal population (about 4 percent).

Of considerable interest is the Marfanoid build or unusually great height attained by several of these patients (12).

Central nervous system. The roentgenographic appearance of the calcification found in nearly all patients with the syndrome is quite different from that noted in the normal population. Its lamellar appearance, with one or more flat sheets, is quite distinctive and usually extends more widely than that in the normal individual (Fig. 99-4). The lamellar form of calcification has also been seen in patients with profound disturbances of calcium and phosphorus metabolism.

Congenital communicating hydrocephaly was noted by a number of authors (10, 12, 28). It has not, however, been established in all cases that this simply represents an abnormality of cranial shape. Kahn and Gordon (19) and Taylor et al. (37) described cysts of the choroid plexus of the third and lateral ventricles and glial nodules projecting into the walls of the lateral ventricles.

Medulloblastoma, which has usually appeared during the first two years of life, has been observed in some patients (12, 15). It would seem likely that medulloblastoma is not commonly recognized as a manifestation of the syndrome, since the affected child usually died of the tumor prior to the development of the rest of

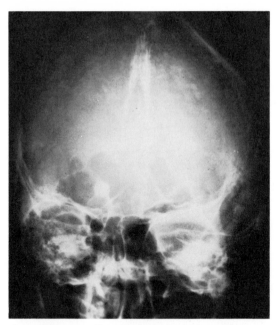

Figure 99-4. Lamellar calcification of falx cerebri.

the syndrome. The number of cases of the disorder having associated medulloblastoma is far too small from which to draw conclusions concerning comparative behavior of the brain tumor. The odds of 1 per 600,000 population for this brain tumor make its occurrence by chance highly unlikely. Meningioma has also been found (34).

Anosmia has been described in one family (40).

Eye. Congenital blindness due to corneal opacity, cataract, glaucoma, and/or coloboma of the choroid and optic nerve, and convergent or divergent strabismus have been recorded by several investigators (5, 12, 40).

Endocrine system. Ovarian fibromas and/or cysts with ovarian or uterine calcification have been noted in a number of cases. Several authors (5, 12, 40) have reported hypogonadism, cryptorchism, missing testicle, female pubic escutcheon in males, and gynecomastia and/or scanty facial hair. Ovarian fibrosarcoma has also been noted (28).

Oral anomalies. Jaw cysts occur in 65 to 75 percent of patients. They have been classified as odontogenic keratocysts. Often appearing initially during the first decade of life, they have been the chief source of complaint in about half the cases. They are scattered throughout both jaws but are about twice as common in the mandible and occur most often in the third molar and canine areas. They vary in size from microscopic to several centimeters in diameter, occasionally being so large as to produce pathologic fracture (Fig. 99-5A, B).

The larger cysts may contain a displaced tooth, may bulge the anterior wall of the maxilla, and may cause elevation of the infraorbital rim. Maxillary teeth may often be displaced immediately beneath the orbit. Following removal, the cysts commonly (in about 40 percent of cases) recur.

Microscopically, the uninfected cyst is lined by a monotonously uniform stratified squamous epithelium covered by keratin or more often parakeratin (Fig. 99-5C). This type of cyst has been designated as "primordial" by Shear (33) and as "odontogenic keratocyst" by Philipsen (24). Some cysts exhibit budding, which may produce further cysts in some instances, and it is likely that some tendency exists for the transformation of these cysts to ameloblastoma (7, 12, 13, 21, 25, 38) or squamous cell carcinoma. Multiple microcysts occur in about 25 percent of cases. Serial sections of keratocysts suggest origin from overlying epithelium (34a).

Fibrosarcoma of the palate or maxillary antrum has been noted in several cases (2, 17, 27, 36). A highly undifferentiated tumor which was called "carcinoma" was noted by Shapiro (32).

Cleft of the lip and/or palate has been seen in several cases (13).

Other findings. Lymphatic cysts of the mesentery of the small intestine has been reported (13). Congenital rhabdomyosarcoma of the anterior chest wall was noted by Schweisguth et al. (31), and one of the authors (R. J. G.). Isolated neurofibroma has also been seen.

Multiple leiomyomas, 0.1 to 3.0 cm in diameter, were distributed over the mesentery of the intestine and beneath the diaphragm in an infant described by Kahn and Gordon (19). Leiomyomas of the esophagus were noted on postmortem examination by Taylor et al. (37).

DIFFERENTIAL DIAGNOSIS

The jaw cysts, if few in number, may be mistaken for conventional dentigerous cysts or isolated keratocysts. Multiple jaw cysts and falx calcification have been noted in association with Charcot-Marie-Tooth disease (35). We have learned (personal communication, 1975) that several of this kindred now manifest typical multiple nevoid basal cell carcinoma syndrome. Dystopia canthorum and mild mandibular prognathism are also seen in the *Waardenburg syndrome*. The incidence of bifid rib, rudimentary rib, and synostosis of ribs unassociated with this syndrome appears to be 6.2, 2.0, and 2.6, respec-

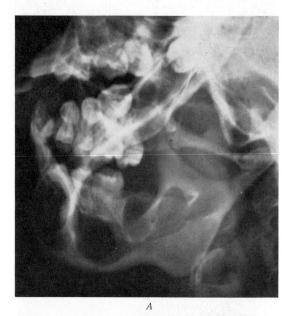

A

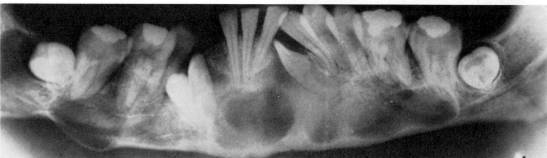

B

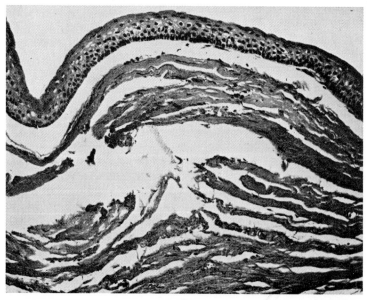

C

Figure 99-5. (*A*). Multiple cysts scattered throughout both jaws. (*From R. J. Gorlin et al.*, Cancer **18**:89, 1965.) (*B*). Extensive involvement of mandible with multiple cysts. (*From J. Mills and J. Foulkes*, Br. J. Radiol. **40**:366, 1967.) (*C*). Photomicrograph of odontogenic keratocyst from forty-year-old female.

tively, per 1,000 live births. The shortened fourth metacarpals and calcification of several organs may suggest *pseudohypoparathyroidism*.

LABORATORY AIDS

Multiple basal cell carcinomas arising in childhood should arouse the suspicion of the observer and should suggest roentgenographic study of the jaws, chest, and spinal column.

Absence of significant phosphorus diuresis (Ellsworth-Howard test) following intravenous injection of parathormone has been noted by some authors [3] but is vigorously denied by Kaufman and Chase [20]. We heartily concur with the latter finding.

Happle and Hoehn [14] found an increased frequency of spontaneous chromosome breaks in fibroblasts from uninvolved skin.

REFERENCES

1 Anderson, D. B., et al., The Nevoid Basal Cell Carcinoma Syndrome. *Am. J. Hum. Genet.* **19**:12–22, 1967.

2 Binkley, G. W., and Johnson, H. H., Jr., Epithelioma Adenoides Cysticum: Basal Cell Nevi, Agenesis of Corpus Callosum and Dental Cysts. *Arch. Dermatol. Syph. (Chic.)* **63**:73–84, 1951.

3 Block, J. B., and Clendenning, W. E., Parathyroid Hormone Hyporesponsiveness in Patients with Basal-cell Nevi and Bone Defects. *N. Engl. J. Med.* **268**:1157–1162, 1963.

4 Bloom, R. A., The Metacarpal Sign. *Br. J. Radiol.* **43**:133–135, 1970.

5 Cernéa, P., et al., Naevomatose baso-cellulaire. *Rev. Stomatol. (Paris)* **70**:181–226, 1969.

6 Clendenning, W. E., et al., Ovarian Fibromas and Mesenteric Cysts; Their Association with Hereditary Basal Cell Cancer of Skin. *Am. J. Obstet. Gynecol.* **87**:1008–1012, 1963.

7 Davidson, F., Multiple Naevoid Basal Cell Carcinomata and Associated Congenital Abnormalities. *Br. J. Dermatol.* **74**:439–444, 1962.

8 van Dijk, E., and Sanderink, J. F. H., Basal Cell Nevus Syndrome. *Dermatologica* **134**:101–106, 1967.

9 Gilhuus-Moe, O., et al., The Syndrome of Multiple Cysts of the Jaws, Basal Cell Carcinomata and Skeletal Anomalies. *Br. J. Oral Surg.* **5**:211–222, 1968.

10 Gorlin, R. J., et al., The Multiple Basal-cell Nevi Syndrome: An Analysis of a Syndrome Consisting of Multiple Nevoid Basal-cell Carcinoma, Jaw Cysts, Skeletal Anomalies, Medulloblastoma, and Hyporesponsiveness to Parathormone. *Cancer* **18**:89–104, 1965.

11 Gorlin, R. J., and Goltz, R. W., Multiple Nevoid Basal-cell Epithelioma, Jaw Cysts and Bifid Rib Syndrome. *N. Engl. J. Med.* **262**:908–912, 1960.

12 Gorlin, R. J., and Sedano, H. O., The Multiple Nevoid Basal Cell Carcinoma Syndrome Revisited. *Birth Defects* **7**(8): 140–148, 1972.

13 Happle, R., Naevobasaliom und Ameloblastom. *Hautarzt* **24**:290–294, 1973.

14 Happle, R., and Hoehn, H., Cytogenetic Studies on Cultured Fibroblast-like cells Derived from Basal Cell Carcinoma Tissue. *Clin. Genet.* **4**:17–24, 1973.

15 Herzberg, J. J., and Wiskemann, A., Die fünfte Phakomatose, Basalzellnaevus mit familiärer Belastung und Medulloblastom. *Dermatologica* **126**:106–173, 1963.

16 Holubar, K., et al., Multiple Basal Cell Epitheliomas in Basal Cell Nevus Syndrome. *Arch. Dermatol.* **101**: 679–682, 1970.

17 Howell, J. B., and Caro, M. R., Basal-cell Nevus: Its Relationship to Multiple Cutaneous Cancers and Associated Anomalies of Development. *Arch. Dermatol.* **79**:67–80, 1959.

18 Jarisch, —, Zur Lehre von den Hautgeschwülsten. *Arch. Dermatol. Syph. (Berl.)* **28**:163–222, 1894.

19 Kahn, L. B., and Gordon, W., Basal Cell Naevus Syndrome. *S. Afr. Med. J.* **41**:832–835, 1967.

20 Kaufman, R., and Chase, L. R., Basal Cell Nevus Syndrome: Normal Responsiveness to Parathyroid Hormone. *Birth Defects* **7**(8):149–155, 1972.

20a Kozlowski, K., et al., Multiple Nevoid Basal Cell Carcinoma Syndrome. *Pediatr. Radiol.* **2**:185–190, 1974.

21 Maddox, W. D., et al., Multiple Nevoid Basal Cell Epitheliomata, Jaw Cysts and Skeletal Defects. *J.A.M.A.* **188**:106–111, 1964.

22 McEvoy, B. F., and Gatzek, H., Multiple Nevoid Basal Cell Carcinoma Syndrome. Radiologic Manifestations. *Br. J. Radiol.* **42**:24–28, 1969.

23 Mills, J., and Foulkes, J., Gorlin's Syndrome: A Radiologic and Cytogenetic Study of 9 Cases. *Br. J. Radiol.* **40**:366–371, 1967.

24 Philipsen, H. P., Om keratocyster (kolesteatomer) i kaeberne. *Tandlaegebladet* **60**:963–980, 1956.

25 Pollard, J. J., and New, P. F. J., Hereditary Cutaneomandibular Polyoncosis: A Syndrome of Myriad Basal Cell Nevi of the Skin, Mandibular Cysts, and Inconstant Skeletal Anomalies. *Radiology* **82**:840–849, 1964.

26 Pollitzer, J., Eine eigentümliche Karzinose der Haut (Carcinoderma pigmentosum-Lang) nebenher: punkt- und strichförmige Defekte im Hornstratum der Palmae und Plantae. *Arch. Dermatol. Syph. (Berl.)* **76**:323–345, 1905.

27 Reed, J. C., Nevoid Basal Cell Carcinoma Syndrome with Associated Fibrosarcoma of the Maxilla. *Arch. Dermatol.* **97**:304–306, 1968.

28 Rittersma, J., Het basocellulaire nevus syndroom. Thesis, Gröningen, 1972.

29 Ryan, D. E., and Burkes, E. J., The Multiple Basal-cell Nevus Syndrome in a Negro Family. *Oral Surg.* **36:**831–840, 1973.

30 Satinoff, M. I., and Wells, C., Multiple Basal Cell Naevus in Ancient Egypt. *Med. Hist.* **13:**294–296, 1969.

31 Schweisguth, O., et al., Naevomatose basocellulaire association à un rhabdomyosarcoma congénital. *Arch. Fr. Pediatr.* **25:**1083–1093, 1968.

32 Shapiro, M. J., Basal Cell Nevus Syndrome: A Case Report with Associated Carcinoma of the Maxilla. *Laryngoscope* **80:**777–787, 1970.

33 Shear, M., Primordial Cysts. *J. Dent. Assoc. S. Afr.* **15:**211–217, 1960.

34 Stoelinga, P., et al., Some New Findings in the Basal Cell Nevus Syndrome. *Oral Surg.* **36:**686–692, 1973.

34a Stoelinga, P., et al., The Origin of Keratocysts in the Basal Cell Nevus Syndrome. *J. Oral Surg.* **33:**675–684, 1975.

35 Swift, M. R., and Horowitz, S. L., Familial Jaw Cysts in Charcot-Marie-Tooth Disease. *J. Med. Genet.* **6:**193–195, 1969.

36 Tamoney, H. J., Jr., Basal Cell Nevoid Syndrome. *Am. Surg.* **35:**279–283, 1969.

37 Taylor, W. B., et al., The Nevoid Basal Cell Carcinoma Syndrome. *Arch. Dermatol.* **98:**612–614, 1968.

38 Thoma, K. H., Polycystoma. *Oral Surg.* **12:**484–488, 1959.

39 Ullman, S., et al., Ultrastructure of Palmar and Plantar Pits in Basal Cell Nevus Syndrome. *Acta Derm. Venereol. (Stockh.)* **52:**329–336, 1972.

40 Wallace, D. C., et al., The Basal Cell Nevus Syndrome: Report of a Family with Anosmia and a Case of Hypogonadotrophic Hypopituitarism. *J. Med. Genet.* **10:**30–33, 1973.

41 Zackheim, H. S., et al., Basal Cell Carcinoma Syndrome. *Arch. Dermatol.* **96:**317–323, 1966.

100

Multiple Pterygium Syndrome

Buried in the literature, most often under the nonspecific diagnosis of arthrogryposis (3, 5, 7, 15) or Bonnevie-Ullrich syndrome (4, 13), is a disorder consisting of (a) growth retardation, (b) multiple pterygia involving the neck, fingers, and antecubital, popliteal, and intercrural areas, and (c) cleft palate. Credit should go to Matolcsy (8) for clearly defining the entity.

Affected sibs (8, 10, 15) as well as parental consanguinity (4) have been reported. The syn-

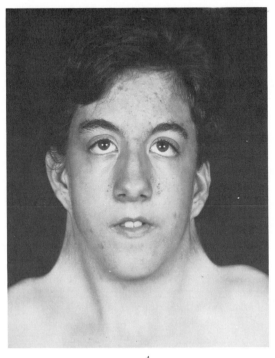
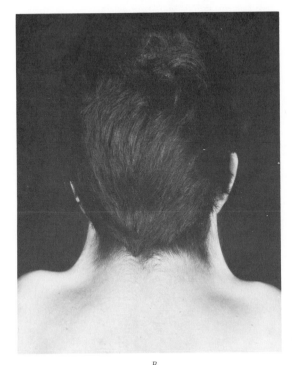

A *B*

Figure 100-1. *Multiple pterygium syndrome.* (*A, B*). Note antimongoloid obliquity of palpebral fissures, pterygium colli, low-set posterior hairline. (*From C. Scott*, Birth Defects **5**(2):231, 1969.)

drome appears to have autosomal recessive inheritance.

SYSTEMIC MANIFESTATIONS

Facies. The palpebral fissures often have mild antimongoloid obliquity, and frequently there is mild ptosis of the lids (Fig. 100-1).

Musculoskeletal alterations. Growth is usually retarded below the 3d percentile, the patient's adult height rarely exceeding 135 cm.

The popliteal pterygia may markedly inhibit walking (8) and, even if only mild, produce a bizarre stance and gait. Pterygia in the cervical area may resemble those in the Turner and Noonan syndromes. Rarely, they may com-

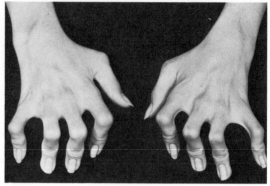

Figure 100-3. Marked flexion deformity of digits. (*From C. Scott*, Birth Defects **5**(2):231, 1969.)

pletely surround the neck (11) (Fig. 100-2). There is often mild soft-tissue syndactyly between the fingers and flexion deformity of the digits, the thumbs being flexed and apposed (1, 3, 6, 10, 14) (Fig. 100-3).

Intercrural webs may be present in both males and females. In the former, the penis and scrotum are retropositioned. This may be associated with cryptorchism (8, 11) and inguinal hernia (10). The labia majora may be absent (1).

Talipes equinovarus, either unilateral or bilateral, has been noted (1, 2, 4, 6, 11), as well as rocker bottom feet [due to vertical talus] (1, 10, 14) and scoliosis and other rib and vertebral anomalies (1, 7, 13).

Oral manifestations. Cleft palate has been found in most affected patients (2, 4, 6, 7, 9, 15).

DIFFERENTIAL DIAGNOSIS

Pterygia about the neck may be seen in the *Turner syndrome*, the *leopard syndrome*, and the *Noonan syndrome*. Pashayan et al. (12) described the multiple pterygium syndrome in a patient with mosaic Klinefelter syndrome who also exhibited cataract and glaucoma.

LABORATORY AIDS

None is known.

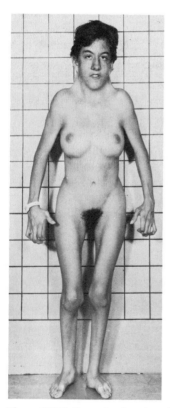

Figure 100-2. Pterygia of neck, axillas, and popliteal areas present. (*From C. Scott*, Birth Defects **5**(2):231, 1969.)

REFERENCES

1 Aarskog, D., Pterygium Syndrome. *Birth Defects* **7**(6):232–234, 1971.

2 Bettman, A. G., Congenital Bands about the Shoulder Girdle. *Plast. Reconstr. Surg.* **1**:205–215, 1946.

3 Gorlin, R. J., and Pindborg, J. J., *Syndromes of the Head and Neck*. McGraw-Hill, New York, 1964, pp. 57–58.

4 Guinand-Doniol, J., Observations nouvelles sur le status Bonnevie-Ullrich (Case 1). *Ann. Paediatr. (Basel)* **169:** 217–234, 1947.

5 Jahn, M., et al., Arthogryposis Multiplex Congenita in a One-month-old Child. *Čs. Pediatr.* **20**:150–153, 1965.

6 Kanof, A., et al., Arthrogryposis: A Clinical and Pathologic Study of Three Cases (Case 1). *Pediatrics* **17**:532–540, 1956.

6a Kroll, W., et al., Beitrag zum Pterygoarthromyodysplasia congenita (Rossi-Syndrom). *Z. Kinderheilkd.* **116**:263–268, 1974.

7 Lang, K., et al., Beitrag zum Bilde der Pterygomyodysplasia arthrogrypotica generalis (Pterygo-Arthromyodysplasia congenita). *Monatsschr. Kinderheilkd.* **108**:248–252, 1960.

8 Matolcsy, T., Über ein chirurgische Behandlung der angeborenen Flughaut. *Arch. Klin. Chir.* **185**:675–681, 1936.

9 McCollum, D. W., Congenital Webbing of the Neck. *N. Engl. J. Med.* **219**:251–254, 1938 (mentioned only).

10 Norum, R. A., et al., Pterygium Syndrome in Three Children in a Recessive Pedigree Pattern. *Birth Defects* **5**(2):233–235, 1969.

11 O'Brien, B., et al., Multiple Congenital Skin Webbing with Cutis Laxa. *Br. J. Plast. Surg.* **23**:329–336, 1970.

12 Pashayan, H., Bilateral Aniridia, Multiple Webs and Severe Mental Retardation in a 47, XXY/48, XXXXY Mosaic. *Clin. Genet.* **4**:126–129, 1973.

13 Rossi, E., and Caflisch, A., Le syndrome du pterygium: Status Bonnevie-Ullrich, dystrophia brevicolli congénita, syndrome de Turner et arthromyodysplasia congénita. *Helv. Paediatr. Acta* **6**:119–148, 1951.

14 Scott, C., Pterygium Syndrome. *Birth Defects* **5**(2): 231–232, 1969.

15 Srivastava, R. N., Arthrogryposis Multiplex Congenita: Case Report of Two Siblings. *Clin. Pediatr.* **7**:691–694, 1968.

101

Myotonic Dystrophy

(Steinert Syndrome)

Myotonic dystrophy, first described by Steinert (46) and Batten and Gibb (2), is characterized by (a) myotonia, (b) progressive muscle wasting, (c) cataracts, (d) hypogonadism, and (e) progressive mental deterioration. Extensive reviews have been provided by Caughey et al. (11) and Pruzanski (40).

The disorder follows an autosomal dominant mode of transmission with complete penetrance and great variation in expression (36, 42). The mutation rate may approach one-third the frequency of affected individuals (7). The incidence has been estimated to range from 1 per 100,000 (45) to 37 per 100,000 (50). Stillbirth and infant mortality rates are high (2, 11, 36). Bunday and Carter (6a) have suggested genetic heterogeneity based on time of onset. The first type has onset in infancy, occasionally after thirty years of age. A second form has its onset from twenty to sixty years and a third type between four and twenty-five years.

Presymptomatic and prenatal detection is feasible, since the gene responsible for myotonic dystrophy is closely linked to the secretor locus (23, 38, 43), the secretor status of the fetus being determined by examination of amniotic fluid (22). While 37.5 percent of matings are theoretically possible for detection by linkage, practically only 5 to 10 percent are detectable (20, 44).

The basic defect originates within muscle and is caused by the association of the aftercontraction with fast repetitive action potentials in af-fected fibers (19). It has been suggested that a disturbance in the ability of the sarcoplasmic reticulum to bind and release calcium occurs, together with disturbed energetics in the muscle fibers (41).

Histologically, both atrophic and swollen muscle fibers are observed in the early stages of the disease. With further degeneration, the site of the fibers is marked solely by long rows of nuclei. These changes may occur in both affected voluntary and involuntary muscle, although they are not always present. Within heart muscle, variability in size of fibers, atrophy, fatty degeneration, and fibrosis have been reported (11, 26, 51).

SYSTEMIC MANIFESTATIONS

The disorder can present protean manifestations, affecting many organ systems. Myotonia usually develops as the first clinical sign. Muscle wasting and weakness are progressive, and there is increasing debility, with death usually occurring during the fifth or sixth decade from cardiac failure, pneumonia, or intercurrent illness.

Although the average age of onset is 27 years (11), recognition of the disorder during infancy has been reported (4, 14, 21). Intrauterine factors may be implicated in these cases, since the mother has almost always been affected (21).

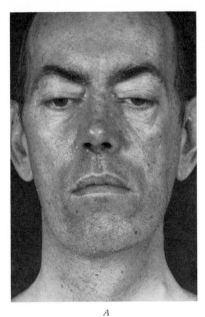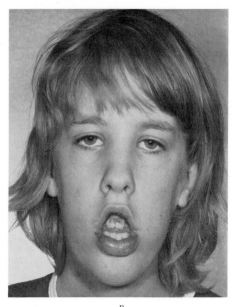

A   *B*

Figure 101-1. *Myotonic dystrophy.* (*A*). Characteristic expressionless face, ptosis of eyelids, temporal and buccal hollows, and slack mandible. (*From H. H. Thayer and J. Crenshaw, J. Am. Dent. Assoc.* **72:**1405, 1966.) (*B*). Compare facies in twelve-year-old girl.

Facies. Progressive atrophy and weakness of facial muscles and muscles of mastication, especially the temporal muscles, produce a narrow, expressionless, masklike facies. Severe wasting of the sternocleidomastoid muscles and exaggerated forward curvature of the neck result in a "swan neck" appearance (11, 40) (Fig. 101-1*A, B*).

Extremities. Wasting of the muscles of the arms, thighs, and anterior lower legs occurs, with progression from proximal to distal. Disturbances of gait and pseudohypertrophy may be observed (24, 40).

Eye. Ptosis of the lids is common. In the early stages of the disease, dustlike blue-green, red, and yellow opacities are localized in the thin zone of the lens cortex and may serve as an aid in presymptomatic detection (20). As the disease progresses, mature cataracts are observed in over 85 percent of patients (13, 39). Other findings may include ophthalmoplegia, blepharitis, keratitis sicca, corneal dystrophy, enoph-

thalmos, microphthalmia, choroidal coloboma, epiphoria, abnormalities of dark adaptation, pigmentary defects of the macula and peripheral retina, and optic atrophy (3, 8, 33, 40).

Hair and skin. Partial alopecia in the frontal and parietal areas may be observed in male patients. Atrophic skin and calcifying epitheliomas of Malherbe may be present (10, 11, 40).

Central nervous system. Hypotonia during infancy has been occasionally recorded. Mental deficiency is common. Various changes, such as persistent morbid cheerfulness, mild grandiosity, lack of initiative, and hypersomia may be noted. Mental deterioration may occur with progression of the disease (2, 35, 37, 40).

Cardiovascular and respiratory systems. Conduction defects with arrhythmias are common (9, 16, 27, 30).

Respiratory distress, pulmonary infection, and chronic pulmonary disease result from weakened chest bellows and inability of the esophagus to empty adequately (18, 40, 52).

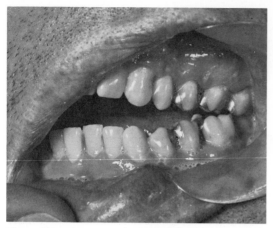

Figure 101-2. Pronounced anterior open bite. (*From H. H. Thayer and J. Crenshaw,* J. Am. Dent. Assoc. **72:**1405, 1966.)

Gastrointestinal tract. Findings may include faulty deglutition with nasal regurgitation of food and spilling of various substances into the bronchial tree, reduced amplitude of peristaltic contractions, esophageal and gastric retention, gastric bezoar, cholelithiasis, abnormal small intestine mobility, dilatation of the colon, malabsorption, steatorrhea, diarrhea, and constipation (18, 25, 29, 31, 34, 47).

Endocrine system. In males, testicular atrophy and pathologic changes similar to those observed in Klinefelter syndrome are common. Decreased urinary excretion of 17-ketosteroids and androgens with an increase in luteinizing hormone has been reported (12, 15, 28). Cryptorchism has been noted in some instances (4, 14, 47). In females, amenorrhea, dysmenorrhea, and ovarian cysts have been reported. Diabetes mellitus, hypothyroidism, and thyroid adenomas have been noted occasionally (11, 40).

Skeletal system. Thickening of the calvaria, hyperostosis frontalis interna, small sella tur-

cica, large paranasal sinuses, ocular hypotelorism, pectus excavatum, kyphoscoliosis, thin ribs in the neonate, and talipes equinovarus have been reported (17, 32, 40, 49).

Other findings. A variety of infrequent abnormalities has been reviewed by Pruzanski (40).

Oral manifestations. Lingual myotonia, resulting in slow, nasal, and indistinct speech, is frequent and, at times, may be the initial sign of the disorder. Retention of saliva in the oral cavity, high dental caries rate, and edentulousness have been reported. Other findings, such as highly arched palate, malocclusion, micrognathia, and prognathism, have been noted in some instances (11, 31, 32, 40) (Fig. 101-2).

DIFFERENTIAL DIAGNOSIS

Myotonia may also be observed in myotonia congenita (Thomsen syndrome), paramyotonia congenita of Eulenburg, generalized myotonia, *osteochondromuscular dystrophy,* Gamstorp-Wohlfart syndrome, and Kok syndrome.

LABORATORY AIDS

Muscle biopsy may be helpful in some cases. Identification of affected individuals before the clinical onset of symptoms is useful for counseling purposes. In this connection, slit lamp examination for "myotonic dust," abnormal electromyographic studies, serum immunoglobulin determinations (decreased IgG and IgM), and insulin secretion studies (excessive insulin response to glucose) may be employed (1, 5, 7, 20, 39, 48, 51) but there is an overlap with normal values (20a). Although not useful as diagnostic aids, a variety of metabolic changes have been reported (40).

REFERENCES

1 Anonymous, Dystrophia Myotonica – Identification of Heterozygotes. *Lancet* **2:**450–451, 1970.
2 Batten, F. E., and Gibb, H. P., Myotonia Atrophica. *Brain* **33:**187–205, 1909.
3 Betten, M. G., et al., Pigmentary Retinopathy of Myotonic Dystrophy. *Am. J. Ophthalmol.* **72:**720–723, 1971.
4 Bell, D. B., and Smith, D. W., Myotonic Dystrophy in the Neonate. *J. Pediatr.* **81:**83–86, 1972.

5 Bird, M., and Tzagournis, M., Insulin Secretion in Myotonic Dystrophy. *Am. J. Med. Sci.* **260:**351–358, 1970.

6 Bundey, S., Detection of Heterozygotes for Myotonic Dystrophy. *Clin. Genet.* **5:**107–109, 1974.

6a Bundey, S., and Carter, C. O., Genetic Heterogeneity for Dystrophia Myotonica. *J. Med. Genet.* **9:**311–315, 1972.

7 Bundey, S., et al., Early Recognition of Heterozygotes for the Gene for Dystrophia Myotonia. *J. Neurol. Neurosurg. Psychiatr.* **33:**279–293, 1970.

8 Burian, H. M., and Burns, C. A., Ocular Changes in Myotonic Dystrophy. *Am. J. Ophthalmol.* **63:**22–34, 1967.

9 Cannon, P. J., The Heart and Lungs in Myotonic Muscular Dystrophy. *Am. J. Med.* **32:**765–775, 1962.

10 Cantwell, A. R., and Reed, W. B., Myotonia Atrophica and Multiple Calcifying Epithelioma of Malherbe. *Acta Derm. Venereol. (Stockh.)* **45:**387–390, 1965.

11 Caughey, J. E., et al., *Dystrophia Myotonica and Related Disorders.* Charles C Thomas, Springfield, Ill., 1963.

12 Clarke, B. B., et al., Myotonia Atrophica with Testicular Atrophy: Urinary Excretion of Interstitial-cell-stimulating (Luteinizing) Hormone, Androgens and 17-Ketosteroids. *J. Clin. Endocrinol.* **16:**1235–1244, 1956.

13 Davidson, S. I., The Eye in Dystrophia Myotonica with a Report on Electromyography of the Extraocular Muscles. *Br. J. Ophthalmol.* **45:**183–196, 1961.

14 Dodge, P. R., et al., Myotonic Dystrophy in Infancy and Childhood. *Pediatrics* **35:**3–19, 1965.

15 Drucker, W. D., et al., The Testis in Myotonic Muscular Dystrophy: A Clinical and Pathologic Study with a Comparison with the Klinefelter Syndrome. *J. Clin. Endocrinol.* **23:**59–75, 1963.

16 Fisch, C., and Evans, P. V., The Heart in Dystrophia Myotonica. *N. Engl. J. Med.* **251:**527–529, 1954.

17 Fried, K., et al., Thin Ribs in Neonatal Myotonic Dystrophy. *Clin. Genet.* **7:**417–420, 1975.

18 Garrett, J. M., et al., Esophageal and Pulmonary Disturbances in Myotonia Dystrophica. *Arch. Intern. Med.* **123:**26–32, 1969.

19 Geschwind, N., and Simpson, J. A., Procaine Amide in the Treatment of Myotonia. *Brain* **78:**81–91, 1955.

20 Harper, P. S., Pre-symptomatic Detection and Genetic Counselling in Myotonic Dystrophy. *Clin. Genet.* **4:**134–140, 1973.

21 Harper, P. S., and P. R. Dyken, Early-onset Dystrophia Myotonica: Evidence Supporting a Maternal Environmental Factor. *Lancet* **2:**53–55, 1972.

22 Harper, P., et al., ABH Secretor Status of the Fetus: A Genetic Marker Identifiable by Amniocentesis. *J. Med. Genet.* **8:**438–440, 1971.

23 Harper, P. S., et al., Genetic Linkage Confirmed between the Locus for Myotonic Dystrophy and the ABH-secretion and Lutheran Blood Group Loci. *Am. J. Hum. Genet.* **24:**310–316, 1972.

24 Harvey, J. C., Myotonic Dystrophica. *Trans. Am. Clin. Climatol. Assoc.* **74:**176–191, 1962.

25 Harvey, J. C., et al., Smooth Muscle Involvement in Myotonic Dystrophy. *Am. J. Med.* **39:**81–90, 1965.

26 Hassin, G. B., and Kesert, B., Myotonia Atrophica: Histologic Considerations. *J. Neuropathol. Exp. Neurol.* **7:**59–64, 1948.

27 Holt, J. M., and Lambert, E. H. N., Heart Disease as the Presenting Feature in Myotonic Atrophica. *Br. Heart J.* **26:**433–436, 1964.

28 Jacobson, W. E., et al., Endocrine Studies in 8 Patients with Dystrophia Myotonica. *J. Clin. Endocrinol.* **15:**801–810, 1955.

29 Kaufman, K. K., and Heckert, E. W., Dystrophia Myotonica with Associated Sprue-like Symptoms. *Am. J. Med.* **16:**614–616, 1954.

30 Kilburn, K. H., et al., Cardiopulmonary Insufficiency Associated with Myotonic Dystrophy. *Am. J. Med.* **26:**929–955, 1959.

31 Kuiper, D. H., Gastric Bezoar in a Patient with Myotonic Dystrophy: A Review of the Gastrointestinal Complications of Myotonic Dystrophy. *Am. J. Dig. Dis.* **16:**529–534, 1971.

32 Lee, K. F., et al., New Roentgenographic Findings in Myotonic Dystrophy, *Am. J. Roentgenol.* **115:**179–185, 1972.

33 Lessell, S., et al., Ophthalmoplegia in Myotonic Dystrophy. *Am. J. Ophthalmol.* **71:**1231–1235, 1971.

34 Ludman, H., Dysphagia in Dystrophia Myotonica. *J. Laryngol.* **76:**234–236, 1962.

35 Maas, O., and Paterson, A. S., Mental Changes in Families Affected by Dystrophia Myotonica. *Lancet* **1:**21–22, 1937.

36 Maas, O., and Paterson, A. S., Genetic and Familial Aspects of Dystrophia Myotonica. *Brain* **66:**55–86, 1943.

37 Maas, O., and Paterson, A. S., Myotonia Congenita, Dystrophia Myotonica and Paramyotonia; Reaffirmation of Their Identity. *Brain* **73:**318–336, 1950.

38 Mohr, J., A Study of Linkage in Man. *Opera Ex Domo Biologiae Hereditariae Humanae Universitatis Hafniensis,* vol. 33. Munksgaard, Copenhagen, 1954.

39 Polgar, J. G., et al., The Early Detection of Dystrophia Myotonica. *Brain* **95:**761–766, 1972.

40 Pruzanski, W., Myotonic Dystrophy—a Multisystem Disease: Report of 67 Cases and a Review of the Literature. *Psychiatr. Neurol. (Basel)* **149:**302–322, 1965.

41 Radu, H., et al., Quantitative Study of the Myotonic State. *Europ. Neurol.* **4:**100–107, 1970.

42 Ravin, A., and Waring, J. J., Studies in Dystrophia Myotonica. I. Hereditary Aspect. *Am. J. Med. Sci.* **197:**593–609, 1939.

43 Renwick, J. H., et al., Confirmation of Linkage of the Loci for Myotonic Dystrophy and ABH Secretion. *J. Med. Genet.* **8:**407–416, 1971.

44 Schrott, H. G., and Omenn, G. S., Myotonic Dystrophy—Opportunities for Prenatal Diagnosis. *Neurology (Minneap.)* **25:**789–791, 1975.

45 Slatt, B., Myotonia Dystrophia: A Review of 17 Cases. *Can. Med. Assoc. J.* **85:**250–261, 1961.

46 Steinert, H., Myopathologische Beitrage: I. Über das klinische und anatomische Bild des Muskelschwundes der Myotoniker, *Dtsch. Z. Nervenheilkd.* **37:**58–104, 1909.

47 Schwindt, W. D., et al., Cholelithiasis and Associated Complications of Myotonia Dystrophica. *Postgrad. Med.* **46:**80–83, 1969.

48 Walsh, J. C., et al., Abnormalities of Insulin Secretion in Dystrophia Myotonica. *Brain* **93:**731–742, 1970.

49 Walton, J. N., and Warrick, C. K., Osseous Changes in Myopathy. *Br. J. Radiol.* **27:**1–15, 1954.

50 Welander, L., Genetic Research in Muscular Disease in Sweden, in *International Congress Series No. 32. Second*

International Conference of Human Genetics, Roma, 1961, p. E88.

51 Wochner, R. O., et al., Accelerated Breakdown of Immunoglobulin G (IgG) in Myotonic Dystrophy: A Hereditary Error in Immunoglobulin Catabolism. *J. Clin. Invest.* **45:**321–329, 1966.

52 Wohlfart, G., Dystrophia Myotonica and Myotonia Congenita. Histopathologic Studies with Special Reference to Changes in the Muscles. *J. Neuropathol. Exp. Neurol.* **10:**109–124, 1951.

102

Neurofibromatosis

(von Recklinghausen Neurofibromatosis)

The syndrome of (a) multiple neurofibromas, (b) cutaneous pigmentation, (c) skeletal anomalies, (d) central nervous system involvement, and (e) predilection to malignancy was classically presented by von Recklinghausen (40) in 1882, although it was described earlier by several authors (5).

The syndrome follows an autosomal dominant mode of transmission, with approximately 50 percent of the cases representing fresh mutations (3). The mutation rate was calculated to be 1×10^{-4} per gamete per generation, the highest rate known in man (11). Genetic aspects of somatic variation and segmental distribution have been discussed by Crowe et al. (11) and by Nicholls (37). Neurofibromatosis appears with a frequency of one case per 2,500 to 3,300 births in the general population and occurs approximately once in 200 mental defectives (11).

The authors object to categorizing the disorder as a neurocutaneous syndrome, because not all defects are attributable to neural crest derivatives. For example, in a careful study, Jaffe (26) found certain bony alterations in the absence of tumors from the region, thus implicating mesenchymal derivatives.

The syndrome has protean manifestations. The complexity of the clinical spectrum is compounded by the fact that the disorder may evolve slowly and may present in a variety of different ways. Over 40 percent of patients demonstrate some manifestations at birth, and over 60 percent by the second year of life (15). Incomplete forms are common and may go unrecognized. A sporadic case without neurofibromas and without the requisite number of cafe-au-lait spots can present great difficulty in diagnosis during childhood.

SYSTEMIC MANIFESTATIONS

Tumors. The most distinctive and common skin tumor is the neurofibroma, especially the plexiform variety (20). Fialkow et al. (14) analyzed neurofibromas from glucose 6-phosphate dehydrogenase A-B heterozygotes and concluded that each tumor had a multiple cell origin, tumorogenesis minimally involving 150 cells.

Tumors may be present at birth or appear during childhood or even later. They vary greatly in size, with localized enlargement of many nerve trunks in larger neurofibromas. They are most striking on the skin, with some patients manifesting hundreds or even thousands of individual neurofibromas and others having large unilateral pendulous masses (Fig. 102-1*A, B*). Many organs may be involved, including stomach, intestine, kidney, bladder, larynx, and heart (4, 6, 7, 13, 15, 18, 30, 43, 47). Neurofibrosarcomatous transformation has been reported in 3 to 12 percent of cases (15, 22, 39).

Schwannomas and fibromas are also known to occur. Meningiomas, neuromas of the cranial nerves (especially optic and acoustic) and spinal nerves, and gliomas (astrocytomas and epen-

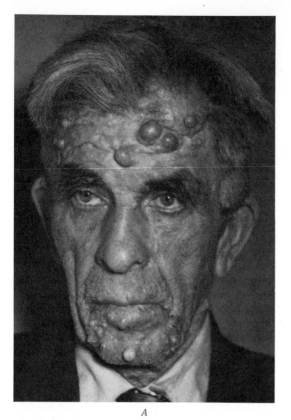
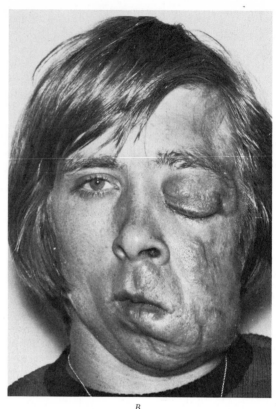

A   *B*

Figure 102-1. *Neurofibromatosis.* (*A*). Patient with hundreds of cutaneous neurofibromas developed a neurofibrosarcoma of the elbow. (*B*). Unilateral neurofibromatosis.
(*From I. Koblin and B. Reil*, J. Maxillofac, Surg. **3**:23, 1975.)

dymomas) have been reported. The incidence of
pheochromocytoma is increased. Various other
low-frequency tumors, both malignant and benign, have been discussed by many authors (5,
6, 11, 12, 15, 20, 21, 24, 29, 36, 44).

Skin. In addition to nodular tumors of the skin,
café-au-lait spots are common, appearing in 90
percent of patients. The smooth-edged pigmented spots usually appear during the first decade, most often preceding the tumors. The color
varies from yellowish to chocolate-brown. Lesions are observed especially on the unexposed
areas of the body (11, 45, 54). The presence of six
or more café-au-lait spots greater than 1.5 cm in
diameter should arouse a strong suspicion of
neurofibromatosis (10, 54). Axillary freckling is
present in approximately one-third of the cases

(9). Pigmented hairy nevi may also be observed
(20, 49).

Central nervous system. Mental deficiency is
usually absent, but retardation may occur, the
stated incidence varying from 8 to 50 percent (2,
53). Seizures frequently accompany the syndrome (7). Hydrocephalus has been noted in
some cases.

In addition to neuromas, gliomas and meningiomas, distortion of cortical architecture from
glial proliferation, and neuronal heterotopias
deep in the cerebral white matter have been
reported (5, 12, 20, 44).

Eyes. Any part of the eye may be involved.
Neurofibromas of the eyelids have been observed
in some cases. Intraorbital lesions may produce

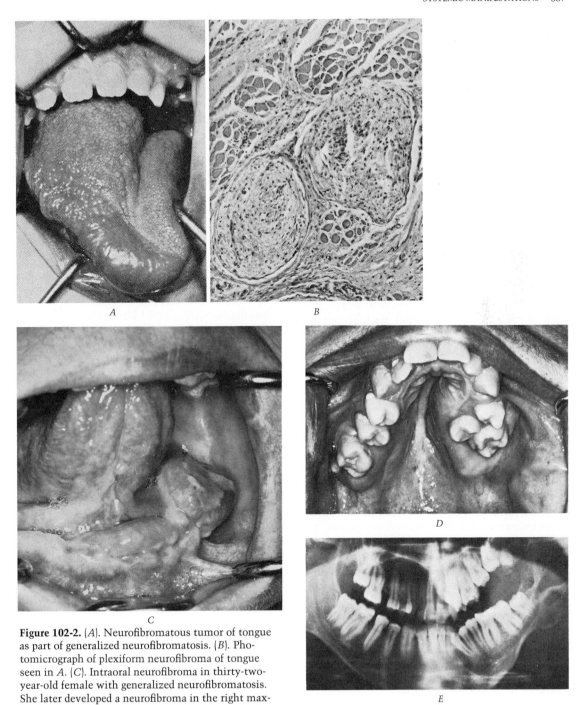

Figure 102-2. (*A*). Neurofibromatous tumor of tongue as part of generalized neurofibromatosis. (*B*). Photomicrograph of plexiform neurofibroma of tongue seen in *A*. (*C*). Intraoral neurofibroma in thirty-two-year-old female with generalized neurofibromatosis. She later developed a neurofibroma in the right maxilla. (*D*). Involvement of maxilla of patient seen in Fig. 102-1*B*. (*E*). Roentgenograph of same patient showing changes in mandibular ramus and angle. (*D, E. From I. Koblin and B. Reil,* J. Maxillofac. Surg. **3**:23, 1975.)

proptosis and muscle palsies. Phakoma, congenital glaucoma, fibroma of the iris, corneal opacity, detached retina, and optic atrophy have been reported (17, 41).

Skeletal system. Bony abnormalities have been particularly well discussed by Holt and Wright (22), Jaffe (26), Hunt and Pugh (23), and Meszaros (34). Commonly observed are subperiosteal erosive changes caused by pressure from proliferating neurofibromatous tissue in the periosteum and overlying soft parts. Central "cystic" lesions of bone result from expansive growth of neurofibromas within the medullary cavity in some cases. In other cases, no cause for central lesions can be found.

Kyphoscoliosis and pseudoarthroses (especially with bowing of the tibia and fibula) are also common. Bony defects of the skull, especially of the posterosuperior orbital wall, have been reported. Overgrowth of cranial bones, craniofacial asymmetry, and macrocephaly have been noted. A variety of other anomalies may be observed, including hemihypertrophy of a limb or digit, spina bifida, absent patella, elevated scapulas, congenital dislocations (especially of the hip, radius, and ulna), clubfoot, syndactyly, and complete or partial absence of limb bones (11, 15, 20, 22, 23, 26, 38, 42).

Endocrine system. Findings have been especially well reviewed by Saxena (46). Pheochromocytoma is the most common endocrine lesion in adult patients. Five percent of patients with pheochromocytoma have neurofibromatosis. In childhood, the most common endocrine abnormality is sexual precocity. Other findings have included hypopituitarism, hypogonadism, gigantism, acromegaly, delayed sexual development, obesity, hypoglycemia, diabetes insipidus, goiter, myxedema, and hyperparathyroidism.

Cardiovascular system. Although this fact is not often appreciated, cardiovascular anomalies may occur in low frequency, including pulmonic valvular stenosis, supravalvular aortic stenosis, coarctation of the aorta, atrial septal defect, congenital heart block, stenotic renal arteries, and other defects (13, 20, 28, 43, 47).

Other findings. The reader is referred to several of the more extensive sources for other low-frequency abnormalities (6, 11, 15).

Oral manifestations. Oral involvement is not common, the incidence probably lying between 4 and 7 percent (3, 8, 33, 39). Tumors may involve any oral soft tissue, although there is some predilection for the tongue (1, 3, 16, 19, 25, 32, 35, 48, 50, 52, 53, 55) (Figs. 102-2A, B). Involvement of the bony maxilla and mandible is also uncommon (3, 33, 42, 55) (Fig. 102D, E), but with marked involvement of the face there may be combined maxillo-zygomatico-temporo-mandibular hypoplasia not from pressure atrophy but from maldevelopment of these bones (28a).

DIFFERENTIAL DIAGNOSIS

Neurofibromatosis should be distinguished from the *multiple mucosal neuroma syndrome, Klippel-Trénaunay-Weber syndrome,* multiple lipomatosis, *leopard syndrome,* and isolated *hemihypertrophy.* The café-au-lait spots of the *McCune-Albright syndrome* tend to be more markedly scalloped (coast of Maine appearance) in contrast to the smooth-edged lesions (coast of California appearance) of neurofibromatosis (45, 54). Café-au-lait spots may also be observed in association with pulmonic stenosis and mental deficiency in the Watson syndrome (31, 51) which in our opinion is an incomplete form of the *leopard syndrome.* One of us (M.M.C.) has observed two sporadic cases of a new distinctive syndrome which shares some features in common with both neurofibromatosis and the Klippel-Trénaunay-Weber syndrome.

It should be carefully noted that isolated neurofibroma or schwannoma without neurofibromatosis is frequently observed by surgeons and pathologists. Bilateral acoustic neuromas without neurofibromatosis are known to follow an autosomal dominant mode of transmission.

LABORATORY AIDS

Biopsy of individual lesions is useful for establishing the diagnosis in questionable cases.

The café-au-lait spots of neurofibromatosis tend to have more large pigmented granules than the melanotic macules in the McCune-Albright syndrome (2). Johnson and Chorneco (27) reported more dopa-positive melanocytes per square millimeter in the café-au-lait spots of neurofibromatosis than in the café-au-lait spots of normal individuals. They also found giant pigment granules in the former but not in the latter.

REFERENCES

1 Baden, E., et al., Multiple Neurofibromatosis with Oral Lesions: Review of the Literature and Report of a Case. *Oral Surg.* **8**:268–280, 1955.

2 Benedict, P. H., et al., Melanotic Macules in Albright's Syndrome and in Neurofibromatosis. *J.A.M.A.* **205**:618–626, 1968.

3 Borberg, A., Clinical and Genetic Investigations in Tuberous Sclerosis and Recklinghausen's Neurofibromatosis. *Acta Psychiatr. Neurol.* (Suppl.) **71**:11–239, 1951.

4 Buntin, P. T., and Fitzgerald, J. F., Gastrointestinal Neurofibromatosis. *Am. J. Dis. Child.* **119**:521–523, 1970.

5 Canale, D., et al., Neurologic Manifestations of von Recklinghausen's Disease of the Nervous System. *Confin. Neurol.* **24**:359–403, 1964.

6 Chao, D. H.-C., Congenital Neurocutaneous Syndromes in Childhood. I. Neurofibromatosis. *J. Pediatr.* **55**:189–199, 1959.

7 Charron, J. W., and Gariepy, G., Neurofibromatosis of the Bladder: Case Report and Review of the Literature. *Can. J. Surg.* **13**:303–306, 1970.

8 Christensen, E., and Pindborg, J. J., A Rare Case of Neurofibromatosis Recklinghausen (Plexiform Type). *Acta Odontol. Scand.* **14**:1–10, 1956.

9 Crowe, F. W., Axillary Freckling as a Diagnostic Aid in Neurofibromatosis. *Ann. Intern. Med.* **61**:1142–1143, 1964.

10 Crowe, F. W., and Schull, W. J., Diagnostic Importance of Café-au-lait Spot in Neurofibromatosis. *Arch. Intern. Med.* **91**:758–766, 1953.

11 Crowe, F. W., et al., *Multiple Neurofibromatosis.* Charles C Thomas, Springfield, Ill., 1956.

12 Davidson, K. C., Cranial and Intracranial Lesions in Neurofibromatosis. *Am. J. Roentgenol.* **98**:550–556, 1966.

13 Diekmann, L., et al., Ungewöhnliche Erscheinungsformen der Neurofibromatose (von Recklinghausensche Krankheit) im Kindesalter. *Z. Kinderheilkd.* **101**:191–222, 1967.

14 Fialkow, P. J., et al., Multiple Cell Origin of Hereditary Neurofibromas. *N. Engl. J. Med.* **284**:298–300, 1971.

15 Fienman, N. L., and Yakovac, W., Neurofibromatosis in Childhood. *J. Pediatr.* **76**:339–346, 1970.

16 Freeman, M. J., and Standish, S. M., Facial and Oral Manifestations of Familial Disseminated Neurofibromatosis. *Oral Surg.* **19**:52–59, 1965.

17 Grant, W. M., and Walton, D. S., Distinctive Gonioscopic Findings in Glaucoma Due to Neurofibromatosis. *Arch. Ophthalmol.* **79**:127–134, 1968.

18 Halpern, M., and Currarino, G., Vascular Lesions Causing Hypertension in Neurofibromatosis. *N. Engl. J. Med.* **273**:248–252, 1965.

19 Hankey, G. T., Von Recklinghausen's Disease with Local Tumors of the Palate. *Proc. R. Soc. Med.* **26**:959–961, 1933.

20 Harkin, J. C., and Reed, R. J., *Tumors of the Peripheral Nervous System*, 2d ser., fasc. 3. Armed Forces Institute of Pathology, Washington, D.C., 1969.

21 Hayes, D. M., et al., Von Recklinghausen's Disease with Massive Intraabdominal Tumor and Spontaneous Hypoglycemia: Metabolic Studies Before and After Perfusion of Abdominal Cavity with Nitrogen Mustard. *Metabolism* **10**:183–199, 1961.

22 Holt, J. F., and Wright, E. M., The Radiologic Features of Neurofibromatosis. *Radiology* **51**:647–663, 1948.

23 Hunt, J. C., and Pugh, D. G., Skeletal Lesions in Neurofibromatosis. *Radiology* **76**:1–20, 1961.

24 Izumi, A. K., et al., Von Recklinghausen's Disease Associated with Multiple Neurilemomas. *Arch. Dermatol.* **104**:172–176, 1971.

25 Jacobs, M. H., Oral Manifestations in von Recklinghausen's Disease (Neurofibromatosis). *Am. J. Orthodont.* (Oral Surg.) **32**:28–33, 1946.

26 Jaffe, H. L., *Tumors and Tumorous Conditions of the Bones and Joints*. Lea & Febiger, Philadelphia, 1958, pp. 242–255.

27 Johnson, B. L., and Chorneco, D. R., Café-au-lait Spot in Neurofibromatosis and in Normal Individuals. *Arch. Dermatol.* **102**:442–446, 1970.

28 Kaufman, R. L., et al., Family Studies in Congenital Heart Disease. IV. Congenital Heart Disease Associated with Neurofibromatosis. *Birth Defects* **8**(5):92–95, 1972.

28a Koblin, I., and Reil, B., Changes in the Facial Skeleton in Cases of Neurofibromatosis. *J. Maxillofac. Surg.* **3**:23–27, 1975.

29 Knight, W. A., et al., Neurofibromatosis Associated with Malignant Neurofibromas. *Arch. Dermatol.* **107**:747–750, 1973.

30 Kragh, L. V., et al., Neurofibromatosis of the Head and Neck. *Plast. Reconstr. Surg.* **25**:565–573, 1960.

31 Kumar, B. B., Watson's Syndrome. *Am. J. Dis. Child.* **123**:612, 1972.

32 LeClerc, G., and Pont, J., Un cas de maladie de Recklinghausen avec tumeur majeure siégeant dans l'espace maxillopharyngien et provoquant des troubles dans le domaine du sympathique cervical. *Rev. Chir. (Paris)* **70**:735–737, 1932.

33 Mertin, H., and Graves, C. L., Plexiform Neurofibroma (von Recklinghausen's Disease) Invading the Oral Cavity. *Am. J. Orthodont.* **28**:694–702, 1942.

34 Meszaros, W. T., et al., Neurofibromatosis. *Am J. Roentgenol.* **98**:557–569, 1966.

35 Muller, H., Makroglossia neurofibromatosa congenita.

Zentralbl. Allg. Pathol. **57**:55–56, 1933.

36 Newell, G. B., et al., Juvenile Xanthogranuloma and Neurofibromatosis. *Arch. Dermatol.* **107**:262, 1973.

37 Nicholls, E. M., Somatic Variation and Multiple Neurofibromatosis. *Hum. Hered.* **19**:473–479, 1969.

38 Norman, M. E., Neurofibromatosis in a Family. *Am. J. Dis. Child.* **123**:159–160, 1972.

39 Preston, F. W., et al., Cutaneous Neurofibromatosis (von Recklinghausen's Disease): Clinical Manifestations and Incidence of Sarcoma in Sixty-one Male Patients. *Arch. Surg.* **64**:813–827, 1952.

40 von Recklinghausen, F., *Über die multiplen Fibroma der Haut und ihre Beziehung zu den multiplen Neuromen.* A. Hirschwald, Berlin, 1882.

41 Reese, A. B., *Tumors of the Eye,* 2d ed. Hoeber, New York, 1963.

42 Rittersma, J., et al., Neurofibromatosis with Mandibular Deformities. *Oral Surg.* **33**:718–727, 1972.

43 Rosenquist, G. C., et al., Acquired Right Ventricular Outflow Obstruction in a Child with Neurofibromatosis. *Am. Heart J.* **79**:103–108, 1970.

44 Rosman, N. P., and Pearce, J., The Brain in Neurofibromatosis. *Brain* **90**:829–838, 1970.

45 Ross, D. E., Skin Manifestations of von Recklinghausen's Disease and Associated Tumors (Neurofibromatosis). *Am. Surg.* **31**:729–740, 1965.

46 Saxena, K., Endocrine Manifestations of Neurofibromatosis in Children. *Am. J. Dis. Child.* **120**:265–271, 1970.

47 Smith, C. J., et al., Renal Artery Dysplasia as a Cause of Hypertension in Neurofibromatosis. *Arch. Intern. Med.* **125**:1022–1026, 1970.

48 Spencer, W. G., and Shattock, S. G., A Case of Macroglossia Neurofibromatosa. *Proc. R. Soc. Med.* **1**:8, 1908 (Path. Sect.).

49 Stein, K. M., et al., Neurofibromatosis Presenting as the Epidermal Nevus Syndrome. *Arch. Derm.* **105**:229–232, 1972.

50 Stillman, F. S., Neurofibromatosis. *J. Oral Surg.* **10**:112–117, 1952.

51 Watson, G. H., Pulmonary Stenosis, Cafe-au-lait Spots and Dull Intelligence. *Arch. Dis. Child.* **42**:303–307, 1967.

52 Weber, F. P., Neurofibromatosis of the Tongue in a Child, Together with a Note on the Classification of Incomplete and Anomalous Cases of Recklinghausen's Disease. *Br. J. Child. Dis.* **7**:13–16, 1910.

53 Whitfield, A., Cutaneous Neurofibromatosis in which Newly Formed Nerve Fibres were Found in the Tumours. *Lancet* **1**:1230–1232, 1903.

54 Whitehouse, D., Diagnostic Value of the Café-au-lait Spot in Children. *Arch. Dis. Child.* **41**:416–419, 1966.

55 Winters, S. E., et al., Neurofibromatosis (von Recklinghausen's Disease) with Involvement of the Mandible. *Oral Surg.* **13**:76–79, 1960.

103

Noonan Syndrome

(XX and XY Turner Phenotype Syndrome)

The Noonan syndrome consists of (*a*) short stature, (*b*) facial anomalies, (*c*) congenital cardiac defects, (*d*) skeletal abnormalities, (*e*) genital malformations, and (*f*) mild mental retardation. Our knowledge of the phenotypic spectrum may be biased by the many case reports that emphasize similarities with the Turner syndrome. Over 50 different major and minor anomalies have been observed in the Noonan syndrome. The use of the term "male Turner syndrome" for this disorder is inaccurate, misleading, and objectionable for the reasons stated by Kaplan et al. (18). In a strict sense, "male Turner syndrome" can be applied only to those disorders in which there are XO/XY mosaicism and ambiguous or male external genitalia.

Although Noonan (23) first clearly distinguished this condition from the Turner syndrome, noting that both males and females could be affected, the disorder was described earlier by Kobylinski (19) and others (8–10, 32). Discussion of the Noonan syndrome in males and females was provided by Summitt et al. (31), Opitz et al. (26), and Char et al. (3). Several reviews have appeared using a variety of criteria for the syndrome (4, 7, 12, 14, 20, 25b, 27, 29). Extensive reviews were carried out by Chaves-Carballo and Hayles (4), Heller (14), and Nora (25b). Over 200 cases have been described (3).

The etiology of the Noonan syndrome has not been resolved. Most cases are sporadic. Buccal smears, karyotypes, and banded karyotypes are normal (2a, 2b, 18, 25b). Undetected XO mosaicism has been suggested (6, 13), but this theory is untenable since no known mechanism of mosaicism can explain involvement in two or more generations affecting approximately half the offspring (24, 25). It has been found in identical twins (18a). Autosomal dominant inheritance is supported by many pedigrees (2a, 24, 25, 25a, 25b, 27b, 27c). X-linked dominant inheritance has been suggested (2, 24, 25) but ruled out by male-to-male transmission (27b). Furthermore, there is no sex predilection. Autosomal recessive inheritance is suggested by affected sibs of normal parentage (1, 17, 21). Some of these instances could be interpreted as being consistent with autosomal dominant inheritance and incomplete penetrance. Multifactorial inheritance has also been suggested. This theory has been proposed on the basis of the relatively common occurrence of the Noonan syndrome, severely affected probands, and less severely affected first-degree relatives, some having only minor stigmata (15, 18). Since different criteria for diagnosis have been applied by different clinicians, a variety of etiologic interpretations is possible. The lack of agreement leads us to suspect that we may be dealing with etiologic heterogeneity.

SYSTEMIC MANIFESTATIONS

Facies. Broad forehead, hypertelorism, mild antimongoloid obliquity, unilateral or bilateral

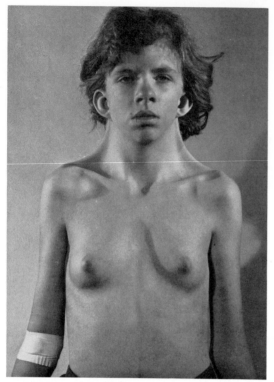

Figure 103-1. *Noonan syndrome.* Pterygium colli and prominent ears. Note normal breast development.

ptosis of the eyelids (in about 60 percent of patients), epicanthal folds, low posterior hairline, prominence or folding of the upper transverse portion of the helix, and low-set, fleshy ears have been observed. Strabismus and saddle nose are present in at least 50 percent of cases (14, 18, 22) (Figs. 103-1, 103-2). Pterygium colli is found in about half of the cases (25).

Central nervous system. Mental retardation has been observed in 50 to 60 percent of patients. Sensorineural deafness and hydrocephaly have been noted rarely (14, 18, 22). Epilepsy has also been documented (27d).

Cardiovascular system. Cardiovascular anomalies are present in 40 to 60 percent of cases (4, 5, 25, 27a, 28). An excellent review was provided by Caralis et al. (2c). The right side of the heart is most frequently involved; valvular pulmonic stenosis, pulmonary artery branch stenosis, supravalvular defect, patent ductus arteriosus, and aortic valve stenosis have been reported in some cases (2d, 3, 5, 22, 25). Eccentric ventricular hypertrophy has been discussed by Ehlers et al. (5a). Multiple cardiac anomalies have also been reported (2c). Coarctation of the aorta (21, 25, 28) and the Ebstein anomaly of the tricuspid valve

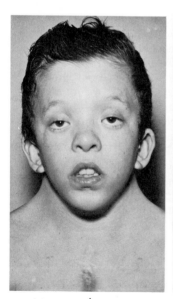

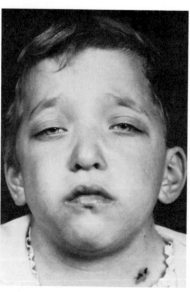

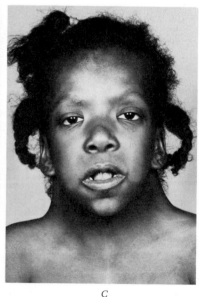

A *B* *C*

Figure 103-2. (*A-C*). Similar facies showing ptosis, widespread eyes, pterygium colli. (*B and C from F. Char et al.,* Birth Defects **8**(5):110, 1972.)

(33) have been documented rarely. Lymphangiectatic edema of the lower extremities is present in about 15 percent of patients (Fig. 103-3). Intestinal lymphangiectasis has also been described (31a).

Genitourinary system. Gonadal differentiation and function may vary from complete absence to normal function and fertility. Puberty may be somewhat delayed (22). Cryptorchism has been noted in 60 to 70 percent of males, but usually a normal or even large phallus has been observed (4, 14, 18, 25). Hypospadias and renal duplication have been noted occasionally (14, 22).

Skeletal system. Short stature is a common feature, adult males and females usually averaging 165 and 152 cm, respectively. Premature fusion of the manubrium and body of the sternum

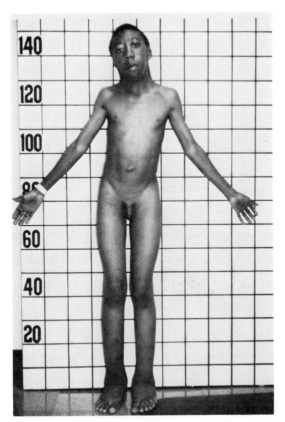

Figure 103-3. Note lymphangiectatic edema of feet and ankles. (*Courtesy of R. L. Summitt, Memphis, Tenn.*)

occurs in 30 percent of patients (3). Proximal pectus carinatum, distal pectus excavatum, cubitus valgus, and short clinodactylous fifth fingers are noted in over 50 percent of cases. Scoliosis, kyphosis, lordosis, spina bifida occulta, Klippel-Feil anomalad, proximal widening of the middle phalanges, and metacarpal modeling defects have been observed (3). Retarded bone age and osteoporosis have also been noted in 50 percent of patients (4, 14, 18).

Integumentary system. Hypoplastic nails, hirsutism, curly hair, low nuchal hairline, hemangiomas, and hypoplastic, inverted, and accessory nipples have been reported (4, 14, 18, 22). The nipples appear widely spaced but this is an illusion (4a).

Other findings. Dermatoglyphic findings are not striking (3). Simian creases are more frequent than normal. Distally placed axial triradius has been observed in some cases (16, 18, 25) but is probably not significant (3). Various other findings have been documented, including inguinal and umbilical hernia, hypotonia, and numerous low-frequency abnormalities (14, 22).

Autoimmune thyroiditis has been reported in six of 10 patients (31b). Hypoparathyroidism has also been noted (27d).

Oral manifestations. Micrognathia, highly arched palate, malocclusion, dental anomalies, bifid uvula, and rarely, cleft palate have been observed (15).

DIFFERENTIAL DIAGNOSIS

The Noonan syndrome should be distinguished from the *Turner syndrome.* Short stature characteristic of the Turner syndrome is variable in the Noonan syndrome. Gonadal dysgenesis is invariably present in the Turner syndrome, but varies from agonadism to normal gonadal function in the Noonan syndrome. In the Turner syndrome, the left side of the heart may be affected (coarctation of the aorta), but in the Noonan syndrome, the right side of the heart is more frequently involved (usually with valvular pulmonic stenosis). Mental retardation is common in the Noonan syndrome but is significantly rare in the Turner syndrome. The total finger ridge count tends to be low in the Noonan syndrome and high in the Turner syndrome. Renal anomalies, which are not generally encountered in the Noonan syndrome, are frequent in the Turner syndrome. Other differences have been noted by Summitt (30). It should be carefully noted, however, that overlap with respect to these features may occur. Several examples of the *Aarskog syndrome* have been confused with the Noonan syndrome in the literature. Also to be excluded is the *leopard syndrome*, an autosomal dominant disorder charac-terized by lentiginosis, electrocardiographic abnormalities, pulmonary stenosis, short stature, pterygium colli, and occasionally sensorineural deafness. The *fetal alcohol syndrome* may occasionally present with a Noonan phenotype (13a).

LABORATORY AIDS

In females, normal karyotype rules out the Turner syndrome.

REFERENCES

1 Abdel-Salam, E., and Temtamy, S. A., Familial Turner Phenotype. *J. Pediatr.* **74**:67–72, 1969.

1a Allen, H. D., et al., The Ullrich-Noonan Syndrome. *Am. J. Dis. Child.* **128**:115–116, 1974.

2 Baird, P. A., and DeJong, B. P., Noonan's Syndrome (XX and XY Turner Phenotype) in Three Generations of a Family. *J. Pediatr.* **80**:110–114, 1972.

2a Bolton, M. R., et al., The Noonan Syndrome: A Family Study. *Ann. Intern. Med.* **80**:626–629, 1974.

2b Borgaonkar, D. S., Normal Banded Karyotype in Noonan Syndrome. *Lancet* **1**:1114, 1973.

2c Caralis, D. G., et al., Delineation of Multiple Cardiac Anomalies Associated with the Noonan Syndrome in an Adult and Review of the Literature. *Johns Hopkins Med. J.* **134**:346–355, 1974.

2d Celermajer, J. M., et al., Pulmonary Stenosis in Patients with the Turner Phenotype. *Am. J. Dis. Child.* **116**:351–358, 1968.

3 Char, F., et al., The Noonan Syndrome—a Clinical Study of Forty-five Cases. *Birth Defects* **8**(5):110–118, 1972.

4 Chaves-Carballo, E., and Hayles, A. B., Ullrich-Turner Syndrome in Males. *Mayo Clin. Proc.* **41**:843–854, 1966.

4a Collins, E., The Illusion of Widely Spaced Nipples in the Noonan and Turner Syndromes. *J. Pediatr.* **83**:557–561, 1973.

5 Collins, E., and Turner, G., The Noonan Syndrome—a Review of the Clinical and Genetic Features of 27 Cases. *J. Pediatr.* **83**:941–950, 1973.

5a Ehlers, K. H., et al., Eccentric Ventricular Hypertrophy in Familial and Sporadic Instances of 46XX,XY Turner Phenotype. *Circulation* **45**:639–652, 1972.

6 Ferguson-Smith, M. A., Karyotype-Phenotype Correlations in Gonadal Dysgenesis and Their Bearing on the Pathogenesis of Malformations. *J. Med. Genet.* **2**:142–155, 1965.

7 Ferrier, P. E., and Ferrier, S. A., Turner's Phenotype in the Male. *Pediatrics* **40**:575–584, 1967.

8 Flavell, G., Webbing of the Neck with Turner's Syndrome in the Male. *Br. J. Surg.* **31**:150–153, 1943.

9 Fraccaro, M., et al., Testicular Germinal Dysgenesis (Male Turner's Syndrome). *Acta Endocrinol.* (Kbh.) **36**:98–114, 1961.

10 Futterweit, W., et al., Multiple Congenital Defects in a Twelve-year-old Boy with Cryptochidism—"Male Turner's Syndrome." *Metabolism* **10**:1074–1084, 1961.

11 Gorlin, R. J., The Leopard (Multiple Lentigines) Syndrome Revisited. *Birth Defects* **7**(4):110–115, 1971.

12 Gustavson, K. H., et al., The Pterygium Colli Syndrome in the Male. *Acta Paediatr. Scand.* **53**:454–464, 1964.

13 Haddad, J. B., Turner's Syndrome: Case Reports and Review of Clinical and Cytogenetic Aspects. *Tulane Med. Fac. Bull.* **21**:139–151, 1962.

13a Hall, B. D., Noonan's Phenotype in Offspring of Alcoholic Mothers. *Lancet* **1**:680, 1974.

14 Heller, R. H., The Turner Phenotype in the Male. *J. Pediatr.* **66**:48–63, 1965.

15 Inhorn, S. L., and Opitz, J. M., Abnormal Sex Development, in J. M. B. Bloodworth, Jr. (ed.), *Endocrine Pathology.* Williams & Wilkins, Baltimore, 1968.

16 Jackson, L. G., and Lefrak, S., Familial Occurrence of the Noonan Syndrome. *Birth Defects* **5**(5):36–38, 1969.

17 Josso, N., et al., Le syndrome de Turner familial: Étude de deux familles avec caryotype XO et XX. *Ann. Pédiatr.* **17**:163–167, 1963.

18 Kaplan, M. S., et al., Noonan's Syndrome. *Am. J. Dis. Child.* **116**:359–368, 1968.

18a Karpouzas, J., and Papaioannou, A. C., Noonan Syndrome in Twins. *J. Pediatr.* **85**:84–86, 1974.

19 Kobylinski, O., Über eine Flughautähnliche Ausbreitung am Halse. *Arch Anthropol.* **14**:342–348, 1883.

20 Lenz, W., Turner Syndrom im männlichen Geschlecht, in P. E. Becker, (ed.), *Handbuch der Humangenetik.* Vol. III. Thieme, Stuttgart, 1964, pp. 371–373.

21 Migeon, B. R., and Whitehouse, D., Familial Occurrence of the Somatic Phenotype of Turner's Syndrome. *Johns Hopkins Med. J.* **120**:78–80, 1967.

22 Noonan, J. A., Hypertelorism with Turner Phenotype. *Am. J. Dis. Child.* **116**:373–380, 1968.

23 Noonan, J. A., and Ehmke, D. A., Associated Noncardiac Malformations in Children with Congenital Heart Disease. *J. Pediatr.* **63**:468–470, 1963.

23a Noonan, J. A., Noonan Syndrome (Comments). *Birth Defects* **8**(5):122–123, 1972.

24 Nora, J. J., and Sinha, A. K., Direct Familial Transmission

of the Turner Phenotype. *Am. J. Dis. Child.* **116:**343–350, 1968.

25a Nora, J. J., et al., Dominant Inheritance of the Noonan Syndrome. *Birth Defects* **8**(5):119–121, 1972.

25b Nora, J. J., et al., The Ullrich-Noonan Syndrome (Turner Phenotype). *Am. J. Dis. Child.* **127:**48–57, 1974.

26 Opitz, J. M., et al., Noonan's Syndrome in Girls: A Genocopy of the Ullrich-Turner Syndrome. *J. Pediatr.* **67:**968, 1965.

27 Overzier, C., Die Nosologie des sogenannten männlichen Turner-Syndroms. *Dtsch. Arch. Klin. Med.* **209:**422–444, 1964.

27a Phornphutkul, C., et al., Cardiomyopathy in Noonan's Syndrome. Report of 3 Cases. *Br. Heart J.* **35:**99–102, 1973.

27b Qazi, Q. H., et al., Familial Occurrence of Noonan Syndrome. *Am. J. Dis. Child.* **127:**696–698, 1974.

27c Rogers, G. L., Noonan's Syndrome and Autosomal Dominant Inheritance. *J. Pediat. Ophthalmol.* **12:**54–56, 1975.

27d Rudge, P., et al., A Case of Noonan's Syndrome and Hypoparathyroidism Presenting with Epilepsy. *J. Neurol. Neurosurg. Psychiat.* **37:**108–111, 1974.

28 Siggers, D. C., and Polani, P. E., Congenital Heart Disease in Male and Female Subjects with Somatic Features of Turner's Syndrome and Normal Sex Chromosomes (Ullrich's and Related Syndromes). *Br. Heart J.* **34:**41–46, 1972.

29 Steiker, D. D., et al., Turner's Syndrome in the Male. *J. Pediatr.* **58:**321–329, 1961.

30 Summitt, R. L., The Noonan Syndrome. *Birth Defects* **5**(5):39–42, 1969.

31 Summitt, R. L., et al., Noonan's Syndrome in the Male. *J. Pediatr.* **67:**936, 1965.

31a Vallet, H. L., et al., Noonan Syndrome with Intestinal Lymphangiectasis. *J. Pediatr.* **80:**269–274, 1972.

31b Vesterhus, P., and Aarskog, D., Noonan's Syndrome and Autoimmune Thyroiditis. *J. Pediatr.* **83:**237–240, 1973.

32 Weissenberg, S., Eine eigentümliche Hautfaltenbildung am Halse. *Anthropol. Anz.* **5:**141–144, 1928.

33 Wright, N. L., et al., Noonan's Syndrome and Ebstein's Malformation of the Tricuspid Valve. *Am. J. Dis. Child.* **116:**367–372, 1968.

104

Oculoauriculovertebral Dysplasia

*(Goldenhar Syndrome, Hemifacial Microsomia,
First and Second Branchial Arch Syndrome, OAV Syndrome)*

The term hemifacial microsomia was used by Gorlin et al. (14) to refer to patients with unilateral (a) microtia, (b) macrostomia, and (c) failure of formation of the mandibular ramus and condyle. They suggested that oculoauriculovertebral dysplasia (Goldenhar syndrome) is a variant of this complex, characterized by (d) vertebral anomalies, most often hemivertebras, and (e) epibulbar dermoids (13, 14).

Terms such as first arch syndrome, first and second branchial arch syndrome, and hemifacial microsomia impart the erroneous impression that involvement is limited to facial structures when, in fact, cardiac, renal, and skeletal anomalies may occur as well (8, 26, 29).

The first recorded case may have been that of von Arlt (1). Grabb (15) suggested an incidence of at least 1 per 5,600 births and Poswillo 1 per 3,500 births (29a). There may be a slight predilection for males (3:2 male/female ratio). Several extensive reviews may be consulted (3, 6, 8, 8a, 11, 15, 17, 23, 27, 34, 38, 40).

The etiology is unresolved and probably complicated. On the one hand, we have seen many transitional forms between hemifacial microsomia and the Goldenhar syndrome, suggesting a continuous spectrum. Invalid nosologic splitting has been discussed by several authors in this connection (8, 16, 28, 37). On the other hand, the great variability observed in sporadic cases and the fact that familial instances do occur, which seem to have different modes of inheritance, suggest etiologic heterogeneity.

The overwhelming majority of cases are sporadic. However, several instances have been observed in successive generations (15, 16, 25, 32, 37). In one family, epibulbar dermoids were documented in two generations, but consanguinity was also noted (30). Affected sibs of normal parentage have been reported (15, 20, 21, 32). Consanguinity was noted in one sporadic instance (28). Autosomal dominant, autosomal recessive, and multifactorial modes of inheritance are all possibilities to consider.

Both concordance (38) and discordance (4, 9, 27a) for the syndrome have been recorded in identical twins. The zygosity of two twin pairs discordant (13, 15) for the syndrome is less certain.

The Goldenhar variant has been seen in association with 5p− karyotype (22).

Poswillo, using an animal model of hemifacial microsomia, was able to show that destruction of differentiating tissues, in the region of the ear and jaw by an expanding hematoma, produced a branchial arch dysplasia. The severity of the dysplasia was related to the degree of local destruction. Thus, a simple branchial arch dysplasia *sui generis* should probably be regarded as a nonspecific symptom complex, whose pathogenesis probably has several different etiologies (29, 29a).

In our present state of knowledge, it is best to evaluate each patient and his or her family on an individual basis. It is important to note that extreme variability of expression is characteristic.

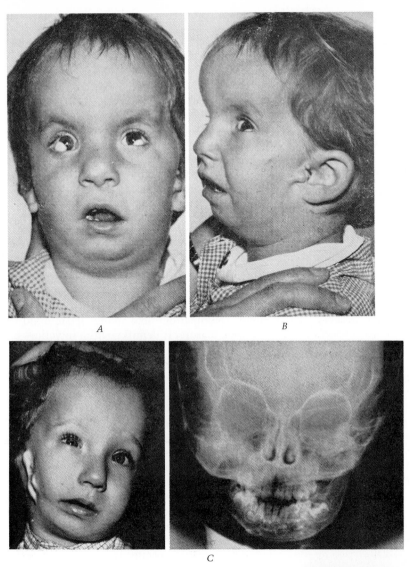

Figure 104-1. (A). *Oculoauriculovertebral dysplasia.* Note bilateral epibulbar dermoids, coloboma of upper right eyelid, small mandible. (B). Lateral view of patient seen in A, showing frontal bossing, extra ear tags. (C). Note facial asymmetry with microtia on right side. Usually there is no ascending ramus or condyle on affected side. Occasionally there is agenesis of part of homolateral lung. (D). Extreme microtia and underdeveloped mastoid area. (*From W. C. Grabb, Plast. Reconstr. Surg.* **36:**485, 1965.)

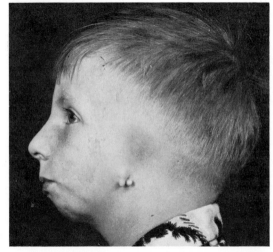

Some patients have an extensive range of anomalies and others have only a single minor anomaly such as a preauricular tag or slightly dysplastic ear. For the purposes of recurrent risk counseling, thorough evaluation for cardiac, skeletal, and renal anomalies should be carried out, the first-degree relatives of the propositus also being carefully scrutinized. A skeletal, cardiac, or renal anomaly in a relative probably has genetic significance, whether or not facial abnormalities are present.

SYSTEMIC MANIFESTATIONS

Not uncommonly the infants are small-for-dates and there are feeding difficulties which may necessitate tube feeding (25a).

Facies. The facies may be striking because of asymmetry; this is partly due to hypoplasia and/or displacement of the pinna, but the degree of involvement is markedly variable. The maxillary, temporal, and malar bones on the involved side are somewhat reduced in size and flattened, and the ipsilateral eye may be at a lower level than that on the opposite side. Further flattening may result from aplasia or hypoplasia of the mandibular ramus and condyle. Some patients manifest mild flattening of the mastoid region. Frequently, there is frontal bossing. About 10 percent of patients have bilateral involvement, but the disorder is nearly always more severe on one side (15). Among 200 cases, the right side was predominantly involved in 62 percent (31a) (Fig. 104-1A–D).

Nervous system. Failure of development or hypoplasia of muscles, such as the masseter, temporalis, pterygoideus, and those of facial expression on the involved side, has been observed. In about 10 percent of cases, lower facial weakness has been noted, possibly being related to bony involvement in the region of the facial canal (15, 23). About 10 percent of patients have been mentally retarded (14). Occipital encephalocele has been noted in several cases (8, 16).

Ear. Malformation of the external ear may vary from complete aplasia to a crumpled, distorted pinna which is displaced anteriorly and in-

feriorly. Occasionally bilateral anomalous pinnas are noted. Longacre (23) estimated that about 40 percent of patients with microtia have varying degrees of the syndrome. Conduction deafness due to middle ear abnormalities and/or absence or deficiency of the external auditory meatus has been noted in 30 to 50 percent of cases (2). Supernumerary ear tags may occur anywhere from the tragus to the angle of the mouth. They are more commonly seen in patients with macrostomia and/or aplasia of the parotid gland. In the presence of epibulbar dermoids, the ear tags tend to be bilateral. Blind-ended fistulas are often found in the same area but not always bilaterally (Fig. 104-1A–D).

Eye. Often the palpebral fissure is somewhat lowered on the affected side, but marked antimongoloid obliquity does not occur in this syndrome. Epibulbar dermoid and/or lipodermoid is a variable feature. It is milky-white to yellow in color, flattened or somewhat ellipsoidal, and usually solid rather than cystic. The surface is usually smooth but may be granular or covered by fine hairs. The dermoid is usually located at the limbus or corneal margin in the lower outer quadrant. The lipodermoid usually is found in the upper outer quadrant. Some patients have a dermoid and lipodermoid in the same eye. Generally, these conditions are bilateral, but about one-third of patients who have epibulbar dermoids have unilateral lesions (2).

Unilateral coloboma of the superior lid is a common finding, occurring in about 50 to 60 percent of those with epibulbar dermoids (2, 40). The defect usually occurs between the middle and inner third of the lid. Rarely, there are colobomas of both upper and lower lids or bilateral involvement of upper lids. Choroidal or iridial coloboma and congenital cystic eye may occasionally be associated with the syndrome (Fig. 104-1A–D).

When unilateral microphthalmia or anophthalmia is present, mental retardation occurs concomitantly (8, 18, 31, 42) (Figs. 104-2A, B 104-3A, B). Infrequent eye findings have been reviewed by Baum and Feingold (2).

Skeletal alterations. Bony anomalies, especially of the vertebral column, are seen in 40 to 60 percent of patients (2). The most common findings

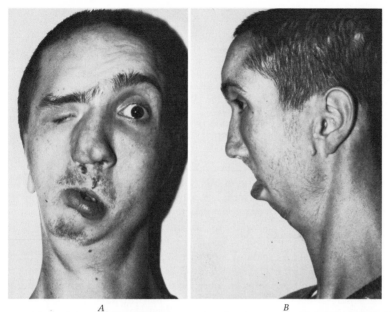

Figure 104-2. (*A, B*). Unilateral anophthalmia, facial asymmetry, ear tags, severe mental retardation, micrognathia. (*From M. M. Cohen, Jr.*, Birth Defects **7**(7):103, 1971.)

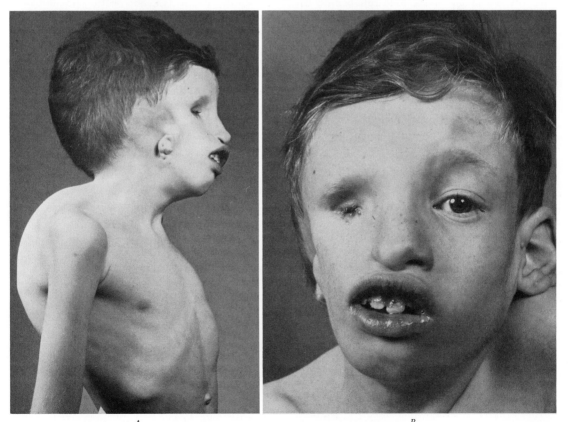

Figure 104-3. (*A, B*). Unilateral anophthalmia, severe kyphoscoliosis in association with hemifacial microsomia. (*From C. H. Ide et al.*, Arch. Ophthalmol. **84**:427, 1970.)

include occipitalization of the atlas, cuneiform vertebra, cervical complete or partial synostosis or block of two or more vertebras, supernumerary vertebras, hemivertebras, spina bifida, and anomalous ribs (10, 38) (Fig. 104-4B). Talipes equinovarus is noted in about 20 percent of cases. Other infrequent peripheral skeletal anomalies have been reviewed (14, 24, 26, 36).

Heart. About 45 to 55 percent of patients have various forms of heart disease: ventricular septal defect and patent ductus arteriosus or a variant of this finding—right-sided aortic arch, connection of the ductus arteriosus with the left subclavian artery which arises from a short but distinct common trunk, coarctation of the descending aorta which occurs immediately distal to the obliterated ductus arteriosus, persistent left superior vena cava and ventricular septal defect. The left subclavian artery may run behind the esophagus. Tetralogy of Fallot or Eisenmenger complex may also be found (15a, 15b, 26, J. Edwards, personal communication, 1975).

Other anomalies. Pulmonary agenesis or hypoplasia has been noted in several cases, the missing lung occurring on the homolateral side (5, 26, 44). A variety of renal abnormalities have been reported as associated findings, including absent kidney, double ureter, crossed renal ectopia, anomalous blood supply to the kidney, and other defects (8, 14, 15, 15b, 16, 36).

Oral manifestations. Patients may have minimal underdevelopment of the condyle to unilateral aplasia of the mandibular ramus and/or condyle with absence of the glenoid fossa (Fig. 104-4A). Kazanjian (19) found microtia in over 70 percent in his series of patients with agenesis of the ramus. Conversely, about 50 percent with microtia had ramus agenesis. The gonial angle is commonly flattened, and the maxilla is narrowed on the involved side. Intraorally, one notes decreased palatal width from the midline palatal raphe to the lingual surface of the teeth on the affected side. The palatal and tongue muscles may be unilaterally hypoplastic and/or paralyzed. About 7 percent have associated cleft lip and/or palate (15, 35). White (43) noted an unusual growth on the anterior maxillary frenum.

At least one-third of the patients with agenesis of the mandibular ramus have associated macrostomia, i.e., lateral facial cleft, usually of mild degree. Occasionally a triangle of skin extends onto the inner surface of the cheek at the angle of the mouth. In the presence of epibulbar dermoids, the incidence of macro-

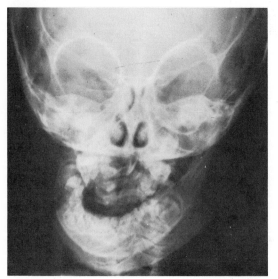

A

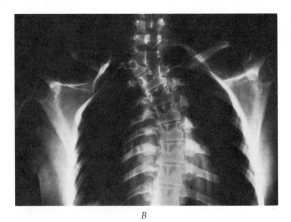

B

Figure 104-4. (*A*). Asymmetry and unilateral hypoplasia of mandibular ramus. (*From W. C. Grabb*, Plast. Reconstr. Surg. **36**:485, 1965.) (*B*). Hemivertebra in thoracic spine.

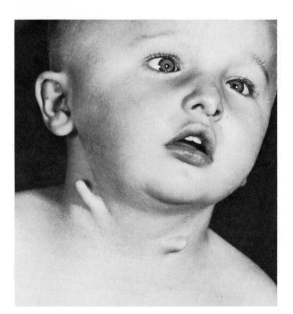

Figure 104-5. Note unusual cervical structures containing cartilage. Observe epibulbar dermoid, strabismus. (*Courtesy of S. Budden, Vancouver, British Columbia.*)

stomia may be somewhat higher. It is nearly always unilateral and on the side of the more affected ear. Occasionally there may be agenesis of the ipsilateral parotid gland, displaced salivary gland tissue (41), or salivary fistulas (12).

DIFFERENTIAL DIAGNOSIS

Epibulbar dermoids may also occur in *frontonasal dysplasia* (7, 33). Oculoauriculovertebral dysplasia differs from *mandibulofacial dysostosis* in several respects. In contrast to the latter, it is asymmetric and there is far less hypoplasia of the malar bones. Colobomas of the lower eyelids do not occur.

Ear anomalies may occur in the *Robin anomalad* but the mandible is symmetrically small. Micrognathia and, at times, hypoplastic pinnas may be observed in the *Moebius syndrome.* Involvement of the seventh cranial nerve may be seen in both conditions. However, the sixth cranial nerve is additionally involved in the Moebius syndrome. Thalidomide embryopathy may sometimes be associated with anomalies of the auricles.

LABORATORY AIDS

None is known.

REFERENCES

1 Arlt, F., von, *Klinische Darstellung der Krankheiten des Auges.* W. Braunmüller, Wien, 1881.

2 Baum, J. L., and Feingold, M., Ocular Aspects of Goldenhar's Syndrome. *Am. J. Ophthalmol.* **75**:250–257, 1973.

3 Berkman, M. D., and Feingold, M., Oculoauriculovertebral Dysplasia (Goldenhar's Syndrome). *Oral Surg.* **25**:408–417, 1968.

4 Bock, R. H., Ein Fall von epibulbärem Dermolipom mit Missbildungen einer Gesichtshälfte. Diskordantes Vorkommen bei einem eineiigen Zwillingspaar. *Ophthalmologica* **122**:86–90, 1961.

5 Booth, J. B., and Berry, C. L., Unilateral Pulmonary Agenesis. *Arch. Dis. Child.* **42**:361–374, 1967 (see Table VII).

5a Budden, S. S., and Robinson, G. C. Oculoauricular Vertebral Dysplasia. *Am. J. Dis. Child.* **125**:431–433, 1973.

6 Cadenati, H., et al., Le syndrome du premier arc branchial. *Rev. Stomatol.* (*Paris*) **67**:359–381, 1966.

7 Christiaens, L., et al., A propos de deux cas de dysplasie oculo-auriculo-vertébrale. *Pédiatrie* **21**:935–942, 1966 (unusual case).

8 Cohen, M. M., Jr., Variability versus "Incidental Findings" in the First and Second Branchial Arch Syndrome: Unilateral Variants with Anophthalmia. *Birth Defects* **7**(7):103–108, 1971.

8a Converse, J. M., et al., On Hemifacial Microsomia. The First and Second Branchial Arch. Syndrome. *Plast. Reconstr. Surg.* **51**:268–279, 1975.

9 Cordier, J., et al., Syndrome de Franceschetti-Goldenhar discordant chez deux jumelles monozygotes. *Arch. Ophthalmol.* (*Paris*) **30**:321–328, 1970.

10 Darling, D. B., et al., The Roentgenological Aspects of Goldenhar's Syndrome (Oculoauriculovertebral Dysplasia). *Radiology* **91**:254–260, 1968.

11 François, J., and Haustrate, L., Anomalies colobomateuses du globe oculaire et syndrome du premier arc. *Ann. Ocul.* **187**:340–368, 1954.

12 Fuchs, G., Doppelseitige Ohrmuschel-sowie Speichelgangsmissbildung mit weiteren Fehlbildungen am Skeletsystem sowie einseitiger Facialislähmung, alles als besondere Form einer Dysostosis cranialis. *Z. Kinderheilkd.* **91**:93–98, 1964.

13 Goldenhar, M., Association malformatives de l'oeil et de l'oreille, en particulier le syndrome dermoide epibulbaire-appendices auriculaires–fistula auris congenita et ses relations avec la dysostose mandibulofaciale. *J. Génét. Hum.* **1**:243–282, 1952.

14 Gorlin, R. J., et al., Oculoauriculovertebral Syndrome. *J. Pediatr.* **63**:991–999, 1963.

15 Grabb, W. C., The First and Second Branchial Arch Syndrome. *Plast. Reconstr. Surg.* **36**:485–508, 1965.

15a Greenwood, R. D., et al., Cardiovascular Malformations in Oculoauriculovertebral Dysplasia (Goldenhar Syndrome). *J. Pediatr.* **85**:816–821, 1974.

15b Gross, W., Ein Fall von Agenesie der linken Lunge. *Beitr. Pathol. Anat.* **37**:487–501, 1905.

16 Herrmann, J., and Opitz, J. M., A Dominantly Inherited First Arch Syndrome. *Birth Defects* **5**(2):110–112, 1969.

17 Hollwich, F., and Verbeck, B., Zur Dysplasia oculo-auricularis (Franceschetti-Goldenhar). *Klin. Monatsbl. Augenheilkd.* **154**:430–443, 1969.

18 Ide, C. H., et al., Familial Facial Dysplasia. *Arch. Ophthalmol.* **84**:427–433, 1970.

19 Kazanjian, V. H., Bilateral Absence of the Ascending Rami of the Mandible. *Br. J. Plast. Surg.* **9**:77–82, 1956–1957.

20 Kirke, D. K., Goldenhar's Syndrome: Two Cases of Oculo-auriculo-vertebral Dysplasia Occurring in Full-blood Australian Aboriginal Sisters. *Aust. Paediatr. J.* **6**:213–214, 1970.

21 Krause, V. H., The Syndrome of Goldenhar Affecting Two Siblings. *Acta Ophthalmol. (Kbh.)* **48**:494–499, 1970.

22 Ladekarl, S., Combination of Goldenhar's Syndrome with the Cri-du-chat Syndrome. *Acta Ophthalmol. (Kbh.)* **46**:605–610, 1968.

23 Longacre, J. J., et al., The Surgical Management of the First and Second Branchial Arch Syndromes. *Plast. Reconstr. Surg.* **31**:507–520, 1963.

24 Mandelcorn, M. S., et al., Goldenhar's Syndrome and Phocomelia. *Am. J. Ophthalmol.* **72**:618–621, 1971.

25 Manfredini, U., Le considett sindrome del primo acro branchiale. *Ann. Ottal.* **91**:689–704, 1965.

25a Mellor, D. H., et al., Goldenhar's Syndrome. *Arch. Dis. Child.* **48**:537–541, 1973.

26 Opitz, J. M., and Faith, G. C., Visceral Anomalies in an Infant with the Goldenhar Syndrome. *Birth Defects* **5**(2):104–105, 1969.

27 Osborne, R., The Treatment of the Underdeveloped Ascending Ramus. *Br. J. Plast. Surg.* **17**:376–388, 1964.

27a Papp, Z., et al., Probably Monozygote Twins with Discordance for Goldenhar Syndrome. *Clin. Genet.* **5**:86–90, 1974.

28 Pashayan, H., et al., Hemifacial Microsomia: Oculo-auriculo-vertebral Syndrome: A Patient with Overlapping Features. *J. Med. Genet.* **7**:185–188, 1970.

29 Poswillo, D., The Pathogenesis of the First and Second Branchial Arch Syndrome. *Oral Surg.* **35**:302–329, 1973.

29a Poswillo, D., Otomandibular Deformity: Pathogenesis as a Guide to Reconstruction. *J. Maxillofac. Surg.* **2**:64–72, 1974.

30 Proto, F., and Scullica, L., Contributo allo studio della ereditarieta dei dermoidi epibulbari. *Acta Med. Genet. (Roma)* **15**:351–363, 1966.

31 Pruett, R. C., Oculovertebral Syndrome. *Am. J. Ophthalmol.* **60**:926–929, 1965.

31a Pruzansky, S., personal communication, 1975.

32 Saraux, H., et al., A propos d'une observation familiale de syndrome de Franceschetti-Goldenhar. *Bull. Soc. Ophthalmol. Fr.* **63**:705–707, 1963.

33 Sitzman, F. C., and Shuch, P., Das Goldenhar-Syndrom. *Z. Kinderheilkd.* **93**:40–45, 1965.

34 Stark, R. B., and Saunders, D. E., The First Branchial Syndrome: The Oral-mandibular-auricular Syndrome. *Plast. Reconstr. Surg.* **29**:229–239, 1967.

35 Sugar, H. S., An Unusual Example of the Oculoauriculovertebral Dysplasia Syndrome of Goldenhar. *J. Pediatr. Ophthalmol.* **4**(2):9–12, 1967.

36 Sugiura, Y., Congenital Absence of the Radius with Hemifacial Microsomia, Ventricular Septal Defect and Crossed Renal Ectopia. *Birth Defects* **7**(7):109–116, 1971.

37 Summitt, R., Familial Goldenhar Syndrome. *Birth Defects* **5**(2):106–109, 1969.

38 Ter Haar, B., Oculo-auriculo-vertebral Dysplasia (Goldenhar's Syndrome). Concordant in Identical Twins. *Acta Med. Genet. (Roma)*, **21**:116–124, 1972.

39 Timm, G., Zur Morphologie des Auges bei Missbildungssyndromen. *Klin. Monatsbl. Augenheilkd.* **137**:557–571, 1960 (unusually severe).

40 Tost, M., Beitrag zur Dysplasie Oculo-auriculo-vertebralis. *Klin. Monatsbl. Augenheilkd.* **154**:183–193, 1969.

41 Valada, A. J., et al., Aberrant Salivary Gland Tissue at the Base of the Tongue. *Laryngoscope* **60**:577–580, 1950.

42 Weyers, H., and Thier, C. J., Malformations mandibulo-faciales et délimitation d'un syndrome oculo-vertebral. *J. Génét. Hum.* **7**:143–173, 1958.

43 White, J. H., Oculo-nasal Dysplasia. *J. Génét. Hum.* **17**:104–114, 1969.

44 Wilson, T. G., A Case of Unilateral Mandibulo-facial Dysostosis Associated with Agenesis of the Homolateral Lung. *J. Laryngol.* **72**:238–249, 1958.

105

Oculodentoosseous Dysplasia

(Oculodentodigital Syndrome)

A lthough recognized as early as 1920 by Lohmann (10), it was not until 1957 that Meyer-Schwickerath et al. (11) fully described a syndrome characterized by (a) narrow nose with hypoplastic alae and thin nostrils, (b) microcornea with iris anomalies, (c) syndactyly and camptodactyly of the fourth and fifth fingers and certain bony anomalies of the middle phalanx of the fifth finger and toes, and (d) enamel hypoplasia, resembling amelogenesis imperfecta. Reisner et al. (15), in 1969, reviewed 43 examples.

The syndrome has autosomal dominant inheritance (15).

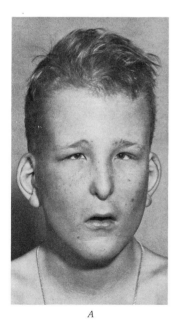 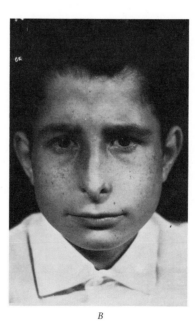 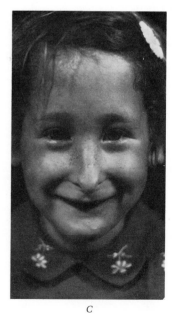

| A | B | C |

Figure 105-1. (*A*). *Oculodentoosseous dysplasia.* Note microphthalmia, thin nose without alar flare. (*B, C*). Note similar facies in seven- and thirteen-year-old sibs unrelated to patient shown in *A*. (*From S. H. Reisner et al., Petah Tikvah, Israel.*)

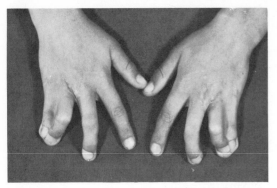

Figure 105-2. Bilateral 4-5 syndactyly with ulnar deviation. (*From S. H. Reisner et al., Petah Tikvah, Israel.*)

SYSTEMIC MANIFESTATIONS

Facies. Ocular hypertelorism, epicanthal folds, and thin nose with absent alar flare produce a characteristic physiognomy (Fig. 105-1*A–C*). Head circumference may be somewhat reduced (8, 15, 16).

Eyes. Eye defects consist of microcornea (6 to 10 mm in diameter), iris anomalies, and, in some cases, secondary glaucoma and small palpebral apertures (2a). Microphthalmos with small orbits has been noted (2, 8). The pupil may be eccentric. The iris consists of fine, porous spongy tissue. Between the frill and the pupillary rim are crypts and lacunas, and the iris frill may overlie the pupillary rim. Remnants of the pupillary membrane are present along the iris margin, rather than across the pupil (2, 3, 6, 11). Narrowing of visual fields has also been observed (11, 16).

Extremities. The most constant finding appears to be camptodactyly of the fifth or, less often, of the fourth and fifth fingers. Clinically, the fifth finger appears to be shortened. Bilateral syndactyly of the fourth and fifth fingers with ulnar clinodactyly and syndactyly of the third and fourth toes are usually present (15) (Fig. 105-2).

Roentgenographic examination reveals the middle phalanx to be cube-shaped or deltoid (Fig. 105-3*A*). The feet, clinically normal, on roentgenographic examination exhibit aplasia or

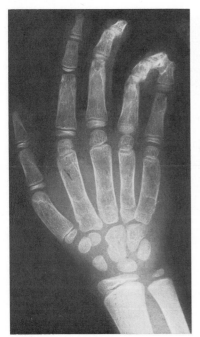

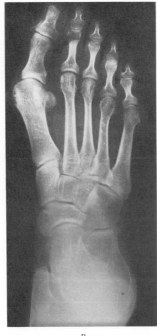

A

B

Figure 105-3. (*A*). Note poor modeling of long bones, bony fusion of terminal phalanges of fourth and fifth fingers. (*B*). Absence of middle phalanges of toes. (*From S. H. Reisner et al., Am. J. Dis. Child. **118**:600, 1969.*)

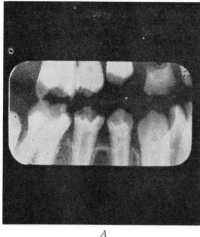 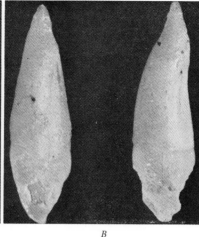

A *B*

Figure 105-4. (*A, B*). Marked enamel hypoplasia.

hypoplasia of the middle phalanx of one or more toes (Fig. 105-3*B*). There is lack of modeling of the metaphyseal area of the long bones (2, 2a, 6, 8, 14).

Hair. Dry, lusterless hair which fails to grow to normal length has been described but is not a constant feature (6, 8, 11, 13, 16).

Other findings. The pinnas may be somewhat abnormally modeled, and conduction deafness has been described (15).

Oral manifestations. Generalized enamel hypoplasia has been noted by a number of investigators (3, 15, 16) (Fig. 105-4). In addition, the alveolar ridge of the mandible may be wider than normal (1, 6, 14). Cleft lip-palate has been noted by Gillespie (5) and by one of the authors (R. J. G.).

DIFFERENTIAL DIAGNOSIS

Although the eye anomalies appear to be similar to those observed in the *Rieger syndrome*, there

is neither microcornea nor enamel hypoplasia in the latter, although tooth formation is suppressed.

In *trisomy 13*, there is a wide collection of abnormalities which include eye anomalies ranging from iridial coloboma to anophthalmia, mental retardation, arhinencephaly, seizures, deafness, digital anomalies such as hyperconvexity of fingernails, trigger thumbs, polydactyly, and cleft lip and/or palate.

Microcornea in combination with glaucoma, epicanthal folds, absent frontal sinuses, and hyperkeratosis of the palms may be inherited as a dominant trait (7).

LABORATORY AIDS

Roentgenographic examination of the femurs, hands, feet, and teeth should aid in the diagnosis.

REFERENCES

1 Cowan, A., Leontiasis Ossea. *Oral Surg.* **12**:983–989, 1959.

2 David, J. E. A., and Palmer, P. E. S., Familial Metaphyseal Dysplasia. *J. Bone Joint Surg.* **40B**:87–93, 1958.

2a Dudgeon, J., and Chisolm, J. A., Oculo-dento-digital Dysplasia. *Trans. Ophthalmol. Soc. U. K.* **94**:203–210, 1974.

3 Duggan, J. W., and Hassard, D. T. R., Familial Microphthal-

mos. *Trans. Can. Ophthalmol. Soc.* **24:**210–216, 1961.

4 Eidelman, E., et al., Orodigitofacial Dysostosis and Oculo-dentodigital Dysplasia. *Oral Surg.* **23:**311–319, 1967.

5 Gillespie, F. D., Hereditary Dysplasia Oculodentodigitalis. *Arch. Ophthalmol.* **71:**187–192, 1964.

6 Gorlin, R. J., et al., Oculodentodigital Dysplasia. *J. Pediatr.* **63:**69–75, 1963.

7 Holmes, L. B., and Walton, D. S., Hereditary Microcornea, Glaucoma and Absent Frontal Sinuses. *J. Pediatr.* **74:**968–972, 1969.

8 Kurlander, G. J., et al., Roentgen Differentiation of the Oculodentodigital Syndrome and the Hallermann-Streiff Syndrome of Infancy. *Radiology* **86:**77–85, 1966.

9 Littlewood, J. M., and Lewis, G. M., The Holmes-Adie Syndrome in a Boy with Acute Juvenile Rheumatism and Bilateral Syndactyly. *Arch. Dis. Child.* **38:**86–88, 1963.

10 Lohmann, W., Beitrag zur Kenntnis des reinen Mikroph-thalmus. *Arch. Augenheilkd.* **86:**136–141, 1920.

11 Meyer-Schwickerath, G., et al., Mikrophthalmussyndrome. *Klin. Monatsbl. Augenheilkd.* **131:**18–30, 1957.

12 Mohr, O. L., Dominant Acrocephalosyndactyly. *Hereditas* **25:**193–203, 1939.

13 Pfeiffer, R. A., et al., Oculo-dento-digitale Dysplasie. *Klin. Monatsbl. Augenheilkd.* **152:**247–262, 1968.

14 Rajic, D. S., and de Veber, L. L., Hereditary Oculodento-osseous Dysplasia. *Ann. Radiol.* **9:**224–231, 1966.

15 Reisner, S. H., et al., Oculodentodigital Dysplasia Syndrome. *Am. J. Dis. Child.* **118:**600–607, 1969.

16 Sugar, H. S., et al., The Oculo-dento-digital Dysplasia Syndrome. *Am. J. Ophthalmol.* **61:**1448–1451, 1966.

106

Oculomandibulodyscephaly

(Hallermann-Streiff Syndrome)

The syndrome consisting of (*a*) dyscephaly, (*b*) beaked nose, (*c*) mandibular hypoplasia, (*d*) proportionate nanism, (*e*) hypotrichosis, and (*f*) blue scleras was probably first described by Aubry (1) in 1893, although he did not observe the complete syndrome. Hallermann (9) and, especially, Streiff (22) separated the symptom complex from progeria and mandibulofacial dysostosis. Extensive recent surveys are those of Suzuki et al. (24) and Steele and Bass (21).

Virtually all cases have been sporadic. There is no sex predilection. The syndrome has been described as concordant (26) and discordant (19) in identical twins, and an affected female has had two normal children (18). Although the disorder has been described in a father and daughter (8), we cannot accept these cases as examples of the syndrome. Chromosome studies with one exception have been normal (13).

SYSTEMIC MANIFESTATIONS

Narrow upper air passages may make for feeding difficulties during infancy (10). Pneumonia and/or severe feeding difficulties have led to the demise of the infant in several instances.

Facies and general appearance. The face is small, with a long, thin, tapering, beaklike nose, receding chin, and an odd-shaped, often bulging skull (Fig. 106-1*A–D*). Brachycephaly is often accompanied by bossing, especially of the frontal or parietal areas. Mild microcephaly and malar bone hypoplasia also occur but are not constant features (14). Gaping or dehiscence of the longitudinal and lambdoidal sutures, as well as delayed closure of fontanels, has been described by nearly all authors.

Body growth is diminished proportionately, being at least 2 to 5 SD below the mean. Adult height for females is about 152.4 cm (5 ft), with males about 2.5 to 5.0 cm taller (21).

Eyes. Patients with previously undiagnosed cases tend to visit ophthalmologists because of visual impairment from congenital cataract. Microphthalmia of variable severity and bilateral congenital cataract are virtually constant features (24). The cataracts are rather unusual, since they often spontaneously resorb (28) (Fig. 106-2). Secondary glaucoma may occur (11, 23). Blue scleras have been described in about 15 to 25 percent of cases (14, 24), as well as posterior synechiae (5, 15), aphakia (2, 7, 9, 17, 26), and prepupillary membrane (26). Because of diminished vision, most patients have manifested nystagmus and/or strabismus. Additional eye findings have been extremely well analyzed (6, 14, 23, 28).

Nose. The nose is thin, pointed, and often curved. Combined with mandibular hypoplasia, these characteristics give the individual an unusual appearance. Several authors have remarked on the tendency to septal deviation (2, 18).

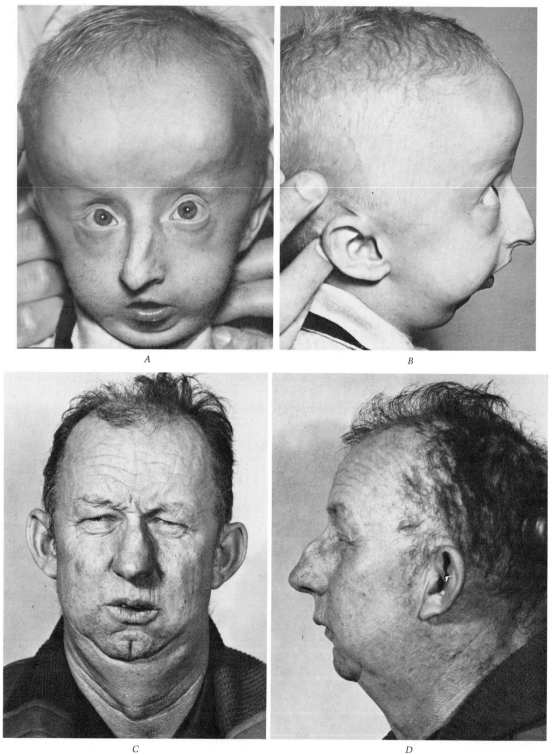

Figure 106-1. *Oculomandibulodyscephaly.* (*A, B*). Micrognathia, posteriorly rotated pinnas, exophthalmos. (*From D. Hoefnagel and K. Benirschke,* Arch. Dis. Child. **40**:57, 1965.) (*C, D*). Compare facies with that in older patient. Also note grooves in chin and balding.

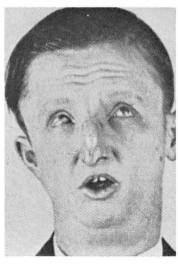
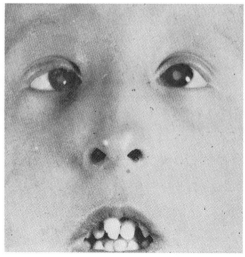

Figure 106-2. Close-up view demonstrating cataracts. (*Courtesy of W. Hallermann.*)

Skin and skin appendages. Hypotrichosis, especially of the scalp, brows, and cilia, has been a frequent feature (24). Axillary and pubic hair may also be scant (5, 6). Alopecia is most prominent about the frontal and occipital areas, but is especially marked along suture lines (23).

Cutaneous atrophy is largely limited to the scalp and nose. The scalp skin is thin and taut, and the scalp veins are prominent. Similar changes, often focal, are observed on the nose.

Mental status. Mental retardation has been noted in about 15 percent of the cases (13, 24).

Other findings. Skeletal anomalies are infrequent and have not been limited to the face and cranium. Osteoporosis (17), syndactyly (26),

lordosis and/or scoliosis (15, 19), and spina bifida have been noted. The scapulas are commonly winglike (13, 18, 24, 26).

Hypogenitalism (10, 20) has also been reported.

Oral manifestations. The most common oral anomaly is hypoplasia of the mandible. This is a constant feature and is often accompanied by a double cutaneous chin with a central cleft or dimple (2, 4, 6, 7, 9, 22). The ascending ramus is usually short, and the condyle may be missing (6) or the fossa hypoplastic (13). Roentgenographic examination of the temporomandibular joint area reveals a characteristic change. The joint is displaced approximately 2 cm forward [normally, the joint is located just in front of the

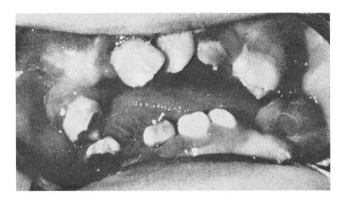

Figure 106-3. Severe dental malocclusion. (*Courtesy of H. Weyers, Cuxhaven, Germany.*)

external auditory meatus (26)]. The palate is high and narrow, and the paranasal sinuses are diminished in size (5). The mouth is usually stated to be small (26).

Dental anomalies are a common feature (6, 12) (Fig. 106-3). Absence of teeth (2, 5, 6, 10), persistence of deciduous teeth (5, 6), malocclusion and open bite (1, 2, 6, 15, 17, 19, 22), malformation of teeth (4, 5, 9, 17), and severe and premature caries (5, 17, 21) have been reported. Supernumerary teeth have been seen, as well as natal teeth (5, 10, 15, 17, 20).

DIFFERENTIAL DIAGNOSIS

Differential diagnosis includes *progeria*, from which oculomandibulodyscephaly differs by the absence of premature arteriosclerosis, nail dystrophy, acromicria, and chronic deforming arthritis. Moreover, the eyes are normal in progeria.

Micrognathia, high palatal vault, and malar hypoplasia are seen also in *mandibulofacial dysostosis*, but there are usually lower-lid colobomas and associated ear anomalies in that syndrome. Brachycephaly with persistently open fontanels and wide sutures, high palatal vault, and malar bone flattening are seen in *cleidocranial dysplasia* and in *pyknodysostosis*.

Oculodentoosseous dysplasia differs from oculomandibulodyscephaly in having an essentially normally developed mandible, no blue scleras, no sutural alopecia, characteristic changes in the middle phalanx of the fifth digits, and amelogenesis imperfecta-like changes in the teeth.

Natal teeth are also found in *chondroectodermal dysplasia*, *pachyonychia congenita*, *type II*, and, at times, *cyclopia*.

LABORATORY AIDS

None is known.

REFERENCES

1 Aubry, M., Variété singulière d'alopécie congénitale; alopécie suturale. *Ann. Dermatol. Syphiligr.* (*Paris*) **4**: 899–900, 1893.

2 Blodi, F. C., Developmental Anomalies of the Skull Affecting the Eye. *Arch. Ophthalmol.* **57**:593–610, 1957.

3 Carones, A. V., Syndrome dyscéphalique de François. *Ophthalmologica* **142**:510–518, 1961.

4 Caspersen, I., and Warburg, M., Hallermann-Streiff Syndrome. *Acta Ophthalmol.* (*Kbh.*) **46**:385–390, 1968.

5 Falls, H. F., and Schull, W. J., Hallermann-Streiff Syndrome: A Dyscephaly with Congenital Cataracts and Hypotrichosis. *Arch. Ophthalmol.* **63**:409–420, 1960.

6 Francois, M. J., A New Syndrome: Dyscephalia with Bird Face and Dental Anomalies, Nanism, Hypotrichosis, Cutaneous Atrophy, Microphthalmia and Congenital Cataract. *Arch. Ophthalmol.* **60**:842–862, 1958.

7 Gregersen, E., Ocular Abnormalities in Progeria. *Acta Ophthalmol.* (*Kbh.*) **34**:347–354, 1956.

8 Guyard, M., et al., Sur deux cas de syndrome dyscéphalique à tête d'oiseau. *Bull. Soc. Fr. Ophtalmol.* **62**:443–447, 1962.

9 Hallermann, W., Vogelgesicht und Cataracta congenita. *Klin. Monatsbl. Augenheilkd.* **113**:315–318, 1948.

10 Hoefnagel, D., and Benirschke, K., Dyscephalia Mandibulo-oculo-facialis (Hallermann-Streiff Syndrome). *Arch. Dis. Child.* **40**:57–61, 1965.

11 Hopkins, D. J., and Horan, E. C., Glaucoma in the Hallermann-Streiff Syndrome. *Br. J. Ophthalmol.* **54**:416–422, 1970.

12 Hutchinson, M., et al., Oral Manifestations of Oculomandibulodyscephaly with Hypotrichosis (Hallermann-Streiff Syndrome). *Oral Surg.* **31**:234–244, 1971.

13 Judge, C., and Chakanovskis, J. E., The Hallermann-Streiff Syndrome. *J. Ment. Defic. Res.* **15**:115–120, 1971.

14 Lamy, M., et al., La dyscéphalie (syndrome de Hallermann-Streiff-François). *Arch. Fr. Pédiatr.* **22**:929–938, 1965.

15 Ludwig, A., and Korting, G., Vogt-Koyanagi-ähnliches Syndrom und mandibulofaciale Dysostosis (Franceschetti-Zwahlen). *Arch. Dermatol. Syph.* (*Berl.*) **190**:307–319, 1950.

16 Marchesani, O., Über Beziehungen zwischen Wachstum und Nervensegmenten. *Dtsch. Ophthalmol. Gesell.* **55**:34–38, 1949.

17 Moehlig, R. C., Progeria with Nanism and Congenital Cataracts in a Five-year-old Child. *J.A.M.A.* **132**:640–642, 1946.

18 Ponte, F., Further Contributions to the Study of the Syndrome of Hallermann and Streiff. *Ophthalmologica* **143**:399–408, 1962.

19 Schondel, A., Two Cases of Progeria Complicated by Microphthalmus. *Acta Paediatr.* **30**:286–304, 1943.

20 Srivastava, S., et al., Mandibulo-oculo-facial Dyscephaly. *Br. J. Ophthalmol.* **58**:543–549, 1966.

21 Steele, R. W., and Bass, J. W., Hallermann-Streiff Syn-

drome: Clinical and Prognostic Considerations. *Am. J. Dis. Child.* **120:**462–465, 1970.

22 Streiff, E. B., Dysmorphie mandibulo-faciale (tête d'oiseau) et alteration oculaires. *Ophthalmologica* **120:**79–83, 1950.

23 Sugar, A., et al., Hallermann-Streiff-François Syndrome. *J. Pediatr. Ophthalmol.* **8:**234–238, 1971.

24 Suzuki, Y., et al., Hallermann-Streiff Syndrome. *Dev. Med. Child. Neurol.* **12:**496–506, 1970.

25 Ullrich, O., and Fremerey-Dohna, H., Dyskephalie mit Cataracta congenita und Hypotrichose als typischer Merk-malskomplex. *Ophthalmologica* **125:**73–90, 144–154, 1953.

26 Van Balen, A. T. M., Dyscephaly with Microphthalmos, Cataract and Hypoplasia of the Mandible. *Ophthalmologica* **141:**53–63, 1961.

27 Walbaum, R., et al., Le syndrome de Hallermann-Streiff-François. *Pédiatrie* **23:**789–794, 1968.

28 Wolter, J. R., and Jones, D. H., Spontaneous Cataract Absorption in Hallermann-Streiff Syndrome. *Ophthalmologica* **150:**401–408, 1965.

107

Oral-Facial-Digital Syndrome I

(OFD I Syndrome)

In 1954, Papillon-Leage and Psaume (18) defined a syndrome of (*a*) abnormally developed frenula, (*b*) cleft tongue, (*c*) hypoplasia of nasal alar cartilages, (*d*) median pseudocleft of upper lip, (*e*) asymmetric cleft palate, (*f*) various malformations of digits, and (*g*) mental retardation.

Similar cases had been reported under a variety of names as early as 1860. To date, approximately 125 cases have appeared in the literature. Comprehensive recent surveys are by Fuhrmann et al. (7), Stahl and Fuhrmann (27), and Gorlin (8). Wahrman et al. (31) suggested that the incidence of the syndrome is probably about 0.0225 per 1,000 live births.

OFD I syndrome is inherited as a dominant X-linked trait limited to females and lethal in males (5–7, 9, 28) and has also been described in a male with the Klinefelter syndrome (31). One of the most perplexing pedigrees is that of Vaillaud et al. (29, 30). In this family the disorder appears to have been transmitted through unaffected males. Several other "affected" males probably had the Mohr syndrome (OFD II syndrome). This syndrome is considered under Differential Diagnosis (*vide infra*) and in Chap. 108.

SYSTEMIC MANIFESTATIONS

Facies. The facies is remarkably distinctive. Usually there is euryopia, but not uncommonly there is dystopia canthorum (lateral displacement of the inner canthi) (16). Some aquiline thinning of the nose, due at least in part to hypoplasia of the alar cartilages, and a pseudocleft in the midline of the upper lip are present in most patients (Fig. 107-1*A, B*). The upper lip is usually short, and the nasal root is broad. One nostril may be smaller than the other, and there may be flattening of the nasal tip. Because of zygomatic hypoplasia, the midfacial region is flattened in about 75 percent of cases.

Skin and skin appendages. Commonly there are evanescent milia of the face and ears (Fig. 107-2). These usually disappear before the third year of life (25). About 65 percent of those affected have dryness and/or alopecia of the scalp (16).

Dermatoglyphics have been studied by Doege et al. (6), Reinwein (19), and Co-Te et al. (2). A preponderance of whorls has been noted. However, Kernohan and Dodge (13) described 10 arches in their patient.

Skeletal manifestations. The nasion-sella-basion, or cranial base, angle is increased, being about 144° and exceeding the normal value of 131° (SD = 4.5°) by almost three standard deviations (1, 4, 9, 25).

On roentgenographic examination, the short tubular bones of the hands and feet appear irregularly short and thick. Irregular reticulated areas of radiolucency or osteoporosis are observed in the metacarpals and, especially, in the phalanges.

Malformations of the fingers, in decreasing

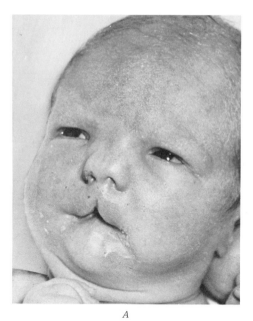
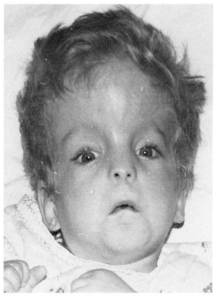

A   *B*

Figure 107-1. *Oral-facial-digital syndrome I.* (*A*). Pseudocleft in midline of upper lip, lack of nasal alar flare. (*From H. Reinwein et al.,* Humangenetik **2:**165, 1966.) (*B*). Note frontal bossing, wide-spaced eyes, hypoplastic alar cartilages, and down-turned mouth.

frequency of appearance, are clinodactyly, syndactyly, and brachydactyly (Fig. 107-3*A*). Toe malformations, which are considerably less common, include *unilateral* hallucal polysyndactyly, syndactyly, and brachydactyly (Fig. 107-3*B*). The hallux is often bent in a fibular direction, with brachydactyly and hypoplasia of the second to fifth toes. Occasionally, there is a postminimus finger or toe (5, 6, 16, 19, 21, 26). Some patients have had cone-shaped epiphyses in the digits. No anomalies have been found in the long bones, pelvis, or spine.

Central nervous system. Mental retardation is seen in over half the patients (16). The intelligence quotient usually ranges from 70 to 90. Various central nervous system alterations have been described, including hydrocephaly, porencephaly, hydranencephaly, and partial agenesis of the corpus callosum (2, 8, 9, 16, 21, 25, 30). Doege et al. (5, 6) noted decreased hearing in their patients.

Oral manifestations. The most striking oral manifestations are the "clefts" associated with

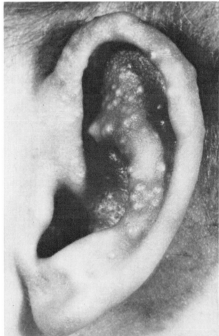

Figure 107-2. Milia of pinna, which ordinarily disappear by the third year of life. (*From F. Majewski et al.,* Z. Kinderheilkd. **112:**89, 1972.)

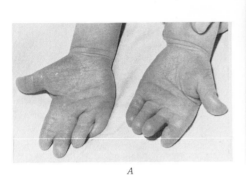
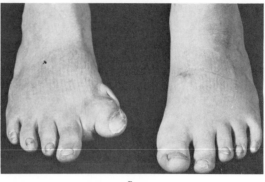

A   *B*

Figure 107-3. (*A*). Asymmetric soft-tissue syndactyly, abbreviation of fingers. (*From H. Reinwein et al.,* Humangenetik **2:**165, 1966.) (*B*). Unilateral preaxial polysyndactyly of hallux. (*From J. W. Curtin,* Plast. Reconstr. Surg. **34:**579, 1964.)

hyperplasia of frenula. There is often (in about 45 percent of cases) a small midline "cleft" in the upper lip extending through the vermilion border (Fig. 107-4*A*). Upon retraction of the short upper lip, a wide, thickened or hyperplastic reduplicated frenum is seen to be associated with the pseudocleft. This, in part, eradicates the mucobuccal fold in the area. Because of these bands, complete retraction is often not possible. Thick frenula are seen in virtually all patients (7, 8, 16).

The palate is cleft laterally, deep bilateral grooves extending medially from the maxillary buccal frenula, dividing the palate into (*a*) an anterior segment containing the incisors and the canines; and (*b*) two lateral palatal processes (Fig. 107-4*D*). The soft palate is completely and asymmetrically cleft in at least 80 percent of patients (7). In some persons, a large bony ridge extends from the alveolar crest medially to the midline in the canine-premolar area, somewhat resembling a misplaced torus.

Numerous thick fibrous bands are evident in the lower mucobuccal fold (Fig. 107-4*E*), eliminating the sulcus, clefting the hypoplastic mandibular alveolar processes, and, by extension, bifurcating, trifurcating, or tetrafurcating the tongue (Fig. 107-4*B, C*). Bifurcation occurs in about 30 percent of cases. Three or more lobes are present in the rest. On the ventral surface of the tongue, between the tongue halves or lobules, a small whitish hamartomatous mass is seen in about 70 percent of those affected (16). This consists of fibrous connective tissue, sali-

vary gland tissue, a few striated muscle fibers, and, rarely, cartilage. Ankyloglossia or tongue-tie of a diffuse nature is present in at least one-third of the cases (16). Correction of these oral anomalies has been discussed extensively by Curtin (3).

Malposition of the maxillary canine teeth, supernumerary maxillary deciduous canines and premolars, and infraocclusion are common. The supernumerary canines are often separated by the clefts. The canine crown form is often T-shaped. Aplasia of mandibular lateral incisors occurs in about half the affected persons and appears to be predicated on the effect of the fibrous bands on the developing tooth germs. The mandible is small or hypoplastic with a short ramus (15).

DIFFERENTIAL DIAGNOSIS

Several of these components may be seen in other syndromes. For example, in the *Ellis-van Creveld syndrome* the upper or, occasionally, the lower lip may be attached to the gingiva, there being no mucobuccal fold anteriorly. Associated with this may be a mild mid-upper lip defect. Alar cartilage hypoplasia and dystopia canthorum occur in the *Waardenburg syndrome,* but to a greater degree.

Most closely related to this syndrome is the *OFD II syndrome,* described by Mohr (17), Rimoin and Edgerton (20), and others (see Table

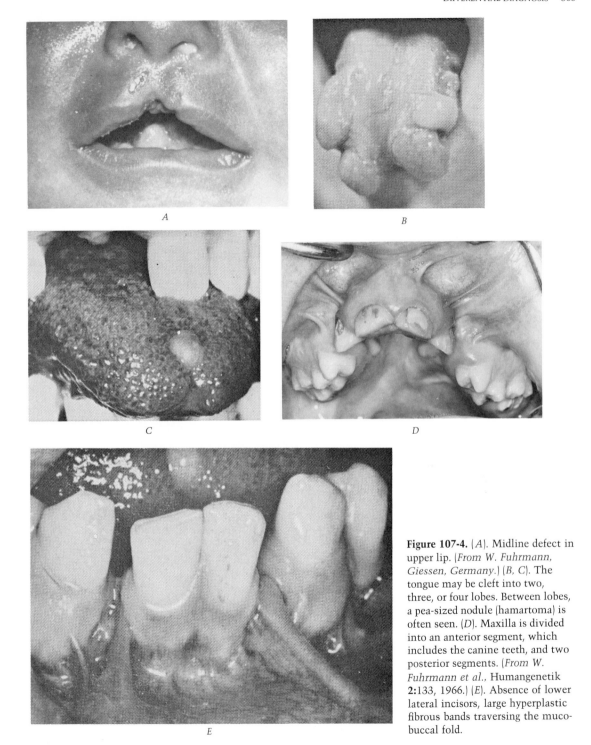

Figure 107-4. (*A*). Midline defect in upper lip. (*From W. Fuhrmann, Giessen, Germany.*) (*B, C*). The tongue may be cleft into two, three, or four lobes. Between lobes, a pea-sized nodule (hamartoma) is often seen. (*D*). Maxilla is divided into an anterior segment, which includes the canine teeth, and two posterior segments. (*From W. Fuhrmann et al., Humangenetik* 2:133, 1966.) (*E*). Absence of lower lateral incisors, large hyperplastic fibrous bands traversing the muco-buccal fold.

Table 107-1. Comparison of OFD I and OFD II syndromes

	OFD I syndrome	OFD II (Mohr) syndrome
Inheritance	X-linked dominant, lethal in male	Autosomal recessive
Hands	Usually five fingers, with variable brachydactyly, syndactyly, clinodactyly. Cystic changes in phalanges in roentgenograms	Bimanual ulnar hexadactyly, unilateral hexadactyly less frequent
Feet	Hallux may exhibit fibular clinodactyly. Occasional unilateral polysyndactyly of hallux. Brachydactyly of second through fourth toes. Rarely postminimus rudimentary supernumerary toes	Bilateral polysyndactyly of halluces. Frequently broad first metatarsal. Postminimus digit common
Hair and skin	Sparse hair. Transient milia of ears and face	Normal
Oral alterations	Bifid, trifid, or tetrafid tongue, cleft plate, multiple hyperplastic frenula, hamartomas of tongue located between tongue lobes	Fatty hamartomas of tongue, often on dorsum

107-1). It is inherited as an autosomal recessive trait. These patients also have a midline cleft of the upper lip, a lobate tongue with small excrescences, bilateral manual hexadactyly, and bilateral polysyndactyly of the halluces. In contrast to patients with OFD I syndrome, these patients may be male. They do not have hyperplastic frenula, the lower central incisors may be absent, and often there is a hearing defect.

The patients described by Helbig (12) and by Koberg and Schettler (14) defy precise classification at this time.

LABORATORY AIDS

None is known.

REFERENCES

1 Aduss, H., and Pruzansky, S., Postnatal Craniofacial Development in Children with the OFD Syndrome. *Arch. Oral Biol.* **9**:193–203, 1954.

2 Co-Te, P., et al., Oral-facial-digital Syndrome. *Am. J. Dis. Child.* **119**:280–283, 1970.

3 Curtin, J. W., Plastic Surgical Correction of the Oral-facial-digital Syndrome. *Plast. Reconstr. Surg.* **34**:579–589, 1964.

4 Dodge, J. A., and Kernohan, D. C., Oral-facial-digital Syndrome. *Arch. Dis. Child.* **42**:214–219, 1967.

5 Doege, T. C., et al., Studies of a Family with the Oral-facial-digital Syndrome. *N. Engl. J. Med.* **271**:1073–1080, 1964.

6 Doege, T. C., et al., Mental Retardation and Dermatoglyphics in a Family with the Oral-facial-digital Syndrome. *Am. J. Dis. Child.* **116**:615–622, 1968.

7 Fuhrmann, W., et al., Das oro-facio-digitale Syndrom. *Humangenetik* **2**:133–164, 1966.

8 Gorlin, R. J., The Oral-facial-digital (OFD) Syndrome. *Cutis* **4**:1345–1349, 1968.

9 Gorlin, R. J., and Psaume, J., Orodigitofacial Dysostosis: A New Syndrome. A Study of 22 Cases. *J. Pediatr.* **61**:520–530, 1962.

10 Grob, M., Dysplasia linguo-facialis (Grob), in *Lehrbuch der Kinderchirurgie.* Thieme, Stuttgart, 1957, pp. 98–100.

11 Hauenstein, P., Beziehungen zwischen Anomalien der bukkalen Frenuli der Kiefer- und Gesichtsdeformitäten. *Fortschr. Kieferorthop.* **22**:100–107, 1961.

12 Helbig, D., Mediane Unterlippenspalte, zugleich ein Beitrag zur Dysplasie linguo-facialis Grob. *Chirurg.* **29**: 509–511, 1958.

13 Kernohan, D. C., and Dodge, J. A., Further Observations on a Pedigree of the Oral-facial-digital Syndrome. *Arch. Dis. Child.* **44**:729–731, 1969.

14 Koberg, W., and Schettler, D., Papillon-Leage-Psaume Syndrom (Vier kasuistische Beiträge zur Dysostosis orodigitofacialis). *Z. Kinderheilkd.* **96**:147–162, 1966.

15 Lauterstein, A., and Pruzansky, S., Tooth Anomalies in the Oral-facial-digital Syndrome. *Teratology* **2**:137–146, 1969.

16 Majewski, F., et al., Das oro-facio-digitale Syndrom. *Z. Kinderheilkd.* **112**:89–112, 1972.

17 Mohr, O. L., A Hereditary Sublethal Syndrome in Man. *Nor. Vidensk.-Akad. Oslo. I. Mat.-naturv. Klasse* **14**:1–18, 1941.

18 Papillon-Leage (Mme) and Psaume, J., Une malformation héréditaire de la muqueuse buccale et freins anormaux. *Rev. Stomatol. (Paris)* **55**:209–227, 1954.

19 Reinwein, H., et al., Untersuchungen an einer Familie mit Oral-facial-digital Syndrom. *Humangenetik* **2**:165–177, 1966.

20 Rimoin, D. L., and Edgerton, M. T., Genetic and Clinical Heterogeneity in the Oral-facial-digital Syndrome. *J. Pediatr.* **71**:94–102, 1967.

21 Romano, C., et al., La sindrome orodigitofacciale. *Minerva Pediatr.* **19**:1288–1295, 1967.

22 Ruess, A. L., et al., The Oral-facial-digital Syndrome. *Pediatrics* **29**:985–995, 1962.

23 Ruess, A. L., Intellectual Development and the OFD Syndrome—a Review. *Cleft Palate J.* **2**:350–356, 1965.

24 Schwarz, E., and Fish, A., Roentgenographic Features of a New Congenital Dysplasia. *Am. J. Roentgenol.* **84**:511–517, 1960.

25 Solomon, L., et al., Pilosebaceous Dysplasia in the OFD Syndrome. *Arch. Dermatol.* **102**:598–602, 1970.

26 Stahl, A., et al., Beitrag zur Genetik des orofazialendigitalen Syndroms. *Fortschr. Kieferorthop.* **26**:455–464, 1965.

27 Stahl, A., and Fuhrmann, W., Oro-facio-digitales Syndrom. *Dtsch. Med. Wochenschr.* **93**:1224–1228, 1968.

28 Thuline, H. C., Current Status of a Family Previously Reported with the Oral-facial-digital Syndrome. *Birth Defects* **5**(2):102–104, 1969.

29 Vaillaud, J. C., et al., Le syndrome oro-facio-digital. Étude clinique et génétique à propos de 10 cas dans une même famille. *Rev. Pédiatr.* **4**:383–392, 1968.

30 Vissian, L., and Vaillaud, J. C., Le syndrome oro-facio-digital. *Ann. Dermatol. Syphiligr. (Paris)* **99**:5–20, 1972.

31 Wahrman, J., et al., The Oral-facial-digital Syndrome: A Male Lethal Condition in a Boy with 47/XXY Chromosomes. *Pediatrics* **37**:812–821, 1966.

108

Oral-Facial-Digital Syndrome II

(Mohr Syndrome, OFD II Syndrome)

In 1941, Mohr (17) described a family later expanded upon by Claussen (6). Several sibs and a cousin exhibited (*a*) lobed tongue, (*b*) manual polydactyly, and (*c*) bilateral polysyndactyly of the halluces. Earlier cases may have been described by Otto (18) in 1841 and by Lyons (15) in 1939. Subsequently, a number of well-defined examples have been published (4, 7, 10, 11, 14, 16, 19, 20). Less certain are several other cases (1, 2, 22). We suspect heterogeneity.

The syndrome is clearly inherited as an autosomal recessive trait. Parental consanguinity has been demonstrated (6) and there have been several examples of the syndrome in sibs (6, 9a, 10, 17, 20, 23). We have seen several affected.

SYSTEMIC MANIFESTATIONS

Facies. Frequently there is a midline cleft of the upper lip (Fig. 108-1).

Skeletal alterations. Bony changes appear to be limited to hands and feet. Bilateral manual ulnar hexadactyly and bilateral polysyndactyly of the halluces are characteristic (4, 7, 10, 11, 14, 16, 20, 23) (Figs. 108-1*B, C, 2B, C*). The hallucal polysyndactyly in the patient described by Beaudry (2) was, however, unilateral. Patients described by several authors (2, 6, 10, 15, 16, 23) also had one or more postminimus digits.

Bimanual hexadactyly apparently is not requisite for diagnosis of the syndrome, since in some cases there have been five fingers with ulnar deviation of the fifth finger, 3-4 syndactyly with extra bones in the web, or hexadactyly of only one hand (6, 15).

Central nervous system. Mental retardation has been reported in several cases (14, 17). Various other neurologic anomalies have been described, including microcephaly (14), porencephaly (14), internal hydrocephaly (7), conduction deafness

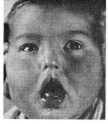
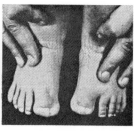

A   *B*   *C*

Figure 108-1. *(A–C). Oral-facial-digital syndrome II.* Note median cleft of upper lip and bimanual hexadactyly. Child also had bilateral polysyndactyly of halluces. *(Courtesy of F. Burian, Prague.)*

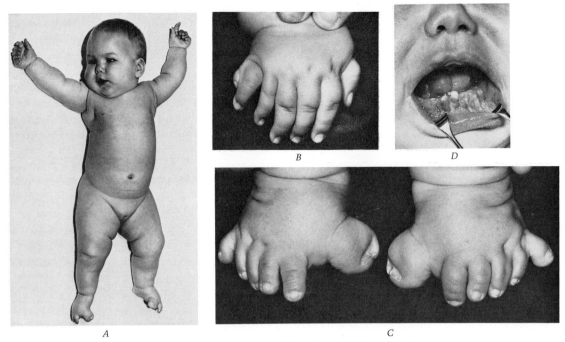

Figure 108-2. (*A–D*). Compare with Fig. 108-1*A–C*. Note bilateral manual hexadactyly, polysyndactyly of halluces, defect in middle of upper lip, hamartoma of tongue. (*From R. A. Pfeiffer et al., Klin. Pediätr.* **185:**224, 1973.)

(9a, 20), choroid coloboma (7), and muscular hypotonia with poor coordination (6, 10, 14, 16).

Other findings. There would appear to be increased susceptibility to respiratory infection, which in several patients has resulted in death during infancy (2, 6, 7, 14–17). Tachypnea has also been reported (6, 10).

Cryptorchism (2, 6, 20) and inguinal hernia have been noted (14).

Oral manifestations. Cleft tongue is probably a constant feature of the syndrome, and several authors have spoken of general ankyloglossia (2, 6, 14, 16, 20). In a few cases, cleft palate (1, 9a, 15, 20) or bifid uvula (5) has been mentioned. However, in most patients the palate has been intact (14, 16, 22). A small median cleft of the upper lip is a relatively common feature (Fig. 108-1) but was missing in the cases described by Mohr (17), Claussen (6), and Gustavson et al. (10). Multiple frenula are occasionally present (9a, 14, 16, 20) but far less frequent than in OFD I syndrome.

Fatty hamartomas on the dorsum of the tongue have been noted in several cases (1, 2, 6, 9a, 10, 16, 17) (Fig. 108-2*D*).

DIFFERENTIAL DIAGNOSIS

Many cases of "median cleft" of the upper lip are not true median clefts but examples of the premaxillary agenesis variant of *holoprosencephaly*, characterized by agenesis of the septum pellucidum and corpus callosum, agenesis of the prolabium, premaxilla, and nasal bones, microcephaly, and ocular hypotelorism (24). True median cleft may be seen in association with bifid nose and ocular hypertelorism as examples of *frontonasal dysplasia* (12, 21). An infant that exhibited certain features of both frontonasal dysplasia and premaxillary agenesis was described by Bell and Van Allen (3). Median cleft of the upper lip is also seen in the OFD I syndrome.

The patients described by Büttner and Eysholdt (5) and by Wolf (25) with bilateral pseudoarthrosis and bending of the tibias have an as yet unclassified syndrome. The cases of Froriep and Froriep (9), Dreibholz (8), and Sugarman et al. (22) probably are examples of other entities.

LABORATORY AIDS

None is known.

REFERENCES

1 Barling, G., Cleft Tongue with Median Lobe and Cleft Palate. *Br. Med. J.* **2:**1061, 1885.

2 Beaudry, G. O., Polydactylisme et malconformation de langue. *Union Méd. Can.* **4:**342–343, 1875.

3 Bell, W. E., and Van Allen, M. W., Agenesis of Corpus Callosum with Associated Facial Anomalies. *Neurology (Minneap.)* **9:**694–698, 1959.

4 Burian, F., *Chirurgie der Lippen und Gaumenspalten.* VEB-Verlag Volk und Gesundheit, Berlin, 1963.

5 Büttner, A., and Eysholdt, K. G., Die angeborenen Verbiegungen und Pseudoarthrosen des Unterschenkels (case 14). *Ergeb. Chir. Orthop.* **36:**165–222, 1950.

6 Claussen, O., Et arveligt syndrom omfattende tungemissdannelse og polydaktyli. *Nord. Med.* **30:**1147–1151, 1946.

7 Dittmer, J., Über 2 Falles des Papillon-Léage-Psaume Syndroms (case 2). *Pädiatr. Grenzgeb.* **6:**35–42, 1967.

8 Dreibholz, E., *Beschreibung einer sogenannten Phokomele.* Thesis, Berlin, 1873.

9 Froriep, L. F., and Froriep, R., Missbildung (Monstrum per excessum). *Neue Notizen Geb. Natur. Heilkd.* **4:**8, 1837.

9a Goldstein, E., and Medina, J. L., Mohr Syndrome or Oral-facial-digital II: Report of Two Cases. *J. Am. Dent. Assoc.* **89:**377–382, 1974.

10 Gustavson, K. H., et al., Syndrome Characterized by Lingual Malformation, Polydactyly, Tachypnea and Psychomotor Retardation (Mohr Syndrome). *Clin. Genet.* **2:**261–266, 1971.

11 Huguet, C., *Contribution à l'étude du syndrome de Papillon-Léage et Psaume: À propos d'un cas chez un enfant de sexe masculin.* Thesis, Nantes, 1967–1968.

12 Kazajian, V. H., and Holmes, E. M., Treatment of Median Cleft Lip Associated with Bifid Nose and Hypertelorism. *Plast. Reconstr. Surg.* **24:**582–587, 1959.

13 Kölliker, T., Über das Os intermaxillare des Menschen und die Anatomie der Hasenscharte und des Wolfsrachens. *Nova Acta Academiae Caesareae Leopoldino-Carolinae Germanicae Naturae Curiosorum.* **43:**325–396, 1882.

14 Kushnick, T., et al., Orofaciodigital Syndrome in a Male. *J. Pediatr.* **63:**1130–1134, 1963.

15 Lyons, D. C., Skeletal Anomalies Associated with Cleft Palate and Harelip. *Am. J. Orthod.* **25:**895–987, 1939.

16 Mandell, F., et al., Oral-facial-digital Syndrome in a Chromosomally Normal Male. *Pediatrics* **40:**63–68, 1967.

17 Mohr, O. L., A Hereditary Sublethal Syndrome in Man. *Nor. Vidensk Akad. Oslo I. Mat. Naturv. Klasse.* **14:**3–18, 1941.

18 Otto, G., *Monstrorum sexcentorum descriptio anatomica.* S. F. Hirt, Vratislaviae, 1841.

19 Pfeiffer, R. A., et al., Das Syndrom von Mohr und Claussen. *Klin. Pediätr.* **185:**224–229, 1973.

20 Rimoin, D. L., and Edgerton, M. T., Genetic and Clinical Heterogeneity in the Oral-facial-digital Syndrome. *J. Pediatr.* **71:**94–102, 1967.

21 Sedano, H. O., et al., Frontonasal Dysplasia. *J. Pediatr.* **76:**906–913, 1970.

22 Sugarman, G. I., et al., See-saw Winking in a Familial Oral-facial-digital Syndrome. *Clin. Genet.* **2:**248–254, 1971.

23 Thurston, E. O., A Case of Median Harelip Associated with Other Malformations. *Lancet* **2:**996–997, 1909.

24 Weaver, D. F., and Bellinger, D. H., Bifid Nose Associated with Midline Cleft of the Upper Lip. *Arch. Otolaryngol.* **44:**480–482, 1946.

25 Wolf, H., Mediane Oberlippspalte mit Persistenz des Frenulum tectolabiale, *Dtsch. Zahnärztl. Z.* **7:**373–379, 1952.

109

Oromandibular-Limb Hypogenesis Syndromes

(Charlie M. Syndrome, Glossopalatine Ankylosis Syndrome,
Hanhart Syndrome, Hypoglossia-Hypodactylia Syndrome,
Moebius Syndrome)

Syndromes of oromandibular limb hypogenesis are confusing. Hall (21) called attention to the number of ambiguous and overlapping entities that exist in the literature on the subject. The problem seems to be twofold. First, because almost all cases reported to date are seemingly sporadic, it has been extremely difficult to define syndrome boundaries among this group. Entities have been delimited on a somewhat arbitrary basis, and cases can be graded with various degrees of overlap between defined syndrome entities. Second, Hall (21) noted that the terminology used to describe these disorders shows many discrepancies, thus compounding the problem. He proposed a classification of syndromes with oromandibular-limb hypogenesis based on the presence of hypoglossia. It should be noted that mild degrees of hypoglossia are difficult to detect and may, in fact, go unnoticed.

This chapter considers five defined syndrome entities, including the Charlie M. syndrome, glossopalatine ankylosis syndrome, Hanhart syndrome, hypoglossia-hypodactylia syndrome, and the Moebius syndrome. Our understanding of this group of conditions is limited for several other reasons besides seemingly sporadic occurrence. First, all except the Moebius syndrome are rare, and relatively few cases have been reported. Second, some authors have emphasized oral manifestations and limb anomalies to the exclusion of other possible abnormalities that may occasionally accompany these conditions. Third, careful family histories and a search for minor anomalies in first-degree relatives of the proband have not been carried out in many cases, resulting in lack of data for genetic analysis.

The etiology of this group of conditions is unknown. However, because sporadicity is seemingly apparent in almost all known cases, and since the clinical features, especially limb anomalies, seem to be remarkably variable, etiologic heterogeneity is likely. Many further reports with extensive documentation are necessary to determine whether these conditions should be regarded as a spectrum of disorders or whether they should be considered separate and distinct entities.

Gorlin and Pindborg (19) first suggested that cases of the hypoglossia-hypodactylia syndrome should be examined carefully for intrauterine environmental factors. Torpin (58) noted that rupture of the amnion during early pregnancy may produce membranous strands which constrict or amputate limbs and which may also lead to oral anomalies by the ingestion of amniotic strands which interfere with orofacial development. Hall (21) noted in his case that Tigan and Bendectin were given to the mother during the critical period of facial and limb development and cited another unpublished case in which the mother received Tigan.

In another case of the hypoglossia-hypodactylia syndrome, Temtamy and McKusick (55) noted that the father and paternal aunt of the proband had hypodontia. They further observed in their study of seven patients with the hypoglossia-hypodactylia syndrome or glosso-palatine ankylosis syndrome that orofacial anomalies were observed in various relatives, but in no instance were limb abnormalities observed in a relative. They suggested either multifactorial inheritance or autosomal dominant transmission with reduced penetrance and extreme variability in expression. Since most cases are seemingly sporadic, the possibility that some examples represent autosomal dominant mutations with reduced genetic fitness cannot be ruled out.

In two published papers on the Hanhart syndrome (22, 39), consanguinity was probable, suggesting the possibility of autosomal recessive inheritance. However, consanguinity was distant, and affected sibs have never been reported.

Spivak and Bennett (53) suggested that the glossopalatine ankylosis syndrome and the hypoglossia-hypodactylia syndrome were, in fact, closely related. One of the authors (M. M. C.) (6) strongly suggested that the glossopalatine ankylosis syndrome, Hanhart syndrome, and hypoglossia-hypodactylia syndrome might really represent the same formal genesis syndrome. Another one of the authors (R. J. G.) regards the Charlie M. syndrome, glossopalatine ankylosis syndrome, Hanhart syndrome and hypoglossia-hypodactylia syndrome as variants of an environmentally induced spectrum of anomalies.

The Moebius syndrome can quite closely mimic other syndromes of oromandibular-limb hypogenesis, but has, in addition, a combined palsy of the sixth and seventh cranial nerves. The basic cause of the Moebius syndrome also remains to be clarified. Postmortem studies have shown nuclear agenesis (27), neuron hypoplasia (50), absence or hypoplasia of various cranial nerve trunks and nerves (1a), and hypoplasia or absence of the facial muscles (47). Electromyograms and muscle biopsies have been of little value in determining etiology, although results have usually indicated a neural deficit (59). The most complete discussion of the pathologic findings and theories of pathogenesis has been presented by Pitner and associates (47).

Although autosomal dominant inheritance (15, 28, 40, 60), autosomal recessive inheritance (2, 2a, 33, 56), affected first cousins (24), and in-

stances of consanguinity (5, 24) have been reported for some cases of the Moebius syndrome, critical review of these cases strongly suggests that they represent entities distinct from the Moebius syndrome. In every instance, with the exception of the questionable mother-son involvement reported by Hicks (28), only the seventh cranial nerve was affected, and none of these patients had other manifestations of the Moebius syndrome (minimally sixth nerve palsy in addition). Furthermore, those in this genetically determined group also had a high incidence of hearing deficit and ear anomalies, and were usually of normal intelligence.

Some cases of thalidomide embryopathy (29, 41) have been noted to mimic the Moebius syndrome (as well as other syndromes of oromandibular-limb hypogenesis), suggesting that environmental factors (i.e., drugs) may be responsible for some cases.

CHARLIE M. SYNDROME

In 1969, Gorlin (18) observed that the Moebius syndrome category had been overworked as a repository for several different disorders and cited the Charlie M. syndrome as an example. The condition is characterized by ocular hypertelorism, facial paralysis in some instances, absent or conically crowned incisors, cleft palate, and variable degrees of hypodactyly of the hands and feet. The authors have observed several cases and, in each instance, the affected individual represented a sporadic occurrence (Fig. 109-1A–E).

GLOSSOPALATINE ANKYLOSIS SYNDROME

This syndrome, first described early in the century by Kettner (32) and Kramer (34), is rare, less than a dozen cases having been recorded (4, 7, 11, 30, 38, 53, 62, 63). All cases are seemingly sporadic.

The tongue is usually attached to the hard palate (4, 30), but may also be adherent to the maxillary alveolar ridge (11). Highly arched palate has been documented in some cases (7). Cleft palate has also been observed (30, 62), and, in

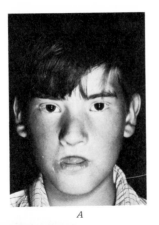

A

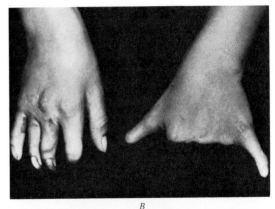

B

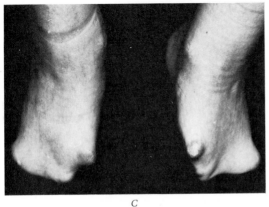

C

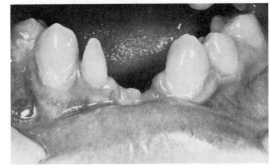

D

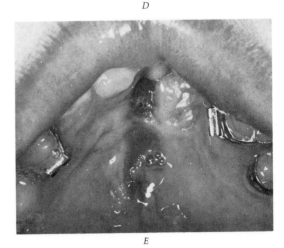

E

Figure 109-1. *Charlie M. syndrome.* (*A*). Mongoloid obliquity of palpebral fissures, ocular hypertelorism, lower facial palsy. (*B, C*). Bizarre digital agenesis and malformations. (*D*). Absence of three lower incisors, conical crown form of remaining incisor. (*E*). Repaired cleft of anterior palate. (*From R. J. Gorlin, Birth Defects 5(2):65, 1969.*)

these cases, the tongue may be attached to the lower edge of the nasal septum (Fig. 109-2).

In glossopalatine ankylosis, palatal attachment usually occurs to the anterior portion of the tongue. The tongue tip has been noted to be mildly cleft (4). Its mobility is reduced, and its extension beyond the teeth is limited (4, 7).

The mandible may be hypoplastic, and the central portion of the upper lip has also been described as hypoplastic (4, 7). Hypodontia principally affects the incisor teeth (4, 7). Ankylosis of the temporomandibular joint has also been recorded (4).

Facial paralysis has been noted by several authors (4, 34, 53).

Limb anomalies are extremely variable and may affect both hands and feet. Oligodactyly, syndactyly, polydactyly, and more severe peromelia have been observed (4, 7, 21, 30, 53, 62, 64).

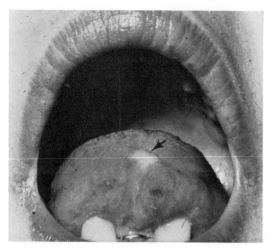

Figure 109-2. *Glossopalatine ankylosis syndrome.* White scar (see arrow) shows point of congenital linguopalatal adhesion. (*From M. Bünnige,* Ann. Paediatr. **195**:175, 1960.)

HANHART SYNDROME

Instances of the Hanhart syndrome were reported by Hanhart (22), Martius and Walter (39), Garner and Bixler (Case 2) (17), Assemany et al. (1), and Wexler and Novark (63). Micrognathia has been a feature in all cases. In Case 2 of Garner and Bixler (17), a fibrous band was noted to connect the maxilla and mandible on both sides but not anteriorly. The tongue was noted to be relatively normal in size in their patient. No other author has commented upon tongue size. The present authors feel that, with the degree of micrognathia expressed in some cases, hypoglossia should certainly be looked for in any suspected case. Hypodontia or delayed eruption occurred in one of Hanhart's cases (Case 2) (22). Assemany et al. (1) reported the Robin anomalad in their case (also see Chap. 29).

Limb anomalies range from stunted digits and oligodactyly to more severe peromelia. Any limb may be affected, and variability of involvement in the same patient and in different patients is well illustrated by Hanhart. Coxa valga was noted in one case (22) (Fig. 109-3A–C).

American clinicians should carefully note that in the European literature, although four conditions are called "Hanhart syndrome" (36), they are nosologically unrelated and are as distinct as von Recklinghausen neurofibromatosis and von Recklinghausen disease of bone. None of the other three conditions named after Hanhart has oligodactyly or partial syndactyly, despite a recent report to the contrary [Case 1 (17)]

HYPOGLOSSIA-HYPODACTYLIA SYNDROME

In a critical review of the literature, Hall (21) was able to confirm only approximately nine cases of the syndrome, including one of his own (2b, 8, 10a, 16, 19, 19a, 28a, 31, 37, 51, 52, 57). Since then, other cases have been observed by Nevin et al. (44), Temtamy and McKusick (55), and Opitz and Pettersen (46). The former term for the syndrome, "aglossia-adactylia," is misleading because the tongue is never completely ab-

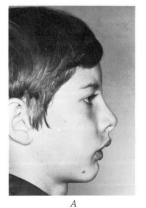
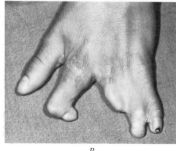
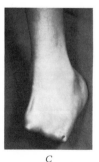

A   *B*   *C*

Figure 109-3. *Hanhart syndrome.* (*A*). Micrognathia. (*B, C*). Oligodactyly of hands and feet.

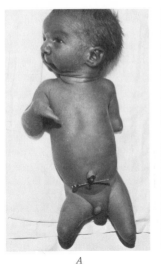
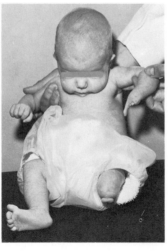
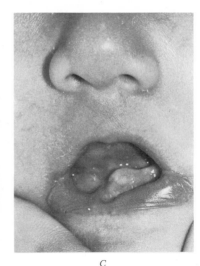

A   *B*   *C*

Figure 109-4. *Hypoglossia-hypodactylia syndrome.* (*A, B*). Small mandible and variable limb deformities. (*A from N. C. Nevin et al.,* Oral Surg. *29:443, 1970; B, courtesy of N. Freire-Maia, Curitiba, Brazil, and J. Opitz, Madison, Wis.*) (*C*). Attachment of anterior oral floor to lower lip. Small tongue was located in posterior part of mouth. (*From W. H. Boon and C. T. Seng,* J. Singapore Paediatr. Soc. **8:**75, 1966.)

sent (53) and "adactylia" does not convey the variation in the limb defects of affected individuals.

The mandible is small and the chin recedes. Hypoglossia is variable in degree, being extreme in the cases of Rosenthal (51), Fulford et al. (16), and Thornton (57), but the tongue was reduced only 25 percent in Hall's case (21). Mandibular incisors have been noted to be absent, with concomitant atrophy of the associated alveolar ridge (10a, 21, 51). Marked enlargement of the sublingual muscular ridges and hypertrophy of the sublingual and submandibular glands have been described (16, 51). A mild defect of the lower lip was noted by Rosenthal (51). Fusion of the anterior alveolar processes and cleft palate were reported in several cases (2b, 28a, 46a). In some patients the size of the oral opening is markedly reduced.

Limb anomalies are extremely variable. Any limb may be affected, and variability may be observed in the same patient as well as in different patients. For example, hemimelia of all four limbs was noted by Temtamy and McKusick (55). Involvement of both left limbs with normal right limbs was reported by Nevin and coworkers (44). Oligodactyly and syndactyly of both hands and complete adactyly of one foot with absence of the hallux on the other foot were observed by Kelln et al. (31) (Fig. 109-4*A*–*C*).

Speech is surprisingly good, and all patients have been of normal intelligence. Other findings have occasionally included fused labia majora (31) and imperforate anus (46). Because of associated abducens and oculomotor palsies, the patient reported by Ernst and Meinhold (10a) represents a nosologic "bridge."

MOEBIUS SYNDROME

Moebius (42, 43), in attempting to classify multiple congenital cranial nerve palsies, created a division in which (*a*) palsies of the sixth and seventh cranial nerves were combined. Subsequent authors have broadened this classification to include involvement of other cranial nerves (26). Additional abnormalities may include (*b*) reductive limb anomalies, (*c*) defects of the chest wall, and (*d*) mental retardation.

If the minimal criteria for the Moebius syn-

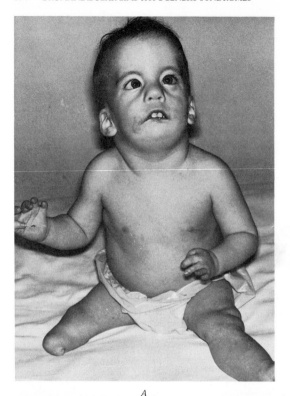

A

Figure 109-5. *Moebius syndrome.* (*A*). Variable degrees of limb hypogenesis. Strabismus, micrognathia, mask-like facies. Child had small tongue. (*From S. M. Harwin and L. C. Lorinsky, New Britain, Conn.*) (*B*). Patient had clubfoot, inability to execute horizontal eye movements, and expressionless face. (*Courtesy of R. Sogg,* Arch. Ophthalmol. **65**:16, 1961.) (*C*). Similar anomalies in a twenty-three-year-old male with defective ocular rotation, bilateral facial paralysis, and atrophy of tongue evident from birth. (*Courtesy of M. W. Van Allen, Fig.* 64, Grinker's Neurology, *Charles C Thomas, Springfield, Ill.,* 1960) (*D*). Severe microglossia. (*From S. M. Harwin and L. C. Lorinsky, New Britain, Conn.*) (*E*). Compare facies with others. (*F*). Observe paralysis of hypoglossal nerve. (E *and* F *from D. Gutman, Haifa, Israel.*)

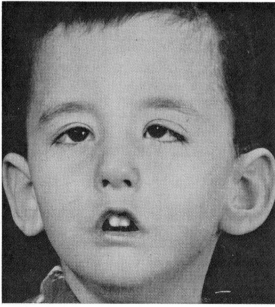

B

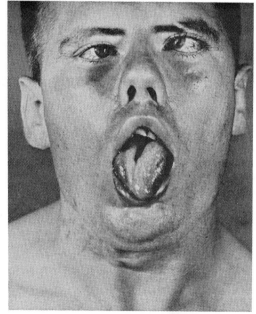

C

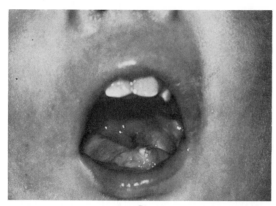

D

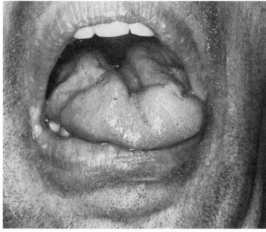

F

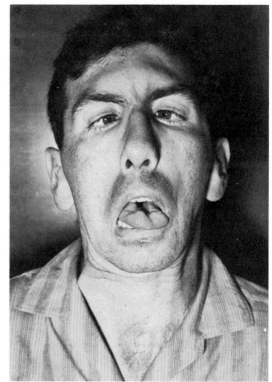

E

drome include (*a*) above, then all examples are apparently sporadic. Approximately 160 cases have been published to date (23). The ratio of affected males to females is equal. Extensive reviews include those of Henderson (26) and Danis (9).

Masklike facies may be obvious in the newborn, but may often go unrecognized at this time (13, 20, 24, 26). Bilateral facial paralysis usually imparts a symmetric appearance to the face, but variance in the degree of involvement on each side of the face or upper and lower portions of the face can cause significant asymmetry. Occasionally, only unilateral facial nerve palsy is present (13). Sixth nerve palsy is the most common ocular finding. Nearly every remaining cranial nerve can be affected in addition, but of these, the third, fifth, ninth, and twelfth nerves predominate (13, 54).

Most patients cannot abduct either eye beyond the midline. However, unilateral palsy does occur (28). Ptosis, nystagmus, or strabismus may accompany the above findings (3, 23, 26). Epicanthal folds are frequent (24). Some patients may be unable to close their eyes either during sleep or while awake, resulting in conjunctivitis or corneal ulceration (28, 40, 48).

The nasal bridge is often high and broad, particularly during infancy and early childhood (48). The broadness of the nasal bridge extends downward in a parallel fashion to include the nasal tip (26). Thus, an upper midfacial prominence usually results.

The mouth aperture is often small. The angles of the mouth droop and may allow saliva to escape (3, 48). Attempts at opening the mouth further result in little change. As the child grows older, a definite but slow improvement can be observed in his ability both to open his mouth and to feed adequately (13, 26). Poor feeding during the first year of life frequently results in poor growth.

Unilateral tongue hypoplasia is frequent (13), but bilateral hypoplasia can occur (13, 23, 48). The degree of hypoplasia may, on occasion, be extreme. One of the authors (M. M. C.) erroneously reported a case of the Moebius syndrome as an example of the hypoglossia-hypodactylia syndrome because of the severe degree of tongue hypoplasia (6). Muscular fasciculations of the tongue may be present (20). Poor palatal mobility, inefficient sucking and swallowing, coarse voice, and speech impairment are often present (48) (Fig. 109-5A–F).

Frequently, the mandible is mildly to moderately hypoplastic (13, 48), and when combined with the small mouth aperture, imparts the appearance of a lower midfacial hypoplasia.

The pinnas may be normal. However, they may be large, may be deficient in cartilage, and may protrude laterally (13). Occasionally, they are hypoplastic, but most instances of severe hypoplasia probably do not represent true examples of the Moebius syndrome (33, 56). Likewise, the hearing deficits which are reported occasionally with these hypoplastic ears are very infrequent findings in the Moebius syndrome (56).

Bilateral, unilateral, or asymmetric hypoplasia or aplasia of the pectoralis major muscle or complete Poland anomalad occurs in 15 percent of cases. Polythelia or athelia may be present (26). Spinal curvatures are occasionally noted but, as a rule, only in those few instances associated with arthrogryposis (23).

Limb defects occur in approximately 50 percent of patients. Thirty percent constitute talipes deformities (26). The remaining 20 percent primarily include hypoplasia of digits, syndactyly, or more severe reduction deformities of the limbs. Clinodactyly, polydactyly, joint contractures, and congenital hip dislocation occur less frequently (26, 40, 49).

Other findings may rarely include congenital heart defects, urinary tract abnormalities, hypogenitalism, and hypogonadism (23, 45). The authors have seen two examples with congenital heart defects.

Ten to 15 percent of patients are mentally retarded (9, 26). The degree of mental retardation is usually mild (24, 26). Estimates of early psychomotor development tend to be erroneously low (3, 13, 24). The severe physical deformities often cause a relative delay in apparent psychomotor development which tends to disappear as the child grows older.

DIFFERENTIAL DIAGNOSIS

As we have already pointed out, there may be variable degrees of overlap between defined syndrome entities of oromandibular-limb hypogenesis. Limb defects have the same range of variability in all five syndromes. Similar limb defects may be observed in the Poland anomalad, amniotic band syndrome, autosomal recessive acheiropody, and other disorders with reductive limb anomalies.

Isolated hypoglossia is known to occur (10, 12). Hypoglossia has also been observed in association with transposed viscera and dextrocardia (61). Hypoglossia has further been noted to occur with intraoral bands (14, 35). Cleft palate has been reported in association with intraoral bands through three generations (25). Such bands have also been documented in some cases of the *popliteal pterygium syndrome.*

Superficially, syndromes of oromandibular-limb hypogenesis (especially the hypoglossia-hypodactylia syndrome and the Moebius syndrome) may be confused with the *Robin anomalad, oculoauriculovertebral dysplasia,* and *mandibulofacial dysostosis.*

Isolated facial palsy may result from birth trauma in some instances, and has also been observed to follow autosomal dominant and autosomal recessive modes of inheritance.

LABORATORY AIDS

None is known.

REFERENCES

1 Assemany, S. R., et al., Syndrome of Phocomelia with Mandibular Hypoplasia. *Helv. Paediat. Acta* **26**:403–409, 1971.

1a Balint, A., Angeborenen Fazialis- und Abducenslähmung. *Arch. Kinderheilkd.* **147**:256–259, 1936.

2 Beetz, P., Beitrag zur Lehre von den angeborenen Beweglichkeitsdefekten im Bereich der Augen-, Gesichts-, und Schultermuskulatur (infantiler Kernschwund Moebius). *J. Psychol. Neurol. (Lpz.)* **20**:137–171, 1913.

2a Becker-Christensen, F., and Lund, H. T., A Family with Möbius Syndrome. *Pediatrics* **84**:115–117, 1974.

2b Bernard, R., et al., Syndrome aglossie adactylie avec synostose bimaxillaire antérieure. *Pédiatrie* **26**:877–883, 1971.

3 Bonar, B. E., and Owens, R. W., Bilateral Congenital Facial Paralysis. *Am. J. Dis. Child.* **38**:1256–1272, 1929.

4 Bünnige, M., Angeborene Zungen-Munddach-Verwachsung. *Ann. Paediatr.* **195**:173–180, 1960.

5 Cadwalader, W. B., A Clinical Report of Two Cases of Agenesis (Congenital Paralysis) of the Cranial Nerves. *Am. J. Med. Sci.* **163**:744–748, 1922.

6 Cohen, M. M., Jr., et al., Nosologic and Genetic Considerations in the Aglossy-Adactyly Syndrome. *Birth Defects* **7**(7):237–240, 1971.

7 Cosack, G., Die angeborene Zungen-Munddach-Verwachsung als Leitmotiv eines Komplexes von multiplen Abartungen (zur Genese des Ankyloglossum superius). *Z. Kinderheilkd.* **72**:240–257, 1952–1953.

8 Cosman, B., and Crikelair, G. F., Midline Branchiogenic Syndromes. *Plast. Reconstr. Surg.* **44**:41–48, 1969.

9 Danis, P., Les paralysies oculo-facialis congénitales (à propos de trois observations nouvelles). *Ophthalmologica* **110**:113–137, 1945.

10 De Jussieu, M., Observation sur la maniere dont une fille sans langue s'acquitte des fonctions qui dependent de cet organe. *Hist. Acad. R. Sci. Paris* Mem. 6–14, 1718–1719.

10a Ernst, T., and Meinhold, G., Ein Beitrag zur angeborenen Aglossie. *Dtsch. Zahn. Mund Kieferheilkd.* **43**:375–384, 1964.

11 Esau, P., Seltene angeborene Missbildungen: Verwachsungen der Zungenspitze mit dem harten Gaumen. *Arch. Klin. Chir.* **118**:817–820, 1921.

12 Eskew, H. A., and Shepard, E. E., Congenital Aglossia. *Am. J. Orthodont.* **35**:116–119, 1949.

13 Evans, P. R., Nuclear Agenesis. Moebius Syndrome: The Congenital Facial Diplegia Syndrome. *Arch. Dis. Child.* **30**:237–243, 1955.

14 Farrington, R. K., Aglossia Congenita: Report of a Case with Other Congenital Manifestations. *North Carolina Med. J.* **8**:24–26, 1947.

15 Fortanier, A. H., and Speijer, N., Eine Erblichkeitsforschung bei einer Familie mit angeborenen Beweglichkeits-störungen der Hirnnerven (infantiler Kernschwund von Moebius). *Genetica* **17**:471–486, 1935.

16 Fulford, G. E., et al., Aglossia Congenita. Cineradiographic Findings. *Arch. Dis. Child.* **31**:400–407, 1956.

17 Garner, L. D., and Bixler, D., Micrognathia, an Associated Defect of Hanhart's Syndrome, Types II and III. *Oral Surg.* **27**:601–606, 1969.

18 Gorlin, R. J., Some Facial Syndromes. *Birth Defects* **5**(2):65–76, 1969.

19 Gorlin, R. J., and Pindborg, J. J., *Syndromes of the Head and Neck.* McGraw-Hill, New York, 1964.

19a Grislain, J., et al., Aglossie-adactylie et syndrome d'Hanhart. *Pédiatrie* **26**:353–364, 1971.

20 Gutman, D., et al., Moebius Syndrome. *Br. J. Oral Surg.* **11**:20–24, 1973.

21 Hall, B. D., Aglossia-adactylia. *Birth Defects* **7**(7):233–236, 1971.

22 Hanhart, E., Über die Kombination von Peromelie mit Mikrognathie: Ein neues Syndrom beim Menschen, entsprechend der Akroteriasis congenita von Wreidt und Mohr beim Rinde. *Arch. Julius Klaus Stift. Vererbungsforsch.* **25**:531–540, 1950.

23 Hanissian, A. S., et al., Moebius Syndrome in Twins. *Am. J. Dis. Child.* **120**:472–475, 1970.

24 Harrison, M., and Parker, N., Congenital Facial Diplegia. *Med. J. Aust.* **1**:650–653, 1960.

25 Hayward, J. R., and Avery, J. K., A Variation in Cleft Palate. *J. Oral Surg.* **15**:320–324, 1957.

26 Henderson, J. L., The Congenital Facial Diplegia Syndrome: Clinical Features, Pathology, and Aetiology. A Review of Sixty-one Cases. *Brain* **62**:381–403, 1939.

27 Heubner, O., Über angeborenen Kernmangel (infantiler Kennschwund, Moebius). *Charite-Ann.* **25**, 211–243, 1900.

28 Hicks, A. M., Congenital Paralysis of Lateral Rotations of Eyes with Paralysis of Muscles of Face. *Arch. Ophthalmol.* **30**:38–42, 1943.

28a Hoggins, G. S., Aglossia Congenita with Bony Fusion of the Jaws. *Br. J. Oral Surg.* **7**:63–65, 1969.

29 Horstmann, W., Hinweise auf zentralnervöse Schäden im Rahmen der Thalidomid-Embryopathie. Pathologisch-anatomische, elektrencephalographische und neurologische Befunde. *Z. Kinderheilkd.* **96**:291–307, 1966.

30 Keith, A., Concerning the Origin and Nature of Certain Malformations of the Face, Head and Foot. *Br. J. Surg.* **28**:173–192, 1940.

31 Kelln, E. E., et al., Aglossia-Adactylia Syndrome. *Am. J. Dis. Child.* **116**:549, 1968.

32 Kettner, —, Kongenitaler Zungendefekt. *Dtsch. Med. Wochenschr.* **33**:532, 1907.

33 Koster (1902), cited by J. L. Henderson, The Congenital Facial Diplegia Syndrome: Clinical Features, Pathology, and Aetiology. *Brain* **62**:381–403, 1939.

34 Kramer, W., Zur Entstehung der angeborenen Gaumenspalte. *Zbl. Chir.* **38**:385–387, 1911.

35 de Lamothe, D., Un cas d'absence congénitale de la langue avec persistance de la membrane orale. *Ann. Mal. Oreil. Larynx* **49**:717–719, 1930.

36 Leiber, B., and Olbrich, G., *Die klinischen Syndrome.* 4th ed., Urban & Schwarzenberg, Munich, Berlin, 1966.

37 Lorinsky, L. C., Aglossia-Adactylia Syndrome. *Am. J. Dis. Child.* **119**:255, 1970.

38 Marden, P., The Syndrome of Ankyloglossia Superior. *Minn. Med.* **49**:1223–1225, 1966.

39 Martius, G., and Walter S., Peromelie und Mikrognathie als Missbildungskombination (Hanhartsches Syndrom).

Geburtsh. Frauenheilkd. **14**:558–563, 1954.

40 Masaki, S., Congenital Bilateral Facial Paralysis. *Arch. Otolaryngol.* **94**:260–263, 1971.

41 Miehlke, A., Anatomy and Clinical Aspects of the Facial Nerve. *Arch. Otolaryngol.* **81**:444–445, 1965.

42 Moebius, P. J., Uber angeborene doppelseitige Abducens-Facialis Lähmung. *Münch. Med. Wochenschr.* **35**:91–94, 108–111, 1888.

43 Moebius, P. J., Über infantilen Kernschwund. *Münch. Med. Wochenschr.* **39**:17–21, 41–43, 55–58, 1892.

44 Nevin, N. C., et al., Aglossia-Adactylia Syndrome. *J. Med. Genet.* **12**:89–93, 1975.

45 Olson, W. H., et al., Moebius Syndrome: Lower Motor Neuron Involvement and Hypogonadotrophic Hypogonadism. *Neurology (Minneap.)* **20**:1002–1008, 1970.

46 Opitz, J. M., and Pettersen, J. C., Personal communication, 1970.

46a Pettersson, G., Aglossia Congenita with Bony Fusion of the Jaws. *Acta Chir. Scand.* **122**:93–95, 1961.

47 Pitner, S. E., et al., Observations on the Pathology of the Moebius Syndrome. *J. Neurol. Neurosurg. Psychiatr.* **28**:362–374, 1965.

48 Reed, H., and Grant, W., Möbius Syndrome. *Br. J. Ophthalmol.* **41**:731–739, 1957.

49 Richards, R. N., The Moebius Syndrome. *J. Bone Joint Surg.* **35A**:437–444, 1953.

50 Richter, R. B., Congenital Hypoplasia of the Facial Nucleus. *J. Neuropathol. Exp. Neurol.* **17**:520A, 1958.

51 Rosenthal, R., Aglossia Congenita: A Report of a Case of the Condition Combined with Other Congenital Malformations. *Am. J. Dis. Child.* **44**:383–389, 1932.

52 Shear, M., Congenital Underdevelopment of the Maxilla Associated with Partial Adactylia, Partial Anodontia, and Microglossia. *J. Dent. Assoc. S. Afr.* **11**:78–83, 1956.

53 Spivak, J., and Bennett, E., Glossopalatine Ankylosis. *Plast. Reconstr. Surg.* **42**:129–136, 1968.

54 Sprofkin, B. E., and Hillman, J. W., Moebius' Syndrome: Congenital Oculofacial Paralysis. *Neurology (Minneap.)* **6**:50–54, 1956.

55 Temtamy, S., and McKusick, V. A., Synopsis of Hand Malformations with Particular Emphasis on Genetic Factors. *Birth Defects* **5**(3):125–184, 1969.

56 Thomas, H. M., Congenital Facial Paralysis. *J. Nerv. Ment. Dis.* **25**:571–593, 1898.

57 Thornton, M., Pierre Robin Syndrome: A Single Clinical History. *J. Dent. Child.* **33**:27–32, 1966.

58 Torpin, R., *Fetal Malformations: Caused by Amnion Rupture during Gestation.* Charles C Thomas, Springfield, Ill., 1968.

59 Van Allen, M. W., and Blodi, F. C., Neurological Aspects of the Möbius Syndrome: A Case Study with Electromyography of the Extraocular and Facial Muscles. *Neurology (Minneap.)* **10**:249–259, 1960.

60 Van der Wiel, H. J., Hereditary Congenital Facial Paralysis. *Acta Genet. (Basel)* **7**:348, 1957.

61 Watkin, H. G., Congenital Absence of the Tongue. *Int. J. Orthodont.* **11**:941–943, 1925, and *Dent. Rec.* **44**:486–488, 1924.

62 Wehinger, H., Kiefermissbildung und Peromelie. *Z. Kinderheilkd.* **108**:46–53, 1970.

63 Wexler, M. R., and Novark, B. W., Hanhart's Syndrome. *Plast. Reconstr. Surg.* **54**:99–101, 1974.

64 Wilson, R. A., et al., Ankyloglossia Superior (Palatoglossal Adhesion in the Newborn Infant). *Pediatrics* **31**:1051–1054, 1963.

110

Osteochondromuscular Dystrophy

(Schwartz-Jampel Syndrome)

In 1962, Schwartz and Jampel (10) described a syndrome characterized by (a) growth retardation, (b) multiple skeletal anomalies, (c) a myotonia-like disorder, and (d) unusual facies. The same children were reported by Aberfeld et al. (1). Additional cases of the disorder were described by a number of authors (2–6, 8–10).

The syndrome appears to be inherited as an autosomal recessive trait. Affected sibs have been described (2, 5, 8, 10). Parental consanguinity has also been noted (9).

SYSTEMIC MANIFESTATIONS

Facies. The facies, essentially normal at birth, develops progressively, because of tonic contraction of facial muscles, into a pinched, immobile mask with puckered lips and narrow palpebral fissures due to medial displacement of the outer canthi (2). There is ptosis of the lids. The neck is short. The facies is usually clinically recognizable at one to three years of age (Figs. 110-1, 110-2).

Musculoskeletal alterations. Height is reduced below the 10th percentile. Limitation of motion at the hips usually is evident within the first six months of life. Gait becomes waddling and progressively difficult because of stiff hips and knees and the child fatigues easily (Figs. 110-1, 110-2). Pectus carinatum, acetabular dysplasia

with fragmentation of femoral heads, coxa vara, and mild platyspondyly are usual features (1, 2, 6, 10) (Fig. 110-3).

Choking on cold liquids and mild muscular hypertrophy have been described during early childhood (2, 8). Weakness is not a prominent

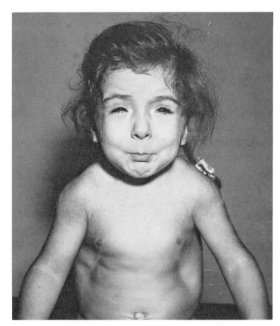

Figure 110-1. *Osteochondromuscular dystrophy.* Three-year-old female. Note blepharophimosis, rigid facial expression, pigeon-breast deformity with lateral chest constriction. (*From O. Schwartz and R. S. Jampel,* Arch. Ophthalmol. **68**:52, 1962.)

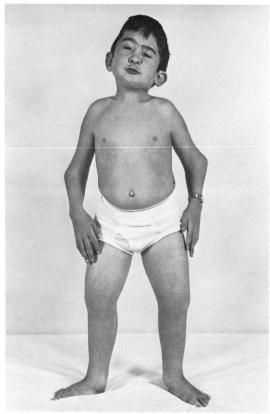

Figure 110-2. Note puckered mouth, mildly narrowed palpebral fissures, flexion at hips, knees, and elbows. (*From W. M. Fowler, Jr., et al.* J. Neurol. Sci. **22:**127, 1974.)

feature. Repetitive contracture decreases the myotonia. Fowler et al. (4) described continuous muscle fiber activity at rest and suggested that the abnormal discharges originated in the muscle component of the neuromuscular junction rather than the nerve. Perhaps the defect rests in the sarcolemmal membrane. They demonstrated that there was no true myotonia since the continuous repetitive discharges were abolished with curare.

Other findings. High-pitched voice, severe myopia, and hypoplastic testicles were noted (1, 2).

Oral manifestations. The palate is highly arched.

DIFFERENTIAL DIAGNOSIS

The facies resembles to some degree that of *craniocarpotarsal dysplasia.*

Growth retardation, platyspondyly, and hip deformity are present in *Morquio syndrome*, but this disorder can be ruled out on other clinical and roentgenographic grounds. Growth retardation, delayed bone age, and muscle hypertrophy may be seen in hypothyroidism. Familial myotonia may be seen in a number of disorders (2).

Marden and Walker (7) described a child with immobility of facial muscles, no Moro response, decreased deep-tendon reflexes, blepharophimosis with antimongoloid palpebral fissures, micrognathia, pectus carinatum, congenital contractures, arachnodactyly, kyphoscoliosis, simian creases, and cleft palate. The child failed to thrive and died at three months of age. On autopsy an abnormal pulmonary return, a common entrance for the superior and inferior vena cava, and microcystic disease of the kidney were found. In contrast to patients with the Schwartz-Jampel syndrome, no myotonia or generalized bone disease were found. Through the courtesy of W. Niosi (Minneapolis, Minn.), one of us (R. J. G.) has seen another example of this disorder with almost identical findings, including cleft palate.

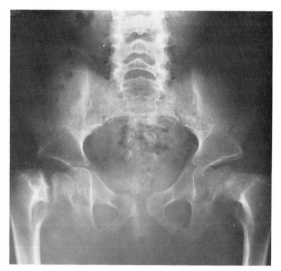

Figure 110-3. Severe coxa vara. (*From P. R. Huttenlocher et al.,* Pediatrics **44:**945, 1969.)

LABORATORY AIDS

Ultrastructural studies of muscle have shown increased glycogen and electron-dense lamellar bodies (8). Aberfeld et al. (2) described extensive vacuolization of muscle fibers.

Standards for normal palpebral fissure size according to age have been established (3a).

REFERENCES

1 Aberfeld, D. C., et al., Myotonia, Dwarfism, Diffuse Bone Disease and Unusual Ocular and Facial Abnormalities (a New Syndrome). *Brain* **88:**313–322, 1965.

2 Aberfeld, D. C., et al., Chondrodystrophic Myotonia: Report of Two Cases. Myotonia, Dwarfism, Diffuse Bone Disease and Unusual Ocular and Facial Abnormalities. *Arch. Neurol.* **22:**455–462, 1970.

3 Catel, W., *Differentialdiagnostische Symptomatologie von Krankheiten des Kindesalters*, 2d ed., Thieme, Stuttgart, 1951, p. 48.

3a Fox, S. A., The Palpebral Fissure. *Am. J. Ophthalmol.* **62:**73–78, 1966.

4 Fowler, W. M., Jr., et al., The Schwartz-Jampel Syndrome. Its Clinical, Physiological and Histological Expressions. *J. Neurol. Sci.* **22:**127–146, 1974.

5 Gellis, S., and Finegold, M., Schwartz-Jampel Syndrome. *Am. J. Dis. Child.* **126:**339–340, 1973.

6 Huttenlocher, P. R., et al., Osteo-chondro-muscular Dystrophy: A Disorder Manifested by Multiple Skeletal Deformities, Myotonia, and Dystrophic Changes in Muscle. *Pediatrics* **44:**945–958, 1969.

6a Kozlowski, K., and Wise, G., Spondylo-epi-metaphyseal Dysplasia with Myotonia. A Radiographic Study. *Radiol. Diagnost. (Berlin)* **15:**817–824, 1974.

7 Marden, P. M., and Walker, W. A., A New Generalized Connective Tissue Syndrome: Association with Multiple Congenital Anomalies. *Am. J. Dis. Child.* **112:**225–228, 1966.

8 Mereu, T. R., et al., Myotonia, Shortness of Stature, and Hip Dysplasia, Schwartz-Jampel Syndrome. *Am. J. Dis. Child.* **117:**470–478, 1969.

9 Saadat, M., et al., Schwartz Syndrome: Myotonia with Blepharophimosis and Limitation of Joints. *J. Pediatr.* **81:**348–350, 1972.

10 Schwartz, O., and Jampel, R. S., Congenital Blepharophimosis Associated with a Unique Generalized Myopathy. *Arch. Ophthalmol.* **68:**52–57, 1962.

11 Van Huffelin, A. C., et al., Chondrodystrophia Myotonica. *Neuropödiatrie* **5:**71–90, 1974 (Case 1).

111

Osteogenesis Imperfecta

The syndrome consists of (*a*) fragile bones, (*b*) clear or blue scleras, (*c*) deafness, (*d*) loose ligaments, and frequently (*e*) dentinogenesis imperfecta–like changes in the teeth. Rarely has a symptom complex been classified under so many eponyms. Credit is usually given to Ekman (11) for performing, in 1788, the first comprehensive study of the syndrome and discussing its inheritance. Lobstein (25) and Vrolik (47), in the early 1800s, described the adult and infantile forms, respectively. Spurway (44) and Eddowes (10) described blue scleras, and van der Hoeve and de Kleijn (46) in the early 1900s mentioned deafness as part of the syndrome. The dental changes were first described by Preiswerk [see (33)].

Osteogenesis imperfecta has been observed in various racial groups and has even been described in an ancient Egyptian mummy (15).

Most reported cases (about 90 percent) represent the "tarda form" with blue scleras (90 percent), brittle bones (60 percent), impaired hearing (60 percent), dentin defect (50 percent), hyperelasticity of joints and ligaments, and capillary fragility (16, 20, 26, 48). This type has autosomal dominant inheritance, with a wide range of expressivity and incomplete penetrance. The incidence varies from about 2 to 5 per 100,000 births in different populations (26, 39, 41).

Since the "congenital form" has been observed in families also exhibiting the "tarda form," clinical distinction based on age of onset of fractures makes little genetic sense (20, 26).

Brittle bones not associated with the other classic signs may be inherited as an isolated autosomal dominant trait (16, 19, 20, 26, 40, 41), with a greater proportion of males being affected (20).

A congenital lethal type seems to exist as an autosomal recessive trait, as suggested by high parental consanguinity (20, 26). A fourth distinct form, also exhibiting autosomal recessive inheritance, most likely represents a renal tubular defect. Anomalies in this type are limited to the skeletal system (8, 9, 20).

The basic defect in osteogenesis imperfecta has been stated to be a generalized mesenchymal change in maturation of collagen beyond the reticulum fiber stage (26). Fine structural study of the cornea suggests that the defect lies in tropocollagen synthesis or in extracellular collagen aggregation (4). It has been suggested that in classic osteogenesis imperfecta, the production of normally cross-linked collagen is reduced, while in the type with only bone involvement, the collagen is unstable but is produced in normal amounts (12a). Bone formation rates have been found to be at least three times the normal rate (22). It is still unknown whether altered levels of tissue mucopolysaccharide and abnormal amino-acid ratios in the collagen are responsible for the defect or simply represent the expression of a metabolic disturbance (29). Bone collagen from

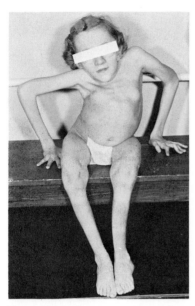

Figure 111-1. *Osteogenesis imperfecta.* Triangular head appears to sit directly on kyphoscoliotic thorax of fourteen-year-old female who has suffered innumerable fractures. (*From B. Buice, St. Paul, Minn.*)

patients with this disorder inhibits calcification in vitro (42). However, Lancaster et al. (23a) found normal biosynthesis, maturation, and excretion of collagen in cultured fibroblasts from patients with classic osteogenesis imperfecta.

SYSTEMIC MANIFESTATIONS

Facies. The facies is similar to that seen in cleidocranial dysplasia. The skull appears disproportionately large, with a temporal bulge that causes the ears to be thrown outward and forward (Fig. 111-1). The forehead is broad and domed, and the occiput is protuberant.

Musculoskeletal system. In the congenital type, intrauterine fractures may be so numerous that the child may be born dead or may survive for only a short time. Micromelia with broad long bones is often quite striking (16, 26, 34, 47). Bones massive at birth may become gracile with age (27). The diagnosis has been made not un-

commonly in utero on roentgenographic examination of the abdomen (18a).

The skull is large, the forehead being especially broad and bossed, with a temporal bulge, an overhanging occiput, decreased vertical dimension, and platybasia, giving the skull a "mushroom" or "soldier's helmet" appearance (26).

Roentgenographic examination may reveal a remarkably thin calvaria (caput membranaceum), these children succumbing from intracranial hemorrhage through birth injury. Numerous Wormian bones are evident in the occipital area, giving rise to a mosaic picture (26, 27, 47). A series of 65 cases was analyzed by Maroteaux and Gilles (27).

The long bones, especially those of the lower extremities, are bowed or unevenly shortened, with thinned cortices (Fig. 111-2). Subperiosteal fractures of the shaft and multiple microfractures at the epiphyses, due to minor trauma or sudden muscle pulls, are frequently observed. Hypercallosity at the site of healing fractures may be erroneously interpreted as osteogenic sarcoma or as a rachitic rosary. Instead of compact cortical bone, there is a thin, loose, poorly formed and arranged, spongy layer. The vertebras are markedly osteoporotic, with a "codfish" appearance.

On histologic section, the bony plates are seen to be small, irregular, and nonanastomosing. They are poorly endowed with osteoblasts and osteoid matrix. The mucoid component of the connective tissue seems to be increased (34), resembling that in ascorbic acid deficiency.

Spinal cord compression resulting from abnormally shaped vertebras, kyphoscoliosis, pectus carinatum and excavatum, and pseudoarthroses are frequently encountered (16, 26).

The tendency toward fractures decreases after puberty, although pregnancy, lactation, or senile involution may enhance their likelihood (26). Laxity of ligaments or rupture of tendons, resulting in habitual dislocation of joints, flatfoot, and distortions, is not uncommon, being seen in at least 25 percent of cases. Hernia occurs with high frequency, sometimes in combination with cryptorchism (26).

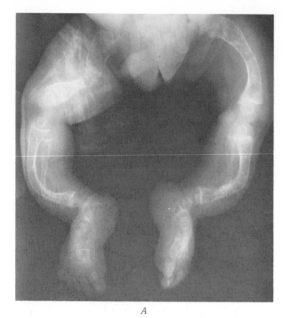 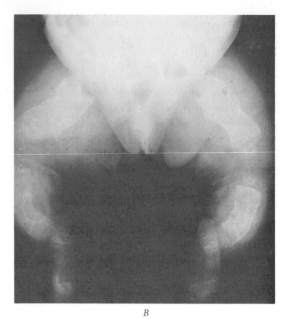

A   *B*

Figure 111-2. (*A*). Osteoporosis and severe bending of bones. (*B*). Multiple intrauterine fractures and callus formation.

Skin. Clinically, the skin may be thin and translucent, resembling that of the aged. Histologically, increased amounts of mucopolysaccharides have been found (18). Healing is often poor, with wide hypertrophic scarring being common (18, 40). Elastosis perforans (Miescher) has been found with increased frequency (28). Subcutaneous hemorrhage tends to occur even after minor trauma (16, 18, 26).

Eyes. Clear (blue) scleras are one of the most common features of the syndrome and may be the only expression. The intensity of the blueness varies from family to family and from case to case. Francis et al. (12a) suggested that those with blue scleras have mild bone disease, and vice versa. Furthermore, patients with blue scleras have reduced amounts of collagen which has normal stability while those with white scleras have a normal amount of collagen with reduced stability due to a defect in cross-linking. The blue color may in part be due to thinning of the sclera, allowing the color of the choroid to be transmitted (2, 26), but also may be due to increased translucency related to a deficiency of collagen fibers or an increase in mucopolysac-

charide content (31, 34). Some reports have, in fact, indicated that the blue sclera may be thicker than that of normal controls (31). The sclera adjacent to the limbus often appears to be whitish, resulting in "Saturn's ring" (26). Hypermetropia, arcus juvenilis, keratoconus, megalocornea, and dislocation of lenses have been encountered (26, 34).

Ears. Severely impaired hearing is found in 60 percent of patients with the tarda type (20, 26). Fewer than half the patients exhibit the classic triad of deafness, blue scleras, and bone disease (20). Rarely is complete deafness observed, but hearing appears to be more severely impaired in patients with marked bone involvement (6). Deafness usually begins in the third decade and increases progressively with time, the footplate of the stapes being slightly fixed with a heavy growth of white chalky material (6, 17, 23, 32), although there may be underlying malformation of the stapes as well (50). The deafness, usually conductive, may be mixed or purely sensorineural. In some patients the tympanic membrane has been found to be thinned and bluish (26). The ears often stand out from the head and

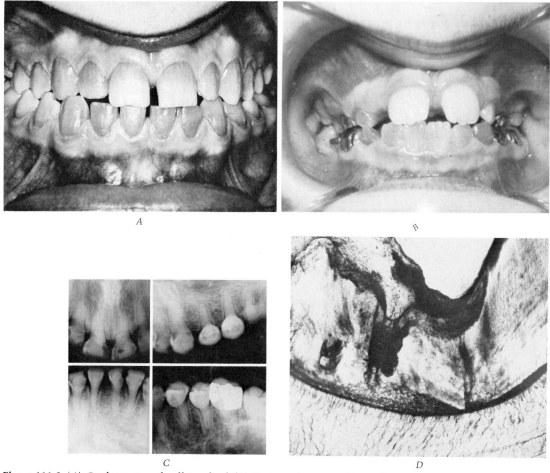

Figure 111-3. (*A*). Opalescent teeth, all involved. (*B*). Note opalescence of lower incisors. Upper incisors are spared. (*C*). Roentgenograms showing reduced root size, obliteration of root canals. (*D*). Photomicrograph of tooth of patient with osteogenesis imperfecta. Note smooth dentinoenamel junction.

are pointed downward, because of the bitemporal bulge.

Cardiovascular system. Premature atherosclerosis has been observed (26). The connective tissue of the myocardium, cardiac valves, and aorta show increased amounts of mucoid material (34). Several patients have had aortic or mitral regurgitation.

Oral manifestations. The dentin is chiefly affected; although the enamel frequently cracks off, it is not considered to be involved (1, 19, 33,

49) (Fig. 111-3*A*). In the tarda type, the deciduous teeth are affected in about 80 percent of the patients, the permanent teeth in only 35 percent (Fig. 111-3*B*). The teeth formed early in life or during fetal development are the more severely affected (49). There seems to be no correlation between dentin impairment and the degree of bone involvement (41).

The tooth crowns may be smaller than normal, especially in the incisivocervical dimension. Upon eruption, they are noted to be translucent or opalescent. The color darkens with age, so that they assume a gray, pink, amber, or bluish color (1, 33, 38, 48, 49). The teeth are liable to pathologic abrasion down to the gingival margin. Hypertrophy of the alveolar bone takes place as a compensatory measure.

On roentgenographic examination, the changes in the teeth are found to be quite striking. The roots are thin, fine, and disproportionately shortened. The pulp chamber and canal are greatly diminished in size or totally obliterated by formation of irregular dentin (Fig. 111-3C).

Microscopically, the dentinoenamel junction seems to be flatter, lacking the normal scalloping (37, 38, 48, 49) (Fig. 111-3D). The normal tubular dentin may partially or totally be replaced by a more laminated dentin which is traversed by tubules of abnormal size and shape. There are comet-shaped structures that appear to be remnants of blood vessels entrapped in the dentin matrix (48, 49). In contrast, in hereditary opalescent dentin all the dentin is abnormal except for the mantle dentin adjacent to the enamel or cementum. In osteogenesis imperfecta, the amount of normal-appearing dentin is quite variable (48). Microscopic evidence of poor calcification of the dentin in the form of interglobular calcification has been corroborated by chemical and physical studies.

DIFFERENTIAL DIAGNOSIS

There are several reports of patients who manifest not only signs of osteogenesis imperfecta but stigmata of the *Ehlers-Danlos syndromes, Marfan syndrome*, etc. (5, 7, 16, 26). These cases currently defy precise classification.

Similar dental changes are seen in hereditary opalescent dentin, which occurs in about 1 in 8,000 persons (33, 36–38, 49) and is inherited as an autosomal dominant trait. When isolated, it occurs in both dentitions, in contrast to the marked variation in dental expression observed in osteogenesis imperfecta, in which only a few teeth may appear to be affected.

Wormian bones are also seen in *cleidocranial dysplasia, pyknodysostosis, progeria, mandibuloacral dysplasia, acroosteolysis,* and Menkes disease. Brittle bones also occur in osteopetrosis, but increased bone density is evident on roentgenographic examination. Osteoporosis, bent legs, and blue sclerae may be seen in hypophosphatasia. Mild cases of osteogenesis imperfecta have been erroneously diagnosed as presenile osteoporosis (26). Osteoporosis, tendency to fracture, and "codfish" vertebras occur in *homocystinuria* and with pseudoglioma (26).

Blue scleras may be seen in normal infants, may be inherited as an isolated autosomal dominant trait, may be observed in other connective tissue disorders such as Ehlers-Danlos syndrome, Marfan syndrome, etc. (26, 31), and may occur with megalokeratoglobus and thin and brittle corneas which rupture after minor trauma (43), as an autosomal recessive trait.

Prenatal bowing of the limbs is seen in *campomelic dwarfism* and hypophosphatasia, as well as idiopathically.

Otosclerosis may be inherited as an isolated autosomal dominant trait with high penetrance and variable expressivity (17, 26).

LABORATORY AIDS

Increased serum alpha-2-globulins and glycoproteins have been found in the tarda type (3, 24). Reports of increased urinary excretion of mucopolysaccharides have been inconsistent (3, 16, 21, 24, 26). Aminoaciduria may express a renal tubular defect in one form of the syndrome (9, 20, 26).

REFERENCES

1 Becks, H., Histologic Study of Tooth Structure in Osteogenesis Imperfecta. *Dent. Cosmos* **73**:437–454, 1931.

2 Berggren, L., et al., Intraocular Pressure and Excretion of Mucopolysaccharides in Osteogenesis Imperfecta. *Arch. Ophthalmol.* (*Kbh.*) **47**:122–128, 1969.

3 Bethge, J. F. J., et al., Biochemische Untersuchungen bei Osteogenesis imperfecta. *Bruns Beitr. Klin. Chir.* **214**:448–458, 1967.

4 Blümcke, S., et al., Histochemical and Fine Structural Studies on the Cornea with Osteogenesis Imperfecta Congenita. *Virchows Arch.* [*Zellpathol.*] **11**:124–132, 1972.

5 Bolletti, M., and Disertori, A., Su di un caso di osteogenesi imperfetta tipo Lobstein associata a sindrome di Ehlers-Danlos, idrocefalia, e piedi torti. *Pediatria* (*Napoli*) **75**:310–330, 1967.

6 Caniggia, A., et al., Fragilitas ossium hereditaria tarda (Ekman-Lobstein Disease). *Acta Med. Scand.* [*Suppl.*] **340:**1-172, 1958.

7 Carey, M. C., et al., Osteogenesis Imperfecta in Twenty-three Members of a Kindred with Heritable Features Contributed by a Non-specific Skeletal Disorder. *Q. J. Med.* **37:**437-449, 1968.

8 Chawla, S., Intrauterine Osteogenesis Imperfecta in Four Siblings. *Br. Med. J.* **1:**99-101, 1964.

9 Chowers, I., et al., Familial Aminoaciduria in Osteogenesis Imperfecta. *J.A.M.A.* **181:**771-775, 1962.

10 Eddowes, A., Dark Sclerotics and Fragilitas Ossium. *Br. Med. J.* **2:**222, 1900.

11 Ekman, O. J., *Dissertatio medica descriptionem et casus aliquot osteomalaciae sistens.* J. Erdman, Uppsala, 1788.

12 Falvo, K. A., and Bullough, P. G., Osteogenesis Imperfecta—a Histometric Analysis. *J. Bone Joint Surg.* **55A:**275-286, 1973.

12a Francis, M. J. O., et al., Instability of Polymeric Skin Collagen in Osteogenesis Imperfecta. *Br. Med. J.* **1:**421-424, 1974.

13 Freda, V. J., et al., Osteogenesis Imperfecta Congenita: A Presentation of 16 Cases and Review of the Literature. *Obstet. Gynecol.* **18:**535-547, 1961.

14 Godfrey, J. L., A Histological Study of Dentin Formation in Osteogenesis Imperfecta Congenita. *J. Oral Pathol.* **2:**85-111, 1973.

15 Gray, P. H. K., A Case of Osteogenesis Imperfecta, Associated with Dentinogenesis Imperfecta, Dating from Antiquity. *Clin. Radiol.* **20:**106-109, 1969.

16 Gremeau, J. L., *La fragilite osseuse héréditaire.* Simep Edit., Lyon, 1968.

17 Gussen, R., The Stapediovestibular Joint: Normal Structure and Pathogenesis of Otosclerosis. *Acta Otolaryngol.* [*Suppl.*] (*Stockh.*) **248:**1-38, 1969.

18 Haebara, H., et al., An Autopsy Case of Osteogenesis Imperfecta Congenita—Histochemical and Electron Microscopical Studies. *Acta Pathol. Jap.* **19:**377-394, 1969.

18a Heller, R. H., et al., The Prenatal Diagnosis of Osteogenesis Imperfecta Congenita. *Am. J. Obstet. Gynecol.* **121:**572-573, 1975.

19 Heys, F. M., et al., Osteogenesis Imperfecta and Odontogenesis Imperfecta: Clinical and Genetic Aspects in Eighteen Families. *J. Pediatr.* **56:**234-245, 1960.

20 Ibsen, K. H., Distinct Varieties of Osteogenesis Imperfecta. *Clin. Orthop.* **50:**279-290, 1967.

21 Janke, D., Klinische und blutchemische Untersuchungen bei der Osteogenesis imperfecta. *Z. Orthop.* **105:**423-430, 1968.

22 Jett, S., et al., Bone Turnover and Osteogenesis Imperfecta. *Arch. Pathol.* **81:**112-116, 1966.

23 Kosoy, J., and Maddox, H. E., Surgical Findings in van der Hoeve's Syndrome. *Arch. Otolaryngol.* **93:**115-122, 1971.

23a Lancaster, G., et al., Dominantly Inherited Osteogenesis Imperfecta in Man: An Examination of Collagen Biosynthesis. *Pediatr. Res.* **9:**83-88, 1975.

24 Langness, U., and Behnke, H., Biochemische Untersuchungen zur Osteogenesis imperfecta. *Dtsch. Med. Wochenschr.* **95:**213-221, 1970.

25 Lobstein, J. B., *Traite de l'anatomie pathologique.* vol. 2. F. G. Lerrault, Paris, 1833, p. 204.

26 McKusick, V. A., *Heritable Disorders of Connective Tissue.* 4th ed. Mosby, St. Louis, 1972, pp. 390-454.

27 Maroteaux, P., and Gilles, M., Etude radiologique de l'osteogenesis imperfecta. *Ann. Radiol.* **8:**571-583, 1965.

28 Mehregan, A. H., Elastosis Perforans Serpiginosa. *Arch. Dermatol.* **97:**381-393, 1968.

29 Niemann, M. W., Aminoacid Composition of Bone Collagen in Osteogenesis Imperfecta. *J. Bone Joint Surg.* **51A:**804, 1969.

30 Nimatti, G. P., and Patriarca, P. L., L'osteogenesi imperfetta. *Minerva Pediatr.* **20:**1543-1554, 1968.

31 Oerkermann, H., and Behnke, H., Untersuchungen an blauen Skleren bei congenitaler Osteogenesis imperfecta. *Frankfurt. Z. Pathol.* **75:**259-268, 1966.

32 Opheim, O., Loss of Hearing Following the Syndrome of Van der Hoeve-de Kleyn. *Acta Otolaryngol.* (*Stockh.*) **65:**337-344, 1968.

33 Pindborg, J. J., Dental Aspects of Osteogenesis Imperfecta. *Acta Pathol. Microbiol. Scand.* **24:**47-64, 1947.

34 Remigio, P. A., and Grinvalsky, H. T., Osteogenesis Imperfecta Congenita. *Am. J. Dis. Child.* **119:**524-528, 1970.

35 Riley, F. C., et al., Osteogenesis Imperfecta: Morphologic and Biochemical Studies of Connective Tissue. *Pediatr. Res.* **7:**757-768, 1973.

36 Roberts, E., and Schour, I., Hereditary Opalescent Dentin. *Am. J. Orthodont.* **25:**267-276, 1939.

37 Rushton, M. A., Structure of the Teeth in Late Cases of Osteogenesis Imperfecta. *J. Pathol. Bacteriol.* **48:**591-603, 1939.

38 Schoenfeld, Y., et al., Osteogenesis Imperfecta. *Am. J. Dis. Child.* **129:**679-687, 1975.

39 Schröder, G., Osteogenesis Imperfecta. *Z. Menschl. Vererb. Konstit. Lehre* **37:**632-676, 1964.

40 Scott, D., and Stiris, G., Osteogenesis Imperfecta Tarda: A Study of Three Families with Special Reference to Scar Formation. *Acta Med. Scand.* **145:**237-257, 1953.

41 Seedorff, K. S., *Osteogenesis Imperfecta: A Study of Clinical Features and Heredity Based on 55 Danish Families Comprising 180 Affected Persons.* Thesis, Munksgaard, Copenhagen, 1949, pp. 1-229.

42 Solomons, C. C., and Styner, J., Osteogenesis Imperfecta: Effect of Magnesium Administration on Pyrophosphate Metabolism. *Calcif. Tissue Res.* **3:**318-326, 1969.

43 Stein, R., et al., Brittle Cornea: A Familial Trait Associated with Blue Sclerae. *Am. J. Ophthalmol.* **66:**67-69, 1968.

44 Spurway, J., Hereditary Tendency to Fracture. *Br. Med. J.* **2:**844, 1896.

45 Stevenson, C. J., et al., Skin Collagen in Osteogenesis Imperfecta. *Lancet* **1:**860, 1970.

46 Van der Hoeve, J., and de Kleijn, A., Blaue Sclerae, Knochenbrüchigkeit und Schwerhörigkeit. *Arch. Ophthalmol.* **95:**91-93, 1918.

47 Vrolik, W., *Tabulae ad illustrandum embryogenesis hominis et mammalium tam naturalem quam abnormen.* Amsterdam, 1849.

48 Weiss, P., Histologische Befund an Kiefergelenk und Zahnkeimen bei Osteogenesis imperfecta congenita. *Dtsch. Zahnärztl. Z.* **17:**329-336, 1962.

49 Witkop, C. J., Jr., and Rao, S., Inherited Defects in Tooth Structure. *Birth Defects* **7**(7):153-184, 1971.

50 Zajtchuk, J. T., and Lindsay, J. R., Osteogenesis Imperfecta Congenita and Tarda: A Temporal Bone Report. *Ann. Otol.* **84:**350-358, 1975.

112

Otocephaly

(Microstomia, Agnathia, and Synotia)

Agnathia, or failure of formation of the mandibular arch, is often associated with synotia or fusion of the external ears in the midline region normally occupied by the mandible. It is doubtful that absolute agenesis of the mandible exists, but its size is so diminished that the symphysis rarely extends anterior to the posterior edge of the hard palate. A remnant of the tongue base is frequently present low in the pharynx. The ears approach each other, may be fused in the midline, and are often deformed, since they arise in part from the first branchial arch (Fig. 112-1A–C). Rarely, the pinnas are missing completely. The condition is incompatible with life.

There are a few reports in which agnathia has been found in combination with cyclopia (cyclopia hypognathus) (6, 11, 14). These cases differ from classic cyclops in that the proboscis-like structure usually located above the central eye is not present (1). Although the oral opening may be absent (astomia), more often it is minute, i.e., 2 to 3 mm in diameter, with the long axis usually rotated 90°. In some cases there

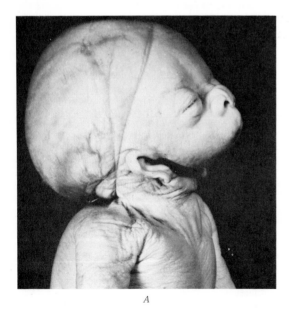

A

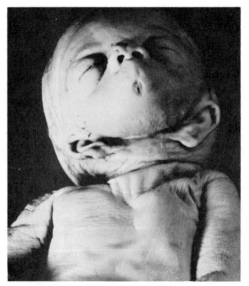

B

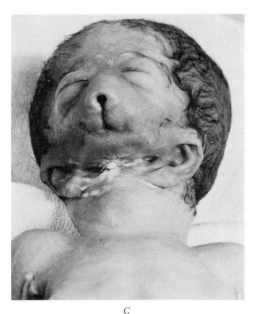

C

is no communication with the pharynx, possibly the result of persistence of the buccopharyngeal membrane. The soft palate may also be deficient. Agnathia may also be associated with talipes equinovarus, vascular malformations, transposition of viscera, and other abnormalities (7).

Figure 112-1. *Otocephaly.* (*A–C*). Note tendency of ears to fuse in midline, absence of mandible. One infant has separate but tiny mouth. Other child has unified nose and mouth. (*Courtesy of H. W. Edmonds, Washington, D.C.*)

REFERENCES

1 Allan, R., Dissection of a Human Astomatous Cyclops. *Lancet* **1:**227–228, 1848.

2 Altman, F., The Ear in Severe Malformations of the Head. *Arch. Otolaryngol.* **66:**7–25, 1957.

3 Arey, L. B., et al., Correlated Defects in Human Agnathus. *Anat. Rec.* **94:**414, 1946.

4 Arnold, J., Beschreibung einer Missbildüng und Hydropsie der gemeinsamen Schlundtrommelhohle. *Virchows Arch. Pathol. Anat.* **38:**145–172, 1867.

5 Blanc, L., Sur l'otocéphalie et la cyclopie. *J. Anat.* (*Paris*) **31:**187–218, 288–309, 1895.

6 Gartner, S., Cyclopia (Case 2). *Arch. Ophthalmol.* **37:**220–231, 1947.

7 Johnson, W. W., and Cook, J. B., Agnathia Associated with Pharyngeal Isthmus Atresia and Hydramnios. *Arch. Pediatr.* **78:**211–217, 1961.

8 Josephy, H., Missbildungen des Halses: Otocephaly, in E. Schwalbe, *Morphologie der Missbildungen der Menschen und der Tiere.* vol. 3. part 1, G. Fischer, Jena, 1909, p. 24.

9 Keen, J. A., A Case of Agnathia with a Note on the Development of the Maxillary Process. *S. Afr. J. Lab. Clin. Med.* **1:**197–202, 1955.

10 Keith, A., Congenital Malformation of Palate, Face and Neck. *Br. Med. J.* **2:**363–367, 1909.

11 Koogler, M. A., A Report of Three Human Monstrosities (Case 1). *Am. J. Med. Sci.* **84:**129–132, 1882.

12 Kuse, —, Über Agnathie und die dabei zu erhabenden Zungenbefunde. *Münch. Med. Wochenschr.* **48:**890–893, 1901.

13 Rogers, R. M. W., A Case of Agnathia or Congenital Absence of the Lower Jaw. *J. Pathol. Bacteriol.* **5:**137–142, 1898.

14 Smith, R. M., and Parker, A. J., Dissection of a Human Otocephalic Cyclops Monstrosity. *Am. J. Med. Sci.* **84:**132–140, 1882.

15 Winckel, F., Aetiologische Untersuchungen über einige sehr seltene fötale Missbildungen. *Münch. Med. Wochenschr.* **43:**423–429, 1896.

113

Otopalatodigital Syndrome

In 1962, Taybi (7) first described the otopalato-digital syndrome. In 1967, Dudding et al. (2) expanded the phenotypic spectrum to include (a) characteristic facies, (b) conduction deafness, (c) short stature, (d) cleft palate, and (e) generalized bone dysplasia.

The inheritance pattern is X-linked recessive (4). Although most patients have been male, affected females have been described (4, 5). A sister of the three male sibs described by Dudding et al. (2) has since been born and exhibits milder stigmata of the syndrome, in accord with the Lyon hypothesis.

SYSTEMIC MANIFESTATIONS

Facies. The facies in the male is rather distinctive, although somewhat difficult to define. Overhanging brow with prominent supraorbital ridges and antimongoloid obliquity of palpebral fissures are noted in all males. The corners of the mouth are often downturned. Ocular hypertelorism with associated broad nasal root gives the patient a pugilistic appearance (Fig. 113-1). A slight notching may be noted at the medial third of the upper eyelid margin in males. Facial features in the female carrier are variable. Most constant is overhanging brow with prominent supraorbital ridges, depressed nasal bridge, and flat midface.

Central nervous system. All male patients have been mildly retarded, their intelligence quotient

ranging between 75 and 90 and perhaps reflecting hearing loss. Speech development has been slow, but this may also be related to bilateral conductive hearing loss (1, 2).

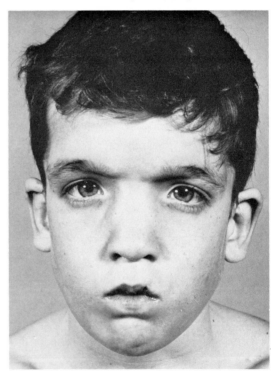

Figure 113-1. *Otopalatodigital syndrome.* Overhanging brow with prominent supraorbital ridge and wide nasal bridge gives pugilistic appearance. (*From B. A. Dudding et al.,* Am. J. Dis. Child. **113**:214, 1967.)

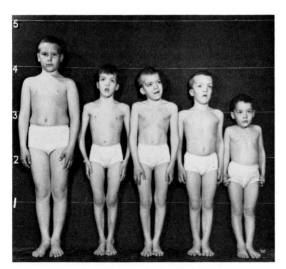

Figure 113-2. Skeletal growth is retarded. Three affected sibs, aged eight, seven, and six years, are flanked by their two normal brothers, aged ten and four years. Note subluxation of elbows of affected. (*From B. A. Dudding et al., Am. J. Dis. Child.* **113:**214, 1967.)

Skeletal anomalies. Skeletal growth is retarded, all patients being below the 10th percentile and often below the 3d percentile (Fig. 113-2). The trunk is small, with pectus excavatum. Limited elbow extension and wrist supination have been noted in several patients, and some have exhibited subluxation of the radial heads.

The appearance of the hands and feet is striking. The thumb and hallux are spatulate and especially abbreviated. The clefting between the hallux and the rest of the toes is exaggerated. The toes and fingers are irregular in form and in direction of curvature, resembling those of a tree frog. The second and third fingers may deviate to the ulnar side, while the fifth finger often bends to the radial side (Fig. 113-3*A*, *B*).

Roentgenographic alterations are marked. Frontal and occipital bossing and thickening give the skull a mushroom-like appearance. The skull base is thick, the facial bones are hypoplastic, and the paranasal sinuses and mastoids are poorly pneumatized. The nasion-sella-basion angle is about 116° (normal mean = 132°), and the mandibular plane angle is increased. The clivus, or basisphenoid, lies further posterior than normal in relation to the cervical spine. These changes are essentially limited to affected males (Fig. 113-4*A*).

The iliac bones are small, with decreased flare. Coxa valga is a common finding. The lower tibia is laterally bowed. Failure of fusion of several vertebral arches is common.

Distinctive changes in the hands of males include shortening of the radial side of the middle phalanx of the fifth finger, clinodactyly, short distal phalanx of thumb, which during development has a cone-shaped epiphysis, accessory ossification center of second metacarpal, teardrop lesser multangular, and transverse capi-

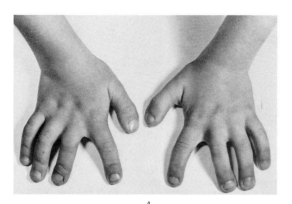

A

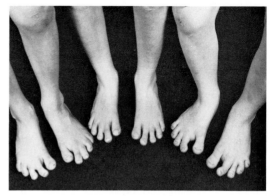

B

Figure 113-3. (*A*). Mild syndactyly and clinodactyly of digits. Note abbreviated and flattened terminal phalanges. (*From A. Prader, Zurich, Switzerland.*) (*B*). Short big toes, variable soft-tissue syndactyly and clinodactyly, gap between hallux and second toes. Toes somewhat resemble those of tree frog. (*From B. A. Dudding et al., Am. J. Dis. Child.* **113:**214, 1967.)

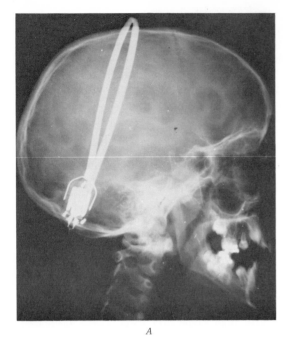

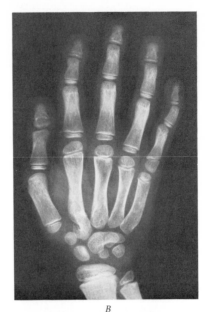

B

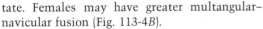

A

Figure 113-4. (*A*). Vertical basisphenoid. (*B*). Abnormal middle phalanx of fifth finger, shortened terminal phalanges, capitate-hamate complex, accessory ossification center of second metacarpal. (*C*). Short hallux, fusion between middle and lateral cuneiforms and corresponding metatarsals, forming paddle-shaped structures. (B, C *from B. A. Dudding et al.,* Am. J. Dis. Child. **113:**214, 1967.)

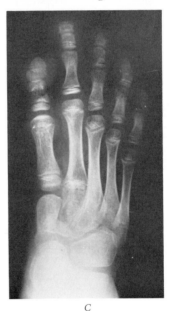

C

tate. Females may have greater multangular–navicular fusion (Fig. 113-4*B*).

In the male, alterations in the feet include short phalanges and metatarsals of the great toes and, because of their fusion with the cuneiform bones, long abnormally shaped second and third metatarsals. The fifth metatarsal may be prominent, with an extra ossification center. Tarsal fusions are common, and males usually have two ossification centers for the navicular bone (Fig. 113-4*C*). For a detailed description, see Langer (6) and Gall et al. (3).

Oral manifestations. All male patients have had cleft palate. The mandible is small, with obtuse angulation.

DIFFERENTIAL DIAGNOSIS

It is difficult to classify the female patient described by Jager and Refior (5). She exhibited features of both the otopalatodigital syndrome and the *Larsen syndrome.* This latter disorder shares a number of features, such as cleft palate and joint dislocations, with the OPD syndrome. However, differentiation should be made on roentgenographic findings of multiple carpal bones, juxtacalcaneal bone, etc. The patients described as having X-linked cleft palate by Weinstein and Cohen (8) are examples of the OPD syndrome.

LABORATORY AIDS

None is known.

REFERENCES

1 Buran, D. J., and Duvall, A. J., The Oto-palato-digital (OPD) Syndrome. *Arch. Otolaryngol.* **85:**394–399, 1967.

2 Dudding, B. A., et al., The Oto-palato-digital Syndrome. *Am. J. Dis. Child.* **113:**214–221, 1967.

3 Gall, J. C., Jr., et al., Oto-palato-digital Syndrome: Comparison of Clinical and Radiographic Manifestations in Males and Females. *Am. J. Hum. Genet.* **24:**24–36, 1972.

4 Gorlin, R. J., et al., The Oto-palato-digital (OPD) Syndrome in Females. Heterozygotic Expression of an X-linked Trait. *Oral Surg.* **35:**218–224, 1973.

5 Jäger, M., and Refior, H. J., Ein Knochendysplasie Syndrom. *Z. Orthop.* **105:**196–208, 1968.

6 Langer, L. O., The Roentgenologic Features of the Oto-palato-digital (OPD) Syndrome. *Am. J. Roentgenol.* **100:**63–70, 1967.

7 Taybi, H., Generalized Skeletal Dysplasia with Multiple Anomalies. *Am. J. Roentgenol.* **88:**450–457, 1962.

8 Weinstein, E. D., and Cohen, M. M., Sex-linked Cleft Palate. *J. Med. Genet.* **3:**17–23, 1966.

114

Pachydermoperiostosis

(Touraine-Solente-Golé Syndrome)

Pachydermoperiostosis is characterized by (*a*) coarsening of facial features with thickening and furrowing of the face, forehead, and scalp and (*b*) clubbing of the digits and periosteal new bone formation, especially over the distal ends of long bones.

Touraine et al. (19), in 1935, first recognized pachydermoperiostosis as a distinct clinical entity, although examples were noted as early as 1868 by Friedreich (6). Other early cases are those of Unna (21) and Grönberg (8).

The syndrome has autosomal dominant inheritance with marked variation in expression, males being more severely affected (15, 23). Only about 15 percent of patients have been females, most of whom had severely affected male sibs (23). Rimoin (15) noted a history of relatives with some or all of the features of the syndrome in about 40 percent of cases.

SYSTEMIC MANIFESTATIONS

The disorder usually appears about puberty and slowly progresses for about 10 years, when it becomes stationary (15, 23). However, there have been several examples with late onset (20, 23).

Facies and skin. Thickening of the skin occurs over the face, forehead, scalp, hands, and feet. The face is drawn into thick folds, producing creasing or furrowing that causes the patient to look worried or angry, as well as prematurely aged (1, 4, 12, 18). The nasolabial folds become deep and sharp (Fig. 114-1*A*, *B*). The thickening of the scalp tends to produce a corrugated surface described as "bulldog scalp," or cutis verticis gyrata (21).

The skin shows widely dilated sebaceous pores filled with plugs of sebum which can be easily expressed (Fig. 114-1*C*). Pseudoptosis, caused by thickening of the eyelids, may be so severe as to obstruct vision. Skin biopsy shows sebaceous gland hyperplasia, thickening of the stratum corneum, and perivascular round-cell infiltrates (15, 23).

The ends of the fingers and toes are bulbous and often grotesque (6, 23) (Fig. 114-2). This clubbing is produced by soft-tissue hyperplasia which stops abruptly at the distal interphalangeal joints. The nails may be thickened and curved. Rimoin (15) and Kerber and Vogl (11) found that peripheral blood flow was reduced. Hyperhidrosis of the hands and feet and, less often, of the face is common (10).

Skeletal alterations. In the early stage of the disease, bony changes tend to be limited to the distal parts of long tubular bones, metacarpals, metatarsals, and proximal phalanges. A diffuse irregular periosteal ossification increases the circumference of the affected bones without altering their shape (23). These minor changes have been noted in clinically unaffected members of a family (15).

In the rare, severely advanced case, all bones

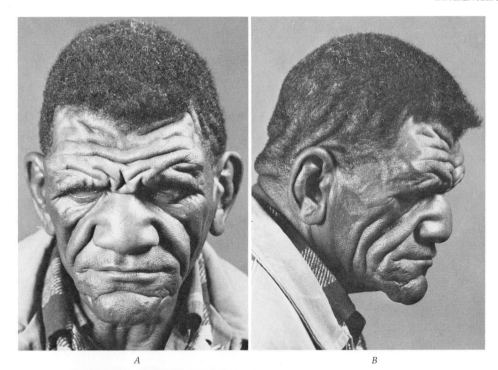

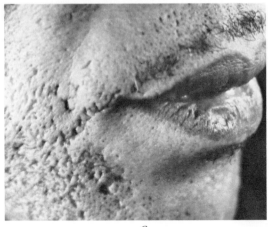

C

Figure 114-1. *Pachydermoperiostosis. (A, B).* Coarse features, cutis gyrata. *(From H. W. Kloepfer, New Orleans, La.) (C).* Oily thickened skin with large sebaceous pores. No history of acne. *(From A. Susmano, Chicago, Ill.)*

DIFFERENTIAL DIAGNOSIS

Several disorders must be excluded: hypertrophic pulmonary osteoarthropathy, acromegaly, thyroid acropachy, hereditary clubbing, and familial idiopathic osteoarthropathy of childhood.

All the clinical aspects of pachydermoperiostosis have been described in secondary (pulmonary) hypertrophic osteoarthropathy, including skin changes (15). Pachydermoperiostosis is suggested by a family history of the disorder and by the absence of a primary lesion, usually bronchogenic carcinoma. There appears to be increased blood flow in pulmonary osteoarthropathy (7), in contrast to reduced flow in pachydermoperiostosis (15).

In acromegaly, there is enlargement of the hands and feet, together with thickening of the

are affected except the skull. Bone thickness is greatly increased. The surface is coarse, but the bones are otherwise not deformed (Fig. 114-3A, B). Joint effusions and ossification of ligaments and tendons occur, leading to ankylosis of joints and spine (10). The clavicles, patellas, and pubis may be affected, but the carpal and tarsal bones, sella turcica, and articular surfaces are spared (10).

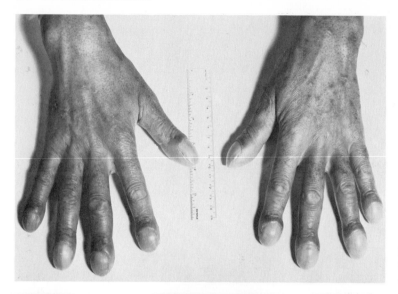

Figure 114-2. Clubbing of terminal phalanges. (*Courtesy of A. Susmano, Chicago, Ill.*)

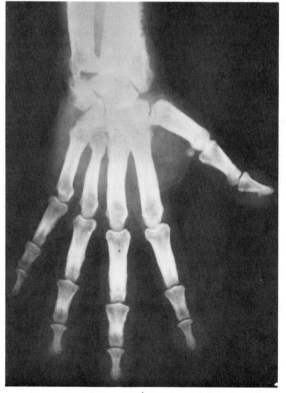

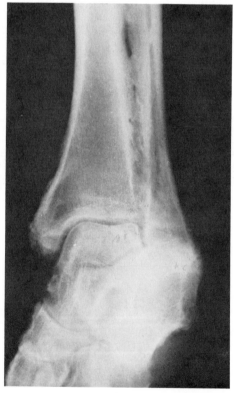

A   *B*

Figure 114-3. (*A*). Note thickening and increased density of proximal phalanges and metacarpals; periosteal thickening of radius. (*From G. Pietruschka et al.*, Klin. Monatsbl. Augenheilkd. **154:**525, 1969.) (*B*). Marked periosteal proliferation along entire length of tibia and fibula. (*Courtesy of A. Susmano, Chicago, Ill.*)

skin, particularly of the face (18, 23). The mandible, nose, sella turcica, supraorbital ridges, and tongue are also enlarged. These findings are not seen in pachydermoperiostosis.

Thyroid acropachy may follow medical or surgical treatment of hyperthyroidism. As in pachydermoperiostosis, the distal parts of the limbs may become enlarged, and clubbing of the fingers and toes may occur (13). There may be subperiosteal new bone formation in the hands. Severe exophthalmos and pretibial myxedema may be present, together with high levels of long-acting thyroid stimulator in the serum of such patients.

Simple hereditary clubbing (acropathy) has been described in many families as an autosomal dominant trait, more often severe in males. Hereditary acropathy may possibly be an incomplete form of pachydermoperiostosis (15).

Rosenthal and Kloepfer (16) described a combination of cutis verticis gyrata, corneal leukoma, and marked supraorbital ridging as an autosomal dominant syndrome in a large kindred, but roentgenographic studies were normal.

Familial idiopathic osteoarthropathy of childhood (2, 3) is an autosomal, recessively inherited disorder characterized by eczema, clubbing of fingers, periosteal new bone formation, and persistent fontanels.

REFERENCES

1 Angel, J. H., Pachydermoperiostosis (Idiopathic Osteoarthropathy). *Br. Med. J.* **2:**789–792, 1957.

2 Chamberlain, D. S., et al., Idiopathic Osteoarthropathy and Cranial Defects in Children. *Am. J. Roentgenol.* **93:**408–415, 1965.

3 Cremin, B. J., Familial Idiopathic Osteoarthropathy. *Br. J. Radiol.* **43:**568–570, 1970.

4 Findlay, G. H., and Oosthuizen, W. J., Pachydermoperiostosis: The Syndrome of Touraine, Solente and Golé. *S. Afr. Med. J.* **25:**747–752, 1951.

5 Fischer, D. S., et al., Clubbing: Review, with Emphasis on Hereditary Acropachy. *Medicine* **43:**459–479, 1964.

6 Friedreich, N., Hyperostose des gesammten Skelettes. *Virchows Arch. Pathol. Anat.* **43:**83–87, 1968.

7 Ginsburg, J., Observations on Peripheral Circulation in Hypertrophic Pulmonary Osteoarthropathy. *Q. J. Med.* **27:**335–532, 1958.

8 Grönberg, A., Is Cutis Verticis Gyrata a Symptom in Endocrine Syndrome Which Has So Far Received Little Attention? *Acta Med. Scand.* **67:**24–42, 1927.

9 Hambrick, G. W., and Carter, D. M., Pachydermoperiostosis. *Arch. Dermatol.* **94:**594–608, 1966.

10 Hammarsten, J. F., and O'Leary, J., The Features and Significance of Hypertrophic Osteoarthropathy. *Arch. Intern. Med.* **99:**431–441, 1957.

11 Kerber, R. E., and Vogl, A., Pachydermoperiostosis. *Arch. Intern. Med.* **132:**245–248, 1973.

12 Lehman, M. A., et al., Idiopathic Hypertrophic Osteoarthropathy (Acropachyderma with Pachyperiostosis). *Bull. Hosp. Joint Dis.* **24:**56–67, 1963.

13 Nixon, D. W., and Samols, E., Acral Changes Associated with Thyroid Diseases. *J.A.M.A.* **212:**1175–1181, 1970.

14 Pietruschka, G., et al., Ein Beitrag zur Pachydermoperiostose. *Klin. Monatsbl. Augenheilkd.* **154:**525–536, 1969.

15 Rimoin, D. L., Pachydermoperiostosis (Idiopathic Clubbing and Periostosis), Genetic and Physiologic Considerations. *N. Engl. J. Med.* **272:**923–931, 1965.

16 Rosenthal, J. W., and Kloepfer, H. W., An Acromegaloid, Cutis Verticis Gyrata, Corneal Leukoma Syndrome: A New Medical Entity. *Arch. Ophthalmol.* **68:**722–726, 1962.

17 Schuster, M. M., et al., Facial Deformity in Pachydermoperiostosis. *Plast. Reconstr. Surg.* **35:**666–674, 1965.

18 Shawarby, K., and Salah Ibrahim, M., Pachydermoperiostosis, a Review of Literature and Report of Four Cases. *Br. Med. J.* **1:**763–766, 1962.

19 Touraine, A., et al., Un syndrome ostéo-dermopathique: La pachydermie plicaturée avec pachypériostose des extrémités. *Presse Méd.* **43:**1820–1824, 1935.

20 Uehlinger, E., Hyperostosis generalisata mit Pachydermie. *Virchows Arch. Pathol. Anat.* **308:**396–444, 1941.

21 Unna, P. G., Cutis verticis gyrata. *Monatsschr. Prakt. Dermatol.* **45:**227–233, 1907.

22 Vague, J., La pachydermopériostose. *Ann. Méd.* **51:**152–164, 1950.

23 Vogl, A., and Goldfischer, S., Pachydermoperiostosis: Primary or Idiopathic Hypertrophic Osteoarthropathy. *Am. J. Med.* **33:**166–187, 1962.

115

Pachyonychia Congenita Syndromes

*(Jadassohn-Lewandowski Syndrome and
Jackson-Lawler Syndrome)*

Pachyonychia congenita is genetically heterogeneous, two distinct syndromes being subsumed under the term. Although the syndromes exhibit some similarities, their differences are never observed within the same pedigree.

JADASSOHN-LEWANDOWSKI SYNDROME

In 1906, Jadassohn and Lewandowski (10) described the syndrome of (a) pachyonychia congenita, (b) palmoplantar keratosis and hyperhidrosis, (c) follicular keratosis, and (d) oral leukokeratosis. The syndrome follows an autosomal dominant mode of transmission.

Skin and skin appendages. In most cases, at birth or soon thereafter, the finger- and toenails become thickened, tubular, and hard, the undersurface being filled with a horny, yellowish-brown material. This substance causes the nail to project upward from the nailbed at the free edge. Commonly, the nails are lost, with similar but more severe involvement appearing on regrowth. Inflammation at the sides of the nails is frequent (1) (Fig. 115-1A).

Hyperhidrosis of the palms and soles nearly always occurs, the rest of the skin being quite dry and often described as "mildly ichthyotic."

Palmar and plantar hyperkeratoses are noted in 40 to 65 percent of the cases during the first few years of life. During warm weather, bullae appear on the feet, especially on the plantar surface of the toes and heels and along the sides. They burst, become infected, and are very painful, often making walking extremely difficult (6) (Fig. 115-1B).

During the first few years of life, pinhead-sized follicular papules appear over the elbows, knees, popliteal areas, and buttocks in over 50 percent of the cases (13). In the center of each papule, a horny plug is seen. Verrucous lesions may also occur in the same areas (6). The skin is thickened, owing to acanthosis and parakeratosis, especially about the pilosebaceous apparatus. The follicles and sweat pores are dilated and plugged with imperfectly cornified and partly degenerated horny material. The hair is frequently noted to be dry, and alopecia has been reported (11, 13).

Ears, nose, and throat. Hoarse voice and thickening of the posterior commissure of the larynx have been noted (8).

Other manifestations. Mental retardation has also been documented (12).

Oral manifestations. The dorsum of the tongue is thickened, presenting a white or grayish-white appearance (7) (Fig. 115-2). Less commonly involved is the buccal mucosa at the interdental line. Oral aphthae are frequent (1, 16).

The oral mucosa is thickened by a uniform acanthosis. There is marked intracellular vacuo-

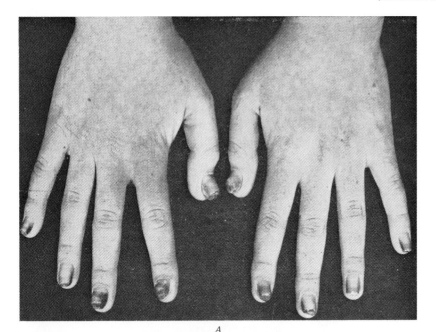

A

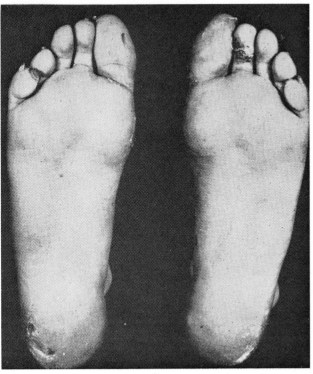

B

Figure 115-1. (*A*). *Pachyonychia congenita.* Note thickening and elevation of fingernails at free edge of thirteen-year-old female. This change is noted in types I and II. (*B*). Note ruptured blisters of toes and heels. Often there is severe hyperkeratosis of soles. (*From A. D. M. Jackson and Lawler,* Ann. Eugen. **16:**141, 1951.)

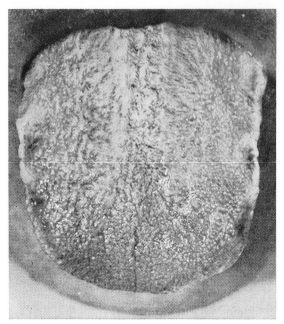

Figure 115-2. Thickening of oral mucosa, especially that of tongue and buccal mucosa, occurs only in type II.

lization. The intercellular bridges in the stratum spinosum are absent. Parakeratosis is marked. No Schiff-positive material is seen in the epithelium. The microscopic picture greatly resembles that seen in white sponge nevus.

Touraine (18) suggested that the incidence of scrotal tongue is high, but we have not been able to support this contention.

JACKSON-LAWLER SYNDROME

In 1951-1952, Jackson and Lawler (9) described a syndrome which has some of the same features observed in the Jadassohn-Lewandowski syndrome, such as (a) pachyonychia congenita, (b) palmoplantar hyperkeratosis and hyperhidrosis, and (c) follicular keratosis. However, (d) oral leu-

kokeratosis is never observed. In addition, patients with the Jackson-Lawler syndrome have (e) large cutaneous epidermoid cysts and (f) natal teeth. Other families have been reported by a number of authors (3, 13, 17, 19–21). Members of the same family were reported by Brain (4), Shrank (16), Besser (2), and possibly by Murray (14). The syndrome follows an autosomal dominant mode of transmission.

Skin and skin appendages. The findings are identical to those observed in the Jadassohn-Lewandowski syndrome. In addition, large epidermoid cysts, especially of the head, neck, and upper chest regions, appear around puberty (2, 5, 9, 13, 16, 17, 19, 20, 21).

Eyes. Corneal dystrophy has been reported by several authors (5, 9, 17).

Ears, nose, and throat. Hoarse voice has been described (9, 13).

Oral manifestations. Natal teeth are poorly calcified (3, 9, 14–17, 19, 20).

DIFFERENTIAL DIAGNOSIS

The nail changes are distinctive, while the oral leukokeratosis is nonspecific, being seen in many disorders, such as *dyskeratosis congenita, hereditary benign intraepithelial dyskeratosis,* and white sponge nevus (7). Isolated natal teeth occur once in 2,000 to 3,000 newborns but may be seen with increased frequency in *Ellis-van Creveld syndrome,* in *Hallermann-Streiff syndrome,* and in cleft lip-palate.

LABORATORY AIDS

None is known.

REFERENCES

1 Andrews, G. C., and Strumwasser, S., Pachyonychia Congenita. *N.Y. J. Med.* **29:**747–749, 1929.
2 Besser, F. S., and Moynahan, E. J., Pachyonychia Congenita

with Epidermal Cysts and Teeth at Birth: 4th Generation. *Br. J. Dermatol.* **84:**95–96, 1971.
3 Boxley, J. D., and Wilkinson, D. S., Pachyonychia

Congenita and Multiple Epidermal Hamartomata. *Br. J. Dermatol.* **85:**298–299, 1971.

4 Brain, R. T., Pachyonychia Congenita with Ectodermal Defect. *Proc. 10th Int. Congr. Dermatol.* London, 1952, pp. 507–508.

5 de Groot, W. P., Pachyonychia Congenita with Sebocystomatosis (Sertoli). *Dermatologica* **133:**344, 1966.

6 Goodman, H., Pachyonychia Congenita. *Urol. Cutan. Rev.* **50:**465–467, 1946.

7 Gorlin, R. J., and Chaudhry, A. P., Oral Lesions Accompanying Pachyonychia Congenita. *Oral Surg.* **11:**541–544, 1958.

8 Hadida, E., and Marill, F. G., Pachyonychie congénitale avec kératodermie et kératoses disseminées de la peau et des muqueuses (syndrome de Jadassohn et Lewandowski). *Bull. Soc. Fr. Dermatol. Syphiligr.* **59:**236–237, 1952.

9 Jackson, A. D. M., and Lawler, S. D., Pachyonychia Congenita: A Report of Six Cases in One Family. *Ann. Eugen.* **16:**142–146, 1951–1952.

10 Jadassohn, J., and Lewandowski, K., in A. Neisser and E. Jacobi, (eds.), *Ikonographia Dermatologica.* Urban & Schwarzenberg, Berlin, 1906, p. 29.

11 Kumer, L., and Loose, H. O., Über Pachyonychia congenita (Typus Riehl). *Wien. Klin. Wochenschr.* **48:**174–178, 1935.

12 Lang, C. R., et al., Pachyonychia Congenita. *Am. J. Dis. Child.* **111:**649–652, 1966.

13 Moldenhauer, E., and Ernst, K., Das Jadassohn-Lewandowsky Syndrom (case 1). *Hautarzt* **19:**441–447, 1968.

14 Murray, F. A., Four Cases of Hereditary Hypertrophy of the Nail Bed Associated with a History of Erupted Teeth at Birth. *Br. J. Dermatol.* **33:**409–411, 1921.

15 Pires De Lima, J. A., Dents à la naissance. *Bull. Soc. Anthropol. Paris* **4**(7):71–74, 1923.

16 Shrank, A. B., Pachyonychia Congenita. *Proc. R. Soc. Med.* **59:**975–976, 1966.

17 Soderquist, N. A., and Reed, W. B., Pachyonychia Congenita with Epidermal Cysts and Other Congenital Dyskeratoses. *Arch. Dermatol.* **97:**31–33, 1968.

18 Touraine, A., Pachyonychie congénitale. *Presse Méd.* **45:**1569–1572, 1937.

19 Velasquez, J. P., and Bustamante, J., Sebocystomatosis with Congenital Pachyonychia. *Int. J. Dermatol.* **11:**77–81, 1972.

20 Vineyard, W. R., and Scott, R. A., Steatocystoma Multiplex with Pachyonychia Congenita. *Arch. Dermatol.* **84:**824–827, 1961.

21 Wolfshaut, A., and Cernaianu, R., Steatocistom si keratodermie familiala. *Derm. Venereol.* (*Bucharest*) **13:**447–454, 1968.

116

Peutz-Jeghers Syndrome

*(Mucocutaneous Melanotic Pigmentation and
Gastrointestinal Polyposis)*

The syndrome of (*a*) mucocutaneous melanotic pigmentation associated with (*b*) intestinal polyposis was probably first described in 1896 by Sir John Hutchinson (14), although he was not aware of the presence of polyposis at the time. Follow-up of one of his patients revealed the cause of death to be intussusception (30). Credit for pointing out the relationship between these ostensibly unrelated conditions goes to Peutz (21), a Dutch physician who, in 1921, described the syndrome in three generations. However, knowledge of the condition did not become widespread until Jeghers et al. (15) published a comprehensive account of 10 cases in 1949. Since that time, nearly 600 cases have been recorded. The surveys of Dormandy (8) and Klostermann (16, 17) furnish current knowledge of the syndrome. For an excellent summary of the history of the syndrome, see Dormandy (8).

The syndrome is transmitted as an autosomal dominant disorder with a high degree of penetrance (8, 15, 17). Bartholomew and Dahlin (4) indicated, in their survey of 117 cases, that 43 percent had a family history of both polyps and pigmentation and another 13 percent of pigmentation alone.

SYSTEMIC MANIFESTATIONS

Gastrointestinal system. Polyposis of the gastrointestinal tract is the clinically more important component of the syndrome. The polyps are hamartomatous in origin (3, 4, 9). Bartholomew and Dahlin (4) suggested that the following sites are involved, with the annotated frequency: jejunum, 63 percent; ileum, 55 percent; large intestine and rectum, 36 percent each; stomach, 23 percent; duodenum, 15 percent. More gastric polyps were found by Utsonomiya et al. (28).

Thus, the polyps may be found anywhere in the mucus-secreting portion of the gastrointestinal tract and may make themselves apparent by producing intussusception. Often the intussusception is self-resolving, but it may lead to serious intestinal obstruction and death. Age of onset of symptoms varies from a few weeks to 77 years (average 25 years). However, about 70 percent of affected persons experience some type of gastrointestinal symptoms–intermittent colicky pain (85 percent) and melena or rectal bleeding (35 percent)–prior to diagnosis; in the majority of patients this period before diagnosis is about 5 years. Hypochromic anemia, due to intestinal bleeding, has been found in about 25 percent of patients (4).

The polyps are usually described as benign adenomatous tumors varying in size from 0.5 to 7.0 cm in diameter. Dormandy (8) suggested that these growths are hamartomatous, arising from primitive adenomatous vesicles embedded in the intestinal wall (Figs. 116-1*A*, *B*, 116-4). This view was supported by other investigations (3, 4, 23, 31). Several authors (20, 28) have described malignant degeneration of a polyp.

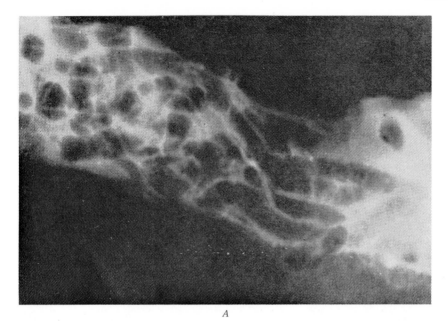

A

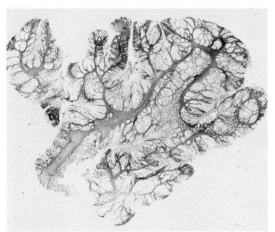

B

Figure 116-1. *Peutz-Jeghers syndrome.* (*A*). Roentgenogram of small intestine demonstrating multiple polyposis on barium swallow. (*B*). Low-power view of polyp from large intestine. Note arborization of nonstriated muscle. (*From J. D. Reid, Cancer* **18:**970, 1965.)

growths. Frequent mitotic figures are also characteristic. The growths may extend to the serosal surface.

Polyps of other organs have been discovered [nose (8, 12, 17, 21, 32), uterus (17, 22, 32), or ureter-bladder, (8, 12, 17, 21, 25)] in a few instances. Bronchial adenosis has also been mentioned (8, 12, 21).

Skin. In about 50 percent of affected persons, numerous, usually discrete, brown to bluish-black macules are present on the skin, especially about the facial orifices — perioral, perinasal, periorbital (Fig. 116-1). Though some patients exhibit only a few pigmented macules, others are severely pigmented. In addition, pigmented spots occur on the extremities in about two-thirds of affected individuals (4, 26, 28), rarely on the palms or soles (22), or, occasionally, in other areas, such as the umbilicus, axilla, or shoulder (11, 32) (Fig. 116-2*A*, *B*). Pigmentation of the nails has also been described (29).

Dozois et al. (9) have reviewed these cases and have found no parallelism between location of the malignant tumor and the general location of polyps in this syndrome, i.e., the most common sites for the adenocarcinomas (stomach and colon) are least likely to be sites of polyps.

Microscopically, the growths represent focal overgrowths in improper proportions of tissues indigenous to that part of the gastrointestinal tract. A branching-tree arrangement of smooth muscle may be seen scattered throughout the

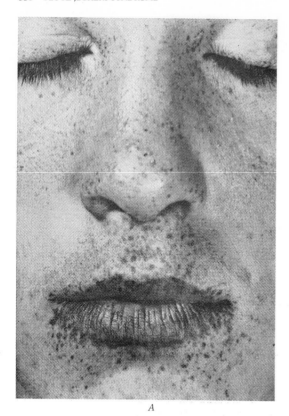

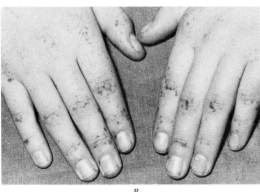

A

B

Figure 116-2. (*A*). Note extensive melanotic pigmentation of lips, numerous very small freckle-like spots about mouth, nose, and eyes. (*Courtesy of J. Calnan, London, England.*) (*B*). Similar deposits on fingers. (*Courtesy of G. P. Klostermann and G. Thieme Verlag, Stuttgart.*)

The pigmentation usually appears in infancy and seems to fade somewhat at about puberty. It may, however, appear as late as in the eighth decade.

Ovarian cysts and tumors. Ovarian tumors occur in about 10 percent of women with Peutz-Jeghers syndrome (7). Granulosa cell tumors, reported by a number of authors (5–7, 9, 12, 15, 22, 27), have effected precocious puberty (7). Brenner tumor, dysgerminoma (28), and cystadenoma (10, 19) have also been found. These cases have been reviewed by Christian (7) and by Scully (24), who suggested that a distinctive ovarian neoplasm, which he called "sex cord tumor with annular tubules," may be associated with Peutz-Jeghers syndrome. Multicentricity and calcification of the tubules are frequently seen. The neoplasm, probably derived from the granulosa cell tumor, produces endometrial hyperplasia (Fig. 116-3).

Other findings. Clubbing of the fingers (5, 18) has been noted, but its significance has not been ascertained.

Oral manifestations. On the lips, especially the lower, and on the oral mucosa, round, oval, or irregular, rarely confluent macules of bluish-gray pigment of variable intensity may be seen (33). They vary in size from 1 to 12 mm and are usually somewhat larger than those on the cutaneous surface. About 98 percent of 117 patients had pigmentation of the lips, and 88 percent had involvement of the buccal mucosa (4). Less frequently pigmented are the palate and gingiva (19). Only rarely are the tongue and the oral floor involved (17, 21, 26). There does not

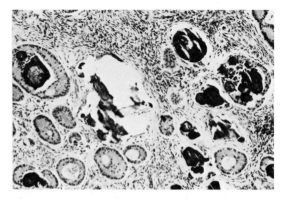

Figure 116-3. Sex cord tumor. Note simple and complex annular tubules with external calcification. (*From R. E. Scully, Cancer* **25:**1107, 1970.)

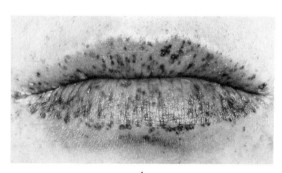
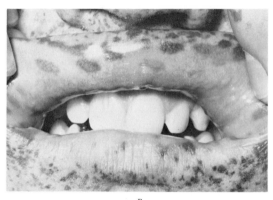

A   *B*

Figure 116-4. (*A*). Labial involvement in Peutz-Jeghers syndrome. (*From M. Zingsheim, Hautarzt* **17**:85, 1966.) (*B*). Melanotic pigmentation of labial mucosal surface. (*From G. P. Klostermann and G. Thieme Verlag, Stuttgart, Germany.*)

appear to be any relationship between the amount of oral pigmentation and the degree or distribution of the visceral polyposis (Fig. 116-4*A*, *B*).

Several investigators have pointed out that labial pigment also tends to fade and that the pigment on the buccal mucosa fades to a lesser degree (17), thus being helpful in diagnosis (3, 4). Rarely, the pigment may be present without polyposis (8, 15, 32).

Pigmentation of other mucosal surfaces, viz., conjunctival (2) and nasal (8), may also be seen. Pigmented oral papillomatosis was noted by Lowe (18a).

DIFFERENTIAL DIAGNOSIS

Similar oral mucosal pigmentation may be seen in Addison disease or, under normal conditions, in blacks or members of other dark-skinned races (33). However, the cutaneous pigmentation in Addison disease is generalized and often increased along body folds. The distribution of freckles does not ordinarily occur about the mouth or on the lips. Lentiginosis profusa (*leopard syndrome*) is generalized over the skin but does not involve the mucosal surfaces.

Oral pigmentation may rarely occur in the *McCune-Albright syndrome*. Polyposis and pigmentation have been described in association with alopecia and nail dystrophy, i.e., Cronkheit-Canada syndrome.

Other forms of polyposis of the intestinal tract are usually limited to the colon. These include familial polyposis, the *Gardner syndrome*, juvenile polyposis, and disseminated polyposis of the colon and rectum. These and other types are discussed in Chap. 59.

LABORATORY AIDS

The presence of labial and/or oral pigmentation should suggest a thorough history and examination of the gastrointestinal tract by proctoscopic and roentgenographic means.

REFERENCES

1 André, R., et al., Syndrome de Peutz-Jeghers avec polypose oesophagienne. *Bull. Soc. Méd. Hôp. Paris* **117**:505–510, 1966.
2 Andrew, R., Generalized Intestinal Polyposis with Melanosis. *Gastroenterology* **23**:495–499, 1953.

3 Bartholomew, L. G., et al., Intestinal Polyposis Associated with Mucocutaneous Melanin Pigmentation: Peutz-Jeghers Syndrome. Review of Literature and Report of Six Cases with Special Reference to Pathologic Findings. *Gastroenterology* **32**:434–451, 1957.

4 Bartholomew, L. G., and Dahlin, D. C., Intestinal Polyposis and Mucocutaneous Pigmentation. *Minn. Med.* **41:**848–852, 1958.

5 Berkowitz, S. B., et al., Syndrome of Intestinal Polyposis with Melanosis of the Lips and Buccal Mucosa: Study of Incidence and Location of Malignancy with Three New Case Reports. *Ann. Surg.* **141:**129–133, 1955.

6 Burdick, D., et al., Peutz-Jeghers Syndrome. *Cancer* **16:**854–867, 1963.

7 Christian, C. D., Ovarian Tumors—an Extension of the Peutz-Jeghers Syndrome. *Am. J. Obstet. Gynecol.* **111:**529–534, 1971.

8 Dormandy, T. L., Gastrointestinal Polyposis with Mucocutaneous Pigmentation: Peutz-Jeghers Syndrome. *N. Engl. J. Med.* **256:**1093–1102, 1141–1146, 1186–1190, 1956.

9 Dozois, R. R., et al., The Peutz-Jeghers Syndrome. *Arch. Surg.* **98:**509–517, 1969.

10 Dozois, R. R., et al., Ovarian Tumors Associated with the Peutz-Jeghers Syndrome. *Ann. Surg.* **172:**233–238, 1970.

11 Fritsche, W., and Fleischhauer, G., Chirurgischen Beitrag zur hereditären Dünndarm-polyposis (Peutz-Jeghers Syndrom). *Chirurg* **28:**266–269, 1957.

12 Hafter, E., Gastrointestinale Polypose mit Melanose der Lippen und Mundschleimhaut (Peutz-Jeghers'sche Syndrom). *Gastroenterologia (Basel)* **84:**341–348, 1955.

13 Humphries, A. L., et al., Peutz-Jeghers Syndrome with Colonic Adenocarcinoma and Ovarian Tumor. *J.A.M.A.* **197:**296–298, 1966.

14 Hutchinson, J., Pigmentation of Lips and Mouth. *Arch. Surg.* **7:**290, 1896.

15 Jeghers, H., et al., Generalized Intestinal Polyposis and Melanin Spots of the Oral Mucosa, Lips, and Digits. *N. Engl. J. Med.* **241:**993–1005, 1031–1036, 1949.

16 Klostermann, G. F., *Pigmentfleckenpolypose. Klinische, histologische und erbbiologische Studien am sogenannten Peutz-Syndrom.* Thieme, Stuttgart, 1960.

17 Klostermann, G. F., Zur Kenntnis der Pigmentfleckenpolypose. Bemerkungen zu Diagnostik, Verlauf und Erbbiologie des sogenannten Peutz-Jeghers—Syndroms auf Grund katamnestischer Daten. *Arch. Klin. Exp. Dermatol.* **226:**182–189, 1966.

18 Kutscher, A. H., et al., Peutz-Jeghers Syndrome. Follow-ups on Patients Reported in the Literature. *Am. J. Med. Sci.* **138:**180–186, 1959.

18a Lowe, N. J., Peutz-Jeghers Syndrome with Pigmented Oral Papillomas. *Arch. Dermatol.* **111:**503–505, 1975.

19 Olansky, S., and Achord, J., The Problem of Carcinoma in the Peutz-Jeghers Syndrome. *South. Med. J.* **62:**827–829, 1969.

20 Papaioannou, A., and Criteselis, A., Malignant Changes in Peutz-Jeghers Syndrome. *N. Engl. J. Med.* **289:**694, 1973.

21 Peutz, J. L. A., Very Remarkable Case of Familial Polyposis of Mucous Membrane of Intestinal Tract and Nasopharynx Accompanied by Peculiar Pigmentation of Skin and Mucous Membrane. *Ned. Maandschr. Geneeskd.* **10:**134–146, 1921.

22 Reid, J. D., Duodenal Carcinoma in the Peutz-Jeghers Syndrome. *Cancer* **18:**970–977, 1965.

23 Rintala, A., The Histological Appearance of Gastrointestinal Polyps in Peutz-Jeghers Syndrome. *Acta Chir. Scand.* **117:**366–373, 1959.

24 Scully, R. E., Sex Cord Tumor with Annular Tubules: A Distinctive Ovarian Tumor of the Peutz-Jeghers Syndrome. *Cancer* **25:**1107–1121, 1970.

25 Sommerhaug, R. G., and Mason, T., Peutz-Jeghers Syndrome and Ureteral Polyposis. *J.A.M.A.* **211:**120–122, 1970.

26 Staley, C. J., and Schwartz, H., Gastrointestinal Polyposis and Pigmentation of the Oral Mucosa (Peutz-Jeghers Syndrome). *Int. Abstr. Surg.* **105:**1–15, 1957.

27 Steenstrup, E. K., Ovarian Tumours and Peutz-Jeghers Syndrome. *Acta Obstet. Gynecol. Scand.* **51:**237–240, 1972.

28 Utsonomiya, J., et al., Peutz-Jeghers Syndrome: Its Natural Course and Management. *Johns Hopkins Med. J.* **136:**71–82, 1975.

29 Valero, A., Pigmented Nails in Peutz-Jeghers Syndrome. *Am. J. Gastroenterol.* **43:**56–58, 1965.

30 Weber, F. P., Patches of Deep Pigmentation of Oral Mucous Membrane not Connected with Addison's Disease. *Q. J. Med.* **12:**404, 1919.

31 Weller, R. O., and McColl, I., Electron Microscope Appearance of Juvenile and Peutz-Jeghers Polyps. *Gut* **7:**265–270, 1966.

32 Zegarelli, E. V., et al., Melanin Spots of the Oral Mucosa and Skin Associated with Polyps: Report of a Case of Peculiar Pigmentation of the Lips and Mouth. *Oral Surg.* **7:**972–978, 1954.

33 Zegarelli, E. V., et al., Atlas of Oral Lesions Observed in the Syndrome of Oral Melanosis with Associated Intestinal Polyposis (Peutz-Jeghers Syndrome). *Am. J. Dig. Dis.* **4:**479–489, 1959.

117

Pfeiffer Syndrome

In 1964, Pfeiffer (10) described a syndrome consisting of (*a*) craniosynostosis resulting in turribrachycephaly, and (*b*) broad thumbs and great toes. (*c*) Partial soft-tissue syndactyly of the hands and feet is a variable feature. Eight affected individuals in three generations with two instances of male-to-male transmission were noted in Pfeiffer's report. Other pedigrees consistent with autosomal dominant transmission were noted by Zippel and Schüler (14), Martsolf et al. (8), and Saldino et al. (12). Penetrance has been complete, and expressivity has been variable. Sporadic cases have also been reported (1, 2, 6, 7, 11).

The Pfeiffer syndrome and Apert-type acrocephalosyndactyly are noteworthy for their close similarity, the former being less severe in degree. It has been suggested that the Pfeiffer syndrome may, in fact, represent a mild form of Apert-type acrocephalosyndactyly. Clinical differences have been explained by later onset of the gene's action (3). However, on the basis of pedigree studies reported to date, no transition from one type to the other has been observed within families, despite the presence of variability in expression. Thus, the two disorders would appear to be nosologically and genetically distinct. An allelic mutant gene to account for the differences between the two disorders was postulated by Pfeiffer (10).

Relatively few reports of the Pfeiffer syndrome have appeared. Other studies are necessary to delineate the syndrome further. It is anticipated that a wide variety of low-frequency visceral abnormalities may be associated with the disorder. Serial documentation of progressive synostosis in the hands, feet, and cervical region of the spine should also be carried out. Other pedigrees would be useful to further study the variability in expression. Finally, a large number of sporadic cases should be studied for possible increased paternal age at the time of conception.

SYSTEMIC MANIFESTATIONS

Craniofacies. The skull is turribrachycephalic. Maxillary hypoplasia with relative mandibular prognathism is observed. The nasal bridge is depressed. Ocular hypertelorism, antimongoloid obliquity, proptosis, and strabismus have been reported (2, 8, 10). Facial asymmetry may be observed in some instances (2). The syndrome has been reported in association with Kleeblattschädel (cloverleaf skull) (2, 4, 5, 13) (Fig. 117-1*A*, *B*).

Central nervous system. Intelligence is usually normal (1, 8, 10), but mental retardation may be observed in some instances (2, 5). Severe retardation and various central nervous system defects may be observed in those cases associated with Kleeblattschädel.

Hands and feet. The thumbs and great toes are broad, usually with varus deformity (10). In

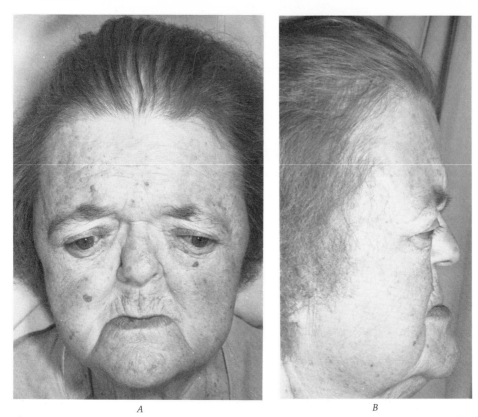

A   *B*

Figure 117-1. *Pfeiffer syndrome.* (*A, B*). Ocular hypertelorism, antimongoloid obliquity of palpebral fissures, and midface hypoplasia.

some instances the great toes may be shortened without varus deformity (2). Mild soft-tissue syndactyly may involve especially digits 2 and 3 and sometimes digits 3 and 4 of both hands and feet (2, 10). Partial soft-tissue syndactyly between toes 1 and 2 has also been reported (2, 10, 14). Syndactyly may be absent in some cases (2). Clinodactyly has also been noted (2) (Fig. 117-2*A, B*).

Skeletal system. Craniosynostosis, especially involving the coronal suture, results in turribrachycephaly, and increased digital markings may be observed with age (1, 2, 10). Maxillary hypoplasia, shallow orbits, and depressed nasal bridge are also seen (2, 8, 10).

Brachymesophalangy of both hands and feet may be observed (8, 10). Middle phalanges may

be absent in some cases (2, 10). The proximal phalanges of both thumbs are trapezoidal, but may be triangular in some instances (10). Pollex varus is commonly found (8, 10) (Fig. 117-3).

The proximal phalanges of both great toes are trapezoid-shaped and hallux varus is usually observed. The first metatarsals are broad, with partial reduplication in some cases (2, 8, 10). Accessory epiphyses in the first and second metatarsals and double ossification centers in the proximal phalanges of the great toes have been reported (1, 8). Talipes calcaneovarus has been noted (1).

Symphalangism of both hands and feet have been reported (2). Fusions of carpals, tarsals, and the proximal ends of metacarpals and metatarsals have also been noted (2, 11, 14). Fused cervical vertebras have been described (2). Radio-

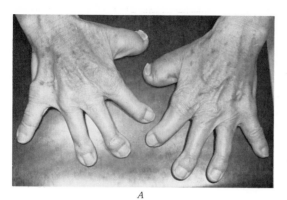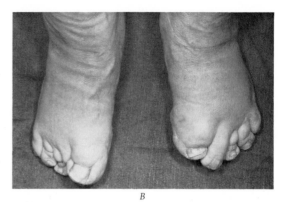

A   *B*

Figure 117-2. (*A*). Broad, radially deviated thumbs, brachydactyly, and clinodactyly of terminal phalanges. (*B*). Broad halluces and crooked toes.

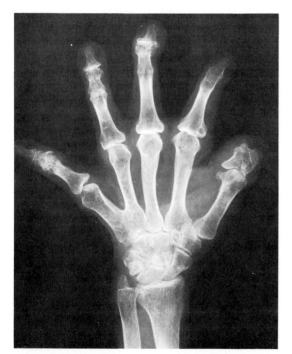

Figure 117-3. Roentgenogram showing malformed fused phalanges of thumbs, brachymesophalangy, symphalangism, fusion of proximal ends of fourth and fifth metacarpals.

humeral and radioulnar synostosis have been reported occasionally (1, 2). Decreased iliac angle was noted in one case (8).

Other findings. Pyloric stenosis (8), bicuspid aortic valve, common mesentery, hypoplastic gallbladder, single umbilical artery (5), umbilical hernia, choanal atresia (9), preauricular tag (8), hearing loss (2, 8), and a variety of other anomalies (2) have been noted.

Oral manifestations. The palate is highly arched (2, 10). Bifid uvula has been noted in one case (1). Class III malocclusion and crowded teeth have been reported (2).

DIFFERENTIAL DIAGNOSIS

The Pfeiffer syndrome should be distinguished from *Apert-type acrocephalosyndactyly* (see Chap. 9), *Saethre-Chotzen syndrome* (see Chap. 130), other *craniosynostosis syndromes* (see Chap. 40), and simple oxycephaly.

LABORATORY AIDS

None is known.

REFERENCES

1 Asnes, R. S., and Morehead, C. D., Pfeiffer Syndrome. *Birth Defects* **5**(3):198–203, 1969.

2 Cohen, M. M., Jr., An Etiologic and Nosologic Overview of Craniosynostosis Syndromes. *Birth Defects* **11**(2):137–189, 1975.

3 Degenhardt, K. U., Zum entwicklungsmechanischen Problem der Akrocephalosyndaktylie. *Z. Menschl. Vererb. Konstit. Lehre* **29**:791–819, 1950.

4 Eaton, A., et al., The Kleeblattschädel Anomaly. *Birth Defects*, **11**(2):238–246, 1975.

5 Hodach, R. J., et al., The Pfeiffer Syndrome, Association with Kleeblattschädel and Multiple Visceral Anomalies. *Z. Kinderheilkd.* **119**:87–103, 1975.

6 Lenz, W., Zur Diagnose und Ätiologie der Akrocephalosyndaktylie. *Z. Kinderheilkd.* **79**:546–554, 1957.

7 Manns, K.-J., and Bopp, K. P., Dysostosis craniofacialis Crouzon mit digitaler Anomalie. *Med. Klin.* **60**:1899–1903, 1965.

8 Martsolf, J. T., et al., Pfeiffer Syndrome. *Am. J. Dis. Child.* **121**:257–262, 1971.

9 Opitz, J. M., Personal communication, 1972.

10 Pfeiffer, R. A., Dominant erbliche Akrocephalosyndaktylie. *Z. Kinderheilkd.* **90**:301–320, 1964.

11 Pfeiffer, R. A., Associated Deformities of the Head and Hands. *Birth Defects* **5**(3):18–34, 1969.

12 Saldino, R. M., et al., Familial Acrocephalosyndactyly (Pfeiffer Syndrome). *Am. J. Roentgenol.* **116**:609–622, 1972.

13 Temtamy, S. A., et al., Limb Malformations in the Cloverleaf Skull Anomaly. *Birth Defects* **11**(2):247–251, 1975.

14 Zippel, H., and Schüler, K.-H., Dominant vererbte Akrozephalosyndaktylie (ACS). *Fortschr. Roentgenstr.* **110**:234–245, 1969.

118

Potter Syndrome

(Oligohydramnios Syndrome)

In 1946, Potter (31, 32) described the characteristic features of infants with bilateral renal agenesis. Abnormalities of the (a) face, (b) limbs, (c) lungs, and (d) skin are now thought to result from oligohydramnios, whatever the cause. Lack of amniotic fluid results in fetal compression, leading to altered facies, abnormal positioning of the hands and feet, wrinkled skin, amnion nodosum, breech presentation, and possibly to (e) pulmonary hypoplasia and (f) growth deficiency (43).

Some authors limit the term Potter syndrome to cases with bilateral renal agenesis. We would like to honor Potter's extensive work in this field by extending the term to include the pattern of abnormalities produced by oligohydramnios, irrespective of cause. We do not like the term "renofacial dysplasia" for the Potter syndrome (oligohydramnios syndrome), nor can we accept confusing the disorder with other malformation syndromes which have renal and facial anomalies not caused by oligohydramnios (7, 16, 17, 18, 27, 28). For example, one such patient (18) had the Saethre-Chotzen syndrome with a renal abnormality.

Bilateral renal agenesis (30, 31), severe polycystic kidneys (12, 17, 27, 32), urinary tract obstruction (2, 21), and amniotic leakage (8, 21, 43) may all cause oligohydramnios. That oligohydramnios per se but not necessarily bilateral renal agenesis is the sine qua non of the Potter syndrome is illustrated by unusual experiments of nature in which infants with renal agenesis do not present the extrarenal features of the syndrome. Fetuses that are unable to excrete urine into the amniotic space may have adequate amniotic fluid in unusual cases. For example, if bilateral renal agenesis occurs in one of monoamniotic twins but urine is excreted by the other twin into the common amniotic space, oligohydramnios is prevented, and the extrarenal features of the Potter syndrome do not occur in the first twin. Various other unusual experiments of nature which fail to produce the extrarenal manifestations of the disorder have been discussed by several authors (2, 21, 25, 43).

It has been established that oligohydramnios may result from any defect in urinary output or by chronic leakage of amniotic fluid. A heterogeneity of causes can be postulated for malunion of the ureteral bud and the metanephric blastema alone. Several embryopathic mechanisms are possible, such as absence of the portion of the mesonephric duct from which the ureteral bud arises, failure of the ureteral bud to form despite the presence of the mesonephric duct, degeneration of the ureteral bud, absence or abnormality of the metanephric blastema, and hypoplasia or degeneration of the embryonic kidney (6, 32). Improper induction and the possibility of unknown circulating factors deserve further investigation.

The incidence of bilateral renal agenesis has been reported to vary from 1 per 3,000 to 1 per 9,000 births (2, 20, 30, 34). It occurs more frequently in males (2:1 to 3:1) (13a, 34, 46).

The overwhelming majority of cases are sporadic, although affected sibs have been reported by several investigators (1, 4, 8, 9, 24, 36, 38). The relatively common occurrence, mostly sporadic and rarely familial instances, preponderance of one affected sex, and discordance in the few reported twin pairs (31) suggest that bilateral renal agenesis sui generis is a multifactorial trait with a threshold effect and very low recurrence risk (8), although genetic heterogeneity with an autosomal recessive type in some families cannot be ruled out.

The incidence and prevalence of unilateral renal agenesis in the general population is not known, although its incidence at necropsy is estimated to vary from 1 per 600 to 1 per 1,000 (46). In women with unilateral renal agenesis, the associated tubal and uterine malformations may be responsible for prematurity and an increased risk of spontaneous abortion (8). Families have been reported in which the proband presented bilateral renal agenesis and relatives of the proband had unilateral renal agenesis (6, 8, 10, 19, 26, 39). Although their clinical effects are dramatically different, unilateral and bilateral renal agenesis should be considered genetically identical in some families. The problem is further complicated by the observation of bilateral renal agenesis, unilateral renal agenesis, and renal dysplasia within the same family (9). Furthermore, since unilateral involvement can be clinically silent and intravenous pyelograms are not routinely carried out on relatives of a severely affected proband, it is not known what the ratio of "sporadic" to "familial" instances might be. Autosomal dominant inheritance with mild expression in females and more severe expression in males has been proposed (8). X-linked inheritance may be ruled out by male-to-male transmission (19), but etiologic heterogeneity in this type of renal agenesis may possibly exist. The term "hereditary renal adysplasia" has been suggested for this type to imply predominantly asymmetric renal involvement and, less commonly, bilateral aplasia or symmetrical degrees of dysplasia (8).

Karyotypes have been normal (29). Masculination of the external genitalia in a patient with 46, XX karyotype has been reported (37).

Occasionally, the Potter syndrome may be part of a more extensive defect in caudal mesoderm, resulting in the Duhamel anomalad which includes a spectrum of abnormalities [sirenomelia, VATER association, caudal regression syndrome, and Rokitansky syndrome (14a, 20, 32, 33, 38a)]. The Potter syndrome may also be observed as part of a true malformation syndrome in which two or more distinct developmental fields are involved. For example, it has been observed in association with ectrodactyly, suggesting a multifocal primary mesodermal defect in which both the metanephros and limb buds are affected (13). The possibility always exists that some true multiple anomaly syndrome, in which the Potter defect is one component, may be caused by a chromosomal aberration.

SYSTEMIC MANIFESTATIONS

Breech presentation (40 percent), intrauterine death (25 percent), and antepartum hemorrhage (15 percent) have been found in a large series (34). Cesarean delivery is required in about 10 percent of cases. About half the infants are small-for-dates (34).

Facies. A prominent semicircular skin fold extends from the inner canthus onto the cheek. When this fold is absent, some functioning kidney tissue may be present. Ocular hypertelorism has been observed. The nose may be blunted, with turned-down tip. A prominent crease is often present on the chin. The ears are low set, posteriorly rotated, large, and floppy, with cartilaginous deficiency (30–33) (Fig. 118-1A–E). Rarely, microphthalmia, absent ears, and hydrocephaly (secondary to vertebral/sacral defects) have been reported (33).

Lungs. The lungs are hypoplastic, with primitive or absent alveoli (32, 34, 38a).

Skeletal and limb abnormalities. Flexion contractures at the knees and hips, spadelike hands, genu varum, and talipes equinovarus are common (29, 32). Hyperextensible knees, webbed knees, vertebral defects, ischial and sacral hypoplasia, sirenomelia, radial defects, and ectrodactyly have been reported (2, 13, 33, 34, 38a).

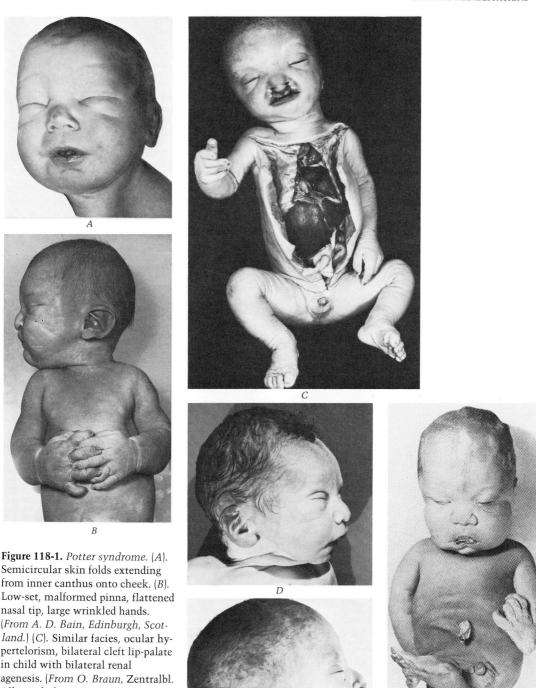

Figure 118-1. *Potter syndrome.* (*A*). Semicircular skin folds extending from inner canthus onto cheek. (*B*). Low-set, malformed pinna, flattened nasal tip, large wrinkled hands. (*From A. D. Bain, Edinburgh, Scotland.*) (*C*). Similar facies, ocular hypertelorism, bilateral cleft lip-palate in child with bilateral renal agenesis. (*From O. Braun,* Zentralbl. Allg. Pathol. **107**:1, 1965.) (*D, E*). Compare with other facies. (*Courtesy of J. Arey, Philadelphia.*) (*F*). Potter facies in sirenomelia. (*From P. J. Carpentier and E. Potter,* Am J. Obstet. Gynecol. **78**:235, 1959.)

Skin. The skin is very dry, loose, and wrinkled, giving a prematurely senile appearance (12, 14, 32).

Genitourinary system. Abnormalities may include bilateral renal agenesis, absent ureters, hypoplastic polycystic kidneys (about 35 percent), absent trigone of the bladder, gonadal hypoplasia, absent ductus deferens, absent seminal vesicles, absent uterus, bicornuate uterus, absent vagina, rectovaginal fistula, and masculinization of the external genitalia with 46, XX karyotype (2, 8, 33, 34, 37, 38a).

Other findings. Imperforate anus, absent rectum, adrenal hypoplasia, cardiovascular anomalies, asplenia, polysplenia, esophageal atresia, diaphragmatic hernia, and single umbilical artery have been reported (20, 32, 33, 38a).

Oral manifestations. Micrognathia has been observed in most cases. Cleft lip and/or palate have been noted in a few instances (32).

DIFFERENTIAL DIAGNOSIS

The association of renal and auricular anomalies independent of the Potter syndrome has been described by several authors (2, 10, 23, 41, 44). In *trisomy 18 syndrome* anomalous low-set ears, micrognathia, and urinary tract malformations have been observed. Although the Duhamel anomalad is one developmental field complex observed with trisomy 18, to our knowledge no patient has ever presented with bilateral renal agenesis. The combination of renal dysgenesis (varying from hypoplasia to agenesis), malformed external genitalia (in particular, vaginal atresia), and defects of the auditory ossicles probably represents a distinct autosomal recessive syndrome (47).

LABORATORY AIDS

Any newborn infant in respiratory distress or with a low Apgar score and other features of the Potter syndrome merits a bladder tap and an excretory pyelogram. If a severe renal defect is discovered, there is little to be gained by maintaining artificial respiration. If the reason for oligohydramnios is nonrenal, however, such management may be indicated (43).

For proper genetic counseling, a careful family history should be taken, with special attention to any abnormalities which are part of the spectrum of the Duhamel anomalad. Intravenous pyelograms may be considered in families where the proband has died of bilateral renal agenesis or severe renal dysplasia.

REFERENCES

1 Arends, N. W., Bilateral Renal Agenesis in Siblings. *J. Am. Osteopath. Assoc.* **56**:681–684, 1957.

2 Ashley, D. J., and Mostofi, F. K., Renal Agenesis and Dysgenesis. *J. Urol.* **83**:211–230, 1960.

3 Bain, A. D., and Scott, J. S., Renal Agenesis and Severe Urinary Tract Dysplasia. A Review of 50 Cases, with Particular Reference to the Associated Anomalies. *Br. Med. J.* **1**:841–846, 1960.

4 Baron, C., Bilateral Agenesis of the Kidneys in Two Consecutive Infants. *Am. J. Obstet. Gynecol.* **67**:667–670, 1954.

5 Blanc, W. A., and Baens, G., Ear Malformations, Abnormal Facies, and Genitourinary Tract Anomalies. *Am. J. Dis. Child.* **100**:781–782, 1960.

6 Bound, J. P., Two Cases of Congenital Absence of One Kidney in the Same Family. *Br. Med. J.* **2**:747, 1943.

7 Braun, O., Weitere Beiträge zum Erscheinungsbild der Dysplasia renofacialis. *Zentralbl. Allg. Pathol.* **107**:175–182, 1965.

8 Buchta, R. M., et al., Familial Bilateral Renal Agenesis and Hereditary Renal Adysplasia. *Z. Kinderheilkd.* **115**:111–129, 1973.

9 Cain, D. R., et al., Familial Renal Agenesis and Total Dysplasia. *Am. J. Dis. Child.* **128**:377–380, 1974.

10 Carpentier, P. J., and Potter, E. L., Nuclear Sex and Genital Malformation in 48 Cases of Renal Agenesis with Especial Reference to Nonspecific Female Pseudohermaphroditism. *Am. J. Obstet. Gynecol.* **78**:235–258, 1959.

11 Davidson, W. M., and Ross, G. I. M., Bilateral Absence of the Kidneys and Related Congenital Anomalies. *J. Pathol. Bacteriol.* **68**:459–474, 1959.

12 Feinzaig, W., Multicystic Dysplastic Kidney. A Clinical and Pathological Study of 29 Cases. Thesis, University of Minnesota, 1964.

13 Fitch, N., and Lachance, R. C., The Pathogenesis of Potter's Syndrome of Renal Agenesis. *Can. Med. Assoc. J.* **107**:653–656, 1972.

13a Fraga, J. R., et al., Association of Pulmonary Hypoplasia

Renal Anomalies and Potter's Facies. *Clin. Pediatr.* **12:**150–153, 1973.

14 François, J., and Marchildon, A., Facies de Potter et agenesie renale. *Ann. Ocul. (Paris).* **197:**347–354, 1964.

14a Gärtner, H., et al., Beitrag zum Problem der renofacialen Dysplasie (Potter-Syndrom). Beziehungen zwischen dem typischen Bild und der Sirenomelie. *Pädiat. Pädiol.* **9:**209–216, 1974.

15 Gorvoy, J. D., et al., Unilateral Renal Agenesis in Two Siblings. *Pediatrics* **29:**270–273, 1962.

16 Gross, H., et al., Familiäre Balkenhypoplasie bei Dysplasia renofacialis. *Zentralbl. Allg. Pathol.* **99:**587–592, 1959.

17 Habedank, M., 18 Beobachtungen von Dysplasia renofacialis. *Z. Kinderheilkd.* **88:**531–547, 1963.

18 Hammar, I., and Roggenkamp, K., Augenveränderungen bei Dysplasia renofacialis (Potter Syndrome). *Klin. Monatsbl. Augenheilkd.* **15:**534–538, 1967.

19 Hilson, D., Malformation of Ears as a Sign of Malformation of Genitourinary Tract. *Br. Med. J.* **2:**785–789, 1957.

20 Källén, B., and Winberg, J., Caudal Mesoderm Pattern of Anomalies: From Renal Agenesis to Sirenomelia. *Teratology* **9:**99–111, 1974.

21 Kohler, H., Fetal Abnormality. *Lancet* **1:**946, 1961.

22 Kohn, G., and Borns, P. K., The Association of Bilateral and Unilateral Renal Aplasia in the Same Family. *J. Pediatr.* **83:**95–97, 1973.

23 Lessen, H. van, and Hintze, A., Aplasie beider Nieren und gleichzeitige Anomalien anderer Organe (Beschreibung dreier Fälle). *Monatsschr. Kinderheilkd.* **111:**57–60, 1963.

24 Longenecker, C. G., et al., Malformation of the Ear as a Clue to Urogenital Anomalies. *Plast. Reconstr. Surg.* **35:**303–309, 1965.

25 Madisson, H., Über das Fehlen beider Nièren. *Zentralbl. Allg. Path.* **60:**1–8, 1934.

26 Mauer, S. M., et al., Unilateral and Bilateral Renal Agenesis in Monoamniotic Twins. *J. Pediatr.* **84:**236–238, 1974.

27 Müntefering, H., and Schlüter, I., Beitrag zur Aetiologie der doppelseitigen Nierenagenesie. *Z. Morphol. Anthropol.* **58:**253–285, 1967.

28 Oppermann, J., Beitrag zur Dysplasia reno-facialis. *Monatsschr. Kinderheilkd.* **114:**397–400, 1966.

29 Oppermann, J., Vier Beobachtungen von Dysplasia renofacialis. *Zentralbl. Gynäkol.* **89:**705–710, 1967.

30 Passarge, E., and Sutherland, J. M., Potter's Syndrome. *Am. J. Dis. Child.* **109:**80–84, 1965.

31 Potter, E. L., Bilateral Renal Agenesis. *J. Pediatr.* **29:**68–76, 1946.

32 Potter, E. L., Facial Characteristics of Infants with Bilateral Renal Agenesis. *Am. J. Obstet. Gynecol.* **51:**885–888, 1946.

33 Potter, E. L., Bilateral Absence of Ureters and Kidneys. *Obstet. Gynecol.* **25:**3–12, 1965.

34 Potter, E. L., *Normal and Abnormal Development of the Kidney.* Year Book Publishers, Chicago, 1972.

35 Ratten G. J., et al., Obstetric Complications when the Fetus has Potter's Syndrome. I. Clinical Considerations. *Am. J. Obstet. Gynecol.* **115:**890–896, 1973.

36 Regnier, C., et al., Agenesie renale bilaterale. *Toulouse Méd.* **64:**539–547, 1963.

37 Rizza, J. M., and Downing, S. E., Bilateral Renal Agenesis in Two Female Siblings. *Am. J. Dis. Child.* **121:**60–63, 1971.

38 Schlegel, R. J., et al., An XX Sex Chromosome Complement in an Infant Having Male-type External Genitals, Renal Agenesis, and Other Anomalies. *J. Pediatr.* **69:**812–814, 1966.

39 Schmidt, E. C. H., et al., Renal Aplasia in Sisters. *Acta Pathol.* **54:**403–406, 1952.

39a Smith, D. W., et al., The Duhamel Anomalad, from Imperforate Anus to Sirenomelia; Including VATER Association, Caudal Regression Syndrome, and Rokitansky Syndrome. *J. Pediatr.,* in press.

40 Stockhausen, H. B. von, Beitrag zur Problematik der Dysplasia renofacialis. *Z. Kinderheilkd.* **105:**303–323, 1969.

41 Sylvester, P. E., and Hughes, D. R., Congenital Absence of Both Kidneys. *Br. Med. J.* **1:**77–79, 1954.

42 Taylor, W. C., Deformity of Ears and Kidneys. *Can. Med. Assoc. J.* **93:**107–110, 1965.

43 Ten Berg, B. S., and Wildervanck, L. S., Familiaire congenitale afwijkingen van uropoëtisch en genitaal systeem. *Ned. Tijdschr. Geneeskd.* **95:**2389–2395, 1951.

44 Thomas, I. T., and Smith D. W., Oligohydramnios, The Cause of the Non-renal Features of Potter's Syndrome, Including Pulmonary Hypoplasia. *J. Pediatr.* **84:**811–814, 1974.

45 Vincent, R. W., et al., Malformation of Ear Associated with Urogenital Anomalies. *Plast. Reconstr. Surg.* **28:**214–220, 1961.

46 Waardenburg, P. J., Einseitige Aplasie der Niere und ihrer Abfuhrwege bei beiden eineiigen Zwillingspaarlingen. *Acta. Genet. Med. (Roma).* **1:**317–320, 1952.

47 Warkany, J., *Congenital Malformations.* Year Book Medical Publishers, Chicago, 1971, pp. 1037–1039.

48 Winter, J. S., et al., A Familial Syndrome of Renal, Genital, and Middle Ear Anomalies. *J. Pediatr.* **72:**88–93, 1968.

119

Prader-Willi Syndrome

(Hypotonia-Hypomentia-Hypogonadism-Obesity Syndrome)

In 1956, Prader et al. (20, 21) described a syndrome, characterized by (a) mental retardation, (b) muscular hypotonia, (c) obesity, (d) short stature, and (e) hypogonadism. In 1961, Prader and Willi (22) noted a marked tendency to develop (f) diabetes mellitus. Forssman and Hagberg (7) added (g) acromicria as a frequent feature. The syndrome is rather common, and over 100 cases have been reported. The preponderance of reported males probably reflects the easy recognition of the rudimentary scrotum. Extensive documentation of the syndrome has been provided by Laurance (15), Dunn (5), and Zellweger and Schneider (27).

The etiology is unknown. Almost all cases are sporadic. The disorder has been reported in sibs, and parental consanguinity has been found in severe cases (8, 12, 25). The syndrome has been observed in cousins (9) and in identical twins (2). Autosomal recessive inheritance (3a, 22), polygenic inheritance (19), and etiologic heterogeneity (9) have been suggested. Karyotypes have been normal in most cases, although various inconsistent chromosomal aberrations have been found (24, 27).

Delivery usually occurs at term, with birth weight being almost always below 3,000 g. Prolonged gestation periods and complicated deliveries have been noted in several instances (6, 7, 10).

Many endocrine and metabolic studies have been carried out with normal or inconsistent results. A hypothalamic-hypophyseal disorder or primary dysfunction of the adrenal cortex or both have been suggested (6, 7, 9, 20). The hyperphagia often manifested in the Prader-Willi syndrome is reminiscent of the behavior of experimental animals with destructive lesions of the ventromedial hypothalamic nucleus (17).

SYSTEMIC MANIFESTATIONS

Generalized obesity becomes apparent during the second and third years of life and in some patients may be less pronounced in later childhood (14). The distribution of fat is particularly marked on the lower part of the trunk and buttocks (Fig. 119-1).

During childhood and adolescence, diabetes mellitus frequently develops; it differs from the usual type by the absence of weight loss and acidosis, the presence of insulin resistance, and good response to oral hypoglycemic drugs (22, 25).

Facies. Bifrontal diameter is reduced (9). Marked obesity is present around the cheeks and under the chin. The palpebral fissures are almond-shaped with slightly overhanging lids. The nose is retroussé, and the mouth, fishlike (15) with a triangular-shaped upper lip (3) (Fig. 119-2).

Nervous system. In the newborn there is noted a marked hypotonia, almost certainly a continuation of the diminished intrauterine movements observed (4, 13, 15, 21) (Fig. 119-3). Laurance (15) commented on the increased frequency of scoliosis. Less common findings include clinodactyly, partial syndactyly (22), genu valgum (11–13), fusion of lumbar vertebras (7), displaced thumbs (18), and poor mineralization (5).

Genitourinary system. In males, the genitalia are poorly developed. The penis is small, the testes are ectopic or infantile, and the scrotum is rudimentary (3, 15, 25) (Fig. 119-4). Pubertal changes are both delayed and diminished. In females, no genital abnormalities have been observed. The menarche is usually normal (22), although puberty may be delayed (10).

Other findings. Hypertelorism, epicanthus, strabismus, astigmatism, dysplastic and/or low-set ears, striae, and acanthosis nigricans have been reported. Dermatoglyphic patterns have shown

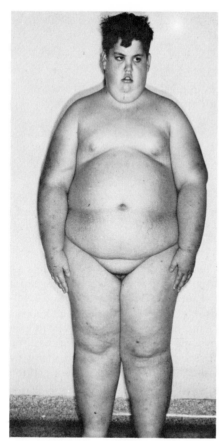

Figure 119-1. *Prader-Willi syndrome.* Marked obesity, small hands, and hypoplastic genitalia.

so frequently observed. There are little spontaneous activity, poor sucking and swallowing reflexes, a weak cry, and sometimes episodes of asphyxia (15, 27). Cortical atrophy has been documented in a few cases by pneumoencephalography (3, 6). Poor thermoregulation with a tendency to hyperpyrexia (3) and convulsions (4, 6, 25) have been reported.

Mental deficiency is almost always observed, although normal intelligence has rarely been reported (9). The friendly, cooperative nature of these patients is striking (15, 26). Psychiatric problems have been noted in the postadolescent period in a number of cases (9). Waddling gait is quite characteristic.

Skeletal system. Short stature, retarded bone age, and small hands and feet are almost always

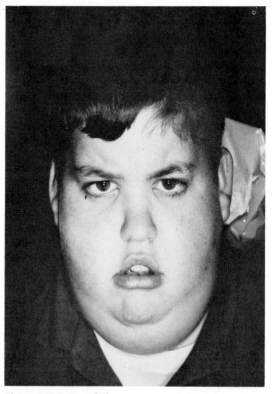

Figure 119-2. Facial obesity, narrow bifrontal diameter, almond-shaped eyes, fishlike mouth.

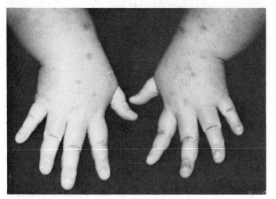

Figure 119-3. Disproportionately small hands.

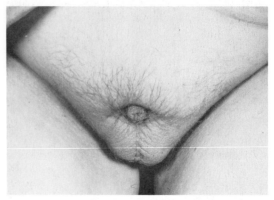

Figure 119-4. Hypoplastic genitalia with penis buried in fat. (*From M. M. Cohen, Jr., and R. J. Gorlin, Am. J. Dis. Child.* **117**:213, 1969.)

considerable variation (3, 7, 10, 11, 14, 15, 18, 22, 23).

Oral manifestations. Marked dental caries, possibly due to xerostomia, has been noted by several authors (6, 7, 10, 13, 22). Hypoplastic enamel (3, 18), supernumerary teeth (6), delayed eruption (10), micrognathia (7, 10, 18), extreme narrowing of the mandibular dental arch (3), and highly arched palate (3, 7, 22) have been observed.

DIFFERENTIAL DIAGNOSIS

Severe congenital muscular dystrophy, neonatal myasthenia, Werdnig-Hoffmann disease with prenatal onset, pathologic conditions of neural structures higher than the peripheral reflex arcs, traumatic brain injuries, intracranial hemorrhage, and cerebral malformations must be distinguished from the Prader-Willi syndrome during the neonatal period. Other disorders in the differential diagnosis include adiposogenital dystrophy, Laurance-Moon syndrome, Biedl-Bardet syndrome, obesity with feminine habitus and small genitalia sometimes observed in prepubertal boys and the *Summitt syndrome.* The disorders described by Lynch et al. (16) and by Alstrøm et al. (1) have some resemblance to the Prader-Willi syndrome.

LABORATORY AIDS

Urinary gonadotropins and 17-hydroxycorticosteroid levels have been inconsistent (7, 18, 22, 26). A glucose tolerance test has revealed a prediabetic or diabetic curve in over 35 percent of the cases (12). Parra et al. (19a) have suggested that the hormonal changes are related to the obesity and not to the syndrome per se.

REFERENCES

1 Alstrøm, C. H., et al., Retinal Degeneration Combined with Obesity, Diabetes Mellitus and Neurogenic Deafness. *Acta Psychiatr. Scand.* [Suppl.] **129**:1–35, 1959.

2 Brissenden, J. E., and Levy, E. P., Prader-Willi Syndrome in Infant Monozygotic Twins. *Am. J. Dis. Child.* **126**:110–112, 1973.

3 Cohen, M. M., Jr., and Gorlin, R. J., The Prader-Willi Syndrome. *Am. J. Dis. Child.* **117**:213–218, 1969.

3a De Fraites, E. B., et al. Familial Prader-Willi Syndrome. *Birth Defects* **11**(4):123–126, 1975.

4 Dubowitz, V., A Syndrome of Benign Congenital Hypotonia, Gross Obesity, Delayed Intellectual Development, Retarded Bone Age, and Unusual Facies. *Proc. R. Soc. Med.* **10**:1006–1008, 1967.

5 Dunn, H. G., The Prader-Labhart-Willi Syndrome: Review of the Literature and Report of Nine Cases. *Acta Paediatr. Scand.* [Suppl.] **186**:1–38, 1968.

6 Evans, P. R., Hypogenital Dystrophy with Diabetic Tendency. *Guy's Hosp. Rep.* **113**:207–222, 1964.

7 Forssman, H., and Hagberg, B., Prader-Willi Syndrome in Boy of 10 with Diabetes. *Acta Paediatr. Scand.* **53**:70–78, 1964.

8 Galiban, J. C., Syndrome de Prader, Labhart et Willi. *J. Pédiatr.* **1**:179, 1962.

9 Hall, B., and Smith, D. W., Prader-Willi Syndrome. *J. Pediatr.* **81**:286–293, 1972.

10 Hoefnagel, D., et al., Prader-Willi Syndrome. *J. Ment. Defic. Res.* **11**:1–11, 1967.

11 Hooft, C., et al., Syndrome de Prader avec diabète sucré. *Acta Paediatr. Belg.* **21**:193–206, 1967.

12 Jancar, J., Prader-Willi Syndrome. *J. Ment. Defic. Res.* **15**:20–29, 1971.

13 Juul, J., and Dupont, A., Prader-Willi Syndrome. *J. Ment. Defic. Res.* **11**:12–22, 1967.

14 Landwirth, J., et al., Prader-Willi Syndrome. *Am. J. Dis. Child.* **116**:211–217, 1968.

15 Laurance, B. M., Hypotonia, Mental Retardation, Obesity, and Cryptorchidism Associated with Dwarfism and Diabetes in Children. *Arch. Dis. Child.* **42**:126–139, 1967.

16 Lynch, H. T., et al., Familial Coexistence of Diabetes Mellitus, Hyperlipemia, Short Stature, and Hypogonadism. *Am. J. Med.* **252**:323–330, 1966.

17 Mayer, J., Some Aspects of the Problem of Regulation of Food Intake and Obesity. *N. Engl. J. Med.* **274**:610–616, 1961.

18 Monnens, L., and Kenis, H., Enkele onderzoekingen bij een patient met het syndroom van Prader-Willi. *Maandschr. Kindergeneeskd.* **33**:482–498, 1965.

19 Opitz, J. M., et al., The Study of Malformation Syndromes in Man. *Birth Defects* **5**(2):1–10, 1969.

19a Parra, A., et al., Immunoreactive Insulin and Growth Hormone Responses in Patients with Prader-Willi Syndrome. *J. Pediatr.* **83**:587–593, 1973.

20 Prader, A., et al., Ein Syndrom von Adipositas, Kleinwuchs, Kryptorchismus und Oligophrenie nach myotonieartigem Zustand in Neugeborenenalter. *Schweiz. Med. Wochenschr.* **86**:1260, 1956.

21 Prader, A., et al., Ein Syndrom von Adipositas, Kleinwuchs, Kryptorchismus und Idiotie bei Kindern und Erwachsenen, die als Neugeborene ein Myotonie-artiges Bild geboten haben. *Proc. Eighth Int. Congr. Pediatr.* **10**:13, 1956.

22 Prader, A., and Willi, H., Das Syndrom von Imbezillität, Adipositas, Muskelhypotonie, Hypogenitalismus, Hypogonadismus und Diabetes Mellitus mit 'Myotonie'-Anamnese. *Proc., Second Int. Congr. Psychic Develop. Defects Child.,* Vienna, 1963, pp. 353–357.

23 Reed, W. B., et al., Acanthosis Nigricans in Association with Various Genodermatoses. *Acta Derm. Venereol. (Stockh.)* **48**:465–473, 1968.

24 Ridler, M. A. C., et al., A Case of Prader-Willi Syndrome in a Girl with a Small Extra Chromosome. *Acta Paediatr. Scand.* **60**:222–226, 1971.

25 Royer, P., Le diabète sucré dans le syndrome de Willi-Prader. *J. Ann. Diabét. Hotel Dieu (Paris)* **4**:91–99, 1963.

25a Rudd, B. T., et al., Adrenal Response to ACTH in Patients with Prader-Willi Syndrome, Simple Obesity and Constitutional Dwarfism. *Arch. Dis. Child.* **44**:244–247, 1969.

26 Stolecke, H., et al., Prader-Labhart-Willi Syndrom. *Monatsschr. Kinderheilkd.* **122**:10–17, 1974.

27 Zellweger, H., and Schneider, H. J., Syndrome of Hypotonia-Hypomentia-Hypogonadism-Obesity (HHHO) or Prader-Willi Syndrome. *Am. J. Dis. Child.* **115**:588–598, 1968.

120

Progeria

(Hutchinson-Gilford Syndrome)

The syndrome first described by Hutchinson (13) and Gilford (10, 11) is a combination of *(a)* dwarfism, and *(b)* pseudosenility. Possibly because of a collagen abnormality, persons with this affliction die of coronary disease during their middle teens.

There are very few reports of the occurrence of this syndrome in sibs (17, 21, 23a). All other cases have been sporadic. Autopsies have been performed on fewer than a dozen patients (3, 10, 18, 19, 25, 28). About 55 cases have been described (6). Though autosomal recessive inheritance is possible, we find it surprising that most cases have been sporadic.

SYSTEMIC MANIFESTATIONS

Birth weight is usually less than 2,500 g. Growth proceeds almost normally until the first year, when it essentially plateaus until about ten years of age. During the second year, scalp hair is lost and replaced by a downy fuzz, giving the child the appearance of a newly hatched bird. Eyebrows and, occasionally, lashes are lost. The voice is high and squeaky (25). By the end of the first decade, the height is approximately that of a three-year-old; only rarely does a patient exceed 110 cm (43.5 in.) in height or 15 kg in weight. Intelligence is normal (19).

Facies and appearance. The appearance has been discussed in part above. The face is dispro-portionately small, giving the head a hydrocephalic appearance, although, in fact, it is usually 2 to 4 cm smaller in circumference than average. There is also frontal and parietal bossing. Prominent scalp veins are quite evident. The ears are small, without lobules (5), and the nose is thin and rather beaked (1, 25), causing a bird facies. The chest is narrow and the abdomen protuberant. On account of mild flexion of the knees there is a "horse-riding" stance (Figs. 120-1, 120-2).

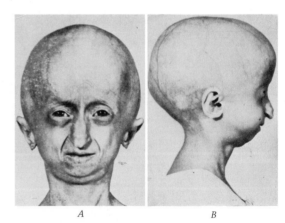

A   *B*

Figure 120-1. *Progeria.* (*A, B*). Face is small in comparison with cranial vault. Lashes are absent, brows are sparse. Note beaklike nose, mandibular hypoplasia, absent earlobes, prominent scalp veins. (*From I. M. Rosenthal et al.,* Pediatrics **18:**565, 1956.)

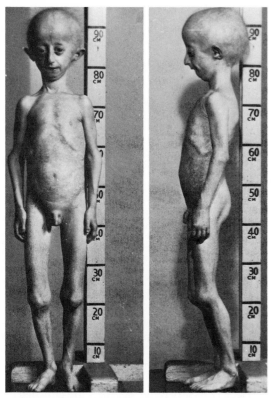

Figure 120-2. Clavicles are short, hands, elbows, and knees contracted, giving "horse-riding" stance. Note senile appearance. (*From L. Atkins,* N. Engl. J. Med. **250:**1065, 1954.)

Musculoskeletal system. The bones are delicate and osteoporotic, although there is normal bone maturation. The small joints of the extremities become thickened and limited in extension because of periarticular fibrosis (3, 25). This appears in some patients as early as the sixth year

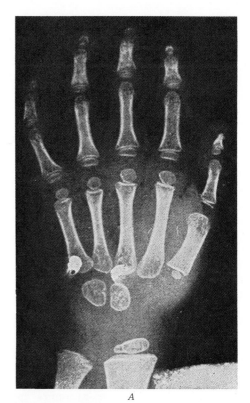

A

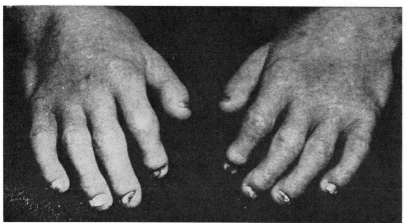

B

Figure 120-3. (*A*). Terminal phalanges are short and taper abruptly. (*B*). Skin of hands is dry, taut, and mottled; fingers are short with enlarged joints. Nails are dry, brittle, and hypoplastic. (*From M. M. Album and J. W. Hope,* Oral Surg. **11:**985, 1958.)

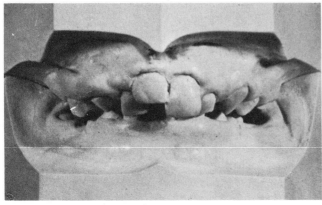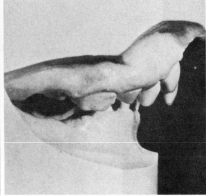

A　　　　　　　　　　　　　　　　　　　　　　　　　　　*B*

Figure 120-4. (*A, B*). Dental casts showing marked retrusion of mandible and malocclusion. (*From M. M. Album and J. W. Hope*, Oral Surg. **11**:985, 1958.)

(25). Less frequently affected are the spine, elbows, and knees. On roentgenographic examination, the terminal phalanges are seen to be abnormally short and to taper abruptly to a pointed end. The calvaria are remarkably thin, the anterior fontanel is open, and there are often no frontal sinuses (3, 16, 19, 25). The neurocranium, however, is relatively normal in size and configuration. Mastoid development is poor. Coxa valga is a constant finding. The terminal phalanges and clavicles undergo progressive osteolysis (1, 8, 20, 23, 29). There may be some predilection for fracture of the humeral shaft (23). There is also loss of muscular and subcutaneous fat.

Cardiovascular system. Cardiac murmurs appear after the age of five years. This is followed by diastolic systemic hypertension and cardiomegaly. Atherosclerosis is early and severe, and anginal attacks and cerebrovascular accidents have been experienced as early as seven years of age (28), but in most cases, death has occurred by approximately fourteen years of age. For a detailed discussion, see Makous et al. (18).

Skin and skin appendages. The skin is thin, atrophic, and often pigmented, with sparse subcutaneous fat (3, 5). Some patients have exhibited scleroderma-like changes (27, 30, 32). The veins are especially prominent over the scalp and thighs (25). The scalp hair and brows are shed at about one year of age and replaced by a downy fuzz. The nails are thin, yellow, atrophic, brittle, or even absent (19) (Fig. 120-3*A, B*).

Oral manifestations. Poor midface development and mandibular hypoplasia are constant features (25) (Fig. 120-4*A, B*). The mandibular angle was 155° (normal, 120°) in the patient described by Album and Hope (1). Because the jaw is small, the teeth, usually of normal size, are crowded (5, 6, 30). However, some authors have found the teeth irregular in form and small or deficient in number (10, 11, 30). In most cases, eruption of the teeth has been delayed (7, 19, 23, 25, 28, 30), and the deciduous dentition is often retained (1, 25). Album and Hope (1) found the teeth to be stained yellowish-brown, with microscopic evidence of senile pulpal changes. The palate has been stated to be high (6).

DIFFERENTIAL DIAGNOSIS

Because the appearance is so characteristic, differential diagnosis is limited. A number of cases of *Hallermann-Streiff syndrome* have been erroneously labeled progeria. The case of Grossman et al. (12) may represent the *Seckel syndrome*. Patients with the *Bloom syndrome* and the *Cockayne syndrome* have also mistakenly been thought to have progeria.

LABORATORY AIDS

Steinberg et al. (26) found aminoaciduria and hypermetabolism in a patient with progeria. Hypermetabolism was also described by Talbot et al. (28) but denied by others (14, 25). Many patients have elevated cholesterol or phospholipid levels (24, 31). Rosenthal et al. (25) have interpreted progeria as a disease of intermediate metabolism of lipoproteins. Keay et al. (14) found the pattern of circulatory lipids and lipo-proteins similar to that of an adult with overt coronary sclerosis. Villee et al. (31) presented evidence for unresponsiveness to growth hormone, relative insulin resistance, and highly cross-linked collagen. They suggested that progeria is a mesenchymal dysplasia in which connective tissue cells respond abnormally to growth influences. This failure to grow may account for "older collagen," which may predispose to atherosclerosis.

REFERENCES

1 Album, M. M., and Hope, J. W., Progeria. Oral Surg. **11**:985–998, 1958.

2 Apert, E., and Robin, P., La progéria (nanisme sénile de Variot). Presse Méd. **28**:433–437, 1927.

3 Atkins, L., Progeria: Report of a Case with Post-mortem Findings. N. Engl. J. Med. **250**:1065–1069, 1954.

4 Bhahoo, O. N., et al., Progeria with Unusual Ocular Manifestation. Indian Pediatr. **2**:164–169, 1965.

5 Cooke, J. V., The Rate of Growth in Progeria, with a Report of Two Cases. J. Pediatr. **42**:26–37, 1953.

6 DeBusk, F. L., The Hutchinson-Gilford Progeria Syndrome. J. Pediatr. **80**:697–724, 1972.

7 Gabr, M., Progeria: Review of the Literature with Report of a Case. Arch. Pediatr. **71**:35–46, 1954.

8 Gabr, M., et al., Progeria, a Pathologic Study. J. Pediatr. **57**:70–77, 1960.

9 Ghosh, S., and Varma, K., Progeria: Report of a Case with Review of the Literature. Indian Pediatr. **1**:146–155, 1964.

10 Gilford, H., On a Condition of Mixed Premature and Immature Development. Trans. Med-Chir. Soc. Edinburgh **80**:17–45, 1897.

11 Gilford, H., Progeria, a Form of Senility. Practitioner **73**:188–217, 1904.

12 Grossman, H. J., et al., Progeroid Syndrome, Report of a Case of Pseudo-senilism. Pediatrics **15**:413–423, 1955.

13 Hutchinson, J., Congenital Absence of Hair with Atrophic Condition of Skin. Trans. Med-Chir. Soc. Edinburgh **69**:473–477, 1886.

14 Keay, A. J., et al., Progeria and Atherosclerosis. Arch. Dis. Child. **30**:410–414, 1955.

15 Keith, A., Progeria and Ateliosis. Lancet **1**:305–313, 1913.

16 Kozlowski, K., Étude radiologique d'un cas de nanisme sénile (progéria). Ann. Radiol. **8**:92–96, 1965.

17 Lejman, K., Progeria in Sibs. Hautarzt **13**:187–188, 1962.

18 Makous, N., et al., Cardiovascular Manifestations in Progeria. Report of Clinical and Pathologic Finding in a Patient with Arteriosclerotic Heart Disease and Aortic Stenosis. Am. Heart J. **64**:334–336, 1962.

19 Manschot, W. A., A Case of Progeronanism (Progeria of Gilford). Acta Paediat. Scand. **39**:158–164, 1950.

20 Margolin, F. R., and Steinbach, H. L., Progeria: Hutchinson-Gilford Syndrome. Am. J. Roentgenol. **103**:173–178, 1968.

21 Mostafa, A. H., and Gabr, M., Heredity in Progeria with Follow-up of Two Affected Sisters. Arch. Pediatr. **71**:163–172, 1954.

22 Nelson, M., Progeria, Audiologic Aspects. Ann. Otol. Rhinol. Laryngol. **74**:376–385, 1965.

23 Ozonoff, M. B., and Clemett, A. R., Progressive Osteolysis in Progeria. Am. J. Roentgenol. **100**:75–79, 1967.

23a Rava, G., Su un nucleo familiare di progeria. Minerva Med. **58**:1502–1509, 1967.

24 Reichel, W., and Garcia-Bunuel, R., Pathologic Findings in Progeria. Am. J. Clin. Pathol. **53**:243–253, 1970.

25 Rosenthal, I. M., et al., Progeria: Report of a Case with Cephalometric Roentgenograms and Abnormally High Concentrations of Lipoproteins in the Serum. Pediatrics **18**:565–577, 1956.

26 Steinberg, A. H., et al., Amino-aciduria and Hypermetabolism in Progeria. Arch. Dis. Child. **32**:401–403, 1957.

27 Strunz, F., Ein Fall von Progeria, beginnend mit ausgedehnter Sklerodermie. Z. Kinderheilkd. **47**:401–416, 1929.

28 Talbot, N. B., et al., Progeria, Clinical, Metabolic and Pathologic Studies on a Patient. Am. J. Dis. Child. **69**:267–279, 1945.

29 Thiers, J., and Nahan, –, Étude radiographique du squelette dans un cas de progéria de Gilford (nanisme sénile), dysostose cléido-crânienne associée. J. Radiol. Électrol. **17**:675–678, 1933.

30 Thomson, J., and Forfar, J. O., Progeria (Hutchinson-Gilford Syndrome): Report of a Case and Review of the Literature. Arch. Dis. Child. **25**:224–234, 1950.

31 Villee, D. B., et al., Metabolic Studies in Two Boys with Classical Progeria. Pediatrics **43**:207–216, 1969.

32 Zeder, E., Über Progerie, eine seltene Form des hypophysären Zwergwuchses mit diffuser Sklerodermie. Monatsschr. Kinderheilkd. **81**:167–205, 1940.

121

Pseudohypoparathyroidism

(Albright Hereditary Osteodystrophy)

Albright and coworkers (1) in 1942 described pseudohypoparathyroidism (PH), a hypocalcemic syndrome having clinical and biochemical similarity to hypoparathyroidism but failing to respond to administered parathormone by normal phosphorus diuresis. Ten years later, Albright and associates (2) defined a normocalcemic variant of PHP, calling it pseudopseudohypoparathyroidism (PPHP).

That PHP and PPHP are different forms of the same disorder is strongly suggested by the occurrence of both forms within the same kindred and by the demonstrable transformation of PHP to PPHP (16).

It has been generally held that the syndrome has X-linked dominant inheritance. The evidence consists of the 2:1 male-to-female ratio and absence of male-to-male transmission. The argument loses its puissance, however, since females are not less but usually more severely affected than males. Perhaps the disorder has a sex-influenced autosomal dominant mode of transmission. A few large kindreds (9, 11, 13a, 19) exhibiting what appears to be PPHP with male-to-male transmission may be examples of another disorder, since neither mental retardation nor cataracts have been found in these kindreds (10). Perhaps they are examples of type E brachydactyly. Cederbaum and Lippe (3a) postulate the existence of an autosomal recessively inherited form. For a rather complete tabulation of cases published prior to 1966, see Gaudier *et al.* (8).

SYSTEMIC MANIFESTATIONS

Patients with PHP are usually short, being 137 to 152 cm tall at maturity. About 60 percent of them exhibit moderate obesity which persists

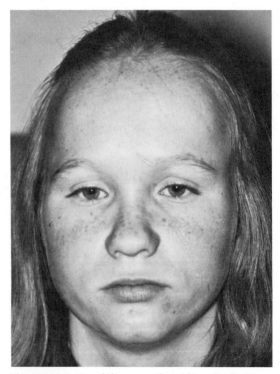

Figure 121-1. *Pseudohypoparathyroidism.* Facies is rounded, with depressed nasal bridge.

from early childhood. Patients with PPHP have a tendency to be taller and less obese (17).

Facies. The face is characteristically rounded, with a depressed nasal bridge. The rounded face is more often seen in PHP (in over 80 percent of cases) than in PPHP (in about 60 percent) (Fig. 121-1).

Musculoskeletal changes. Most striking is shortening of one or more fingers or toes due to abbreviation of the corresponding metacarpals or metatarsals. This has been noted in about 70 percent of patients. Shortened metacarpals are manifested when the patient makes a fist (Fig. 121-2A). The fourth and fifth metacarpals are nearly always involved, less often the first, third,

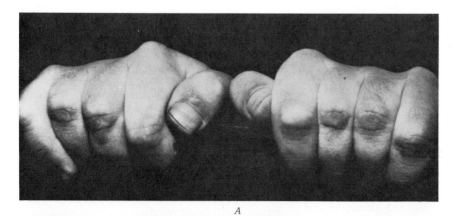

A

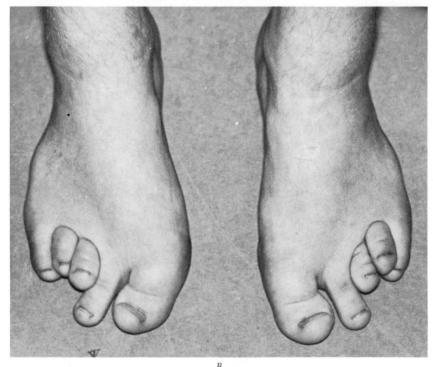

B

Figure 121-2. (*A*). Note absence of knuckles. (*From J. Jancar, J. Med. Genet.* **2**:32, 1965.) (*B*). Severe shortening of toes due to abbreviated metatarsals.

and second, in that order. The fourth and, less often, the third metatarsals are shortened (16) (Fig. 121-2B). The phalanges are also abbreviated, with cone-shaped epiphyses. The radius may be mildly to severely curved, with displacement of the distal epiphyses and carpal bones (Fig. 121-3A, B).

Skull changes include thickening of the calvaria in about one-third of the patients. Brachycephaly and premature suture closure are frequent.

Central nervous system. Mental retardation has been noted in about 65 percent of patients with PHP but in less than half of those with the normocalcemic variant (14).

Eye. Cataracts develop in about 25 percent of those with PHP but in fewer than 10 percent with PPHP (16).

Skin. Calcifications are often found in subcutaneous tissues of the scalp and along the extremities, especially in periarticular areas of the hands and feet. The deposits, composed of true bone or amorphous calcium salts, are not symmetrically arranged and do not involve muscles, blood vessels, cartilage, or viscera (3, 7, 17).

Oral manifestations. Enamel hypoplasia, widened root canals, and delayed eruption have been noted in over one-third of the patients with PHP (3, 6, 13, 15, 18).

DIFFERENTIAL DIAGNOSIS

In idiopathic hypoparathyroidism, one may find tetanic and epileptiform convulsions, increased thickness of the skull, hypoplasia of the enamel, and cataracts. However, shortening of the metacarpals and other skeletal defects are not present. Shortened metacarpals may be seen in about 10 percent of normal individuals and in a variety of conditions: *multiple nevoid basal cell carcinoma syndrome, Turner syndrome, acrodysostosis,* and peripheral dysostosis.

LABORATORY AIDS

Biochemical alterations, confined by definition to PHP, consist of hypocalcemia, hyperphosphatemia, diminished renal excretion of phosphate,

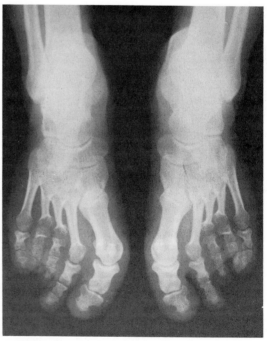

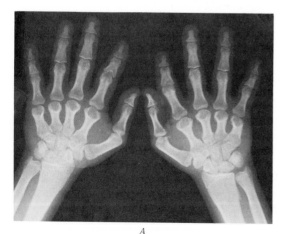

A   B

Figure 121-3. (*A*). All metacarpals shortened; also observe cone-shaped epiphyses in index fingers. (*B*). Markedly shortened third and fourth metatarsals.

and virtual lack of renal response to exogenous parathormone, i.e., failure to exhibit phosphorus diuresis. Presumably the biochemical differences between PHP and PPHP depend upon the ability of patients with the latter to compensate for the tubular phosphate reabsorption, perhaps through some degree of secondary hyperparathyroidism.

In normal persons, parathormone causes rapid excretion of cyclic AMP, which mediates the phosphaturic action of the hormone. This effect is totally absent in patients with PHP (4).

REFERENCES

1 Albright, F., et al., Pseudo-hypoparathyroidism–Example of "Seabright Bantam" Syndrome. *Endocrinology* **30:**922–932, 1942.

2 Albright, F., et al., Pseudo-pseudohypoparathyroidism. *Trans. Assoc. Am. Physicians* **65:**337–350, 1952.

3 Arnstein, A. R., et al., Albright's Hereditary Osteodystrophy. *Ann. Intern. Med.* **64:**996–1008, 1966.

3a Cederbaum, S. D., and Lippe, B. M., Probable Autosomal Recessive Inheritance in a Family with Albright's Hereditary Osteodystrophy and an Evaluation of the Genetics of the Disorder. *Am. J. Hum. Genet.* **25:**638–645, 1973.

4 Chase, L. R., et al., Pseudohypoparathyroidism: Defective Excretion of 3',5'-AMP in Response to Parathyroid Hormone. *J. Clin. Invest.* **48:**1832–1844, 1969.

5 Cranin, A. N., and Katz, H. E., Pseudohypoparathyroidism. *J. Am. Dent. Assoc.* **74:**741–746, 1967.

6 Croft, L. K., et al., Pseudohypoparathyroidism. *Oral Surg.* **20:**758–770, 1965.

7 Elrich, H., et al., Further Studies on Pseudohypoparathyroidism: Report of Four New Cases. *Acta Endocrinol.* **5:**199–225, 1950.

8 Gaudier, B., et al., Osteodystrophie héréditaire d'Albright. *Pédiatrie* **21:**273–298, 1966.

9 Goeminne, C., Albright's Hereditary Poly-osteochondro-dystrophy (Pseudo-pseudohypoparathyroidism with Diabetes, Hypertension, Arteritis and Polyarthrosis). *Acta Genet. Med.* (*Roma*) **14:**226–281, 1966.

10 Gorlin, R. J., and Sedano, H. O., Cryptodontic Brachymeta-carpalia. *Birth Defects* **7**(7):200–203, 1971.

11 Hermans, P. E., et al., Pseudo-pseudoparathyroidism (Albright's Hereditary Osteodystrophy): A Familial Study. *Mayo Clin. Proc.* **39:**81–91, 1964.

12 Lee, J. B., et al., Familial Pseudohypoparathyroidism. *N. Engl. J. Med.* **276:**1179–1184, 1968.

13 Mackler, H., et al., Familial Pseudohypoparathyroidism. *Calif. Med.* **77:**332–334, 1952.

13a Minozzi, M., et al., Su un caso di osteodistrofia ereditaria de Albright varieta normocalcemia con documenta transmissione da maschio a maschio. *Folia Endocrinol.* (*Roma*) **16:**168–188, 1963.

14 Papaivannoa, A. C., and Matsas, B. E., Albright's Hereditary Osteodystrophy (without Hypocalcemia). *Pediatrics* **31:**599–607, 1963.

15 Ritchie, G. M., Dental Manifestations of Pseudohypoparathyroidism. *Arch. Dis. Child.* **40:**565–573, 1965.

16 Spranger, J. W., Skeletal Dysplasias and the Eye: Albright's Hereditary Osteodystrophy. *Birth Defects* **5**(4):122–128, 1969.

17 Steinbach, H. L., and Young, D. A., The Roentgen Appearance of Pseudohypoparathyroidism (PH) and Pseudo-pseudohypoparathyroidism (PPH). *Am. J. Roentgenol.* **97:**49–66, 1966.

18 Trevathan, T. H., Delayed Eruption of Teeth in Pseudohypoparathyroidism. *N.Z. Dent. J.* **57:**20–23, 1961.

19 Weinberg, A. G., and Stone, R. T., Autosomal Dominant Inheritance in Albright's Hereditary Osteodystrophy. *J. Pediatr.* **79:**996–999, 1971.

122

Pseudothalidomide Syndrome

Herrmann et al. (3) described a syndrome consisting of (*a*) symmetric reductive limb defects, (*b*) flexion contractures of various joints, and (*c*) characteristic facies. Other examples include the patients reported by Hall and Greenberg (2), Herrmann et al. (4), Levy et al. (7), O'Brien and Mustard (8), and Lenz et al. (6). Less certain are the cases of Keutel et al. (5).

Affected sibs of normal parentage and consanguinity are consistent with an autosomal recessive mode of transmission (3, 7, 8).

SYSTEMIC MANIFESTATIONS

There is intrauterine growth retardation (birth weight usually being less than 2,250 g), with continued growth failure postnatally.

Facies. The hair is scant and silvery blond. The cartilages of the nose are hypoplastic, producing a pinched, pointed nose. Auricular and ear canal cartilages are also hypoplastic. The ears may be rotated, with hypoplastic lobes. Superficial capillary hemangiomas are present on the midface, forehead, and ears (2, 3, 7). The corneas are cloudy and the scleras blue. Convergent strabismus has also been noted (7) (Fig. 122-1).

Musculoskeletal system. The skull is microbrachycephalic, with Wormian bones in the occipital region. Various joints exhibit flexion contractures, especially at the elbows and knees.

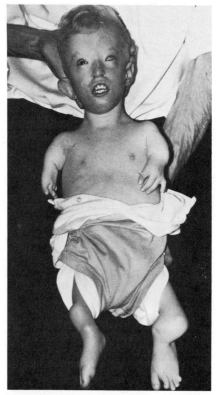

Figure 122-1. *Pseudothalidomide syndrome.* Thin, pinched nose, abnormal pinnas, convergent strabismus, symmetric reduction of arms and legs with decreased number of fingers. (*From J. Herrmann et al.,* Birth Defects **5**(3):81, 1969.)

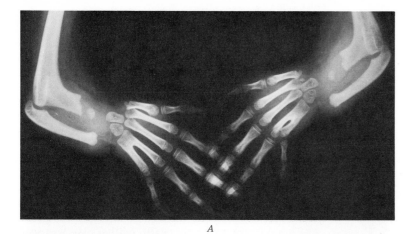

A

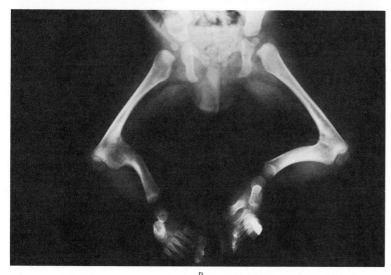

B

Figure 122-2. (*A, B*). Radiohumeral synostosis with marked shortening of humerus, synmetacarpalism, femorotibial fusion. (*From M. Levy et al.*, Ann. Pediatr. **19**:313, 1972.)

Shortening of the extremities, especially the arms, is striking. There may be absence or severe hypoplasia of the radius, ulna, thumb phalanges, and the first and, less often, fifth metacarpals. The fifth finger, if present, is often hypoplastic or clinodactylous. Radiohumeral synostosis, talipes calcaneovalgus, and absence or posterior displacement and/or bilateral deformity of the fibulas are commonly observed. Less frequently, shortened or curved humerus and tibia, syndactyly of the fourth and fifth toes, synostosis of the fourth and fifth toes, synostosis of the fourth and fifth metacarpals, and femorotibial synostosis have been found (3, 8) (Fig. 122-2*A, B*). Scoliosis has been noted (8).

Central nervous system. Mental retardation and seizures may be present (3), although normal intelligence has been reported (2).

Other findings. Inguinal hernia, horseshoe kidney (4), and absent foreskin (8) have been noted.

Oral manifestations. Cleft lip-palate has been observed (3, 8).

ceral (especially renal) anomalies in association with cleft lip-palate and tetraphocomelia.

The relationship between these two entities is not completely resolved. Lenz [see (3)] and Freeman et al. (1) believe that the two disorders are nosologically and genetically distinct. Herrmann et al. (4) and B. D. Hall and D. W. Smith (personal communication, 1972) opt for the two disorders as representing mild and severe forms of the same genetic condition.

That the two conditions may be identical is supported by two clear-cut instances of the pseudothalidomide syndrome in which a more severely affected sib with clefting was mentioned (3, 6). However, because of retrospective ascertainment and early death, neither case was well documented and facial photographs were not included.

Herrmann et al. (4) have suggested that sparse, silvery blond hair and midfacial hemangioma may not be useful distinguishing features. Since infant mortality seems to be high in cleft lip-palate and tetraphocomelia, patients may not live long enough to develop silvery blond, sparse hair. Herrmann et al. (4) also noted that cleft lip-palate might prevent the development of a hemangioma in the upper lip area. Thus, hemangioma of the upper lip and cleft lip-palate might be manifestations of the same pathogenetic process.

Other well-documented studies to delineate further the phenotypic spectrum and intrafamilial variability are necessary to resolve the relationship between these two disorders with certainty.

In thalidomide embryopathy, limbs are usually asymmetrically malformed.

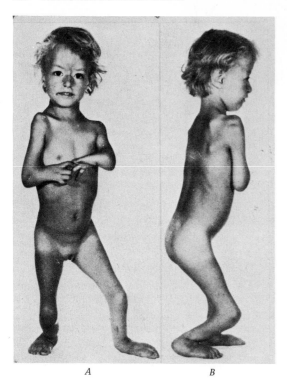

A   *B*

Figure 122-3. (*A, B*). Compare with other cases. (*From B. D. Hall and M. H. Greenberg,* Am. J. Dis. Child. **123:**602, 1972.)

DIFFERENTIAL DIAGNOSIS

In the present edition, we have separated the pseudothalidomide syndrome from *cleft lip-palate and tetraphocomelia.* The limb abnormalities are similar in both conditions, although they are usually more severe in cleft lip-palate and tetraphocomelia. Differences include midline facial hemangioma, silvery blond sparse hair, and dysplastic alar and auricular cartilages in the pseudothalidomide syndrome, and cleft lip-palate, ocular proptosis, hypertelorism, genital abnormalities, and a higher frequency of vis-

LABORATORY AIDS

None is known.

REFERENCES

1 Freeman, M. V. R., et al., The Roberts Syndrome. *Clin. Genet.* 5:1–16, 1974.
2 Hall, B. D., and Greenberg, M. H., Hypomelia-Hypotrichosis-Facial Hemangioma Syndrome. *Am. J. Dis. Child.* 123:602–604, 1972.

3 Herrmann, J., et al., A Familial Dysmorphogenetic Syndrome of Limb Deformities, Characteristic Facial Appearance and Associated Anomalies: The "Pseudothalidomide" or SC-syndrome. *Birth Defects* 5(3):81–89, 1969.
4 Herrmann, J., et al., The SC Phocomelia (Pseudothalido-

mide) Syndrome: Report of an Additional Case, and Nosologic Considerations of the Roberts Syndrome, to be published.

5 Keutel, J., et al., Eine wahrscheinlich autosomal recessiv
vererbte Skeletmissbildung mit Humeroradialsynostose.
Humangenetik **9**:43–53, 1970.

6 Lenz, W. D., et al., Pseudo-Thalidomide Syndrome. *Birth
Defects* **10**(8):97–107, 1974.

7 Levy, M., et al., Malformations graves des membres et
oligophrenie dans une famille (avec études chromosomiques). *Ann. Pédiatr.* **19**:313–320, 1972.

8 O'Brien, H. R., and Mustard, H. S., An Adult Living Case
of Total Phocomelia. *J.A.M.A.* **77**:1964–1967, 1921.

9 Schröder, C. H., Familiäre kongenitale Luxationen. *Z.
Orthopäd. Chir.* **57**:580–596, 1932.

123

Pseudoxanthoma Elasticum

(Grönblad-Strandberg Syndrome)

Originally described by Rigal (23) in 1881 and Balzer (2) in 1884, and grouped with the xanthomatoses, the syndrome of (a) alterations of the skin, (b) recurrent severe gastrointestinal hemorrhages, (c) weak peripheral pulses, and (d) failing vision was identified as a separate nonxanthomatous entity and named by Darier (9) in 1896. The (e) angioid streaks were added to the syndrome by Grönblad (14) and Strandberg (28) in 1929, although they had been described as early as 1889 by Doyne (10). The most thorough review to date is that of McKusick (18).

Pseudoxanthoma elasticum is a genetic heterogeneity but in most cases it has autosomal recessive inheritance (18). There are two recessive and two dominant forms (7, 21, 22, 22a, 31). The differences are delineated in Table 123-1. The data presented below represent the average of the various types. About 65 percent of patients have been females (11) if ascertainment is made from skin changes. However, if angioid streaks are used for discernment, there is no sex predilection. Many families have been surveyed in which the syndrome has occurred in sibs (18, 27). Consanguinity has been found in at least 20 percent of cases. The combined prevalence of the four types has been estimated at 1 per 40,000 (1).

The primary alteration in pseudoxanthoma elasticum is calcification of elastic fibers possibly due to the accumulation of polyanions within the fibers which may play a role in increased calcium binding (17a). Elevated lysine and hydroxylysine levels in collagen (3) and raised glutamine content in the elastin (3a) have been discovered. There is some evidence that a relationship may exist between chronic idiopathic hyperphosphatasia and pseudoxanthoma elasticum (19). Also see Differential Diagnosis.

SYSTEMIC MANIFESTATIONS

Skin. The skin becomes thickened and the markings are accentuated by raised, yellowish, flat papules, especially about the mouth, neck, axillas, elbows, groin, and perimbilical area. From a few yellowish papules on the neck or axilla to virtually general cutaneous involvement has been described in association with calcification of the subcutis (15, 25). These changes are usually recognized after the second decade, although they may appear as early as the third or fourth year of life. The thickened, yellowish skin becomes inelastic, redundant, thickened, and grooved, the normal skin marking becoming accentuated so that the skin resembles coarse-grained leather, especially on the neck and axilla (Fig. 123-1). Miescher elastoma has also been noted (18, 24).

Eyes. Visual disturbances have been noted in almost 30 percent of older patients (11). Funduscopic examination has demonstrated brownish or gray streaking (angioid streaks) in over 85 percent of cases. The streaks probably appear in the

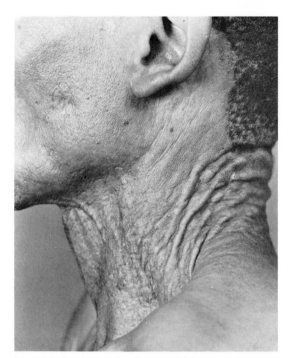

Figure 123-1. *Pseudoxanthoma elasticum.* Skin becomes thickened and markings are accentuated by yellowish papules, especially around neck, axilla, elbows, and groin. (*From T. Heyl,* Arch. Dermatol. **96:**528, 1967.)

second decade or later. They resemble vessels but actually represent involvement of the Bruch membrane (Fig. 123-2). Retinal hemorrhage, followed by organization, results in loss of visual acuity. Less often there is senile macular degeneration or central chorioretinitis (4, 18, 30).

Cardiovascular system. By the third decade, there may be weakness or absence of pulses in the arms and legs, accompanied by variable degrees of intermittent claudication in about 20 percent of cases (5). Roentgenographic examination has revealed calcification of peripheral arteries, especially those of the lower extremities, in about 15 percent (11). Hypertension has been noted in about 20 percent (11). Angina pectoris is seen in at least half the patients (5), and abdominal angina due to stenosis of the celiac artery is common (18).

Hemorrhage, especially gastrointestinal, occures in 15 percent of patients (6, 8) because of involvement of small blood vessels. A number of patients have had peptic ulcer (1). Bleeding may also occur in the retina, kidney, uterus, or bladder (1). Epistaxis (5) and hemarthrosis have been recorded, and subarachnoid hemorrhage has been a cause of death.

Other findings. Psychiatric disorders have been seen in about 5 percent of cases (5, 11). Calcification of the falx cerebri has also been described. Hypothyroidism was noted in a few patients (1).

Oral manifestations. The skin about the mouth may become redundant, the nasolabial folds and skin creases becoming accentuated and producing a "hound dog" appearance. The mucosal surface of the lips, especially the lower one, may exhibit yellowish intramucosal nodules (9, 18) in about 10 percent of involved persons. The buccal mucosa, soft or hard palate, and tonsillar

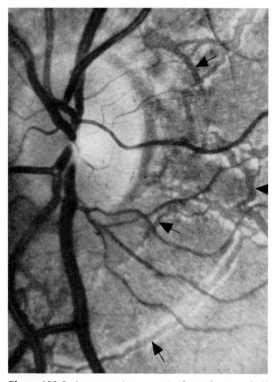

Figure 123-2. Arrows point to angioid streaks. Egg shell "fractures" in Bruch membrane, usually grouped around optic disks, mimic appearance of blood vessels. (*Courtesy of W. F. Hoyt, San Francisco, Calif.*)

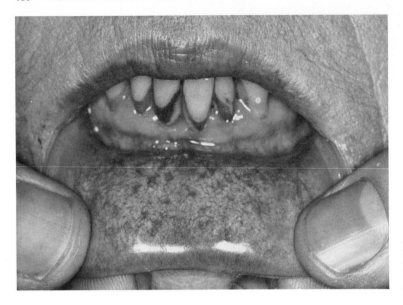

Figure 123-3. Mucosal surface of lower lip exhibits yellowish intramucosal nodules. (*Courtesy of R. Goodman, Baltimore, Md.*)

areas may be similarly affected (5, 20–22) (Fig. 123-3). The vaginal, gastric, and rectal mucosas have also been involved (5, 12).

Ultrastructural study of oral lesions showed large numbers of thickened and twisted collagen fibers (7a).

DIFFERENTIAL DIAGNOSIS

Angioid streaks may also be seen in Paget disease of bone. A combination of Paget disease and pseudoxanthoma elasticum has been described by Woodcock (32), Shaffer et al. (25), and others

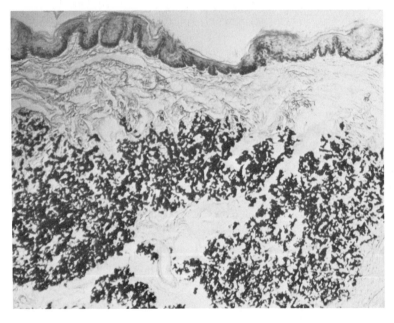

Figure 123-4. Elastic tissue appears fragmented and granular because of presence of calcium salts (von Kossa stain). (*From T. Heyl,* Arch. Dermatol. **96:**528, 1967.)

Table 123-1. Comparison of clinical findings of autosomal dominant and recessive forms of pseudoxanthoma elasticum*

Characteristics	Dominant I, percent	Dominant II, percent	Recessive I, percent	Recessive II, percent
Cutaneous changes				
Classical peau d'orange and flexural rash	100	25	75	
Macular rash		70	15	
General increase of extensibility	10	65	10	
General cutaneous PXE				100
Vascular disease				
Angina	55			
Claudication	55			
Hypertension	75	10	20	
Hematemesis	10	5	15	
Opthalmic abnormalities				
Severe choroiditis	75	10	35	
Angioid streaks	35	50	50	
Washed-out pattern		15	2	
Prominent choroidal vessels		20		
Myopia	25	50	5	
Blue sclerae	10	40	10	
Other findings				
High-arched palate		55	15	
Joint hypermobility		35	5	

*Based on data presented by F. M. Pope, *Arch. Dermatol.* **110:**209, 1974.

(18). Angioid streaks have also been seen in sickle cell disease, possibly because of iron deposits in Bruch membrane (14), and in osteoectasia with macrocranium (hyperphosphatasia) (13). Angioid streaks in combination with tumoral calcinosis and hyperphosphatemia have been noted in several families (1a). The clinical skin changes in senile elastosis somewhat resemble those in pseudoxanthoma elasticum.

LABORATORY AIDS

The involved skin or mucous membrane presents a characteristic microscopic picture. The changes are observed in the middle and lower part of the corium. The elastic tissue appears as fragmented masses, presenting a granular structure which is due at least in part to the presence of calcium salts demonstrated by von Kossa staining (Fig. 123-4). The amount of normal collagen fibers is reduced, while reticulum fibers are present in large amounts. The finding of calcium salts in ostensibly normal elastic fibers indicates that calcification is the primary event in pseudoxanthoma elasticum (8). Increased amounts of calcium have also been found in the skin on microincineration (17). Photographs of the fundus following injection of fluorescent dye clearly demonstrate the angioid streaks (26).

REFERENCES

1 Altman, L. K., et al., Pseudoxanthoma Elasticum. *Arch. Intern. Med.* **134:**1048–1054, 1974.

1a Baldursson, H., et al., Tumoral Calcinosis with Hyperphosphatemia. *J. Bone Joint Surg.* **51A:**913–925, 1969.

2 Balzer, F., Recherches sur les caractères anatomiques du xanthelasma. *Arch. Physiol.* **4:**65–80, 1884.

3 Blumenkrantz, N., et al., Biosynthesis of Collagen in Pseudoxanthoma Elasticum. *Acta Derm. Venereol.* (*Stockh.*) **53:**429–434, 1973.

3a Blumenkrantz, N., et al., Biosynthesis of Elastin in Pseudoxanthoma Elasticum. *Acta Derm. Venereol.* (*Stockh.*) **53:**435–438, 1973.

4 Britten, M. J., Unusual Traumatic Retinal Haemorrhage Associated with Angioid Streaks. *Br. J. Ophthalmol.* **50**:540–542, 1966.

5 Carlborg, V., et al., Vascular Studies in Pseudoxanthoma Elasticum with a Series of Color Photographs of the Eyeground Lesions. *Acta Med. Scand.* [Suppl.] **350**:1–84, 1959.

6 Cocco, A. E., et al., The Stomach in Pseudoxanthoma Elasticum. *J.A.M.A.* **210**:2381–2382, 1969.

7 Coffman, J. D., and Sommers, S. C., Familial Pseudoxanthoma Elasticum and Valvular Heart Disease. *Circulation* **19**:252–260, 1959.

7a Danielsen, L., and Kobayasi, T., Pseudoxanthoma Elasticum. *Acta Derm. Venereol.* (*Stockh.*) **54**:121–128, 173–176, 1974.

8 Danielsen, L., et al., Pseudoxanthoma Elasticum, a Clinico-pathological Study. *Acta Derm. Venereol.* (*Stockh.*) **50**:355–373, 1970.

9 Darier, J., Pseudoxanthoma elasticum. *Monatsh. Prakt. Dermatol.* **23**:609–617, 1896.

10 Doyne, R. W., Choroidal and Retinal Changes: The Result of Blows on the Eyes. *Trans. Ophthalmol. Soc. U.K.* **9**:128, 1889.

11 Eddy, D. D., and Farber, E. M., Pseudoxanthoma Elasticum: Internal Manifestations. A Report of Cases and a Statistical Review of the Literature. *Arch. Dermatol.* **86**:729–740, 1962.

12 Goodman, R. M., et al., Pseudoxanthoma Elasticum: A Clinical and Histopathological Study. *Medicine* (*Baltimore*) **42**:297–334, 1963.

13 Gorlin, R. J., and Goldman, H. M., *Thoma's Oral Pathology.* 6th ed. Mosby, St. Louis, 1970.

14 Grönblad, E., Angioid Streaks—Pseudoxanthoma Elasticum: Vorläufige Mitteilung. *Acta Ophthalmol.* (*Kbh.*) **7**:329, 1929.

15 James, A. E., et al., Roentgen Findings in Pseudoxanthoma Elasticum (PXE). *Am. J. Roentgenol.* **106**:642–647, 1969.

16 Kaplan, L., and Hartman, S. W., Elastica Disease: Case of Grönblad-Strandberg Syndrome with Gastrointestinal Hemorrhage. *Arch. Intern. Med.* **94**:489–492, 1954.

17 Lobitz, W. C., Jr., and Osterberg, A. E., Pseudoxanthoma Elasticum: Microincineration. *J. Invest. Dermatol.* **15**:297–298, 1950.

17a Martinez-Hernandez, A., and Huffer, W. E., Pseudoxanthoma Elasticum: Dermal Polyanions and Mineralization of Elastic Fibers. *Lab. Invest.* **31**:181–186, 1974.

18 McKusick, V. A., *Heritable Disorders of Connective Tissue.* 4th ed. Mosby, St. Louis, 1972.

19 Mitsudo, S. M., Chronic Idiopathic Hyperphosphatasia Associated with Pseudoxanthoma Elasticum. *J. Bone Joint Surg.* **53A**:303–314, 1971.

20 Miyaka, H., et al., A New Finding in Oral Cavity in Pseudoxanthoma Elasticum. *Nagoya J. Med. Sci.* **29**:251–259, 1967.

21 Pope, F. M., Autosomal Dominant Pseudoxanthoma Elasticum. *J. Med. Genet.* **11**:152–157, 1974.

22 Pope, F. M., Two Types of Autosomal Recessive Pseudoxanthoma Elasticum. *Arch. Dermatol.* **110**:209–212, 1974.

22a Pope, F. M., Historical Evidence for the Genetic Heterogeneity of Pseudoxanthoma Elasticum. *Br. J. Dermatol.* **92**:493–510, 1975.

23 Rigal, –, Observation pour servis à l'histoire de la chéloide diffuse xanthélasmique. *Ann. Dermatol. Syphiligr.* (*Paris*) **2**:491–501, 1881.

24 Schutt, D., Pseudoxanthoma Elasticum and Elastosis Perforans Serpiginosa. *Arch. Dermatol.* **91**:151–152, 1965.

25 Shaffer, B., et al., Pseudoxanthoma Elasticum: A Cutaneous Manifestation of a Systemic Disease: Report of a Case of Paget's Disease and a Case of Calcinosis with Arteriosclerosis as Manifestations of this Syndrome. *Arch. Dermatol. Syph.* (*Chic.*) **76**:622–633, 1957.

26 Smith, J. L., et al., Fluorescein Fundus Photography of Angioid Streaks. *Br. J. Ophthalmol.* **48**:517–521, 1964.

27 Stegmaier, O. C., Pseudoxanthoma Elasticum (Associated with Angioid Streaks of the Retina). *Arch. Dermatol. Syph.* (*Chic.*) **70**:530–532, 1954.

28 Strandberg, J., Pseudoxanthoma elasticum. *Z. Haut. Geschlechtskr.* **31**:689, 1929.

29 Syzmanski, F. J., and Caro, M. D., Pseudoxanthoma Elasticum: Review of Its Relationship to Internal Diseases and Report of an Unusual Case. *Arch. Dermatol. Syph.* (*Chic.*) **71**:184–189, 1955.

30 Van Balen, A. T., and Houtsmuller, A. J., Syndrome of Grönblad-Strandberg-Touraine. *Ophthalmologica* **149**:246–247, 1965.

31 Wise, D., Hereditary Disorders of Connective Tissue, in H. Gottron and V. Schnyder (eds.), *Vererbung von Hautkrankheiten.* Springer-Verlag, Berlin, 1966.

32 Woodcock, C. W., Pseudoxanthoma Elasticum, Angioid Streaks of Retina and Osteitis Deformans. *Arch. Dermatol. Syph.* (*Chic.*) **65**:623, 1952.

124

Pyknodysostosis

Maroteaux and Lamy (12), in 1962, defined pyknodysostosis as a syndrome consisting of (a) dwarfism, (b) osteopetrosis, (c) abbreviated terminal phalanges, (d) cranial anomalies, such as persistence of fontanels and failure of closure of cranial sutures, and (e) hypoplasia of the angle of the mandible. Several cases of this syndrome have been published as examples of other disorders, chiefly osteopetrosis and cleidocranial dysplasia. The first documented case is that of Montanari (14) in 1923. About 80 cases have been reported (9a, 24).

Affected sibs have been noted in many instances (1, 6, 11, 14, 16–18, 21, 25–27). The syndrome has also been seen in identical twins (2). Parental consanguinity has been noted in more than 30 percent of cases (19), and autosomal recessive inheritance is clearly indicated. There is good evidence to suggest that Toulouse-Lautrec had this syndrome (13).

SYSTEMIC MANIFESTATIONS

Facies. The head appears large, because of occipital bulging. Characteristic are parrot-like nose with mild exophthalmos and micrognathia (Fig. 124-1A, B).

Skeletal alterations. Because of shortness of the extremities, adult height is reduced, being 134 to 152 cm (53 to 60 in.). The trunk is not shortened but often exhibits marked pectus excavatum,

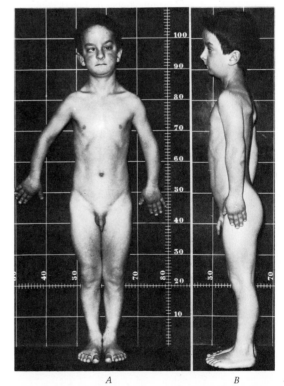

A   B

Figure 124-1. *Pyknodysostosis.* (A, B). Dwarfed eight-year-old boy. Note mild exophthalmos and small mandible. (*From A. Giedion and M. Zachmann,* Helv. Paediatr. Acta **21**:412, 1966.)

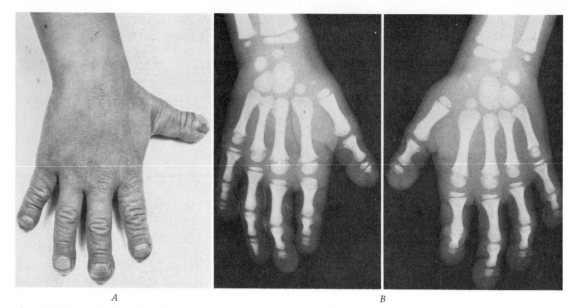

A   *B*

Figure 124-2. (*A, B*). Terminal digits of fingers reduced and widened. Nails often overlap ends of fingers. Note increased bone density, acroosteolysis of terminal phalanges, also pointed terminal phalanx. (*From S. E. Shuler*, Arch. Dis. Child. **38**:620, 1963.)

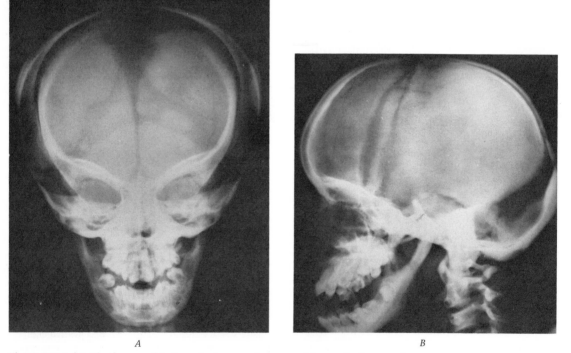

A   *B*

Figure 124-3. (*A, B*). Absence of fusion of sutures and closure of fontanels. Increased bone density and absence of mandibular angle. (*From S. E. Shuler*, Arch. Dis. Child. **38**:620, 1963.)

with underdeveloped breasts in women. The terminal digits of the fingers and toes are reduced and widened, often presenting a drum-stick appearance (Fig. 124-2A, B). The nails may be thin and hypoplastic.

The acromial end of the clavicle has been noted to be somewhat hypoplastic (2, 20, 24, 26). Bilateral genu valgum is frequent.

On roentgenographic examination, there is increased radiopacity of all bones, but especially of the long bones, spine, and skull base. Bone fragility is increased, many patients having a history of prior fracture. The terminal phalanges of the fingers and toes are markedly bizarre, exhibiting fragmentation of the heads with preservation of the bases, osteolysis of the unguiculate portions, or narrowing of the ends of otherwise normal terminal phalanges. Brachymesophalangy of the fifth fingers, less often the index finger, is a common finding. The fourth metatarsal is occasionally abbreviated (24).

The skull is dolichocephalic with frontal and occipital bossing (1, 8, 11, 25). Most cranial sutures and fontanels are open, especially the parietooccipital. The bones of the calvaria are thin, dense, and without diploic markings. Wormian bones are commonly observed (2, 18, 19, 21). The frontal sinuses are consistently absent, and other paranasal sinuses are hypoplastic or missing. The mastoid air cells are often not pneumatized (2, 17, 18, 19, 26) (Fig. 124-3A, B).

Microscopic studies of the involved bones carried out by Shuler (20), Taracena del Piñal (25), and Soto (21) have shown reduction in osteoclastic and osteoblastic activity, with a reduced rate of bone formation and resorption.

Eyes. The eyes may be somewhat exophthalmic (1, 24–26) with blue scleras (17, 28).

Oral anomalies. Obtuse mandibular angle is a constant feature. Facial bones are often underdeveloped, with relative mandibular prognathism (2, 8, 9, 17, 26, 28).

Oral and dental anomalies include premature or delayed eruption (1, 7, 8, 24, 28), enamel hypoplasia (16, 25), malposition of teeth (4, 7, 24, 25), and grooved palate (8, 9, 24, 25). The soft palate tends to be long (15).

DIFFERENTIAL DIAGNOSIS

Differential diagnosis would include osteopetrosis and *acroosteolysis*. The open cranial fontanels and sutures might suggest *cleidocranial dysplasia*.

Acroosteolysis is associated with progressive reduced height, kyphosis, bathrocephaly, basalar impression, numerous Wormian bones, absence of frontal sinuses, and fusion of the spinous processes of the cervical vertebras. The terminal phalanges are shortened and often exhibit tenderness, pain, and paresthesia. The alveolar process often is markedly atrophic, but the angle is not missing as in pyknodysostosis. It is inherited as an autosomal dominant trait. So-called industrial acroosteolysis has been described in workers synthesizing polyvinyl chloride (11). Lamy and Maroteaux (10) described isolated autosomal dominant acroosteolysis.

Stanesco et al. in 1963 (22) described a rare form of craniofacial dysostosis, inherited as an autosomal dominant trait, characterized by small skull, thin cranial bone, depressions over the frontoparietal and occipitoparietal sutures, poorly developed mandible with obtuse angle, exophthalmos, and very short limbs with massive thick cortices.

Mandibuloacral dysplasia resembles pyknodysostosis in delayed closure of skull sutures, Wormian bones, and hypoplasia of terminal phalanges, but there is no increase in bone density or aplasia of the mandibular angle. Instead there is antegonial mandibular notching, stiff joints, and cutaneous atrophy (5, 29).

LABORATORY AIDS

Reduced serum alkaline phosphatase has been found in a few cases (8, 25, 27). Baker et al. (3) described intermittently high plasma calcitonin levels.

REFERENCES

1 Abboud, M. S., et al., Albers-Schonberg Disease with Report of Two Cases in an Egyptian Family. *Arch. Pediatr.* **71**:131–138, 1954.

2 Andrén, L., et al., Osteopetrosis Acro-osteolytica: A Syndrome of Osteopetrosis, Acro-osteolysis and Open Sutures of the Skull. *Acta Chir. Scand.* **124**:496–507, 1962.

3 Baker, R. K., et al., Plasma Calcitonin in Pycnodysostosis. *J. Clin. Endocrinol. Metab.* **37**:46–55, 1973.

4 Braun, J. P., and Peterschmitt, J., L'aspect radiologique de la pycnodysostose. *J. Radiol. Électrol.* **46**:509–512, 1965.

5 Cavallazzi, C., et al., Su di un caso di disostosi cleidocrania. *Riv. Clin. Pediatr.* **65**:312–326, 1960.

6 Dusenberry, J. F., and Kane, J. J., Pycnodysostosis: Report of Three New Cases. *Am. J. Roentgenol.* **99**:717–723, 1967.

7 Elmore, S. M., et al., Pycnodysostosis with a Familial Chromosome Anomaly. *Am. J. Med.* **40**:273–282, 1966.

8 Giedion, A., and Zachmann, M., Pyknodysostose. *Helv. Paediatr. Acta* **21**:612–621, 1966.

9 Janečka, J., and Bruna, J., Pyknodysostosis im Röntgenbild. *Fortschr. Röntgenstr.* **118**:298–305, 1973.

9a Kemperdick, H., and Lehr, H. J., Die Pyknodysostose. *Monatschr. Kinderhielkd.* **123**:52–57, 1975.

10 Lamy, M., and Maroteaux, P., Acro-ostéolyse dominante. *Arch. Fr. Pédiatr.* **18**:693–702, 1961.

11 Markowitz, S. S., et al., Occupational Acroosteolysis. *Arch. Dermatol.* **106**:219–223, 1972.

12 Maroteaux, P., and Lamy, M., La pycnodysostose. *Presse Méd.* **70**:999–1002, 1962.

13 Maroteaux, P., and Lamy, M., The Malady of Toulouse-Lautrec. *J.A.M.A.* **191**:715–717, 1965.

14 Montanari, U., Acondroplasia e disostosi cleidocrania digitale. *Chir. Organi Mov.* **7**:379–391, 1923.

15 Nielsen, E. L., Pycnodysostosis. *Acta Paediatr. Scand.* **63**:437–442, 1974.

16 Perez-Cuadra, E., and Galvez-Galan, F., Enfermedad de Albers-Schönberg: Dos casos en la misma familia. *Bol. Inst. Pat. Med. (Madr.)* **15**:322–332, 1960.

17 Roca, J., Osteosclerosis y disostosis craneal. *Prensa Med. Argent.* **44**:1875–1879, 1957.

18 Sandomenico, C., and Del Vecchio, E., La picnodisostosi. Inquadramento classificativo e patogenico. *Radiol. Med. (Torino)* **53**:160–181, 1967.

19 Sedano, H. O., et al., Pycnodysostosis: Clinical and Genetic Considerations. *Am. J. Dis. Child.* **116**:70–77, 1968.

20 Shuler, S. E., Pycnodysostosis. *Arch. Dis. Child.* **38**: 620–625, 1963.

21 Soto, R. J., et al., Pycnodysostosis: Metabolic and Histologic Studies. *Birth Defects* **5**(4):109–116, 1969.

22 Stanesco, V., et al., Syndrome héréditaire dominant, reunissant une dysostose cranio-faciale de type particulièr, une insuffisance de croissance d'aspect chondrodystrophique et une épaississement massif de la corticale des os longs. *Rev. Fr. Endocrinol. Clin.* **4**:221–231, 1963.

23 Stanesco, V., et al., Une nouvelle observation de pycnodysostose avec étude métabolique. *Arch. Fr. Pédiatr.* **21**:135–142, 1964.

24 Sugiura, Y., et al., Pycnodysostosis in Japan: Report of Six Cases and a Review of Japanese Literature. *Birth Defects* **10**(12):78–98, 1974.

25 Taracena del Piñal, B., Cuatro casos de una enfermedad nueva, la picnodisostosis. *Ann. Med. Quirg. Cruz. Roja Esp.* **6**:5–24, 1964.

26 Thoms, J., Cleido-cranial Dysostosis: Report of Two Cases with Special Characteristics. *Acta Radiol. (Stockh.)* **50**:514–520, 1958.

27 Weismann-Netter, R., and Lorch, P., Nanisme familial avec densification generalisée du squelette et dysgénesies polytopiques. *Sem. Hôp. Paris* **32**:2713–2719, 1956.

28 Wiedemann, H. R., Pyknodysostose. *Fortschr. Roentgenstr.* **103**:590–597, 1965.

29 Young, L. W., et al., Mandibular Hypoplasia, Acroosteolysis, Stiff Joints and Cutaneous Atrophy. *Birth Defects* **7**(7):291–297, 1971.

125

Reiter Syndrome

The classic triad, described by Reiter (16), in 1916, consists of (a) arthritis, (b) conjunctivitis, and (c) urethritis. However, cases of the syndrome had appeared in the literature almost 100 years prior to his report. Brodie (4), in 1818, reported on six patients suffering from the same symptoms. In 1904, Markwald (9) described a patient having urethritis, conjunctivitis, and arthritis following dysentery. In 1916, Fiessinger and Leroy (5) described a "syndrome conjunctivo-uretrosynovial" in four postdysenteric patients. Comprehensive studies are those of Paronen (11) and Weinberger et al. (25). The original concept of a triad has been expanded to include a variety of other signs, primarily of the skin, mucous membranes, and viscera (10).

The etiology is still unclear. There is suggestive evidence that a pleuropneumonia-like organism may be etiologically related (18, 22, 24, 25). The organism has been recovered from synovial fluid but not carried in subculture. Symptoms suggest gonorrhea, but smears of the urethral discharge are always negative for *Neisseria*. However, venereal origin has been suggested (6, 20). A chlamydial agent has also been implicated (5a).

SYSTEMIC MANIFESTATIONS

The syndrome usually occurs in young men between twenty and thirty years of age, although it has been seen in a two-year-old boy (11). Above the age of fifty years, the disease is seldom documented. Though Paronen (11) found that 10 percent of patients were women, Weinberger and Bauer (23) postulated that no authentic instance of the complete triad in females had been reported. Specific geographic distribution has not been demonstrated.

Reiter syndrome is a self-limited disorder associated with fever in the initial stages. The onset of the characteristic symptoms may be preceded by weight loss, fatigability, and, in one-third of the patients, a mild, nonbloody diarrhea. Sometimes the disease is ushered in by nausea and vomiting. In most patients, the onset is monosymptomatic. There is some disagreement as to which organ is affected first. According to Paronen (11), the sequence is urethritis, arthritis, and conjunctivitis. In 70 percent of patients, the complete syndrome evolves during the first 10 days of the disease.

Genitourinary system. Urethral involvement consists of itching and burning associated with discharge and reddening of the meatus. This discharge may be mucoid or purulent; microscopic examination reveals numerous leukocytes but no bacteria. The duration of the urethritis may vary from a day to several months. One may also note circinate balanitis (Fig. 125-1). In a number of patients, cystitis develops, leading to dysuria, abacterial pyuria, and hematuria. Cystoscopic examination shows superficial membranous

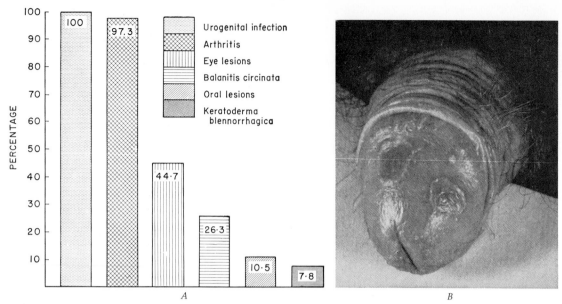

Legend:
- ▦ Urogenital infection
- ▧ Arthritis
- ▥ Eye lesions
- ▤ Balanitis circinata
- ▨ Oral lesions
- ▩ Keratoderma blennorrhagica

Bar values: 100, 97.3, 44.7, 26.3, 10.5, 7.8

A

B

Figure 125-1. (A). *Reiter syndrome.* (B). Penis with circinate balanitis. Note similarity to oral changes in Fig. 125-4.

sloughs and petechial bleeding in the bladder mucosa (23). Nephritis has also been described.

Arthritis. Articular involvement, almost always polyarticular, is the most disabling feature. The joints most frequently affected are the weight-bearing ones of the lower extremities. Next in frequency are the shoulder, fingers, and sacrum (11) (Fig. 125-2). The articular manifestations comprise tenderness, pain, and swelling. In a number of cases, the skin covering the joints is changed in color. In severe cases, roentgenographic examination shows bone atrophy and flecky decalcification (23). Surveys of patients with well-documented Reiter syndrome have demonstrated a tendency toward asymmetric arthritic involvement, most commonly in the sacroiliac joints, toes, and heels. The distribution of these findings will often permit a presumptive roentgenographic diagnosis in the absence of a classic clinical history (19, 25). Very high hemolytic complement activity and macrophages containing neutrophils have been found in the synovial fluid (13). In addition to joints, muscles and tendons may also be affected.

Eyes. The most frequent ocular manifestation is conjunctivitis which, in most patients, is bilateral, at times so mild that the condition may be overlooked (Fig. 125-3). The first symptoms of conjunctivitis are smarting, photophobia, and

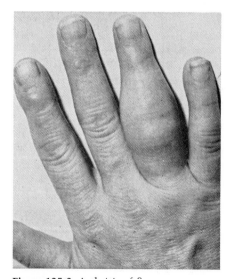

Figure 125-2. Arthritis of finger.

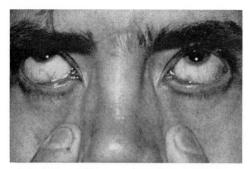

Figure 125-3. Conjunctivitis and early circumcorneal flush.

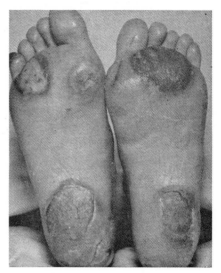

Figure 125-4. Extensive keratoderma blennorrhagica–like lesions on soles of feet.

epiphora, followed by redness of the conjunctiva and mucopurulent discharge. The duration of the conjunctivitis varies from a few days to several months, but in most cases the inflammation subsides within 1 to 4 weeks (12). Recovery without loss of vision is the rule. Besides conjunctivitis, eye involvement includes nongranulomatous iridocyclitis, most often unilateral, and keratitis.

Skin. Lesions similar to keratosis blennorrhagica or pustular psoriasis are frequently observed (10). However, Paronen (11) found only 10 of 344 patients to have skin involvement. The skin lesions, usually found on the palms and soles and occasionally on the trunk and extremities, exhibit striking symmetry (Fig. 125-4). The skin manifestations begin as small, red to yellowish macules or papules, which become confluent and hyperkeratotic. After several weeks, the hyperkeratotic crust falls off. The skin lesions are usually seen in patients with severe arthritis, appear 4 to 6 weeks after onset of the syndrome, and may last 2 to 4 months (8). The nails of the fingers and toes are affected in many patients, subungual keratoses and abscesses with loss of nails being commonly observed.

Because of the similarity between the penile and oral lesions and their simultaneous occurrence, the incidence in these two locations is given in Table 125-1. The penile lesions are mainly limited to the foreskin and glans and are of a superficial and painless nature. They are small erythematous papules surrounded by a slightly elevated grayish-whitish border (balanitis circinata). The configuration may be map-

Table 125-1. Incidence of oral and penile lesions in patients with Reiter syndrome

Author	Year	No. of cases	Country	Incidence of penile lesions, %	Incidence of oral lesions, %
Paronen (11)	1948	344	Finland	26	3
Hancock (8)	1960	76	England	26	10
Montgomery et al. (10)	1959	38	United States	79	37
Hall and Finegold (6)	1953	23	United States	78	48

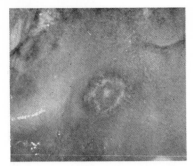

Figure 125-5. Oral lesion on left buccal mucosa of twenty-seven-year-old man with Reiter syndrome.

like. At times they become covered with scales. Occasionally, ulcers are found on the scrotum and on the shaft of the penis.

Other findings. Among his 344 patients, Paronen [11] found 23 with carditis and 26 with pleurisy. Aortic insufficiency of rapid onset (3, 12, 22) has been described in patients with a high incidence of spondylitis, iritis, and atrio-ventricular conduction defects. The nasal mucosa may also be involved. Rare complications include thrombophlebitis, encephalitis, lacrimitis, parotitis, epididymitis, orchitis, mastitis, and amyloidosis (2, 4a).

Oral manifestations. From Table 125-1, it may be seen that the incidence of oral manifestations apparently shows pronounced variation in different surveys. Some larger studies do not even mention oral complications; the lesions may be overlooked because of their painlessness. A number of cases with oral manifestations have been described as "blennorrhagic balanitiform keratoderma with oral involvement" (1, 7, 14, 17, 25). Particularly, Montgomery et al. (10) and Hancock (8) have been concerned with oral manifestations in the Reiter syndrome.

The lesions seen on the buccal mucosa, lips, and gingiva are usually red, slightly elevated areas, varying from 1 mm to 1 cm in diameter and sometimes surrounded by a whitish circinate line resembling circinate balanitis (Fig. 125-5). They may also have the appearance of small, opaque vesicles or areas of glistening erythema exhibiting a granular surface. Multiple, small, bright-red purpuric spots, which

later darken and coalesce, may be seen on the palate. The tongue may exhibit superficial erosions similar to those of geographic tongue or to those seen in pustular psoriasis. They are most prominent when the tongue is coated (8, 14, 25) (Fig. 125-6A). Rarely, the palate is involved (Fig. 125-6B).

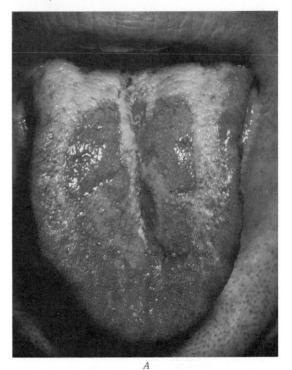

A

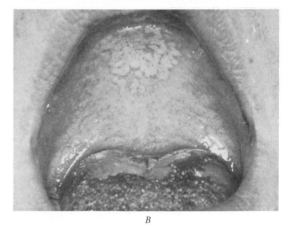

B

Figure 125-6. (*A*). Tongue lesions resemble glossitis migrans ("geographic tongue"). (*B*). Erosive lesions of palate. (*Courtesy of H. C. Sturde, Koblenz, Germany.*)

PATHOLOGY

The histopathologic findings in the penile and oral lesions and in the skin are essentially the same, the epithelium showing parakeratosis, acanthosis, and elongation of the rete ridges. The epithelium is infiltrated with polymorphonuclear leukocytes, and intraepithelial microabscesses may be found. The underlying connective tissue is infiltrated with lymphocytes and smaller numbers of plasma cells and leukocytes. The synovial tissues exhibit hyperemia and edema, and acute and chronic inflammation may be seen.

DIFFERENTIAL DIAGNOSIS

Because of the clinical symptoms of urethral discharge, conjunctivitis, and arthralgia, gonorrhea should be considered. However, the negative urethral cultures, the failure of response to antibodies, and the rather specific oral changes are evidence that the condition is not gonorrhea.

Erythema multiforme also presents conjunctivitis, skin lesions, urethritis, and oral involvement. In contrast to those of the Reiter syndrome, the oral lesions are much more extensive and the lips, particularly, are severely affected. The skin lesions also differ from those in Reiter syndrome by their iris-like appearance.

Another mucocutaneous-ocular disorder, *Behçet syndrome,* may have features resembling those of Reiter syndrome. In the former, however, the oral lesions are typical aphthae, the eye lesions are more severe, and the occurrence of urethritis is quite rare.

Undoubtedly, incomplete forms of Reiter syndrome may occur in which only two members of the triad or tetrad are present, thus giving rise to diagnostic difficulties.

LABORATORY AIDS

There are no specific tests for the Reiter syndrome. However, a few laboratory findings seem to be constantly present in this disease, such as mild to moderate leukocytosis, increased blood sedimentation rate, and pyuria. Secondary anemia has also been described.

REFERENCES

1 Berman, L., Über einen Fall von gonorrhöischer Keratose der Haut und Mundschleimhaut. *Dermatol. Z.* **51:** 420–423, 1928.

2 Bleehen, S. S., et al., Amyloidosis Complicating Reiter's Syndrome. *Br. J. Vener. Dis.* **42:**88–93, 1966.

3 Block, S. R., Reiter's Syndrome and Acute Aortic Insufficiency. *Arthritis Rheum.* **15:**218–220, 1972.

4 Brodie, B. C., *Pathological and Surgical Observations on Disease of the Joints.* Longman, London, 1818.

4a Csonka, G., Thrombophlebitis in Reiter's Syndrome. *Br. J. Vener. Dis.* **42:**93–95, 1966.

5 Fiessinger, N., and Leroy, E., Contribution à l'étude d'une épidémie de dysenterie dans la somme (juillet-octobre 1916). *Bull. Soc. Méd. Hôp. Paris* **40:**2030–2069, 1916.

5a Gordon, F. B., et al., Chlamydial Isolates from Reiter's Syndrome. *Br. J. Vener. Dis.* **49:**376–380, 1973.

6 Hall, W. H., and Finegold, S., A Study of 23 Cases of Reiter's Syndrome. *Ann. Intern. Med.* **38:**533–550, 1953.

7 Hamner, J. E., and Graykowski, E. A., Oral Lesions Compatible with Reiter's Disease: A Diagnostic Problem. *J. Am. Dent. Assoc.* **69:**560–564, 1964.

8 Hancock, J. A., Surface Manifestations of Reiter's Disease in the Male. *Br. J. Vener. Dis.* **36:**36–39, 1960.

9 Markwald, B., Über seltene Complicationen der Ruhr. *Z. Klin. Med.* **53:**321–325, 1904.

10 Montgomery, M. M., et al., The Mucocutaneous Lesions of Reiter's Syndrome. *Ann. Intern. Med.* **51:**99–109, 1959.

11 Paronen, I., Reiter's Disease: A Study of 344 Cases Observed in Finland. *Acta Med. Scand.* [Suppl.] **212:**1–114, 1948.

12 Paulus, H. E., et al., Aortic Insufficiency in Five Patients with Reiter's Syndrome. *Am. J. Med.* **53:**464–472, 1972.

13 Pekin, T. J., Jr., et al., Unusual Synovial Fluid Findings in Reiter's Syndrome. *Ann. Intern. Med.* **66:**677–684, 1967.

14 Pindborg, J. J., et al., Reiter's Syndrome. *Oral Surg.* **16:**551–560, 1963.

15 Popert, A. J., A Prospective Study of Reiter's Syndrome: An Interim Report on the First 82 Cases. *Br. J. Vener. Dis.* **40:**160–165, 1964.

16 Reiter, H., Über eine bisher unerkannte Spirochäten-Infektion (Spirochaetosis arthritica). *Dtsch. Med. Wochenschr.* **42:**1535–1536, 1916.

17 Schirren, H., and Sturde, H. C., Morbus Reiter mit "symptomatischer" Exfoliatio areata linguae. *Hautarzt* **21:** 283–284, 1970.

17a Sharp, J. T., Reiter's Syndrome. *Curr. Probl. Dermatol.*

5:157–179, 1973.

18 Shepard, M. C., Nongonococcal Urethritis Associated with Human Strains of "T" Mycoplasmas. *J.A.M.A.* **211:** 1335–1340, 1970.

19 Sholkoff, S. D., et al., Roentgenology of Reiter's Syndrome. *Radiology* **97:**497–503, 1970.

20 Steinmetz, P. R., and Green, J. P., Reiter's Syndrome. *U.S. Armed Forces Med. J.* **10:**1185–1193, 1959.

21 Walther, G., Beiträge zur Klinik der Bacillenruhr. *Z. Klin. Med.* **138:**663–673, 1940.

22 Warthin, T. A., Reiter's Syndrome. *Am. J. Med.* **4:**827–835, 1948.

23 Weinberger, H. J., Reiter's Syndrome Re-evaluated. *Arthritis Rheum.* **5:**202–210, 1962.

24 Weinberger, H. J., et al., Clinical Features and Bacteriologic Studies in Reiter's Syndrome, in C. Slocumb (ed.), *Rheumatic Diseases,* American Rheumatism Association. Saunders, Philadelphia, 1952, pp. 73–77.

25 Weinberger, H. W., et al., Reiter's Syndrome, Clinical and Pathologic Observations: A Long Term Study of 16 Cases. *Medicine* **41:**35–91, 1962.

26 Wright, V., and Reed, W. B., The Link Between Reiter's Syndrome and Psoriatic Arthritis. *Ann. Rheum. Dis.* **23:**12–21, 1964.

126

Rieger Syndrome

(Oligodontia and Primary Mesodermal Dysgenesis of the Iris)

Oligodontia was described as occurring in combination with malformation of part of the anterior chamber of the eye as early as 1883 by Vossius (13). However, the condition was not recognized as a heritable syndrome until 1935 by Rieger (8). Its frequency has been estimated as 1 per 200,000 population (1). The disorder has been thoroughly reviewed by Alkemade (1).

The syndrome has an autosomal dominant pattern of inheritance (1–6, 14), with almost complete penetrance and variable expressivity (1).

SYSTEMIC MANIFESTATIONS

Facies. A number of patients have had a broad flat nasal root, prominent supraorbital ridges,

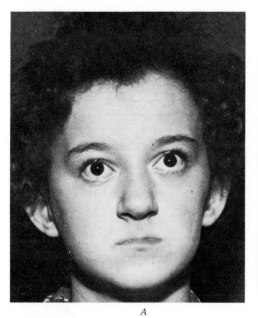
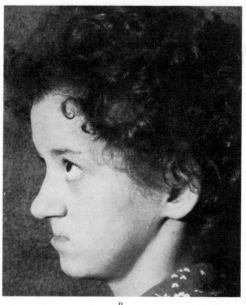

A   B

Figure 126-1. *Rieger syndrome.* (A, B). Note midfacial hypoplasia with relative mandibular prognathism. (*From E. Frandsen,* Acta Ophthalmol. (Kbh.) **41:**757, 1963.)

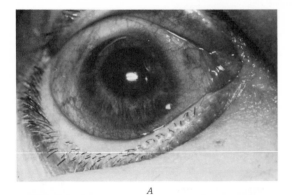

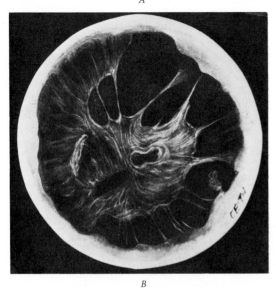

Figure 126-2. (A). Corectopia and dyscoria. Note blending of iris and sclera, iris stromal hypoplasia. (*From W. Lemmingson, Klin. Monatsbl. Augenheilkd.* **138:**96, 1961.) (B) Complex developmental abnormalities involve the limbus, cornea, anterior chamber angle, stroma of iris, and pupils. (*From G. Busch et al., Klin. Monatsbl. Augenheilkd.* **136:**512, 1960.)

and relative prognathism due to underdevelopment of the maxilla or to loss of vertical height because of oligodontia. Mild telecanthus with or without ocular hypertelorism is present in about 40 percent of patients (1) (Fig. 126-1).

Eyes. There are hypoplasia of the iris and anterior synechiae running from the iris to the cornea across the anterior chamber. Slitlike pupils (dyscoria) result from traction of these synechiae in over 70 percent of the cases (1) (Fig. 126-2*A*, *B*). Posterior embryotoxon (thickening of the Schwalbe line) is also a constant feature. Microcornea, megalocornea, corneal opacity, iris coloboma, blue scleras, aniridia, glaucoma, and strabismus are common.

Other findings. A wide spectrum of incidental findings has been tabulated by Alkemade (1), but they form no pattern and appear to represent aleatory association.

Oral manifestations. The premaxillary area is relatively underdeveloped (1–3, 6, 10), and a reduced number of teeth (oligodontia) is frequent (2, 5, 14). The maxillary incisors and second premolars are most commonly missing (3, 6, 10). Conical crown form has been recorded by several authors (3, 6, 7, 13, 14) (Fig. 126-3).

DIFFERENTIAL DIAGNOSIS

Suppression of dentition and teeth with conical crown form are seen in several other disorders such as *hypohidrotic ectodermal dysplasia, chondroectodermal dysplasia,* and *incontinentia pigmenti.*

We have seen brothers with the Rieger anomaly, severe growth retardation, inguinal hernia, joint hypermobility, deep-set eyes, and delayed teething. Sensenbrenner et al. (11) have reported a similarly affected child. This definitely represents a distinct syndrome with autosomal recessive inheritance (3a). The patients reported by

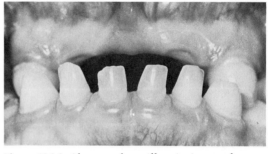

Figure 126-3. Absence of maxillary incisors and peg-shaped crowns of lower incisors and canines. (*From M. Feingold et al., Pediatrics* **44:**564, 1969.)

Sedeghi-Najar and Senior (10) have some resemblance to our cases but their disorder was dominantly inherited.

LABORATORY AIDS

None is known.

REFERENCES

1 Alkemade, P. P. H., *Dysgenesis Mesodermalis of the Iris and the Cornea.* Van Gorcum, The Netherlands, 1969.
2 Busch, G., et al., Dysgenesis mesodermalis et ectodermalis Rieger oder Rieger'sche Krankheit. *Klin. Monatsbl. Augenheilkd.* **136:**512–523, 1960.
3 Feingold, M., et al., Rieger's Syndrome. *Pediatrics* **44:** 564–569, 1969.
3a Gorlin, R. J., et al., Rieger Anomaly and Growth Retardation (the S-H-O-R-T Syndrome). *Birth Defects* **11**(2):46–48, 1975.
4 Henkind, P., et al., Mesodermal Dysgenesis of the Anterior Segment: Rieger's Anomaly. *Arch. Ophthalmol.* **73:** 810–817, 1965.
5 Langdon, J. D., Rieger's Syndrome. *Oral Surg.* **30:**788–795, 1970.
6 Lemmingson, W., and Riethe, P., Beobachtungen bei Dysgenesis mesodermalis corneae et iridis in Kombination mit Oligodontie. *Klin. Monatsbl. Augenheilkd.* **133:** 877–891, 1958.
7 Rejchrt, B., and Miska, J., Dysgenesis mesodermalis corneae et iridis. *Excerpta Med. (Amst.)* **7**(12):287–288, 1953.
8 Rieger, H., Beiträge zur Kenntnis seltener Missbildungen der Iris. *Albrecht von Graefes Arch. Klin. Ophthalmol.* **133:**602–635, 1935.
9 Rieth, P., and Lemmingson, W., Zur Kombination von Oligodontie mit Dysgenesis mesodermalis corneae et iridis. *Stoma (Heidelb.)* **15:**11–25, 1962.
10. Sedeghi-Najar, A., and Senior, B., Autosomal Dominant Transmission of Isolated Growth Hormone Deficiency in Iris-Dental Dysplasia (Rieger's Syndrome). *J. Pediatr.* **85:**644–648, 1974.
11 Sensenbrenner, J. A., et al., A Low-Birthweight Syndrome; Rieger Syndrome. *Birth Defects* **11**(2):423–426, 1975.
12 Unger, L., Beitrag zur sogen. Dysgenesis mesodermalis corneae et iridis (Rieger). *Ophthalmologia* **132:**27–35, 1956.
13 Vossius, A., Kongenitale Anomalie der Iris. *Klin. Monatsbl. Augenheilkd.* **21:**233–237, 1883.
14 Wilson, J. P., A Case of Partial Anodontia. *Br. Dent. J.* **99:**199–200, 1955.

127

Rothmund-Thomson Syndrome

(*Poikiloderma Congenita*)

The syndrome of (*a*) poikiloderma appearing from the third to sixth month of life, (*b*) bilateral cataracts which appear from the fourth to the seventh year, and (*c*) hypogonadism was described independently by several authors. Rothmund (23), in 1868, and Thomson (28), in 1923, delineated the same syndrome. At least 65 cases have been described.

The syndrome has autosomal recessive inheritance, although over 70 percent of patients have been female (11, 18, 27). Consanguinity has been present in several cases (2, 17, 18, 21, 23, 25), and the syndrome has occurred in identical twins (8). The case of Hallman and Patiala (13), in which a mother and son had similar findings, raises the question of genetic heterogeneity.

SYSTEMIC MANIFESTATIONS

Facies. Not enough data are available concerning the facies. However, a few authors have noted a large head with frontal bossing and a broad depressed nasal bridge (26, 28, 29). Microcephaly has also been mentioned (6, 14, 21, 28, 29).

Skin and skin appendages. The skin of the cheeks and ears, uninvolved at birth, becomes red and swollen about the third to sixth month of life (Figs. 127-1, 127-2, 127-3). Then the extensor surfaces of the hands, forearms, legs and thighs, and the buttocks become involved but usually to a lesser degree, the exposed surfaces being more severely affected (Fig. 127-1). The trunk is often spared. The inflammatory phase soon subsides and leaves areas which appear to be varying combinations of pigmentation, depigmentation, atrophy, and telangiectasia. The dull-brown, irregular macular or reticular pigmentation usually follows the appearance of the atrophy and telangiectasia.

Sensitivity to sunlight in the form of blister production is seen in at least 35 percent of patients (5, 6, 8, 17, 21, 26, 27). It is usually more severe in early life.

Scalp, pubic, and axillary hair is often somewhat sparse, and may be almost absent in some patients (21). The eyebrows and lashes have frequently been missing or severely diminished (2, 8, 15, 17, 18, 21, 26–29).

Warty hyperkeratosis, especially over the joints (21, 28, 29, 31), with late developing squamous cell carcinoma and palmoplantar keratoses (6, 13) has been found. Nail dystrophy has been noted in at least one-quarter of the cases (2, 15, 17, 18, 26, 27).

Endocrine system. An endocrine disorder appears to be present in about one-fourth of the patients, most frequently hypogonadism (2, 15, 18, 21, 24, 26). Scanty menstruation is common, and few affected women have borne children.

Skeletal system. Over half the patients have been of markedly short stature, with short ter-

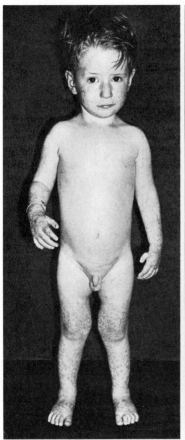
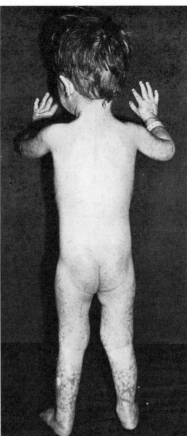

Figure 127-1. *Rothmund-Thomson syndrome.* Skin of cheeks and ears, uninvolved at birth, assumes a poikilodermatous appearance about the third to sixth month of life. There is similar involvement of legs, thighs, and buttocks.

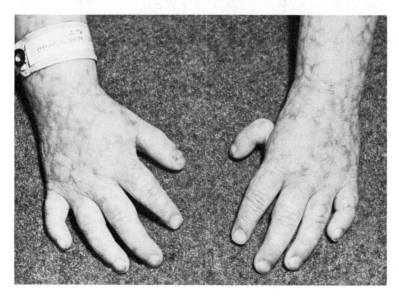

Figure 127-2. Similar involvement of hands with hypoplasia of thumbs. (*From R. K. Oates et al.,* Aust. Paediatr. J. **7**:103, 1971.)

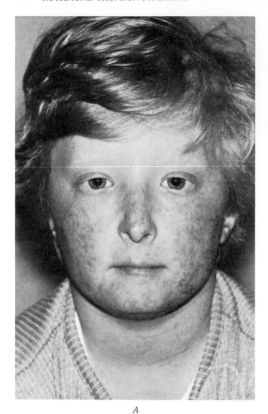 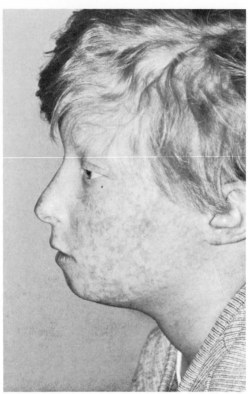

A   B

Figure 127-3. (*A, B*). Similar facial involvement in another patient. (*Courtesy of D. W. Smith, Seattle, Wash.*)

minal phalanges. The dwarfism has been proportionate (2, 5, 6, 13, 15, 21, 23, 24, 26). The limbs are often slender or delicate, and acrocyanosis may be severe.

Absence of thumbs and rudimentary ulnas and radiuses have been noted by Thomson (28, 29) and by Rook et al. (21) (Fig. 127-2). Jäckli (15) described bipartite patella and bone sclerosis. Taylor (27) noted cystic areas similar to fibrous dysplasia.

Eyes. Anterior subcapsular, perinuclear, and posterior stellate cataracts have been described in 50 to 75 percent of the cases (2, 10, 15a, 17, 18, 23, 26, 27). The cataracts are bilateral and usually appear between the fourth and seventh years (18), though they may appear earlier (26). They are complete and semisolid and produce loss of vision within weeks.

Various eye anomalies less frequently encountered include band keratopathy, microcornea, and strabismus (15a).

Oral manifestations. Microdontia, multiple crown malformations, delayed and ectopic eruption, and supernumerary and congenitally missing teeth have been mentioned. Bifid uvula has also been noted (14, 16).

DIFFERENTIAL DIAGNOSIS

A somewhat similar syndrome in adults has been called the *Werner syndrome* (7). It consists of shortness of stature, premature graying of hair (canities), scleropoikiloderma, trophic ulcers of legs, arteriosclerosis, juvenile cataracts, hoarse, high-pitched voice, hypogonadism, osteoporosis,

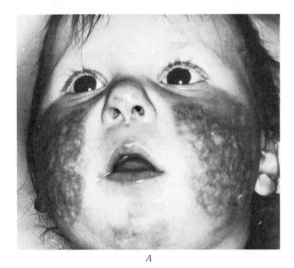

A

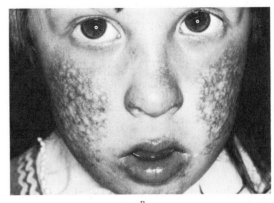

B

Figure 127-4. (*A, B*). Affected two- and four-year-old sibs showing characteristic facial poikiloderma. (*Courtesy of S. Alexander, Barking, Essex, England.*)

and diabetic tendency. It is somewhat more common in males (11) and has autosomal recessive inheritance. There does not appear to be characteristic oral involvement, other than possibly small oral aperture. In contrast to the Rothmund-Thomson syndrome, patients with the Werner syndrome are essentially normal until twenty to thirty years of age, when the hair becomes gray. The skin changes and cataracts develop after the canities has appeared. Shortness of stature and atrophy of muscle and subcutaneous fat of the distal extremities are more pronounced in the Werner syndrome. Arteriosclerosis, diabetic tendency, and osteoporosis are not seen in the Rothmund-Thomson syndrome.

The skin involvement in the Werner syndrome is different from that in the Rothmund-Thomson syndrome. In the former, the forearms, hands, and face are chiefly involved. Hyperkeratotic areas are present on the soles, and ulcers are present over the heels, toes, and ankles.

In *geroderma osteodysplastia* there is premature senescence of the skin, nanism, various anomalies of the eye (including microcornea and congenital corneal opacities), bony anomalies, and yellowish color of the teeth, presumably due to an enamel defect (1).

The *Cockayne syndrome* consists of primordial dwarfism, flexion deformities, kyphosis, hyperostosis of skull bones, sensitivity to sunlight, and various eye anomalies such as optic atrophy, retinal degeneration, and cataract (5, 20, 32). The child appears prematurely senile, with sunken eyes, prognathic mandible, and carious teeth. The *Bloom syndrome* (3) is characterized by dwarfism, sunlight sensitivity, chromosomal breakage, a tendency to develop leukemia and autosomal recessive inheritance.

LABORATORY AIDS

Low vitamin A blood levels have been found by Sexton (25) and Whittle (31). Taylor (27) found an abnormal peak in the α_2-globulin fraction of the blood.

REFERENCES

1 Bamatter, F., et al., Gérodermie ostéodysplastique héréditaire. *Ann. Paediatr.* **174:**126–127, 1950.
2 Bloch, B., and Stauffer, H., Skin Diseases of Endocrine Origin (Dyshormonal Dermatosis). *Arch. Dermatol. Syph.* (*Chic.*) **19:**22–34, 1929.
3 Bloom, D., Congenital Telangiectatic Erythema Resem-

bling Lupus Erythematosus in Dwarfs. Probably a Syndrome Entity. *Am. J. Dis. Child.* **88:**754–758, 1954.

4 Braun, W., and Unger, C., Zur Frage des Rothmund-Thomson Syndroms. *Dermatol. Wochenschr.* **151:** 1189–1198, 1965.

5 Cockayne, E. A., Dwarfism with Retinal Atrophy and Deafness. *Arch. Dis. Child.* **11:**1–8, 1936, and **21:**52–54, 1946.

6 Dowling, C. B., Congenital Developmental Malformations. *Br. J. Dermatol.* **48:**645–647, 1936.

7 Epstein, C. J., et al., Werner's Syndrome. *Medicine (Baltimore)* **45:**177–221, 1966.

8 Feldreich, H.: Poikiloderma Congenitale in Twins. *Acta Derm. Venereol. (Stockh.)* **35:**86–87, 1955.

9 Fischer, H., and Friederich, H., Rothmund-Thomson Syndrom. *Hautarzt* **16:** 359–364, 1965.

10 Franceschetti, A., Les dysplasies ectodermiques et les syndromes héréditaires apparantes. *Dermatologica* **106:** 145–156, 1953.

11 Franceschetti, A., and Maeder, G., Cataracte et affections cutanées du type poikilodermie (syndrome de Rothmund) et du type sclérodermie (syndrome de Werner). *Schweiz. Med. Wochenschr.* **79:**657–663, 1949.

12 Greither, A., and Dyckerhoff, D., Über das Rothmund und das Werner Syndrom. *Arch. Klin. Exp. Dermatol.* **201:**411–445, 1955.

13 Hallman, N., and Patiala, R., Congenital Poikiloderma Atrophicans Vasculare in a Mother and Son. *Acta Derm. Venereol. (Stockh.)* **31:**401–406, 1951.

14 Heuyer, G., et al., Nanisme avec infantilisme, microcephalie, malformations osseuse et cutanées du type de nanisme sénile ou progéria chez deux fréres. *Bull. Soc. Pédiatr.* **34:**159–170, 1936.

15 Jäckli, W., Ein Fall von infantiler Poikilodermie (Atrophodermia reticularis cum Incontinentia pigmenti kombiniert mit Alopecie, Mikrodontie und frühzeitiger Cataracta complicata). *Monatsschr. Kinderheilkd.* **78:**73–81, 1939.

15a Kirkham, T. H., and Werner, E. B., The Ophthalmic Manifestations of Rothmund's Syndrome. *Canad. J. Ophthalmol.* **10:**1–14, 1975.

16 Kraus, B. S., et al., The Dentition in Rothmund's Syndrome. *J. Am. Dent. Assoc.* **81:**894–915, 1970.

17 Lutz, W., Poikiloderma atrophicans. *Schweiz. Med. Wochenschr.* **45:**1118-1119, 1928.

18 Maeder, G., Le syndrome de Rothmund et le syndrome de Werner. *Ann. Ocul. (Paris)* **182:**809–854, 1949.

19 Maurer, R. M., and Langford, O. L., Rothmund's Syndrome: A Cause of Resorption of Phalangeal Tufts and Dystrophic Calcification. *Radiology* **89:**706–708, 1967.

20 McDonald, W. B., et al., Cockayne's Syndrome: A Heredofamilial Disorder of Growth and Development. *Pediatrics* **25:**997–1007, 1960.

21 Rook, A., and Whimster, I., Congenital Cutaneous Dystrophy (Thomson's Type). *Br. J. Dermatol.* **61:**197–205, 1949.

22 Rook, A., et al., Poikiloderma Congenitale: Rothmund-Thomson Syndrome. *Acta Derm. Venereol. (Stockh.)* **39:**392–420, 1959.

23 Rothmund, A., Über Cataracten in Verbindung mit einer eigentümlichen Hautdegeneration. *Albrecht von Graefes Arch. Klin. Ophthalmol.* **14:**159–182, 1868.

24 Schneider, W. F., Über Katarakt im Kindesalter bei gleichzeitigem Vorkommen von Poikilodermia atrophicans. *Schweiz. Med. Wochenschr.* **65:**719–721, 1935.

25 Sexton, G., Thomson's Syndrome. *Can. Med. Assoc. J.* **70:**622–665, 1954.

26 Silver, H. K., Rothmund-Thomson Syndrome: An Oculocutaneous Disorder. *Am. J. Dis. Child.* **111:**182–190, 1966.

27 Taylor, W. B., Rothmund's Syndrome – Thomson's Syndrome. *Arch. Dermatol.* **75:**236–244, 1957.

28 Thomson, M. S., A Hitherto Undescribed Familial Disease. *Br. J. Dermatol.* **35:**455–461, 1923.

29 Thomson, M. S., Poikiloderma Congenitale. *Br. J. Dermatol.* **48:**221–234, 1936.

30 Wahl, J. W., and Ellis, P. P., Rothmund-Thomson Syndrome. *Am. J. Ophthalmol.* **60:**722–726, 1965.

31 Whittle, C. H., Poikiloderma Congenitale (Thomson). *Proc. R. Soc. Med.* **40:**499–500, 1947.

32 Windmiller, J., et al., Cockayne's Syndrome with Chromosomal Analysis. *Am. J. Dis. Child.* **105:**204–208, 1963.

33 Wolfram, C., et al., Zum Werner Syndrom. *Dtsch. Med. Wochenschr.* **84:**2125–2130, 1959.

Rubinstein-Taybi Syndrome

(Broad Thumbs and Great Toes Syndrome)

In 1963, Rubinstein and Taybi (25) observed the constellation of (a) broad thumbs and great toes, (b) growth retardation, (c) mental deficiency, and (d) characteristic facial features. Over 120 cases have been recorded to date (1–5, 8–15, 19–26, 29–32). An extensive review was provided by Rubinstein (23). The incidence in the general population is unknown. In various diagnostic clinics and mental retardation groups, the frequency has ranged from one in 300 to one in 700 individuals. The syndrome has been observed in patients of African and Oriental extraction (24).

Etiology is unknown. No affected individual has reproduced. Almost all cases have been sporadic. Affected sibs were noted by Johnson (11) and Takeuchi (29). Male twins were observed (12, 17a). We have also seen the disorder in female identical twins. Consanguinity was reported in two instances (9, 17). Simpson and Brissenden (26a) reported a recurrence risk of about 1 percent. Normal karyotypes have been observed in almost all cases, although inconsistent chromosomal variations have been noted occasionally (4, 33).

SYSTEMIC MANIFESTATIONS

Major reported medical difficulties include neonatal distress, recurrent respiratory infections, feeding difficulties during infancy, and various allergic states including hay fever, asthma, and eczema (23).

Facies. The facial appearance is striking, with microcephaly, prominent forehead, antimongoloid obliquity of palpebral fissures, epicanthal folds, strabismus, broad nasal bridge, beaked nose with the nasal septum extending below the alae, and mild micrognathia (Fig. 128-1). Grimacing or unusual smile has been observed frequently. Other findings may include long eyelashes, nasolacrimal duct obstruction, ptosis of the eyelids, refractive error, and minor abnormalities in the shape, position, and degree of rotation of the pinnas (1, 2, 5, 21, 24, 25). Various other low-frequency anomalies have been discussed by Rubinstein (23).

Central nervous system. Mental deficiency has been present in all reported cases, the intelligence quotient usually being less than 50 (23, 24). In several cases (13, 25), language and speech were retarded to a greater extent than expected on the basis of IQ. Electroencephalographic abnormalities, seizures, absence of the corpus callosum, and hyperactive deep-tendon reflexes have been noted (16, 23, 24).

Hands and feet. Broad thumbs and great toes have been present in all reported cases (Fig. 128-2). In most instances, the terminal phalanges of the fingers are also broad. Clinodactyly of the fifth fingers and overlapping of the toes

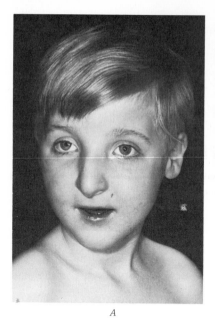

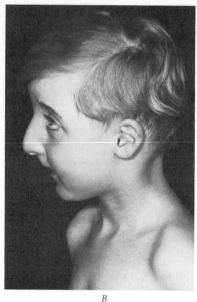

A

B

Figure 128-1. *(A, B). Rubinstein-Taybi syndrome.* Note aquiline nose with broad nasal bridge and septum extending below alae. Head circumference usually reduced below 10th percentile. (*From R. Weiland,* Arch. Kinderheilkd. **179:**78, 1969.)

are present in over half the cases. Angulation deformities of the thumbs and halluces, together with abnormally shaped proximal phalanges, occur in some instances. Abnormally shaped first metatarsals and duplication of the proximal or distal phalanx of the halluces have also been reported. Rarely, hexadactyly of the feet, partial cutaneous syndactyly involving the toes, and absence of the distal phalanx of the hallux have been noted (1–3, 5, 8, 22–25, 30, 31).

Alterations in the frequency of various fingerprint patterns have been observed, but the findings have been inconsistent. Increased frequencies of loops, whorls, or arches have been reported. Significant dermatoglyphic findings have included an increased frequency of thenar, interdigital, and hypothenar patterns. Simian creases have been observed in many cases. Thumb tip triradius, thumb double pattern, distally placed axial triradius, deep plantar crease, and large hallucal loop with laterally displaced f triradius with or without associated e^1 triradius have also been reported (4–7, 19, 22–25, 26a, 27).

Skeletal system. Growth retardation and delayed bone age have been observed. Large anterior fontanel or delay in its closure, large foramen magnum, and parietal foramens have

been reported in some cases. Other skeletal anomalies have included pectus excavatum, other sternal abnormalities, rib defects, scoliosis, kyphosis, lordosis, spina bifida, flat acetabular angles, flaring of ilia, and notched ischia (23, 24). Various other low-frequency anomalies have been discussed by Rubinstein (23).

The gait has been stated to be stiff. Hypotonia, lax ligaments, and hyperextensible joints have also been noted (23, 24).

Genitourinary system. Incomplete or delayed descent of the testes has been reported in most males. Anomalies of the urinary tract, including duplication of the kidney and ureter, renal agenesis, and other abnormalities, have been recorded in a number of cases. Rarely, angulated penis and hypospadias have been noted (2, 21, 27, 31).

Other findings. A variety of congenital heart defects, abnormal lung lobulation, supernumerary nipples, nevus flammeus of the forehead, nape, or back, hirsutism, and other abnormalities have been reported (1, 2, 11, 23, 31, 32).

Oral manifestations. Micrognathia and highly arched palate with malocclusion have been ob-

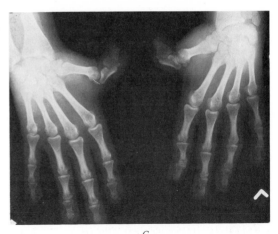

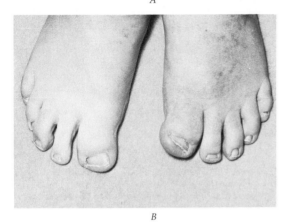

A

B

C

Figure 128-2. (*A*). Broad and radially deviated thumbs. (*B*). Broad and tibially deviated halluces. (*C*). Roentgenogram showing broad short terminal phalanges and triangular proximal phalanges of thumbs. (A, B *from J. M. Berg et al.,* J. Ment. Defic. Res. **10:**204, 1966.)

served in most instances. Low-frequency abnormalities have included bifid uvula, bifid tongue, macroglossia, short lingual frenum, and thin upper lip (2, 9, 23, 26).

DIFFERENTIAL DIAGNOSIS

Although many components of the syndrome may occur as isolated findings or as features of various other syndromes, the overall pattern of anomalies is sufficiently distinctive to permit diagnosis in most instances. The authors have seen numerous patients who have exhibited only some of the stigmata of the Rubinstein-Taybi syndrome. Some of these may represent in-

complete forms, but, because no pathognomonic clinical or laboratory finding has been discovered, questionable cases are probably best not diagnosed as instances of the syndrome at the present time. We cannot, for example, accept the case reported by Spencer (28). The family with broad thumbs and mental deficiency observed by Robinow (18) probably represents a separate condition.

Differential diagnosis has also been a problem in the newborn period. Occasionally, some cases have been confused with the *de Lange syndrome* (12) or with *trisomy 13* (34). Broad thumbs may be observed in the *Apert syndrome* and the *Pfeiffer syndrome,* and short thumbs and fingers are seen in type D brachydactyly.

LABORATORY AIDS

None is known.

REFERENCES

1 Berg, J. M., et al., On the Association of Broad Thumbs and First Toes with Other Physical Peculiarities and Mental Retardation. *J. Ment. Defic. Res.* **10:**204–220, 1966.

2 Coffin, G. S., Brachydactyly, Peculiar Facies, and Mental

Retardation. *Am. J. Dis. Child.* **108**:351–359, 1964.

3 Coffin, G. S., Three Retarded Children with Unusual Face and Hands: A Variant of the Wide-thumbs Syndrome? Symposium 10: Rubinstein-Taybi Syndrome, in B. W. Richards (ed.), *Proceedings, First Congress of the International Association for the Scientific Study of Mental Deficiency*, Montpellier, France, 1967, pp. 600–605.

4 Davison, B. C. C., et al., Mental Retardation with Facial Abnormalities, Broad Thumbs and Toes and Unusual Dermatoglyphics. *Dev. Med. Child Neurol.* **9**:588–593, 1967.

5 Filippi, G., The Rubinstein-Taybi Syndrome: Report of 7 Cases. *Clin. Genet.* **3**:303–319, 1972.

6 Giroux, J., and Miller, J. R., Dermatoglyphics of the Broad Thumb and Great Toe Syndrome. *Am. J. Dis. Child.* **113**:207–209, 1967.

7 Herrmann, J., and Opitz, J. M., Dermatoglyphic Studies in a Rubinstein-Taybi Patient, Her Unaffected Dizygous Twin Sister and Other Relatives. *Birth Defects* **5**(2):22–24, 1969.

8 Jancar, J., Rubinstein-Taybi's Syndrome. *J. Ment. Defic. Res.* **9**:265–270, 1965.

9 Jeliu, G., and Saint-Rome, G., Le syndrome de Rubinstein-Taybi: à propos d'une observation. *Union Med. Can.* **96**:22–29, 1967.

10 Job, J. C., et al., Études sur les nanismes constitutionnels. II. Le syndrome de Rubinstein et Taybi. *Ann. Pédiatr.* **11**:646–650, 1964.

11 Johnson, C. F., Broad Thumbs and Broad Great Toes with Facial Abnormalities and Mental Retardation. *J. Pediatr.* **68**:942–951, 1966.

12 Kroth, H. von, Cornelia de Lange-Syndrom I bei Zwillingen. *Arch. Kinderheilkd.* **173**:273–283, 1966.

13 Kushnick, T., Brachydactyly, Facial Abnormalities and Mental Retardation. Rubinstein-Taybi Syndrome. *Am. J. Dis. Child.* **111**:96–98, 1966.

14 Lamy, M., et al., Le syndrome de Rubinstein-Taybi. *Arch. Fr. Pédiatr.* **24**:472, 1967.

15 McArthur, R. G., Rubinstein-Taybi Syndrome: Broad Thumbs and Great Toes, Facial Abnormalities and Mental Retardation: A Presentation of Three Cases. *Can. Med. Assoc. J.* **96**:462–466, 1967.

16 Neuhäuser, G., Pneumoencephalographic Findings in the Rubinstein-Taybi Syndrome, Symposium 10: Rubinstein-Taybi Syndrome, in B. W. Richards (ed.), *Proceedings, First Congress of the International Association for the Scientific Study of Mental Deficiency*, Montpellier, France, 1967, pp. 615–617.

17 Padfield, C. J., et al., The Rubinstein-Taybi Syndrome. *Arch. Dis. Child.* **43**:94–106, 1967.

17a Pfeiffer, R. A., Rubinstein-Taybi Syndrom bei wahrscheinlich eineiigen Zwillingen. *Humangenetik* **6**:84–87, 1968.

18 Robinow, M., A Familial Syndrome of Mental Deficiency and Broad Thumbs. *Birth Defects* **5**(2):42, 1969.

19 Robinson, G. C., et al., Broad Thumbs and Toes and Mental Retardation: Unusual Dermatoglyphic Observa-

tions in Two Individuals. *Am. J. Dis. Child.* **111**:287–290, 1966.

20 Rohling, B., et al., Rubinstein-Taybi Syndrome. *Am. J. Dis. Child.* **121**:71–74, 1971.

21 Roy, F. H., et al., Ocular Manifestations of the Rubinstein-Taybi Syndrome: Case Report and Review of the Literature. *Arch. Ophthalmol.* **79**:272–278, 1968.

22 Rubinstein, J. H., A Syndrome of Broad Thumbs and First Toes, Mental Retardation, and Characteristic Facial Features—a Follow-up Report, Symposium 10: Rubinstein-Taybi Syndrome, in B. W. Richards (ed.), *Proceedings, First Congress of the International Association for the Scientific Study of Mental Deficiency*, Montpellier, France, 1967, pp. 589–595.

23 Rubinstein, J. H., The Broad Thumbs Syndrome—Progress Report 1968. *Birth Defects* **5**(2):25–41, 1969.

24 Rubinstein, J. H., Broad Thumb-Hallux Syndrome, in D. Bergsma (ed.), *Birth Defects Compendium and Atlas.* National Foundation, Williams & Wilkins, 1973, pp. 218–219.

25 Rubinstein, J. H., and Taybi, H., Broad Thumbs and Toes and Facial Abnormalities. *Am. J. Dis. Child.* **105**:588–603, 1963.

26 Salmon, M. A., The Rubinstein-Taybi Syndrome: A Report of Two Cases. *Arch. Dis. Child.* **43**:102–106, 1968.

26a Simpson, N. E., and Brissenden, J. E., The Rubinstein-Taybi Syndrome. *Am. J. Hum. Genet.* **25**:225–229, 1973.

27 Smith, G. F., and Berg, J. M., Dermatoglyphics in Rubinstein-Taybi Syndrome, Symposium 10: Rubinstein-Taybi Syndrome, in B. W. Richards (ed.), *Proceedings, First Congress of the International Association for the Scientific Study of Mental Deficiency*, Montpellier, France, 1967, pp. 606–612.

28 Spencer, D. A., Partial Rubinstein-Taybi Syndrome. *Lancet* **2**:713–714, 1971.

29 Takeuchi, M., Rubinstein's Syndrome in Two Siblings. *Gann J. Med. Sci.* **15**:17, 1966.

30 Taybi, H., and Rubinstein, J. H., Broad Thumbs and Toes, and Unusual Facial Features: A Probable Mental Retardation Syndrome. *Am. J. Roentgenol.* **93**:362–366, 1965.

31 Taybi, H., Broad Thumbs and Great Toes, Facial Abnormalities, and Mental Retardation Syndrome, Symposium 10: Rubinstein-Taybi Syndrome, in B. W. Richards (ed.), *Proceedings, First Congress of the International Association for the Scientific Study of Mental Deficiency*, Montpellier, France, 1967, pp. 596–599.

32 True, C. W., and Rubinstein, J. H., Pathological Findings in a Case of the Rubinstein-Taybi Syndrome, Symposium 10: Rubinstein-Taybi Syndrome, in B. W. Richards (ed.), *Proceedings, First Congress of the International Association for the Scientific Study of Mental Deficiency*, Montpellier, France, 1967, pp. 613–614.

33 van Gelderen, H. H., et al., Trisomy G/Normal Mosaics in Non-mongoloid Mentally Deficient Children. *Acta Paediatr. Scand.* **56**:517–525, 1967.

34 Wilson, M. G., Rubinstein-Taybi and D₁ Trisomy Syndromes. *J. Pediatr.* **73**:404–408, 1968.

129

Russell-Silver Syndrome

The syndrome of (a) short stature of prenatal onset, (b) triangular facies, (c) asymmetry, (d) variation in the pattern of sexual development, and (e) other abnormalities including café-au-lait pigmentation and clinodactyly was independently described by Silver (16) in 1953 and by Russell (13a) in 1954. Many authors regard the Russell-Silver syndrome as a single entity (7), although Szalay (22) separates the Russell syndrome from the Silver syndrome.

The etiology is unknown. Approximately 70 cases have been reported. Almost all have been sporadic, although a few familial instances have been noted (2, 5, 8). In two instances, the mother was stated to be short. Autosomal dominant inheritance with most cases representing fresh mutations is possible. Monozygotic twins were reported by Rimoin (13). The syndrome has been observed with 45,X/46,XY mosaicism (25) with XXY karyotype (15), and in an 18 trisomy mosaic (9).

SYSTEMIC MANIFESTATIONS

Birth weight is usually less than 2,200 g at full term. The placenta is small (1). Short stature is maintained throughout childhood, height usually being below the 3d percentile level. There is catch-up growth, adult height not being grossly retarded (147 to 153 cm) (7, 13, 23).

Facies. The facies is characterized by pseudohydrocephaly, due to relative smallness of the face, the almost normal-sized calvaria appearing

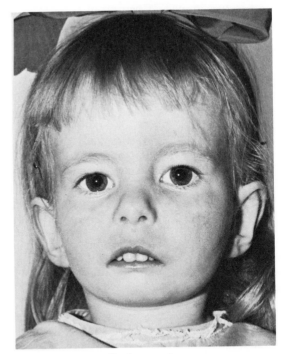

Figure 129-1. *Russell-Silver syndrome.* Pseudohydrocephaly with normal-sized cranium but disproportionately small facial bones. Note downturned angles of mouth. (*Courtesy of A. Russell, London, England.*)

large (4, 20, 23). The forehead is prominent, sometimes bossed, with the face triangular and the chin small and pointed. The corners of the mouth are often turned downward. Appearance becomes markedly less striking with age (20) (Figs. 129-1, 129-2).

Musculoskeletal. Congenital asymmetry has been noted in 65 to 80 percent of patients (1) (Fig. 129-2). While occasionally total, it may involve only the head, trunk, or limbs. Rarely, the asymmetry becomes evident only with growth (17). There are poor muscular development and delay in early gross motor performance.

Delayed closure of the anterior fontanel is common (10). Bone age is usually retarded in relation to sexual development and chronologic age (19, 26). Occasionally, there is hip or elbow dislocation.

The humerus may be somewhat shortened. The fifth fingers are abbreviated and exhibit clinodactyly in over 75 percent of cases (1, 10, 13a, 23) (Fig. 129-3).

Roentgenographically, there is hypoplasia of the middle phalanges of the fifth fingers. Pseudoepiphyses are found more often at the base of the second metacarpal than in the normal population (23). Soft-tissue syndactyly between the second and third toes is seen in about one-third of the cases.

Genital anomalies. Variation in sexual development has been found in over 30 percent of patients (17). There is usually normal puberty (23) and, rarely, cryptorchism (12), enlarged clitoris (21), or hypospadias. Urinary gonadotropin levels have been elevated in about 10 percent of those affected. Curi (3) noted elevation in levels of both FSH and LH. In other cases, there has been premature estrogenation of the urethral or vaginal mucosa (11, 26).

Other findings. Café-au-lait spots have been noted in about 45 percent of cases. Rarely there is mild mental retardation (20). Hyperhidrosis is a common finding (7). Renal and/or ureteral anomalies have been reported (1, 5).

Oral manifestations. Turned-down corners of the mouth have been observed in over 60 percent of patients (17). The maxilla and mandible

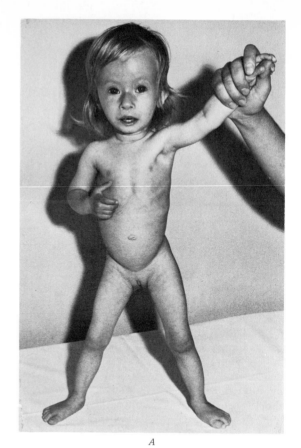

A

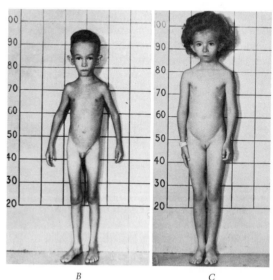

B   *C*

Figure 129-2. (*A–C*). Similar facies. Note leg asymmetry. (A *from* G. Schumacher and H. Niederhoff, Helv. Paediatr. Acta **22:**404, 1967. B, C, *from* R. H. Haslam et al., Pediatrics **51:**216, 1973.)

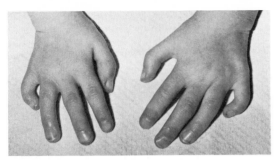

Figure 129-3. Clinodactyly of fifth fingers, noted in over 75 percent of cases. (*Courtesy of A. Russell, London, England.*)

are small, the palate is high and narrow, and the teeth are crowded. The total and posterior cranial base are reduced in length (11, 24).

DIFFERENTIAL DIAGNOSIS

Russell-Silver syndrome is one of a large group of conditions which have been categorized as "intrauterine growth retardation" or "low birth weight dwarfism." Differential diagnosis includes a plethora of conditions with short stature and precocious sexual development (17). Café-au-lait pigmentation may be seen with *neurofibromatosis, hemihypertrophy, McCune-Albright syndrome,* and various vascular abnormalities of the blood vessel or lymphatic system (*Klippel-Trénaunay-Weber syndrome,* lymphedema, etc.).

LABORATORY AIDS

Urinary gonadotropin levels have been elevated in about 10 percent of cases (1, 11, 16, 17). Hypoglycemia following short periods of fasting has been described (7). Relative lack of growth hormone secretion has been discussed (23). An increased number of chromosome breaks has been observed, but this needs confirmation (6, 14).

Pseudohydrocephaly does not merit pneumoencephalographic study (20–22).

REFERENCES

1 Anoussakis, C., et al., Le nanisme congénitale avec dysmorphie crânio-faciale et asymetrie corporelle (type Silver-Russell). *Pédiatrie* **29**:249–260, 1974.

2 Callaghan, K. A., Asymmetrical Dwarfism, or Silver's Syndrome, in Two Male Siblings. *Med. J. Australia* **2**:789–792, 1970.

3 Curi, J. F. J., et al., Elevated Serum Gonadotrophin in Silver's Syndrome. *Am. J. Dis. Child.* **114**:658–661, 1967.

4 Fitch, N., and Pinsky, L., The Lateral Facial Profile of the Russell-Silver Dwarf. *J. Pediatr.* **80**:827–829, 1972.

5 Fuleihan, D. S., et al., The Russell-Silver Syndrome: Report of Three Siblings. *J. Pediatr.* **78**:654–657, 1971.

6 Ganner, E., and Schwingshackl, A., Neigung zu Chromosomenbrüchen bei Russell-Syndrom. *Klin. Wochenschr.* **48**:629–632, 1970.

7 Gareis, F. J., et al., The Russell-Silver Syndrome without Asymmetry. *J. Pediatr.* **79**:775–781, 1971.

8 Gray, O. P., Dwarfism? Cockayne? Russell Type. *Proc. R. Soc. Med.* **52**:304–305, 1959.

9 Haslam, R. H., et al., Renal Abnormalities in the Russell-Silver Syndrome. *Pediatrics* **51**:216–222, 1973.

10 Lässker, G., and Reich, J., Das Russell-Syndrom-eine Form des kindlichen Zwergwuchses. *Arch. Kinderheilkd.* **178**:303–315, 1969.

11 Moseley, J. E., et al., The Silver Syndrome: Congenital Asymmetry, Short Stature and Variations in Skeletal Development. *Am. J. Roentgenol.* **97**:74–81, 1966.

12 Reister, H. C., and Scherz, R. G., Silver Syndrome. *Am. J. Dis. Child.* **107**:410–416, 1964.

13 Rimoin D. L., The Silver Syndrome in Twins. *Birth Defects* **5**(2):183–187, 1969.

13a Russell, A., A Syndrome of "Intra-Uterine" Dwarfism Recognizable at Birth with Cranio-Facial Dysostosis, Disproportionately Short Arms, and Other Anomalies (5 Examples). *Proc. R. Soc. Med.* **47**:1040–1044, 1954.

14 Schwingshackl, A., et al., Familiäres Russellsyndrom. *Pädiat. Pädol.* **9**:130–137, 1974.

15 Severi, F., et al., Comment on Russell-Silver Syndrome. *Pediatrics* **54**:119, 1974.

16 Silver, H. K., et al., Syndrome of Congenital Hemihypertrophy, Shortness of Stature, and Elevated Urinary Gonadotropins. *Pediatrics* **12**:368–376, 1953.

17 Silver, H. K., Asymmetry, Short Stature and Variations in Sexual Development: A Syndrome of Congenital Malformations. *Am. J. Dis. Child.* **107**:495–515, 1964.

18 Spirer, Z., et al., Renal Abnormalities in the Russell-Silver Syndrome. *Pediatrics* **54**:120, 1974.

19 Stool, S., and Cohen, P., Silver's Syndrome. *Am. J. Dis. Child.* **105**:199–203, 1963.

20 Szalay, G. C., Pseudohydrocephalus in Dwarfs: The Russell Dwarf. *J. Pediatr.* **63**:622–633, 1963.

21 Szalay, G. C., Intrauterine Growth Retardation versus Silver's Syndrome. *J. Pediatr.* **64**:234–240, 1964.

22 Szalay, G. C., Russell Dwarf versus Silver Syndrome. *J.*

Pediatr. **80:**1066–1068, 1972.

23 Tanner, J. M., et al., The Natural History of the Silver-Russell Syndrome: A Longitudinal Study of Thirty-nine Cases. *Pediatr. Res.* **9:**611–623, 1975.

24 Taussig, L. M., et al., Silver-Russell Dwarfism and Cystic Fibrosis in a Twin. *Am. J. Dis. Child.* **125:**495–503, 1973.

25 Tulinius, H., et al., 45,X/46,XY Chromosome Mosaic with Features of the Russell-Silver Syndrome. *Dev. Med. Child. Neurol.* **14:**161–172, 1972.

26 Vestermark, S., Silver's Syndrome. *Acta Paediatr. Scand.* **59:**435–439, 1970.

130

Saethre-Chotzen Syndrome

(Acrocephalosyndactyly, Type 3)

S aethre-Chotzen syndrome is characterized by (a) craniosynostosis, (b) low frontal hairline, (c) beaked nose or absent frontonasal angle, (d) ptosis of the eyelids, (e) deviated nasal septum, (f) tear-duct stenosis, (g) dermatoglyphic alterations, and (h) brachydactyly. The syndrome was first recognized and described in 1931 by Saethre (11) and in 1932 by Chotzen (3). A number of other cases have since been reported under a variety of different terms (1, 2, 5-7, 9, 12, 13). The most extensive discussion of the disorder was published by Pantke et al. (8).

The syndrome is transmitted as an autosomal dominant trait with full penetrance and variable expressivity.

The Saethre-Chotzen syndrome is relatively common among craniosynostosis syndromes (8). A large number of unrecognized cases have been found in the literature, but many incompletely documented examples are omitted from the present review.

SYSTEMIC MANIFESTATIONS

Facies. The time of onset and degree of craniosynostosis (most commonly involving coronal sutures) are variable. Involvement is often asymmetric, producing plagiocephaly and facial asymmetry (Fig. 130-1). This appears to be more frequent on the left side. Acrocephaly is most frequently observed, but scaphocephaly has been

noted in some instances. Frontal and parietal bossing and flattened occiput have been reported in various cases. Head circumference is reduced. Low frontal hairline (1-3, 5, 8, 11-13) as well as eyelid ptosis and strabismus are common (3, 8, 12, 13). In some instances, lacrimal duct abnormalities have been noted. Optic atrophy has also been observed (1, 8). Cephalometric study has been carried out by Pruzansky et al. (10).

Nose. The nose tends to be beaked, with deviation of the nasal septum. In some cases, the nasofrontal angle may be flattened (2, 3, 8, 11-13).

Ears. The ears may be low-set, small, or posteriorly rotated, or they may have folded helices or prominent antihelices (1-3, 8). A minor degree of hearing loss is common (2, 3, 8).

Central nervous system. Intelligence is usually normal. However, mild-to-moderate mental retardation has been observed (2, 3, 8). Moderate dilatation of the lateral ventricles has been demonstrated in one case (2). Epilepsy and schizophrenia have also been noted (2, 3, 11).

Hands and feet. Some degree of brachydactyly may be observed (3, 8, 11, 13). Partial cutaneous syndactyly is present in some instances, most frequently between the second and third fingers, but sometimes extending from the second to the fourth fingers (2, 3, 6, 7, 11-13) (Fig. 130-2). Clino-

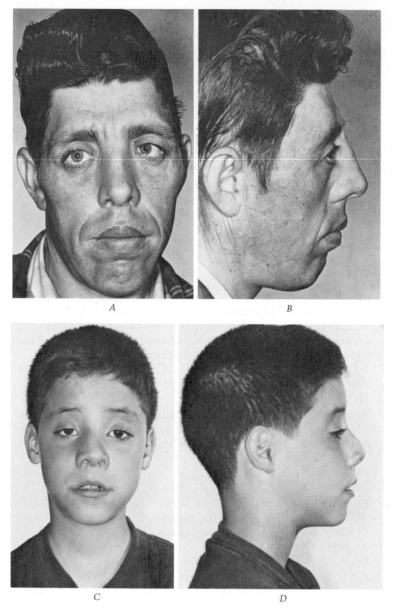

Figure 130-1. *Saethre-Chotzen syndrome.* (*A, B*). Acrocephaly, facial asymmetry, low hairline. (*C, D*). Son of man seen in *A* and *B*. Note eyelid ptosis.

dactyly, especially of the fifth finger, has been noted (1, 8, 11).

Dermatoglyphic findings have included simian creases, distally placed axial triradii, increased frequency of thenar and hypothenar patterns, and low total ridge count (1, 2, 8).

Partial cutaneous syndactyly between the second and third toes, but occasionally involving other toes, has been reported (2, 3, 11). Hallux valgus has been noted in some instances (8, 10).

Skeletal system. Short stature (3, 11), defects of the cervical and lumbar regions of the spine (3, 8, 11), radioulnar synostosis (2), shortened fourth metacarpals (1) have been reported.

Cranial changes include reduced length of

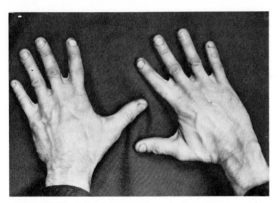

Figure 130-2. Soft-tissue syndactyly between second and third fingers. (*From C. S. Bartsocas et al.*, J. Pediatr. **77**:267, 1967.)

posterior cranial base, low position of sella turcica, steep mandibular plane angle, reduced facial depth, and absence or reduced size of cranial sinuses (4a).

Genitourinary system. Cryptorchism (2, 3, 8) and renal abnormalies (2) have been described.

Cardiovascular system. Congenital heart disease has been noted in two instances (1).

Oral manifestations. Peg-shaped or missing maxillary lateral incisors have been noted in almost half the cases reported by Pantke et al. (8). Narrow or highly arched palate (1–3, 8) and cleft palate (1, 8, 11, 12) have been documented, as well as relative mandibular prognathism, class III malocclusion, and enamel hypoplasia (2, 3, 8).

DIFFERENTIAL DIAGNOSIS

Because syndactyly is not an obligatory anomaly of Saethre-Chotzen syndrome, an isolated case without this finding may be confused with simple craniosynostosis, *Crouzon syndrome, Apert syndrome, Pfeiffer syndrome,* or *Weiss syndrome.* Many cases have been reported as "pseudo-Crouzon syndrome."

LABORATORY AIDS

None is known.

REFERENCES

1 Aase, J. M., and Smith, D. W., Facial Asymmetry and Abnormalities of Palms and Ears: A Dominantly Inherited Developmental Syndrome. *J. Pediatr.* **76**:928–930, 1970.

2 Bartsocas, C. S., et al., Acrocephalosyndactyly Type III: Chotzen's Syndrome. *J. Pediatr.* **77**:267–272, 1970.

3 Chotzen, F., Eine eigenartige familiäre Entwicklungsstörung. (Akrocephalosyndaktylie, Dysostosis craniofacialis und Hypertelorismus.) *Monatsschr. Kinderheilkd.* **55**:97–121, 1932.

4 Cohen, M. M., Jr., An Etiologic and Nosologic Overview of Craniosynostosis Syndromes. *Birth Defects* **11**(2):137–189, 1975.

4a Evans, C. A., and Christiansen, R. L., Cephalic Malformations in Saethre-Chotzen Syndrome. *Radiology,* in press.

5 Gellis, S. S., and Feingold, M., *Atlas of Mental Retardation Syndromes.* U.S. Dept. Health, Education, and Welfare, 1968, p. 26, Figs. 3 and 4.

5a Gordon, I. R. S., et al., Polysynostosis. The Association of Extracranial Synostosis and Craniostenosis. *Clin. Radiol.* **25**:253–259, 1974.

6 Kreiborg, S., et al., The Saethre-Chotzen Syndrome. *Teratology* **6**:287–294, 1972.

7 Moffie, D., Une famille avec oxycéphalie et acrocéphalosyndactylie. *Rev. Neurol.* **83**:306–312, 1950.

8 Pantke, O. A., et al., The Saethre-Chotzen Syndrome. *Birth Defects* **11**(2):190–225, 1975.

9 Pfeiffer, R. A., Associated Deformities of the Head and Hands. *Birth Defects* **5**(3):18–34, 1969.

10 Pruzansky, S., et al., Roentgencephalometric Studies of the Premature Craniofacial Synostoses: Report of a Family with the Saethre-Chotzen Syndrome. *Birth Defects* **11**(2):226–237, 1975.

11 Saethre, H., Ein Beitrag zum Turmschädelproblem. (Pathogenese, Erblichkeit und Symptomatolgie). *Dtsch. Z. Nervenheilkd.* **117**:533–555, 1931.

12 Waardenburg, P. J., Verschillende torenschedelvormen en daarbij vorkomende oogkas- en oogverschijnselen. *Ned. Tijdschr. Geneeskd.* **78**:1700–1705, 1934.

13 Waardenburg, P. J., et al., *Genetics and Ophthalmology,* part 1. Charles C Thomas, Springfield, Ill., 1961.

Seckel Syndrome

(Nanocephalic Dwarfism)

Although Virchow (13) defined nanocephalic dwarfism, the classic study was carried out by Seckel (11) in 1960. The Seckel syndrome is characterized by (*a*) low-birth weight proportionate dwarfism, (*b*) adult head circumference of 39 to 45 cm, with head circumference in newborns being as small as 27 cm, (*c*) mental retardation (less severe than that of the microcephalic idiot), and (*d*) beaklike protrusion of the central part of the face. Probably fewer than 25 well-documented cases have been reported to date.

There have been several cases in sibs (5, 6, 8, 11, 15). In 2 of 13 families there was a history of consanguinity (4). Autosomal recessive inheritance appears likely. The reader is referred to the comprehensive survey of Seckel (11) for a detailed presentation. These patients may represent a heterogeneous group of disorders, some possibly having had Fanconi syndrome (8).

SYSTEMIC MANIFESTATIONS

Gestation is prolonged to 42 weeks or longer and birth weight is usually below 1800 g.

Facies. Beaklike protrusion of the nose, mild antimongoloid obliquity of palpebral fissures, large eyes, and receding chin produce an "Aztec-like" appearance (Fig. 131-1). The eyeballs appear large. The ears are often lobeless.

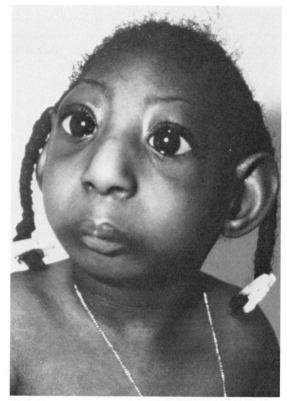

Figure 131-1. *Seckel syndrome.* Characteristic facies, with small head circumference and micrognathia, lending prominence to the midface. *(Courtesy of J. J. Sauk, Minneapolis, Minnesota.)*

Central nervous system. Intelligence rarely surpasses that of the five-year-old level. An intelligence quotient of 70 to 90 is attained at one to two and one-half years of age but decreases to 50 or less by school age. The Seckel dwarf is generally cheerful but rapidly changes moods. Cranial capacity has been estimated to be 400 to 640 ml. Autopsy findings have revealed a small, simplified cerebrum resembling the chimpanzee brain (pongidoid microencephaly).

Skeletal system. Study has shown premature closure of cranial sutures, ocular hypertelorism, zygomatic and mandibular hypoplasia, dislocation of joints (especially radial head and/or hips), kyphoscoliosis, sacralization of lumbar vertebras, absent inferior pubic rami and horizontal ischia, sternal anomalies, incurving of distal phalanges, clubbing of fingers, absence of patella, proximal shortening of the fibula muscle hypotrophy, and hypotonicity. Maximal adult height is less than 120 cm (1a).

In addition to the autopsy findings mentioned above, several patients have had hypoplasia of clavicles, clinodactyly of fingers with hypoplasia of distal phalanges and hypoplastic ribs.

Skin. Abnormalities in pigmentation, hypertrichosis, and anomalous hand creases have been recorded.

Eye, ear, nose, and throat. Antimongoloid obliquity of palpebral fissures, epicanthus, strabismus, absence of anterior chamber, chorioretinopathy, lobeless ears, and bizzare colobomas of the epiglottis have been seen. Strabismus and ocular hypertelorism have been commonly observed (5, 7).

Genitourinary system. Bilateral cryptorchism, clitoromegaly, and other anomalies of the genitalia and urinary tract are common (12). However, normal sexual maturation has been reported to occur.

Oral manifestations. In contrast to the diminished size of the patient, the teeth are of normal size (11). Hypodontia, malalignment, and enamel hypoplasia have been reported. Diminished mandibular size results in a class II malocclusion.

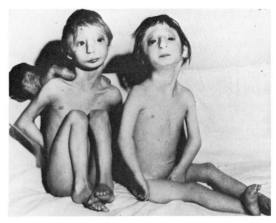

Figure 131-2. *Seckel syndrome (Harper type).* Affected female sibs. (*From R. Harper, et al.* J. Pediatr. **70:**299, 1967.)

High palatal vault and cleft lip and/or palate have also been noted (1a, 5, 10, 14).

DIFFERENTIAL DIAGNOSIS

Intrauterine growth retardation (15) and normocephalic "primordial dwarfism" can be considered in differential diagnosis. *Progeria* is sufficiently different to be excluded easily. A microcephalic idiot resembles a Seckel dwarf in several respects, but the head is disproportionately small in contrast to that of the nanocephalic dwarf and intelligence is more severely retarded. Microcephaly may be an isolated autosomal recessively inherited condition, it may be a component of several syndromes (*cri-du-chat*, phenylketonuria), or it may be due to radiation injury, rubella, cytomegalovirus, etc. The reader is referred to the monograph of Seckel (11) for an excellent discussion of other conditions to be considered, and to that of Cowrie (3) for consideration of the differential diagnosis of microcephaly.

Fitch et al. (4a) reported a child with microcephaly, mental retardation, premature senility (premature greying and loss of scalp hair, wrinkled palmar skin), eyelid ptosis, and cryptorchism. McKusick (personal communication, 1974) examined similarly affected sibs and suggested autosomal recessive inheritance.

LABORATORY AIDS

None is known.

REFERENCES

1 Arons, P., Vogelkopdwergen. *Maandschr. Kindergeneeskd.* **32**:386–394, 1964.

1a Bixler, D., and Antley, R. M., Microcephalic Dwarfism in Sisters. *Birth Defects* **10**(7):161–165, 1974.

2 Black, J., Low Birth Weight Dwarfism. *Arch. Dis. Child.* **36**:633–644, 1961.

3 Cowrie, V., Genetics and Subclassification of Microcephaly. *J. Ment. Defic. Res.* **4**:42–47, 1960.

4 De La Cruz, F. F., Bird-headed Dwarf. *Am. J. Ment. Defic.* **68**:54–62, 1963.

4a Fitch, N., Pinsky, L., and Lachance, R., A Form of Bird-headed Dwarfism with Features of Premature Senility. *Am. J. Dis. Child.* **120**:260–264, 1970.

5 Harper, R. G., et al., Bird-headed Dwarfs (Seckel's Syndrome). *J. Pediatr.* **70**:799–804, 1967.

6 Maass, K., and Virchow, R., Birmesischen Zwerge (mit einem Salzburger Riesen). *Z. Ethnol.* **28**:524–528, 1896.

7 McKusick, V. A., et al., Chorioretinopathy with Hereditary Microcephaly. *Arch. Ophthalmol.* **75**:597–600, 1966.

8 McKusick, V. A., et al., Seckel's Bird-headed Dwarfism. *N. Engl. J. Med.* **277**:279–286, 1967.

9 Panos, T. C., Observations on Siblings with Primordial Dwarfism Associated with Hypersplenism. *Soc. Pediatr. Res.*, 1951, cited by Seckel (11).

10 Sauk, J. J., Familial Bird-headed Dwarfism (Seckel's Syndrome). *J. Med. Genet.* **10**:196–198, 1973.

11 Seckel, H. P. G., *Bird-headed Dwarfs.* Charles C Thomas, Springfield, Ill., 1960 (Cases 1, 2).

12 Szalay, G., Intrauterine Growth Retardation versus Silver's Syndrome. *J. Pediatr.* **64**:234–240, 1964.

13 Virchow, R., Zwergenkind. *Z. Ethnol.* **14**:215, 1882.

14 Virchow, R., Vorstellung des Knaben Dobos Janos. *Berl. Klin. Wochenschr.* **29**:517, 1892.

15 Warkany, J., et al., Intrauterine Growth Retardation. *Am. J. Dis. Child.* **102**:249–279, 1961.

132

Sideropenic Dysphagia

(Plummer-Vinson Syndrome, Paterson-Kelly Syndrome)

The syndrome comprising (*a*) dysphagia and (*b*) hypochromic anemia occurring in women between forty and fifty years of age received its first thorough description in 1919 when Paterson (24) and Kelly (19) independently reported cases. Inspired by an oral communication by Plummer some years before, Vinson (29), in 1922, gave an account of the same disease. Since that time, the condition has been called either "Paterson-Kelly" or "Plummer-Vinson syndrome." However, in 1938–1939, Waldenström (30, 31) suggested "sideropenic dysphagia," a term subsequently widely employed. Ahlbom (1) published an investigation of 150 cases of carcinoma of the upper part of the alimentary tract in women and showed that about 70 percent of them suffered from sideropenic dysphagia.

The syndrome is found almost exclusively in middle-aged women, who have a typically pale, "shrunken" appearance. There is often a history of fatigability, anemia, and difficulty in swallowing, together with a variety of other symptoms. The symptoms usually begin between fifteen and thirty years of age (16). Incomplete forms of the syndrome have been reported in which anemia and other signs have been absent (20). Bothwell and Thomas (6) explained the absence of the anemia by noting that the iron stores have been depleted but that there is enough iron available from the breakdown of red cells to supply erythropoiesis. However, there is insufficient iron to maintain the normal status of the epithelium in the upper part of the alimentary tract.

For many years it was thought that the syndrome was seen only in the United States, England, and Scandinavia. Subsequently, however, the occurrence of the disorder in most European countries and in North and South America was documented (3, 18, 23).

Etiology is unclear, although investigations have clarified the significance of some factors. Waldenström (30, 31) pointed out that iron deficiency was responsible for the various symptoms observed in the syndrome: changes in the mucosa, dysphagia, anemia, angular cheilosis, and koilonychia. He also found improvement of the dysphagia upon iron therapy. This view was bolstered by the studies of Jones (18). On the other hand, Jacobs and Kilpatrick (15) suggested that the syndrome is associated with genetically determined gastric atrophy found in patients with pernicious anemia and that iron deficiency is a secondary feature.

SYSTEMIC MANIFESTATIONS

General appearance. Patients are usually pale, with dry skin and untidy hair. The facial skin is smooth and atrophic, giving the patient a characteristic asthenic appearance. The nails, particularly of the thumb and first three fingers, are brittle and spoon-shaped (koilonychia) (30) (Figs. 132-1, 132-2).

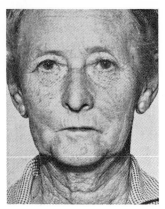

Figure 132-1. *Sideropenic dysphagia* in seventy-year-old woman. Note atrophic skin, asthenic appearance, angular cheilosis, and narrow vermilion border.

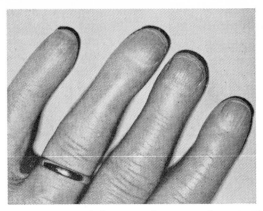

Figure 132-2. Nail changes in the patient shown in Fig. 132-1.

Esophagus. Dysphagia is the outstanding symptom found in all patients (18). Difficulties in swallowing are usually of long duration. Some patients may date the onset of symptoms to choking on a pill. The patient may try to avoid solids and thus becomes subjected to a monotonous diet of soft consistency. Fatigue and blood loss, as from menstruation, seem to aggravate dysphagia. The difficulties in swallowing have been attributed to formation of webs stated to occur at the level of the fifth or sixth cervical vertebra (27). The web has been described as a thin, crescentic membrane usually arising from the anterior esophageal wall. Roentgenographic examination of barium swallowing (31) has revealed a characteristic change in the form of a thin shadow extending from the anterior wall of the esophagus into the barium-distended lumen. Not all patients suffering from dysphagia show roentgenographic changes, and Moersch and Conner (22) found no webs in any of their 65 patients. A comparative study (9) has demonstrated marked differences in the roentgenographic diagnosis of webs by skilled observers, thus casting doubt on the significance of this factor in various surveys. The dysphagia may be relieved by iron therapy (19, 30).

Pharynx. The mucous membrane of the pharynx is drier, shinier, and apparently thinner than normal. Fissures and superficial ulcerations may be present (18). The pharynx may also be the seat of web formation (Fig. 132-3).

Hematology. A hypochromic microcytic anemia with the hemoglobin as low as 30 percent is present in the majority of patients (1, 18, 30). The number of erythrocytes is not correspondingly decreased (31). The serum iron con-

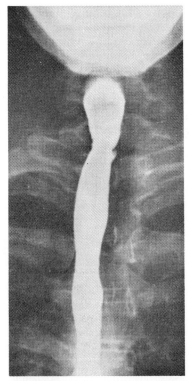

Figure 132-3. Web formation in esophagus in forty-six-year-old woman with sideropenic dysphagia.

centration may be lowered (16). The patients often suffer from achlorhydria.

Other findings. The eyes may be dry and present a burning sensation; the conjunctivas are pale. In the genital region, burning and itching of the vulva have been described (30), as well as atrophy of the vaginal and anal mucosa (11, 27). Splenomegaly has been observed in a number of patients (29). Jones (18) found 23 percent of patients with enlargement of the spleen.

Sideropenic dysphagia as a precancerous condition. The precancerous nature of sideropenic dysphagia was recognized by Paterson in 1931 (25). Subsequently, several references were made to its precancerous nature (32). Ahlbom (1), in 1936, showed definite correlation between sideropenic dysphagia and cancer of the upper part of the alimentary tract in Swedish women, findings later confirmed by several investigators (2, 18). Wynder et al. (35) found the most significant relationship for cancer of the upper and lower regions of the pharynx. Jacobsson (16) found that 35 percent of 126 women with tongue cancer had sideropenia. Eleven of these patients later developed another primary cancer in the upper part of the alimentary tract. In contrast, it should be noted that among 236 Austrian women with cancer in the upper alimentary tract, Laub (21) found fewer than 1 percent suffering from sideropenic dysphagia, and Videbaek (28) found 2.3 percent with the syndrome among 235 Danish women with cancer in the same region.

The precancerous nature of sideropenic dysphagia can also be established when patients with the syndrome are followed over a longer period of time. Thus, several reports have shown a 10 to 50 percent incidence of cancer in the upper alimentary tract. The carcinoma in the majority of cases is located in the postcricoid region of the cervical esophagus. Jones (18) followed 76 cases of sideropenic dysphagia (half of them for more than 10 years) and found that only one developed a postcricoid carcinoma. The low incidence is explained as a result of intensive iron therapy. In Sweden, iron was introduced into bread in 1940, and 20 years later a striking reduction of cases of hypopharyngeal carcinoma was reported (18).

Oral manifestations. Patients suffering from sideropenic dysphagia have a very thin vermilion border of the lip and, often, angular cheilosis. The width of the mouth is narrowed (Fig. 132-4) (20). Patients with this condition are almost always edentulous; however, dentures are poorly tolerated. If teeth are present, they are severely carious. The oral mucosa is pale and atrophic. Characteristic lingual findings are seen in 50 to 70 percent of patients (18). The tongue is

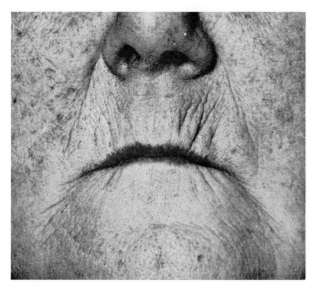

Figure 132-4. Circumoral changes in fifty-seven-year-old woman with sideropenic dysphagia.

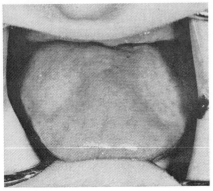

Figure 132-5. Atrophy of tongue papillae and angular cheilosis in patient seen in Fig. 132-1.

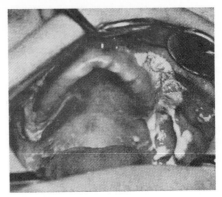

Figure 132-6. Incipient carcinoma in upper left vestibule of patient seen in Fig. 132-1.

smooth, devoid of papillae, usually red (Fig. 132-5), and often painful and edematous. Fissuring of the tongue surface has also been described (7). Dyskeratosis of the oral mucosa has been reported in a number of cases, especially on the dorsum of the tongue (7, 33). The normal papillary pattern of the tongue may be restored by iron therapy (7, 31, 36). The oral changes may also be conceived as a precancerous condition, as mentioned above, and multiple oral carcinomas often develop in patients with sideropenic dysphagia (17) (Fig. 132-6).

PATHOLOGY

Reports concerning the histopathologic findings in the affected mucous membranes have been scarce. In his first paper dealing with the syndrome, Paterson (24) examined histologic sections from the altered buccal mucosa and tongue and found thinning of the superficial epithelium and thickening of the underlying lamina propria. In the tongue, hypopharynx and esophagus, hyperkeratinization of the epithelium with areas of desquamation and atrophic degeneration of the underlying muscle have been noted. In the esophagus, local atrophic changes in the epithelium and marked atrophy of the muscular wall may be seen. The atrophic tongue shows a very thin keratinized layer. The epithelium in the affected regions has shown evidence of increased cellular activity in the basal layers (10, 33). In

the postcricoid region, most webs consist of normal mucosa.

DIFFERENTIAL DIAGNOSIS

Since dysphagia is an outstanding feature, it is important to rule out conditions such as carcinoma and chronic esophagitis that cause dysphagia but are not associated with sideropenia. Angular cheilosis, atrophic glossitis, and nail changes may be found in ariboflavinosis, but dysphagia is lacking. The atrophic glossitis is indistinguishable from that seen in other types of iron deficiency anemias and pernicious anemia. Although the *Sjögren syndrome* has certain features in common with some cases of sideropenic dysphagia (eye changes, dryness of the skin, and atrophic oral mucosa), the latter syndrome never presents articular signs (12). Cricopharyngeal web may be seen in thyroid disease (4).

LABORATORY AIDS

The diagnosis of sideropenic dysphagia is mainly supported by laboratory findings, such as levels of hemoglobin and serum iron. Gastric secretion should also be tested in patients suspected of having the syndrome.

REFERENCES

1 Ahlbom, H. E., Simple Achlorhydric Anaemia, Plummer-Vinson Syndrome and Carcinoma of the Mouth, Pharynx and Oesophagus in Women. *Br. Med. J.* **2**:331–333, 1936.

2 Akerlund, A., and Welin, S., Roentgen Diagnosis of Malignant Tumors within the Boundary Region between the Pharynx and Esophagus. *Acta Radiol.* (*Stockh.*) **25**:883–911, 1944.

3 Beauregard, J. M., et al., La dysphagie sidéropénique. Syndrome dit de Plummer-Vinson. *Union Méd. Can.* **90**:9–15, 1961.

4 Blendis, L. M., et al., The Aetiology of "Sideropenic Web." *Br. J. Radiol.* **38**:112–115, 1965.

5 Botet, J. M. F., Consideration sur le syndrome de Plummer-Vinson. *Ann. Otolaryngol.* (*Paris*) **66**:23–30, 1949.

6 Bothwell, T. H., and Thomas, R. G., Sideropenic Dysphagia. *S. Afr. Med. J.* **32**:614–617, 1958.

7 Cahn, L. R., A Case of Plummer-Vinson Syndrome. *Oral Surg.* **5**:325–329, 1952.

8 Darby, W. J., The Oral Manifestations of Iron Deficiency. *J.A.M.A.* **130**:830–835, 1946.

9 Elwood, P. C., and Pitman, R. G., Observed Error in the Radiological Diagnosis of Paterson-Kelly Webs. *Br. J. Radiol.* **39**:587–589, 1966.

10 Entwistle, C. C., and Jacobs, A., Histological Findings in the Paterson-Kelly Syndrome. *J. Clin. Pathol.* **18**:408–413, 1965.

11 Ezes, H., Syndrome de Plummer-Vinson observé au 7e mois de la grossesse. *Bull. Féd. Soc. Obstét. Gynecol. Fr.* **3**:780–782, 1951.

12 Godtfredsen, E., Relation between Sjögren's Disease, the Plummer-Vinson Syndrome and Ariboflavinosis. *Acta Ophthalmol.* **25**:95–109, 1947.

13 Howell, J. T., and Monto, R. W., Syndrome of Anemia, Dysphagia and Glossitis (Plummer-Vinson Syndrome). *N. Engl. J. Med.* **249**:1009–1012, 1953.

14 Hutton, C. F., Plummer-Vinson Syndrome. *Br. J. Radiol.* **29**:81–85, 1956.

15 Jacobs, A., and Kilpatrick, G. S., The Paterson-Kelly Syndrome. *Br. Med. J.* **2**:79–82, 1964.

16 Jacobsson, F., Carcinoma of the Tongue. *Acta Radiol.* (*Stockh.*) [Suppl.] **68**:1–184, 1948.

17 Jones, R. F., Multiple Primary Malignant Neoplasms in the Upper Respiratory and Alimentary Tracts. *J. Laryngol.* **71**:49–55, 1957.

18 Jones, R. F., The Paterson-Brown Kelly Syndrome: Its Relationship to Iron Deficiency and Postcricoid Carcinoma. I-II. *J. Laryngol.* **75**:529–561, 1961.

19 Kelly, A. B., Spasm at Entrance to the Esophagus. *J. Laryngol.* **34**:285–289, 1919.

20 Kruisinga, R. J. H., and Huizinga, E., The Too Small Mouth in Patients with "Plummer-Vinson" Syndrome. *Ann. Otol. Rhinol. Laryngol.* **68**:115–121, 1959.

21 Laub, R., Ein klinischer Beitrag zum Plummer-Vinsonschen Syndrom. *Acta Otolaryngol.* **26**:668–679, 1938.

22 Moersch, H. J., and Conner, H. M., Hysterical Dysphagia. *Arch. Otolaryngol.* **4**:112–119, 1926.

23 Moutier, F., La dysphagie sidéropénique: du syndrome de Kelly-Paterson (ex syndrome de Plummer-Vinson) au cancer hypopharyngé. *Arch. Mal. App. Dig.* **40**(5):85–87, 1952.

24 Paterson, D. R., A Clinical Type of Dysphagia. *J. Laryngol.* **34**:289–291, 1919.

25 Paterson, D. R., Obstruction at the Upper End of the Oesophagus. *J. Laryngol.* **46**:532–535, 1931.

26 Paterson, D. R., Upper Dysphagia. *J. Laryngol.* **52**:75–86, 1937.

27 Terracol, J., and Sweet, R. H., *Diseases of the Esophagus.* Saunders, Philadelphia, 1958.

28 Videbaek, A., Solitary and Multiple Carcinomas of the Upper Alimentary Tract: Their Location, Age and Sex Incidence and Correlation with the Plummer-Vinson Syndrome. *Acta Radiol.* (*Stockh.*) **25**:339–350, 1944.

29 Vinson, P. P., Hysterical Dysphagia. *Minn. Med.* **5**:107–108, 1922.

30 Waldenström, J., Iron and Epithelium: Some Clinical Observations. *Acta Med. Scand.* [Suppl.] **90**:380–397, 1938.

31 Waldenström, J., and Kjellberg, S. R., The Roentgenological Diagnosis of Sideropenic Dysphagia (Plummer-Vinson's Syndrome). *Acta Radiol.* (*Stockh.*) **20**:618–638, 1939.

32 Wassink, W. F., Voorzetting van het onderzoek betreffende de typologie van vrouwen met kranker van den slokdarmmond. *Ned. Tijdschr. Geneeskd.*, **79**:1491–1492, 1935.

33 Watts, J. McK., The Importance of the Plummer-Vinson Syndrome in the Aetiology of Carcinoma of the Upper Gastro-intestinal Tract. *Postgrad. Med. J.* **37**:523–533, 1961.

34 Welin, S., Diagnostic Radiological Aspects of Hypopharyngeal Cancer. *Br. J. Radiol.* **26**:218–223, 1953.

35 Wynder, E. L., and Fryer, J. H., Etiologic Considerations of Plummer-Vinson (Paterson-Kelly) Syndrome. *Ann. Intern. Med.* **49**:1106–1128, 1958.

36 Wynder, E. L., et al., Environmental Factors in Cancer of the Upper Alimentary Tract: A Swedish Study with Special Reference to Plummer-Vinson (Paterson-Kelly) Syndrome. *Cancer* **10**:470–487, 1957.

133

Sjögren Syndrome

In 1933, Sjögren (33) found xerostomia, pharyngolaryngitis sicca, rhinitis sicca, enlarged salivary glands, and polyarthritis in patients with keratoconjunctivitis sicca. Most authors have employed Sjögren's name to describe the condition, although it had already been described in 1925 by Gougerot (18) and by several still earlier investigators (31). Because of the dryness of several mucous membranes, it has also been called the "sicca syndrome," but some investigators (44) define the sicca syndrome as keratoconjunctivitis sicca and xerostomia with or without salivary gland enlargement, but *not* with rheumatoid arthritis or other connective tissue disease. An animal model in NZB mice has been described (24). An excellent recent review is that of Shearn (31).

The syndrome occurs most frequently in women of middle age, the female-to-male ratio being greater than 9:1. Mean age is about fifty-seven years (45). However, an affected twelve-year-old female has been reported (11). Theories of etiology abound. Jones (22) and Sjögren (35) considered the sicca syndrome an autoimmunopathy, a concept which has been borne out by recent studies demonstrating antibodies in serum of patients with the Sjögren syndrome which react specifically with antigens present in the salivary duct epithelium (3b). These antibodies have been found in 50 to 70 percent of patients (4, 5, 22, 27). Söborg and Bertram (37) demonstrated in vitro that cellular hypersensi-tivity against salivary glands was present in over 60 percent of patients with the syndrome.

The Sjögren syndrome is often associated with other autoimmune disorders. In a series of 62 patients with Sjögren syndrome studied at the National Institutes of Health, 32 had rheumatoid arthritis, and 23 had sicca syndrome without a clinically definable connective tissue disease (8). Similar findings were noted by Whaley et al. (45). Patients with coexisting Sjögren syndrome and systemic lupus erythematosus have been discussed by Steinberg and Talal (38), Whaley et al. (45), and Alarcón-Segovia et al. (3). A similar association has been made in patients with scleroderma, primary biliary cirrhosis, and chronic active hepatitis (3). It has been shown that lacrimal and parotid secretion is significantly reduced in a group of patients with rheumatoid arthritis compared with a group of healthy individuals (13).

In some cases, malignant lymphoma (principally reticulum cell sarcoma) has developed late in the course of the Sjögren syndrome (3a, 26, 40). It is important for the clinician to be aware of this rare complication.

SYSTEMIC MANIFESTATIONS

Facies. There may be unilateral or bilateral enlargement of the parotid salivary glands (Fig. 133-1).

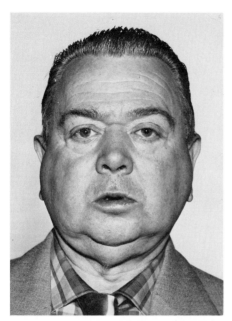

Figure 133-1. *Sjögren syndrome.* Swelling of parotid salivary glands. (*From U. Bertram,* Acta Odontol. Scand. **25:***Suppl.* 49, 1967.)

Eyes. Typical eye changes consist of dryness, burning sensation, and photophobia. The symptoms are caused by failure of the lacrimal and conjunctival glands to maintain adequate secretion. Instead of normal tears, the eye may be covered by a thick, sticky, mucous material which can be drawn out into fine threads. The corneal epithelium is thinner than normal. Ulceration is superficial. Marked ulcerative disease of the conjunctiva and cornea is rare, even in the full-blown syndrome. The lacrimal glands exhibit the same histopathologic changes as the salivary glands (15) and may be enlarged in about 5 percent of cases (45). Tear lysozyme levels are reduced (39).

Other mucous membranes. Dryness of the pharynx and larynx may be experienced, and the nasal passages may be the seat of atrophic rhinitis. Smell is reduced (21). The vagina is dry or atrophic in about 5 percent of female patients (45).

Arthritis. Rheumatoid arthritis is the most commonly recognized extraocular sign. In most surveys, the frequency of arthritis is about 40 to 60 percent (8, 20, 24). Those with rheumatoid arthritis are more frequently males (39). Silberger and Peterson (32) emphasized juxtaarticular bone destruction.

Other findings. Numerous other associated symptoms have been described, including weakness and fatigue, myopathy, loss of weight, dryness of skin, mental disturbances, purpura, chronic or recurrent pulmonary infection, dysphagia, gastrointestinal disturbances, thyroid disease, Raynaud phenomenon, and lymphadenopathy (10, 40). Peripheral neuropathy, involving the trigeminal nerve, has been reported by several authors (23). Interstitial nephritis is common (43).

ORAL MANIFESTATIONS

Oral Cavity. Next to eye symptoms, the chief complaint is dry mouth and lack of saliva (xerostomia) in about 50 percent of patients (45). The symptoms have often been present over a long period of time. The dryness often leads to disturbances in speaking (dysphonia), swallowing (dysphagia), and masticating. Since most of the patients are edentulous, such dry mucous membranes produce great problems in wearing dentures. Small, sticky, ropy accumulations of saliva may be seen on the oral mucosa, particularly on the dorsum of the tongue. The sense of taste is reduced (21). Clinically, the oral mucosa is often so dry that the mirror used for the oral examination sticks to the buccal mucosa. The color of the mucosa may vary from pale pink to fiery red, giving an atrophic appearance (4).

On the dorsum of the tongue, a sequence of changes occurs (4). At first the tongue is dry and slightly furrowed. Later, marked atrophy of the papillae is noted. After many years, the surface of the tongue characteristically becomes smooth and lobulated (Fig. 133-2). According to Bertram et al. (7), this can be an important diagnostic sign.

Angular cheilosis is often observed. In many cases the cheilosis is combined with dryness of

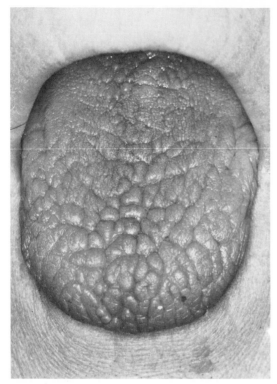

Figure 133-2. Characteristic lobulation of dorsum of tongue. (*From U. Bertram*, Acta Odontol. Scand. **25:***Suppl.* 49, 1967.)

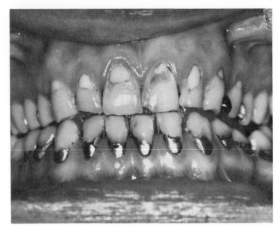

Figure 133-3. Extensive cervical dental caries. (*From U. Bertram*, Acta Odontol. Scand. **25:***Suppl.* 49, 1967.)

Cylindric peripheral sialectasis, the most prevalent pattern, represents a criterion for early diagnosis of the syndrome. It should be pointed out, however, that sialectasis is not pathognomonic for the Sjögren syndrome and may be seen in the lips. This symptom may be noticed long before the development of xerostomia (12).

If a patient has teeth at the onset of the syndrome, rapid carious destruction is likely to follow, for without the cleansing, diluting, and buffering action of saliva, food debris accumulates around the cervices of the teeth, with resultant cervical caries (Fig. 133-3).

Salivary glands. According to Bertram (4), swelling of the parotid glands is observed in two-thirds of the patients (Fig. 133-1). Our experience, like that of Chisholm and Mason (9), suggests that about 30 percent of patients have salivary gland enlargement. The swelling is most often unilateral, nontender, and putty-like in consistency. Swelling is frequently intermittent. Sialography may be used to demonstrate the characteristic sialectatic changes in the glands (9, 17, 32) (Fig. 133-4). Peripheral sialectasis has been found in about 95 percent of cases (17).

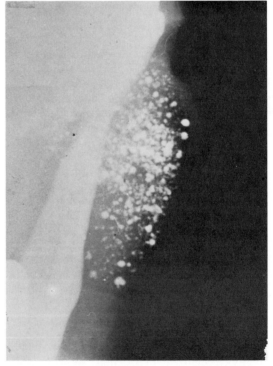

Figure 133-4. Sialogram showing sialectasia. (*From U Bertram*, Acta Odontol. Scand. **25:***Suppl.* 49, 1967.)

other chronic inflammatory conditions of the parotid glands.

PATHOLOGY

Three types of histopathologic changes are found in the salivary glands as described by Wohl and Bloch (47): (a) Infiltration with lymphocytes may be so extensive as to replace lobules of the gland. However, the lobular architecture is preserved. (b) Atrophy and partial or complete disappearance of secretory acini, which is generally parallel to the extent of the lymphoid infiltration. (c) Proliferation of epithelial and epimyoepithelial lining of the duct walls. This change, when fully developed, leads to formation of epimyoepithelial islands. The minor salivary glands, particularly those in the lower labial mucosa and nasal mucous membrane, present similar alterations (6, 29a). Plasma cells, found in mild cases, are replaced by lymphocytes in severe cases (18a). The ultrastructural changes in the acinar cells consist of decreased number of secretory granules and endoplasmic reticulum. Some acinar cells contain droplets and amorphous material which probably represent neutral fat and necrotic debris (25). Ultrastructural studies have also been carried out both before and after immunosuppressive therapy (29).

DIFFERENTIAL DIAGNOSIS

Xerostomia may occur as a result of drugs, radiation, etc. (4).

Because of the inconstant picture of the Sjögren syndrome, differential diagnosis may be difficult. Swelling of the parotid and lacrimal glands is seen in Mikulicz disease, which may be a variant of the Sjögren syndrome. This concept was strongly supported by the so-called benign lymphoepithelial lesion of Godwin, because this latter condition is histologically similar to that observed in Sjögren and Mikulicz disease. In *Heerfordt syndrome*, the parotid glands are enlarged, but lacrimation is normal. Eye changes consist of iritis (28). The Sjögren syndrome also has a number of signs, such as dryness and atrophy of the upper part of the alimentary tract, achylia, and anemia, in common with *Plummer-Vinson syndrome*. Simultaneous occurrence of Plummer-Vinson syndrome and Sjögren syndrome has been described (16). Isolated absence of lacrimal secretion may be developmental (36).

LABORATORY AIDS

The syndrome is associated with leukopenia in one-third of the patients. Nearly all have hypergammaglobulinemia. Some exhibit macroglobulinemia (4). Immunoelectrophoresis shows diffuse increase in concentration of IgA, IgG, and IgM (14, 19, 45) which may lead to hyperviscosity (8a). Most patients have rheumatoid factor in their serum (24, 47).

Talal et al. (41) found an increase in B lymphocytes and a decrease in T lymphocytes in the peripheral blood and a mixed infiltrate in salivary gland tissues.

A quantitative estimate of lacrimal gland secretion using the Schirmer test may be helpful (7). Keratoconjunctivitis sicca can be diagnosed by use of rose bengal or fluorescein, a positive result being highly suggestive of, but not pathognomonic for, Sjögren syndrome (33).

Immunofluorescence technique employed on sections of salivary gland tissue using serum from patients with Sjögren syndrome reveals cytoplasmic fluorescence in the salivary gland ducts and nuclear fluorescence.

The deficiency of salivary secretions may be measured by sialometry, the majority having values between 0 and 0.2 ml per 15 minutes (4, 9). Scintillation scanning utilizing a radioisotope of technetium has been used to demonstrate decreased salivary glandular function (1, 2, 9, 30).

Labial salivary gland biopsy has also been employed to demonstrate acinar atrophy, focal lymphocytic sialadenitis, and ductal hyperplasia in over 70 percent of patients with Sjögren syndrome. There is correlation between severity of ocular findings and labial histology (39). About 20 percent of individuals with rheumatoid arthritis exhibit focal lymphocytic adenitis of labial salivary glands (9). Tarpley (42) and Whaley et al. (44) noted correlation of symptoms with presence or absence of antisalivary duct antibody.

REFERENCES

1 Abramson, A. L., et al., Sjögren Syndrome: Additional Diagnostic Tools. *Arch. Otolaryngol.* **88**:91–94, 1968.

2 Alarcón-Segovia, D., et al., Radioisotopic Evaluation of Salivary Gland Dysfunction in Sjögren's Syndrome. *Am. J. Roentgenol.* **112**:373–379, 1971.

3 Alarcón-Segovia, D., et al., Sjögren's Syndrome in Systemic Lupus Erythematosus. *Ann. Intern. Med.* **81**:577–583, 1974.

3a Anderson, L. G., and Talal, N., The Spectrum of Benign to Malignant Lymphoproliferation in Sjögren's Syndrome. *Clin. Exp. Immunol.* **10**:199–221, 1972.

3b Anderson, L. G., et al., Cellular-versus-Humoral Autoimmune Responses to Salivary Gland in Sjögren's Syndrome. *Clin. Exp. Immunol.* **13**:335–342, 1973.

4 Bertram, U., Xerostomia. *Acta Odontol. Scand.* **25**:Suppl. 49, Copenhagen, 1967.

5 Bertram, U., and Halberg, P., A Specific Antibody against the Epithelium of the Salivary Ducts in Sera from Patients with Sjögren's Syndrome. *Acta Allergol.* (*Kbh.*) **19**:458–466, 1964.

6 Bertram, U., and Hjörting-Hansen, E., Punch-biopsy of Minor Salivary Glands in the Diagnosis of Sjögren's Syndrome. *Scand. J. Dent. Res.* **78**:295–300, 1970.

7 Bertram, U., et al., On Sjögren's Syndrome with Special Reference to Oral Symptoms. *Ugeskr. Laeger* **123**:1085–1092, 1961.

8 Bloch, K. J., et al., Sjögren's Syndrome. *Arthritis Rheum.* **3**:287–297, 1960.

8a Blaylock, W. M., et al., Sjögren's Syndrome: Hyperviscosity and Intermediate Complexes. *Ann. Intern. Med.* **80**:27–34, 1974.

9 Chisholm, D. M., and Mason, D. K., Salivary Gland Function in Sjögren's Syndrome. *Br. Dent. J.* **135**:393–399, 1973.

10 Denko, C. W., and Old, J. W., Myopathy in the Sicca Syndrome (Sjögren's Syndrome). *Am. J. Clin. Pathol.* **51**:631–637, 1969.

11 Duncan, H., et al., Sjögren's Syndrome in Childhood: Report of a Case. *Henry Ford Hosp. Med. J.* **17**:35–42, 1962.

12 Ehrlich, J. C., and Greenberg, D., Sicca Syndrome: Gougerot-Sjögren Disease. *Arch. Intern. Med.* **93**:731–741, 1954.

13 Ericson, S., and Sundmark, E., Studies on the Sicca Syndrome in Patients with Rheumatoid Arthritis. *Acta Rheumatol. Scand.* **16**:60–80, 1970.

14 Fischer, C. J., et al., Sjögren's Syndrome: Electrophoretic and Immunological Observations on Serum and Salivary Proteins of Man. *Arch. Oral Biol.* **13**:257–270, 1968.

15 Font, R. L., et al., Benign Lymphoepithelial Lesion of the Lacrimal Gland and Its Relationship to Sjögren's Syndrome. *Am. J. Clin. Pathol.* **48**:365–376, 1967.

16 Godtfredsen, E., Relation between Sjögren's Disease, the Plummer-Vinson Syndrome and Ariboflavinosis. *Acta Ophthalmol.* (*Kbh.*) **25**:95–109, 1947.

17 Gonzales, L., et al., Parotid Sialography in Sjögren's Syndrome. *Radiology* **97**:91–93, 1970.

18 Gougerot, M., Insuffisance progressive et atrophie des glandes salivares et muqueuses de la bouche des conjonctives (et parfois des muqueuses nasale, laryngée, vulvaire). *Bull. Soc. Fr. Dermatol. Syphiligr.* **32**:376–379, 1925.

18a Greenspan, J. S., et al., The Histopathology of Sjögren's Syndrome in Labial Salivary Gland Biopsies. *Oral Surg.* **37**:217–229, 1974.

19 Gumpel, J. M., and Hobbs, J. R., Serum Immune Globulins in Sjögren's Syndrome. *Ann. Rheum. Dis.* **29**:681–683, 1970.

20 Heaton, J. M., Sjögren's Syndrome and Systemic Lupus Erythematosus. *Br. Med. J.* **1**:466–469, 1959.

21 Henkin, R. T., et al., Abnormalities of Taste and Smell in Sjögren's Syndrome. *Ann. Intern. Med.* **76**:375–383, 1972.

22 Jones, B. R., Lacrimal and Salivary Precipitating Antibodies in Sjögren's Syndrome. *Lancet* **11**:773–776, 1958.

23 Kaltreider, H. B., and Talal, N., The Neuropathy of Sjögren's Syndrome: Trigeminal Nerve Involvement. *Ann. Intern. Med.* **70**:751–762, 1969.

24 Kessler, H. S., A Laboratory Model for Sjögren's Syndrome. *Am. J. Pathol.* **52**:671–686, 1968.

25 Kitamura, T., et al., Parotid Gland of Sjögren's Syndrome. *Arch. Otolaryngol.* **91**:64–70, 1970.

26 Kuffer, R., and Szpirglas, H., Syndrome de Gougerot-Sjögren et hémopathies lymphoïdes. *Rev. Stomatol.* (*Paris*) **73**:318–323, 1972.

27 Nacsween, R. N. M., et al., Occurrence of Antibody to Salivary Duct Epithelium in Sjögren's Disease, Rheumatoid Arthritis and Other Arthritides. *Ann. Rheum. Dis.* **26**:402–411, 1967.

28 Morgan, A. D., and Raven, R. W., Sjögren's Syndrome: A General Disease. *Br. J. Surg.* **40**:154–162, 1952–1953.

29 Pirsig, W., and Donath, K., Zur Ultrastructur der Parotis beim Sjögren-Syndrom vor und nach immunosuppresiver Therapie. *Arch. Klin. Exp. Ohren Nasen Kehlkopfheilkd.* **201**:309–323, 1972.

29a Powell, R. D., et al., Nasal Mucous Membrane Biopsy in Sjögren's Syndrome. *Ann. Intern. Med.* **81**:25–31, 1974.

30 Schall, G., et al., Xerostomia in Sjögren's Syndrome. *J.A.M.A.* **216**:2109–2116, 1971.

31 Shearn, M. H., *Sjögren's Syndrome.* Saunders, Philadelphia, 1971.

32 Silberger, M. L., and Peterson, C. C., Sjögren's Syndrome: Its Roentgenographic Features. *Am. J. Roentgenol.* **100**:554–558, 1967.

33 Sjögren, H., Zur Kenntnis der Keratoconjunctivitis sicca. *Acta Ophthalmol.* (*Kbh.*) [Suppl.] **2**, 1933.

34 Sjögren, H., Zur Kenntnis der Keratoconjunctivitis sicca. VI. Das Siccasyndrom und ähnliche Zustände: Dacryosialo-adenopathia atrophicans. *Acta Ophthalmol.* (*Kbh.*) **18**:369–382, 1940.

35 Sjögren, H., Some New Investigations Concerning the Sicca-Syndrome. *Acta Ophthalmol.* (*Kbh.*) **39**:619–622, 1961.

36 Sjögren, H., and Eriksen, A., Alacrima Congenita. *Br. J. Ophthalmol.* **34**:691–694, 1950.

37 Söborg, M., and Bertram, U., Cellular Hypersensitivity in Sjögren's Syndrome. *Acta Med. Scand.* **184**:319–322, 1968.

38 Steinberg, A., and Talal, N., The Coexistence of Sjögren's Syndrome and Systemic Lupus Erythematosus. *Ann. Intern. Med.* **74**:55–61, 1971.

39 Tabbara, K. F., et al., Sjögren's Syndrome: A Correlation Between Ocular Findings and Labial Salivary Gland His-

tology. *Trans. Am. Acad. Ophthalmol. Otolaryngol.* **78:**OP467–478, 1974.

40 Talal, N., et al., Extra Salivary Lymphoid Abnormalities in Sjögren's Syndrome (Reticulum Cell Sarcoma, "Pseudolymphoma," Macroglobulinemia). *Am. J. Med.* **43:**50–65, 1967.

41 Talal, N., et al., T and B Lymphocytes in Peripheral Blood and Tissue Lesions in Sjögren's Syndrome. *J. Clin. Invest.* **53:**180–189, 1973.

42 Tarpley, T. M., Jr., Minor Salivary Gland Involvement in Sjögren's Syndrome. *Oral Surg.* **37:**64–74, 1974.

43 Tu, W. H., et al., Interstitial Nephritis in Sjögren's Syndrome. *Ann. Intern. Med.* **69:**1163–1170, 1968.

44 Whaley, K., et al., Salivary Duct Antibody in Sjögren's Syndrome: Correlation with Focal Sialoadenitis in the Labial Mucosa. *Clin. Exp. Immunol.* **4:**273–282, 1969.

45 Whaley, K., et al., Sjögren's Syndrome. *Q. J. Med.* **42:**279–304, 513–548, 1973.

46 Whitehouse, A. C., et al., Macroglobulinemia and Vasculitis in Sjögren's Syndrome. *Am. J. Med.* **43:**609–619, 1967.

47 Wohl, M. J., and Bloch, K. J., Sjögren's Syndrome. *Postgrad. Med.* **45:**108–111, 1969.

134

Smith-Lemli-Opitz Syndrome

In 1964, Smith et al. (27) described a syndrome consisting of (*a*) broad nasal tip with anteverted nostrils, (*b*) ptosis of the eyelids, (*c*) slanted, low-set pinnas, (*d*) micrognathia, (*e*) broad maxillary alveolar ridges, (*f*) cutaneous syndactyly of the second and third toes, (*g*) hypospadias and cryptorchism, (*h*) growth retardation, and (*i*) mental deficiency. Over 40 cases have been reported to date (1, 2, 4–7, 9–18, 22–29). The diagnosis of some cases is questionable (8, 25). Males have been reported far more frequently than females, but this probably reflects ascertainment bias of the genital anomaly. The syndrome has rarely been described in adults (7a, 13).

The syndrome has autosomal recessive inheritance. Affected sibs (1, 1a, 2a, 5, 6, 13a, 15, 22, 25, 27) have been reported. Parental consanguinity has been noted in only a few instances (3, 19), suggesting that the disorder may be relatively common in the general population. Thus, the frequency of heterozygous carriers in the population may be high, which could explain the affected first cousins reported by Dallaire (5).

SYSTEMIC MANIFESTATIONS

Decreased fetal movements and breech presentation are encountered in some cases. Birth weight may be less than 2,500 g in approximately 30 percent of the cases. During the neonatal period, vomiting with variable frequency, irritability generally associated with intense, prolonged and high-pitched screaming, failure to thrive, and resultant short stature are characteristic (22, 24, 27).

Facies. The facial appearance may be quite striking, with microcephaly, eyelid ptosis, strabismus, epicanthal folds, upturned nares, broad nasal tip, micrognathia, low-set and/or slanted pinnas, and short neck (5, 22, 27). Cataracts have been noted in some instances (4, 9, 23). Occasionally, findings such as plagiocephaly, ocular hypertelorism, mild antimongoloid slant, and minor ear anomalies have been described (2, 22) (Fig. 134-1*A, B*).

Central nervous system. During the neonatal period, hypotonicity may be followed by hypertonicity. All patients exhibit mental deficiency. Ventricular dilatation, abnormal electroencephalographic findings, epilepsy, partial agenesis of the cerebellar vermis and/or corpus callosum, and hypoplasia of the frontal lobes have been reported (2, 2a, 22, 24, 25).

Hands and feet. Camptodactyly and rudimentary postaxial polydactyly may be observed in some instances. Simian creases are common. An increased number of digital whorls has been reported, although increased arches may be observed, especially when severe camptodactyly is present. Occasionally, the axial triradius may be distally placed (2, 5, 22).

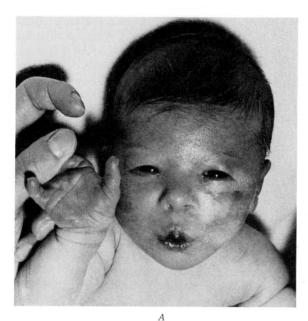
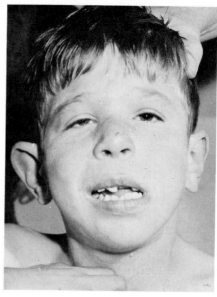

A   B

Figure 134-1. *Smith-Lemli-Opitz syndrome.* (*A*). Ptosis of eyelids, epicanthal folds, broad nasal tip, anteverted nostrils, and micrognathia. Note simian crease. (*From H. Schumacher,* Z. Kinderheilkd. **105**:88, 1969.) (*B*). Ptosis of eyelids, broad nasal tip, anteverted nostrils, and asymmetric, low-set pinnas. (*From C. G. Judge et al.,* Med. J. Aust. **2**:145, 1971.)

Cutaneous syndactyly between the second and third toes is common (Fig. 134-2). Metatarsus adductus, pes equinovarus, metatarsus varus, and other anomalies have been observed (5, 12, 22, 27).

Other findings have included clinodactyly of fingers, hallucal hammertoe, short fingers and toes, and proximally placed thumbs (2, 22, 24, 27).

Genitalia. In affected males, the genitalia may range from relative normality with descended but small testes to severe perineoscrotal hypospadias with perineal urethral opening, cleft scrotum, and bilateral cryptorchism (22) (Fig. 134-3).

Other findings. Sacral dimple and a deep cutaneous pit anterior to the anus have been re-

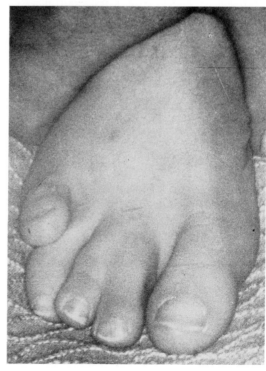

Figure 134-2. Soft-tissue syndactyly of second and third toes. Note short fifth toes with tibial clinodactyly. (*From C. G. Judge et al.,* Med. J. Aust. **2**:145, 1971.)

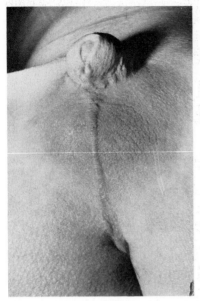

Figure 134-3. Hypospadias and hypoplastic scrotum. (*From C. G. Judge et al.,* Med. J. Aust. **2**:145, 1971.)

ported (27). Cardiovascular anomalies have included patent ductus arteriosus, ventricular septal defect, tetralogy of Fallot, and aberrant right subclavian artery (4, 5, 12, 22, 23, 24a).

Pyloric stenosis (4, 22) and renal abnormalities (12, 22) have been noted. Occasional findings have included dislocated hips, coxa valga, cubitus valgus, premature fusion of sternal ossification centers, short terminal phalanges secondary to stippled epiphyses, widely spaced nipples, and inguinal hernia (2, 11, 12, 25).

Oral manifestations. The maxillary alveolar ridges are broad. The palate may be highly arched, and in some cases, cleft palate or bifid uvula may occur (5, 7a).

DIFFERENTIAL DIAGNOSIS

The syndrome may occasionally be confused with the *Meckel syndrome* or *trisomy 13.* Differential diagnosis and discussion of the spurious entity known as the Ullrich-Feichtiger syndrome have been especially well discussed by Opitz and Howe (21).

LABORATORY AIDS

None is known.

REFERENCES

1 Blair, H. R., and Martin, J. K., A Syndrome Characterized by Mental Retardation, Short Stature, Craniofacial Dysplasias, and Genital Anomalies Occurring in Siblings. *J. Pediatr.* **69**:457–459, 1966.

1a Bundey, S., and Smyth, H. G., Three Sisters with the Smith-Lemli-Opitz Syndrome. *J. Ment. Defic. Res.* **18**:51–61, 1974.

2 Chakanovskis, J. E., and Sutherland, G. R., The Smith-Lemli-Opitz Syndrome in a Profoundly Retarded Epileptic Boy. *J. Ment. Defic. Res.* **15**:153–161, 1971.

2a Cherstroy, E. D., et al., The Pathological Anatomy of the Smith-Lemli-Opitz Syndrome. *Clin. Genet.* **7**:382–387, 1975.

3 Chicoine, L., cited by L. Dallaire, Syndrome of Retardation with Urogenital and Skeletal Anomalies (Smith-Lemli-Opitz Syndrome). *J. Med. Genet.* **6**:113–120, 1969.

4 Cotlier, E., and Rice, P., Cataracts in the Smith-Lemli-Opitz Syndrome. *Am. J. Ophthalmol.* **72**:955–959, 1971.

5 Dallaire, L., Syndrome of Retardation with Urogenital and Skeletal Anomalies (Smith-Lemli-Opitz Syndrome): Clinical Features and Mode of Inheritance. *J. Med. Genet.* **6**:113–120, 1969.

6 Dallaire, L., and Fraser, F. C., The Syndrome of Retardation with Urogenital and Skeletal Anomalies in Siblings. *J. Pediatr.* **69**:459–460, 1966.

7 Dallaire, L., and Fraser, F. C., The SLO Syndrome of Retardation, Urogenital and Skeletal Anomalies. *Birth Defects* **5**(2):180–182, 1969.

7a Deaton, J. G., and Mendoza, L. O., Smith-Lemli-Opitz Syndrome in a 23-year-old Man. *Arch. Intern. Med.* **132**:422–426, 1973.

8 Fine, R. N., et al., Smith-Lemli-Opitz Syndrome. *Am. J. Dis. Child.* **115**:483–488, 1968.

9 Finley, S. C., et al., Cataracts in a Girl with Features of the Smith-Lemli-Opitz Syndrome. *J. Pediatr.* **75**:706–707, 1969.

10 Gellis, S. S., and Feingold, M., Smith-Lemli-Opitz Syndrome. *Am. J. Dis. Child.* **115**:603, 1968.

11 Gibson, R., A Case of the Smith-Lemli-Opitz Syndrome of Multiple Congenital Anomalies in Association with Dysplasia Epiphysialis Punctata. *Can. Med. Assoc. J.* **92**:574–575, 1965.

12 Hanissian, A. S., and Summitt, R. L., Smith-Lemli-Opitz Syndrome in a Negro Child. *J. Pediatr.* **74**:303–305, 1969.

13 Hoefnagel, D., et al., The Smith-Lemli-Opitz Syndrome in an Adult Male. *J. Ment. Defic. Res.* **13**:249–257, 1969.

13a Johnson, V. P., Smith-Lemli-Opitz Syndrome. Review and Report of Two Affected Siblings. *Z. Kinderheilkd.* **119**:221–234, 1975.

14 Judge, C. G., et al., The Smith-Lemli-Opitz Syndrome. *Med. J. Aust.* **2**:145–147, 1971.

15 Kenis, H., and Hustinx, Th. W. J., A Familial Syndrome of Mental Retardation in Association with Multiple Congenital Anomalies Resembling the Syndrome of Smith-Lemli-Opitz. *Maandschr. Kindergeneeskd.* **35**:37–48, 1967.

16 Kiss, P., Smith-Lemli-Opitz Syndroma. *Gyermekgyógyászat (Budapest)* **21**:95–99, 1970.

17 Kunze, J., Das Ullrich-Feichtiger-Syndrom. *Arch. Kinderheilkd.* **179**:182–186, 1969.

18 Lowry, R. B., et al., Micrognathia, Polydactyly and Cleft Palate. *J. Pediatr.* **72**:859–861, 1968.

18a Metzke, H., et al., Das Smith-Lemli-Opitz Syndrom. *Pädiatr. Pädiol.* **7**:259–266, 1972.

19 Nevo, S., et al., Smith-Lemli-Opitz Syndrome in an Inbred Family. *Am. J. Dis. Child.* **124**:431–433, 1972.

20 Opitz, J. M., Personal communication, 1972.

21 Opitz, J. M., and Howe, J. J., The Meckel Syndrome (Dysencephalia splanchnocystica, the Gruber Syndrome). *Birth Defects* **5**(2):167–179, 1969.

22 Opitz, J. M., et al., The RSH Syndrome. *Birth Defects* **5**(2):43–52, 1969.

23 Park, S. C., et al., Congenital Heart Disease in an Infant with the Smith-Lemli-Opitz Syndrome. *J. Pediatr.* **73**:896–902, 1968.

24 Pinsky, L., and DiGeorge, A. M., A Familial Syndrome of Facial and Skeletal Anomalies Associated with Genital Abnormality in the Male and Normal Genitals in the Female. *J. Pediatr.* **66**:1049–1054, 1965.

24a Robinson, C. D., et al., Smith-Lemli-Opitz Syndrome with Cardiovascular Abnormality. *Pediatrics* **47**:844–847, 1971.

25 Ruvalcaba, R. H. A., et al., Smith-Lemli-Opitz Syndrome. *Arch. Dis. Child.* **43**:620–623, 1968.

26 Schumacher, H., Das Smith-Lemli-Opitz-Syndrom. *Z. Kinderheilkd.* **105**:88–98, 1969.

27 Smith, D. W., et al., A Newly Recognized Syndrome of Multiple Congenital Anomalies. *J. Pediatr.* **64**:210–217, 1964.

28 Wasz-Höckert, O., et al., El sindrome de Smith-Lemli-Opitz en dos niñas, con especial atención a los patrones de sus gritos de dolor. *Rev. Mex. Pediatr.* **38**:63–68, 1969.

29 Zucker, J. M., et al., Une nouvelle variete de nanisme intrautérin dystrophique: le syndrome de Smith, Lemli et Opitz. *Ann. Pédiatr.* **43**:2404–2411, 1967.

135

Sturge-Weber Anomalad

(Encephalofacial Angiomatosis)

The Sturge-Weber anomalad is characterized by (*a*) venous angiomatosis of the leptomeninges. Other findings most often include (*b*) ipsilateral facial angiomatosis, (*c*) ipsilateral gyriform calcifications of the cerebral cortex, (*d*) seizures, (*e*) mental deficiency, (*f*) hemiplegia, and (*g*) ocular defects. Many eponyms have been used to denote the disorder, and priority of discovery has been debated. Several references are of historical interest (11, 17–19, 30, 32, 37). The most extensive study of the Sturge-Weber anomalad was provided by Alexander and Norman (2).

All cases reported to date have been sporadic. Although a few histories have suggested incomplete forms in first-degree relatives who presented single features such as seizures, mental deficiency, or vascular nevi, no instance of full-blown Sturge-Weber anomalad has ever been recorded in more than one individual within the same family. Neither sex preponderance nor predilection for left- or right-sided involvement has been found (2).

The Sturge-Weber anomalad can be explained on the basis of an embryologic anomaly with secondary consequences. During the sixth week of normal intrauterine development, a vascular plexus develops around the cephalic portion of the neural tube and under the ectoderm destined to become facial skin. Normally, this vascular plexus regresses during the ninth week, but in the Sturge-Weber anomalad, it persists, resulting in angiomatosis of the leptomeninges overlying the cerebral cortex, together with facial angiomatosis on the ipsilateral side. Variation in the degree of persistence or regression of the vascular plexus accounts for cases of bilateral involvement and also for cases with unilateral occurrence in which angioma of the leptomeninges occurs in the absence of facial involvement (3).

Other features of the association seem to be secondary to the leptomeningeal lesion. A poorly understood alteration in the vascular dynamics of the angioma results in the precipitation of calcium deposits in the cerebral cortex underlying the angioma. Seizures and mental deficiency are probably secondary to this process. Thus, it is unnecessary to insist on multiple criteria for the Sturge-Weber anomalad. However, a single obligatory defect — angioma of the leptomeninges — can be said to constitute a minimum criterion for the disorder.

Since angiomas of the skin and, in some cases, the viscera may be observed in the Klippel-Trénaunay-Weber syndrome, it is not surprising that the Sturge-Weber anomalad occurs in association with this syndrome. In our literature review, over 20 such cases were noted (e.g., 14, 33). One of us (M. M. C.) has observed this association in several patients. Since angiomas may occur anywhere in the Klippel-Trénaunay-Weber syndrome, it is possible that this syndrome and the Sturge-Weber anomalad represent

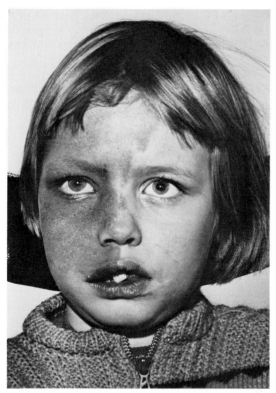

Figure 135-1. *Sturge-Weber anomalad.* Angiomatosis of face (usually upper two-thirds), epilepsy, contralateral hemiplegia, and cerebral calcification; mental retardation is common. Note distribution of angioma in eight-year-old girl.

the same basic disorder, the latter occurring whenever an angioma happens to be present in the leptomeninges.

SYSTEMIC MANIFESTATIONS

Face. A nevus flammeus lesion occurs on the ipsilateral side of the face in approximately 90 percent of patients (25) (Fig. 135-1). In some instances, the nevus may extend onto the neck, chest, and back. Occasionally, bilateral facial nevus or no facial nevus may occur (2, 3). The color varies from pink to purplish-red and may decrease in intensity with age in some cases. The lesion is sharply demarcated and usually flat. One of us (M. M. C.) has observed two patients with distinctly elevated lesions. In one case, pronounced saccular outpouchings of the nevus occurred with age.

Cushing (10) noted a correlation between the distribution of the nevus flammeus and the course of the trigeminal nerve. However, Alexander and Norman (2) found the trigeminal relationship to be secondary and fortuitous. They assumed that the distribution of the facial nevus was determined, in part, by the position of the processes and fissures in the developing face.

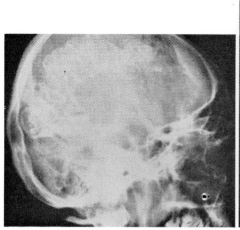

A

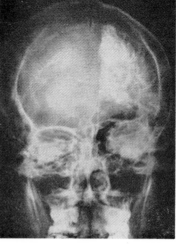

B

Figure 135-2. (*A, B*). The "tram-line" calcification seen in skull roentgenograms is a characteristic of the syndrome. Note unilateral limitation.

Brain. The characteristic lesion consists of a unilateral, thin-walled angioma in the leptomeninges overlying the posterior temporal, posterior parietal, and occipital areas. Occasionally, bilateral involvement may be present (2, 21, 23, 35, 38). An abnormal cerebral venous drainage pattern, caused by lack of functioning superficial cortical veins beneath the angioma, has been reported. Whether these veins become thrombosed or are truly absent remains to be determined (6).

Gyriform, double-contoured lines of calcification develop in the underlying cerebral cortex usually after the second year of life (Fig. 135-2*A*, *B*). Rarely, they may be present at birth (23). The roentgenographic appearance is pathognomonic for the disorder (2, 9). Calcific deposition becomes stationary usually by the end of the second decade (2). Asymmetry of the skull has been noted (16).

Nervous system. Seizures were observed in 90 percent of cases in one series (25), symptoms appear during infancy; seizures occurring contralateral to the angiomatosis. They are most often focal, but generalized convulsions may occur. Hemiparesis is less frequent, and the paretic limb is sometimes hypotrophic (2).

Mental status. At least 30 percent of patients exhibit mental deficiency. With extensive cerebral changes, retardation may be pronounced (2, 25).

Eyes. Choroidal angioma is common, and buphthalmos, glaucoma, and hemianopia have been reported (2, 20).

Other findings. Any of the various findings associated with the Klippel-Trénaunay-Weber syn-

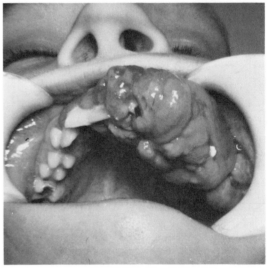

A

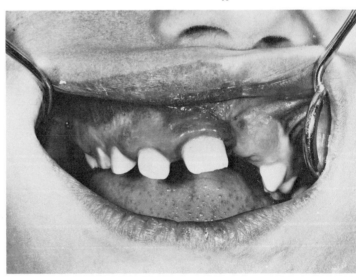

Figure 135-3. (*A*). Gingival hypertrophy and angiomatosis are commonly on the same side as the facial angiomatosis. (*From H. E. Royle,* Oral Surg. **22:**490, 1966.) (*B*). Intraoral hemangioma in eight-year-old girl with encephalofacial angiomatosis. Eruption of teeth on the affected side is more advanced than on the normal side.

B

drome may be observed with the Sturge-Weber anomalad, including macrocephaly (31a). Oculo-cutaneous melanosis has been reported (14, 24).

Oral manifestations. Intraoral angiomatosis occurs most frequently on the buccal mucosa and lips-macrocheilia occurring when the lips are involved (1, 2, 7, 36) (Fig. 135-3*A, B*). The palate is less frequently affected. Tongue involvement may be accompanied by hemihypertrophy (4, 25, 29). Gingival lesions, when present, may range from slight vascular hyperplasia to monstrous overgrowth, making closure of the mouth impossible (5, 12, 13, 15, 27). Vascular gingival hyperplasia, which blanches on pressure, should be distinguished from fibrous hyperplasia, which may accompany medication with diphenylhydantoin. Multiple pyogenic granulomas of the gingiva were reported in one case by Thoma (34).

Both unilateral hypertrophy and hypotrophy of the alveolar process have been reported (2, 16, 22). Ipsilateral premature eruption of permanent teeth (22, 31), ipsilateral delayed eruption (13), and ipsilateral normal eruption (36) have been noted. Unilateral premature eruption causes irregular positioning of teeth, leading to malocclusion. The size of the teeth may vary in the affected area, macrodontia being most frequently observed (2, 8).

DIFFERENTIAL DIAGNOSIS

The relationship between the Sturge-Weber anomalad and the *Klippel-Trénaunay-Weber*
syndrome has been discussed above. Transitory nevus flammeus lesions during the neonatal period are extremely common. However, in many cases, they may not be as intense in color as the Sturge-Weber lesion, which tends to be darker and most frequently unilateral in distribution. Although the facial nevus in the Sturge-Weber anomalad varies considerably in extent, dark, supraocular involvement should arouse suspicion (2).

The association of macrocephaly and angiomatosis may occur in disseminated hemangiomatosis, *neurofibromatosis, Beckwith-Wiedemann syndrome, Klippel-Trénaunay-Weber syndrome*, and cutis marmorata telangiectatica congenita (31a).

DIAGNOSTIC AIDS

Because severe brain damage can exist, it is important to establish the presence of leptomeningeal angiomatosis as soon as possible by means of angiography. However, once cerebral calcification occurs, the chances of obtaining a positive angiogram are considerably diminished (2, 26). Roentgenograms after two years of age usually reveal the pathognomonic, gyriform, double-contoured, calcification lines. Electroencephalographic studies are abnormal, usually revealing unilateral depression of cortical activity (2, 28).

REFERENCES

1 Achslogh, J., Hémisphérectomie dans un cas de maladie de Sturge-Weber. *Acta Neurol. Belg.* **58**:837–847, 1958.

2 Alexander, G. L., and Norman, R. M., *The Sturge-Weber Syndrome.* John Wright and Sons, Bristol, 1960.

3 Andriola, M., and Stolfi, J., Sturge-Weber Syndrome. *Am. J. Dis. Child.* **123**:507–510, 1972.

4 Arendt, A., Sturge-Webersche Erkrankung. *Dtsch. Gesundheitsw.* **8**:137–141, 1953.

5 Baer, P. N., et al., Gingival Hemangioma Associated with Sturge-Weber Syndrome. *Oral Surg.* **14**:1383–1390, 1961.

6 Bentson, J. R., et al., Cerebral Venous Drainage Pattern of the Sturge-Weber Syndrome. *Am. J. Roentgenol.* **101**:111–118, 1971.

7 Born, E., Über die Sturge-Weber Angiomatose. *Zentralbl. Allg. Pathol.* **97**:569–576, 1957–1958.

8 Brushfield, T., and Wyatt, W., Sturge-Weber Disease. *Br. J. Child. Dis.* **24**:98–106, 209–213, 1927; **25**:96–101, 1928.

9 Chao, D. H.-C., Congenital Neurocutaneous Syndromes of Childhood: III. Sturge-Weber Disease. *J. Pediatr.* **55**:635–649, 1959.

10 Cushing, H., Cases of Spontaneous Intracranial Hemorrhage Associated with Trigeminal Nevi. *J.A.M.A.* **47**:178–183, 1906.

11 Dimitri, V., Tumor cerebral congenito (angioma cavernoso). *Rev. Med. Argent.* **36**:1029, 1923.

12 El Mostehy, M. R., and Stallard, R. E., The Sturge-Weber

Syndrome: Its Periodontal Significance. *J. Periodontol.* **40:**243–246, 1969.

13 Falk, W., Beitrag zur Aetiologie und Klinik den Sturge-Weberschen Krankheit. *Oest. Z. Kinderheilkd.* **5:**175–185, 1950.

14 Furukawa, T., et al., Sturge-Weber and Klippel-Trénaunay Syndrome with Nevus of Ota and Ito. *Arch. Dermatol.* **102:**640–645, 1970.

15 Gyarmati, I., Oral Change in Sturge-Weber's Disease. *Oral Surg.* **13:**795–801, 1960.

16 Höring, H., Zur Lokalisation mesenchymaler Dysplasien bei Sturge-Weber Krankheit. *Arch. Klin. Exp. Dermatol.* **209:**615–624, 1960.

17 Kalischer, S. Demonstration des Gehirns eines Kindes mit Teleangiectasie der linksseitigen Gesichts-Kopfhaut und Hirnoberfläche. *Berl. Klin. Wochenschr.* **34:**1059, 1897.

18 Krabbe, K. H., Facial and Meningeal Angiomatosis Associated with Calcifications of Brain Cortex: Clinical and Anatomo-pathologic Contribution. *Arch. Neurol. Psychiatr.* **32:**737–755, 1934.

19 Krabbe, K. H., and Wissing, O., Calcifications de la pie-mère du cerveau (d'origine angiomateuse) demontrée par la radiographie. *Acta Radiol.* **10:**523–532, 1929.

20 Miller, S. J. N., Ophthalmic Aspects of the Sturge-Weber Syndrome. *Proc. R. Soc. Med.* **56:**419–421, 1965.

21 Morgan, G., Pathology of the Sturge-Weber Syndrome. *Proc. R. Soc. Med.* **56:**422–423, 1963.

22 Myle, G., Sémiologie de l'angiomatose encéphalotri-géminée ou encéphalo-cranio-faciale. *Acta Neurol. Belg.* **50:**713–785, 1950.

23 Nellhaus, G., et al., Sturge-Weber Disease with Bilateral Intracranial Calcifications at Birth and Unusual Pathologic Findings. *Acta Neurol. Scand.* **43:**314–347, 1967.

24 Noriega-Sanchez, A., et al., Oculocutaneous Melanosis Associated with the Sturge-Weber Syndrome. *Neurology* **22:**256–262, 1972.

25 Peterman, A. F., et al., Encephalotrigeminal Angiomatosis (Sturge-Weber Disease): Clinical Study of Thirty-five Cases. *J.A.M.A.* **167:**2169-2176, 1958.

26 Poser, C. M., and Taveras, J. M., Cerebral Angiography in Encephalotrigeminal Angiomatosis. *Radiology* **68:**327–336, 1957.

27 Protzel, M. S., Sturge-Weber Syndrome. *Oral Surg.* **10:** 388–399, 1957.

28 Radermecker, J., L'électroencéphalographie dans l'angiomatose encéphalo-trigéminée de Sturge-Weber-Krabbe. *Acta Neurol. Belg.* **51:**427–451, 1951.

29 Roizin, L., et al., Congenital Vascular Anomalies and Their Histopathology in Sturge-Weber-Dimitri Syndrome (Naevus Flammeus with Angiomatosis and Encephalosis Calcificans). *J. Neuropathol. Exp. Neurol.* **18:**75–97, 1959.

30 Schirmer, R., Ein Fall von Telangiektasie. *Albrecht von Graefes Arch. Ophthalmol.* **7:**119–121, 1860.

31 Schuermann, H., *Krankheiten der Mundschleimhaut und der Lippen,* 2d ed., Urban & Schwarzenberg, Berlin, 1958.

31a Stephan, M. J., et al., Macrocephaly in Association with Unusual Cutaneous Angiomatosis. *J. Pediatr.* **87:**353–359, 1975.

32 Sturge, W. A., Case of Partial Epilepsy Apparently Due to Lesion of One of Vasomotor Centres of Brain. *Trans. Clin. Soc. London* **12:**162–167, 1879.

33 Teller, H., and Lindner, B., Über Mischformen der phakotösen Syndrome von Sturge-Weber und Klippel-Trénaunay. *Z. Haut. Geschlechtskr.* **13:**113–120, 1952.

34 Thoma, K. H., Sturge-Kalischer-Weber Syndrome with Pregnancy Tumors. *Oral Surg.* **5:**1124–1131, 1952.

35 Tönnis, W., and Friedmann, G., Roentgenographische und klinische Befunde bei 23 Patienten mit Sturge-Weber Erkrankung. *Zentralbl. Neurochir.* **25:**1–10, 1964.

36 Wannenmacher, M. F., and Forck, G., Mundschleimhaut-veränderungen beim Sturge-Weber-Syndrom. *Dtsch. Zahnärztl. Z.* **25:** 1030–1035, 1970.

37 Weber, F. P., Right-sided Hemi-hypotrophy Resulting from Right-sided Congenital Spastic Hemiplegia, with Morbid Condition of Left Side of Brain, Revealed by Radiograms. *J. Neurol. Psychopathol.* **3:**134–139, 1922.

38 Wohlwill, F. J., and Yakovlev, P. I., Histopathology of Meningofacial Angiomatosis (Sturge-Weber's Disease): Report of Four Cases. *J. Neuropathol. Exp. Neurol.* **16:**341–364, 1957.

136

Temporomandibular Joint Syndrome

The syndrome consists of (a) temporomandibular crepitation, (b) decreased temporomandibular joint mobility, (c) preauricular and auricular pain, pain on movement, headache, tenderness of the jaws on palpation, and sometimes (d) head and nasopharyngeal symptoms. Following a series of papers by other authors between 1918 and 1934, Costen (4) attributed a syndrome consisting of otologic symptoms, head and neck pain, temporomandibular joint symptoms, and nasopharyngeal symptoms to overclosure of the mandible. However, Shapiro and Truex (23), Sicher (24, 25), and Zimmermann (35) disproved the anatomic premises and clinical conclusions described by Costen. It is clear, though, that since the temporomandibular joint, the muscles of mastication, and the dentition form a mutually interdependent system, organic or functional derangement in any one component necessarily affects the others.

In nearly all studies, between 80 and 90 percent of patients are female (1, 6, 21, 26, 27, 32). Although age of onset has ranged from six (1) to seventy years (21), in the majority of cases the patient is under forty years of age (1, 6, 9, 32).

SYSTEMIC MANIFESTATIONS

In Posselt's compilation of symptoms from five patient series (18), the following were found in decreasing order of frequency: clicking of the joint on movement, limited joint mobility, pain in or about the ears, pain on movement, headache, and tenderness on palpation. Less frequently found were tinnitus, excessive mandibular movement, mild catarrhal deafness, pain over the vertex, occiput, or postauricular areas, and neuralgia in the maxillary, mandibular, or cervical areas. Very few patients in any series reviewed by Shapiro and Gorlin (22) had the signs or symptoms listed by Costen, i.e., ear symptoms were extremely rare.

The basis of symptoms is obscure. Numerous hypotheses have been in vogue at different times, the essential ones being (a) overclosure of the mandible, (b) occlusal abnormalities, (c) internal derangement of the joint, and (d) spasm of muscles of mastication. Recent investigators usually acknowledge involvement of the teeth, the musculature, and the joint in production of the symptoms. Differences of opinion usually do not reflect clearly distinct mechanisms but rather the emphasis of one or another component. The history of attempts to elucidate an etiologic and pathogenic basis for the syndrome has been documented by Schwartz (21), Freese and Scheman (8), and Ramfjord and Ash (19).

Schwartz (21) and others (2, 30, 35) stated that most cases of temporomandibular joint disturbances constitute a pain dysfunction syndrome involving the muscles of mastication, rather than the joints themselves, and result from spasms in these muscles. Accordingly, Schwartz (21) hypothesized that individuals subjected to stress or anxiety manifest increased muscular tension, particularly in the jaw musculature. Secondarily, muscle forces are exerted against the teeth and malocclusion may result. There is little evidence to support the notion of a relationship between degenerative changes within the joint and the symptoms (21, 29, 30). Travell (30) suggested that noxious stimuli (mechanical, emotional, infectious, metabolic, nutritional, or a combination of these) result in spasm and shortening of the muscles of mastication. They lose the capacity for voluntary relaxation and resist passive lengthening. In most cases reviewed by her, muscle spasm as recorded with electromyography was relieved by occlusal adjustment.

The role of emotional factors in predisposing an individual to symptoms of this syndrome has frequently been noted (28). Kydd (11) reported 30 patients with the syndrome who were examined by personality tests. Twenty-three were significantly emotionally disturbed, and in 22, it was possible to establish a relationship between the onset of acute symptoms and the immediate premenstrual period.

PATHOLOGY

There is no general agreement concerning pathologic alterations. The syndrome may result in organic joint changes or may be the result of such changes. The view that joint changes, when they do occur, are secondary to primary muscle spasm is not universally held. Foged (5) and Nörgaard (17) believed that the primary disorder was within the joint itself and together with Boman (1) considered the primary problem due to arthrosis, i.e., a degenerative, noninfectious, condition of the joint. Sicher (24) suggested that the pain, cracking of the joint, and restriction of its movements, are simply those of arthritis. In 1955, Sicher (25) stated that the pathologic changes are mainly degenerative and are localized to the fibrous covering of the articular eminence and condylar head and to the fibrous articular disk. However, Coleman and Weisengreen (3) examined microscopically 90 temporomandibular joints from 45 cadavers ranging in age from thirty-nine to ninety-five years. In

about one-quarter of the cases, either one or both articular disks exhibited maximal degenerative changes, yet a history of temporomandibular joint disturbances was not given by these patients prior to death.

There seems to be no doubt that locking and clicking of the joint may result in joint disease, whether or not the disease is primary or secondary. It is quite possible that the pain dysfunction syndrome may be etiologically heterogeneous, the pathologic alterations in the joint being primary in some cases and secondary in others.

DIFFERENTIAL DIAGNOSIS

Until more is known about the syndrome, diagnosis must rest upon exclusion. Conditions that may simulate the disorder include neoplasms, deceleration injury to the cervical region of the spine, cervical traction, temporal arteritis, rheumatoid arthritis, osteoarthritis, nonspecific cervicitis, fibrositis of the masseter muscle, tonsillitis, parotitis, middle ear disease, old fractured condyle, migraine, cluster, hypertensive, or posttraumatic headaches, and atypical neuralgias (9, 12). Kiehn and Des Prez (10) suggested that pain on pressure from the examining finger on the ramus was absent in tic douloureux, parotid disease, trigeminal neuralgia, and temporal arteritis. Trigeminal neuralgia or atypical toxic neuritis may be distinguished from the temporomandibular joint syndrome by detecting a trigger point, its fulminating character, and neurologic findings. Pain resulting from disorders of the ear, teeth, paranasal sinuses, parotid gland, and cervical area of the spine must be excluded, as well as conversion hysteria (26).

DIAGNOSTIC AIDS

According to Wooten (33), diagnosis of the pain dysfunction syndrome is established when it can be demonstrated that the symptoms arise from spastic areas within one or more muscles of mastication. He listed the following criteria useful in diagnosis: "(a) knowledge of the syndrome and consideration of it in the diagnosis of facial pain, (b) limitation of mandibular function with increased pain upon attempts to stretch the elevating muscles of the mandible, (c) the ability to palpate unusually tender areas in one or more of the mastication muscles, and (d) demonstration of patient anxiety or habits of anxiety, such as bruxism or clamping."

In most cases of the temporomandibular joint syndrome, no relevant roentgenographic changes are noted (14, 17). Negative results, however, are essential in ruling out organic disease. In addition to standard lateral and anteroposterior views, a variety of special techniques has been applied to the joint (7, 13, 15–17, 20, 31). Evaluation of dental occlusion and electromyography of the muscles of mastication may contribute to diagnosis.

REFERENCES

1 Boman, K., Temporomandibular Joint Arthrosis and Its Treatment by Extirpation of the Disc. *Acta Chir. Scand.* [*Suppl.*] **118:**1–225, 1947.

2 Campbell, J., Distribution and Treatment of Pain in Temporomandibular Arthroses. *Br. Dent. J.* **105:**393–408, 1958.

3 Coleman, R. D., and Weisengreen, H. H., Degenerative Changes in the Articular Disc in Later Maturity. *J. Dent. Res.* **34:**679–680, 1955.

4 Costen, J. B., Syndrome of Ear and Sinus Symptoms Dependent on Disturbed Function of the Temporomandibular Joint. *Ann. Otol. Rhinol. Laryngol.* **43:**1–15, 1934.

5 Foged, J., Temporomandibular Arthrosis. *Lancet* **2:**1209–1211, 1949.

6 Franks, A. S. T., The Social Character of Temporomandibular Joint Dysfunction, *Dent. Pract. Dent. Rec.* **15:**94–100, 1964.

7 Freese, A. S., Temporomandibular Joint Pain; Etiology, Symptomatology, and Diagnosis. *J. Prosthet. Dent.* **10:**1078–1086, 1960.

8 Freese, A. S., and Scheman, P., *Management of Temporomandibular Joint Problems.* Mosby, St. Louis, 1962.

9 Hankey, G., Temporomandibular Arthrosis. *Br. Dent. J.* **97:**249–270, 1954.

10 Kiehn, C. L., and Des Prez, J. D., Meniscectomy for Internal Derangement of the Temporomandibular Joint. *Br. J. Plast. Surg.* **15:**199–204, 1962.

11 Kydd, W. L., Psychosomatic Aspects of Temporomandibular Joint Dysfunction. *J. Am. Dent. Assoc.* **59:**31–44, 1959.

12 Kydd, W. L., Cranial Arthritis Simulating Temporomandibular Joint Arthrosis. *Oral Surg.* **15:**677–679, 1962.

13 Lindbloom, G., On the Anatomy and Function of the Temporomandibular Joint. *Acta Odontol. Scand.* [*Suppl.*] **28:**1–287, 1960.

14 Madsen, B., Normal Variations in Anatomy, Condylar Movements, and Arthrosis Frequency of the Temporomandibular Joints. *Acta Radiol.* [*Diagn.*] (*Stockh.*) **4:**273–288, 1966.

15 Mallett, S. R., Special Considerations of Temporomandibular Joint Disturbances with Particular Emphasis on Myositis and X-ray Determination of Changes in the Head of the Condyle. *Oral Surg.* **16:**788–789, 1963.

16 Markowitz, H. S., and Gerry, R. G., Temporomandibular Joint Disease. *Oral Surg.* **3:**75–117, 1950.

17 Nörgaard, F., *Temporomandibular Arthrography.* Munksgaard, Copenhagen, 1947.

18 Posselt, U., *Physiology of Occlusion and Rehabilitation.* Blackwell Scientific Publications, Oxford, 1962, pp. 59–96.

19 Ramfjord, S. P., and Ash, M. M., *Occlusion.* Saunders, Philadelphia, 1966, pp. 160–179.

20 Ricketts, R. M., Variations of the Temporomandibular Joint as Revealed by Cephalometric Laminographs. *Am. J. Orthodont.* **36:**887–898, 1950.

21 Schwartz, L., *Disorders of the Temporomandibular Joint.* Saunders, Philadelphia, 1959.

22 Shapiro, B. L., and Gorlin, R. J., Disorders of the Temporomandibular Joint, in R. J. Gorlin and H. M. Goldman (eds.), *Oral Pathology,* 6th ed. Mosby, St. Louis, 1970, pp. 577–606.

23 Shapiro, H. H., and Truex, R. C., The Temporomandibular Joint and the Auditory Function. *J. Am. Dent. Assoc.* **30:**1147–1168, 1943.

24 Sicher, H., Temporomandibular Articulation in Mandibular Overclosure. *J. Am. Dent. Assoc.* **36:**131–139, 1948.

25 Sicher, H., Structural and Functional Basis for Disorders of the Temporomandibular Articulation. *J. Oral. Surg.* **13:**275–279, 1955.

26 Silver, C. M., and Simon, S. D., Meniscus Injuries of the Temporomandibular Joint; Further Experience. *J. Bone Joint Surg.* **45A:**113–124, 1963.

27 Silver, C. M., et al., Meniscus Injuries of the Temporomandibular Joint. *J. Bone Joint Surg.* **38A:**541–552, 1956.

28 Taylor, R. C., et al., The Importance of Determining the End Point in Treatment of Patients with Temporomandibular Joint Syndrome. *J. Oral Med.* **22:**3–6, 1967.

29 Thomson, H., Temporomandibular Joint Problems; Conservative Treatment. *Br. Dent. J.* **111:**422–423, 1961.

30 Travell, J., Temporomandibular Joint Pain Referred from Muscles of the Head and Neck. *J. Prosthet. Dent.* **10:**745–763, 1960.

31 Updegrave, W. J., Interpretation of Temporomandibular Joint Radiographs. *Dent. Clin. North Am.* 567–586, 1966.

32 Vero, D., Facial Pain in Association with Temporomandibular Joint Dysfunction. *J. Laryngol.* **79:**707–723, 1965.

33 Wooten, J. W., Temporomandibular Joint–Diagnosis of the Pain-dysfunction Syndrome. *J. Prosthet. Dent.* **14:**961–966, 1964.

34 Worth, H. M., *Principles and Practice of Oral Radiologic Interpretation.* Year Book, Chicago, 1963, pp. 691–695.

35 Zimmermann, A. A., An Evaluation of Costen's Syndrome from an Anatomic Point of View, in B. G. Sarnat (ed.), *The Temporomandibular Joint.* Charles C Thomas, Springfield, Ill., 1951, pp. 82–110.

137

Thanatophoric Dwarfism

Described by Maroteaux et al. (27, 28) in 1967 as a new form of chondrodystrophy, thanatophoric ("death-bringing") dwarfism is incompatible with life. The disorder is characterized by (a) marked shortness and bowing of the extremities, with numerous skin folds, and (b) narrow trunk of normal length. Most examples of so-called lethal achondroplasia of the newborn represent cases of thanatophoric dwarfism.

The frequency of thanatophoric dwarfism is probably about 1 per 6,000 births (15); it appears to be the most common form of lethal micromelic dwarfism. Combining our own survey and that of Lenz et al. (24), at least 70 cases have been identified (3a, 5–7, 8, 9, 11–14, 16–18, 24a, 30–43). A propensity of births during the summer and early fall has been noted (14a). There appears to be male predilection.

There is no question that what has been called "thanatophoric dwarfism" in the literature represents a heterogeneous group of disorders. All familial examples cited either seem to represent disorders that are not quite "classic" or are insufficiently documented radiographically to be certain. We believe that the affected sibs reported by Harris and Patton (15) and Graff et al. (13) probably do not represent thanatophoric dwarfism. Affected sibs have also been reported by Partington et al. (30). While the postcranial skeletons were completely compatible with thanatophoric dwarfism, both sibs had the Kleeblattschädel anomalad. Many cases of thanatophoric dwarfism have this finding (3a, 16a, 42,

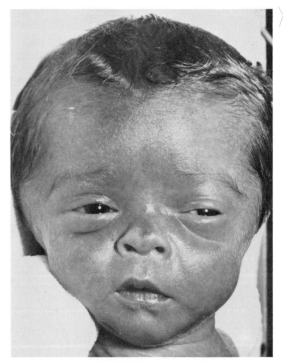

Figure 137-1. *Thanatophoric dwarfism.* Enlarged head circumference with frontal bossing, ocular hypertelorism, proptosis. (*From A. Giedion*, Helv. Paediatr. Acta **23**:175, 1968.)

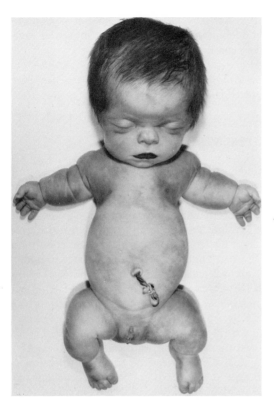

Figure 137-2. Short neck, short bowed extremities with shortened digits, constricted upper part of chest, large abdomen.

SYSTEMIC MANIFESTATIONS

The child either is born dead or survives at most a few days, usually succumbing with respiratory distress and cardiac failure. The respiratory distress can be explained in most cases by the thoracic form, muscular hypotonia, and alterations in the bronchial cartilages (24). Survival beyond one year has rarely been noted (33a). In about 70 percent there is a history of hydramnios (15, 41). At least one-third of these infants are premature and born by breech presentation (40). In the past, most examples of thanatophoric dwarfism were misdiagnosed as examples of achondroplasia.

Facies. There is considerable frontal bossing. The skull circumference may be as large as 40 cm. In some cases there is Kleeblattschädel

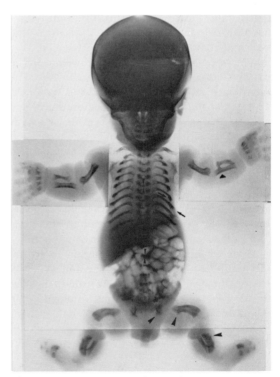

Figure 137-3. Note narrow thorax, short ribs flared at costochondral junctions, platyspondyly, narrow sacrosciatic notches, horizontal acetabular roof with spurring, shortening of long bones with especially bent femurs. (*From A. Giedion*, Helv. Paediatr. Acta **23**:175, 1968.)

43). However, the possibility still exists that it represents further heterogeneity. The reported triplets (36) are incompletely documented. Thus, familial examples reported to date are somewhat questionable in our opinion. All classic cases described thus far are seemingly sporadic. We cannot accept the suggestion that thanatophoric dwarfism is polygenic (31). Some cases may be autosomal recessive, but the genetics are poorly understood at the present time because of heterogeneity (7b, 14a, 18a, 24a).

In classic thanatophoric dwarfism, there is generalized disruption of endochondral bone formation. There is little attempt at column formation and no orderly progression of chondrocytes at the growth plates (34). Cultured fibroblasts can be distinguished from achondroplasia and the normal on the basis of total intracellular mucopolysaccharide content and the relative proportion of dermatan sulfate (7a).

anomalad (3, 3a, 30, 38, 42, 43). The nasal bridge is depressed, and the eyes may bulge (Fig. 137-1).

Skeletal alterations. All four extremities are severely shortened and bowed. Numerous redundant skin folds are evident in the arms. The chest is narrow, contrasting with a large abdomen (Figs. 137-2, 137-3). The extremities extend outward from the trunk, with the thighs abducted and externally rotated in a froglike position. Total body length has ranged from 29 to 47 cm (average, 40 cm). The diagnosis has been made in utero (4, 7).

Roentgenographically, the thorax is narrow, the clavicles are high, and the ribs are very short and flared at the costochondral junctions. The height of the vertebral bodies is considerably reduced, with the midpoint being narrowest. The interpediculate distance of the lower lumbar vertebras is reduced, and the intervertebral spaces are greatly enlarged, in some cases between two and three times the height of the vertebral body (24).

The scapulas are incompletely developed. The ilia are larger horizontally than vertically. The sacrosciatic notches are narrow and beaklike. The ischial and pubic bones are short and thick, with normal ossification. The acetabular roof is horizontal, with formation of internal and external spurs. The humerus has little metaphyseal widening. The diaphysis of the femur is bowed and deformed. The epiphysis at the knee is absent. The proximal femur exhibits a triangular area of increased radiolucency. There are bony thorns at the proximal end of the tibia.

The development of the vault of the skull is excessive, contrasting with reduction in size of the skull base and foramen magnum (37, 40). Histopathologic study has revealed disorganization of endochondral ossification (19, 20, 34, 39).

Other findings. Rhombencephalon hypoplasia and adenomyosis of the pyloric muscular layer have been described (39).

Oral manifestations. Cleft lip-palate has been reported (14).

DIFFERENTIAL DIAGNOSIS

Though the condition resembles heterozygotic *achondroplasia* and other short-limbed dwarfism to some extent, the abbreviation of the ribs, the reduction in height of the vertebral bodies, and the extreme shortening of the extremities should make it possible to differentiate these conditions with ease. There is closer resemblance to homozygous achondroplasia, but in the latter, the skull is more markedly hydrocephalic, the vertebral bodies are less flat, and the extremities and ribs are less abbreviated. *Achondrogenesis*, also a form of lethal short-limbed dwarfism, can be distinguished both clinically and roentgenographically. The head is larger; ossification is deficient in the vertebral bodies, especially in the lumbar region, and absent in the sacral, pubic, and ischial bones (37).

The so-called thanatophoric dwarfism II (11a), in our opinion, is a well-mineralized example of achondrogenesis.

Another short-limbed dwarfism characterized by lymphopenic agammaglobulinemia and ectodermal changes was described by McKusick and Cross (29), Davis (7b), Gatti et al. (10), Gotoff et al. (12), and Amman et al. (1).

LABORATORY AIDS

None is known.

REFERENCES

1 Amman, J., et al., Antibody-mediated Immunodeficiency in Short-limbed Dwarfism. *J. Pediatr.* **84:**200–203, 1974.

2 Beaudoing, A., et al., Thanatophoric Dwarfism. *Pédiatrie* 24:459–462, 1969.

3 Bloomfield, J. A., Cloverleaf Skull and Thanatophoric Dwarfism. *Aust. Radiol.* **14:**429–434, 1970.

3a Bonucci, E., and Nardi, F., The Cloverleaf Skull Syndrome—Histological, Histochemical and Ultrastructural Findings. *Virchows Arch. Pathol. Anat.* **357:**199–212, 1972.

4 Campbell, R. E., Thanatophoric Dwarfism in Utero. *Am. J. Roentgenol.* **112:**198–200, 1971.

5 Canton, E., Sobre tres fetos acondroplásticos y sus radio-

grafiás respectivos (Cases 1, 3) *Sem. Med. (B. Aires)* **10**:489–505, 1903.

6 Centa, A., and Camera, G. Il considetto "nanismo tanatoforo." *Minerva Pediatr.* **21**:447–453, 1969.

7 Cronenberg, N. E., A Case of Chondrodystrophia Foetalis. Discovered by X-ray Examination before Delivery. *Acta Obstet. Gynecol. Scand.* **13**:275–282, 1933.

7a Danes, B. S., Achondroplasia and Thanatophoric Dwarfism. A Study of Cell Culture. *Birth Defects* **10**(12):37–42, 1974.

7b Davis, J. A., A Case of Swiss-type Agammaglobulinemia and Achondroplasia. *Br. Med. J.* **2**:1371–1374, 1966.

8 Edwards, J. A., et al., Lethal Short-Limbed Dwarfism. *Birth Defects* **10**(12):18–20, 1974.

9 Franceschini, P., et al., Le nanisme thanatophore dans le cadres des nanismes pseudo-achondroplastiques. *Ann. Radiol.* **13**:399–404, 1970.

10 Gatti, R. A., et al., Hereditary Lymphopenic Agammaglobulinemia Associated with a Distinctive Form of Short-limbed Dwarfism and Ectodermal Dysplasia. *J. Pediatr.* **75**:675–684, 1969.

11 Giedion, A., Thanatophoric Dwarfism. *Helv. Paediatr. Acta* **23**:175–183, 1968.

11a Goard, K. E., and Kozlowski, K., Thanatophoric Dwarfism II. *Pediatr. Radiol.* **1**:8–11, 1973.

12 Gotoff, S. P., et al., Granulomatous Reaction in an Infant with Combined Immunodeficiency Disease and Short-limbed Dwarfism. *J. Pediatr.* **80**:1010–1017, 1972.

13 Graff, G., et al., Familial Recurring Thanatophoric Dwarfism. *Obstet. Gynecol.* **39**:515–520, 1972.

14 Gwinn, J. L., et al., Thanatophoric Dwarfism. *Am. J. Dis. Child.* **120**:141–142, 1970.

14a Hall, J. G., Thanatophoric Dwarfism May Be Genetic but not Polygenic. *Pediatrics* **52**:469–470, 1973.

15 Harris, R., and Patton, J. T., Achondroplasia and Thanatophoric Dwarfism in the Newborn. *Clin. Genet.* **2**:61–72, 1971.

16 Huguenin, M., et al., Two Different Mutations within the Same Sibship. *Helv. Paediatr. Acta* **24**:239–245, 1969.

16a Iannaccone, G., and Gerlini, G., The So-called "Cloverleaf Skull Syndrome." *Pediatr. Radiol.* **2**:175–184, 1974.

17 Jeannin, C., and Surun, —, Foetus achondroplastique (présentation) de pièces. *Bull. Soc. Obstét. Gynécol. Paris* **13**:181–184, 1910.

18 Jurczok, F., and Schollmeyer, R., Zur Frage des gehäuften Auftretens von Extremitätenmissbildungen bei Neugeborenen. *Geburtshilfe Frauenheilkd.* **22**:400–421, 1962 (Case 4).

18a Kaufman, H. J., "New" Skeletal Dysplasias in the Newborn: New X-ray Findings. *Birth Defects* **10**(12):1–9, 1974.

19 Kaufman, R. L., et al., Thanatophoric Dwarfism. *Am. J. Dis. Child.* **120**:53–57, 1970.

20 Keats, T. E., et al., Thanatophoric Dwarfism. *Am. J. Roentgenol.* **108**:473–480, 1970.

21 Kozlowski, K., et al., Thanatophoric Dwarfism. *Br. J. Radiol.* **43**:565–568, 1970.

22 Langenbach, E., Ein Fall von Chondrodystrophia foetalis mit Asymmetrie des Schädels. *Virchows Arch. Pathol. Anat.* **189**:12–17, 1907.

23 Langer, L. O., et al., Thanatophoric Dwarfism: A Condition Confused with Achondroplasia in the Neonate, with Brief Comments on Achondrogenesis and Homozygous Achondroplasia. *Radiology* **92**:285–294, 1969.

24 Lenz, W., et al., Thanatophoric Zwergwuchs. *Z. Kinderheilkd.* **111**:162–174, 1971.

24a Leroy, J. G., et al., Fatal Neonatal Dwarfism: Examples of Thanatophoric Dwarfism and of Hypophosphatasia. *Birth Defects* **10**(12):21–30, 1974.

25 Levi, L., and Bouchacourt, L., Radiographies de foetus achondroplases (Case 1). *Rev. Hyg. Méd. Inf.* **3**:517–528, 1904.

26 Magrier, C., Présentation d'un foetus achondroplastique. *Bull. Soc. Obstét. Gynécol. Paris* **1**:248–256, 1898.

27 Maroteaux, P., et al., Le nanisme, thanatophore. *Presse Méd.* **75**:2519–2524, 1967.

28 Maroteaux, P., and Lamy, M., Le diagnostic des nanismes chondrodystrophiques chez les nouveau-nés. *Arch. Fr. Pédiatr.* **25**:241–242, 1967.

29 McKusick, V. A., and Cross, H. E., Ataxia-telangiectasia and Swiss-type Agammaglobulinemia. *J.A.M.A.* **195**:739–745, 1966.

30 Partington, M. W., et al., Cloverleaf Skull and Thanatophoric Dwarfism. Report of Four Cases, Two in the Same Sibship. *Arch. Dis. Child.* **46**:656–664, 1971.

31 Pena, S. D. J., and Goodman, H. O., The Genetics of Thanatophoric Dwarfism. *Pediatrics* **51**:104–109, 1973.

32 Porak, C., and Durante, G., Les micromélies congénitales. Achondroplasie vraie et dystrophie périostale. *Nouv. Iconogr. Salpêt.* **18**:481–538, 1905.

33 Raffele, F., diL'achondroplasia nel feto. Considerazione cliniche e anatomopatologische. *Chir. Organi Mov.* **5**:467–502, 1921.

33a Ramos, M. G., Personal communication, 1975.

34 Rimoin, D. L., et al., Histologic Studies in the Chondrodystrophies. *Birth Defects* **10**(12):274–295, 1974.

35 Rischbieth, H., and Barrington, A., Dwarfism (Fig. 31-2). *Treas. Hum. Inherit.* 7–8, 559, 1921.

36 Sabry, A., Thanatophoric Dwarfism in Triplets. *Lancet* **2**:533, 1974.

37 Saldino, R. M., Lethal Short-limbed Dwarfism: Achondrogenesis and Thanatophoric Dwarfism. *Am. J. Roentgenol.* **112**:185–197, 1971.

38 Shah, K., Thanatophoric Dwarfism. *J. Med. Genet.* **10**:243–252, 1973.

39 Shrseň, Š., et al., Thanatophorer Zwergwuchs *Nanismus Thanatophorus* bei vier Neugeborenen. *Pädiatr. Pädiol.* **9**:336–343, 1974.

40 Southion, C. L., Thanatophoric Dwarfism. *Aust. Radiol.* **16**:316–319, 1972.

41 Thompson, B. H., and Parmley, T. H., Obstetric Features in Thanatophoric Dwarfism. *Am. J. Obstet. Gynecol.* **109**:396–401, 1971.

42 Widdig, K., et al., Beitrag zum Kleeblattschädel-Syndrom. *Zentralbl. Allg. Path.* **118**:358–366, 1974.

43 Young, R. S., et al., Thanatophoric Dwarfism and Cloverleaf Skull. *Radiology* **106**:401–406, 1973.

138

Trichorhinophalangeal Syndromes

(Including the Langer-Giedion Syndrome)

W hile studying conditions associated with cone-shaped epiphyses, Giedion (7, 8) described a disorder which he called the trichorhinophalangeal syndrome, consisting of (*a*) cone-shaped epiphyses, (*b*) sparse fine hair, (*c*) bulbous nose with tented alae, and (*d*) variable growth retardation.

The syndrome is genetically heterogeneous, both autosomal dominant (1a, 5, 5a, 6, 10, 17–19, 20, 26, 27) and autosomal recessive (15, 16, 25) forms occurring. Several cases have been isolated examples (3, 21, 24a). The present authors cannot distinguish dominant and recessive forms either clinically or roentgenographically. Differentiation is made on the basis of pedigree data. In sporadic cases, parents should be counseled as having a 0 (dominant mutation) to 25 percent (recessive) risk of recurrence.

A third disorder with multiple exostoses and many features of the trichorhinophalangeal syndrome was first recognized by Langer (18) and Giedion (11). To date, all cases have been sporadic. Twins have been noted by one of the authors (M. M. C.) (13). The disorder was termed the "Langer-Giedion syndrome" by Hall et al. (13), who published the most extensive study of the syndrome to date. Other examples were described by Alè and Calò (1) and by Gorlin et al. (12). The Langer-Giedion syndrome is described later in this chapter and compared with trichorhinophalangeal syndrome.

AUTOSOMAL DOMINANT AND RECESSIVE FORMS

Facies. The hair is sparse. The nose is bulbous with tented alae, and the cartilaginous framework has been described as flabby. The philtrum is elongated and prominent. The upper lip is thin. Mild micrognathia has been described. The ears may be large and outstanding. Midface hypoplasia has been noted in some instances (7, 8, 17, 24) (Fig. 138-1*A*, *B*).

Hair and nails. Scalp hair is sparse from the time of birth (23), being especially scant in the frontotemporal areas, somewhat simulating the male baldness pattern. Its texture is fine and brittle, and growth is slow. The eyebrows are broad medially and narrow laterally (16, 23). The cilia and pubic and axillary hair may be scant (7, 16) and the nails thin (7, 14).

Skeletal system. Growth retardation is variable, height being below the 3d percentile in 40 percent of patients and seldom above the 25th percentile (7, 11, 15, 25). Bone age is often several years behind chronologic age.

The fingers tend to become progressively deformed during midchildhood, but these changes tend to plateau at puberty. Characteristically, there is swelling of the proximal interphalangeal joints, resulting in clinobrachydactyly (Fig. 138-1*C*). The distal phalanges in both thumbs

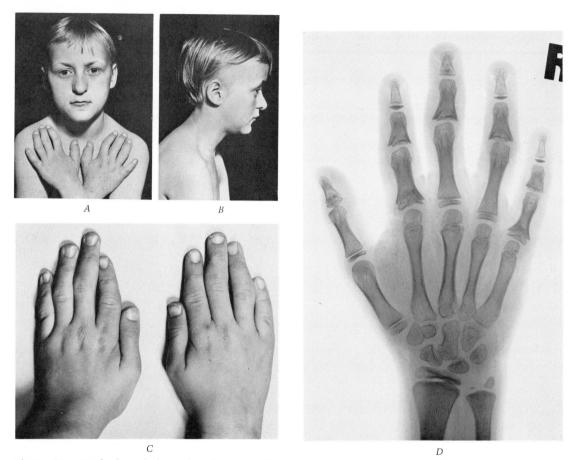

Figure 138-1. *Trichorhinophalangeal syndrome.* (*A, B*). Pear-shaped nose, frontal bossing with high lateral hairline, fingers deviated at proximal interphalangeal joints. (*C*). Close-up of hands showing deviation of fingers at proximal interphalangeal joints. (*D*). Cone-shaped epiphyses (type 12) and eburnated epiphyses. (*A, B, and D from A. Giedion,* Fortschr. Roentgenstr. **110:**507, 1969; *C from A. Giedion,* Helv. Paediatr. Acta **21:**475, 1966.)

and halluces are usually short. Toes as well as fingers may be abbreviated. Pes planus has been noted in several cases (7, 16).

Roentgenographically, cone-shaped epiphyses (type 12) are usually present in the middle phalanges of the second, third, and fourth fingers (9) (Fig. 138-1*D*). Metacarpals, especially the fourth and fifth, are shortened (5) in about half the cases. Elimination of some epiphyses before phalangeal epiphyseal fusion is seen in about 65 percent of cases (11). Multiple cone-shaped epiphyses may also be noted in the toes. Scoliosis and lordosis have been described by several authors (7, 14, 15). The scapulas are often winged.

Other findings. Increased susceptibility to upper respiratory tract infections has been noted in several cases (7, 14, 16), and Hussels (15) cited repeated cyanotic attacks caused by glossoptosis during infancy. Giedion et al. (11) suggested possible increased incidence of congenital heart disease and renal disorders.

Table 138-1. Comparison of the features of the dominant and recessive forms of the trichorhinophalangeal syndrome and the Langer-Giedion syndrome

Features	Trichorhinophalangeal syndrome (dominant and recessive forms)	Langer-Giedion syndrome
Features in common:		
Recurrent respiratory infections	+	+
Sparse scalp hair	+	+
Large, laterally protuding ears	+	+
Bulbous nose with tented alae	+	+
Prominent elongated philtrum	+	+
Thin upper lip	+	+
Apparent mandibular micrognathia	+	+
Clinobrachydactyly	+	±
Cone-shaped epiphyses (type 12) of the hands	+	+
Winged scapula	+	+
Short stature	+	+
Additional features of the Langer-Giedion syndrome:		
Multiple exostoses	−	+
Redundant and/or loose skin in infancy and early childhood	−	+
Laxity or hypermobility at joints	−	+
Microcephaly	−	+
Mental retardation	−	+
Significantly delayed onset of speech	−	+
Skin nevi	−	+

SOURCE: Modified after B. D. Hall et al., *Birth Defects* **10**(12):147, 1974.

Oral manifestations. Malocclusion (5) and supernumerary incisors (7, 14) have been described.

LANGER-GIEDION SYNDROME

The Langer-Giedion syndrome has many features in common with both the autosomal dominant and autosomal recessive forms of the trichorhinophalangeal syndrome, although there are differences (Table 138-1). Findings have been thoroughly discussed by Hall et al. (13). All cases have been sporadic.

Facies. The craniofacial appearance is similar to that in the trichorhinophalangeal syndrome, but the nose tends to be less bulbous and the philtral area tends to be more prominent (Fig. 138-2A–D). Mild microcephaly has been a feature of all cases. Exotropia has been documented in several instances. The eyebrows are not as sparse as in trichorhinophalangeal syndrome.

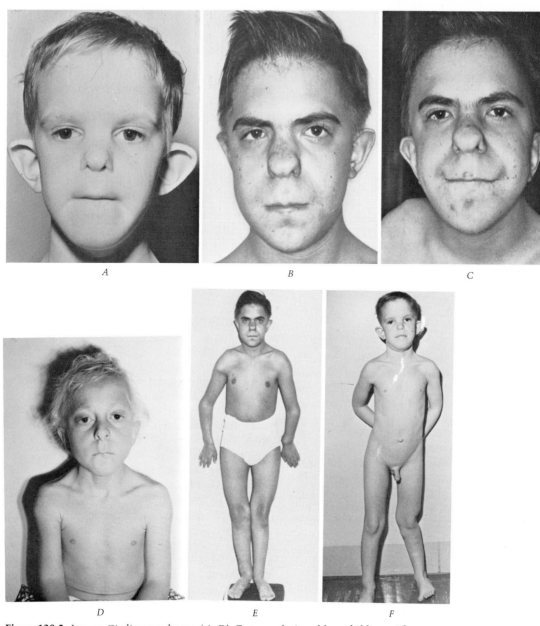

Figure 138-2. *Langer-Giedion syndrome.* (*A–D*). Compare facies of four children with the disorder. Note less pear-shaped nose and more prominent philtrum than in tricho-rhinophalangeal syndrome. All have mild microcephaly, outstanding ears. (*E, F*). Multiple exostoses become evident by the fourth year of life. (A–C, E, *and* F, *from B. D. Hall et al.,* Birth Defects **10**(12):147, 1974; D *from R. J. Gorlin et al.,* Am. J. Dis. Child. **118**:595, 1969.)

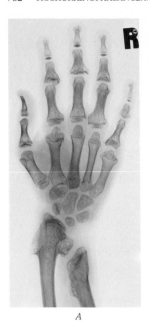

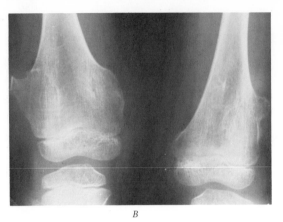

B

Figure 138-3. (*A, B*). Multiple exostoses, cone-shaped epiphyses. (A *from A. Giedion*, Fortschr. Roentgenstr. **110:**507, 1969; B *from R. J. Gorlin et al.*, Am. J. Dis. Child. **118:**595, 1969.)

A

Central nervous system. Mild to moderate mental retardation has been present in all cases. Significantly delayed onset of speech and, less frequently, hearing deficit have been reported.

Skeletal system. Multiple exostoses are present by the third or fourth year of life, and may contribute to abnormalities such as winged scapulas, spinal curvature, clinobrachydactyly, and limb asymmetry (Figs. 138-2*E*, *F*, 138-3*A*, *B*). Growth retardation is of postnatal onset and seems to antedate the presence of multiple exostoses. Fractures have been documented in some cases. Laxity or hypermobility of joints has also been observed.

Skin. During infancy and early childhood, the skin is loose or redundant. This feature disappears with age. Brown to black maculopapular nevi are frequently located on the upper part of the trunk, neck, scalp, and face. They are not present before four years and increase in numbers with age.

Other findings. Upper respiratory tract infections are common in infancy but they abate in childhood.

DIFFERENTIAL DIAGNOSIS

Cruz and Frances (4) described patients with abnormalities similar to those observed in the trichorhinophalangeal syndrome but without the characteristic nasal alterations. The disorder described by Bellini and Bardare (2) represents a completely different entity, with cone-shaped epiphyses (not type 12) and involvement of the epiphyses of both knees.

The combination of short stature, sparse hair, and short fingers may be observed in *cartilage-hair hypoplasia*.

Cone-shaped epiphyses may occur in the general population as an isolated finding, or they may be associated with a plethora of disorders: *de Lange syndrome, cleidocranial dysplasia,* asphyxiant thoracic dystrophy, *chondroectodermal dysplasia, cartilage-hair hypoplasia, pseudohypoparathyroidism,* etc.

Multiple cartilaginous exostoses in the absence of other abnormalities constitute a well-established autosomal dominant entity.

LABORATORY AIDS

Hypoglycemia was reported by Parkhurst et al. (22).

REFERENCES

1 Alè, G., and Calò, S., Su di un caso di disostosi periferica associata con esostosi osteogeniche multiple ed iposomia disuniforme e disarmonica. *Ann. Radiol. Diagn. (Bologna)* **34**:376–385, 1961.

1a Beals, R. K., Tricho-rhino-phalangeal Dysplasia. *J. Bone Joint Surg.* **55A**:821–826, 1973.

2 Bellini, F., and Bardare, M., Su un caso di disostosi periferica. *Minerva Pediatr.* **18**:106–110, 1966.

3 Cesarani, F., and Jucker, C., Aspetti radiologici insoliti delle epifisi falangee delle mani e dei piedi. *Ann. Radiol. Diagn. (Bologna)* **32**:89–97, 1959.

4 Cruz, M., and Frances, J. M., Le syndrome trichophalangien: Une forme nouvelle de dysostose peripherique. *Arch. Fr. Pédiatr.* **27**:649–656, 1970.

5 Fontaine, G., et al., Le syndrome tricho-rhino-phalangien. *Arch. Fr. Pédiatr.* **27**:635–647, 1970.

5a Frisch, H., and Vormittag, W., Trico-rhino-phalangeales Syndrom mit autosomal dominantem Erbgang. *Z. Kinderheilkd.* **120**:141–150, 1975.

6 Fruchter, Z., et al., Radiodiagnostic et pathogenie de la dysostose phalangienne. *J. Radiol. Électrol.* **47**:653–656, 1966.

7 Giedion, A., Das tricho-rhino-phalangeale Syndrom. *Helv. Paediatr. Acta* **21**:475–482, 1966.

8 Giedion, A., Cone-shaped Epiphyses of the Hands and Their Diagnostic Value: The Tricho-rhino-phalangeal Syndrome. *Ann. Radiol.* **10**:322–329, 1967.

9 Giedion, A., Zapfenepiphysen. *Ergeb. Med. Radiol.* **1**:59–124, 1968.

10 Giedion, A., Die periphere Dysostoses (PD)–ein Sammelbegriff. *Fortschr. Roentgenstr.* **110**:507–524, 1969.

11 Giedion, A., et al., Autosomal Dominant Transmission of the Tricho-rhino-phalangeal Syndrome. *Helv. Paediatr. Acta* **28**:249–259, 1973.

12 Gorlin, R. J., et al., Tricho-rhino-phalangeal Syndrome. *Am. J. Dis. Child.* **118**:595–599, 1969.

13 Hall, B. D., et al., Langer-Giedion Syndrome. *Birth Defects* **10**(12):147–164, 1974.

14 Hobolth, N., and Mune, D., Dyostosis epiphysarea peripherica. *Acta Rheumatol. Scand.* **9**:269–276, 1963.

15 Hussels, I., Trichorhinophalangeal Syndrome in Two Sibs. *Birth Defects* **7**(7):301–302, 1971.

16 Klingmüller, G., Über eigentümliche Konstitutionsanomalien der zwei Schwestern und ihre Beziehungen zu neueren entwicklungspathologischen Befunden. *Hautarzt* **7**:105–113, 1956.

17 Lamont Murdoch, J., Tricho-rhino-phalangeal Dysplasia with Possible Autosomal Dominant Transmission. *Birth Defects* **5**(3):218–219, 1969.

18 Langer, L. O., Jr., The Thoracic-pelvic-phalangeal Dystrophy. *Birth Defects* **5**(4):55–64, 1969.

19 Lemaitre, G., et al., Syndrome tricho-rhino-phalangien. Étude de deux fratries, *J. Radiol. Électrol.* **51**:429–432, 1970.

20 Liess, G., Λ-förmige Epiphysen an Händen und Füssen (periphere Dysotosen) (Case 2). *Fortschr. Roentgenstr.* **81**:173–191, 1954.

21 Liévre, J. A., and Camus, J. P., Maladie de Thiemann. *Rev. Rhum.* **39**:39–43, 1967.

22 Parkhurst, R. D., et al., Tricho-rhino-phalangeal Syndrome with Hypoglycemia. *South. Med. J.* **65**:457–459, 1972.

23 Patzer, H., Periphere Dysostosen an den Fingern. *Kinderärztl. Prax.* **32**:231–235, 1964.

24 Senechal, G., and Lambert, H., Les malformations faciales du syndrome tricho-rhino-phalangien. *Ann. Chir. Plast.* **19**:169–173, 1974.

24a Theile, U., et al., Tricho-rhino-phalangeal Syndrome – A Seldom Constitutional Disorder. *Humangenetik* **22**:267–269, 1974.

25 Van der Werff ten Bosch, J. J., The Syndrome of Brachymetacarpal Dwarfism ("Pseudo-pseudo-hypoparathyroidism") with and without Gonadal Dysgenesis. *Lancet* **1**:69–71, 1959 (Cases 5 and 8).

26 Verona, R., and Zoratto, E., La sindrome di Giedion. *Minerva Pediat.* **26**:313–321, 1974.

27 Weaver, D. D., et al., The Tricho-rhino-phalangeal Syndrome. *J. Med. Genet.* **11**:312–314, 1974.

139

Tuberous Sclerosis

(Bourneville-Pringle Syndrome, Epiloia)

Tuberous sclerosis is characterized by (*a*) epilepsy, (*b*) mental retardation, and (*c*) cutaneous angiofibromas. Although it was possibly first recorded by von Recklinghausen, credit is usually given to Bourneville (3) and Pringle (29) for their classic descriptions.

The components of the triad may appear in any order. Some patients may manifest signs at birth, but in the majority of cases, seizures and skin changes first appear in the two- to six-year-old.

The syndrome is found in about 0.1 to 0.6 percent of persons institutionalized for epilepsy and mental retardation (5), and in about 1 in 100,000 to 200,000 in the general population (8). Possibly 850 cases have been reported.

Autosomal dominant inheritance with variable expressivity has been demonstrated. About 70 percent of cases are isolated examples (4, 34), representing fresh mutations (4, 9, 26, 34, 38). However, paternal age is not increased in the isolated case (26).

SYSTEMIC MANIFESTATIONS

Most patients die before they are twenty years old, but some survive into middle age. The usual cause of death is pneumonia, cachexia, status epilepticus, or acute heart failure.

Facies. The facies, with characteristic angiofibromas, may be so evident that the clinician will experience little difficulty in diagnosing the condition after the fourth or fifth year of life (Fig. 139-1*A*–*C*). The term "adenoma sebaceum," so long used, is a misnomer and should be discarded.

Skin and skin appendages. The skin lesions are of several types. Most common are the small, reddish, flat or rounded, seedlike masses composed of hyperplastic connective and vascular tissues (angiofibromas) that are located over the nose, cheeks, nasolabial furrows, and chin. There is a tendency for the upper lip to be spared except on the philtrum. These lesions are present in 90 percent of patients over four years of age. The number seems to increase at puberty. Less common are soft polypoid fibromatous masses over the dorsal area of the trunk or scalp, or beneath or along the nail beds (subungual fibromas) (Fig. 139-2). Round, flat plaques of fibrous connective tissue (shagreen patches) may be noted in the lumbar area in over 20 percent of patients (23, 30).

Many other types of cutaneous lesions may be seen, including oval areas of pigment loss (in about 70 percent of patients) and café-au-lait spots in about 7 percent (27). The white leukodermic areas shaped like the leaf of a mountain ash may be an extremely helpful diagnostic sign at birth or in early infancy (7, 11, 12). They may be evident only under ultraviolet light. The fingernails may be discolored and misshapen (5, 27, 28, 30) because of the subungual fibromas.

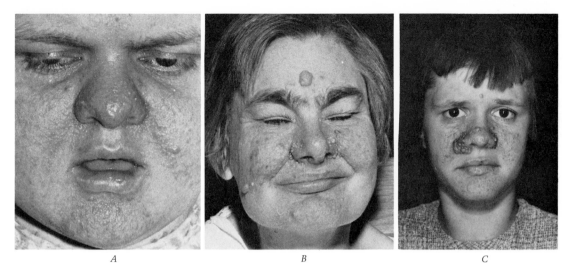

A   *B*   *C*

Figure 139-1. (*A–C*). *Tuberous sclerosis.* Mental retardation and epilepsy, characteristic distribution of skin lesions. Compare severity of facial lesions. B *and* C *from R. Goodman and R. Gorlin,* The Face in Genetic Disease, *Mosby, St. Louis, 1970.*

Central nervous system. The name "tuberous sclerosis" is derived from the numerous smooth, hard, "potato-like" masses of proliferated glial elements and ganglion cells located throughout the cerebral cortex, ependymal lining of the ventricles, and other areas of the brain (36). Rarely, there will be an associated malignancy arising in the glial tissue (19).

About 50 percent of those affected manifest intracranial calcification (23) (Fig. 139-3).

Only about 60 percent of the patients with facial angiofibromas are mentally retarded (8, 23), but when mentality is affected, these pa-

tients are often idiots or low-grade imbeciles (6). Seizures of petit mal, grand mal, or Jacksonian-type epilepsy usually begin within the first two years of life and occur with variable frequency in over 90 percent of cases (23). The degree of severity seems to increase with time.

Eyes. Present in about 50 percent of patients is unilateral or, less often, bilateral retinal tumor ("phakoma"), which may be large and nodular or, more commonly, flat and oval (6, 23, 30). These tumors are gray or yellowish-gray and composed of glial cells, nerve cells, and vascular

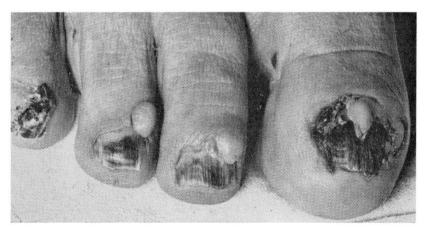

Figure 139-2. Subungual fibromas. (*Courtesy of A. Lodin, Stockholm, Sweden.*)

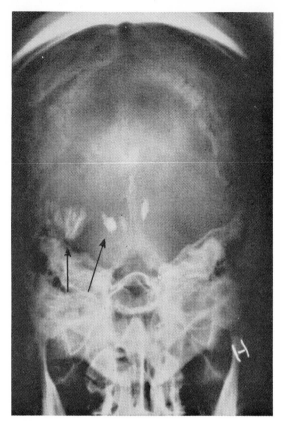

Figure 139-3. Intracranial calcification. (*Courtesy of A. Lodin, Stockholm, Sweden.*)

Genitourinary system. About 40 percent of those affected have renal hamartomas of the mixed type (angiomyolipomas). Rarely is there malignant change (11, 24).

Other findings. Rhabdomyomas of the heart are common (1, 8). Hamartomas may be noted in many organs (lungs, liver, thyroid, testicles, pancreas, etc.) (10, 25).

Oral manifestations. The oral mucosa may be the site of fibrous growths (Fig. 139-5). Schuermann (33) found 11 percent of 186 patients to have such lesions. Most frequently they are located on the anterior gingiva, but they may occur on the oral mucosa (5, 12, 23, 29). They are

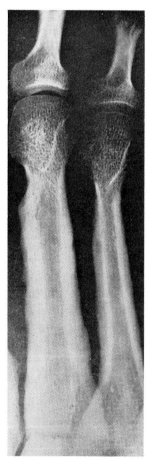

Figure 139-4. Lytic lesions of hand bones. (*Courtesy of T. D. Hawkins,* Br. J. Radiol. **32:**157, 1959.)

tissue (21). Epicanthus is also common (6). The eye anomalies are thoroughly discussed by Reese (31).

Skeletal system. In about half the cases, the skull exhibits thickened calvaria, with an irregular outer table, and exostoses are often seen on the inner table of the frontal bone (23). Areas of increased density appear throughout the skull, especially in the parietal region after puberty (14).

About 65 percent of patients have cystlike areas in the phalanges and irregular periosteal new bone formation along the shafts of the metacarpals and metatarsals (16, 17, 35). Less frequently, long bones are involved (37) (Fig. 139-4).

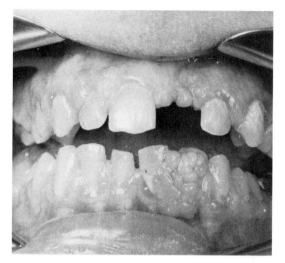

Figure 139-5. Gingival fibromas.

usually the color of normal oral mucosa but occasionally are bluish, red, or yellow, ranging in size from that of a pinpoint to that of a small pea. Enamel defects have been reported (15).

DIFFERENTIAL DIAGNOSIS

Most frequently mistaken for facial angiofibromas are multiple trichoepitheliomas, syringocystadenomas, colloid milia, atypical xanthomas, or, occasionally, intradermal nevi.

Roentgenographic differential diagnosis of the skull should include *Sturge-Weber anomalad*, calcifying subdural hematoma and calcifying neoplasms, cytomegalic inclusion disease, toxoplasmosis, and *hyalinosis cutis et mucosae*. Long-bone changes in tuberous sclerosis should be differentiated from those of *neurofibromatosis*, fibrous dysplasia, enchondromatosis, gout, sarcoid, and hypertrophic arthritis (2). Shagreen patches may also be seen in association with osteopoikilosis.

LABORATORY AIDS

Biopsy of the cutaneous angiofibromas, electroencephalography, and Wood's lamp examination for depigmentation of the skin may be useful (27).

REFERENCES

1 Ackermann, A. J., Pulmonary and Osseous Manifestations of Tuberous Sclerosis. *Am. J. Roentgenol.* **51**:315–325, 1944.

2 Berland, H. I., Roentgenological Findings in Tuberous Sclerosis. *Arch. Neurol. Psychiatr.* **69**:669–683, 1953.

3 Bourneville, D., Sclereuse tubereuse des circonvolutions cérébrales. Idiotie et épilepsie hemiplégique. *Arch. Neurol. (Paris)* **1**:81–91, 1880.

4 Bundey, S., and Evans, K., Tuberous Sclerosis: A Genetic Study. *J. Neurol. Neurosurg. Psychiatr.* **32**:591–603, 1969.

5 Butterworth, T., and Wilson, M., Jr., Dermatologic Aspects of Tuberous Sclerosis. *Arch. Dermatol. Syphiligr. (Chic.)* **43**:1–41, 1941.

6 Chao, D. H.-C., Congenital Neurocutaneous Syndromes in Childhood. II. Tuberous Sclerosis. *J. Pediatr.* **55**:447–459, 1959.

7 Crichton, J. V., Infantile Spasms and Skin Anomalies. *Dev. Med. Child. Neurol.* **8**:273–278, 1966.

8 Dawson, J., Pulmonary Tuberous Sclerosis and Its Relationship to Other Forms of the Disease. *Q. J. Med.* **23**:113–145, 1954.

9 Dickerson, W. W., Characteristic Roentgenographic Changes Associated with Tuberous Sclerosis. *Arch. Neurol. Psychiatr.* **65**:683–702, 1951.

10 Dwyer, J. M., et al., Pulmonary Tuberous Sclerosis. Report of Three Patients and a Review of the Literature. *Q. J. Med.* **40**:115–126, 1971.

11 Fitzpatrick, T. B., et al., White Leaf-shaped Macules. *Arch. Dermatol.* **98**:1–6, 1968.

12 Gold, A. P., and Freeman, J. M., Depigmented Naevi: The Earliest Sign of Tuberous Sclerosis. *Pediatrics* **35**:1003–1005, 1965.

13 Gorlin, R. J., et al., Oral Manifestations of the Fitzgerald-Gardner, Pringle-Bourneville, Robin, Adrenogenital and Hurler-Pfaundler Syndromes. *Oral Surg.* **13**:1233–1244, 1960.

14 Hawkins, T. D., Radiological Bone Changes in Tuberous Sclerosis. *Br. J. Radiol.* **32**:157–161, 1959.

15 Hoff, M. F., et al., Enamel Defects Associated with Tuberous Sclerosis. *Oral Surg.* **40**:261–269, 1975.

16 Holt, J. F., and Dickerson, W. W., The Osseous Lesions of Tuberous Sclerosis. *Radiology* **58**:1–7, 1952.

17 Hornstein, O., Über Skelettveränderungen beim Morbus Bourneville-Pringle. *Dtsch. Med. Wochenschr.* **83**:214–218, 1958.

18 Hurwitz, S., and Braverman, I., White Spots in Tuberous Sclerosis. *J. Pediatr.* **77**:587–594, 1970.

19 Jervis, G. A., Spongioneuroblastoma and Tuberose Sclero-

sis. *J. Neuropathol. Exp. Neurol.* **13:**105–116, 1954.

20 Jordan, W. M., Familial Tuberous Sclerosis. *Br. Med. J.* **2:**132–135, 1956.

21 Kirby, T. J., Ocular Phakomatosis. *Am. J. Med. Sci.* **222:**227–239, 1951.

22 Koch, G., Tuberöse Sklerose. *Ärztl. Fortsch.* **6:**471–480, 1952.

23 Lagos, J. C., and Gomez, M. R., Tuberous Sclerosis. Reappraisal of a Clinical Entity. *Mayo Clin. Proc.* **42:**26–49, 1967.

24 Lebrun, H. I., et al., Renal Hamartoma. *Br. J. Urol.* **27:**394–407, 1955.

25 Milledge, R. D., et al., Pulmonary Manifestations of Tuberous Sclerosis. *Am. J. Roentgenol.* **98:**734–738, 1966.

26 Nevin, N. C., and Pearce, W. G., Diagnostic and Genetical Aspects of Tuberous Sclerosis. *J. Med. Genet.* **5:**273–280, 1968.

27 Nickel, W. R., and Reed, W. B., Tuberous Sclerosis. *Arch. Dermatol.* **85:**209–226, 1962.

28 Pagenstecher, W. J., Tuberous Sclerosis. Historical Review and Report of Two Cases. *Am. J. Ophthalmol.* **39:**663–676, 1955.

28a Papanayotou, P., and Vezirtzi, E., Tuberous Sclerosis with Gingival Lesions. *Oral Surg.* **39:**578–582, 1975.

29 Pringle, J. J., A Case of Congenital Adenoma Sebaceum. *Br. J. Dermatol.* **2:**1–14, 1890.

30 Reed, W. B., et al., Internal Manifestations of Tuberous Sclerosis. *Arch. Dermatol.* **87:**715–728, 1963.

31 Reese, A. B., *Tumors of the Eye.* Hoeber, New York, 1951.

32 Rushton, M. A., Some Less Common Bone Lesions Affecting the Jaws: Tuberous Sclerosis with Jaw Lesions. *Oral Surg.* **9:**289–304, 1956.

33 Schuermann, H., *Krankheiten der Mundschleimhaut und der Lippen,* 2d ed., Urban & Schwarzenberg, Munich, 1958.

34 Singer, K., Genetic Aspects of Tuberous Sclerosis in a Chinese Population. *Am. Jt Hum. Genet.* **23:**33–40, 1971.

35 Smith, T. K., et al., Orthopaedic Problems Associated with Tuberous Sclerosis. *J. Bone Joint Surg.* **51A:**97–102, 1969.

36 Thibault, J. H., and Manuelidis, E. E., Tuberous Sclerosis in a Premature Infant. *Neurology* **20:**139–146, 1970.

37 Whitaker, P. H., Radiological Manifestations in Tuberose Sclerosis. *Br. J. Radiol.* **32:**152–156, 1959.

38 Zaremba, J., Tuberous Sclerosis. A Clinical and Genetical Investigation. *J. Ment. Defic. Res.* **12:**63–80, 1968.

140

Waardenburg Syndrome

The syndrome so precisely described by Waardenburg in 1948 (35) was reported earlier by Mende (19a), van der Hoeve (34), and others (8, 21). The main features include (a) lateral displacement of the medial canthi and lacrimal punctas with a broad nasal root, (b) poliosis, (c) heterochromia irides, (d) hyperplasia of the medial portions of the eyebrows, and (e) congenital sensorineural deafness. Features such as vitiligo, pigmentary changes of the fundi, nasal alar hypoplasia, mild mandibular prognathism, cleft lip-palate, and skeletal deformities have been recognized as other expressions of the Waardenburg syndrome (5, 9–11, 21, 36).

Approximately 80 pedigrees with over 500 affected individuals and about 50 isolated cases have been reported (21). The genetic evidence is consistent with autosomal dominant transmission, complete penetrance, and variable expressivity. Estimates of prevalence suggest that the syndrome is found in approximately 2 percent of all congenitally deaf persons in the United States (5). Between two and three per 100,000 in the general population are affected in the Netherlands (35). However, since most probands have been recognized because of impaired hearing, there is ascertainment bias (21). There may be linkage with the ABO blood groups (28).

The association of cutaneous albinism and deafness is also known to occur in dogs, cats, mice, mink, cattle, and horses (8, 13, 21).

SYSTEMIC MANIFESTATIONS

Facies. The broad nasal root, apparent even in infancy, when combined with other features such as poliosis, synophrys, heterochromia irides, hypoplastic alar cartilages, and mild mandibular prognathism, produces a remarkably striking appearance (Figs. 140-1, 140-2).

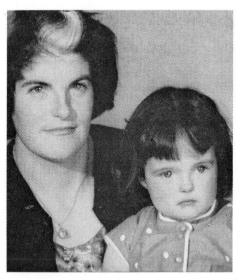

Figure 140-1. *Waardenburg syndrome.* Note white forelock in both mother and daughter, lack of alar flare, dystopia canthorum, mild prognathism. (*From M. W. Partington,* Arch. Dis. Child. **34**:154, 1959.)

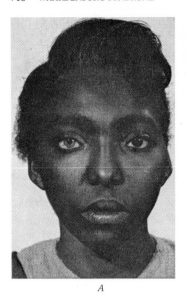
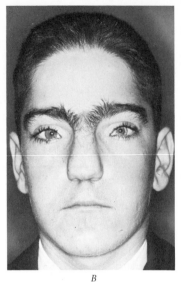

A

B

Figure 140-2. (*A*). Similar findings in an Afro-American patient. Note heterochromia irides. (*From A. M. DiGeorge et al.*, J. Pediatr. **57**:649, 1960.) (*B*). Note marked synophrys, dystopia canthorum, heterochromia irides, and severe hypoplasia of the nasal alae. (*From M. W. Partington*, Canadian Med. Assoc. J. **90**:1008, 1964.)

Eyes. Although the interpupillary and outer canthal distances are normal in most affected individuals, an increased distance between the inner canthi (dystopia canthorum) is evident, resulting in blepharophimosis (Fig. 140-1). This appears to be the most frequent finding (in about 85 percent of cases) in the syndrome. Scleras may be covered medially, giving a false impression of esotropia. True ocular hypertelorism is present in about 10 percent of the cases (21, 33). Normal inner canthal, outer canthal, and interpupillary values have been discussed by Pryor (25) and others (16, 20).

The inferior lacrimal points are displaced laterally, sometimes as far as the cornea. There is an increased susceptibility to dacryocystitis (21). Hyperplasia of the medial portions of the eyebrows, or even confluence (synophrys), is present in more than half the cases. [This characteristic may be less evident in women, who often pluck these hairs (5, 21) (Figs. 140-1, 140-2).] Heterochromia irides, or, more accurately, hypoplasia of the irides, is seen in more than one-third of the cases. It may be partial or total, both irides ranging from a mottled to blue appearance. Especially striking is the presence of one blue and one brown eye or of two pale-blue eyes in an Afro-American (5). DiGeorge et al. (5) noted pigmentary mottling at the periphery of the fundi (10). Other eye anomalies such as cataracts, mi-

crophthalmia, and ptosis have been reported (10, 26, 33, 35, 36).

Hair and skin. White forelock (poliosis) is present in more than 40 percent of patients. In some cases, only a few white hairs are evident. This feature may be present at birth but tends to disappear with age (6). [In females, poliosis may not be evident because of the tendency to mask it by dyeing the hair (5).] Premature graying of eyebrows, lashes, and hair may also occur. Hypertrichosis has been observed in several cases (1, 20, 25). Pigmentary anomalies, such as vitiligo, may be found in about 15 percent of affected persons (21).

Ears and nose. Waardenburg (35) noted that congenital sensorineural deafness occurred in 20 percent of affected individuals. A recent review article (21) indicated a higher frequency. Little residual hearing is present for the lower frequencies. Some patients have unilateral deafness, rarely of severe degree, in which moderate uniform hearing loss for the lower and middle ranges occurs with improvement in the higher range—often with normal hearing for 6,000 to 8,000 cycles per second (7). In both man and animals, this deafness has been shown to be due to absence of the organ of Corti and demyelinization of the acoustic nerve (7, 8, 13). Malformations of the external ear have also been reported (20, 26, 35).

The nasal root is broad, often with loss of the frontonasal angle. The alar cartilages are usually hypoplastic, resulting in narrow nostrils (Fig. 140-2B). The tip of the nose tends to be rounded and slightly upturned, revealing the columella (15, 26).

Skeletal system. Few cases have been reported in which full roentgenographic surveys were carried out. Of the cases reported, a variety of skeletal anomalies such as the Sprengel deformity, skull anomalies, bony defects of the thorax, abnormal upper limb length, abnormal carpal bones, syndactyly, sacralization of the fifth lumbar vertebra, and spina bifida have been noted (3, 17, 21, 24, 35).

Oral manifestations. Oral findings have not been well documented. The lower lip is especially full and protrudes, with shortened interangular distance. The mandible seems to be prognathic in most patients, although this feature has been studied cephalometrically in few instances (5, 21, 33, 35, 36). At least 13 cases of cleft lip-palate have been reported (9–11, 24, 26, 29, 35) (Fig. 140-3). Highly arched palate is frequently observed (1, 9–11, 20, 21, 24, 26). Roentgenographic examination of the skull in a small series of patients has demonstrated marked lateral winging of the angle of the mandible, increasing the bigonial distance.

DIFFERENTIAL DIAGNOSIS

Klein (15) described a patient with primary telecanthus, synophrys, partial albinism of skin and hair, and blue irides. However, there was also osseous dysplasia — aplasia of the first two ribs and carpal bones, cystic alterations of the sacrum, cutaneous union of the thorax and upper arm, and syndactyly. A patient described by Wilbrandt (36) who also had arthromyodysplasia was noted in a family having otherwise typical Waardenburg syndrome.

Dystopia canthorum and hypertelorism may be seen in a variety of disorders (23). Synophrys is a feature of the *de Lange syndrome* and may also occur with pilonidal cyst (27). Hypoplastic

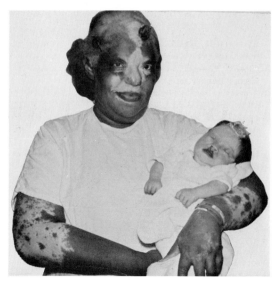

Figure 140-3. Note similar facies, vitiligo, cleft lip in infant. (*Courtesy of M. Goldberg, Chicago, Ill.*)

alar cartilages may be seen in the *OFD I syndrome.* Poliosis, with or without piebaldness, may be inherited as an autosomal dominant trait (8, 29). Poliosis, vitiligo, and dysacousia may be seen in combination with alopecia and uveitis in the Vogt-Koyanagi syndrome (12). Heterochromia irides may be acquired, inherited as an autosomal dominant trait (7, 8), or associated with the *Romberg syndrome.* Partial albinism with deafness is known to occur as an X-linked trait (38). An autosomal dominant syndrome of white forelock, leukoderma, cerebellar ataxia, poor motor coordination, and mild mental retardation was described by Telfer et al. (31). An autosomal recessive disorder similar to the Waardenburg syndrome but with black instead of white forelock has been reported to occur in South America (2).

LABORATORY AIDS

See Appendix for normal inner canthal and interpupillary distances. A rough estimate of whether a person has dystopia canthorum may be made either on the person or on a photograph employing an inexpensive caliper. The inner canthal distance divided by the interpupillary is greater than 0.6 with dystopia canthorum.

REFERENCES

1 Ahrendts, H., Das Waardenburg-Syndrom, dargestellt an fünf Familien. *Z. Kinderheilkd.* **93**:295–313, 1965.

2 Arias, S., Genetic Heterogeneity in the Waardenburg Syndrome. *Birth Defects* **7**(4):87–101, 1971.

3 Arnvig, J., The Syndrome of Waardenburg. *Acta Genet. (Basel)* **9**:41–46, 1959.

4 Basile, R., A Pedigree of Binocular Heterochromia Iridis Associated with Other Anomalies (Waardenburg-Klein Syndrome). *J. Génét. Hum.* **14**:87–91, 1965.

5 DiGeorge, A. M., et al., Waardenburg's Syndrome. *J. Pediatr.* **57**:649–669, 1960.

6 Feingold, M., et al., Waardenburg's Syndrome During the First Year of Life. *J. Pediatr.* **71**:874–876, 1967.

7 Fisch, L., Deafness as Part of an Hereditary Syndrome. *J. Laryngol. Otol.* **73**:355–383, 1959.

8 François, J., and Verriest, G., Anomalies of Pigmentation, in J. François (ed.), *Heredity in Ophthalmology*. Mosby, St. Louis, 1961, pp. 519–541.

9 Giacoia, J. P., and Klein, S. W., Waardenburg's Syndrome with Bilateral Cleft Lip. *Am. J. Dis. Child.* **117**:344–347, 1969.

10 Goldberg, M. F., Waardenburg's Syndrome with Fundus and Other Anomalies. *Arch. Ophthalmol.* **76**:797–810, 1966.

11 Gorlin, R. J., et al., Facial Clefting and Its Syndromes. *Birth Defects* **7**(7):3–49, 1971.

12 Hague, E. B., Uveitis, Dysacousia, Alopecia, Poliosis and Vitiligo. *Arch. Ophthalmol.* **31**:520–538, 1944.

13 Innes, J. R. M., and Saunders, L. Z., Diseases of the Central Nervous System of Domesticated Animals and Comparison with Human Neuropathology. *Adv. Vet. Sci.* **3**:33–196, 1957.

14 Johr, P., Valeurs moyennes et limites normales, en fonction de l'âge de quelques mesures de la tête et de la région orbitaire. *J. Génét. Hum.* **2**:247–282, 1953.

15 Klein, D., Albinisme partiel (leucisme) avec surdi-mutité, blepharophimosis et dysplasia myo-ostéo-articulaire. *Helv. Paediatr. Acta* **5**:35–58, 1950.

16 Laestadius, N. D., et al., Normal Inner Canthal and Outer Orbital Dimensions. *J. Pediatr.* **74**:465–468, 1969.

17 Lavergne, M. G., Problème d'eugénisme posé par une famille atteinte du syndrome de Waardenburg-Klein. *Bull. Soc. Belg. Ophthalmol.* **122**:403–407, 1959.

18 McDonald, R., and Harrison, V. C., The Waardenburg Syndrome. *Clin. Pediatr.* **4**:739–744, 1965.

19 McKenzie, J., The First Arch Syndrome. *Arch. Dis. Child.* **33**:477–486, 1958.

19a Mende, I., Über eine Familie hereditär-degenerativer Taubstummer mit mongoloidem Einschlag und teilweisen Leukismus der Haut und Haare. *Arch. Kinderheilkd.* **79**:214–222, 1926.

20 Metres, K., and Kutzvegli, F., Inner Canthal and Intermamillary Indices in the Newborn Infant. *J. Pediatr.* **85**:90–92, 1975.

21 Pantke, O. A., and Cohen, M. M., Jr., The Waardenburg Syndrome. *Birth Defects* **7**(7):147–152, 1971.

22 Partington, M. W., Waardenburg's Syndrome and Heterochromia Iridum in a Deaf School Population. *Canadian Med. Assoc. J.* **90**:1008–1017, 1964.

23 Peterson, M. A., et al., Comments on Frontonasal Dysplasia, Ocular Hypertelorism and Dystopia Canthorum. *Birth Defects* **7**(7):120–124, 1971.

24 Pirodda, A., et al., Contributo alla conoscenza della sindrome di Waardenburg e Klein. *Ann. Ottalmol. Clin. Ocul.* **87**:401–426, 1961.

25 Pryor, H. B., Objective Measurement of Interpupillary Distance. *Pediatrics* **44**:973–977, 1969.

26 Reed, W. B., et al., Pigmentary Disorders in Association with Congenital Deafness. *Arch. Dermatol.* **95**:176–186, 1967.

27 Sebrechts, P. H., A Significant Sign of Pilonidal Cyst. *Dis. Colon Rectum* **4**:56–59, 1961.

28 Simpson, J. L., et al., Analysis for Possible Linkage Between the Loci for the Waardenburg Syndrome and Various Blood Groups and Serological Traits. *Humangenetik* **23**:45–50, 1974.

29 Sundfor, H., A Pedigree of Skin-spotting in Man. *J. Hered.* **30**:67–77, 1939.

30 Tay, C. H., Waardenburg's Syndrome and Familial Periodic Paralysis. *Postgrad. Med. J.* **47**:354–360, 1971.

31 Telfer, M. A., et al., Dominant Piebald Trait (White Forelock and Leukoderma) with Neurological Impairment. *Am. J. Hum. Genet.* **23**:383–389, 1971.

32 Tietz, W., A Syndrome of Deaf-mutism Associated with Albinism Showing Dominant Autosomal Inheritance. *Am. J. Hum. Genet.* **15**:259–264, 1963.

33 Ulivelli, A., and Silenzi, M., Hypertelorism and Waardenburg's Syndrome. *Helv. Paediatr. Acta* **24**:123–126, 1969.

34 Van der Hoeve, J., Abnorme Länge der Tränenröhrchen mit Ankyloblepharon. *Klin. Monatsbl. Augenheilkd.* **56**:232–238, 1916.

35 Waardenburg, P. J., A New Syndrome Combining Developmental Anomalies of the Eyelids, Eyebrows and Nose Root with Congenital Deafness. *Am. J. Hum. Genet.* **3**:195–253, 1951.

36 Wilbrandt, H. R., and Ammann, F., Nouvelle observation de la forme grave du syndrome de Klein-Waardenburg. *Arch. Julius Klaus Stift. Vererbungsforsch.* **39**:80–92, 1964.

37 Witkop, C. J., Jr., Albinism, in H. Harris and K. Hirschhorn (eds.). *Adv. Hum. Genet.* **2**:61–141, 1971.

38 Ziprkowski, L., et al., Partial Albinism and Deafmutism, Due to a Recessive Sex-linked Gene. *Arch. Dermatol.* **86**:530–536, 1962.

39 Ziprkowski, L., and Adam, A., Recessive Total Albinism and Congenital Deaf-mutism. *Arch. Dermatol.* **89**:151–155, 1964.

141

Werner Syndrome

The syndrome, first delineated by Werner (17) in 1904, consists of (a) shortness of stature, (b) premature graying of hair (canities) and baldness, (c) scleropoikiloderma, (d) trophic leg ulcers, (e) juvenile cataracts, (f) hypogonadism, (g) diabetes mellitus, (h) calcification of blood vessels, and (i) osteoporosis.

Confusion with Rothmund-Thomson syndrome (13) occurred until Oppenheimer and Kugel (9), Thannhauser (15), and Greither (4) clearly separated the syndromes.

Autosomal recessive inheritance for the disorder has clearly been established (2, 11).

SYSTEMIC MANIFESTATIONS

The disorder becomes apparent in the third and fourth decades of life—graying of the hair occurs at about age twenty, skin changes and loss of hair at age twenty-five, cataracts at age thirty, and diabetes mellitus at about thirty-five years of age.

Shortness of stature due to arrest of growth at puberty is a constant feature. The mean height is 157 cm for males and 146 cm for females (2, 18). The thinness of the arms and legs and the diminution in the size of the hands and feet are striking. Patients characteristically develop an abnormally high-pitched, sometimes squeaky or, less often, hoarse voice.

Facies. The combination of atrophic skin changes, baldness, and graying hair gives these patients, even while young, an appearance of being 20 to 30 years older than their age. Although the cheeks are full, the nose assumes a pinched or beaked appearance (Fig. 141-1).

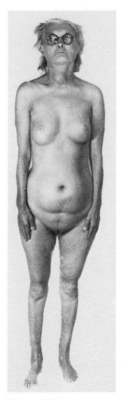

Figure 141-1. *Werner syndrome.* Aged appearance together with marked thinness of arms and legs. (*From S. Jablonska, Warsaw, Poland.*)

Skin. The principal areas of skin involvement are the face and distal legs, especially the feet. There is atrophy of the skin over areas depleted of adipose tissue, connective tissue, and musculature. This results in shiny smooth skin which adheres to the underlying tissue, giving a sclerodermoid appearance (15). Commonly there is ischemic ulceration. The eyes appear protuberant because of loss of circumorbital tissue. The ears may become stiff and inelastic. Circumscribed hyperkeratoses develop over bony prominences and on the soles, and may become ulcerated, with slow or no healing (12). Shortly after adolescence, the patient develops premature graying, baldness, and loss of pubic and axillary hair.

Localized or, less common, generalized hyperpigmentation, depigmentation, and telangiectasia have occurred on the arms and legs in some patients, the term "poikilodermatous" then being applied (16).

Eyes. Senile cataracts, another cardinal feature, are invariably bilateral and are usually posterior, cortical, or subcapsular. They have an abrupt onset during the third or fourth decade. Retinitis pigmentosa, senile macular degeneration, and chorioretinitis have also been described (6, 11, 12, 17).

Hair. Loss and graying of scalp hair is characteristic (Fig. 141-2). Generalized hair loss involving the scalp, eyebrows, eyelashes, and body hair may be secondary to hypogonadism.

Musculoskeletal. Osteoporosis and profound wasting of the musculature of the legs, feet, and hands are characteristic (Fig. 141-3*A, B*). Soft-tissue calcification has been observed in one-third of the cases, especially in the tendons and ligaments of the knees, elbows, and ankles (2). The tissues adjacent to these areas may also exhibit soft-tissue calcification similar to that observed in scleroderma (11).

Cardiovascular system. Patients develop severe, often generalized vascular disease. Calcification occurs in both peripheral (Mönckeberg) vessels and in the aortic valve and coronary vessels (2, 11). Peripheral vascular disease further compli-

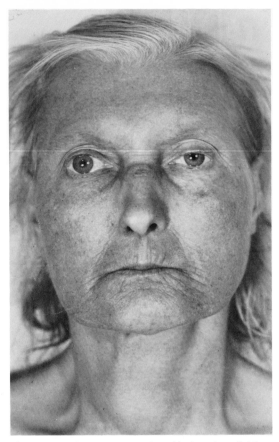

Figure 141-2. Premature graying of hair, aging of skin. (*From S. Jablonska, Warsaw, Poland.*)

cates or promotes atrophy and ulceration of the skin.

Endocrine system. Diabetes mellitus has been recognized in 45 percent of patients (2). However, the usual complications of diabetes (nephropathy, retinopathy, neuropathy) have not been observed. Neither the vascular disease nor the cataracts are well correlated with the diabetes mellitus.

Hypogonadism occurs in both males and females with the Werner syndrome. Most males have small testes and penis, with diminished pubic hair. Women have poorly developed genitalia and breasts, and some never develop secondary sex characteristics. Menses are sparse and irregular. However, there are valid reports of

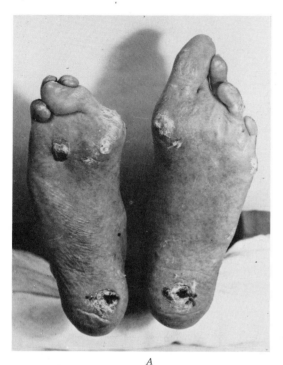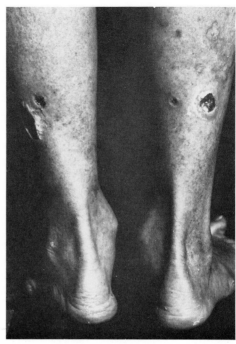

A   B

Figure 141-3. (A). Hyperkeratosis and ulceration of soles. (*From S. Jablonska, Warsaw, Poland.*) (B). Ulceration and pigmentation of ankles. (*From W. Knoth et al.,* Hautarzt **14:**145, 1963.)

men who have sired children and women who have borne children.

Central nervous system. Some patients may be mentally retarded (11), and about one-third may have mild neurologic deficits, such as loss of deep-tendon reflexes, paresthesias, and dizziness (2).

Neoplasia. Despite the profound skin changes, there have been no reports of cutaneous carcinoma. However, a striking preponderance of other neoplasms does occur: hepatoma, breast carcinoma, thyroid adenocarcinoma, and osteosarcoma (12). About 10 percent of those affected have had tumors of mesenchymal derivation (2, 11).

Oral manifestations. The skin around the mouth is often radially ridged, and Frenkel (3) described atrophy of the oral mucosa.

DIFFERENTIAL DIAGNOSIS

In the *Rothmund-Thomson syndrome,* the onset of skin changes and cataracts occurs during the first 10 years of life and photosensitivity is present in about one-third of the patients. The skin also shows telangiectasia, scaling, and pigmentary changes, and skin cancer is a prominent feature (Table 141-1).

Progeria, in contrast to the Werner syndrome progeria, has a very early onset. There are severe dwarfing, nearly complete alopecia, absence of subcutaneous fat, and characteristic facies. Generalized atherosclerosis leads to early death.

Gilkes et al. (3a) described an autosomal recessively inherited disorder which is apparent at birth which they called metageria. It was characterized by normal height, diabetes mellitus of early onset, no loss of hair, and no cataracts. The skin was dry, atrophic, and mottled. The face was pinched with a beaked nose.

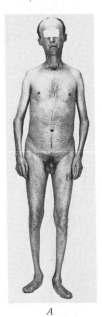

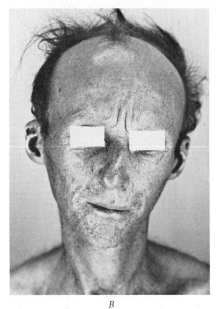

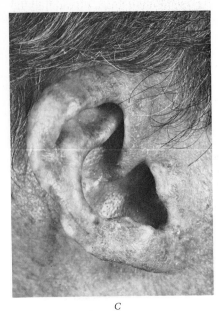

A   *B*   *C*

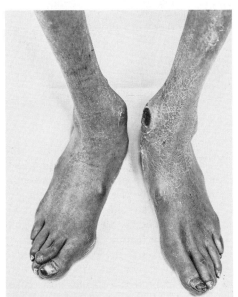

D

Figure 141-4. (*A–D*). Compare with appearance of patients seen in Figs. 141-1 to 141-3. (*From G. Bohnenstengel, Postock, East Germany.*)

Myotonic dystrophy frequently has its onset in the second and third decades (1). Cataracts, diabetes, premature frontal baldness, and atrophy of the skin are all features of this disorder. Testicular atrophy occurs, but the external genitalia are otherwise normal. Inheritance is autosomal dominant.

Acrogeria refers to senile changes largely limited to the distal extremities (4a). The subcutaneous vascular pattern is usually evident over the chest. Mulvihill et al. (7a) reported a syndrome of microcephaly, short stature, bird facies, mental retardation, and premature aging.

LABORATORY AIDS

Nienhaus et al. (8) demonstrated reduced tritiated thymidine uptake in cultured fibroblasts. A marked increase in the dermatan sulfate content of the ground substance of the skin has been found (2a).

Table 141-1. Comparison of Werner Syndrome with Rothmund-Thomson syndrome

Characteristic	Werner syndrome	Rothmund-Thomson syndrome
Habitus	Small, thin extremities, plump trunk	Short, proportional
Face	Moon face	Not characteristic
Cataracts	After 20 years, rapid development, less often resulting in blindness	3-6 years, rapid development, frequent blindness
Hypoplastic teeth	+/0	+/0
Premature graying	+++	0
Premature baldness	+++	0
High voice	+++	0
Skin	Atrophy of skin, subcutaneous connective tissue, and muscle, with pigmentation	Poikiloderma
Fingers	Sclerodactyly	Short, stumpy
Nail changes	++	+/0
Hyperkeratoses	Extremities	0
Skin ulcers	+++	0
Diabetes	+/0	0
Osteoporosis	+++	0
Arteriosclerosis	+++	0
Hypogenitalism	++	+
Late sexual maturation	++	+
Sterility	++	+++
Psychic disturbance, intelligence	Retarded	Normal
Sex	60% males	80% females
Age of predilection	20-30 yr	1-6 yr

SOURCE: Modified from A. Greither, *Arch. Klin. Exp. Dermatol.* **201**:431-445, 1955.

REFERENCES

1 Caughey, E., and Myrianthopoulos, N. C., *Dystrophia Myotonia and Related Disorders.* Charles C Thomas, Springfield, Ill., 1963.

2 Epstein, C. J., et al., Werner's Syndrome. *Medicine (Baltimore)* **45**:177-221, 1966.

2a Fleischmajer, R., and Nedwich, A., Werner's Syndrome. *Am. J. Med.* **54**:111-118, 1973.

3 Frenkel, G., Schleimhautatrophie unter besonderer Berücksichtigung des Werner-Syndroms. *Dtsch. Zahnärztl. Z.* **25**:1026-1029, 1970.

3a Gilkes, J. J. H., et al., The Premature Ageing Syndromes. Report of Eight Cases and Description of a New Entity Named Metageria. *Br. J. Derm.* **91**:243-262, 1974.

4 Greither, A., Über das Rothmund und das Werner-Syndrom. *Arch. Klin. Exp. Dermatol.* **201**:431-445, 1955.

4a Grüneberg, T., Die Akrogerie (Gottron). *Arch. Klin. Exp. Dermatol.* **210**:409-417, 1960.

5 Kansky, A., and Franzot, J., Werner's Syndrome. *Acta Derm. Venereol. (Stockh.)* **43**:441-450, 1963.

6 Kleeberg, J., A Case of Werner's Syndrome. *Acta Med. Orient. (Tel-Aviv)* **8-9**:145-148, 1949.

7 Müller, L., and Andersson, B., Werner's Syndrome. *Acta Med. Scand. [Suppl.]* **283**:1-17, 1953.

7a Mulvihill, J. J., and Smith, D. W., Another Disorder with Premature Shortness of Stature and Premature Aging. *Birth Defects* **11**(2):368-371, 1975.

8 Nienhaus, A. J., et al., Fibroblast Culture in Werner's Syndrome. *Humangenetik* **13**:244-246, 1971.

9 Oppenheimer, B. S., and Kugel, V. H., Werner's Syndrome: Report of the First Necropsy and of Findings in a New

Case. *Am. J. Med. Sci.* **202:**629–642, 1941.

10 Petrohelos, M. A., Werner's Syndrome. *Am. J. Oph-thalmol.* **56:**941–953, 1963.

11 Riley, T. R., et al., Werner's Syndrome. *Ann. Intern. Med.* **63:**285–294, 1965.

12 Rosen, R. S., et al., Werner's Syndrome. *Br. J. Radiol.* **43:**193–198, 1970.

13 Rothmund, A., Über Kataract in Verbindung mit einer eigentümlichen Hautdegeneration. *Albrecht von Graefes Arch. Klin. Ophthalmol.* **14:**159–182, 1868.

14 Smith, R. C., et al., Werner's Syndrome. *Arch. Dermatol.* **71:**197–204, 1955.

15 Thannhauser, S. J., Werner's Syndrome (Progeria of the Adult) and Rothmund's Syndrome: Two Types of Closely Related Heredo-familial Atrophic Dermatosis with Juvenile Cataracts and Endocrine Features. *Ann. Intern. Med.* **23:**559–626, 1945.

16 Valero, A., and Gellei, B., Retinitis Pigmentosa, Hypertension and Uraemia in Werner's Syndrome. *Br. Med. J.* **2:**351–356, 1960.

17 Werner, O., *Über Katarakt in Verbindung mit Sklerodermie.* Thesis, 1904, Kiel, Schmidt & Klaunig, Kiel.

18 Zucker-Franklin, D., et al., Werner's Syndrome. An Analysis of Ten Cases. *Geriatrics* **23**(8):123–135, 1968.

142

Williams Syndrome

(Elfin Facies Syndrome, Idiopathic Hypercalcemia-Supravalvular Aortic Stenosis Syndrome)

The syndrome of (*a*) characteristic facial appearance, (*b*) mental retardation, (*c*) growth deficiency, (*d*) cardiovascular anomalies, and (*e*) infantile hypercalcemia was described independently by Fanconi and Girardet (13) and Schlesinger et al. (39) in 1952. A good historical review of the condition has been presented by Myers and Willis (33).

Naming the syndrome has been problematical. The disorder is probably best known as the idiopathic hypercalcemia–supravalvular aortic stenosis syndrome despite the fact that both features are frequently absent (24). Furthermore, the term is cumbersome. The "elfin face" syndrome (10) presents a problem in naming the disorder after a mythical being. The currently accepted designation, Williams syndrome (44), ignores the historical precedent mentioned earlier.

Delineating the phenotypic spectrum of abnormalities has also been problematical. Defining a syndrome on the basis of sporadic occurrence when the basic defect is unknown truncates the phenotype toward the severe end of the spectrum. Thus, reported frequencies of various findings are not especially meaningful. The problem is further compounded by ascertainment on the basis of cardiovascular anomalies in some reports (3) and on the basis of facial features in others (24). It has been suggested that the syndrome may represent a spectrum which overlaps with hypercalcemia with and without mental retardation and supravalvular aortic stenosis with and without mental retardation

(3). However, few families have been reported in which more than one of these phenotypes is present.

All "severe" cases reported to date are seemingly sporadic. The etiology and pathogenesis are unknown. Friedman and associates (16–18) have produced similar craniofacial, dental, and cardiovascular anomalies in the offspring of rabbits treated with excessive vitamin D during pregnancy. Hypotheses for the human syndrome have included vitamin D hypersensitivity or excess, an abnormality of cholesterol metabolism, and delayed turnover or degradation of vitamin D (16, 17, 19). Forbes et al. (14) demonstrated an impaired ability of normocalcemic children with the Williams syndrome to handle large intravenous calcium loads efficiently and suggested a deficiency of calcitonin. All available human studies to date are limited by the inability to evaluate vitamin D or calcium metabolism during early fetal development.

SYSTEMIC MANIFESTATIONS

Facies. Facial features are distinctive and become more striking with age. The combination of flat midface, depressed nasal bridge, anteverted nostrils, long philtrum, thick lips, wide intercommissural distance, and open mouth is characteristic (Fig. 142-1*A–D*). Ocular findings may include medial eyebrow flaring, short palpebral fissures, ocular hypotelorism, epicanthal

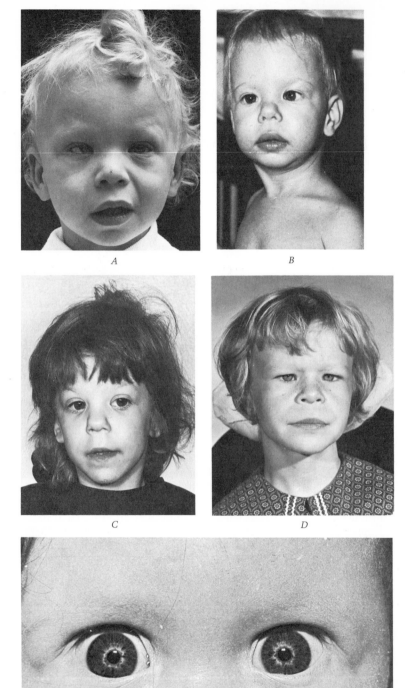

A

B

C

D

E

Figure 142-1. *Williams syndrome.* (*A–D*). Compare facies for anteverted nostrils, long philtrum, mild midface hypoplasia, epicanthal folds, strabismus. (A, *from A. Dupont,* Dan. Med. Bull. **17:**33, 1970; B, *from F. Ray,* J. Pediatr. Ophthalmol. **8:**188, 1971.) (*E*). Stellate iris pattern. (*From F. O. Jensen and A. C. Begg,* N. Z. Med. J. **68:**364, 1968.)

folds, periorbital fullness, strabismus (especially esotropia), and a high percentage of blue-eyed individuals with a stellate iris pattern (Fig. 142-1E) (3–5, 13, 24, 27, 38, 39, 40, 44). Uncommonly, corneal and/or lenticular opacities (38) and ptosis of the eyelids (personal observation) may be observed. In some cases, the ears may be prominent. The thyroid cartilage becomes more prominent with age (Fig. 142-1A–D).

Hypercalcemia. Hypercalcemia has not been documented in most cases (24). When present, it usually disappears during the second year of life. Retrospective interviewing may reveal a history of failure to thrive, hypotonia, anorexia, constipation, or renal impairment (1, 7, 28).

Skeletal and limb abnormalities. Mild to moderate growth deficiency of prenatal onset with more striking growth deficiency during the postnatal period is a feature in most cases (24).

The hypercalcemic phase may result in widespread osteosclerotic changes which regress in time (39, 40). Craniosynostosis (secondary to microcephaly), retarded bone age, and increased density of the metaphyses, epiphyses, and skull base may be present in some instances (10, 13, 27a, 39, 40).

Pectus excavatum, hallux valgus, fifth finger clinodactyly, and hypoplastic deep-set nails have been reported (24).

Central nervous system. Mild microcephaly (most striking in bifrontal diameter), mental retardation, mild neurologic dysfunction, and unusual personality are characteristic features. Intelligence quotients have varied from 41 to 80 with an average of 56 among 14 noninstitutionalized patients (24). In childhood, patients have been described as friendly or loquacious or as having a "cocktail party manner" (2, 24).

Cardiovascular system. Findings have included supravalvular aortic stenosis, valvular aortic stenosis, aortic hypoplasia, coarctation of the aorta, pulmonary artery stenosis, peripheral artery stenoses (cardiac, celiac, subclavian, mesenteric, and renal), atrial septal defect, ventricular septal defect, anomalous pulmonary venous return, arteriovenous fistula (lung), interruption of the aortic arch, and aplasia of the

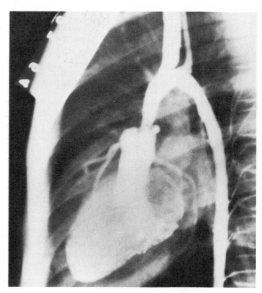

Figure 142-2. Note area of stenosis and hypoplasia of entire aorta distal to obstruction. (*From K. Jue et al.,* J. Pediatr. **67:**1130, 1965.)

portal vein (1, 7–10, 20, 29, 36, 37). Arterial hypertension and heart murmur have been noted frequently (1, 13, 24, 28, 36) (Fig. 142-2). There is no apparent correlation between the degree of mental retardation and the severity of the cardiovascular abnormalities.

Other findings. Small penis, inguinal hernia, and umbilical hernia have also been reported (24).

Oral manifestations. Thick lips, wide intercommissural distance, and long philtrum are characteristic. The voice is often hoarse (3–5, 11, 24, 28). The maxillary arch has been described as being too broad for the mandibular arch. Hypodontia, microdontia, small slender roots, and dens invaginatus have been reported (3–5, 7, 10, 12, 15, 44). Hypoplastic bud-shaped maxillary deciduous second molars and mandibular permanent first molars have been noted by some authors (4, 5) (Fig. 142-3). In a series of 17 patients studied metrically, microdontia was not observed nor were hypoplastic bud-shaped teeth present in any patient. However, absent teeth, especially the lower second premolars, were observed in some (22). Mild micrognathia, widened

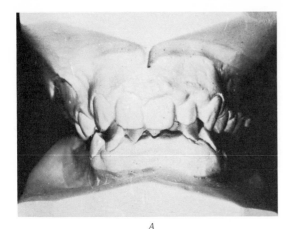

A

Figure 142-3. (*A*). Upper dental arch completely overlaps lower arch. (*B*). Note expanded upper arch, hypoplastic upper second deciduous molar on right. (*C*). Detail showing bud-shaped maxillary teeth. (*From A. J. Beuren et al., Am. J. Cardiol.* **13**:471, 1964.)

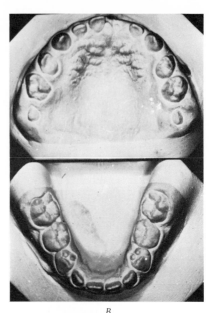

B

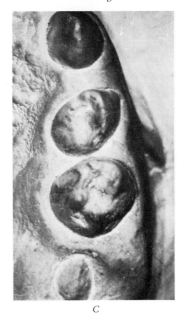

C

mandibular angle, osteosclerotic changes in the lamina dura (especially in the premolar-molar region), delayed mineralization of teeth, folding and thickening of the buccal mucous membranes, and prominent and accessory labial frenula have also been noted (4, 5, 10, 11, 27a).

DIFFERENTIAL DIAGNOSIS

Lightwood (30) described a mild form of idiopathic hypercalcemia which is not associated with osteosclerosis, mental deficiency, or cardiovascular anomalies. However, anorexia, vomiting, weight loss, and failure to thrive may occur. Hooft et al. (23) reported familial occurrence of idiopathic hypercalcemia. Isolated supravalvular aortic stenosis has been reported to follow an autosomal dominant mode of transmission (31, 41), but occurs most frequently as a sporadic defect.

LABORATORY AIDS

Hypercalcemia may be present during the first three years of life in some cases.

REFERENCES

1 Antia, A. U., et al., Pathogenesis of the Supravalvular Aortic Stenosis Syndrome. *J. Pediatr.* **71:**431–441, 1967.

2 Arnim, V. G., and Engel, P., Mental Retardation Related to Hypercalcaemia. *Dev. Med. Child. Neurol.* **6:**366–377, 1964.

3 Beuren, A. J., Supravalvular Aortic Stenosis: A Complex Syndrome with and without Mental Retardation. *Birth Defects* **8**(5):45–56, 1972.

4 Beuren, A. J., et al., Supravalvular Aortic Stenosis in Association with Mental Retardation and a Certain Facial Appearance. *Circulation* **26:**1235–1240, 1962.

5 Beuren, A. J., et al., The Syndrome of Supravalvular Aortic Stenosis, Peripheral Pulmonary Stenosis, Mental Retardation and Similar Facial Appearance. *Am. J. Cardiol.* **13:**471–483, 1964.

6 Blancquaert, A., et al., Stenoses pulmonaires et aortiques postvalvulaires avec facies particulier et retard intellectuel. *Acta Cardiol.* (Brux.) **21:**611–643, 1966.

7 Chantler, C., et al., Cardiovascular and Other Associations of Infantile Hypercalcaemia. *Guy's Hosp. Rep.* **115:**221–241, 1966.

8 Char, F., Williams Facies with Portal Vein Aplasia and Mental Retardation. *Birth Defects* **8**(5):262–263, 1972.

9 Char, F., and Rowe, R. D., Infantile Hypercalcemia Syndrome with Mitral Regurgitation and Hypoplasia of Aorta. *Birth Defects* **8**(5):258–261, 1972.

10 Dupont, B., et al., Idiopathic Hypercalcemia of Infancy: The Elfin Face Syndrome. *Dan. Med. Bull.* **17:**33–46, 1970.

11 Ebeling, J., et al., Ein weiterer Beitrag zu den kardiovaskulären Veränderungen und der Klinik defektgeheilter infantiler Hyperkalzämien. *Arch. Kinderheilkd.* **180:**1–14, 1969.

12 Faivre, G., et al., Le rétrécissement aortique sus-valvulaire avec malformations multiples. *Arch. Mal. Coeur* **58:**977–996, 1965.

13 Fanconi, G., and Girardet, P., Chronische Hypercalcämie, kombiniert mit Osteosklerose, Hyperazotämie, Minderwuchs und kongenitalen Missbildungen. *Helv. Paediatr. Acta* **7:**314–334, 1952.

14 Forbes, G. B., et al., Impaired Calcium Homeostasis in Infantile Hypercalcemic Syndrome. *Acta Paediatr. Scand.* **61:**305–309, 1972.

15 Frank, R. M., et al., Aspects odonto-stomatologiques de la stenose aortique susvalvulaire. *Rev. Stomatol.* (Paris) **67:**223–232, 1966.

16 Friedman, W. F., Vitamin D and the Supravalvular Aortic Stenosis Syndrome. *Adv. Teratol.* **3:**85–96, 1968.

17 Friedman, W. F., and Mills, L. F., The Relationship between Vitamin D and the Craniofacial and Dental Anomalies of the Supravalvular Aortic Stenoses Syndrome. *Pediatrics* **43:**12–18, 1969.

18 Friedman, W. F., and Roberts, W. C., Vitamin D and the Supravalvular Aortic Stenosis Syndrome. The Transplacental Effects of Vitamin D on the Aorta of the Rabbit. *Circulation* **34:**77–86, 1966.

19 Gorin, R., et al., Un nouveau cas d'hypercalcémie idiopathique grave. *Ann. Pédiatr.* **13:**20–42, 1966.

20 Harris, L. L., and Nghiem, Q. X., Idiopathic Hypercalcaemia of Infancy with Interruption of the Aortic Arch. *J. Pediatr.* **73:**84–88, 1968.

21 Härtel, G., et al., Supravalvular Pulmonic Stenosis, Abnormal Facial Appearance and Mental Retardation. *Am. Heart J.* **75:**540–544, 1968.

22 Heinemann, M. R., and Cohen, M. M., Jr., Personal observations, 1974.

23 Hooft, C., et al., Familial Incidence of Hypercalcaemia. *Helv. Paediatr. Acta* **16:**199–210, 1961.

24 Jones, K. L., and Smith, P. W., The Williams Elfin Facies Syndrome: A New Perspective. *J. Pediatr.* **86:**718–723, 1975.

25 Jörgensen, G., and Beuren, A. J., Genetische Untersuchungen bei supravalvulären Aortenstenosen. *Humangenetik* **1:**497–515, 1965.

26 Joseph, M. C., and Parrott, D., Severe Infantile Hypercalcemia with Special Reference to the Facies. *Arch. Dis. Child.* **33:**385–395, 1958.

27 Jue, K. L., et al., The Syndrome of Idiopathic Infancy with Associated Congenital Heart Disease. *J. Pediatr.* **67:**1130–1140, 1965.

27a Kelly, J. R., and Barr, E. S., The Elfin Facies Syndrome. *Oral Surg* **40:**205–218, 1975.

28 Kivalo, E., et al., Mental Retardation, Typical Facies and Aortic Stenosis Syndrome. *Ann. Med. Intern. Fenn.* **54:**81–87, 1965.

29 Levy, E. P., Infantile Hypercalcemia Facies and Mental Retardation Associated with Atrial Septal Defect and Anomalous Pulmonary Venous Return. *Birth Defects* **8**(5):73–74, 1972.

30 Lightwood, R., Idiopathic Hypercalcaemia with Failure to Thrive. *Arch. Dis. Child.* **27:**302–303, 1952.

31 McCue, C. M., et al., Familial Supravalvular Aortic Stenosis. *J. Pediatr.* **73:**889–895, 1968.

32 Murgeon, –, Anomalies dento-maxillo-faciales et stenose aortique susvalvulaire. Thesis, Paris, 1970.

33 Myers, A. R., and Willis, P. W., Clinical Spectrum of Supravalvular Aortic Stenosis. *Arch. Intern. Med.* **118:**553–561, 1966.

34 Ottesen, O. E., et al., Peripheral Vascular Anomalies Associated with the Supravalvular Aortic Stenosis Syndrome. *Radiology* **86:**430–435, 1966.

35 Page, H. L., et al., Supravalvular Aortic Stenosis. *Am. J. Cardiol.* **23:**270–277, 1969.

36 Rashkind, W. J., et al., Cardiac Findings in Idiopathic Hypercalcaemia of Infancy. *J. Pediatr.* **58:**464–469, 1961.

37 Roberts, N. K., and Moes, C. A. F., Supravalvular Pulmonary Stenosis and Unusual Facial Appearance. *Birth Defects* **8**(5):57–59, 1972.

38 Roy, F. H., et al., Infantile Hypercalcemia and Supravalvular Aortic Stenosis. *J. Pediat. Ophthalmol.* **8:**188–193, 1971.

39 Schlesinger, B. E., et al., Chronische Hypercalcämie mit Osteosklerose. *Helv. Paediatr. Acta* **7:**335–349, 1952.

40 Schlesinger, B. E., et al., Severe Type of Infantile Hypercalcaemia. *Br. Med. J.* **1:**127–134, 1956.

41 Schmidt, R. E., et al., Generalized Arterial Fibromuscular Dysplasia and Myocardial Infarction in Familial Supravalvular Aortic Stenosis Syndrome. *J. Pediatr.* **74:**576–584, 1969.

42 Singleton, E. B., et al., The Radiographic Features of Severe Idiopathic Hypercalcemia of Infancy. *Radiology* **68:**721–726, 1957.

43 Sutcliffe, J., Severe Infantile Hypercalcaemia and Stenosis of Major Arteries. *Ann. Roentgenol.* **8:**277–278, 1965.

44 Williams, J. C. P., et al., Supravalvular Aortic Stenosis. *Circulation* **24:**1311–1318, 1961.

143

Xerodermic Idiocy

(De Sanctis-Cacchione Syndrome)

Although Kaposi described classical xerodermia pigmentosum over 100 years ago, the syndrome of (a) xeroderma pigmentosum with (b) somatic and mental retardation was first identified by De Sanctis and Cacchione (7) in 1934. Fewer than 50 examples of the syndrome have been described to date.

Both the classical skin disorder, which in itself is a genetic heterogeneity, and the syndrome manifest autosomal recessive inheritance. Classical xeroderma pigmentosum is possibly more common in individuals of Arabic and Jewish origin (11, 12, 16, 18, 24, 32) and has been estimated to occur in 1 per 250,000 in the general population (31).

There is a good evidence, on the basis of cell fusion techniques, to suggest that four or more different genes are involved (intergenic complementation) (8, 32). Affected family members have similar clinical symptoms and repair rates (3, 32). There is no correlation between severity of clinical symptoms and DNA repair rate (32). Prenatal diagnosis is possible (29).

SYSTEMIC MANIFESTATIONS

About 60 percent of patients have developed cutaneous malignancies resulting in death before the fifteenth year of life.

Facies and skin. Many but not all patients exhibit in early infancy an acute sun sensitivity, which subsides later in life. Although the skin appears normal at birth, erythema of exposed parts usually occurs within the first few months of life (11, 12, 18, 24, 25, 33). As the erythema subsides, freckling, increased pigmentation, atrophy, dryness, scaliness, and telangiectasia are noted usually before two years of age, in sun-exposed areas of the skin (Figs. 143-1, 143-2). Electronmicroscopic changes in the skin were described by Guerrier (17).

Basal cell carcinoma and squamous cell carcinoma are the most common cutaneous lesions to appear in childhood or adolescence following the degenerative skin changes. Some patients have more than 100 tumors. Melanoma, keratoacanthoma, and various benign and malignant angiomatous neoplasms have also been reported (26, 32). Squamous cell carcinoma and melanoma arising in xeroderma pigmentosum patients rapidly metastasize.

The basic defect is a failure of DNA excision repair of ultraviolet-induced thymine dimers (5, 30, 32).

Eyes. Photophobia, lacrimation, and conjunctivitis are early and constant manifestations. The bulbar conjunctiva may exhibit pigmentation and telangiectasia and may undergo malignant degeneration. The cornea may cloud and ulcerate with secondary iritis, which may result in synechiae or iris atrophy. Neoplasms, usually intraepithelial or squamous cell carcinomas, may develop at the limbus. With severe involvement,

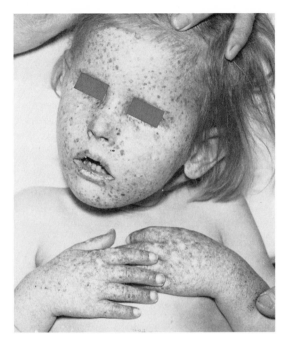

Figure 143-1. *Xerodermic idiocy.* Note skin lesions. (*Courtesy of O. P Hornstein, Erlangen, Germany.*)

the eyelids may lose their cilia, and ectropion, entropion, or symblepharon may complicate the clinical picture (10, 11, 18).

Central nervous system. It has been estimated that about 15 percent of patients with xeroderma pigmentosum have mental and somatic retardation (13). Intelligence is usually within the idiot or imbecile range (20, 31, 34). Autopsy findings include microcephaly with a small brain and a diffuse mild cerebral and olivopontocerebellar neuronal loss (6, 13, 20, 24, 30, 35).

Clinically, there may be spastic-ataxic gait and athetoid movement of the head and arms (20, 30). Areflexia has been described in several patients; it is apparently due to lower motor neuron involvement (32, 33). Pyramidal and extrapyramidal signs are common, and speech is often disturbed (7, 20). Neural deafness has been noted in several cases (34). Abnormal electroencephalographic changes (diffuse dysrhythmia with poorly developed alpha rhythm and with occasional paroxysmal burstlike slow-wave discharges) have been noted (6, 20, 34).

Other findings. Nuclear atypia of hepatic and pancreatic cells (12, 35) and gonadal hypoplasia (7, 20) have been described.

Oral manifestations. Squamous or basal cell carcinoma of the lips is common (19, 31).

DIFFERENTIAL DIAGNOSIS

Pigmented xerodermoid is a distinct but similar disorder characterized by lesions appearing after the age of thirty years. In this disorder, there is no evidence for defective DNA excision repair. However, enhanced ultraviolet ray depression of mitotic activity has been reported (21, 22). Another variant, clinically indistinguishable from classical xeroderma pigmentosum, has no defect in DNA repair (4, 32). A dominant form of xero-

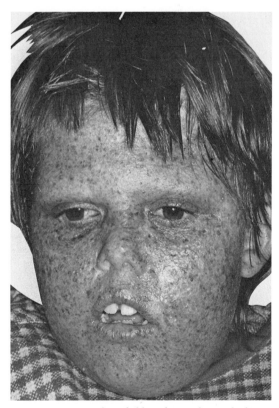

Figure 143-2. Another child with xerodermoid idiocy. Her brother was similarly involved. (*Courtesy of W. Reed, Burbank, Calif.*)

derma pigmentosum has been described in a Scottish family (2).

Thrush et al. (35) reported sibs with an unclassified form of xeroderma pigmentosum characterized by progressive dementia, chorea, sensorineural deafness, corticospinal tract degeneration, peripheral neuropathy, and skeletal abnormalities.

LABORATORY AIDS

Study of excision repair of DNA in fibroblasts of homozygotes and heterozygotes following ultraviolet exposure has been elegantly discussed by Cleaver (5).

There is a higher than expected (about 80 percent) association with blood group O (12). Increased chromosomal breakage has been described in cultured fibroblasts (29). Prenatal diagnosis by means of autoradiography has been described (5).

Elevation of IgE level has been noted (29). While El-Hefnawi and El-Hawary (9) suggested elevated blood glutathione and serum copper levels, others (16, 20, 29) have failed to confirm this finding. Aminoaciduria was reported by some investigators (6, 9, 15, 27), but denied by others (20).

Afifi et al. (1) noted massive accumulation of glycogen and subsarcolemmal mitochondrial aggregates in muscle.

REFERENCES

1 Afifi, A. K., et al., Muscle Abnormality in Xeroderma Pigmentosum. *J. Neurol. Sci.* **17:**435–442, 1972.

2 Anderson, T. E., and Begg, M., Xeroderma Pigmentosum of Mild Type. *Br. J. Dermatol.* **62:**402–407, 1950.

3 Botsma, D., et al., Different Inherited Levels of DNA Repair Replication in Xeroderma Pigmentosum Cell Strains after Exposure to Ultraviolet Irradiation. *Mutat. Res.* **9:**507–516, 1970.

4 Burk, P. G., et al., Ultraviolet Stimulated Thymidine Incorporation in Xeroderma Pigmentosum Lymphocytes. *J. Lab. Clin. Med.* **77:**759–767, 1971.

5 Cleaver, J. E., Xeroderma Pigmentosum – Progress and Regress. *J. Invest. Dermatol.* **60:**374–380, 1973.

6 Clodi, P. H., et al., Xeroderma pigmentosum mit körperlichem sowie geistigem Entwicklungsrückstand und intermittierender Aminoacidurie. Ein neues Syndrom? *Z. Kinderheilkd.* **93:**223–225, 1965.

7 De Sanctis, C., and Cacchione, A., L'idiozia xerodermica. *Riv. Sper. Freniatr.* **56:**269, 1932.

8 DeWeerd-Kastelein, E. A., et al., Genetic Heterogeneity of Xeroderma Pigmentosum Demonstrated by Somatic Cell Hybridization. *Nature* [*New Biol.*] **238:**80–83, 1972.

9 El-Hefnawi, H., and El-Hawary, M. F. S., Chromatographic Studies of Amino Acids in Sera and Urine of Patients with Xeroderma Pigmentosum and Their Normal Relatives. *Br. J. Dermatol.* **75:**235–244, 1963.

10 El-Hefnawi, H., and Mortada, A., Ocular Manifestations of Xeroderma Pigmentosum. *Br. J. Dermatol.* **77:**261–276, 1965.

11 El-Hefnawi, H., et al., Xeroderma Pigmentosum. *Br. J. Dermatol.* **74:**201–221, 1962.

12 El-Hefnawi, H., et al., Xeroderma Pigmentosum – Its Inheritance and Relationship to the ABO Blood Group System. *Ann. Hum. Genet.* **28:**273–290, 1965.

13 Elsässer, G., et al., Das Xeroderma pigmentosum und die xerodermische Idiotie. *Arch. Dermatol. Syph.* (*Berl.*) **188:**651–655, 1950.

14 Festoff, B. W., and Kraemer, K. H., Xeroderma Pigmentosum; Neurologic and Cutaneous Abnormalities Associated with a Defect in DNA Repair. *Neurology* (*Minneap.*) **22:**420, 1972.

15 Feuerstein, M., and Langhof, H., Untersuchungen über die freien Aminosäuren im Harn und Aminosäurengehalt der Haare bei Xeroderma pigmentosum. *Arch. Klin. Exp. Dermatol.* **220:**486–491, 1964.

16 Friedman, A., et al., Xerodermic Idiocy or De Sanctis-Cacchione Syndrome. *Clin. Pediatr.* **12:**56–58, 1973.

17 Guerrier, C. J., et al., An Electron Microscopical Study of the Skin in 18 Cases of Xeroderma Pigmentosum. *Dermatologica* **146:**211–221, 1973.

18 Hadida, E., et al., Xeroderma pigmentosum. *Ann. Dermatol. Syphiligr.* (*Paris*) **90:**467–496, 1963.

19 Haim, S., and Zonis, S., Squamous Cell Carcinoma of the Conjunctiva in Xeroderma Pigmentosum. *Israel J. Med. Sci.* **1:**431–434, 1965.

20 Hokkanen, E., et al., Zu den neurologischen Manifestationen des Xeroderma pigmentosum. *Dtsch. Z. Nervenheilkd.* **196:**206–216, 1969.

21 Jung, E. G., Bedeutung und Heterogenität des Syndroms Xeroderma pigmentosum. *Hautarzt* **24:**175–179, 1973.

22 Jung, E. G., and Schnyder, U. W., Xeroderma pigmentosum und pigmentiertes Xerodermoid. *Schweiz. Med. Wochenschr.* **100:**1718–1726, 1970; and *Birth Defects* **7**(8): 126–128, 1972.

23 Kraemer, K. H., et al., Cell-fusion Analysis of Different Inherited Mutations Causing Defective DNA Repair in Xeroderma Fibroblasts. *J. Cell Biol.* **59:**176a, 1973.

24 Mehregan, A. H., Dermatitis Solaris Related to Xeroderma Pigmentosum. *Arch. Dermatol.* **87:**469–474, 1963.

25 Mendoza, H. R., Sindrome de Sanctis-Caccione (Xeroderma pigmentoso deficiencia mental y enanismo). *Rev. Dominicana Dermatol.* **3:**38–40, 1969.

26 Moore, C., and Iverson, P. C., Xeroderma Showing Common Skin Cancer Plus Melanocarcinoma Controlled

by Surgery. *Cancer* **7:**377–382, 1954.

27 Moss, H. V., Xeroderma Pigmentosum, Clinical and Laboratory Investigation of Its Basic Defect. *Arch. Dermatol.* **92:**638–642, 1965.

28 Noojin, R. O., Xeroderma Pigmentosum Treated with Oral Methoxsalen. *Arch. Dermatol.* **92:**422–423, 1965.

29 Ramsay, C. A., et al., Prenatal Diagnosis of Xeroderma Pigmentosum. *Lancet* **2:**1109–1112, 1974.

30 Reed, W. B., Xeroderma Pigmentosum, Clinical and Laboratory Investigation of Its Basic Defect. *J.A.M.A.* **207:**2073–2079, 1969.

31 Reed, W. B., et al., Xeroderma Pigmentosum with Neurological Complications: The De Sanctis-Cacchione Syndrome. *Arch. Dermatol.* **91:**224–226, 1965.

32 Robbins, J. H., et al., Xeroderma Pigmentosum: An Inherited Disease with Sun Sensitivity, Multiple Cutaneous Neoplasms, and Abnormal DNA Repair. *Ann. Intern. Med.* **80:**221–248, 1974.

33 Silberstein, A. G., Xeroderma Pigmentosum with Mental Deficiency. *Am. J. Dis. Child.* **55:**784–791, 1938.

34 Strian, F., Kausistischer Beitrag zur xerodermalen Idiotie. De Sanctis-Cacchione-Syndrom. *Dtsch. Z. Nervenheilkd.* **189:**218–230, 1966.

35 Thrush, D. C., et al., Neurologic Manifestations of Xeroderma Pigmentosum in Two Siblings. *J. Neurol. Sci.* **22:**91–104, 1974.

36 Yano, K., Xeroderma pigmentosum mit Störungen des Zentralnervensystems. *Folia Psychiatr. Neurol. Jap.* **44:**55, 1950.

144

Miscellaneous Syndromes

A section dealing with miscellaneous syndromes was inevitable. Since our cutoff date for new chapters in 1972, many reports of striking new syndromes have appeared. In general, four types of syndromes are included in this section. First, there are many recent and incompletely delineated disorders. Second, there are some recent but fairly well defined disorders such as the Coffin-Lowry syndrome. Third, there are a few well-limned but extremely rare syndromes that have been known for a long time, such as the Böök syndrome. Finally, there are a few recently delineated but apparently common disorders, such as the fetal alcohol syndrome. In the third edition, many of these will assume a position in the book in alphabetical order, only to have their space occupied by still newer entities.

TUBULAR STENOSIS
(KENNEY SYNDROME)

Caffey (1) and Kenney and Linarelli (3) first described autosomal inheritance of a disorder of proportional dwarfism, transient hypercalcemia, and retardation in skeletal maturation. The shafts of the long bones are narrow, with stenosis of the medullary cavities. Large anterior fontanel and wide metopic suture with lack of differentiation of the calvaria into its three zones have been reported (2).

The facies shows frontal bossing, a high hair line, and diminished eyebrows and lashes (Fig. 144-1A–E).

We cannot cite the case of Wilson et al. (4) as an example of the disorder.

MENTAL AND SOMATIC RETARDATION AND CRANIODIGITAL ANOMALIES (SCOTT SYNDROME)

Scott et al. (1) described what may be a new X-linked recessive syndrome characterized by mental and somatic retardation, hirsutism, and mild cutaneous syndactyly between the second, third, and fourth fingers.

The head was brachycephalic, the nose pointed, and the mandible small. The lashes were long. The eyebrows were prominent and arched, giving the children a startled expression (Fig. 144-2).

FRONTODIGITAL SYNDROME

Frontal bossing with scaphocephaly, broad thumb and hallux, variable soft-tissue syndactyly of fingers and toes, polysyndactyly of halluces with postaxial polydactyly of toes were described in a family as an autosomal dominant syndrome by Marshall and Smith (1) (Fig. 144-3A, B).

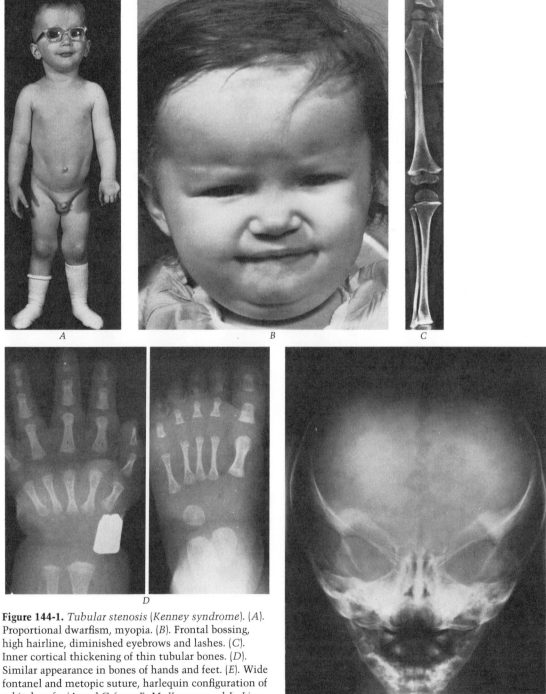

Figure 144-1. *Tubular stenosis (Kenney syndrome).* (*A*).
Proportional dwarfism, myopia. (*B*). Frontal bossing,
high hairline, diminished eyebrows and lashes. (*C*).
Inner cortical thickening of thin tubular bones. (*D*).
Similar appearance in bones of hands and feet. (*E*). Wide
fontanel and metopic suture, harlequin configuration of
orbital roofs. (A and C *from F. M. Kenney and L. Linarelli,* Am. J. Dis. Child. **111**:201, 1967; D and E *from
R. Frech and W. McAlister,* Radiology **91**:457, 1968.)

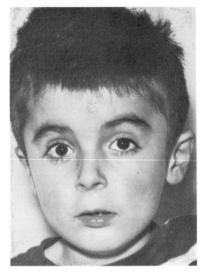

Figure 144-2. *Mental and somatic retardation and craniodigital anomalies.* Brachycephaly, pointed nose, and startled expression. (*From C. R. Scott et al., J. Pediatr.* **78**:658, 1971.)

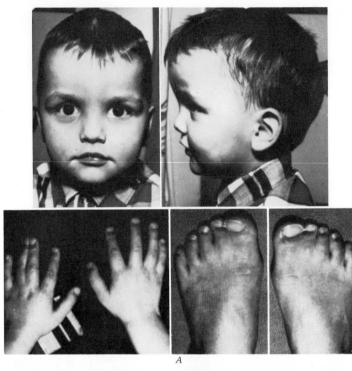

A

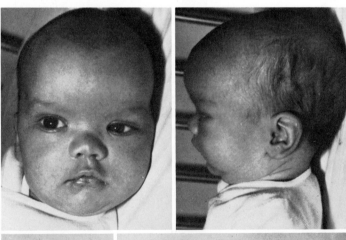

B

Figure 144-3. *Frontodigital syndrome.* (*A, B*). Frontal bossing, variable soft-tissue syndactyly, polysyndactyly of halluces with postaxial polydactyly of toes. (*From R. E. Marshall and D. W. Smith, J. Pediatr.* **77**:126, 1970.)

FAMILIAL POLYSYNDACTYLY AND CRANIOFACIAL ANOMALIES (HOOTNICK-HOLMES SYNDROME)

Hootnick and Holmes (1) reported a father and son with polysyndactyly, hypertelorism, broad nose, and scaphocephaly. They thought the disorder was similar to the *frontodigital syndrome.* However, the degree of polysyndactyly was much more severe in their patients (Fig. 144-4*A–C*).

A patient with similar features was described by Korting and Ruther (2). In addition, this patient had mild ichthyosis vulgaris and tapetoretinal degeneration.

PYRAMIDAL MOLAR ROOTS, JUVENILE GLAUCOMA, AND UNUSUAL MORPHOLOGY OF UPPER LIP (ACKERMAN SYNDROME)

Ackerman et al. (1) described a family in which several members in two generations exhibited pyramidal, taurodont, or fused molar roots with a single root canal, a finding noted on both sides of the kindred. Three of six sibs had only pyramidal molar roots.

Juvenile glaucoma was noted in two of three affected sibs, and all had sparse body hair. The upper lip was full without a cupid's bow, and there was thickening and widening of the philtrum. One of the three sibs also had entropion of both lower eyelids, 3-4 soft-tissue syndactyly of the left hand, indurated hyperpigmented skin over the interphalangeal joints of the fingers, and clinodactyly of the fifth fingers (Fig. 144-5*A–C*).

OLIGODONTIA, ABSENT NASAL ALAE, MENTAL AND SOMATIC RETARDATION, HYPOTHYROIDISM, AND MALABSORPTION (JOHANSON-BLIZZARD SYNDROME)

Johanson and Blizzard (1) described three unrelated female children with severe mental and somatic retardation, sensorineural deafness, hypothyroidism, and malabsorption apparently due to trypsinogen deficiency (1–4). Hypotonia with hyperextensibility of joints was a common feature. Pitting edema of the hands and feet was

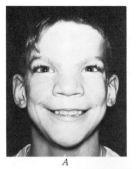

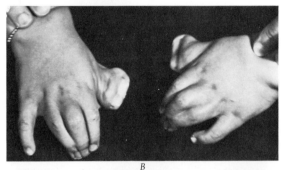

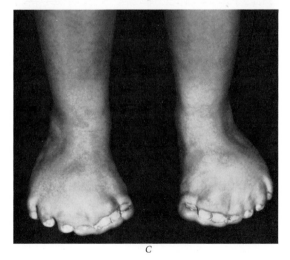

Figure 144-4. *Familial polysyndactyly and craniofacial anomalies* (Hootnick-Holmes syndrome). (*A*). Broad nose, ocular hypertelorism. (*B*). Deviated and duplicated thumbs with 2-4 soft-tissue syndactyly. Postaxial digit removed earlier. (*C*). Preaxial duplication or triplication and syndactyly. (*From D. Hootnick and L. B. Holmes,* Clin. Genet. 3:128, 1972.)

also noted (2, 3). A single urogenital orifice with infantile ovaries and double or septate vagina and imperforate anus were described (1, 2). Severe oligodontia was seen in the permanent dentition (1, 2). Aplasia of lacrimal puncta was noted in one child, and hypoplastic nipples and areolas in another (1). Striking was absence of the nasal alae (1–4). Skin dimples and defects were also noted over the fontanels (1) (Fig. 144-6A–C).

ABSENT FIFTH FINGER- AND TOENAILS, UNUSUAL FACIES, AND MENTAL DEFICIENCY (COFFIN-SIRIS SYNDROME)

In 1970, Coffin and Siris (2) reported three patients with coarse facial features and hypoplastic to absent fifth finger- and toenails. Other cases appear to be those of Weiswasser et al. (5) and Bartsocas and Tsiantos (1). Less certain are the patients of Senior (4) and Mace and Gotlin (3), patients not as severely affected who may possibly represent a separate entity. To date, all cases of the Coffin-Siris syndrome have been sporadic except for one instance of affected sibs (B. D. Hall, personal communication, 1974). Perhaps some examples really had *fetal hydantoin syndrome.*

Feeding problems and recurrent respiratory infections are common during infancy. Findings

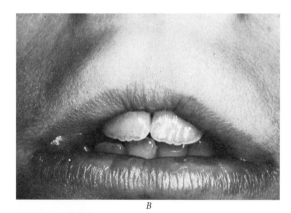

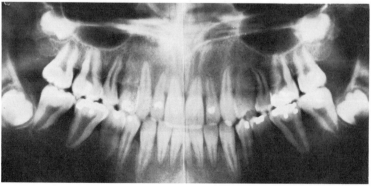

Figure 144-5. *Pyramidal molar roots, juvenile glaucoma, and unusual morphology of upper lip (Ackerman syndrome). (A). Widened philtrum. (B). Full upper lip, lack of cupid's bow. (C). Pyramidal molar roots. (From J. Ackerman et al., Am. J. Phys. Anthropol.* **38**:681, 1973.)

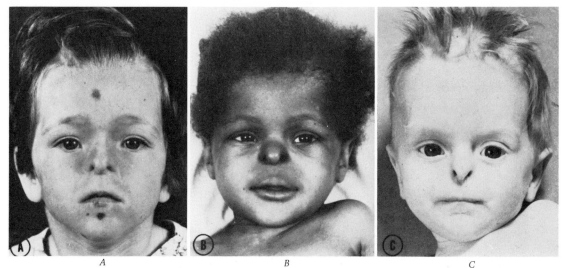

A   B   C

Figure 144-6. *Oligodontia, absent nasal alae, mental and somatic retardation, hypothyroidism, and malabsorption* (Johanson-Blizzard syndrome). (*A–C*). Children exhibiting similiar faces characterized by hypoplasia of nasal alae. They also have hypotonia, genital anomalies, and trypsinogen deficiency. (*From A. Johanson and R. Blizzard*, J. Pediatr. **79:**982, 1971.)

include coarse facial features, sparse scalp hair, thick lips, mild microcephaly, mental deficiency, hypotonia, growth deficiency of prenatal onset, hypoplastic to absent fifth finger- and toenails with less severe involvement of other digits, hirsutism, lax joints, dislocation of the radial heads, coxa valga, and small to absent patellas (Fig. 144-7*A–D*). Various low-frequency anomalies have included eyelid ptosis, cleft palate, cardiac defect, Dandy-Walker malformation, and other abnormalities.

MICROCEPHALY, GROWTH RETARDATION, AND FLEXION DEFORMITIES (NEU SYNDROME)

Laxova et al. (1) and Neu et al. (2) each described three sibs with a lethal syndrome of intrauterine growth retardation, marked microcephaly, flexion deformities, overlapping fingers, edematous, rocker bottom feet with protruding heels, and syndactyly of toes.

Craniofacial anomalies included brain atrophy, absence of corpus callosum, ocular hypertelorism, absent eyelids, short neck, and enlarged pinnas. Two infants had absent eyelids and almost absent nose (Fig. 144-8).

Inheritance appears to be autosomal recessive.

SOMATIC AND MENTAL RETARDATION, CORNEAL OPACITIES, SHORT ULNA AND RADIUS, AND UNUSUAL FACIES (MIETENS-WEBER SYNDROME)

Four of six children of consanguineous normal parents were reported by Mietens and Weber (1) to have a syndrome of marked growth retardation (3 S.D. below the mean) and mild mental retardation (intelligence quotient of 70 to 80).

Clinical appearance was striking, the facies being marked by convergent strabismus and a small, narrow, pointed nose. Disklike central opacities of the cornea, located mainly in the superficial layers, were noted bilaterally. Short forearms and flexion of the elbows with proliferation and contraction of the connective tissues on the volar aspect were also marked. Calf muscles were atrophic, and pes valgus planus was evident (Fig. 144-9*A–C*).

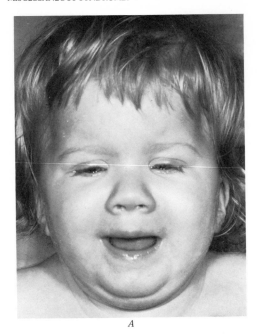

A

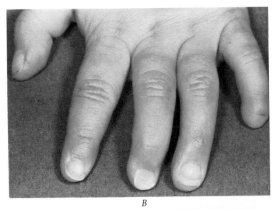

B

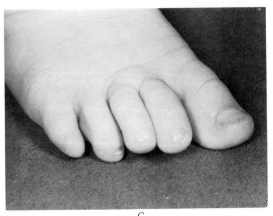

C

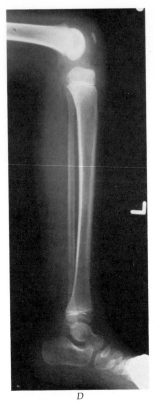

D

Figure 144-7. *Absent fifth terminal phalanges, mental retardation, and unusual facies* (Coffin-Siris syndrome). (*A*). Broad nose with anteverted nostrils. (*B*, *C*). Hypoplasia of terminal fifth phalanges. (*D*). Hypoplastic patella. (*From E. Siris, Eldridge, Calif.*)

Roentgenographically, the ulna and radius were abbreviated. The head of the radius was dislocated, and its epiphysis was absent bilaterally.

The disorder apparently has autosomal recessive inheritance.

GERODERMA OSTEODYSPLASTICA (BAMATTER SYNDROME)

The disorder, first described by Bamatter et al. (1), is characterized by generalized hyperlaxity, hypotonia, kyphosis, and winged scapulas. There are also microcephaly, severe myopia, and chorioretinitis.

ACROFACIAL DYSOSTOSIS (WEYERS SYNDROME)

Weyers (1, 2) reported several unrelated children with postaxial hexadactyly, bony cleft of

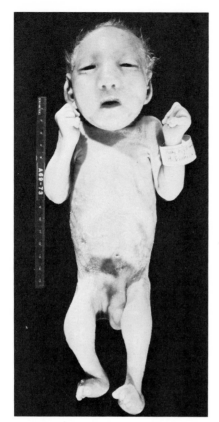

Figure 144-8. *Microcephaly, growth retardation, and flexion deformities* (Neu syndrome). Microcephaly, short neck, wide-spaced eyes, flexion deformities, rocker bottom feet. (*From R. L. Neu et al.,* Pediatrics **47:**64, 1971.)

Figure 144-9. *Somatic and mental retardation, corneal opacities, short ulna and radius, and unusual facies* (Mietens-Weber syndrome). (*A, B*). Two of four affected sibs with convergent strabismus, narrow pointed nose, short forearms, contraction at elbows, atrophic calves. (*C*). Short radius and ulna; radial head dislocated, its epiphysis absent. (*From C. Mietens and H. Weber,* J. Pediatr. **69:**624, 1966.)

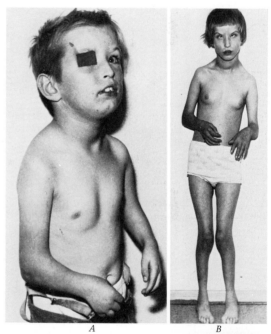

A   B

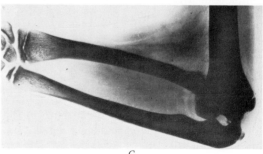

C

atrophy and aging of the skin, hyperlaxity of joints, predisposition to fracture of bones, growth retardation, and muscular hypotonia with associated hernias, flatfoot, and dislocated hips. The facial features are distinctive (2) (Fig. 144-10*A, B*).

Platyspondyly with biconcave vertebral bodies and generalized osteoporosis have been frequent (3).

Inheritance is X-linked, with variable but less severe manifestations in female heterozygotes.

The syndrome should be differentiated from the wrinkly skin syndrome reported by Gazit et al. (4). The autosomal recessively inherited disorder is characterized by wrinkled skin of the anterior chest and/or dorsal surfaces of the hands,

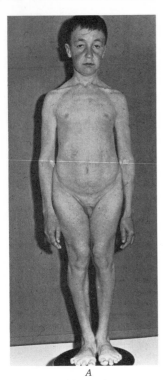 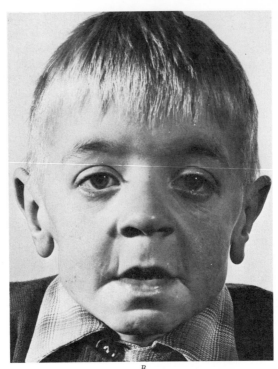

A   B

Figure 144-10. *Geroderma osteodysplastica.* (*A*). Hyperlaxity, atrophy and aging of the skin, dislocated hips, and flat foot. (*B*). Facies showing premature aging. (*Courtesy of D. Klein, Geneva, Switzerland.*)

the mandibular symphysis, and anomalies of the lower central incisors and oral vestibule.

Autosomal dominant transmission was suggested.

Postaxial hexadactyly with partial or complete fusion of the fifth and sixth metacarpals was noted in all cases. In one patient, hexadactyly was limited to a postminimus digit. The feet also exhibited postaxial hexadactyly, with complete or partial fusion of the proximal phalanges of the fifth and sixth toes and with a single fifth metatarsal.

Bony cleft of the mandibular symphysis was a constant finding. The lower central and lateral incisors were malformed, ranging from peg-shaped crowns to complete absence in the primary and permanent dentitions. In some children, the oral vestibule was absent both in the anterior maxillary and mandibular region (Fig. 144-11*A*–*C*).

HYPODONTIA AND NAIL DYSGENESIS SYNDROME (WITKOP SYNDROME)

The tooth-nail syndrome, characterized by (*a*) fine hair, (*b*) oligodontia, and (*c*) hypoplasia or koilonychia of fingernails and especially toenails, has been infrequently documented (1–5). Microscopic examination of the hair has not revealed any obvious abnormality (Fig. 144-12*A*–*C*).

The teeth most often missing are the mandibular incisors, second molars, and maxillary canines.

Evidence suggests that the syndrome is inherited as an autosomal dominant trait (3). However, there may also be an autosomal recessive form (personal observations, 1975). It has been observed in Canada among Dutch Mennonites (5) and in a family of Dutch extraction (2, 3).

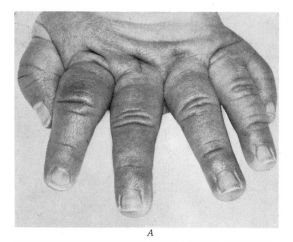

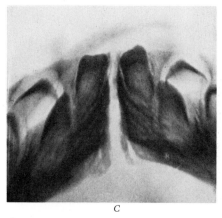

A

C

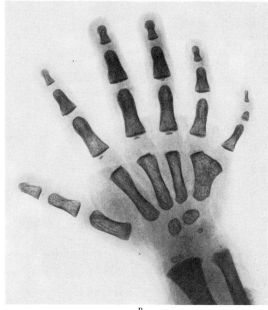

B

Figure 144-11. *Acrofacial dysostosis* (Weyers syndrome). (*A*). Postaxial hexadactyly. (*B*). Postaxial hexadactyly with fusion of metacarpals V and VI. (*C*). Cleft of mandibular symphysis. (A–C *from H. Weyers,* Ann. Paediatr. (Basel) **181**:45, 1953.)

CONGENITAL MUSCULAR TORTICOLLIS, MULTIPLE KELOIDS, CRYPTORCHISM, AND RENAL ABNORMALITIES (GOEMINNE SYNDROME)

Goeminne (1) described an apparently unique family in which males had congenitally progressive muscular torticollis with facial asymmetry, multiple spontaneous keloids which appear at puberty, cryptorchism, chronic pyelonephritis, varicose veins of the legs, and multiple pigmented cutaneous nevi (Fig. 144-13). Female carriers of this apparently X-linked disorder were less severely affected.

OPHTHALMOMANDIBULOMELIC DYSPLASIA (PILLAY SYNDROME)

Pillay (1), in 1964, reported a father and his son and daughter with corneal opacities, short forearms due to radiohumeral and proximal radioulnar dislocations, aplasia of lateral humeral condyle, head of radius, and lower third of ulna. The radius was bowed and short, articulating solely with the lunate. There were temporomandibular fusion, absent coronoid process, and obtuse mandibular angle (Fig. 144-14*A–D*).

The disorder has autosomal dominant inheritance.

FISTULAS OF LATERAL SOFT PALATE AND ASSOCIATED ANOMALIES

A number of cases of bilateral symmetrical defects of the soft palate have been reported (1–12). The reader is referred to the paper of Campbell (2) for review of early cases. Several examples have been found in association with other anom-

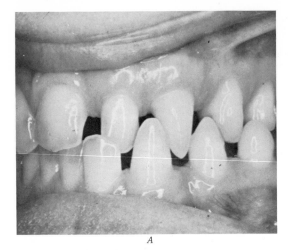

A

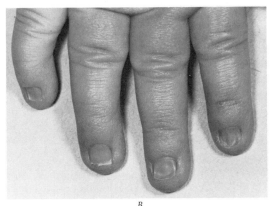

B

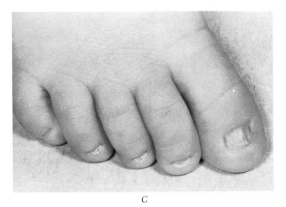

C

Figure 144-12. *Hypodontia and nail dysgenesis* (Witkop syndrome). (*A*). Oligodontia and conical tooth crown form. No evidence of hypohidrosis. (*From J. S. Giansanti*, Oral Surg. **37**:576, 1974.) (*B, C*). Hypoplasia of fingernails and toenails.

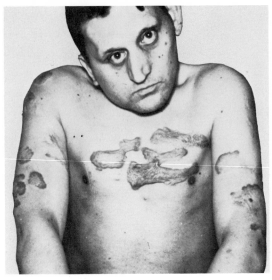

Figure 144-13. *Congenital muscular torticollis, multiple keloids, cryptorchism, and renal dysplasia* (Goeminne syndrome). Facial asymmetry, torticollis, numerous keloids of arms and thorax. (*From L. Goeminne*, Acta Genet. Med. (Roma) **17**:439, 1968.)

alies such as absent or hypoplasia of one or both palatine tonsils (2, 4, 6, 7, 12), preauricular fistulas (7), deafness (3), and strabismus (2).

Though usually bilateral, the defect may be unilateral (2, 6, 7, 11). It may be familial, having been seen in two brothers (7) (Fig. 144-15).

The defect appears to be related to irregularity in development of the second branchial pouch (9).

FLEXION AND EXTENSION DEFORMITIES OF THE HANDS AND UNUSUAL FACIES (EMERY-NELSON SYNDROME)

Mild mental and somatic retardation, increased US/LS ratio, flexion deformities of the first three metacarpophalangeal joints, and extension deformity of the interphalangeal joints of both thumbs, clawed toes, and an unusual facies (long philtrum, flat midface) were described in a mother and daughter by Emery and Nelson (1). We have seen the same anomalies in a mother and her two sons (Fig. 144-16).

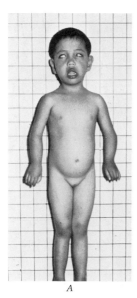

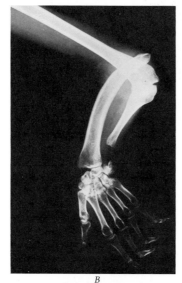

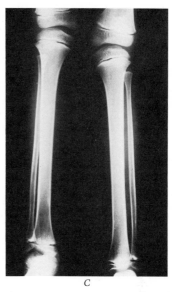

A   B   C

Figure 144-14. *Ophthalmomandibulomelic dysplasia* (*Pillay syndrome*). (*A*). Seven-year-old girl with bilateral complete corneal opacities, shortened forearms. Father and brother similarly affected. (*B*). Lateral humeral condyle aplastic, abnormal trochlea, olecranon. Coronoid processes absent, as are radial heads. Both radial shaft heads end in points that are located posterolateral to lower end of humerus. Radius bowed and short, ulna short with distal third absent. Articulation of radius only with lunate. Distal interphalangeal fusion. (*C*). Lateral malleolus higher than medial malleolus. Fibula shorter than tibia. (*D*). Temporomandibular joint ankylosis, lack of mandibular angle, and absence of coronoid process. (*From V. K. Pillay*, J. Bone Joint Surg. **46A:**858, 1964.)

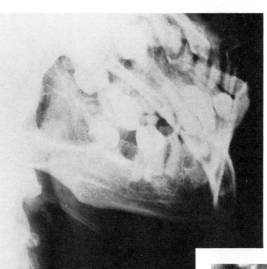

D

Figure 144-15. *Fistulas of lateral soft palate.* This anomaly is often associated with agenesis of one, or both, of the palatine tonsils. (*From O. Neuss, Z. Laryngol. Rhinol.* **35:**411, 1956.)

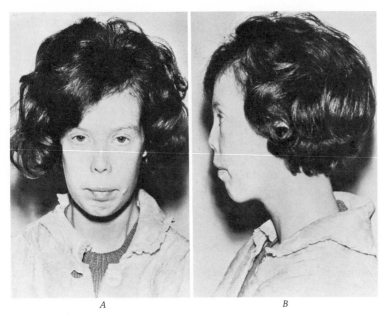

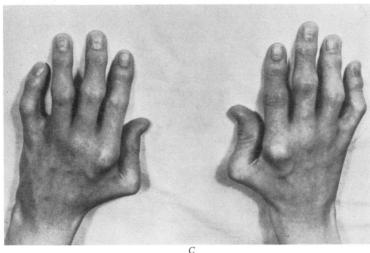

Figure 144-16. *Flexion and extension deformities of the hands, and unusual facies* (Emery-Nelson Syndrome). (*A, B*). Flat midface with long philtrum. (*C*). Flexion deformity of first three metacarpophalangeal joints, extension deformity of interphalangeal joints of thumbs. (*From A. Emery and M. Nelson,* J. Med. Genet. **7:**379, 1970.)

BRACHYMETAPODY, ANODONTIA, HYPOTRICHOSIS, AND ALBINOID TRAIT (TOUMAALA-HAAPANEN SYNDROME)

Toumaala and Haapanen (1) reported three sibs affected with short stature and shortening of all digits other than thumbs and halluces due to brachymetapody. Hypoplastic maxilla, anodontia, generalized hypotrichosis, hypoplastic breasts and genitalia, convergent strabismus, distichiasis, hypoplastic tarsus, cataracts, myopia, irregular nystagmus, and albinoid skin were also present (Fig. 144-17*A–D*).

The syndrome presumably has autosomal recessive inheritance.

MESIODENS AND CATARACT (NANCE-HORAN SYNDROME)

Nance et al. (2) described a syndrome comprising supernumerary central incisor (mesiodens), screwdriver-shaped incisors, congenital posterior suture cataract, short fourth metacarpals, and elevated serum alkaline phosphatase. The facies was not striking, but most affected patients had anteverted pinnas with folded lobes. A similar family was reported by Horan and Billson (1). We have seen a similarly affected family (Fig. 144-18A–C).

The disorder is inherited as an X-linked trait. Female heterozygotes exhibit posterior Y-sutural, punctate cataracts and marked diastemas, the incisor teeth having incisal edges which are narrower than the necks of the teeth and resembling those of congenital syphilis (Hutchinson incisors).

ORAL AND CONJUNCTIVAL AMYLOIDOSIS AND MENTAL RETARDATION (HORNOVÁ-DLUHOSOVÁ SYNDROME)

Hornová and Dluhosová (1) reported a boy and his mentally retarded sister. Within the first year of life, the eyelids were noted to be swollen, with nodular deposits of amyloid in the conjunctiva. Congenital cataracts, atrophy of the ocular bulb, and amaurosis were also present. Amyloid deposits found in the enlarged boggy gingiva imparted the appearance of icing (Fig. 144-19A, B).

BRACHYMETAPODY, HYPOPLASTIC GENITALIA, AND SOMATIC AND MENTAL RETARDATION (RUVALCABA SYNDROME)

Male sibs who exhibited severe mental and somatic retardation, hypoplastic skin, microcephaly, hypoplastic genitalia with delayed adolescence, various skeletal anomalies, and peculiar facies were described by Ruvalcaba et al. (1).

The facies was characterized by antimongoloid palpebral fissures, narrow small nose, and narrow maxilla with crowded teeth (Fig. 144-20).

Musculoskeletal anomalies included narrow trunk with pectus carinatum, kyphoscoliosis osteochondritis of spine, limitation of elbows,

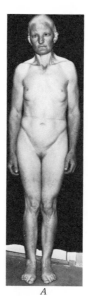
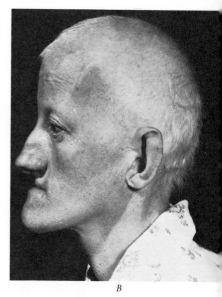

A   *B*

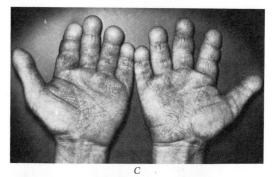

C

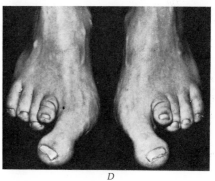

D

Figure 144-17. *Brachymetapody, anodontia, hypotrichosis, and albinoid trait.* (A). Albinoid skin, hypoplastic breasts, generalized hypotrichosis. (B). Sunken midface with loss of vertical height due to anodontia. (C, D). Shortening of all digits except thumbs and halluces. (*From P. Toumaala and E. Haapanen,* Acta Ophthalmol. (Kbh.) **46:**365, 1968.)

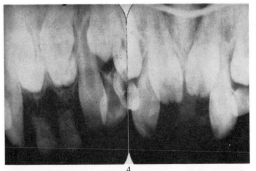

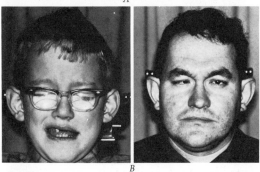

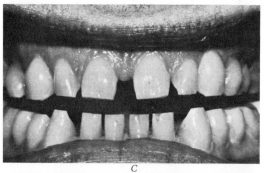

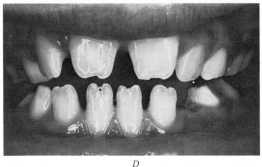

Figure 144-18. *Mesiodens and cataract.* (*A*). Mesiodens, before and after surgical removal. (*B*). Affected males. Note similar pinnas. (*C*). Heterozygote showing diastemas, screwdriver-shaped incisors. (*From D. Bixler, Indianapolis.*) (*D*). Compare with *C*. (*From M. B. Horan and F. A. Billson.* Aust. Paediat. J. **10:**98, 1974.)

shortened metacarpals and metatarsals, and inguinal hernia.

Though autosomal recessive transmission appears likely, X-linked inheritance cannot be excluded.

UNUSUAL FACIES, MENTAL AND SOMATIC RETARDATION, AND SKELETAL AND LIMB DEFECTS (COFFIN-LOWRY SYNDROME)

Coffin (1) and Lowry (2) independently reported a syndrome of mental and somatic retardation, large soft hands with distally tapering fingers, and facial alterations. Additional cases were re-

Figure 144-19. *Oral and conjunctival amyloidosis and mental retardation.* (*A*). Atrophy of bulb, amyloid deposits in conjunctiva. (*B*). Amyloid deposits in gingiva, imparting appearance of icing. (*From J. Hornová and O. Dluhosová,* Oral Surg. **25:**457, 1968.)

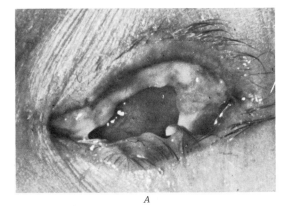

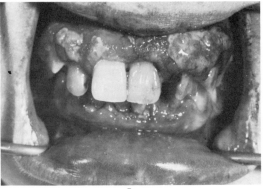

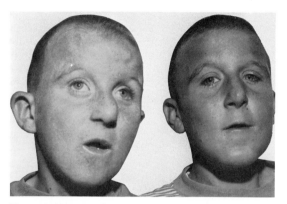

Figure 144-20. *Brachymetapody, hypoplastic genitalia, and somatic and mental retardation* (Ruvalcaba syndrome). Antimongoloid palpebral fissures, small narrow nose. (*From R. Ruvalcaba et al.*, J. Pediatr. **79:**450, 1971.)

ported by other authors (3, 4). However, it was Temtamy and coworkers (5) who recognized the unity of the reports and coined the name Coffin-Lowry syndrome.

The severity of expression in males and transmission of the syndrome through mildly affected females suggest either X-linked or sex-influenced autosomal dominant inheritance. There has been no male-to-male transmission.

The facies, which becomes progressively worse with age, is characterized by a square forehead with bitemporal narrowing, prominent supraorbital ridges, ocular hypertelorism with antimongoloid obliquity of palpebral fissures, thickened upper eyelids, poor midfacial development with relative mandibular prognathism, thick pouting lips, anteverted nostrils, and large prominent pinnas (Fig. 144-21A, B).

Musculoskeletal changes include reduced stature, clumsy broad-based gait, hypotonia and/or lax ligaments with pes planus and inguinal hernia, thickened calvaria, large anterior fontanel with delayed suture closure, pectus carinatum or excavatum, short bifid sternum, and intervertebral disk changes which eventuate in kyphosis or scoliosis in affected males (1, 4, 5). Bone age is retarded in both sexes, and pseudoepiphyses may be seen at the base of each metacarpal in males during childhood. The hands are large and soft with tapering fingers (Fig. 144-21C, D). The distal phalanges of the fingers are short with prominent tufting and there is lack of modeling of the bases of the middle phalanges. The hallux is often short. The iliac wings are narrow. Affected females tend to be obese.

Mental and motor deterioration is progressive, especially in males. Internal communicating hydrocephalus was found in a few cases (1, 2).

The skin in males is loose and easily stretched. Cutis marmorata, dependent acrocyanosis, and varicose veins are common. The hair is straight and coarse in males. Dermatoglyphic changes include a characteristic transverse hypothenar crease (1, 4, 5). The "atd" angle is increased and simian or Sydney lines are frequent. All patients have thick lips with a pouting lower lip. The tongue exhibits a deep midline furrow (Fig. 144-21E). Malocclusion with overjet and/or overbite is present in nearly all patients. Oligodontia is present in male patients, especially absence of one or both lower central incisors. Torus palatinus was present in all patients described by Temtamy et al. (5).

FAMILIAL OSTEODYSPLASIA (ANDERSON SYNDROME)

Under this unfortunately nonspecific title, Anderson et al. (1) reported sibs with an autosomal recessive disorder.

The facies was characterized by marked midfacial hypoplasia with resultant relative mandibular prognathism, pointed chin, and large earlobes (Fig. 144-22A, B).

Roentgenographically, kyphoscoliosis, thinning of calvaria, pointed configuration of mastoids and spinous processes of the cervical vertebras, abnormal ribs, and thinning of the superior pubic ramus were noted. Most remarkable, however, was alteration in the form of the mandible, which had a widened angle, increased body length, reduced ramus height, and severely decreased bigonial width (Fig. 144-22C).

BRANCHIOSKELETOGENITAL SYNDROME (ELSAHY-WATERS SYNDROME)

Elsahy and Waters (1) described three male sibs who exhibited seizures, mental retardation,

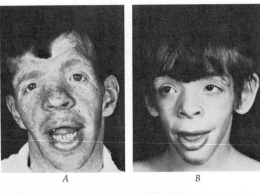

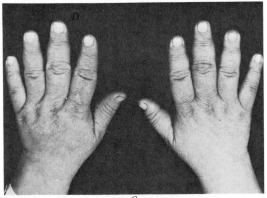

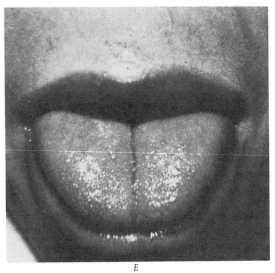

Figure 144-21. (*A, B*). *Coffin-Lowry syndrome.* Twenty-three- and ten-year-old affected males. Note facial similarities: marked hypertelorism, prominent supraorbital ridges and outer margins, short upturned nostrils, open mouth with pouty lower lip, thick bulging chin, and enlarged protruberant ears. Facial features are more coarse in the older affected male. All males had straight coarse hair. (*C, D*). Hands are spadelike; digits are thick at base and taper distally. (*E*). Exaggerated median furrow of tongue. (*From S. A. Temtamy et al.,* J. Pediatr. **86:**724, 1975.)

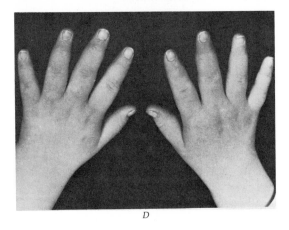

pectus excavatum, and penoscrotal hypospadias. Roentgenographic study showed fusion of the second and third cervical vertebras.

The facies was characterized by brachycephaly, marked midfacial hypoplasia, ocular hypertelorism, divergent strabismus, nystagmus, and mild ptosis. The nasal bridge was broad with a wide nasal tip and flared alae (Fig. 144-23*A*).

Penoscrotal hypospadias was present in all three sibs but to a variable degree (Fig. 144-23*B*).

Oral manifestations included submucous palatal cleft, multiple jaw cysts, and teeth having dysplastic dentin.

The disorder is probably transmitted as an autosomal recessive trait, but X-linked inheritance cannot be excluded. There was parental consanguinity.

MENTAL RETARDATION, MICROCEPHALY, MICROCORNEA, AND UNUSUAL FACIES (KAUFMAN SYNDROME)

Kaufman et al. (1) documented four of seven sibs with mental retardation, microcephaly, ear tags, microcornea, strabismus, myopia, and micrognathia. The columella was especially low (Fig. 144-24). Autosomal recessive inheritance was likely.

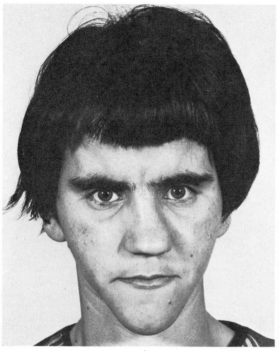

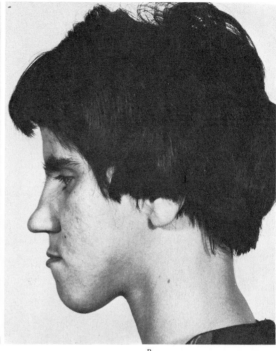

A   *B*

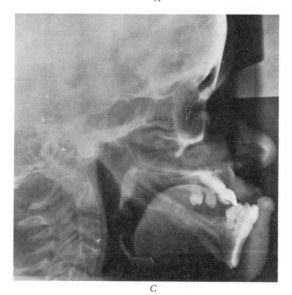

C

Figure 144-22. *Familial osteodysplasia* (Anderson syndrome). (*A, B*). Triangular face with pointed chin and hypoplastic midface. (*C*). Mandible with widened angle, increased body length, reduced ramus height. (*From L. G. Anderson et al.*, J.A.M.A. **220:**1687, 1972.)

AMELOGENESIS IMPERFECTA, TAURODONTISM, CURLY HAIR, AND SCLEROTIC BONES (TRICHODENTOOSSEOUS SYNDROME)

Robinson et al. (5), Lichtenstein et al. (4), and Crawford (1) described what is probably the same syndrome in different families. Winter et al. (8) likely observed a different condition.

The scalp hair is curly but not woolly, and the lashes and eyebrows are long. In some cases, the hair tends to straighten with age.

The patients described by Lichtenstein and coworkers (3, 4) had somewhat sclerotic bones, were dolichocephalic, and had multiple depressed, well-demarcated brown circular lesions on the ankles, pretibial areas, hips, and forearms. The nails were thinned and likely to peel or fracture.

The teeth, which often became abscessed within the first few years of life, exhibited very thin, pitted, yellowish-brown hypoplastic and/or hypocalcified enamel. The molars, both deciduous and permanent, were taurodont in form.

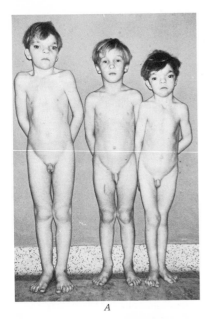

A

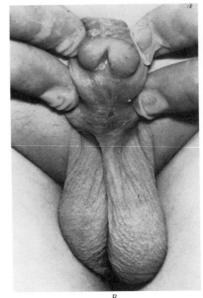

B

Figure 144-23.
Branchioskeletogenital syndrome. (A). Brachycephaly, wide-set eyes, midface hypoplasia, divergent strabismus, broad nasal bridge with wide nasal tip, flared alae, and pectus carinatum in two affected male sibs flanking normal male sib. *(B).* Penoscrotal hypospadias. *(From N. I. Elsahy and W. Waters,* Plast. Reconstr. Surg. **48:**542, 1971.)

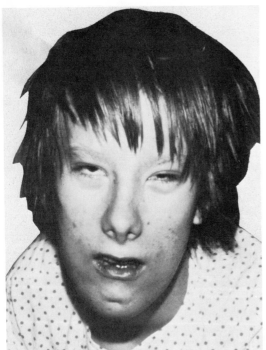

Figure 144-24. *Mental retardation, microcephaly, microcornea, and unusual facies* (Kaufman syndrome). Note microcornea and unusual nasal configuration. *(From R. Kaufman et al.,* Birth Defects 7(1):135, 1971.)

Formation and eruption were, in general, delayed (2) (Fig. 144-25*A, B*).

The syndrome clearly has autosomal dominant inheritance.

Taurodontism may be seen in syndromal association with oligodontia and sparse hair growth (1a, 7), microcephalic dwarfism and diminished root formation (6), and in X-chromosomal aneuploidy. There are many genetic forms of simple amelogenesis imperfecta (9) (Fig. 144-25*C, D*).

HYPOTONIA, OBESITY, MENTAL DEFICIENCY, AND FACIAL, ORAL, OCULAR, AND LIMB ANOMALIES

Cohen et al. (1) reported a syndrome consisting of obesity with midchildhood onset, hypotonia, mental deficiency, tapering extremities with narrow hands and feet, lumbar lordosis with compensatory dorsal kyphosis, mild dorsal scoliosis, cubitus valgus, genu valgum, hyperextensibility at the elbows and proximal interphalangeal joints, characteristic facial appearance, ocular defects, and oral anomalies.

The facies was characterized by mild microcephaly, antimongoloid obliquity of palpebral fissures, mild maxillary hypoplasia, short phil-

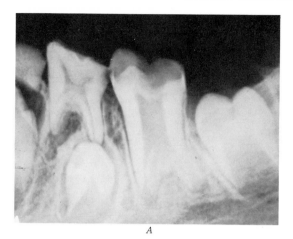

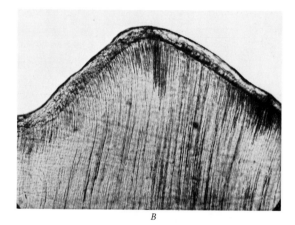

A

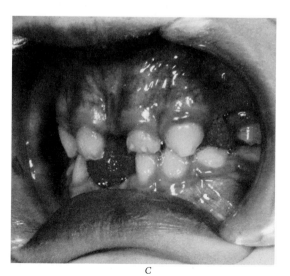

B

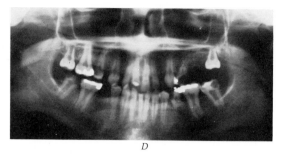

D

Figure 144-25. *Amelogenesis imperfecta, taurodontism, curly hair, and sclerotic bones.* (*A*). Taurodontism of first molar. Note generally thin enamel. (*From J. L. Crawford,* J. Dent. Child. **37**:171, 1970.) (*B*). Ground section of tooth, showing hypoplastic enamel. (*C*). *Taurodontism and oligodontia syndrome.* (*D*). Note normal amount of enamel in roentgenogram of syndrome noted in *C*.

trum, open mouth with prominent central incisors, and micrognathia. The palate was narrow and highly arched, and the teeth were crowded.

Ocular anomalies were variable and included mottled retina, strabismus, myopia, microphthalmia, and coloboma of the iris, retina, and choroid. Other findings included mild shortening of various metacarpals and metatarsals. Two patients had simian creases. In one case, mild cutaneous 2–3 syndactyly was present in both hands and feet (Fig. 144-26*A*–*C*).

Affected sibs with normal parents suggested autosomal recessive transmission.

TEMPORAL "FORCEPS-MARKS" SCARRING AND UNUSUAL FACIES (SETLEIS SYNDROME)

Congenital temporal ("forceps-marks") scarring, vertical grooving below the lower lip, multiple rows of lashes on upper eyelids but lower lids devoid of lashes and meibomian glands, widow's peak, eyebrows which angled sharply upward and outward but were deficient laterally were noted in two sets of sibs (2). Similarly affected individuals were seen by Rudolph (1) and D. Daentel (personal communication, 1975).

In addition, the skin about the eyes appeared wrinkled, and the nose and chin felt rubbery. The thenar and hypothenar areas were somewhat flattened. Inheritance is presumably autosomal recessive (Fig. 144-27).

C

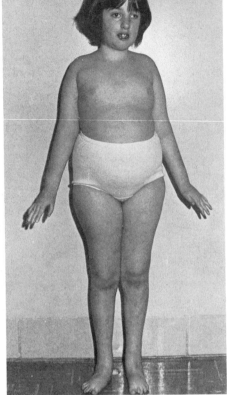

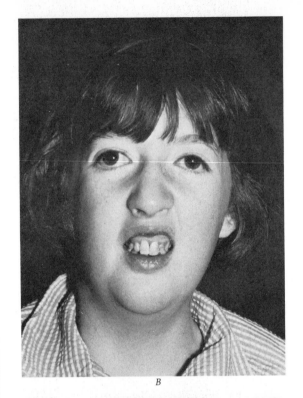

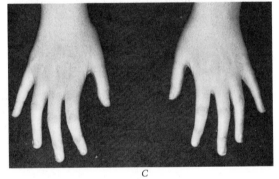

Figure 144-26. *Hypotonia, obesity, mental deficiency, and facial, oral, ocular and limb anomalies. (A). Obesity and tapering hands and feet. (B). Mild microcephaly, antimongoloid obliquity of palpebral fissures, short philtrum, and open mouth. (C). Narrow hands and fingers. (From M. M. Cohen, Jr., et al., J. Pediatr.* **83:**280, 1973.)

MILD MENTAL RETARDATION, RIGHT-SIDED AORTIC ARCH, AND FACIAL DYSMORPHIA

Strong (1) described right-sided aorta, mild mental retardation, and abnormal facies characterized by beaklike nose, antimongoloid obliquity of palpebral fissures, large posteriorly angulated pinnas, small carplike mouth, and nasal septum deviation in a mother and three children.

HYPERHIDROSIS, PREMATURE GRAYING OF THE HAIR, AND PREMOLAR HYPODONTIA (PHC SYNDROME, BÖÖK SYNDROME)

Böök (1) in 1950 reported the PHC syndrome: P–premolar aplasia, H–hyperhidrosis, and C–canities prematura.

The syndrome was transmitted as an autosomal dominant condition with complete penetrance.

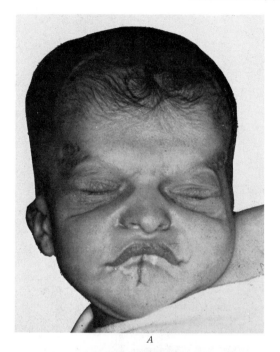

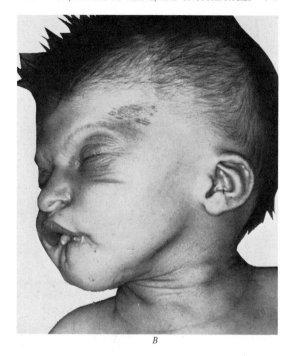

A   *B*

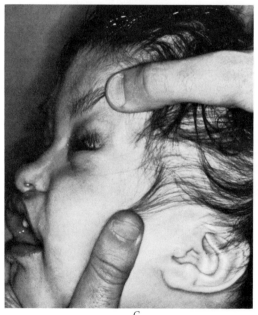

C

Figure 144-27. *Temporal "foreceps-marks" scarring and unusual facies (Setleis syndrome). (A, B).* Temporal defects, eyelash abnormalities, central defect of chin. *(C).* Multiple rows of lashes on upper lids, absence on lower lids. *(From H. Setleis et al., Pediatrics* **32:**540, 1963.*)*

Canities prematura (early, diffuse whitening of the hair) was the most common sign. It appeared usually between the sixth and twenty-third years of life and progressed slowly. About one-third of the patients presented whitening of the hair in other parts of the body.

Two-thirds of the patients had marked functional hyperhidrosis. Although often palmoplantar, it involved the axillas and forehead less severely. One or more premolars were absent, with corresponding retention of their deciduous precursors.

ACCELERATED SKELETAL MATURATION, FAILURE TO THRIVE, AND UNUSUAL FACIES

Marshall et al. (1), Tipton et al. (3), Visveshwara et al. (4), and Perrin et al. (2) described several children with mental and somatic retardation but markedly accelerated skeletal maturation. Noisy respiration, pneumonia, and failure to thrive were also noted. Perrin et al. (2) found pulmonary hypertension in their infant.

Facial features included bulging eyes, blue

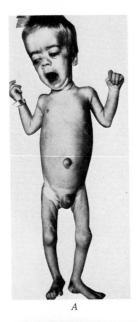

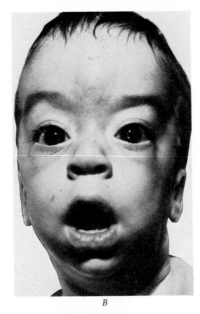

A *B*

Figure 144-28. *Accelerated skeletal maturation, failure to thrive, and unusual facies.*
(*A*). Bulging eyes, coarse eyebrows, depressed
nasal bridge, umbilical hernia. (*B*). Compare
facies in another child with the same disorder. (*C*). Prominent calvaria, small facial
bones, and hypoplastic mandibular rami.
(*D*). Bone age is six to seven years at chronologic age of ten months. (*From R. E. Marshall et al., J. Pediatr. **78**:95, 1971.*)

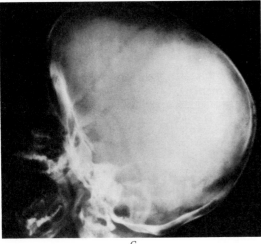

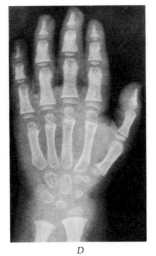

C *D*

scleras, megalocornea, bushy eyebrows with synophrys, and small nose with anteverted nostrils.
Umbilical hernia was present in both children.

Roentgenographically, carpal bone age was
markedly advanced. The proximal and middle
phalanges were thicker and terminal phalanges
smaller than normal. The frontal bone was
prominent, with shallow orbits and hypoplastic
facial bones. The mandibular rami were hypoplastic with absence of normal angle. (Fig.
144-28*A–D*).

This syndrome should be distinguished from
the disorder described by Weaver et al. (4) (vide
infra).

MIRROR HANDS AND FEET, TALIPES EQUINOVARUS, AND NASAL ALAR COLOBOMAS

Supernumerary digits of hands and feet with
syndactyly and duplication of carpal and tarsal

bones (mirror hands and feet) in combination with talipes equinovarus, dislocated knees, and colobomas of the nasal alae were documented in a father and daughter by Sandrow et al. (1).

AMELOGENESIS IMPERFECTA AND TERMINAL ONYCHOLYSIS

Witkop and colleagues (1, 2) described a kindred exhibiting hypoplastic hypocalcified enamel, terminal onycholysis, seborrheic dermatitis of scalp, xerosis, and functional hypohidrosis (Fig. 144-29A, B).

Inheritance was autosomal dominant.

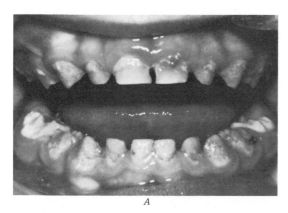

A

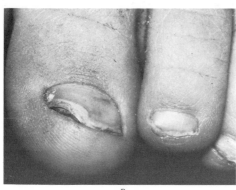

B

Figure 144-29. *Amelogenesis imperfecta and terminal onycholysis.* (*A*). Enamel, largely missing on some teeth, is hypomineralized. (*B*). Terminal onycholysis. (*From C. J. Witkop, Jr.,* Schweiz. Monatsschr. Zahnheilkd. **82**:917, 1972.)

INCREASED BONE DENSITY AND SYNDACTYLY (BRAHAM-LENZ SYNDROME)

Braham (1) reported a child with progeroid skin, dilated veins, a large open anterior fontanel, increased bone density, large ears, soft-tissue syndactyly of all fingers and toes, hyperflexible joints and hypoplastic enamel. Roentgenographic studies showed increased density of the skull base and mandible, thickened clavicles, ribs and diaphyses of long bones. The vertebras exhibited central notching. Although the child was stated to have Camurati-Engelmann disease, we cannot accept that diagnosis. Lenz and Majewski (2) reported a similarly affected child.

BLEPHARONASOFACIAL SYNDROME

Pashayan et al. and Putterman et al. (1, 2) described autosomal dominant inheritance of a syndrome of telecanthus and lateral displacement and stenosis of lacrimal puncta, bulky nose with broad nasal bridge, masklike face, midfacial hypoplasia, longitudinal cheek furrows, and trapezoidal upper lip (Fig. 144-30).

Joints were hyperextensible. All patients exhibited a positive Babinski reflex, poor coordination, torsion dystonia, mild soft-tissue syndactyly of the fingers, and mental retardation.

MULTIPLE ODONTOMAS, ESOPHAGEAL STENOSIS, AND CHRONIC INTERSTITIAL CIRRHOSIS OF THE LIVER

Herrmann (3) reported a young male with huge tumors of the maxilla and mandible containing 1,200 and 900 teeth, respectively, in various stages of development, including geminated and invaginated teeth. In 1973, Schmidseder and Hausamen (5) studied the same patient, noting that his two sons (one dying from pneumonia soon after birth) also manifested multiple odontomas of both jaws in infancy (Fig. 144-31). The surviving infant was found to have a liver disorder and pulmonary stenosis. Subsequently, a daughter was born who again manifested odontomas. The boy experienced recurrences of odon-

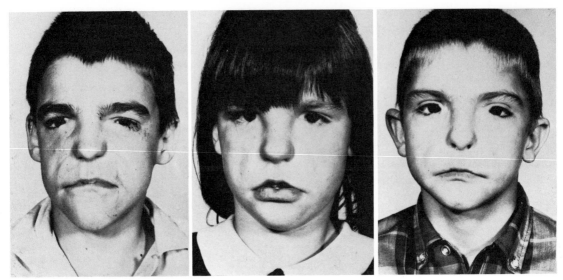

Figure 144-30. *Blepharonasofacial syndrome.* Facies of three mentally retarded sibs with torsion dystonia, showing telecanthus with temporal displacement of puncta, antimongoloid slant of palpebral fissures. Nose is fleshy, midface hypoplastic, upper lip trapezoidal, lower lip pouty. (*From H. Pashayan et al.,* Am. J. Dis. Child. **125:**389, 1973.)

tomas, exhibiting a higher degree of differentiation. He also exhibited esophageal stenosis, as did his father (7).

Bader (1) reported multiple odontomas of both jaws in a female infant with calcified aortic stenosis, congenital cylindric bronchiectasis, leiomyomatosis of the esophagus with stenosis

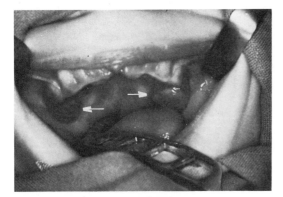

Figure 144-31. *Multiple odontomas, esophageal stenosis, and chronic interstitial cirrhosis of the liver.* Arrows point to congenital bilateral odontomas of posterior maxilla. (*From R. Schmidseder and J. R. Hausamen,* Oral Surg. **39:**249, 1975.)

and hyperplasia of the myenteric plexus and chronic interstitial cirrhosis of the liver. G. L. Barnes (personal communication, 1974) observed sibs with odontomas in four quadrants, malrotation of the bowel, anal stenosis, and iris colobomas.

Multiple odontomas were documented in male sibs by Schmitz and Witzel (6), but associated anomalies were not mentioned. Beisser (2) and Malik and Khalid (4) also reported multiple bilateral odontomas in both jaws.

In view of the occurrence of what appears to be a syndrome of multiple odontomas, chronic interstitial cirrhosis of the liver, and esophageal stenosis in two generations, it must be assumed that the disorder is inherited as an autosomal dominant trait. In the case of Schmitz and Witzel, the parents of the male sibs were normal.

BROAD TERMINAL PHALANGES AND FACIAL ABNORMALITIES (KEIPERT SYNDROME)

Male sibs with severe sensorineural hearing loss, unusual facies, and broad terminal phalanges were described by Keipert et al. (1973).

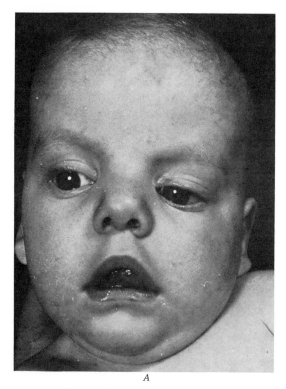

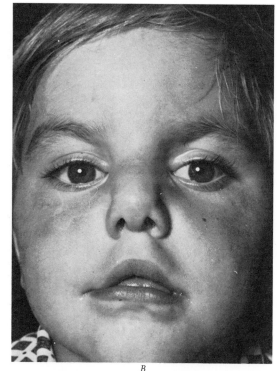

A   *B*

Autosomal or X-linked recessive inheritance is likely.

The facies was marked by a large nose with a high bridge, large rounded columella, and prominent nasal alae. The upper lip protruded, with a cupid's bow configuration overlapping the rather straight lower lip laterally (Fig. 114-32*A, B*).

The distal phalanges of the thumbs, the first, second, and third fingers, and all the toes were remarkably broad. The fifth fingers were short and clinodactylous. The toes were rotated medially (Fig. 144-32*C, D*).

Roentgenographically, one sib had bifid terminal phalanges in both index fingers. In the halluces of both patients, the proximal phalanges were short and the terminal phalanges were short with large, rounded epiphyses.

EXCESSIVE OVERGROWTH, ACCELERATED SKELETAL MATURATION, CAMPTODACTYLY, AND UNUSUAL FACIES (WEAVER SYNDROME)

Weaver et al. (1) reported two sporadic instances of a striking syndrome with excessive persistent

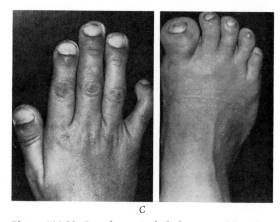

C

Figure 144-32. *Broad terminal phalanges and facial abnormalities (Keipert syndrome). (A, B).* Nine-month and three-year-old sibs exhibiting large nose with high bridge, large rounded columella, and prominent alae. Upper lip protrudes with cupid's bow configuration. *(C).* Terminal phalanges are short and broad. Fifth fingers are short and clinodactylous. *(D).* Toes short and broad, especially hallux. *(From J. A. Keipert et al., Aust. Paediatr. J.* **9:**10, 1973.)

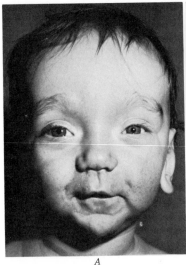 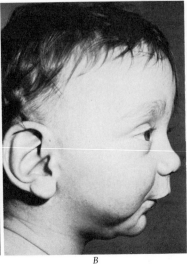

A   *B*

Figure 144-33. (*A, B*). *Excessive overgrowth, hypertonia, and unusual facies* (Weaver syndrome). Note broad forehead, ocular hypertelorism, large ears, long philtrum, and micrognathia. (*From D. D. Weaver et al., J. Pediatr.* **84:**547, 1974.)

overgrowth of prenatal onset, accelerated osseous maturation, hypertonia, hoarse, low-pitched cry, and voracious appetite. Craniofacial features included broad forehead, hypertelorism, large ears, long philtrum, and micrognathia (Fig. 144-33). Camptodactyly, prominent finger pads with thin deeply set nails, broad thumbs, talipes equinovarus, and clinodactyly of the toes were observed. Excessive loose skin, umbilical hernia, and other abnormalities were noted. Roentgenographic abnormalities included remarkably advanced bone age (especially carpal maturation) and widened distal femurs and ulnas.

HEREDITARY OSTEOLYSIS (THIEFFRY-KOHLER SYNDROME)

Kohler et al. (1) reported a syndrome in a father and in his two sons and daughter characterized by a marfanoid appearance, frontal bossing, micrognathia, mild scoliosis, pes cavus, overlapping toes, and plantar cysts (Fig. 144-34A). Bone destruction of the wrists and ankles, beginning with the carpal and tarsal bones and spreading to involve adjacent bones, occurred during childhood and progressed, with painless, at times asymmetric, osteolysis (Fig. 144-34B). Serum alkaline phosphatase and hydroxyproline levels were elevated. Similar cases were reported by Thieffry and Sorell-Dejerine (2).

MANDIBULOACRAL DYSPLASIA (CRANIOMANDIBULAR DERMATODYSOSTOSIS)

Cavallazzi (1) reported a female child with mandibular hypoplasia, delayed cranial suture closure, numerous Wormian bones, narrow shoulders, dysplastic outer clavicles, and abbreviated terminal club-shaped phalanges associated with acroosteolysis. No mention was made of cutaneous atrophy. Two unrelated male children with the same syndrome were documented by Young et al. (5). Their patients were older and had been followed for several years. In addition, progressive stiffness of the joints was noted. Fat deposits were increased over the abdomen and absent or decreased over the distal limbs. The skin over the hands and feet was atrophic and a mottled brown skin rash was distributed over the trunk. Height was at the 3d percentile (Fig. 144-35A–E).

McKusick (3, 4) reported an isolated example of the syndrome in a young boy. Although he did not mention cutaneous atrophy, it is evident from the photographs. Danks et al. (2) coined the name *craniomandibular dermatodysostosis* to describe a condition seen in a boy with what we believe is the same disorder, although the former authors argue that it is a separate entity. Their child also had prominent eyes and a sharp nose (seen in all affected), open cranial sutures, nu-

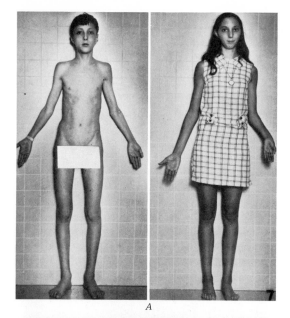

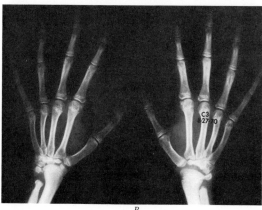

Figure 144-34. *Hereditary osteolysis* (Thieffry-Kohler syndrome). (*A*). Affected sibs manifesting similar facies, micrognathia, marfanoid appearance, and foot deformities. (*B*). Roentgenograms of sixteen-year-old showing bilateral dissolution of distal ulnas with ulnar deviation of the distal radii. The carpus is shortened, with the carpal bones small, dense, and eroded. (*From E. Kohler et al.,* Radiology **108**:99, 1973.)

merous Wormian bones, mandibular hypoplasia, stiff joints, brown atrophic cutaneous macules on the trunk, arms, legs, and face, short terminal bullous phalanges with acroosteolysis, and short stature. Calcium deposits were extruded from the scalp, ears, elbows, and fingertips. Modeling of the femur and humerus was abnormal with patchy areas of central sclerosis and defects.

Oral manifestations include mandibular hypoplasia with inability to open the mouth widely. Danks et al. (2) demonstrated crowding of the mandibular teeth and absence of cellular cementum on the roots.

All these patients were isolated examples. The inheritance pattern, if any, is unknown.

HAPPY PUPPET SYNDROME

The syndrome was first described by Angelman (1) in 1965. Over a dozen examples have been described to date (1–7). All examples to date are sporadic.

Patients resemble one another markedly. They are microcephalic or brachycephalic with a horizontal occipital depression. Prognathism and frequent extrusion of the tongue are characteristic (Fig. 144-36*A–C*).

Ophthalmologic examination shows decreased pigmentation of the choroid in 70 percent and optic atrophy in over 40 percent. About 30 percent have Brushfield spots.

Patients have severe mental retardation with intelligence quotients below 40. They appear happy, exhibiting unprovoked and prolonged bursts of laughter. Motor development is retarded and muscular tone decreased. One is impressed by their constant useless activity and ataxic uncoordinated movements like that of a puppet, hence the name. They exhibit epilepsy in the form of hypsarrhythmia or grand mal seizures.

Pathologic alterations are unknown, but the symptoms suggest brain damage, probably involving the cerebellum. Electroencephalographic studies have shown slow wave or spike activity. Pneumoencephalography has demonstrated cortical atrophy or dilation of the ventricular system.

Roentgenographically, there is flattening in the occipital region and tilting of the cranial base so that the sella turcica is obliquely positioned.

Nonspecific aminoaciduria has been found in some cases.

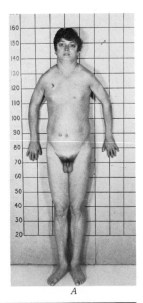

A

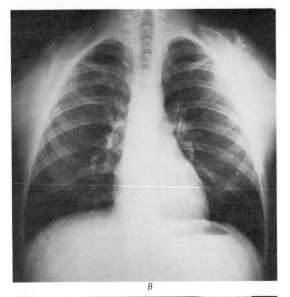

B

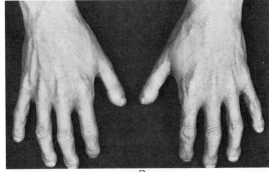

D

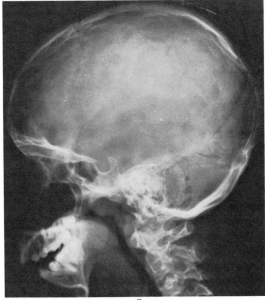

C

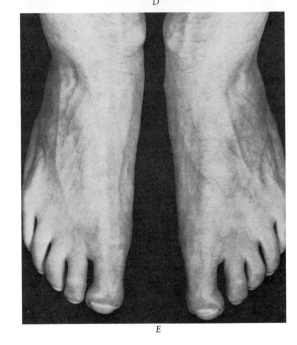

E

Figure 144-35. *Mandibuloacral dysplasia.* (*A*). Short stature, sloping shoulders, thick trunk and neck, and micrognathia. (*B*). Hypoplastic clavicles. (*C*). Wide sagittal sutures and hypoplastic body and ramus of mandible. (*D*). Short terminal phalanges and stiffness of interphalangeal joints. (*E*). Similar acroosteolytic alterations in toes. (A to E *from V. A. McKusick et al.,* Birth Defects **7**(7):291, 1971.)

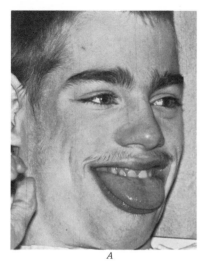
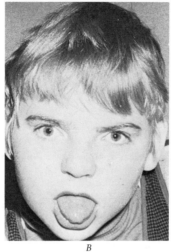
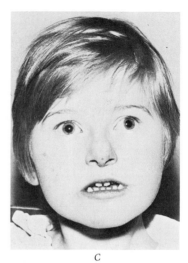

A   B   C

Figure 144-36. *Happy puppet syndrome. (A–C).* Note protruding tongue, mandibular prognathism. Patients exhibit pointless activity, ataxic uncoordinated puppetlike movements, and unprovoked prolonged paroxyms of laughter. (A *from C. Howry, Yakima, Washington;* B *from M. Warburg, Gentofte, Denmark;* C *from O. Mayo et al.,* Develop. Med. Child. Neurol. **15:**63, 1973.)

MULIBREY NANISM

The mnemonic employed by Perheentupa et al. (2, 3) refers to a form of prenatal growth retardation associated with anomalies of muscle, liver, brain and eye. Most cases reported to date stem from Finland (1, 2, 3). The disorder possibly has autosomal recessive inheritance.

Birth weight and length are usually 2 SD or greater below or above the mean. With age, growth becomes progressively retarded. Adult male height varies from 136 to 161 cm while adult females range from 126 to 151 cm. Bone age is normal. The extremities are thin and short. The patients are mildly hypotonic.

The face is triangular, the forehead prominent and high, and the nasal bridge deep and broad. There is mild ocular hypertelorism (Fig. 144-37A–C). Ocular changes consist of aggregation and dispersion of pigment in the mid-periphery and characteristic yellowish dots. The choroid appears hypoplastic (Fig. 144-37D).

Cardiovascular anomalies include pericardial constriction due to thickened and adherent pericardium, elevated venous pressure, enlarged heart, dilated neck veins, and in some cases, ascites with congestive failure (5, 6). The liver is enlarged in the neonatal period, possibly due to congestion (3).

Intelligence is mildly retarded and pneumoencephalography has shown abnormally large cerebral ventricles and cisternae. The voice is highly pitched.

About 65 percent have cutaneous nevus flammeus.

Roentgenographically there is frontal and occipital bossing. The sella is long and shallow. The frontal and sphenoidal sinuses are absent or hypoplastic (Fig. 144-37E, F). Fibrous dysplastic lesions of the tibia have been found in about 30 percent of patients.

Dental malocclusion has been found in about half the patients, hypodontia in about one-quarter. The tongue appears small in most patients.

MYOPIA, CATARACTS, SADDLE NOSE, AND SENSORINEURAL DEAFNESS (MARSHALL SYNDROME)

Seven members in four generations of a family studied by Marshall (2) had a syndrome including saddle-nose defect, congenital and juve-

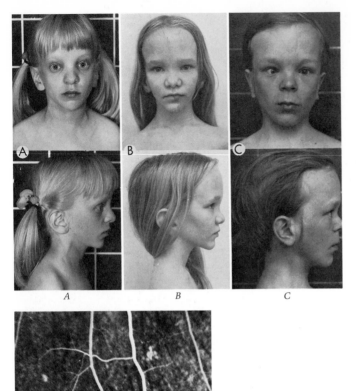

A   B   C

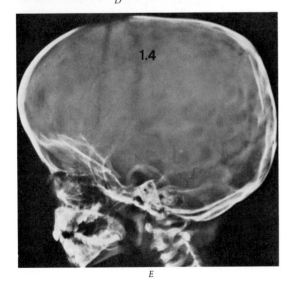

E

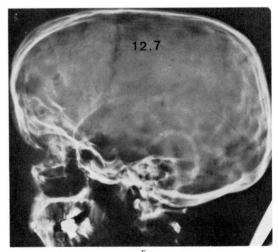

F

Figure 144-37. *Mulibrey nanism.* (*A–C*). Three unrelated adolescent patients exhibiting similar facies. Two of the patients had pericardial calcification. (*D*). Fluorescein angiogram of fundus showing conglomerate of dots and severe hypoplasia of choroid. (*E, F*). Typical skull radiographs at 1.4 and 12.7 years exhibiting abnormal cranial form, J-shaped sella, and increased basilar angle. (A to F *from J. Perheentupa et al.*, Lancet **2:**351, 1973.)

nile cataracts, myopia, and sensorineural hearing loss. Other kindred were reported by Ruppert et al. (4) and Zellweger et al. (5). The cases of Keith et al. (1) are less-certain examples.

The facies is characterized by a markedly small nose with a sunken nasal bridge, anteverted nostrils, and hypoplastic midface (Fig. 144-38A, B). Failing vision usually occurs in the second decade but within the first six months of life in a few cases. Posterior polar cortical and subcapsular opacities which spontaneously resorb have been noted in the second, third, and fourth decades. Severe myopia (10 diopters or more) and fluid vitreous have been evident from birth. Retinal detachment has occurred in a few patients (2, 3).

Affected family members have reported hearing loss in early childhood. Audiometric tests have shown a 30 to 60 dB mixed or mostly sensorineural deafness.

Roentgenographic studies have demonstrated thickened calvaria, intracranial calcifications (falx, tentorium, meninges), hypoplastic nasal bones, hypoplastic maxilla, absent frontal sinuses, beaked or bullet-shaped vertebras in children, concave vertebral margins in adults, small irregular pelvis with delayed closure of pubic and ischial bones, coxa valga, mild bowing of radius and ulna, and irregular epiphyses of extremities (3).

The disorder, occurring in several generations, is clearly dominant. However, since there have been no examples of male-to-male transmission, X-linkage cannot be presently excluded.

Hereditary arthroophthalmopathy (Stickler syndrome) must be excluded.

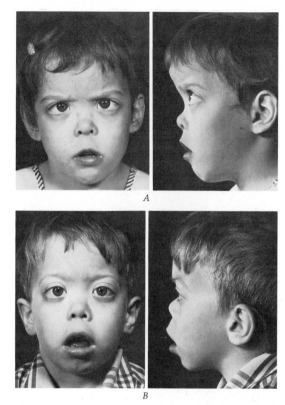

A

B

Figure 144-38. *Myopia, cataracts, saddle nose, and sensorineural deafness. (A, B).* Affected sibs exhibiting growth retardation, frontal bossing, small upturned saddle nose, small maxilla, mild ocular hypertelorism, severe myopia, decreased visual acuity, esotropia, and sensorineural hearing loss. Mother and younger sister similarly affected. (A and B *courtesy of H. Zellweger et al., Iowa City, Iowa.*)

CALCIFICATION OF AORTIC ARCH, OSTEOPOROSIS AND HYPOPLASIA OF TOOTH BUDS (SINGLETON-MERTEN SYNDROME)

A syndrome consisting of calcification of the aortic arch and aortic valve, hypoplastic tooth buds, and osteoporosis and widening of the metacarpals, carpals, and phalanges was described in two unrelated female children by Singleton and Merten (2). Two additional female patients were reported by McLoughlin et al. (1).

The teeth were reduced in number, were probably severely hypoplastic, and failed to erupt in at least three of the girls. In one of these, the teeth were stated to have exfoliated (Fig. 144-39A, B).

Cardiac enlargement with calcification of the aortic arch was seen in all four children (Fig. 144-39C). Death resulted in two of the children from ventricular fibrillation.

Muscular weakness and poor development were present in at least two of the children. There was osteoporosis of the cranial vault and all long bones, being most markedly involved in the hand bones (Fig. 144-39D). Subungual soft tissue calcification was observed in one hand.

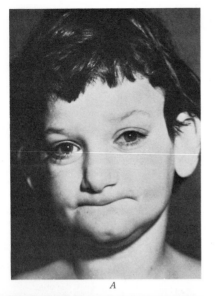

A

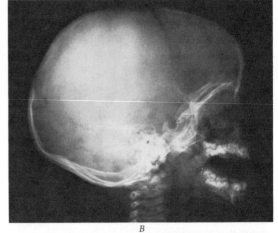

B

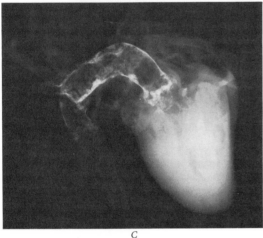

C

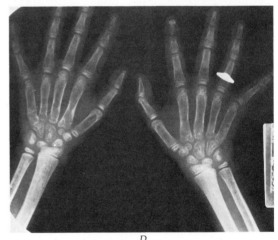

D

Figure 144-39. *Calcification of aortic arch, osteoporosis and hypoplasia of tooth buds (Singleton-Merten syndrome).* (*A*). Loss of vertical height in lower face due to unerupted teeth make child look older than ten years of age. (*B*). Radiograph showed mild maxillary hypoplasia, mild diffuse osteoporosis, and multiple unerupted teeth. (*C*). Extensive calcification of aortic arch and aortic valve. (*D*). Marked osteoporosis of hand bones, subungual calcification of second finger. (*From E. B. Singleton and D. F. Merten, Pediatr. Radiol.* **1**:2, 1973.)

DOLICHOCEPHALY, UNUSUAL FACIES, WITH HAIR, DENTAL, AND SKELETAL ANOMALIES (SENSENBRENNER SYNDROME)

Sensenbrenner et al. (1) described male and female sibs with dolichocephaly, short thorax, and mild shortening of limbs with oddly shaped distal phalanges. Height was below the 3d percentile.

The facies was marked by frontal bossing, epicanthal folds, hypertelorism, antimongoloid obliquity of palpebral fissures, full cheeks, and everted lower lip (Fig. 144-40*A–D*). Hair was short and reduced in diameter. The pinnae were

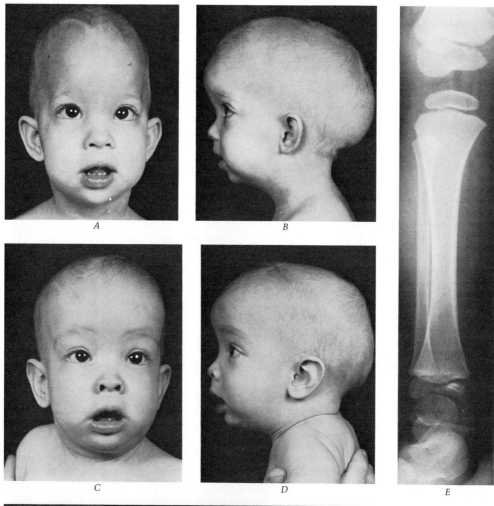

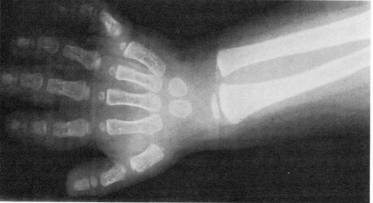

Figure 144-40. *Dolichocephaly, unusual facies, with hair, dental, and skeletal anomalies (Sensenbrenner syndrome).* (*A–D*). Sibs exhibiting dolichocephaly, frontal bossing, epicanthal folds, ocular hypertelorism, and everted lower lip. (*E*). Radiograph shows flat irregular epiphyses and shortening of fibulas, both proximally and distally. (*F*). All hand bones shortened, many epiphyses flattened. Shortened middle phalanges and clinodactyly of fifth finger. (A to E *from J. Sensenbrenner et al.*, Birth Defects **11**(2):372, 1975.)

posteriorly angulated. The teeth were small, greyish, and widely spaced. Multiple frenula were present.

The upper arms and hands were especially shortened. Roentgenographic studies showed flattening of the epiphyses of all long bones. The fibulas were abbreviated. All hand bones were short, especially the middle and distal phalanges. The fifth fingers were clinodactylous (Fig. 144-40E, F). Bilateral simian creases were present.

Presumably the syndrome has autosomal recessive inheritance. S. Levin (personal communication, 1975) has seen two similarly affected sibs.

CONGENITAL BLEPHAROPHIMOSIS, JOINT CONTRACTURES, AND MUSCULAR HYPOTONIA (MARDEN-WALKER SYNDROME)

Marden and Walker (4), Fitch et al. (2), Temtamy et al. (7), and Passarge (5) described infants or children with multiple congenital irreducible joint contractures which disappear during the first year of life, muscular hypotonia, pectus excavatum, arachnodactyly, widely set nipples, depressed nasal bridge, and pursed lips with eversion of the low lip. The face was immobile with sagging cheeks. Strabismus, blepharophimosis, microstomia, and micrognathia were also noted (Fig. 144-41A, B). The patients reported by Marden and Walker (4) and Passarge (5) had cleft palate. Possibly other examples were reported by Ealing (1) and Simpson and Degnan (6). We are uncertain about how to classify the patient of Younessian and Ammann (8).

Temtamy et al. (7) reported the disorder in first cousins. Parental consanguinity suggests autosomal recessive inheritance.

Fitch et al. (2) found reduction in the size of scattered muscle fibers of both histochemical types. No percussion myotonia or myotonic discharges on the electromyogram were elicitable. Pneumoencephalographic study indicated partial or complete agenesis of the cerebellum and brainstem. There were decreased deep tendon reflexes.

The condition must be differentiated from *Schwartz-Jampel* syndrome.

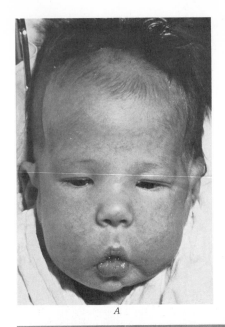

A

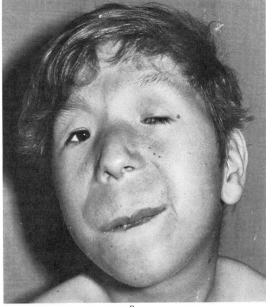

B

Figure 144-41. *Marden-Walker syndrome.* (A). Note blepharophimosis unusual facies and ptosis of lids. (*From N. Fitch et al.*, Neurology (Minneap.) **21**:1214, 1971.) (B). Older patient having similar characteristics. (*From E. Passarge*, Birth Defects **11**(2):470, 1975.)

MALFORMATION/RETARDATION SYNDROME WITH DISTINCTIVE FACIAL APPEARANCE

One of us (M.M.C.) has observed an X-linked recessive malformation/retardation syndrome with unusual facial appearance (Fig. 144-42) (1). Findings include broad flat nose, prominent philtrum, synophrys, long eyelashes, microcephaly, mental deficiency, growth deficiency, cryptorchism, foot deformities, and other abnormalities.

FETAL WARFARIN SYNDROME

Anticoagulant therapy of the coumarin type administered during the first trimester of preg-

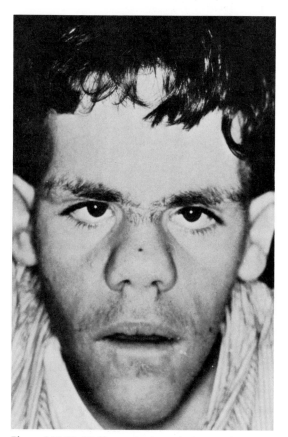

Figure 144-42. *Malformation/retardation syndrome with distinctive facial appearance.* Broad flat nose, prominent philtrum, synophrys, and triangular face.

nancy may result in a characteristic phenotype: (*a*) hypoplasia of nasal bones, (*b*) stippled epiphyses, and (*c*) hypoplasia of the terminal phalanges (6).

Hypoplasia of the nasal bones leading in some cases to upper airway obstruction was first reported in association with anticoagulant therapy by DiSaia (2) and Kerber et al. (3). Other reports are those of Pettifor and Benson (4) and Shaul et al. (5). There is apparent mild ocular hypertelorism. The neck is short (Fig. 144-43*A–C*).

General manual brachydactyly with radial deviation of index fingers, short halluces, intermediate fontanel (4), and prominent occiput (5) were evident. Roentgenographic examination has revealed hypoplasia and stippling of the terminal phalanges of the hands with radial deformities of the proximal phalanges of the index fingers in about half the cases. Stippling of carpal bones, vertebral bodies (especially sacral and cervical), proximal femur, calcaneus, and cuboids has been reported in infancy. The proximal metacarpals have been noted to be deformed (Fig. 144-43*D, E*).

Mild mental retardation and optic atrophy (1, 2, 4) have been reported as well as dysplastic fingernails (4) and simian creases (5).

Similarity to *chondrodysplasia punctata* of the dominant type is striking.

FETAL HYDANTOIN SYNDROME

Diphenylhydantoin taken during pregnancy has been shown to be teratogenic, producing a two- to threefold increase in congenital anomalies (1–9). There is also evidence that its effect may be potentiated by barbiturates (2, 4, 9).

Growth deficiency is usually of prenatal onset and is apparently permanent. Psychomotor retardation is common.

Craniofacial features include metopic sutural ridging, low posterior hairline, broad depressed nasal bridge with retroussé nose, epicanthal folds, ocular hypertelorism, ptosis, strabismus, various minor ear anomalies, wide mouth with prominent lips, and short neck which may be somewhat webbed (Fig. 144-44*A, B*).

Musculoskeletal anomalies include large open fontanel, hypoplasia of distal phalanges and nails, digitalization of the thumb (2–4), and inguinal hernia (Fig. 144-44*C, D*).

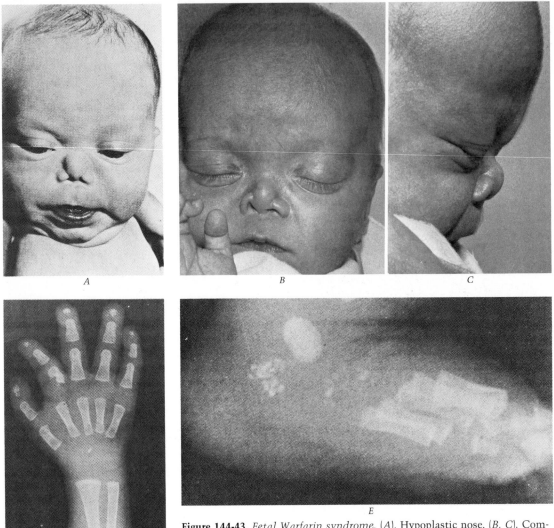

Figure 144-43. *Fetal Warfarin syndrome.* (*A*). Hypoplastic nose. (*B, C*). Compare facies with child seen in *A*. (*D*). Hypoplastic terminal phalanges and proximal phalanx of index finger. Stippled carpal bones. (*E*). Stippled calcaneus and cuboid bones. (A, D, E *from J. M. Pettifor and R. Benson, J. Pediatr.* **86:**459, 1975.) (B, C *courtesy of J. G. Hall, Seattle, Wash.*)

Dermatoglyphic alterations include simian or Sydney palmar creases and an increase in the number of fingertip arches. Hirsutism may be marked.

Cleft lip and/or palate and cardiac defects (ventricular septal defect, tetralogy of Fallot) while emphasized in many reports are *not* among the most common features of the disorder (1, 5, 6, 7). Broad alveolar ridges have been noted in about 30 percent of the cases.

The syndrome has been mistaken for *Coffin-Siris syndrome* and *Noonan syndrome*.

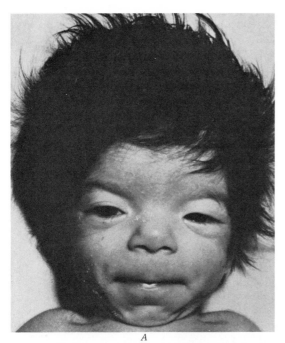

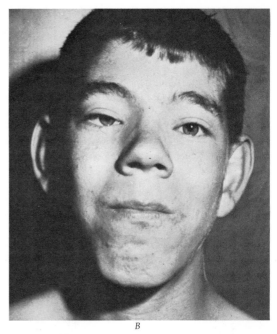

A

B

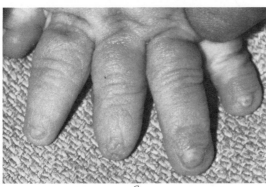

C

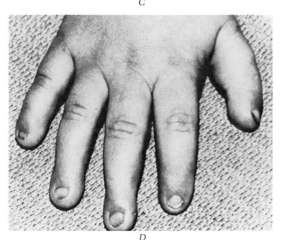

D

Figure 144-44. *Fetal hydantoin syndrome.* (*A*). Note ocular hypertelorism, depressed nasal bridge, low hairline, marked hypertrichosis, and wide mouth. (*B*). Ocular hypertelorism, strabismus, ptosis, depressed nasal bridge, and anteverted nostrils. (*C*). Terminal digit and nail hypoplasia. (*D*). Compare digital and nail changes with those seen in *C*. (A *from R. Hill et al.,* Am. J. Dis. Child. **127**:645, 1974; B *from J. W. Hanson and D. W. Smith,* J. Pediatr. **87**:285, 1975; D *from R. Hill et al.,* Am. J. Dis. Child. **127**:645, 1974.)

FETAL TRIMETHADIONE SYNDROME

Several reports have indicated that trimethadione and paramethadione taken during pregnancy can produce multiple defects in the offspring (1, 2, 4–7). The risk of abnormalities in the offspring of mothers taking either drug may be as high as 65 percent. Significant findings include mild midface hypoplasia, short upturned nose, broad low nasal bridge, V-shaped eyebrows, strabismus, ptosis of the eyelids, epicanthal folds, and dysplastic ears (Fig. 144-45). Cleft lip and palate, micrognathia, and the Robin anomalad (3) have been observed in some instances. Other abnormalities include somatic and mental retardation, speech disorder, cardiac septal defects, tetralogy of Fallot, and genital anomalies.

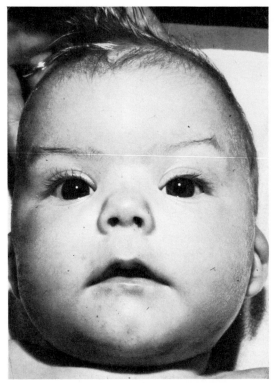

Figure 144-45. *Fetal trimethadione syndrome.* V-shaped eyebrows and dysplastic ears. (*Courtesy of J. Hanson, Iowa City, Iowa.*)

Occasionally, facial hemangiomas, webbed neck, and various other defects may be observed.

FETAL ALCOHOL SYNDROME

The fetal alcohol syndrome has been described in several reports (1–9). The frequency of adverse outcome of pregnancy for chronically alcoholic women is 43 percent (7) and the condition is relatively common. The infant may manifest prenatal and postnatal growth deficiency, fine motor dysfunction, mental retardation, microcephaly, short palpebral fissures, prominent ear crus, maxillary hypoplasia, joint anomalies, altered palmar creases, and cardiac anomalies. Other findings may include epicanthal folds, ptosis of eyelids, strabismus, cleft palate, micrognathia, hypoplastic labia majora and clitoromegaly, capillary hemangiomas, and various miscellaneous defects (Fig. 144-46A, B). Clinical

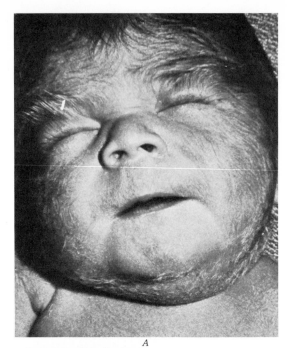

A

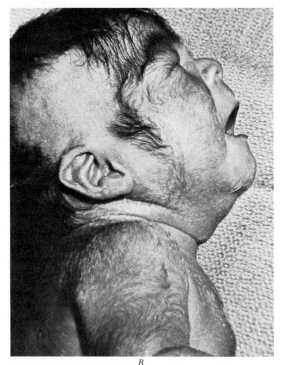

B

Figure 144-46. *Fetal alcohol syndrome.* (*A, B*). Note short palpebral fissures and hirsutism. (*From K. L. Jones and D. W. Smith, Lancet* **2**:999, 1973.)

findings in 41 cases have been reported by Hanson et al. (4).

The fetal alcohol syndrome may simulate the *Noonan syndrome* (*1, 3*). and has been mistaken for the *de Lange syndrome* and *trisomy 18 syndrome* (6).

RIEGER ANOMALY AND GROWTH RETARDATION

Gorlin et al. (1) and Sensenbrenner et al. (2) independently reported a new syndrome characterized by severe growth retardation, disproportionately small face, deep sunken eyes, Rieger anomaly, delayed tooth eruption, delayed speech development, bilateral inguinal hernia, joint hypermobility, and diminished subcutaneous fat (Fig. 144-47*A, B*). Feeding difficulties were experienced during early infancy.

Inheritance is probably autosomal recessive.

EPILEPSY, MENTAL DETERIORATION, AND AMELOGENESIS IMPERFECTA

Kohlschütter et al. (1) reported five male sibs with a sudden generalized seizure disorder that had its onset between one and four years. The infants had normal development until the appearance of the epilepsy, but subsequently mental deterioration followed, the degree being correlated with the frequency and severity of the seizures. Death occurred between four and nine years.

All affected males had marked amelogenesis imperfecta.

Associated findings, established only in the survivor, included hypohidrosis, mildly elevated sodium, and chloride but markedly increased potassium in the sweat, and myopia.

Inheritance is either X-linked or autosomal recessive.

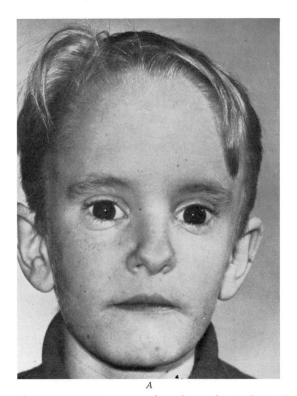
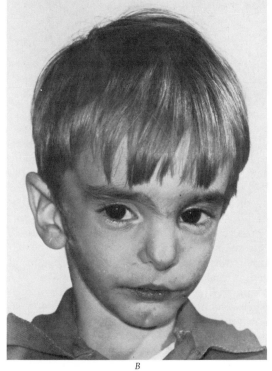

A	*B*

Figure 144-47. *Rieger anomaly and growth retardation.* (*A, B*). Brothers exhibiting severe growth retardation, disproportionately small face, sunken eyes, Rieger anomaly, and delayed tooth eruption. (*From R. J. Gorlin et al.*, Birth Defects **11**(2):46, 1975.)

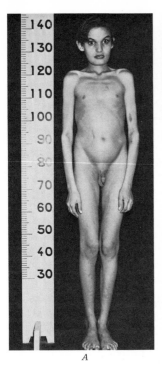

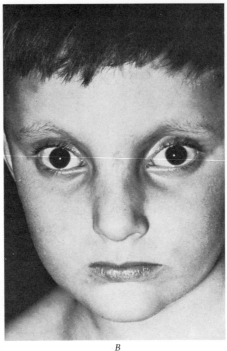

A   *B*

Figure 144-48. *Hepatic ductular hypoplasia, characteristic facies, mental, somatic, and sexual retardation, and cardiac murmur.* (*A*). Note prominent forehead, deeply set eyes, mongoloid obliquity of palpebral fissures, mild ocular hypertelorism, straight nose, and lack of sexual maturity in sixteen-year-old male. (*B*). Observe similar facial features. (*From D. Alagille et al.,* J. Pediatr. **86:**63, 1975.)

HEPATIC DUCTULAR HYPOPLASIA, CHARACTERISTIC FACIES, MENTAL, SOMATIC, AND SEXUAL RETARDATION, VERTEBRAL MALFORMATIONS, AND CARDIAC MURMUR

Alagille and coworkers (1) described 15 children having chronic cholestasis due to intrahepatic ductular hypoplasia which appeared during the first three postnatal months. It was accompanied by hepatosplenomegaly and intense pruritus with moderate elevation in serum bilirubin concentration. The urine was dark and the stools clay-colored. In some cases, xanthomas were distributed over the palms, extensor surfaces, and body creases. Toward the second year of life, serum triglycerides and cholesterol rose to high levels. Electrophoretic studies showed depressed or absent alpha-lipoprotein and sharply increased beta-lipoprotein peaks. Patients with similar features were reported by Watson and Miller (2).

The facies is characterized by a prominent forehead, deeply set eyes, mongoloid obliquity of palpebral fissures, mild ocular hypertelorism, and a straight nose (Fig. 144-48*A*, *B*). A harsh mesosystolic murmur heard most intensely in the third interspace at the left sternal border over the pulmonary valve area was found in 12 of 15 patients. However, cardial function was unimpaired. Vertebral defects (spina bifida) were found in 8 of 15 patients. Growth retardation was present in all children with spina bifida. Mild to moderate mental retardation (60 to 80 IQ) was evident in nine patients. Hypogonadism was suspected in six males.

Parental consanguinity and the occurrence of the disorder in sibs suggest autosomal recessive inheritance.

OLIGODONTIA, HYPOTRICHOSIS, PALMOPLANTAR HYPERKERATOSIS, AND CYSTS OF EYELID MARGINS

Schöpf et al. (1) described two sisters with oligodontia, palmar-plantar hyperkeratosis which began at puberty, hair loss at twenty-five years of age, rosacea at fifty years, and cysts of both eyelid margins at sixty years. Their parents were consanguineous. Presumably the disorder has autosomal recessive inheritance.

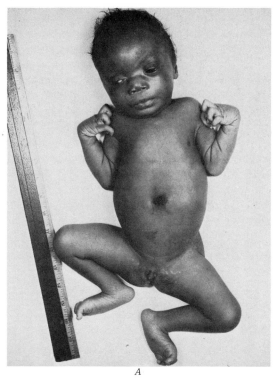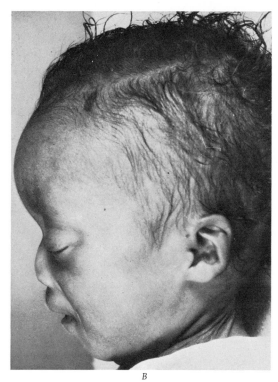

A   *B*

Figure 144-49. (*A*). *Multiple ankyloses, pulmonary hypoplasia, camptodactyly, and unusual facies.* Note ocular hypertelorism, camptodactyly, fixed joints, rocker-bottom feet. (*B*). Profile showing flattened nasal tip. (*From P. Bowen et al.,* Johns Hopkins Med. Bull. **114:**402, 1964.)

MULTIPLE ANKYLOSES, PULMONARY HYPOPLASIA, CAMPTODACTYLY AND UNUSUAL FACIES (PENA-SHOKEIR SYNDROME)

Pena and Shokeir (2) reported sisters with a syndrome comprising intrauterine growth retardation, severe camptodactyly of the fingers, talipes equinovarus, knee and hip ankylosis, and pulmonary hypoplasia. The knees were fixed in extension; the hips in semiflexion. Each died in the perinatal period. Two males described by Punnett et al. (3) exhibited cryptorchism. Bowen et al. (1) probably reported the same disorder.

The ears are malformed. Ocular hypertelorism, depressed nasal tip, and micrognathia characterized the facies.

Inheritance is autosomal recessive.

This syndrome should be differentiated from *Potter syndrome* and *trisomy 18 syndrome.*

REFERENCES

TUBULAR STENOSIS (KENNEY SYNDROME)

1 Caffey, J., Congenital Stenosis of Medullary Spaces in Tubular Bones and Calvaria in Two Proportional Dwarfs—Mother and Son. *Am. J. Roentgenol.* **100:**1–11, 1967.

2 Frech, R. S., and McAlister, W. H., Medullary Stenosis of the Tubular Bones Associated with Hypocalcemic Convulsions and Short Stature. *Radiology* **91:**457–461, 1968.

3 Kenney, F. M., and Linarelli, L., Dwarfism and Cortical Thickening of the Tubular Bones: Transient Hypercalcemia in a Mother and Son. *Am. J. Dis. Child.* **111:**201–207, 1968.

4 Wilson, M. G.,et al., Dwarfism and Congenital Medullary Stenosis (Kenney Syndrome). *Birth Defects* **10**(12):128–132, 1974.

MENTAL AND SOMATIC RETARDATION AND CRANIODIGITAL ANOMALIES (SCOTT SYNDROME)

1 Scott, C. R., et al., A New Craniodigital Syndrome with Mental Retardation. *J. Pediatr.* **78:**658–663, 1971.

FRONTODIGITAL SYNDROME

1 Marshall, R. E., and Smith, D. W., Frontodigital Syndrome: A Dominantly Inherited Disorder with Normal Intelligence. *J. Pediatr.* **77:**129–133, 1970.

FAMILIAL POLYSYNDACTYLY AND CRANIOFACIAL ANOMALIES (HOOTNICK-HOLMES SYNDROME)

1 Hootnick, D., and Holmes, L. B., Familial Polysyndactyly and Craniofacial Anomalies. *Clin. Genet.* **3:**128–134, 1972.
2 Korting, G. W., and Ruther, H., Ichthyosis vulgaris und akro-faciale Dysostose. *Arch. Dermatol. Syph.* (*Berl.*) **197:**91–104, 1954.

PYRAMIDAL MOLAR ROOTS, JUVENILE GLAUCOMA, AND UNUSUAL MORPHOLOGY OF UPPER LIP (ACKERMAN SYNDROME)

1 Ackerman, J. L., et al., Taurodont, Pyramidal, and Fused Molar Roots Associated with Other Anomalies in a Kindred. *Am. J. Phys. Anthropol.* **38:**681–694, 1973.

OLIGODONTIA, ABSENT NASAL ALAE, MENTAL AND SOMATIC RETARDATION, HYPOTHYROIDISM, AND MALABSORPTION (JOHANSON-BLIZZARD SYNDROME)

1 Johanson, A., and Blizzard, R., A Syndrome of Congenital Aplasia of the Alae Nasi, Deafness, Hypothyroidism, Dwarfism, Absent Permanent Teeth and Malabsorption. *J. Pediatr.* **79:**982–987, 1971.
2 Morris, M. D., and Fisher, D. A., Trypsinogen Deficiency Disease. *Am. J. Dis. Child.* **114:**203–208, 1967.
3 Park, I. J., et al., Special Female Hermaphroditism Associated with Multiple Disorders. *Obstet. Gynecol.* **39:**100–106, 1972.
4 Townes, P. L., Trypsinogen Deficiency and Other Proteolytic Deficiency Diseases. *Birth Defects* **8**(2):95–101, 1972.

ABSENT FIFTH FINGER- AND TOENAILS, UNUSUAL FACIES, AND MENTAL DEFICIENCY (COFFIN-SIRIS SYNDROME)

1 Bartsocas, C. S., and Tsiantos, A. K., Mental Retardation with Absent Fifth Fingernail and Terminal Phalanx. *Am. J. Dis. Child.* **120:**493–494, 1970.
2 Coffin, G. S., and Siris, E., Mental Retardation with Absent Fifth Fingernail and Terminal Phalanx. *Am. J. Dis. Child.* **119:**433–439, 1970.
3 Mace, J. W., and Gotlin, R. W., Short Stature and Onychodysplasia. *Am. J. Dis. Child.* **125:**114–116, 1973.
4 Senior, B., Impaired Growth and Onychodysplasia. *Am. J. Dis. Child.* **122:**7–9, 1971.
5 Weiswasser, W. H., et al., Coffin-Siris Syndrome. *Am. J. Dis. Child.* **125:**838–840, 1973.

MICROCEPHALY, GROWTH RETARDATION, AND FLEXION DEFORMITIES (NEU SYNDROME)

1 Laxova, R., et al., Further Example of a Lethal Autosomal Recessive Condition in Sibs. *J. Ment. Defic. Res.* **16:**139–143, 1972.
2 Neu, R. L., et al., A Lethal Syndrome of Microcephaly with Multiple Congenital Anomalies in Three Siblings. *Pediatrics* **47:**611–612, 1971.

SOMATIC AND MENTAL RETARDATION, CORNEAL OPACITIES, SHORT ULNA AND RADIUS, AND UNUSUAL FACIES (MIETENS-WEBER SYNDROME)

1 Mietens, C., and Weber, H., A Syndrome Characterized by Corneal Opacity, Nystagmus, Flexion Contraction of the Elbows, Growth Failure and Mental Retardation. *J. Pediatr.* **69:**624–629, 1966.

GERODERMA OSTEODYSPLASTICA (BAMATTER SYNDROME)

1 Bamatter, F., et al., Gérodermie ostéodysplastique héréditaire. Un nouveau biotype de la "progeria." *Confin. Neurol.* **9:**397, 1949; *Ann. Paediat.* **174:**126–127, 1950.
2 Boreux, G., La gérodermie ostéodysplastique à hérédite liée au sexes, nouvelle entité clinque et génétique. *J. Génêt. Hum.* **17:**137–178, 1969.
3 Brocher, J. E. W., et al., Roentgenologische Befunde bei Geroderma osteodysplastica hereditaria. *Fortschr. Roentgenstr.* **109:**185–198, 1968.
4 Gazit, E., et al., The Wrinkly Skin Syndrome: A New Heritable Disorder of Connective Tissue. *Clin. Genet.* **4:**186–192, 1973.

ACROFACIAL DYSOSTOSIS (WEYERS SYNDROME)

1 Weyers, H., Über eine korrelierte Missbildung der Kiefer und Extremitätenakren (Dysostosis acro-facialis). *Fortschr. Roentgenstr.* **77:**562–567, 1952.
2 Weyers, H., Hexadactylie, Unterkieferspalt und Oligodontie, ein neuer Symptomenkomplex. Dysostosis acrofacialis. *Ann. Paediatr.* (*Basel*) **181:**45–60, 1953.

HYPODONTIA AND NAIL DYSGENESIS SYNDROME (WITKOP SYNDROME)

1 Giansanti, J. S., et al., The "Tooth and Nail" Type of Autosomal Dominant Ectodermal Dysplasia. *Oral Surg.* **37:**576–582, 1974.
2 Gorlin, R. J., et al., A Selected Miscellany. *Birth Defects*, **11**(2):39–50, 1975.
3 Hudson, C. D., and Witkop, C. J., Autosomal Dominant Hypodontia with Nail Dysgenesis. *Oral Surg.* **39:**409–423, 1975.
4 Redpath, T. H., and Winter, G. S., Autosomal Dominant Ectodermal Dysplasia with Significant Dental Defects. *Br. Dent. J.* **126:**123–128, 1969.
5 Witkop, C. J., Jr., Genetic Diseases of the Oral Cavity, in R. W. Tiecke (ed.), *Oral Pathology.* McGraw-Hill, New York, 1965.

CONGENITAL MUSCULAR TORTICOLLIS, MULTIPLE KELOIDS, CRYPTORCHISM, AND RENAL ABNORMALITIES (GOEMINNE SYNDROME)

1 Goeminne, L., A New Probably X-linked Inherited Syn-

drome: Congenital Muscular Torticollis, Multiple Keloids, Cryptorchidism, and Renal Dysplasia. *Acta Genet. Med. (Roma)* **17:**439–467, 1968.

OPHTHALMOMANDIBULOMELIC DYSPLASIA (PILLAY SYNDROME)

1 Pillay, V. K., Ophthalmo-mandibulo-melic Dysplasia: An Hereditary Syndrome. *J. Bone Joint Surg.* **46A:**858–862, 1964.

FISTULAS OF LATERAL SOFT PALATE AND ASSOCIATED ANOMALIES

1 Bumba, J., Symmetrische Defekte in den vorderen Gaumenbögen. *Z. Hals-, Nas.-Ohrenheilkd.* **1:**245–247, 1922.
2 Campbell, E. H., Perforation of the Faucial Pillars. *Arch. Otolaryngol.* **1:**503–509, 1925.
3 Chiari, O., Symmetrische Defecte in den vorderen Gaumembögen. *Z. Hals-, Nas.- Ohrenheilkd.* **1:**245–247, 1922.
4 Claiborne, J. H., Jr., Hiatus in the Anterior Pillar of the Fauces of the Right Side with Congenital Absence of the Tonsil on Either Side. *Am. J. Med. Sci.* **89:**490–491, 1885.
5 Cohen, J. S., A Case of Separate Investment of Palato-glossi Muscles. *Med. Rec.* **14:**44–45, 1878.
6 Friedenberg, P., Congenital Detachment of Faucial Pillars and Isolation of Palatoglossus Muscle. *Laryngoscope* **18:**567–571, 1908.
7 Levinstein, O., Unvollständige innere Halskiemenfistel in Verbindung mit doppelseitiger Fistula preauricularis congenita. *Arch. Laryngol. Rhinol. (Berl.)* **23:**128–142, 1910.
8 Miller, A. S., et al., Lateral Soft Palate Fistula. *Arch. Otolaryngol.* **91:**200, 1970.
9 Neuss, O., Anatomische Varianten und Fehlbildungen der Mundhöhle. *Z. Laryngol. Rhinol.* **35:**411–413, 1956.
10 Rouqet, J., Perforations multiples des pilière du voile du palais. *Arch. Intern. Laryngol.* **2:**643–644, 1923.
11 Schapringer, A., Ein weiterer Fall von symmetrischen Defekten in den vorderen Gaumenbögen. *Monatsschr. Ohrenheilkd.* **18:**204, 1884.
12 Töplitz, M., Symmetrische congenitale Defekte in den vorderen Gaumenbögen. *Z. Ohrenheilkd.* **23:**268–270, 1892.

FLEXION AND EXTENSION DEFORMITIES OF THE HANDS AND UNUSUAL FACIES (EMERY-NELSON SYNDROME)

1 Emery, A. E. H., and Nelson, M. M., A Familial Syndrome of Short Stature, Deformities of the Hands and Feet and an Unusual Facies. *J. Med. Genet.* **7:**379–382, 1970.

BRACHYMETAPODY, ANODONTIA, HYPOTRICHOSIS, AND ALBINOID TRAIT (TOUMAALA-HAAPANEN SYNDROME)

1 Toumaala, P., and Haapanen, E., Three Siblings with Similar Anomalies in the Eyes, Bones and Skin. *Acta Ophthalmol. (Kbh.)* **46:**365–371, 1968.

MESIODENS AND CATARACT (NANCE-HORAN SYNDROME)

1 Horan, M. B., and Billson, F. A., X-linked Cataract and Hutchinsonian Teeth. *Aust. Paediat. J.* **10:**98–102, 1974.
2 Nance, W. E., et al., Congenital Sex-linked Cataract,

Dental Anomalies, and Brachymetacarpalia. *Birth Defects,* **10**(4):285–291, 1974.

ORAL AND CONJUNCTIVAL AMYLOIDOSIS AND MENTAL RETARDATION (HORNOVÁ-DLUHOSOVÁ SYNDROME)

1 Hornová, J., and Dluhosová, O., Primary Amyloidosis of Gingiva and Conjunctiva and Mental Disorder in a Brother and Sister. *Oral Surg.* **25:**457–464, 1968.

BRACHYMETAPODY, HYPOPLASTIC GENITALIA, AND SOMATIC AND MENTAL RETARDATION (RUVALCABA SYNDROME)

1 Ruvalcaba, R. H. A., et al., A New Familial Syndrome with Osseous Dysplasia and Mental Deficiency. *J. Pediatr.* **79:**450–455, 1971.

UNUSUAL FACIES, MENTAL AND SOMATIC RETARDATION, AND SKELETAL AND LIMB DEFECTS (COFFIN-LOWRY SYNDROME)

1 Coffin, G. S., et al., Mental Retardation with Osteocartilaginous Anomalies. *Am. J. Dis. Child.* **112:**205–213, 1966.
2 Lowry, B., et al., A New Dominant Gene Mental Retardation Syndrome. *Am. J. Dis. Child.* **121:**491–500, 1971.
3 Martinelli, B., and Campailla, E., Contributo alla conoscenze della sindrome di Coffin, Siris and Wegienka. *G. Psichiat. Neuropatol.* **97:**449–451, 1969.
4 Procopis, P. G., and Turner, B., Mental Retardation, Abnormal Fingers, and Skeletal Anomalies, Coffin's Syndrome. *Am. J. Dis. Child.* **124:**258–265, 1972.
5 Temtamy, S. A., et al., The Coffin-Lowry Syndrome: An Inherited Faciodigital Mental Retardation Syndrome. *J. Pediatr.* **86:**724–731, 1975.

FAMILIAL OSTEODYSPLASIA (ANDERSON SYNDROME)

1 Anderson, L. G., et al., Familial Osteodysplasia. *J.A.M.A.* **220:**1687–1693, 1972.
2 Buchignani, J. S., et al., Roentgenographic Findings in Familial Osteodysplasia. *Am. J. Roentgenol.* **116:**602–608, 1972.

BRANCHIOSKELETOGENITAL SYNDROME (ELSAHY-WATERS SYNDROME)

1 Elsahy, N. I., and Waters, W. R., The Branchio-skeletogenital Syndrome. *Plast. Reconstr. Surg.* **48:**542–550, 1971.

MENTAL RETARDATION, MICROCEPHALY, MICROCORNEA, AND UNUSUAL FACIES

1 Kaufman, R. L., et al., An Oculocerebrofacial Syndrome. *Birth Defects* **7**(1):135–138, 1971.

AMELOGENESIS IMPERFECTA, TAURODONTISM, CURLY HAIR, AND SCLEROTIC BONES (TRICHODENTOOSSEOUS SYNDROME)

1 Crawford, J. L., Concomitant Taurodontism and Amelogenesis Imperfecta in an American Caucasian. *J. Dent. Child.* **37:**171–175, 1970.
1a Gorlin, R. J., A Selected Miscellany. Oligodontia, Tauro-

dontia and Sparse Hair Growth. *Birth Defects* **11**(2):39–50, 1975.

2 Jorgenson, R. J., and Warson, R. W., Dental Abnormalities in the Tricho-dento-osseous Syndrome. *Oral Surg.* **36**:693–700, 1973.

3 Lichtenstein, J. R., and Warson, R. W., Syndrome of Dental Anomalies, Curly Hair and Sclerotic Bones. *Birth Defects* **7**(7):308–311, 1971.

4 Lichtenstein, J., et al., The Tricho-dento-osseous (TDO) Syndrome. *Am. J. Hum. Genet.* **24**:569–582, 1972.

5 Robinson, G. C., et al., Hereditary Enamel Hypoplasia: Its Association with Characteristic Hair Structure. *Pediatrics* **37**:498–502, 1966.

6 Sauk, J. J., Jr., and Delaney, J. R., Taurodontism, Diminished Root Formation and Microcephalic Dwarfism. *Oral Surg.* **36**:231–235, 1973.

7 Stenvik, A., et al., Taurodontism and Concomitant Hypodontia in Siblings. *Oral Surg.* **33**:841–845, 1972.

8 Winter, G. B., et al., Hereditary Amelogenesis Imperfecta: A Rare Autosomal Dominant Type. *Br. Dent. J.* **127**:157–164, 1970.

9 Witkop, C. J., Jr., and Rao, S., Inherited Defects in Tooth Structure. *Birth Defects* **7**(7):153–184, 1971.

HYPOTONIA, OBESITY, MENTAL DEFICIENCY, AND FACIAL, ORAL, OCULAR, AND LIMB ANOMALIES

1 Cohen, M. M., Jr., et al., A New Syndrome with Hypotonia, Obesity, Mental Deficiency and Facial, Oral, Ocular, and Limb Anomalies. *J. Pediatr.* **83**:280–284, 1973.

TEMPORAL "FORCEP-MARKS" SCARRING AND UNUSUAL FACIES (SETLEIS SYNDROME)

1 Rudolph, R. I., et al., Bitemporal Aplasia Cutis Congenita. *Arch. Dermatol.* **110**:615–618, 1974.

2 Setleis, H., et al., Congenital Ectodermal Dysplasia of the Face. *Pediatrics* **32**:540–548, 1963.

MILD MENTAL RETARDATION, RIGHT-SIDED AORTIC ARCH, AND FACIAL DYSMORPHIA

1 Strong, W. D., Familial Syndrome of Right-Sided Aortic Arch, Mental Deficiency and Facial Dysmorphism. *J. Pediatr.* **73**:882–888, 1968.

HYPERHIDROSIS, PREMATURE GRAYING OF THE HAIR, AND PREMOLAR HYPODONTIA (PHC SYNDROME, BOÖK SYNDROME)

1 Böök, J. A., Clinical and Genetical Studies of Hypodontia: I. Premolar Aplasia, Hyperhidrosis, and Canities Prematura: A New Hereditary Syndrome in Man. *Am. J. Hum. Genet.* **2**:240–263, 1950.

ACCELERATED SKELETAL MATURATION, FAILURE TO THRIVE, AND UNUSUAL FACIES

1 Marshall, R. E., et al., Syndrome of Accelerated Skeletal Maturation and Relative Failure to Thrive: A Newly Recognized Clinical Growth Disorder. *J. Pediatr.* **78**:95–101, 1971.

2 Perrin, J. C. S., et al., Accelerated Skeletal Maturation Syndrome with Pulmonary Hypertension. *Birth Defects*, in press.

3 Tipton, R. E., et al., Accelerated Skeletal Maturation Syndrome. Report of a Third Case. *J. Pediatr.* **83**:829–832, 1973.

4 Visveshwara, N., et al., Syndrome of Accelerated Skeletal Maturation in Infancy, Peculiar Facies and Multiple Congenital Anomalies. *J. Pediatr.* **84**:553–556, 1974.

MIRROR HANDS AND FEET, TALIPES EQUINOVARUS, AND NASAL ALAR COLOBOMAS

1 Sandrow, R. E., et al., Hereditary Ulnar and Fibular Dimelia with Peculiar Facies. *J. Bone Joint Surg.* **52A**:367–370, 1970.

AMELOGENESIS IMPERFECTA AND TERMINAL ONYCHOLYSIS

1 Witkop, C. J., Jr., Genetics. *Schweiz. Monatsschr. Zahnheilkd.* **82**:917–941, 1972.

2 Witkop, C. J., Jr., et al., Hypoplastic Enamel, Onycholysis and Hypohidrosis Inherited as an Autosomal Dominant Trait. *Oral Surg.* **39**:71–86, 1975.

INCREASED BONE DENSITY AND SYNDACTYLY (BRAHAM-LENZ SYNDROME)

1 Braham, R. L., Multiple Congenital Abnormalities with Diaphyseal Dysplasia (Camurati-Englemann's Syndrome). *Oral Surg.* **27**:20–26, 1969.

2 Lenz, W. D., and Majewski, F., A Generalized Disorder of the Connective Tissues with Progeria, Choanal Atresia Symphalangism, Hypoplasia of Dentine and Craniodiaphyseal Hypostosis. *Birth Defects* **10**(12):133–136, 1974.

BLEPHARONASOFACIAL SYNDROME

1 Pashayan, H., et al., A Family with Blepharo-naso-facial Malformation. *Am. J. Dis. Child.* **125**:389–393, 1973.

2 Putterman, A. M., et al., Eye Findings in the Blepharo-naso-facial Malformation Syndrome. *Am. J. Ophthalmol.* **76**:825–831, 1973.

MULTIPLE ODONTOMAS, ESOPHAGEAL STENOSIS, AND CHRONIC INTERSTITIAL CIRRHOSIS OF THE LIVER

1 Bader, G., Odontomatosis (Multiple Odontomas). *Oral Surg.* **23**:770–773, 1967.

2 Beisser, V., Ein seltene Fall von selbständigem, multiplen Odontom beiderseits im Ober- und Unterkiefer und ein Literaturstudium über diese Geschwülste des Zahn-, Mund- und Kieferbereiches. Thesis, Düsseldorf, 1964.

3 Herrmann, M., Über von Zahnsystem ausgehende Tumoren bei Kindern. *Fortschr. Kiefer Gesichtschir.* **4**:226–229, 1958.

4 Malik, S. A., and Khalid, M., Odontomatosis – A Case Report. *Br. J. Oral Surg.* **11**:262–264, 1974.

5 Schmidseder, R., and Hausamen, J. R., Multiple Odontogenic Tumors and Other Anomalies. *Oral Surg.* **39**:249–258, 1975.

6 Schmitz, –, and Witzel, A., Neubildung von Zahnen und zahnähnlichen Gebilden. *Dtsch. Monatsschr. Zahnkeilkd.* **19**:126–130, 1901.

7 Schonberger, W., Angeborene multiple Odontome und

Dysphagie bei Vater und Sohn—eine syndromhafte Verknüpfung? *Z. Kinderheilkd.* **117**:101–108, 1974.

BROAD TERMINAL PHALANGES AND FACIAL ABNORMALITIES (KEIPERT SYNDROME)

1   Keipert, J. A., et al., A New Syndrome of Broad Terminal Phalanges and Facial Abnormalities. *Aust. Paediatr. J.* **9**:10–13, 1973.

EXCESSIVE OVERGROWTH, ACCELERATED SKELETAL MATURATION, CAMPTODACTYLY, AND UNUSUAL FACIES (WEAVER SYNDROME)

1   Weaver, D. D., et al., A New Overgrowth Syndrome with Accelerated Skeletal Maturation, Unusual Facies and Camptodactyly. *J. Pediatr.* **84**:547–552, 1974.

HEREDITARY OSTEOLYSIS (THIEFFRY-KOHLER SYNDROME)

1   Kohler, E., et al., Hereditary Osteolysis. *Radiology* **108**:99–105, 1973.
2   Thieffry, S., and Sorrell-Dejerine, J., Forme spéciale d'ostéolysis essentielle héréditaire et familiale à stabilization spontanée, survenant dans l'enface. *Presse Méd.* **66**:1858–1861, 1958.

MANDIBULOACRAL DYSPLASIA (CRANIOMANDIBULAR DERMATODYSOSTOSIS)

1   Cavallazzi, C., et al., Su di un caso di disostosi cleidocranica. *Riv. Clin. Pediatr.* **65**:312–326, 1960.
2   Danks, D. M., et al., Craniomandibular Dermatodysostosis. *Birth Defects* **10**(12):99–105, 1974.
3   McKusick, V. A., *Heritable Disorders of Connective Tissue.* 4th ed., C. V. Mosby, St. Louis, 1972, pp. 822–823.
4   McKusick, V. A., et al., *Medical Genetics, 1961–1963.* Pergamon Press, New York, 1966, p. 447.
5   Young, L. W., et al., A New Syndrome Manifested by Mandibular Hypoplasia, Acroosteolysis, Stiff Joints, and Cutaneous Atrophy (Mandibuloacral Dysplasia) in Two Unrelated Boys. *Birth Defects* **7**(7):291–297, 1971.

HAPPY PUPPET SYNDROME

1   Angelman, H., "Puppet" Children. A Report on 3 Cases. *Develop. Med. Child. Neurol.* **7**:681–685, 1965.
2   Berg, J. M., and Pakula, Z., Angelman's "Happy Puppet" Syndrome. *Am. J. Dis. Child.* **123**:72–74, 1972.
3   Elian, M., Fourteen Happy Puppets. *Clin. Pediatr.* **14**:902–908, 1975.
4   Kibel, M. A., and Burness, F. R., The "Happy Puppet" Syndrome. *Cent. Afr. J. Med.* **19**:91–93, 1973.
5   Massey, J. Y., and Roy, F. A., Ocular Manifestations of the Happy Puppet Syndrome. *J. Pediat. Ophthalmol.* **10**:282–284, 1973.
6   Mayo, O., et al., Three More Happy Puppets. *Dev. Med. Child. Neurol.* **15**:63–69, 1973.
7   Moore, J. R., and Jeavons, P. M., The "Happy Puppet" Syndrome? Two New Cases and a Review of Five Previous Cases. *Neuropädiatrie* **4**:172–179, 1973.

MULIBREY NANISM

1   Myllärniemi, S., et al., Craniofacial and Dental Study of Mulibrey Nanism. *Am. J. Dis. Child.*, in press.

2   Perheentupa, J., et al., Mulibrey-Nanism, An Autosomal Recessive Syndrome with Pericardial Constriction. *Lancet* **2**:351–355, 1973.
3   Perheentupa, J., et al., Mulibrey-Nanism: Review of 23 Cases of a New Autosomal Recessive Syndrome. *Birth Defects* **11**(2):3–17, 1975.
4   Raitta, C., and Perheentupa, J., Mulibrey-Nanism; An Inherited Dysmorphic Syndrome with Characteristic Ocular Findings. *Acta Ophthalmol.* **52**:162–171, 1974.
5   Thorén, L., The So-called Mulibrey-Nanism with Pericardial Constriction. *Lancet* **2**:731, 1973.
6   Tuuteri, L., et al., The Cardiopathy of Mulibrey Nanism, A New Inherited Syndrome. *Chest* **65**:628–631, 1974.

MYOPIA, CATARACTS, SADDLE NOSE, AND SENSORINEURAL DEAFNESS (MARSHALL SYNDROME)

1   Keith, C. G., et al., Abnormal Facies, Myopia and Short Stature. *Arch. Dis. Child.* **47**:787–793, 1972.
2   Marshall, D., Ectodermal Dysplasia. Report of Kindred and Ocular Abnormalities and Hearing Defect. *Am. J. Ophthalmol.* **45**(2):143–156, 1958.
3   O'Donnell, J. J., et al., Generalized Osseous Abnormalities in Marshall's Syndrome. *Birth Defects*, in press.
4   Ruppert, E. S., et al., Hereditary Hearing Loss with Saddlenose and Myopia. *Arch. Otolaryngol.* **92**:95–98, 1970.
5   Zellweger, H., et al., The Marshall Syndrome: Report of a New Family. *J. Pediatr.* **84**:868–871, 1974.

CALCIFICATION OF AORTIC ARCH, OSTEOPOROSIS AND HYPOPLASIA OF TOOTH BUDS (SINGLETON-MERTEN SYNDROME)

1   McLoughlin, M. J., et al., Idiopathic Calcification of the Ascending Aorta and Aortic Valve in Two Young Women. *Br. Heart J.* **36**:96–100, 1974.
2   Singleton, E. B., and Merten, D. F., An Unusual Syndrome of Widened Medullary Cavities of the Metacarpals and Phalanges, Aortic Calcification and Abnormal Dentition. *Pediatr. Radiol.* **1**:2–7, 1973.

DOLICHOCEPHALY, UNUSUAL FACIES, WITH HAIR, DENTAL, AND SKELETAL ANOMALIES (SENSENBRENNER SYNDROME)

1   Sensenbrenner, J. A., et al., New Syndrome of Skeletal Dental and Hair Anomalies. *Birth Defects* **11**(2):372–379, 1975.

CONGENITAL BLEPHAROPHIMOSIS, JOINT CONTRACTURES, AND MUSCULAR HYPOTONIA (MARDEN-WALKER SYNDROME)

1   Ealing, M., Amyoplasia Congenita Causing Malpresentation of the Foetus. *J. Obstet. Gynaecol. Br. Emp.* **51**:144–146, 1944.
2   Fitch, N., et al., Congenital Blepharophimosis, Joint Contractures and Muscular Hypotonia. *Neurology (Minneap.)* **21**:1214–1220, 1971.
3   Gellis, S. S., *The Year Book of Pediatrics.* Year Book Med. Pub., Inc., 1963–1964, Chicago, p. 193.
4   Marden, P. M., and Walker, W. A., A New Generalized Connective Tissue Syndrome. *Am. J. Dis. Child.* **112**:225–228, 1966.
5   Passarge, E., Marden-Walker Syndrome. *Birth Defects* **11**(2):470–471, 1975.

6 Simpson, J. L., and Degnan, M., A Child with Facial and Skeletal Dysmorphia Reminiscent of Schwartz Syndrome. *Birth Defects* **11**(2):456–458, 1975.

7 Temtamy, S. A., et al., Probable Marden-Walker Syndrome: Evidence for Autosomal Recessive Inheritance. *Birth Defects* **11**(2):104–108, 1975.

8 Younessian, S., and Ammann, F., Deux cas de malformations crânio-faciales. *Ophthalmologica* **147**:108–117, 1964 (Case 1).

MALFORMATION/RETARDATION SYNDROME WITH DISTINCTIVE FACIAL APPEARANCE

1 Cohen, M. M., Jr., personal observation, 1973.

FETAL WARFARIN SYNDROME

1 Becker, M. H., et al., Chondrodysplasia Punctata. Is Maternal Warfarin Therapy a Factor? *Am. J. Dis. Child.* **129**:356–359, 1975.

2 DiSaia, P. J., Pregnancy and Delivery of a Patient with a Starr-Edwards Mitral Valve Prosthesis. *Obstet. Gynecol.* **28**:469–472, 1966.

3 Kerber, V. J., et al., Pregnancy in a Patient with a Prosthetic Mitral Valve. *J.A.M.A.* **203**:223–225, 1968.

4 Pettifor, J. M., and Benson, R., Congenital Malformations Associated with the Administration of Oral Anticoagulants During Pregnancy. *J. Pediatr.* **86**:459–462, 1975.

5 Shaul, W. L., et al., Chondrodysplasia Punctata and Maternal Warfarin Use During Pregnancy. *Am. J. Dis. Child.* **129**:360–362, 1975.

6 Warkany, J., A Warfarin Embryopathy? *Am. J. Dis. Child.* **129**:287–288, 1975.

FETAL HYDANTOIN SYNDROME

1 Elshove, J., and Van Eck, J. H. M., Congenital Malformations, Cleft Lip and Palate in Particular, in Children of Epileptic Women. *Nederl. Maandschr. Geneeskd.* **115**:1371–1374, 1971.

2 Fedrick, J., Epilepsy and Pregnancy: A Report from the Oxford Record Linkage Study. *Br. Med. J.* **2**:442–448, 1973.

3 Hanson, J. W., and Smith, D. W., The Fetal Hydantoin Syndrome. *J. Pediatr.* **87**:285–291, 1975.

4 Hill, R. M., et al., Infants Exposed in Utero to Antiepileptic Drugs. *Am. J. Dis. Child.* **127**:645–653, 1974.

5 Lowe, C. R., Congenital Malformations Among Infants Born to Epileptic Women. *Lancet* **1**:9–10, 1973.

6 Meadow, S. R., Anticonvulsant Drugs and Congenital Abnormalities. *Lancet* **2**:1296, 1968.

7 Mirkin, B. L., Diphenylhydantoin: Placental Transport, Fetal Localization, Neonatal Metabolism, and Possible Teratogenic Effects. *J. Pediatr.* **78**:329–337, 1971.

8 Monson, R. R., et al., Diphenylhydantoin and Selected Congenital Malformations. *N. Engl. J. Med.* **289**:1049–1052, 1973.

9 Speidel, B. D., and Meadow, S. R., Maternal Epilepsy and Abnormalities of the Fetus and Newborn. *Lancet* **2**:839–843, 1972.

FETAL TRIMETHADIONE SYNDROME

1 German, J., et al., Possible Teratogenicity of Trimethadione and Paramethadione. *Lancet* **2**:261–262, 1970.

2 German, J., et al., Trimethadione and Human Teratogenesis. *Teratology* **3**:349–362, 1970.

3 Hanson, J. W., and Smith, D. W., U-Shaped Palatal Defect in the Robin Anomalad: Developmental and Clinical Relevance. *J. Pediatr.* **87**:23–29, 1975.

4 Nichols, M. M., Fetal Anomalies Following Maternal Trimethadione Ingestion. *J. Pediatr.* **82**:885–886, 1973.

5 Rutman, J. Y., Anticonvulsants and Fetal Damage. *N. Engl. J. Med.* **289**:696–697, 1973.

6 Zachai, E. H., et al., Trimethadione Teratogenic Syndrome. *J. Pediatr.* **87**:280–284, 1975.

7 Zellweger, H., Anticonvulsants During Pregnancy: A Danger to the Developing Fetus? *Clin. Pediat.* **13**:338–346, 1974.

FETAL ALCOHOL SYNDROME

1 Char, F., Fetal Alcohol Syndrome with Noonan Phenotype. *Birth Defects,* in press.

2 Green, H. G., Infants of Alcoholic Mothers. *Am. J. Obstet. Gynecol.* **118**:713–716, 1974.

3 Hall, B. D., Noonan's Phenotype and the Fetal Alcohol Syndrome. *Lancet* **1**:933, 1974.

4 Hanson, J. W., et al., Fetal Alcohol Syndrome: Experience with Forty-One Cases. *J. Pediatr.,* in press.

5 Jones, K. L., et al., Pattern of Malformation in Offspring of Chronic Alcoholic Mothers. *Lancet* **1**:1267–1271, 1973.

6 Jones, K. L., and Smith, D. W., Recognition of the Fetal Alcohol Syndrome in Early Infancy. *Lancet* **2**:999–1001, 1973.

7 Jones, K. L., and Smith, D. W., The Fetal Alcohol Syndrome. *Teratology* **12**:1–10, 1975.

8 Palmer, R. H., Ouellette, E. M., Warner, L., and Leichtman, S. R., Congenital Malformations in Offspring of a Chronic Alcohol Mother. *Pediatrics* **53**:490–494, 1974.

9 Saule, H., Fetales Alcohol-Syndrom. *Klin. Pädiatr.* **186**:452–455, 1974.

RIEGER ANOMALY AND GROWTH RETARDATION

1 Gorlin, R. J., et al., Rieger Anomaly and Growth Retardation (The S-H-O-R-T Syndrome). *Birth Defects* **11**(2):46–48, 1975.

2 Sensenbrenner, J. A., et al., A Low-Birthweight Syndrome? Rieger Syndrome. *Birth Defects* **11**(2):423–426, 1975.

EPILEPSY, MENTAL DETERIORATION, AND AMELOGENESIS IMPERFECTA

1 Kohlschütter, A., et al., Familial Epilepsy and Yellow Teeth—A Disease of the Central Nervous System Associated with Enamel Hypoplasia. *Helv. Paediat. Acta* **29**:283–294, 1974.

HEPATIC DUCTULAR HYPOPLASIA, CHARACTERISTIC FACIES, MENTAL, SOMATIC AND SEXUAL RETARDATION, VERTEBRAL MALFORMATIONS, AND CARDIAC MURMUR

1 Alagille, D., et al. Hepatic Ductular Hypoplasia Associated with Characteristic Facies, Vertebral Malformations, Retarded Physical, Mental, and Sexual Development and Cardiac Murmur. *J. Pediatr.* **86**:63–71, 1975.

2 Watson, G. H., and Miller, V., Arteriohepatic Displasia. Familial Pulmonary Arterial Stenosis with Neonatal Liver Diseases. *Arch. Dis. Child.* **48**:459–466, 1973.

OLIGODONTIA, HYPOTRICHOSIS, PALMOPLANTAR HYPERKERATOSIS, AND CYSTS OF EYELID MARGINS

1 Schöpf, E., et al., Syndrome of Cystic Eyelids, Palmoplantar Keratosis, Hypospadias and Hypotrichosis as a Possible Autosomal Recessive Trait. *Birth Defects* **7**(8):219–221, 1971.

MULTIPLE ANKLYOSES, PULMONARY HYPOPLASIA, CAMPTODACTYLY AND UNUSUAL FACIES (PENA-SHOKEIR SYNDROME)

1 Bowen, P., et al., A Familial Syndrome of Multiple Congenital Defects. *Johns Hopkins Hosp. Bull.* **114**:402–414, 1964.

2 Pena, S. D. J., and Shokeir, M. H. K., Syndrome of Camptodactyly, Multiple Ankyloses, Facial Abnormalities, and Pulmonary Hypoplasia: A Lethal Condition. *J. Pediatr.* **85**:373–375, 1974.

3 Punnett H. H., et al., Syndrome of Ankylosis, Facial Anomalies and Pulmonary Hypoplasia. *J. Pediatr.* **85**:375–377, 1974.

Appendix

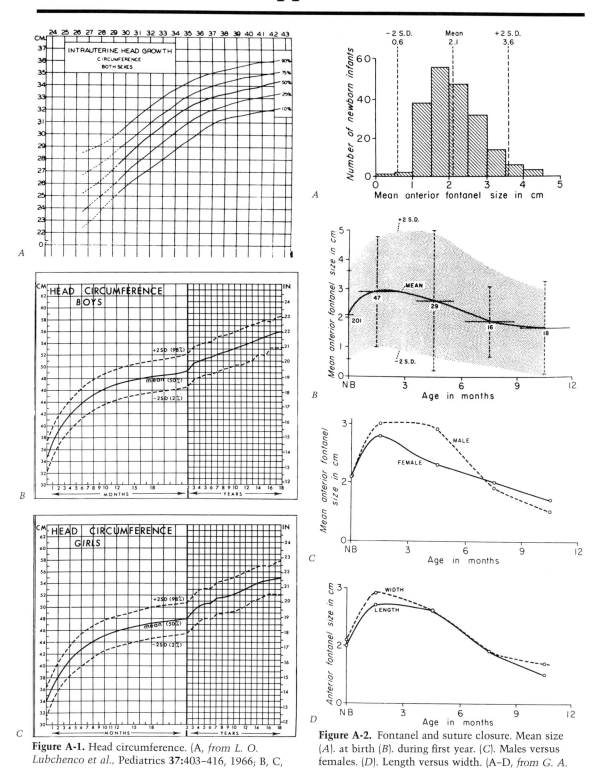

Figure A-1. Head circumference. (A, *from L. O. Lubchenco et al.*, Pediatrics **37**:403–416, 1966; B, C, *from G. Nelhaus*, Pediatrics **41**:106–114, 1968.)

Figure A-2. Fontanel and suture closure. Mean size (A). at birth (B). during first year. (C). Males versus females. (D). Length versus width. (A–D, *from G. A. Popich and D. W. Smith*, J. Pediatr. **80**:749–752, 1972.)

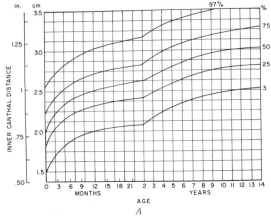

A

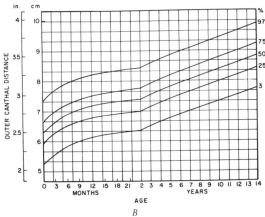

B

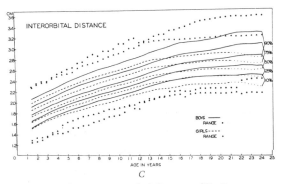

C

Figure A-3. (*A*). Inner canthal distance. (*B*). Outer canthal distance. (*C*). Bony interorbital distance. [A, B, *from M. Feingold*, Birth Defects **10**(13):1–16, 1974; C, *from C. F. Hansman*, Radiology **86**:87–96, 1966.]

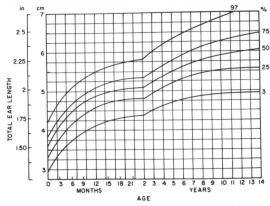

Figure A-4. Ear length. [*From M. Feingold and W. H. Bossert*, Birth Defects **10**(13):1–16, 1974.]

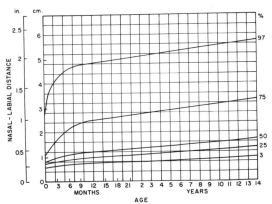

Figure A-5. Nasal-labial length. [*From M. Feingold and W. H. Bossert*, Birth Defects **10**(13):1–16, 1974.]

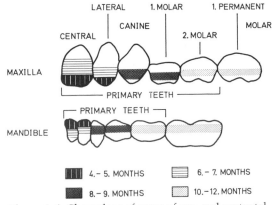

Figure A-6. Chronology of onset of pre- and postnatal enamel hypoplasia. Time is indicated in months from the onset of gestation. (*From W. F. Via and J. A. Churchill*, J. Am. Dent. Assoc. **59**:702–707, 1959.)

Table A-1. Cephalic index*

Index	Skull type
x–75.9	Dolichocephaly
76.0–80.9	Mesocephaly
81.0–85.4	Brachycephaly
85.5–x	Hyperbrachycephaly

Source: M. F. A. Montagu, *An Introduction to Physical Anthropology*, 3d ed., Thomas, Springfield, 1960, pp. 570–571.
* Cephalic index = [(maximum head breadth)/(maximum head length)](100).

Table A-3. Intercommissural distance of white American children and adults

Age, yr	Males, mm	Females, mm
0–1	32	27
2–3	35	30
4–5	39	36
6–7	42	40
8–9	44	42
10–11	46	43
12–13	48	45
14–15	50	47
Adult	55	52

Source: J. Cervenka et al., Cranio-carpo-tarsal Dysplasia or the Whistling Face Syndrome. *Am. J. Dis. Child.* **117:**434–435, 1969.

Table A-2. Fontanel and suture closure

Closure	Time
Anterior fontanel	1 year ± 4 months
Posterior fontanel	Birth ± 2 months
Anterolateral fontanel	By third month
Posterolateral fontanel	During second year
Metopic suture	By third year (10%, never)
Clinical closure of sutures	6–12 months
Anatomic closure of sutures	By thirtieth year

Source: Robert J. Gorlin and Jens J. Pindborg, *Syndromes of the Head and Neck*, 1st ed., McGraw-Hill Book Company, New York, 1964.

Table A-4. Normal chronologic development of primary teeth

Tooth	Initiation, week in utero	Calcification begins, week in utero	Crown completed, month	Eruption, month	Root completed, year	Root resorption begins, year	Tooth shed, year
Central incisor	7	14 (13–16)	1–3	6–9	$1\frac{1}{2}$–2	5–6	7–8
Lateral incisor	7	16 ($14\frac{1}{2}$–$16\frac{1}{2}$)	2–3	7–10	$1\frac{1}{2}$–2	5–6	7–9
Canine	$7\frac{1}{2}$	17 (15–18)	9	16–20	$2\frac{1}{2}$–$3\frac{1}{4}$	6–7	10–12
First molar	8	$15\frac{1}{2}$ ($14\frac{1}{2}$–17)	6	12–16	2 –$2\frac{1}{2}$	4–5	9–11
Second molar	10	$18\frac{1}{2}$ (16–$23\frac{1}{2}$)	10–12	20–30	3	4–5	11–12

Sources: Logan, W. H. G., and Kronfeld, R., Development of the Human Jaws and Surrounding Structures from Birth to the Age of 15 Years. *J. Am. Dent. Assoc.* **20:**379–427, 1933; Lunt, R. C., and Law, D. B., A Review of the Chronology of Calcification of the Deciduous Teeth. *J. Am. Dent. Assoc.* **89:**599–606, 1974; Schour, I., and Massler, M., Studies in Tooth Development. The Growth Pattern of Human Teeth. *J. Am. Dent. Assoc.* **27:**1918–1931, 1940.

Table A-5. Normal chronologic development of secondary teeth

Tooth	Initiation, month	Calcification begins	Crown completed, year	Eruption, year	Root completed, year
Maxilla:					
Central incisor	5–5¼ in utero	3–4 months	4–5	7–8	10
Lateral incisor	5–5¼ in utero	1 year	4–5	8–9	11
Canine	5½–6 in utero	4–5 months	6–7	11–12	13–15
First premolar	Birth	1½–1¾ years	5–6	10–11	12–13
Second premolar	7½–8	2–2½ years	6–7	10–12	12–14
First molar	3½–4 in utero	Birth	2½–3	6–7	9–10
Second molar	8½–9	2½–3 years	7–8	12–13	14–16
Third molar	3½–4 (yr)	7–9 years	12–16	17–25	18–25
Mandible:					
Central incisor	5–5¼ in utero	3–4 months	4–5	6–7	9
Lateral incisor	5–5¼ in utero	3–4 months	4–5	7–8	10
Canine	5½–6 in utero	4–5 months	6–7	9–11	12–14
First premolar	Birth	1¾–2 years	5–6	10–12	12–13
Second premolar	7½–8	2¼–2½ years	6–7	11–12	13–14
First molar	3½–4 in utero	Birth	2½–3	6–7	9–10
Second molar	8½–9	2½–3 years	7–8	11–13	14–15
Third molar	3½–4 (yr)	8–10 years	12–16	17–25	18–25

SOURCES: Logan, W. H. G., and Kronfeld, R., Development of the Human Jaws and Surrounding Structures from Birth to the Age of 15 Years. *J. Am. Dent. Assoc.* **20:**379–427, 1933; Schour, I., and Massler, M., Studies in Tooth Development. The Growth Pattern of Human Teeth. *J. Dent. Assoc.* **27:**1918–1931, 1940.

Table A-6. Mean palatal dimensions of Minnesota children and adults

Sex	Age group	Number of measurements	Mean height	SD*	Mean width	SD	Mean length	SD	Mean index	SD
Male	6–7	60	8.0	1.38	30.8	2.26	43.6	2.41	26.3	4.65
Female	6–7	68	7.9	1.47	29.9	2.37	43.0	2.63	26.4	5.03
Male	8–9	124	8.7	1.48	31.7	2.83	45.3	2.87	27.5	5.27
Female	8–9	98	8.4	1.56	30.5	2.06	44.9	2.65	27.6	5.27
Male	10–11	78	9.5	1.83	32.5	2.33	48.1	2.38	29.4	5.97
Female	10–11	71	9.3	1.61	32.1	2.62	46.9	3.08	29.0	5.29
Male	12–13	67	11.0	2.24	32.4	3.03	50.5	3.30	34.2	7.41
Female	12–13	58	10.1	2.01	32.3	2.84	48.3	3.11	31.5	6.22
Male	14–15	116	12.3	2.36	33.9	2.60	51.4	3.25	36.5	7.54
Female	14–15	105	11.2	1.90	31.8	2.46	49.0	2.79	35.3	6.31
Male	16–18	130	13.8	2.64	33.7	2.92	51.6	3.03	41.0	8.78
Female	16–18	123	12.1	2.24	32.3	2.69	49.8	3.10	37.7	7.31
Male	Adult	101	14.9	2.93	34.6	3.03	51.8	3.28	43.4	9.68
Female	Adult	123	12.7	2.45	32.6	2.80	49.6	3.03	39.0	7.04

SOURCE: B. L. Shapiro et al., Measurement of Normal and Reportedly Malformed Palatal Vaults. I. Normal Adult Measurements, *J. Dent. Res.* **42:**1039, 1963; R. S. Redman et al., Measurements of Normal and Reportedly Malformed Palatal Vaults. II. Normal Juvenile Measurements. *J. Dent. Res.* **45:**266–269, 1966.

* SD = standard deviation. All measurements were made to the nearest millimeter. Each index was computed from the formula: Height/width × 100.

Table A-7. Cephalometric measurements

Measurement or relationship	Abbreviation	Mean	SD	Range	Comment
Cranial base angle	N-S-Ba	131°	4.8	. . .	Age 19 and over
Anterior cranial base length	N-S	73.7	3.7	. . .	Age 19 and over
Length of clivus	S-Ba	48.5	2.7	. . .	Age 19 and over
Maxilla to cranial base	S-N-A	81°	. . .	75–87	
Mandible to cranial base	S-N-Po	80°	. . .	72–88	
Maxilla to mandible	A-N-B	+2	. . .	(−1)–(5)	
Maxillary base angle	N-S/ANS-Ptm	6.2°	3.2	. . .	Age 19 and over
Mandibular plane angle	N-S/mandibular tangent through gnathion	27.5°	5.8	. . .	Age 19 and over
Prominence of bony chin	Po/N-B	3 mm	. . .	2–5 mm	

Adapted from various sources. See W. M. Krogman and V. Sassouni, *Syllabus of Roentgencephalometry*, mimeographed booklet, Philadelphia, 1958.

Table A-8. Frequency of nondental oral anomalies

Anomaly	Frequency in ostensibly normal population, approximate percent
Cheek biting (39)	2
Cleft:	
Lip-palate	
Caucasian (12, 14)	0.06–0.15
Afro-American (3, 4, 10, 24)	0.04
Japanese (20, 33)	0.17
Amerindian (33, 44)	0.3
Palate, isolated	
Caucasian (10, 12)	0.04–0.05
Oriental (33)	0.06–0.07
Afro-American (3, 4)	0.02–0.04
Uvula	
Amerindian (8, 40)	10–20
Inuit (16)	3–6
Japanese (16)	1–2
Caucasian (30, 43)	1–2
Afro-American (36, 38)	0.25–0.50
Cysts, eruption (12)	0.2
Fordyce granules (sebaceous glands):	
Lips	
Caucasian (15, 25, 39a)	50–80
Buccal mucosa	
Caucasian (15, 25, 39a)	60–95
Afro-American (29)	55
Lip pits	
Paramedian (45)	1:200,000
Commissural	
Afro-American (5, 38)	20
Caucasian (5)	12
Oriental (5)	6
Amerindian (8)	9
Inuit (19)	8
Tongue	
Ability to touch nose with (personal observation)	7–10
Ankyloglossia (7, 28, 47)	1:300 to 1 per 2,000
Fissured	
5–18 years (9, 35)	
Overall (1, 15, 47)	2–5
Folding of tip	
Within mouth	1–2
Outside mouth (46)	1 per 600
Geographic	
Caucasian (9, 15)	1.0–2.5
Median rhomboid "glossitis"	
Caucasian (15, 47)	0.2–0.3
Inuit (19)	0.6
Rolling or tubing	
Caucasian (13, 41)	60–75
Afro-American (23)	80
Japanese (22)	25–30

Table A-8. (*Continued*)

Anomaly	Frequency in ostensibly normal population, approximate percent
Tongue—Continued	
Thyroid gland inclusion	
Microscopic evidence (6, 37)	10
Clinical evidence (6)	1 per 10,000
Torus mandibularis	
Caucasian and Afro-American (17, 21, 42)	3–16
Inuit (17, 18, 19, 26, 27)	10–80
Oriental (38)	20–30
Torus palatinus	
Caucasian and Afro-American (21, 31, 38, 42)	20 (F-2, M-15)
Amerindian and Inuit (17, 19, 32)	25–75
Oriental (2, 38)	40–90

1 Aboyans, V., and Ghaemmaghami, A., The Incidence of Fissured Tongue Among 4,009 Iranian Dental Outpatients. *Oral Surg.* **36**:34–38, 1973.

2 Akabori, E., Torus Mandibularis. *J. Shanghai Sci. Inst.* **4**:239–255, 1939.

3 Altemus, L. A., and Ferguson, A. D., Comparative Incidence of Birth Defects in Negro and White Children. *Pediatrics* **36**:56–61, 1965.

4 Altemus, L. A., The Incidence of Cleft Lip and Palate Among North American Negroes. *Cleft Palate J.* **3**:357–361, 1966.

5 Baker, W. R., Pits of the Lip Commissures in Caucasoid Males. *Oral Surg.* **21**:56–60, 1966.

6 Baughman, R. A., Lingual Thyroid and Lingual Thyroglossal Tract Remnants. *Oral Surg.* **34**:781–799, 1972.

7 Catlin, F. I., and De Haas, V., Tongue-Tie. *Arch. Otolaryngol.* **94**:548–557, 1971.

8 Cervenka, J., Unpublished data, 1970.

9 Chosack, A., et al., The Prevalence of Scrotal Tongue and Geographic Tongue in 70,359 Israeli School Children. *Community Dent. Oral Epidemiol.* **2**:253–257, 1974.

10 Chung, C. E., and Myrianthopoulos, N. C., Racial and Prenatal Factors in Major Congenital Malformations. *Am. J. Hum. Genet.* **20**:44–60, 1968.

11 Clark, C. A., A Survey of Eruption Cysts in the Newborn. *Oral Surg.* **15**:917, 1962.

12 Drillien, C. M., et al., *The Causes and Natural History of Cleft Lip and Palate.* E. & S. Livingston, Ltd., Edinburgh, 1966.

13 Gahres, E. E., Tongue Rolling and Tongue Folding and Other Hereditary Movements of the Tongue. *J. Hered.* **43**:221–225, 1952.

14 Greene, J. C., et al., Epidemiologic Study of Cleft Lip and Cleft Palate in Four States *J. Am. Dent. Assoc.* **68**:387–404, 1964.

15 Halperin, V., et al., The Occurrence of Fordyce Spots, Benign Migratory Glossitis, Median Rhomboid Glossitis and Fissured Tongue in 2,478 Dental Patients. *Oral Surg.* **6**:1072–1077, 1953.

16 Heathcote, G. M., The Prevalence of Cleft Uvula in an Inuit Population. *Am. J. Phys. Anthropol.* **41**:433–438, 1974.

17 Hooton, E. A., On Certain Eskimoidal Characters in Icelandic Skulls. *Am. J. Phys. Anthropol.* **1**:53–76, 1918.

18 Hrdlička, A., Mandibular and Maxillary Hyperostoses. *Am. J. Phys. Anthropol.* **27**:1–55, 1940.

19 Jarvis, A., and Gorlin, R. J., Minor Orofacial Anomalies in an Eskimo Population. *Oral Surg.* **33**:417–427, 1972.

20 Kobayashi, Y., A Genetic Study of Harelip and Cleft Palate. *Jap. J. Hum. Genet.* **3**:73–107, 1958.

21 Kolas, S., et al., The Occurrence of Torus Palatinus and Torus Mandibularis in 2,478 Dental Patients. *Oral Surg.* **6**:1134–1141, 1953.

22 Komai, T., Notes on Lingual Gymnastics. *J. Hered.* **42**:293–297, 1951.

23 Lee, J. W., Tongue-Folding and Tongue-Rolling in an American Negro Population Sample. *J. Hered.* **46**:289–291, 1955.

Table A-8. *(Continued)*

24 Longenecker, C. G., et al., Cleft Lip and Cleft Palate, Incidence at a Large Charity Hospital. *Plast. Reconstr. Surg.* **35:**548–550, 1965.

25 Martin, E. A., and Wales, R. T., Sebaceous Glands in the Mouth. *Irish J. Med. Sci.* **6:**481–486, 1964.

26 Mayhall, J. T., Torus Mandibularis in an Alaskan Eskimo Population. *Am. J. Phys. Anthropol.* **33:**57–60, 1970.

27 Mayhall, J. T., and Mayhall, M. F., Torus Mandibularis in Two Northwest Territories Villages. *Am. J. Phys. Anthropol.* **34:**143–148, 1971.

28 McEnery, E. T., and Gaines, F. P., Tongue-Tie in Infants and Children. *J. Pediatr.* **18:**252–255, 1941.

29 McGoodwin, R. C., Fordyce's Granules in Pigmented Oral Mucosa. *J. Dent. Res.* **43:**773, 1964.

30 Meskin, L. H., et al., The Prevalence of Cleft Uvula. *Cleft Palate J.* **1:**342–346, 1964.

31 Miller, S. C., and Roth, H., Torus Palatinus: A Statistical Study. *J. Am. Dent. Assoc.* **27:**1950–1957, 1940.

32 Moorrees, C. F. A., The Dentition as a Criterion of Race with Special Reference to the Aleut. *J. Dent. Res.* **30:**815–821, 1951.

33 Neel, J. V., A Study of Major Congenital Defects in Japanese Infants. *Am. J. Hum. Genet.* **10:**398–445, 1958.

34 Niswander, J., and Adams, M. S., Oral Clefts in the American Indians. *Public Health Rep.* **82:**807–812, 1967.

35 Redman, R. S., The Prevalence of Geographic Tongue, Fissured Tongue, Median Rhomboid Glossitis and Hairy Tongue Among 3,611 Minnesota School Children. *Oral Surg.* **30:**390–395, 1970.

36 Richardson, E. R., Cleft Uvula in Negroes. *Cleft Palate J.* **7:**669–672, 1970.

37 Sauk, J. J., Jr., Ectopic Lingual Thyroid. *J. Pathol.* **102:**239–243, 1970.

38 Schaumann, B. F., et al., Minor Craniofacial Anomalies Among a Negro Population. *Oral Surg.* **29:**566–575, 729–734, 1970.

39 Sewerin, I., The Prevalence of Morsicatio Buccarum/Labiorum in 841 Copenhagen School Children. *Tandlaegebladet* **77:**861–864, 1973.

39a Sewerin, I., The Sebaceous Glands in the Vermilion Border of the Lips and in the Oral Mucosa of Man. *Acta Odontol. Scand.* **33:**Suppl. 68:1–226, 1975.

40 Shapiro, B. L., et al., Cleft Uvula: A Microform of Facial Clefts and Its Genetic Basis. *Birth Defects* **7**(7):80–82, 1971.

41 Sturtevant, A. H., A New Inherited Character in Man. *Proc. Nat. Acad. Sci. (Wash.)* **26:**100–102, 1940.

42 Summers, C. J., Prevalence of Tori. *J. Oral Surg.* **26:**718–720, 1968.

43 Tolarova, M., et al., Distribution of Signs Considered to be a Microform of Cleft Lip and/or Cleft Palate in a Population of Normal 18- to 21-year-old Subjects. *Acta Chir. Plast. (Praha)* **9:**1–14, 1967.

44 Tretsven, V. E., Incidence of Cleft Lip and Palate in Montana Indians. *J. Speech Hearing Dis.* **28:**52–57, 1963.

45 Van der Woude, A., Fistula Labii Inferioris Congenita and Its Association with Cleft Lip and Palate. *Am. J. Hum. Genet.* **6:**244–256, 1954.

46 Whitney, D. D., Tongue Tip Overfolding. *J. Hered.* **40:**19–21, 1949.

47 Witkop, C. J., and Barros, L., Oral and Genetic Studies of Chileans. Oral Anomalies. *Am. J. Phys. Anthropol.* **21:**15–24, 1963.

Table A-9. Frequency of dental anomalies

Teeth	Percent
Congenitally missing, primary, Caucasian (10, 19, 22)	0.1–0.7
Congenitally missing, secondary, Caucasian	
Maxillary central incisors (24, 27)	0.05
Maxillary lateral incisors (7, 8, 10, 20, 24, 25, 27)	1.0–2.0
Maxillary canines (7, 24, 27)	0.3
Maxillary first premolars (7, 24, 27)	0.3
Maxillary second premolars (7, 8, 10, 24, 27)	1.0–2.0
Maxillary first molars (24, 27)	0.3
Maxillary second molars (7, 24, 27)	0.1
Mandibular central incisors (7, 24, 27)	0.3
Mandibular lateral incisors (7, 24, 27)	0.3
Mandibular canines (24)	0.1
Mandibular first premolars (7, 24, 27)	0.3
Mandibular second premolars (7, 8, 10, 24, 27)	1.2–2.5
Mandibular first molars (24, 27)	0.3
Mandibular second molars (7, 24, 27)	0.3
Secondary teeth, other than third molars	
Caucasian (4, 5, 7, 8, 10, 27)	3.0–7.5
Japanese (21, 26)	5.8–9.2
Third molars, one or more absent (10, 12, 14)	2.5–35.0
One absent	7–10
Two absent	10–12
Three absent	4–6
Four absent	4–7
Defects, hereditary	
Dentin (31)	1:8,000
Enamel (31)	1:15,000
Dens invaginatus	
Maxillary lateral incisors (1, 9, 13, 28)	1.2–6.6
Maxillary central incisors (13)	0.6
Double formations (fusion or gemination)	
Primary dentition	
Caucasian (5, 11, 17, 19, 22)	0.2–0.5
Japanese (21, 26)	2.5
Secondary dentition	
Caucasian (27)	0.2
Impacted	
Teeth, primary (6, 18)	17.0
Maxillary canines, secondary (6)	0.9
Natal teeth (2)	0.03–0.05
Pegged	
Primary teeth (26)	0.2
Secondary maxillary lateral incisors	
Caucasian (27)	1.0–2.0
Japanese (30)	6.2
Shovel-shaped incisors	
Amerindian, Inuit, Oriental (15)	60–75
Supernumerary teeth	
Primary dentition (10, 16, 19, 22)	0.3–0.8
Secondary dentition	
Caucasian (4, 5, 16, 23, 29)	1.0–3.5
Japanese (21)	2.2–5.3
Maxillary incisors, secondary (2, 3, 23)	0.3–0.5
Fourth molars, secondary (29)	0.2

Table A-9. (*Continued*)

1 Amos, E. R., Incidence of the Small Dens in Dente. *J. Am. Dent. Assoc.* **51:**31–33, 1955.

2 Bodenhoff, J., Dentitio connatalis et neonatalis. *Odontol. Tidskr.* **67:**645–695, 1959.

3 Boyne, P. J., Supernumerary Maxillary Incisors. *Oral Surg.* **7:**901–905, 1954.

4 Castaldi, C. R., et al., Incidence of Congenital Anomalies in Permanent Teeth of a Group of Canadian Children Aged 6–9. *J. Can. Dent. Assoc.* **32:**154–159, 1966.

5 Clayton, J. M., Congenital Dental Anomalies Occurring in 3,557 Children. *J. Dent. Child.* **23:**206–208, 1956.

6 Dachi, S. F., and Howell, F. V., A Survey of 3,874 Routine Full Mouth Radiographs. II. A Study of Impacted Teeth. *Oral Surg.* **14:**1165–1169, 1961.

7 Dolder, E., Deficient Dentition. *Dent. Rec.* **57:**142–143, 1937.

8 Glenn, F. B., Incidence of Congenitally Missing Permanent Teeth in a Private Pedodontic Practice. *J. Dent. Child.* **28:**317–320, 1961.

9 Grahnén, H., et al., Dens Invaginatus. I. A Clinical Roentgenological and Genetical Study of Permanent Upper Lateral Incisors. *Odont. Revy* **10:**115–137, 1959.

10 Grahnén, H., and Granath, L. E., Numerical Variation in Primary Dentition and their Correlation with the Permanent Dentition. *Odont. Revy* **4:**348–357, 1961.

11 Grahnén, H., and Lindahl, B., Supernumerary Teeth in the Permanent Dentition. A Frequency Study. *Odont. Revy* **12:**290–294, 1961.

12 Gravely, J. F., A Radiographic Survey of Third Molar Development. *Br. Dent. J.* **119:**397–401, 1965.

13 Hallett, G. E. M., The Incidence, Nature and Clinical Significance of Palatal Invaginations in Maxillary Incisor Teeth. *Proc. Roy. Soc. Med.* **46:**491–499, 1953.

14 Hellman, M., Our Third Molar Teeth: Their Eruption, Presence and Absence. *Dent. Cosm.* **78:**750–762, 1936.

15 Hrdlička, A., Shovel-shaped Teeth. *Am. J. Phys. Anthropol.* **3:**429–465, 1920.

16 Luten, J. R., The Prevalence of Supernumerary Teeth in Primary and Mixed Dentitions. *J. Dent. Child.* **34:**346–353, 1967.

17 McKibben, D. R., and Brearley, L. J., Radiographic Determination of the Prevalence of Selected Dental Anomalies in Children. *J. Dent. Child.* **38:**390–398, 1971.

18 Mead, S. V., Incidence of Impacted Teeth. *Int. J. Orthodont.* **16:**885–890, 1930.

19 Menczer, L. F., Anomalies of the Primary Dentition. *J. Dent. Child.* **22:**57–62, 1955.

20 Miller, T. P., et al., A Survey of Congenitally Missing Permanent Teeth. *J. Am. Dent. Assoc.* **81:**101–107, 1970.

21 Niswander, J. D., and Sajuku, C., Congenital Anomalies of Teeth in Japanese Children. *Am. J. Phys. Anthropol.* **21:**569–574, 1963.

22 Plaetschke, J., Okklusionsanomalien im Milchgebiss. *Deutsche Zahn Mund Kieferheilk.* **5:**435–451, 1938.

23 Ravin, J. J., and Nielsen, L. A., An ortopantomografisk undersøgelse af overtal og aplasier hos 1,530 Kobenhavnske skolebørn. *Tandlaegebladet* **77:**12–22, 1973.

24 Ringqvist, M., and Thilander, B., The Frequency of Hypodontia in an Orthodontic Material. *Svensk. Tandläk. Tidskr.* **62:**535–541, 1969.

25 Rose, J. S., A Survey of Congenitally Missing Teeth, Excluding Third Molars, in 6,000 Orthodontic Patients. *Dent. Pract.* (*Bristol*) **17:**107–111, 1966.

26 Saito, T., A Genetic Study on the Degenerative Anomalies of Deciduous Teeth. *Jap. J. Hum. Genet.* **4:**27–53, 1959.

27 Schulze, C., Developmental Abnormalities of the Teeth and Jaws, in R. J. Gorlin and H. M. Goldman (eds.). *Thoma's Oral Pathology,* 6th ed., C. V. Mosby, St. Louis, 1970.

Table A-9. *(Continued)*

28 Shafer, W. C., Dens in Dente. *NY Dent. J.* **19:**220–223, 1953.
29 Stafne, E. C., Supernumerary Teeth. *Dent. Cosm.* **74:**653–659, 1932.
30 Sumiya, Y., Statistical Study on Dental Anomalies in the Japanese. *J. Anthropol. Soc. Nippon.* **67:**171–172, 1959.
31 Witkop, C. J., and Rao, S., Inherited Defects in Tooth Structure. *Birth Defects* **7**(7):153–184, 1971.

Index